Ultrasound of the Eye and Orbit

Ultrasound of the Eye and Orbit

SANDRA FRAZIER BYRNE
Visiting Research Scholar
Mars Hill College
Mars Hill, North Carolina

RONALD L. GREEN, MD
Professor
Doheny Eye Institute
Department of Ophthalmology
University of Southern California Keck School of Medicine
Los Angeles, California

SECOND EDITION
Illustrations by **Timothy G. Hengst, FAHI**

JAYPEE

JAYPEE BROTHERS MEDICAL PUBLISHERS
The Health Sciences Publisher
New Delhi | London

Jaypee Brothers Medical Publishers (P) Ltd.

Headquarters
Jaypee Brothers Medical Publishers (P) Ltd
EMCA House
23/23-B, Ansari Road, Daryaganj
New Delhi - 110 002, India
Landline: +91-11-23272143, +91-11-23272703
+91-11-23282021, +91-11-23245672
Email: jaypee@jaypeebrothers.com

Corporate Office
Jaypee Brothers Medical Publishers (P) Ltd
4838/24, Ansari Road, Daryaganj
New Delhi 110 002, India
Phone: +91-11-43574357
Fax: +91-11-43574314
Email: jaypee@jaypeebrothers.com

Overseas Office
J.P. Medical Ltd
83 Victoria Street, London
SW1H 0HW (UK)
Phone: +44 20 3170 8910
Fax: +44 (0)20 3008 6180
Email: info@jpmedpub.com

Website: www.jaypeebrothers.com
Website: www.jaypeedigital.com

Ultrasound of the Eye and Orbit

Second Edition : 2010

Reprint : **2025**

ISBN: 978-81-8448-899-9

Printed at Replika Press Pvt. Ltd.

Contributors

PAUL T. FINGER, MD, FACS
Associate Professor of Ophthalmology
New York Eye and Ear Infirmary
New York University School of Medicine
New York, New York
Chapter 9: Three-Dimensional Imaging of the Eye

F. STUART FOSTER, PhD
Professor and Associate Chair
Department of Medical Biophysics
Faculty of Medicine
University of Toronto
Sunnybrook and Women's Health Sciences Centre
Toronto, Ontario
Canada
Chapter 8: Ultrasound Biomicroscopy of the Eye

WOLFGANG E. LIEB, MD
Associate Professor
Department of Ophthalmology
Julius-Maximilians-University
Würzburg, Germany
Chapter 14: Color Doppler Imaging of the Eye and Orbit

CHARLES J. PAVLIN, MD
Professor
Department of Ophthalmology
Faculty of Medicine
University of Toronto
Toronto, Ontario
Canada
Chapter 8: Ultrasound Biomicroscopy of the Eye

Foreword

Almost 10 years have passed since the publication of the first edition of *Ultrasound of the Eye and Orbit* by Sandra Frazier Byrne and Dr. Ron Green. Many new developments in ultrasonography have occurred, and the ophthalmic community looks forward to the authors' updated information regarding the new techniques and available instrumentation. In addition to their own new observations, they have included three new chapters by guest authors. These concern ultrasound biomicroscopy, color Doppler imaging, and three-dimensional ultrasound.

Ultrasonography has established itself as one of our most important diagnostic tools in ophthalmology. Perhaps more than any other such tool the value of the information obtained is highly dependent on the skill, technique, experience, interpretation, and dedication of the ultrasonographer. When it comes to examination of difficult diagnostic cases, the busy practitioner doing only a few ultrasound studies a week cannot compete with those devoting most of their time to ultrasonography.

The authors have used detailed, clearly written, and illustrated instructions on proper ultrasonographic techniques that will be invaluable to those wishing to master any one or all phases of ultrasonography. They have included a comprehensive collection of ultrasound images for most of the neoplastic, hamartomatous, inflammatory, metabolic, traumatic, and degenerative disorders of the uveal tract, macula, retina, vitreous, sclera, optic nerve, and orbit. This book serves as an excellent reference for students, residents, ophthalmologists, and those who are not involved in doing ultrasonography. A culmination of more than 50 years of combined experience of two world-recognized authorities, this beautifully illustrated classic provides the reader with a clear understanding of the physics, techniques, instrumentation, and interpretation of ultrasound.

J. Donald M. Gass, MD
Professor of Ophthalmology
Department of Ophthalmology
Vanderbilt University Medical School
Nashville, Tennessee

Foreword

This second edition of *Ultrasound of the Eye and Orbit* extends the collaborative voice and experience of Sandra Frazier Byrne and Ronald Green to 50 years. Their balanced view of the role of echography in the armamentarium of the orbital specialist is evident throughout the book. In addition, the careful correlation of diagnostic images using different technology allows the reader to contextualize the spectrum of orbital processes delineated herein. The range and specificity of examples also provides a ready reference for the student of ultrasonography and orbital disease. They have added sections on color Doppler imaging and three-dimensional ultrasound, which add to the dynamic spectrum of techniques emphasized.

Throughout, the reader is able to incorporate the basic knowledge of ultrasound and apply it to a range of lesions in a meaningful manner. Most people who recognize the complex constellation of clinical signs and symptoms of orbital disease enjoy the challenge of piecing the investigative findings to sort out the appropriate management of their patients. The study of these patients requires the clinician to draw upon vast clinical, investigative, pathologic, and systemic knowledge. This book, with its lucid text and illustrations, is essential to the comprehensive investigation and management of the orbital patient.

Jack Rootman, MD, FRCSC
Professor, Departments of Ophthalmology and Pathology
Head, Department of Ophthalmology
University of British Columbia and the Vancouver General Hospital;
Associate Member, Division of Neurosurgery
Vancouver General Hospital
Vancouver, British Columbia
Canada

Preface to the Second Edition

Since the first publication of this book in 1992, numerous advances have occurred in the field of ophthalmic ultrasound. Many new observations have been made, and over the past decade, new technologies have emerged that have greatly enhanced the practice of echography. As a result, a second edition was necessary to update the body of knowledge in ophthalmic ultrasound and to describe new instrumentation and examination techniques.

We are grateful to our guest contributors who have written three new chapters for this book. These chapters describe the most important technologic advances in ophthalmic ultrasound in the last ten years: ultrasound biomicroscopy (Chapter 8), three-dimensional ultrasound (Chapter 9), and color Doppler imaging (Chapter 14).

We have written new chapters on inflammatory diseases of the eye (Chapter 6) and glaucoma (Chapter 7). These chapters reflect our increased experience and demonstrate additional indications for ophthalmic ultrasound.

In Chapter 2, *Examination Techniques for the Eye*, three-dimensional drawings have been created to better illustrate the examination techniques. This chapter also includes a more detailed explanation of the anterior segment evaluation.

Chapter 3, *Vitreoretinal Disease*, has been greatly expanded. It contains a new section on macular disease, as well as additional illustrations of vitreoretinal disorders. Significant new material regarding the sclera and its abnormalities has also been added. Chapter 4 has been updated to include additional examples of trauma and post-surgical findings.

Major revisions have been made to Chapter 5, *Intraocular Tumors*. These include new observations and illustrations for both the diagnosis and measurement of choroidal melanoma. In addition, the discussion of other types of intraocular tumors has been expanded and a new section for anterior segment lesions has been created.

With the growing interest in IOL calculations, it was necessary to significantly enhance the explanation and illustration of axial eye length measurements in Chapter 10.

Chapters 11 through 17 cover examination techniques and disorders of the orbital soft tissue, extraocular muscles, optic nerves, and periorbital region. These chapters demonstrate the use of ultrasound as an important adjunct to CT scan and MRI for the detection and diagnosis of orbital and periorbital disease.

Chapter 18 has been updated to provide a more thorough explanation of the artifacts that are usually encountered in ophthalmic ultrasound.

We are indebted to many individuals for their assistance in the preparation of this second edition.

We wish to thank Nilo Davila and Tracy Nichols of the Photography Department at the Doheny Eye Institute and Richard Stratton of the Photography Department at the Bascom Palmer Eye Institute for their efforts in the preparation of the illustrations. Thanks are additionally extended to Rhonda Waldron, MMSc, COMT, and Cynthia Kendall, BMET, RDMS, for providing us with numerous illustrations for the book. Furthermore, we wish to acknowledge contributions from Barbara Blodi, MD; Diane Chialant, RN, COT; Cathy DiBernardo, RN, RDMS; Eileen Gendron, ROUB; Linda Kelley, CRA, COA; and Kathleen Meyer, RDMS, ROUB.

Special thanks go to Susan Clarke for her expertise in editing the manuscript. In addition, we are very appreciative of the administrative assistance provided by Sylvia Rea that greatly facilitated the preparation of this edition. Ann Dawson also provided advice and useful suggestions.

A number of colleagues were very helpful in reviewing portions of the manuscript. Thanks are extended to Culver Boldt, MD; Kari Boyce, PhD; Brian Francis, MD; Warren Hill, MD; Mark Johnson, MD; Gregg Kokame, MD; Tom Prager, PhD; and Russell Read, MD.

We also wish to thank Bernie Byrne for all of his support, encouragement, and many other contributions.

Sandra Frazier Byrne
Ronald L. Green, MD

Preface to the First Edition

In recent years, echography has become an essential component in the clinical practice of ophthalmology, and has increased greatly our ability to detect and differentiate a wide variety of ocular and orbital disorders. This diagnostic imaging modality, however, can be used reliably only when the echographer understands the basic principles of ultrasound and utilizes appropriate examination techniques. Our goal in writing this book is to provide a comprehensive overview of ultrasound as it applies to the eye and orbit. We emphasize those techniques that have been found to be of greatest value in our own practices, and we describe and illustrate the most common ophthalmic disorders that one might expect to encounter.

The reader will note that the terms echography, ultrasonography, and ultrasound are used interchangeably throughout the text. All three terms are commonly used to describe the use of diagnostic ultrasound in medicine. In the book, our lack of consistent use of this terminology is due primarily to our different customary usages of these terms.

The first chapter reviews the physical principles of diagnostic ultrasound and describes the instrumentation used in ophthalmic echography. Chapters 2 through 6 describe echography of the eye. This section is an outgrowth of a chapter that we co-authored in Stephen Ryan's textbook, *Retina*, but we have greatly expanded our description of vitreoretinal disorders, ocular trauma, and intraocular tumors. Chapters 7 through 12 are devoted to orbital echography. Many readers may be surprised by our extensive coverage of this subject, but these chapters reflect the importance that we place on ultrasound for orbital diagnosis. At our institutions, echography is considered to be an important adjunct to computed tomographic scanning and magnetic resonance imaging.

It is important to emphasize that the techniques described in this book are based primarily on the pioneering work of Dr. Karl Ossoinig. We both studied with Dr. Ossoinig at the University of Iowa, and are very grateful to him for his instruction and for his major contributions to the field of ophthalmic echography.

This book also would have not been possible without the support and vision of Dr. Edward W.D. Norton, Chairman Emeritus of the Bascom Palmer Eye Institute, and Dr. Stephen J. Ryan, Chairman of the Doheny Eye Institute. By establishing echography departments in their institutions, they have recognized the importance of ophthalmic ultrasound, and we are very grateful for their continued support and encouragement.

This book is the result of our combined experience of more than 30 years in the field of ophthalmic echography. Over those years we have learned that, although proper instrumentation and examination techniques are essential, nothing is more important than experience. New findings and applications for ultrasound in ophthalmology continue to make echography an exciting and challenging field. We hope that this book will allow the reader to benefit from our experience and that this text will serve as a useful reference.

Sandra Frazier Byrne
Ronald L. Green, MD

Contents

1

Physics and Instrumentation

This chapter reviews the physical principles of diagnostic ultrasound and describes the instrumentation used to perform ophthalmic echography. It is important to be aware of the variety of available instrumentation and to have an understanding of basic ultrasound physics. A general overview of ultrasound physics as it applies to ophthalmology is provided. For a more in-depth understanding of this subject, a suggested reading list is provided at the end of this chapter.

HISTORY

Ultrasound was first used in ophthalmology in 1956 by two American ophthalmologists, Mundt and Hughes.[17] Using time amplitude-mode (A-scan) to evaluate an intraocular tumor, they showed that ultrasound had potential as a diagnostic tool in ophthalmology. Soon afterward, Oksala and associates, in Finland, greatly expanded the use of A-scan for the diagnosis of intraocular disorders[18] and published data regarding the sound velocities of various components of the eye.[19]

In 1958, Baum and Greenwood[1] co-developed the first two-dimensional (immersion) brightness-mode (B-scan) ultrasound instrument for ophthalmology. In the early 1960s, Jansson and associates,[11,12] in Sweden, used ultrasound to measure the distances between structures in the eye.

Further pioneering work with immersion B-scan was carried out by Purnell,[38] followed later by Coleman et al.[4] In the early 1970s, Coleman and associates[5-7] developed the first commercially available immersion B-scan instrument. In 1977, Coleman and investigators first described a method of ultrasonic tissue characterization using spectrum analysis.[8,16]

Shortly thereafter, Bronson[2] introduced a contact B-scan machine for ophthalmology. This portable instrument allowed placement of the probe on the closed eyelids. With the development of this instrument, ultrasound began to be a useful component of the everyday practice of ophthalmology.

In the 1960s, Ossoinig[20-23] an Austrian ophthalmologist, first emphasized the importance of standardizing instrumentation and techniques so that echographers could rely on the results of fellow investigators using similar instrumentation and techniques. To this end, he developed the first standardized A-scan instrument, the Kretztechnik 7200 MA. This machine was carefully designed to allow reliable differentiation of tissue.[24-28] Later, Ossoinig further expanded his diagnostic method by adding the use of a contact B-scan instrument and then devised meticulous examination techniques for use with the two instruments. This concept eventually evolved into what is known today as Standardized Echography,[31,32] a method that has proved to be highly accurate for the detection and differentiation of both intraocular and orbital disorders.

In the early 1990s, Pavlin and associates popularized the use of high frequency ultrasound instrumentation for evaluation of the anterior segment.[34-37] This new instrumentation greatly enhanced the resolution of anterior segment structures and lesions and added a better understanding of the pathophysiology of anterior segment disorders.

Doppler ultrasound has been used in ophthalmology since the early 1970s.[7,13,31] In the late 1980s, color Doppler imaging (CDI) began to be used for the assessment of ocular and orbital disorders.[9,10,14,15]

In recent years, the digitization of ultrasound has greatly enhanced its potential and clinical applications. This computerization has made possible the development of three-dimensional ultrasound imaging in ophthalmology.[40]

PHYSICS

Ultrasound is an acoustic wave that consists of an oscillation of particles within a medium. By definition, ultrasound waves have frequencies greater than 20 KHz (i.e., 20,000 oscillations/sec), rendering them inaudible to humans. In contrast, frequencies of less than 20 KHz are audible to persons with normal hearing. Frequencies used in diagnostic ophthalmic ultrasound are in the range of 8 to 10 MHz (1 megahertz = 1,000,000 cycles/sec). These very high frequencies produce short wavelengths (less than 0.2 mm),

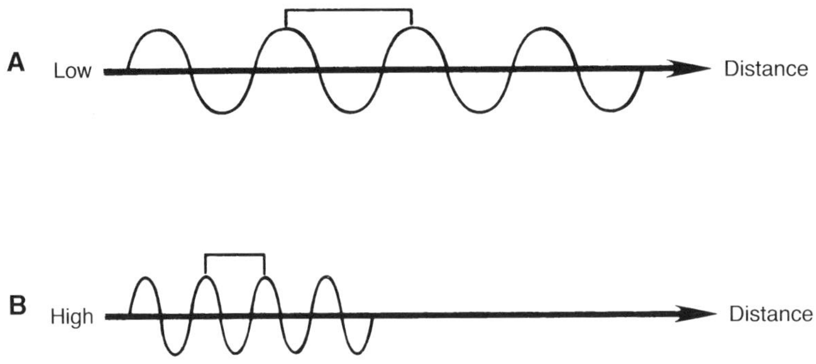

Figure 1-1 Low-frequency vs. high-frequency ultrasound. Lower frequency **(A)** produces longer wavelength than higher frequency **(B).** The wavelength *(bracket)* corresponds to one oscillation of the sound wave.

TABLE 1-1
Sound Wave Velocities

Medium	Velocity (m/sec)
Water	1,480
Aqueous/vitreous	1,532
Soft tissue	1,550
Crystalline lens	1,641
Bone	3,500

which allow resolution of minute ocular and orbital structures. Conversely, abdominal and obstetric ultrasound examinations usually require frequencies in the range of 1 to 5 MHz. The wavelengths produced by these lower frequencies are longer, allowing much deeper penetration of tissue (Figure 1-1). Although the longer wavelengths result in decreased resolution, this lower resolution is not critical because the abdominal and pelvic structures examined are much larger than those of the eye and orbit.

Ultrasound is propagated as a longitudinal wave that consists of alternating compressions and rarefactions of molecules as the wave passes through a medium. The velocity of the ultrasound wave is primarily dependent on the medium through which it passes. Water, for example, is very compressible; sound waves are transmitted through water at a slower velocity than through more solid media, which are less compressible. As a result, sound travels faster through a solid lens than it does through liquid vitreous (Table 1-1).

The behavior of longitudinal waves produced by ultrasonic energy is similar to that of light rays in that these longitudinal waves can be refracted and reflected predictably. It is this property that makes ultrasound useful for diagnostic purposes. As a longitudinal wave travels through a tissue, part of the wave may be reflected back toward the source of the emitted energy (i.e., the transducer or probe); this reflected wave is referred to as an echo.

Echoes

Echoes are produced by acoustic interfaces created at the junction of two media that have different acoustic impedances. The acoustic impedance of a medium is determined by its sound velocity and density (acoustic impedance = sound velocity × density). The greater the difference in the acoustic impedance of the two media that produce the interface, the stronger the reflection of the ultrasound wave (i.e., echo) (Figure 1-2). For example, the anterior lens surface produces a stronger echo when bordered by aqueous media than when it is bordered by blood (i.e., hyphema) because the difference in the impedance between lens and aqueous is greater than the difference in impedance between lens and hemorrhage (Figure 1-3).

The returning echoes are affected by many factors, including absorption and refraction, the angle of sound incidence, and the size, shape, and smoothness of acoustic interfaces. An understanding of these principles is necessary for the performance of accurate ultrasound examinations.

Angle of Sound Incidence

The acoustic wave directed by an ultrasound transducer is referred to as the sound beam. The angle at which the sound beam strikes an interface is an important factor in the strength of the returning echo. It is important to note that the angle of incidence is equal to the angle of reflection. Therefore, when the beam strikes an interface in a perpendicular manner, the echo is reflected back toward the direction from which it originated (e.g., the probe). If, however, the incident sound beam strikes an interface at an oblique angle, some of the reflected energy is diverted away from the direction of its origin, resulting in a weaker echo than when the sound incidence is perpendicular (Figure 1-4).

Acoustic Interfaces

The size, shape, and smoothness of an interface also play important roles in the character of the returning echo.

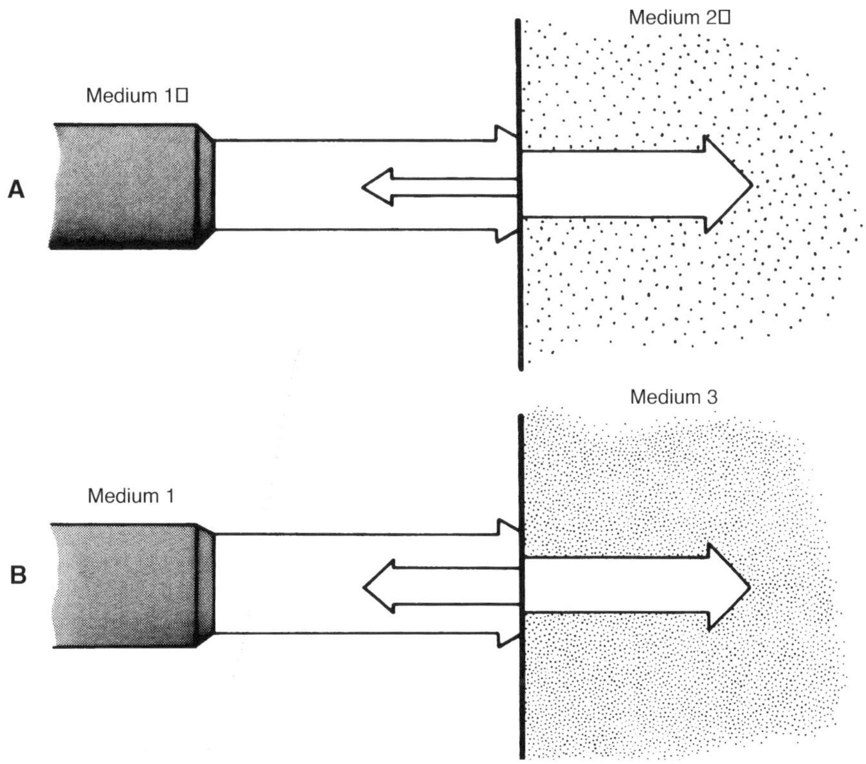

Figure 1-2 Acoustic impedance. The strength of the echo produced at the interface between the two media depicted is dependent on the acoustic impedance of the two media. In these examples, acoustic impedance is lower in **A,** resulting in less energy returning to the probe.

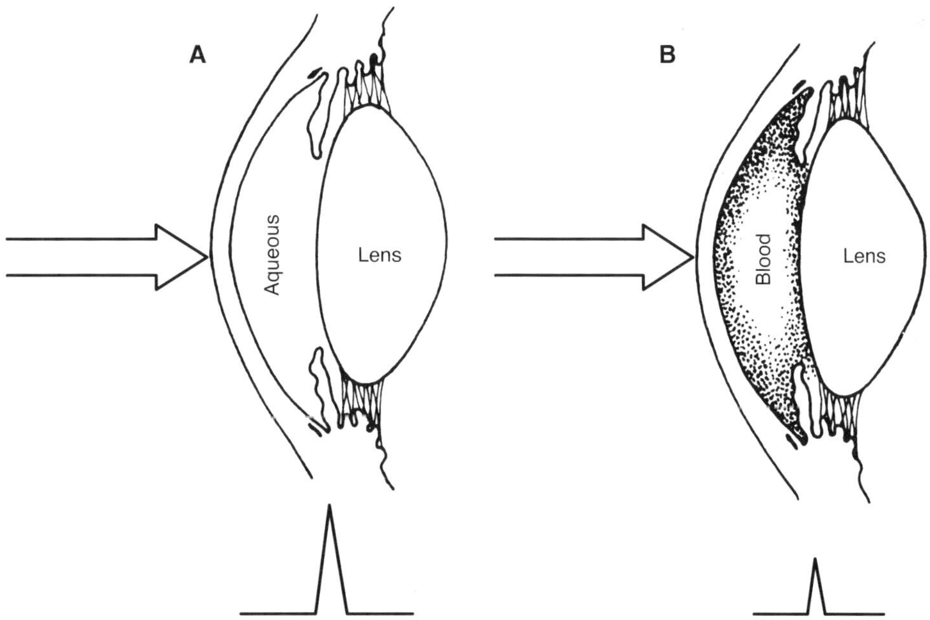

Figure 1-3 Acoustic impedance. The echo produced from the interface between aqueous and the anterior lens capsule **(A)** is stronger (higher acoustic impedance) than that produced by hemorrhage and the anterior lens capsule **(B).**

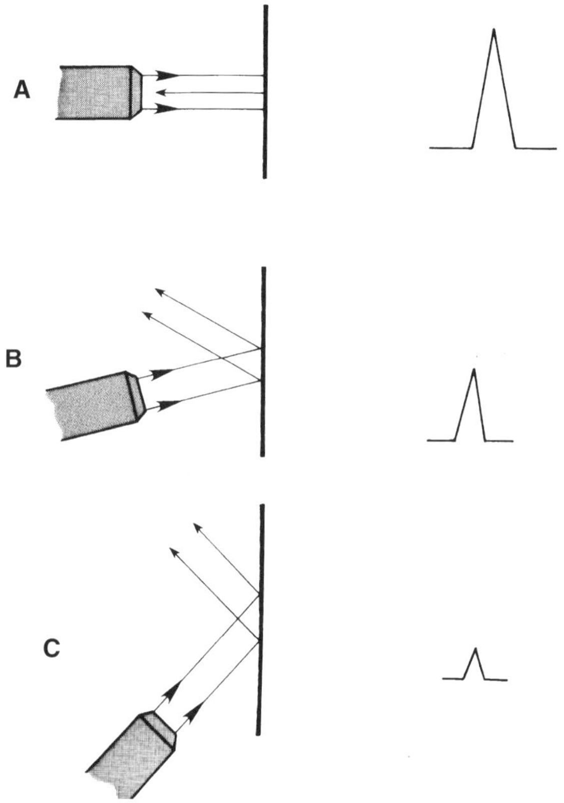

Figure 1-4 Perpendicular vs. oblique incidence. Oblique sound incidence results in a weaker echo than perpendicular sound incidence because less energy is returned to the transducer. Note that the angle of the reflected wave always equals that of the incident wave.

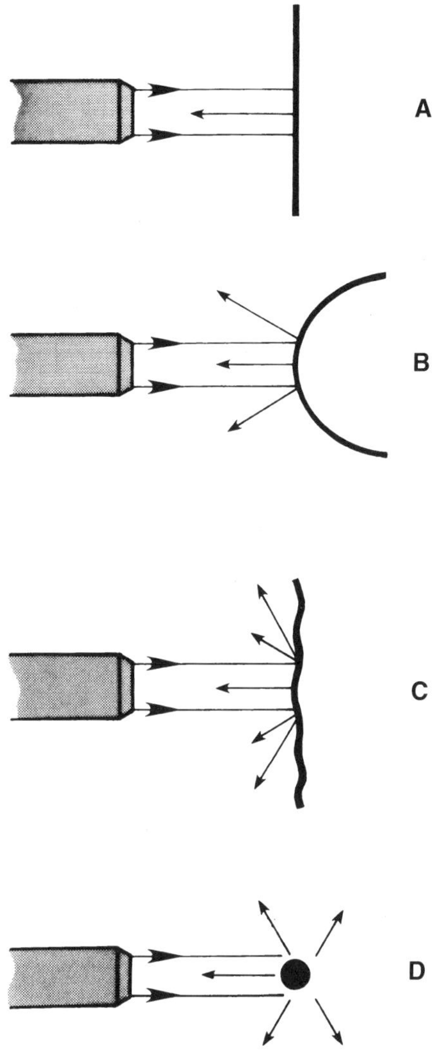

Figure 1-5 Different types of acoustic interfaces. **A,** When interface is smooth and flat, most of the reflected sound returns to the probe. **B,** At smooth, concave interface, a portion of the reflected sound is diverted away from the probe. **C,** When interface is coarse, a large portion of the reflected sound is diverted away from the probe (scattering). **D,** When interface is small, most of the echo is diverted away from the source (scattering).

Assuming that sound beam incidence is perpendicular, a smooth, straight interface (e.g., retinal surface) reflects nearly all of an echo wave back to its source (e.g., the probe); this is referred to as specular or mirror-like reflection (Figure 1-5, *A*). If, on the other hand, the interface is smooth but convex (e.g., a collar button-shaped melanoma), some of the echo will be reflected away from its origin, resulting in a weaker echo (Figure 1-5, *B*).

If an interface is not smooth, but has an irregular or coarse surface (e.g., ciliary body), part of the echo will be scattered (Figure 1-5, *C*). As a result, the echo wave returning to its origin will be weakened, even if sound beam incidence is perpendicular. Even more pronounced scattering is produced by very small interfaces (e.g., clumps of cells) (Figure 1-5, *D*). Consequently, these types of interfaces return only a small amount of the echo back in the direction of the transducer. This means that the echoes displayed from small or coarse interfaces are less dependent on the direction of the incident sound wave than are those displayed from larger, smooth interfaces.

Absorption

Ultrasound energy is gradually absorbed and converted to heat as it passes through a medium, although the amount of heat generated by diagnostic ultrasound is extremely low

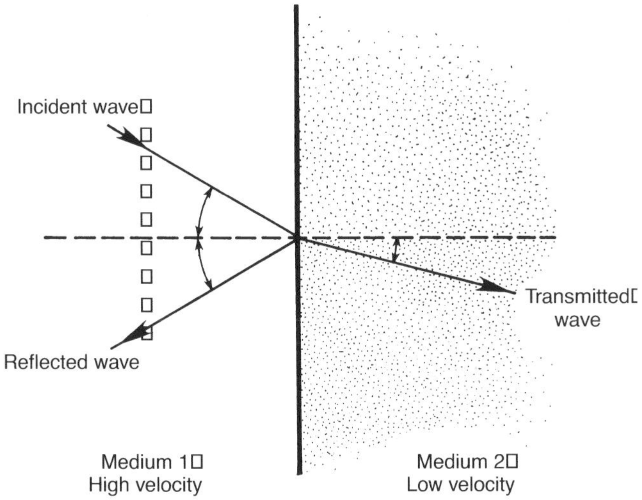

Figure 1-6 Refraction of the sound wave. With oblique incidence, the *incident wave* and *reflected wave* have the same angle. The angle of the *transmitted wave*, however, varies according to the sound velocity of the second media compared with the first media. In this example, the angle of the transmitted wave decreases because the sound velocity of *medium 1* is higher than that of *medium 2.*

and has no harmful effects on tissues.[13] Higher frequency sound waves are absorbed to a greater degree than are lower frequency sound waves, which is why a wave of higher frequency cannot penetrate as deeply into a tissue as can a wave of lower frequency. Absorption is also related directly to sound velocity, as well as to the thickness of the tissue through which it passes. Consequently, higher sound velocities and greater tissue thickness result in greater absorption of the sound wave.

Refraction

Another important factor that affects the appearance of echoes is refraction. As with light rays, refraction can be undesirable, producing artifacts, or it may be beneficial, contributing to the display of desired interfaces. Refraction occurs when a sound beam is directed obliquely to an interface that demarcates two media of different sound velocities. Conversely, no refraction occurs when a sound beam is directed perpendicular to an interface or when the velocity of the two media is the same.

When sound beam incidence is oblique and travels from a medium of lower sound velocity into another medium with higher sound velocity, the transmitted beam is refracted away from the perpendicular. Conversely, if the sound beam travels from a medium of higher velocity into a medium of lower sound velocity, the transmitted beam is refracted toward the perpendicular (Figure 1-6).

Refraction can be useful in certain situations, such as when examining the optic nerve and the extraocular muscles. In these circumstances, refraction can bend the sound beam in such a way that the surfaces of the nerve or of an extraocular muscle may be struck in a relatively perpendicular manner. Also, it is refraction that allows an acoustic lens to focus a sound beam, as is the case with B-scan probes.

Pulse-Echo System

Clinical echography depends on technology that emits an ultrasound wave and then detects and processes the returning echoes. This technique, known as pulse-echo, requires the production of multiple short pulses of ultrasound energy with a brief interval between pulses; the interval allows returning echoes to be detected, processed, and displayed.

Probe/Transducer

The basis of the pulse-echo system is the piezoelectric element, typically a quartz or ceramic crystal, which is the key component of the ultrasound transducer. The piezoelectric crystal, located near the face of the probe, undergoes a mechanical vibration when stimulated by electrical energy (i.e., voltage pulse) from the instrument. This vibration causes a longitudinal ultrasound wave (i.e., the sound beam) to be propagated through the medium (e.g., ocular and orbital tissues). A pause of several microseconds then occurs, which allows the transducer time to receive returning echoes. Returning energy creates another mechanical vibration as it strikes the crystal. The vibration, in turn, produces an electrical signal that is transmitted to the receiver and the display screen. This process of generating a sound wave, alternating with receiving an echo, is repeated a thousand or more times per second to produce a "real-time" display.

Another important component of the ultrasound probe is the damping material that is attached to the back of the crystal. This material, consisting of metal powder mixed with plastic or epoxy, serves to limit the vibrations of the crystal that produce the pulses of ultrasonic energy, thus shortening the pulse (Figure 1-7). This factor, in addition to the frequency, relates directly to the axial resolution of an ultrasound system. Axial resolution is the minimum distance between two interfaces (echo sources) along the direction of the sound beam that can be displayed. The shorter the pulse, the better the axial resolution.

The sound beam is made up of two zones: the near field and the far field. The near field is the portion of the sound beam located closest to the probe face. In the near field, the sound beam diameter generally decreases slightly with increasing distance from the transducer. The far field is the portion of the sound beam that is located beyond the near field. In the far field, the sound beam diameter generally increases with increasing distance from the transducer. Resolution of echoes is greatest when the echo source is located within the near field. The length of the near field depends on both the diameter and the frequency of the transducer crystal. Transducers with a larger diameter and/or higher frequency will have a longer near field.

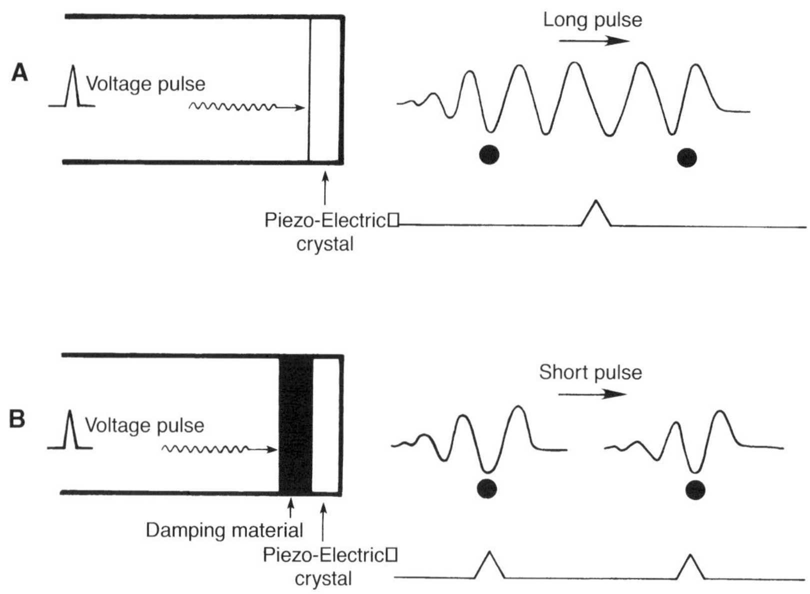

Figure 1-7 Damping material within probe shortens the emitted pulse and improves axial resolution. **A,** Probe without damping material emits long pulses. The two spherical objects are not resolved individually; thus, only one echo is produced. **B,** Probe with damping material emits shorter pulses. The two spherical objects are resolved individually; hence, two echoes are produced (improved axial resolution).

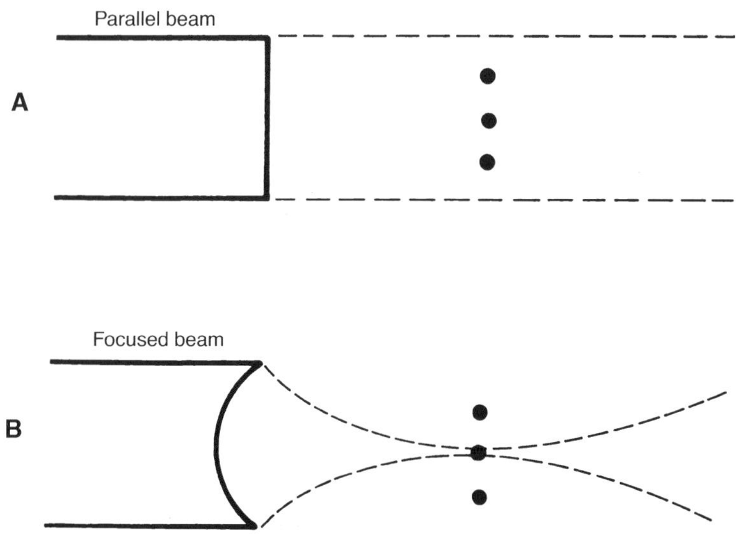

Figure 1-8 *Parallel* vs. *focused* sound beam. A focused sound beam improves lateral resolution. **A,** Wide, parallel sound beam does not permit resolution of the three spherical objects as separate echoes. **B,** Narrow, focused sound beam allows resolution of the three spherical objects as separate echoes.

The shape of the crystal is an important factor in determining the character of the sound beam. A planar crystal results in a relatively parallel sound beam, whereas a concave crystal or the addition of an acoustic lens can focus the sound beam. The focal distance of a focused lens system can vary from one instrument to another. The focal distance corresponds to the point where the sound beam is most narrow. The resolution of echo sources is greatest within the focal zone (an area just anterior and posterior to the focal point). Focusing increases both axial and lateral resolution of an ultrasound instrument. Lateral resolution is the minimum separation between two echo sources

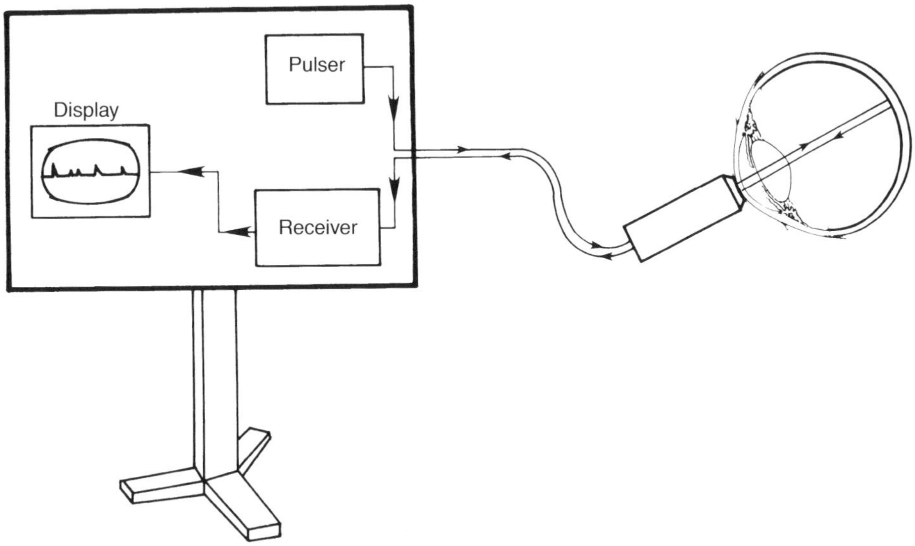

Figure 1-9 Schematic diagram of an ultrasound system.

aligned perpendicular to the direction of a scanning sound beam (Figure 1-8).

Signal Processing

An ultrasound system must be able to create a pulse of ultrasound energy propagated from its transducer. The unit also must be able to receive the returning echo and display it as a signal on a screen. Therefore, an instrument must have four components: a pulser, a transducer, a receiver, and a display screen (Figure 1-9).

The electrical signal produced by the returning echoes is initially received by the ultrasound instrument as a very weak radio frequency signal. This signal then undergoes complex processing that can include amplification, compensation, compression, demodulation, and rejection.

Although all of these parameters are important, amplification plays a particularly prominent role in the methods described in this textbook. In ophthalmic ultrasound instruments, one of three different types of amplification is generally used: linear, logarithmic, or S-shaped.[28] The type of amplification used affects the ability of the ultrasound system to display differences in the strengths of various echo signals. This is indicated by the range of echo intensities that can be displayed by the system (i.e., the dynamic range). The dynamic range is described in units of decibels, a measure of ultrasound intensity. A small dynamic range, characteristic of linear amplifiers, can display minor differences in echo strength between echo sources, but the range of echo intensities that can be displayed is very limited. In contrast, a large dynamic range, characteristic of logarithmic amplifiers, can display a wide range of echo intensities, but it cannot show slight differences between echo signals. These two amplification curves are used in various ultrasound systems, depending on the specific requirements of the instrument. The S-shaped amplification curve, developed by Ossoinig, is used in some systems to combine the wide range of the logarithmic amplifier and the great sensitivity of the linear amplifier (Figure 1-10). This special type of amplification enhances tissue differentiation and has proved to have unique diagnostic capabilities in ophthalmology.[29-32]

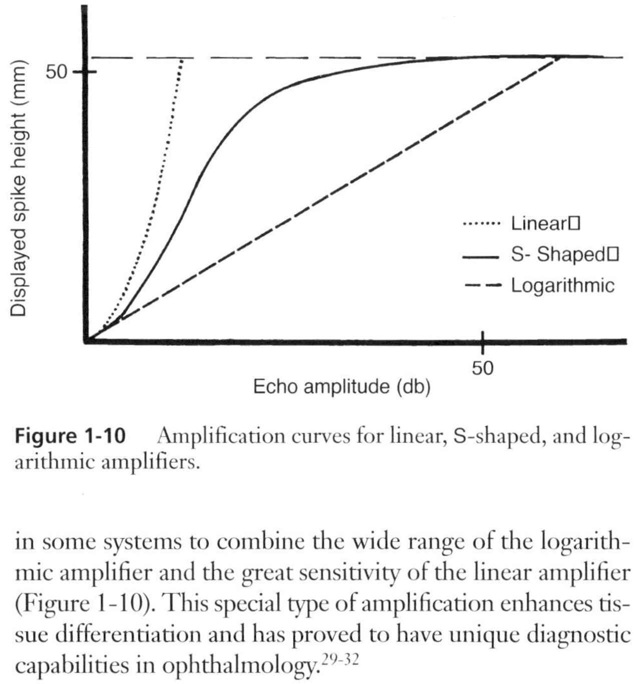

Figure 1-10 Amplification curves for linear, S-shaped, and logarithmic amplifiers.

Gain

All ultrasound instruments allow the examiner to adjust the amplification of the echo signals (overall gain control) displayed on the instrument screen. This adjustment, which is similar to turning the volume up or down on a radio, is referred to as the gain or sensitivity setting of the instrument. Gain is measured in decibels (db), which represent relative units of ultrasound intensity. It is important to realize that adjusting the gain does not change the amount of energy emitted from the transducer; it changes only the intensity of the returning echo that is displayed on the screen. The higher the gain level, the greater the ability of the instrument to display weaker echoes (e.g., vitreous opacities).

Conversely, as the gain is lowered, only the stronger echoes will continue to be displayed (e.g., retina and sclera). Because the strongest echoes are located along the central axis of the returning sound wave, lowering the gain effectively (not actually) narrows the sound beam, and thus improves both axial and lateral resolution. Also, lowering the gain effectively decreases the depth of sound beam penetration, because weaker echoes originating from deeper layers of tissue are not sufficiently amplified to be displayed (see Figures 2-13 and 5-16).

Many instruments incorporate time gain compensation (TGC) to enhance weak echoes displayed from deeper tissue layers. This process allows greater amplification of these more distant, weaker echoes than of the stronger echoes originating close to the transducer. This control has the effect of equalizing echo signals from similar tissues located at varying distances from the transducer. Although most current instruments have an automatic, internal TGC control, some instruments offer a manual TGC mode.

INSTRUMENTATION

Specific details regarding signal processing, as well as the manner in which the echoes are finally displayed, vary among the different types of ultrasound instruments. A- and B-scan echography are the types of ultrasound display systems most commonly used in ophthalmology, although Doppler ultrasound is sometimes also used.

A-Scan

A-scan echography is a one-dimensional acoustic display in which echoes are represented as vertical spikes from a baseline. Spacing of the spikes is dependent on the time required for the sound beam to reach a given interface and for its echo to return to the probe. The time between any two echo spikes can then be converted into distance by knowing the sound velocity of the medium from which the echoes are received. This is expressed by the formula, distance = velocity × time ($D = V \times T$; see Appendix A). The height of the displayed spikes indicates the strength (i.e., amplitude) of the echoes (Figure 1-11).

There are various types of A-scan displays used in ophthalmology. These include the A-scan that is used primarily for axial eye length measurements, the vector A-scan that can occur simultaneously on a B-scan echogram, and the standardized A-scan. The characteristics of these various A-scan

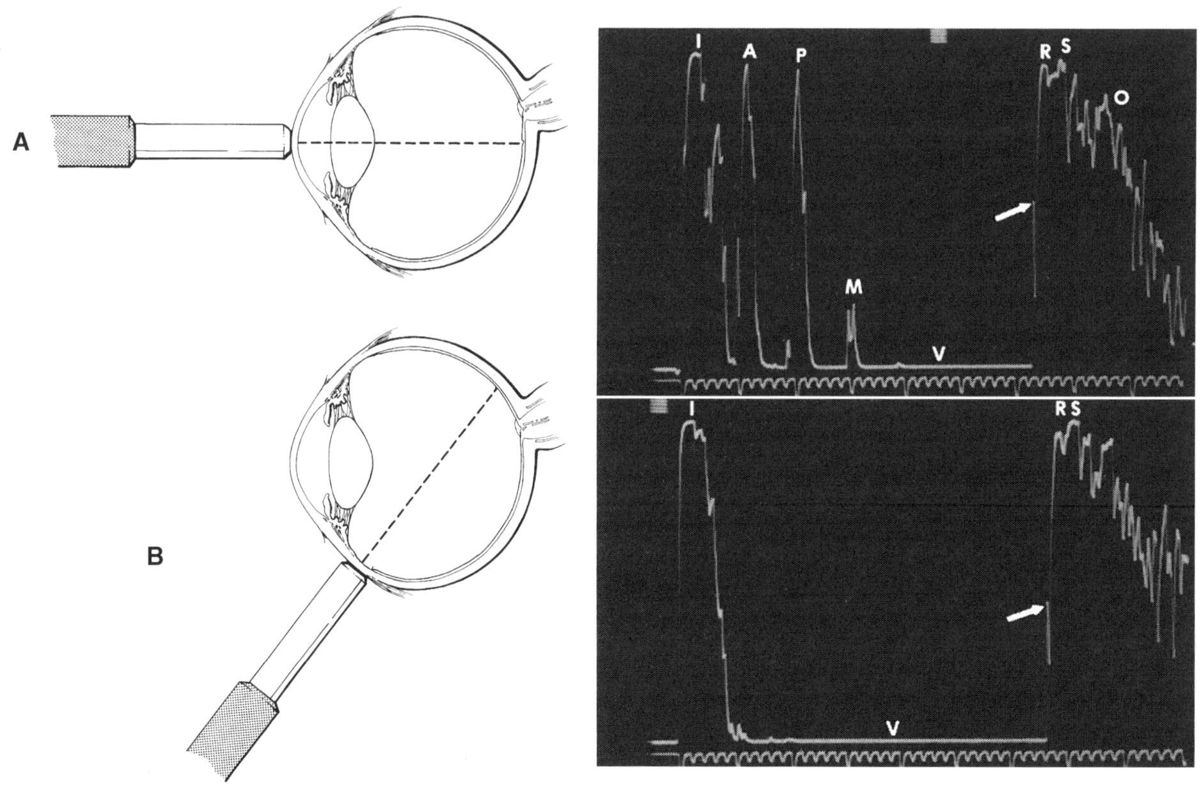

Figure 1-11 Normal standardized A-scan echograms. **A,** Probe placed on cornea with sound beam directed through lens. *I*, Initial spike corresponding to probe tip (corneal spike hidden by initial spike); *A*, anterior lens capsule; *P*, posterior lens capsule; *M*, multiple signal; *V*, vitreous cavity; *R*, retina; *S*, sclera; *O*, orbital soft tissue. Steeply rising spikes from lens and retina indicate sound beam perpendicularity. *Arrow*, Thin artifact spike, which indicates perpendicularity. **B,** Sound beam bypassing lens. (From Green RL, Byrne SF: Diagnostic ophthalmic ultrasound, in Ryan SJ [ed]: *Retina*. ed 3, St Louis, Mosby, 2001, p 226.)

displays differ somewhat. The A-scan used for most axial eye length measurements employs linear amplification, a focused transducer, and a frequency of between 10 and 15 MHz. The vector A-scan (see Figures 5-11 and 10-26) incorporates the same characteristics as the B-scan from which it is derived. These characteristics usually include logarithmic amplification, a focused transducer, and a frequency of 10 MHz.

The standardized A-scan, pioneered by Ossoinig, was developed as a diagnostic tool for ophthalmology.[31,32] Standardized A-scan instruments incorporate the previously described S-shaped amplification curve, as well as other unique characteristics designed to enhance tissue differentiation. The standardized A-scan, according to Ossoinig's criteria, requires the use of a nonfocused 8-MHz transducer that emits a parallel sound beam. External standardization is performed for each probe/instrument combination with a Tissue Model[41,42] (Figure 1-12). This determines the standard decibel setting, referred to as Tissue Sensitivity, which is the setting used for both detection and differentiation of lesions.

B-Scan

B-scan echography produces a two-dimensional acoustic section (similar to a photograph) by using both the vertical and the horizontal dimensions of the screen to indicate configuration and location. A section of tissue is examined by an oscillating transducer that emits a sound beam that "slices" through a tissue, much like the slice of a knife. Most ophthalmic B-scan instruments use logarithmic amplification and require a focused, narrow sound beam to display a two-

A

B

C

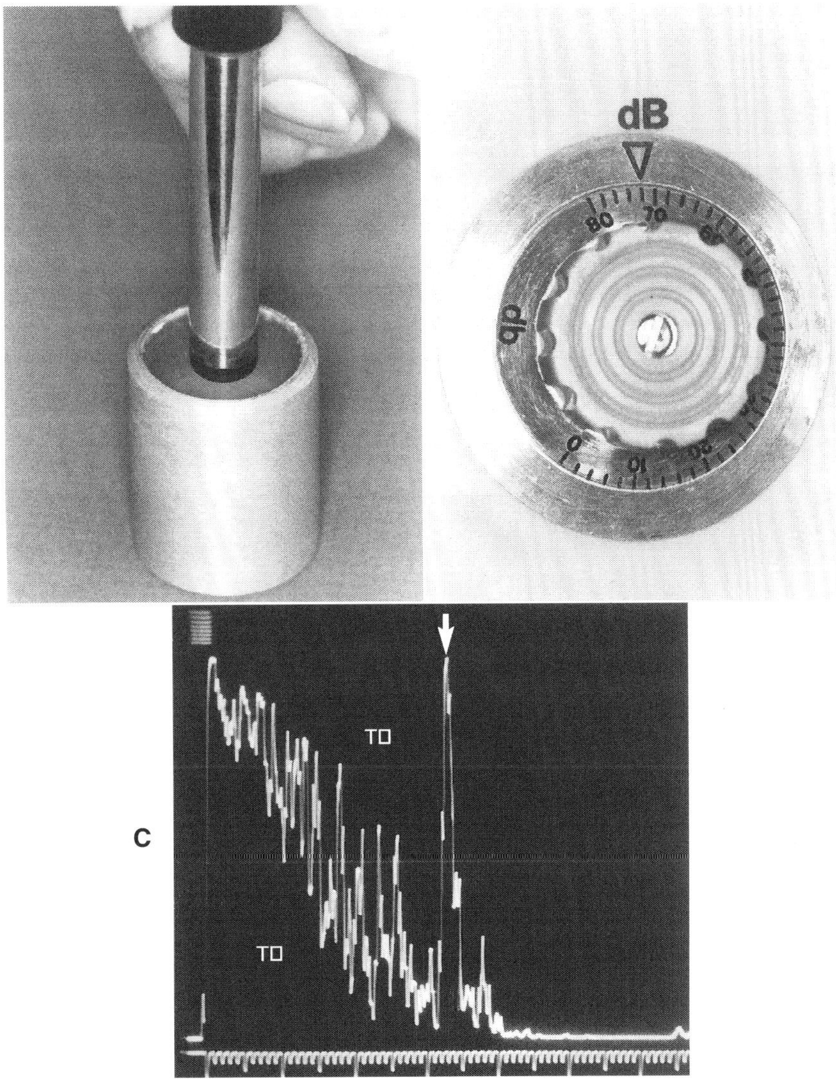

Figure 1-12 Calibration of standardized A-scan probe and instrument to obtain Tissue Sensitivity. **A,** With probe on Tissue Model, decibel dial **(B)** is adjusted until correct echogram is displayed **(C).** The spike chain *(T)* creates echo-free triangles that are of equal size above and below. *Arrow,* Bottom of Tissue Model; spikes to right are artifacts. (From Green RL, Byrne SF: Diagnostic ophthalmic ultrasound, in Ryan SJ [ed]: *Retina.* ed 3, St Louis, Mosby, 2001, p 227.)

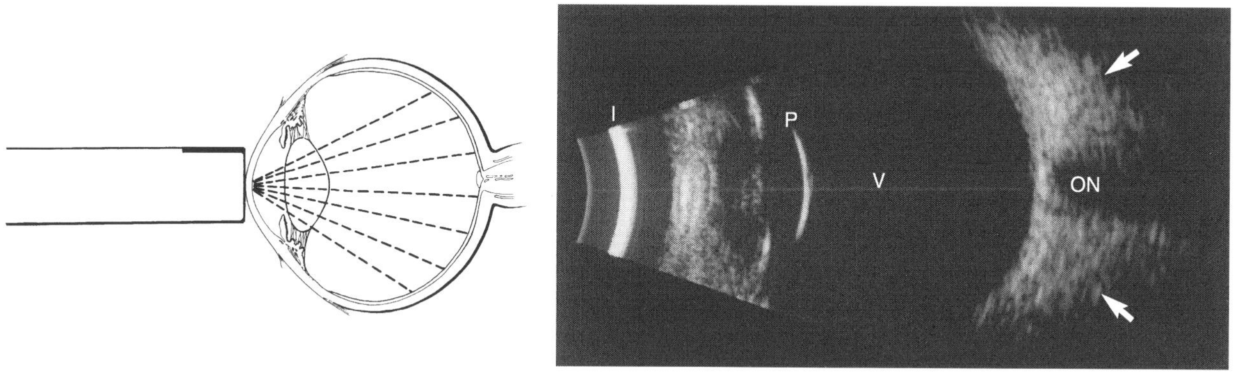

Figure 1-13 Oscillating transducer within B-scan probe creates two-dimensional acoustic section through normal eye. *I,* Initial line corresponding to transducer; *P,* posterior lens capsule; *V,* vitreous cavity; *ON,* optic nerve; *arrows,* orbital soft tissue. (From Green RL, Byrne SF: Diagnostic ophthalmic ultrasound, in Ryan SJ [ed]: *Retina.* ed 3, St Louis, Mosby, 2001, p 227.)

dimensional sector image. In addition, the majority of ophthalmic B-scan transducers operate at a frequency in the range of 10 MHz. An echo is represented as a dot on the screen, and the strength of the echo is depicted by the brightness of the dot. The coalescence of multiple dots on the screen forms a two-dimensional representation of the examined tissue section (Figure 1-13). Several factors in addition to signal processing affect the B-scan image. These include the angle of the scanning section, the speed of the transducer oscillation, and the gray scale.

The area of the eye and orbit that can be imaged on the echogram at any one time is related directly to the sector angle of the moving transducer. This angle can vary anywhere from 45 to 60 degrees, depending on the instrument used. Another important factor is the rate of transducer oscillation. To obtain a real-time image, the B-scan probe must produce multiple "slices" through a tissue each second (frame rate). This frame rate usually varies from 10 to 60 frames/sec. Finally, gray scale is the continuous range of brightness between white and black. Instruments differ in their ability to display levels of gray scale, but the greater the number of gray levels an instrument can display, the greater its ability to quantitate differences in echo intensity (see Chapter 2).

Three-dimensional B-scan imaging has also been developed.[40] This involves obtaining multiple sections using a mechanically rotated probe and software that reconstructs two-dimensional images into a three-dimensional format. The instrumentation and clinical application of this technology are described in Chapter 9. In addition to the conventional 10 MHz B-scan, newer high frequency B-scan instrumentation has been developed. The high frequencies used range from 20 MHz (see p 39) to greater than 50 MHz (see Chapter 8).

Doppler

A Doppler instrument emits a beam of pulsed or continuous ultrasound that is used to detect blood flow by means of the Doppler shift (i.e., Doppler effect),[13] which is defined as a change in the frequency of the sound wave caused by movement of a reflector (i.e., echo source). If reflector motion is toward the transducer, the frequency of the returning echo is greater than that of the emitted frequency. Conversely, if reflector motion is away from the transducer, the frequency of the returning echo is lower than that of the emitted sound beam. The greater the velocity of the reflector (e.g., the faster the blood flow), the greater the difference between the reflected and emitted frequencies. In orbital echography, Doppler ultrasound is helpful for assessing the direction of flow within orbital blood vessels and for the detection of blood flow within orbital lesions. For more details, see Chapter 14.

Recent advances have incorporated the use of color Doppler instruments with conventional B-scan imaging. This allows for the two-dimensional presentation of ocular and orbital images, with simultaneous Doppler evaluation indicated by color changes in the echogram. This color-flow Doppler technique allows the demonstration of blood flow through specific vessels within the eye and orbit. Frequency shifts that occur from blood flow toward the probe are generally coded in red, whereas blood flow away from the probe is colored blue. Spectrum analysis can be used to quantitate the velocity of the blood flow. CDI appears to be useful for the study of vascular disorders of the eye and orbit, as well as for the study of blood flow characteristics of tumors.[15]

Intravenous contrast agents are now being used in an attempt to enhance Doppler signals from blood flow.[3] A more detailed discussion of color Doppler and its clinical applications in ophthalmology is provided in Chapter 14.

Standardized Echography

The combined use of standardized A-scan and contact B-scan (along with Doppler for the orbit) is referred to as Standardized Echography.[31,32] B-scan echography, with its two-dimensional display, yields information primarily about the topographic nature of intraocular and orbital structures and lesions. A-scan* echography provides a variety of information regarding a lesion's character, as well as its size. The optimal echographic examination results from the appropriate combination of both A- scan and B-scan.

REFERENCES

1. Baum G, Greenwood I: The application of ultrasonic locating techniques to ophthalmology. II. Ultrasonic slit lamp in the ultrasonic visualization of soft tissues. *Arch Ophthalmol* 1958;60:263.
2. Bronson NR: Development of a simple B-scan ultrasonoscope. *Trans Am Ophthalmol Soc* 1972;70:365.
3. Cennamo G, Rosa N, Vallone GF, et al: First experience with a new echographic contrast agent. *Br J Ophthalmol* 1994;78:823.
4. Coleman DJ, Konig WF, Katz L: A hand-operated, ultrasound scan system for ophthalmic evaluation. *Am J Ophthalmol* 1969;68:256.
5. Coleman DJ: Reliability of ocular and orbital diagnosis with B-scan ultrasound. 1. Ocular diagnosis. *Am J Ophthalmol* 1972;73:501.
6. Coleman DJ: Reliability of ocular tumor diagnosis with ultrasound. *Trans Am Acad Ophthalmol Otolaryngol* 1973;77:677.
7. Coleman DJ, Lizzi FL, Jack RL: *Ultrasonography of the Eye and Orbit.* Philadelphia, Lea & Febiger, 1977, p 3.
8. Coleman DJ, Lizzi FL: Computer-processed acoustic spectral analysis. *Trans Am Acad Ophthalmol Otolaryngol* 1977;83:725.
9. Erickson SJ, Hendrix LE, Massaro BM, et al: Color Doppler flow imaging of the normal and abnormal orbit. *Radiology* 1989;173:511.
10. Flaharty PM, Lieb WE, Sergott RC, et al: Color Doppler imaging: A new noninvasive technique to diagnose and monitor carotid cavernous sinus fistulas. *Arch Ophthalmol* 1991;109:522.
11. Jansson F, Sundmark E: Determination of the velocity of ultrasound in ocular tissues at different temperatures. *Acta Ophthalmol* 1961;39:899.
12. Jansson F, Kock E: Determination of the velocity of ultrasound in the human lens and vitreous. *Acta Ophthalmol* 1962;40:420.
13. Kremkau FW: *Diagnostic Ultrasound. Principles and Instruments.* ed 5, Philadelphia, WB Saunders Co, 1998.
14. Lieb WE, Flaharty PM, Sergott RC, et al: Color Doppler imaging provides accurate assessment of orbital blood flow in occlusive carotid artery disease. *Ophthalmology* 1991;98:548.
15. Lieb WE: Color Doppler imaging of the eye and orbit. *Radiol Clin North Am* 1998;36:1059.
16. Lizzi FL, Coleman DJ: Computer-processed acoustic spectral analysis in ophthalmology, in White DN (ed): *Recent Advances in Ultrasound in Biomedicine.* vol 1. Forest Grove, Research Studies Press, 1977, p 117.
17. Mundt GH Jr, Hughes WF Jr: Ultrasonics in ocular diagnosis. *Am J Ophthalmol* 1956;41:488.
18. Oksala A: The clinical value of time-amplitude ultrasonography. *Am J Ophthalmol* 1964;57:453.
19. Oksala A, Lehtinen A: Diagnostics of detachment of the retina by means of ultrasound. *Acta Ophthalmol* 1957;35:461.
20. Ossoinig KC, Seher K: Echographische Untersuchungen feingeweblicher Strukturen zur Klärung des Echo-Ursprunges in Tumoren. I. Theoretische Uberlegungen. *Albrecht von Graefes Arch Klin Exp Ophthalmol* 1966;171:17.
21. Ossoinig K, Steiner H: Zum Problem der Normung in der ultraschalldiagnostik des auges. *Albrecht von Graefes Arch Clin Exp Ophthalmol* 1966;169:241.
22. Ossoinig K, Seher K: Einige Erkenntnisse über das histologische Substrat der Echogramme, in Oksala A, Gernet H (eds): *Ultrasonics in Ophthalmology.* Basel, S. Karger, 1967, p 103.
23. Ossoinig K, Seher K, Kaufmann F: Echographische Untersuchungen feingeweblicher strukturen. II. über ein bei der Ultraschalluntersuchung von Citratblut beobachtetes Phänomen. *Albrecht von Graefes Arch Klin Exp Ophthalmol* 1967;173:327.
24. Ossoinig KC: Basics of clinical echo-ophthalmography. IV: Clinical standardization of equipment and techniques, in Bock J, Ossoinig KC (eds): *Ultrasonographia Medica.* Vienna, Wiener Med Akademie, 1971, p 83.
25. Ossoinig KC: Basics of echographic tissue differentiation. II: Acoustic behavior of biological structures, in Bock J, Ossoinig KC (eds): *Ultrasonographia Medica.* Vienna, Wiener Med Akademie, 1971, p 419.
26. Ossoinig KC: Basics of echographic tissue differentiation. I. Experimental and clinical examinations of the influence of system parameters on the diagnostic value of echograms, in Bock J, Ossoinig KC (eds): *Ultrasonographia Medica.* Vienna, Wiener Med Akademie, 1972, p 155.
27. Ossoinig KC: The first standardized system for echo-ophthalmography, in Massin M, Poujol J (eds): *Diagnostica Ultrasonica in Ophthalmologia.* Paris, Centre National d'Ophthalmologie des Quinze-Vingts, 1973, p 131.
28. Ossoinig KC: Quantitative echography—the basis of tissue differentiation. *J Clin Ultrasound* 1974;2:33.
29. Ossoinig KC, Patel JH: A-scan instrumentation for acoustic tissue differentiation. II: Clinical significance of various technical parameters of the 7200 MA unit of Kretztechnik, in White D, Brown RE (eds): *Ultrasound in Medicine.* New York, Plenum Press, 1977, p 3B:1949.
30. Ossoinig KC, Patel JH: A-scan instrumentation for acoustic tissue differentiation. III: Testing and calibration of the 7200 MA unit of Kretztechnik, in White D, Brown RE (eds): *Ultrasound in Medicine.* New York, Plenum Press, 1977, p 3B:1955.
31. Ossoinig KC: Standardized echography: Basic principles, clinical applications, and results. *Int Ophthalmol Clin* 1979;19(4):127.
32. Ossoinig KC: *Standardized Ophthalmic Echography of the Eye, Orbit and Periorbital Region. A comprehensive slide set and study guide.* ed 3, Iowa City, Goodfellow, 1985, p 1.
33. Patel JH, Ossoinig KC: A-scan instrumentation for acoustic tissue differentiation. I: Signal processing in the 7200 MA unit of Kretztechnik, in White D, Brown RE (eds): *Ultrasound in Medicine.* New York, Plenum Press, 1977, p 3B:1949.
34. Pavlin CJ, Sherar MD, Foster FS: Subsurface ultrasound microscopic imaging of the intact eye. *Ophthalmology* 1990;97:244.
35. Pavlin CJ, Harasiewicz KA, Sherar MD, et al: Clinical use of ultrasound biomicroscopy. *Ophthalmology* 1991;98:287.
36. Pavlin CJ, Foster FS: *Ultrasound Biomicroscopy of the Eye.* New York, Springer-Verlag, 1995.
37. Pavlin CJ, Foster FS: Ultrasound Biomicroscopy: high-frequency ultrasound imaging of the eye and microscopic resolution. *Radiol Clin North Am* 1998;36:1047.
38. Purnell EW: Ultrasound in ophthalmological diagnosis, in Grossman CC (ed): *Diagnostic Ultrasound.* New York, Plenum Press, 1965, p 95.
39. Purnell EW: Intensity modulated (B-scan) ultrasonography, in Goldberg RE, Sarin LK (eds): *Ultrasonics in Ophthalmology. Diagnostic and Therapeutic Applications.* Philadelphia, WB Saunders Co, 1967, p 102.
40. Shammas HJ, Dunne S, Fisher YL: *Three-Dimensional Ultrasound Tomography of the Eye.* Eden Mills, Ontario, Canada, 1999.
41. Till P: Solid tissue model for the standardization of the echo-ophthalmograph 7200 MA (Kretztechnik). *Doc Ophthalmol* 1976;41:205.
42. Till P, Ossoinig KC: First experience with a new solid tissue model for the standardization of A- and B-scan instruments used in tissue diagnosis, in White D, Brown RE (eds): *Ultrasound in Medicine.* New York, Plenum Press, 1977, p 3B:2167.

Suggested Reading

Bioeffects considerations for the safety of diagnostic ultrasound. American Institute of Ultrasound in Medicine. Bioeffects Committee. *J Ultrasound Med* 1988;7(suppl.):S4.

Bushong S, Archer B: *Diagnostic Ultrasound Physics, Biology, and Instrumentation.* St Louis, Mosby, 1991.

Hedrick WR, Hykes DL, Starchman D: *Ultrasound Physics and Instrumentation.* ed 3, St Louis, Mosby, 1994.

McDicken WN: *Diagnostic Ultrasonics. Principles and Use of Instrument.* ed 3, Edinburgh, Churchill Livingstone, 1990.

Zagzebski AA: *Essentials of Ultrasound Physics.* St Louis, Mosby, 1996.

*The term "A-scan" indicates standardized A-scan throughout the book except in Chapter 10.

THE GLOBE

INTRODUCTION

Echography has become the most important method for evaluating an eye with opaque ocular media. It provides an instantaneous "glimpse" into the eye and, in many instances, can yield information not obtainable by any other method. Echography has also proven to be indispensable in the differentiation and measurement of intraocular tumors, even in the presence of clear ocular media. It is a painless, noninvasive method that can be performed easily in the clinic, at the patient's bedside, or in the operating room. Furthermore, ultrasound can be readily performed on children, often without sedation. Recent advances in technology have vastly improved the ability of ultrasound to accurately display the small structures and lesions within the eye. Also, the wealth of experience and data that has been accumulated throughout the years provides the echographer with a large reference base that allows accurate and reliable diagnoses. It is important to emphasize, however, that in many cases accurate interpretation of echographic findings is possible only when they are correlated with the history and clinical findings.

INDICATIONS

The indications for echographic examination of the eye have become more numerous with the accumulation of experience and the improvement of instrumentation and examination techniques. Ultrasound is indicated whenever the anterior or posterior segments cannot be visualized due to opaque ocular media and is indicated also in the presence of clear ocular media for the evaluation of ocular tumors and for biometry (Table I-I).

TABLE I-I

Indications for Intraocular Examination

Opaque Ocular Media

Anterior segment
- Corneal opacification
- Hyphema or hypopyon
- Miosis
- Cataract
- Pupillary or retrolenticular membrane

Posterior segment
- Vitreous hemorrhage or inflammation

Clear Ocular Media

Anterior segment
- Iris lesions
- Ciliary body lesions

Posterior segment
- Tumors
- Choroidal detachment: serous versus hemorrhagic
- Retinal detachment: rhegmatogenous versus exudative
- Optic disc abnormalities
- Unexplained retinitis and/or choroditis

Intraocular Foreign Bodies
- Detection
- Localization

2

William D. Bates

Examination Techniques for the Globe

Specific examination techniques have been carefully designed to allow thorough evaluation of the anterior and posterior segments of the globe.[1-10] The type of examination performed is determined by the indication for examination. The contact method, in which the probe is placed directly on the globe, is used to evaluate the posterior segment. In those cases in which the anterior segment also must be evaluated, an easy immersion technique has been developed that can be performed with the same instruments used for the contact examination. In addition, new higher resolution B-scan technology has been developed for the anterior segment examination. One of these instruments, the ultrasound biomicroscope (UBM),[9,10] is discussed in Chapter 8. This chapter will address A- and B-scan examination techniques for the detection and differentiation of intraocular lesions.

POSITIONING THE PATIENT

A- and B-scan instruments may be placed on one large or two separate, small carts. The patient is seated in a reclinable examination chair of adjustable height. While most examinations are performed with the patient reclined, it is occasionally helpful to examine the patient in a sitting position (see Figure 3-12). The echographer is seated on an examining stool of adjustable height, usually to the patient's right. A fixation light, suspended from the ceiling, is useful to facilitate steady gaze. The patient's head and the instruments to be used are situated close together, so that the probe position and the screen may be viewed simultaneously (Figure 2-1). Topical anesthetic drops are applied to the eye before the examination.

B-SCAN EXAMINATION TECHNIQUES

An adequate evaluation of the eye depends on the ability of the echographer to think three-dimensionally while examining the globe with instruments that have only a one- or two-dimensional display. Once proper examination techniques are mastered, lesions can be reliably localized in relationship to one another and to ocular structures. The two-dimensional B-scan is the primary modality for determining lesion topography (i.e., location and configuration). By obtaining echograms from a variety of probe positions in a systematic fashion, the echographer may construct a mental three-dimensional picture of a lesion's topography.

Characteristics of B-Scan Probes

All B-scan probes contain a transducer that oscillates rapidly back and forth near the face (i.e., tip) of the probe. Each probe has a marker, usually a dot, line or logo, that indicates the side of the probe that is represented on the upper portion of the B-scan screen display. The oscillating movement of the transducer within the probe always occurs away from and toward the marker (Figure 2-2).

The probe face is always represented by the initial line that appears on the left side of the echogram. The right side of the echogram indicates the region of the eye located opposite the probe face. The upper part of the echogram corresponds to the portion of the globe where the probe marker is directed. The center of the screen corresponds to the central portion of the probe face. Furthermore, because the best resolution of the echogram is in this central region, the area of interest should be centered within the echogram whenever possible.

Methylcellulose is applied to the face of the B-scan probe as a coupling medium. The probe is then placed directly on the eye (i.e., conjunctiva or cornea). Examination through the lids is generally less desirable because of sound attenuation produced by the lid tissues. In addition, with the lids closed, the echographer cannot be certain of which portion of the globe is being evaluated. The particular section of ocular tissue displayed on the screen is dependent on where the probe is positioned and how the marker is directed.

B-Scan Probe Orientations

The three basic probe orientations that are used to evaluate intraocular lesions are transverse, longitudinal, and axial.

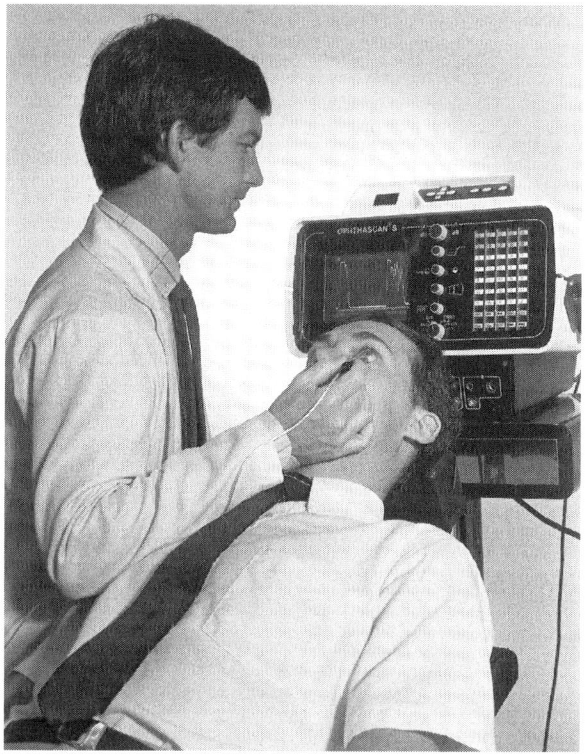

Figure 2-1 Patient positioned properly for echographic examination. Patient is in a reclined position. Examined eye is near screen, so that echogram and probe position may be monitored simultaneously.

A

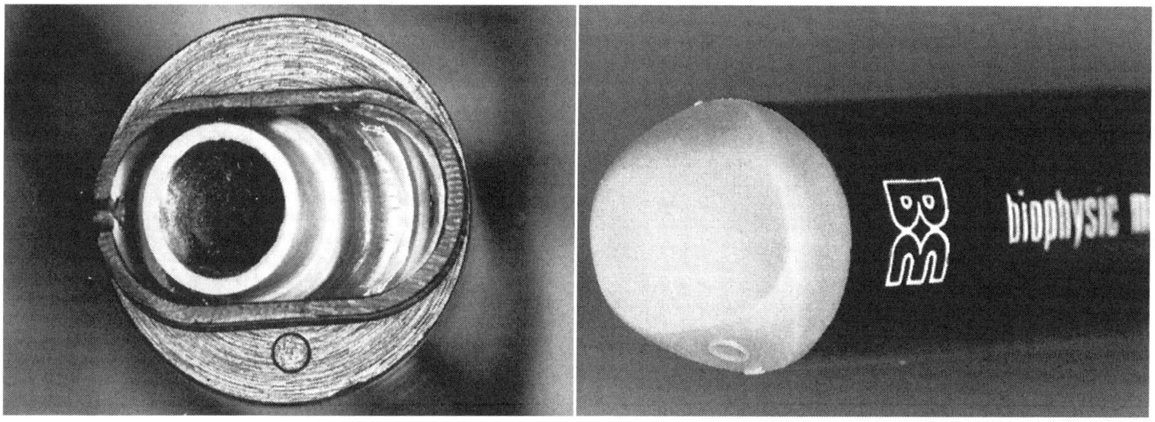

B

Figure 2-2 B-scan probe. **A,** Transducer is shown with cap removed. Transducer oscillates near face of probe to produce a two-dimensional acoustic section. **B,** Cap in place after probe is filled with distilled water. Note probe marker (i.e., insignia on this probe) that designates upper portion of echogram. (From Green RL, Byrne SF: Diagnostic ophthalmic ultrasound, in Ryan SJ [ed]: *Retina*. ed 3, St Louis, Mosby, 2001, p 231.)

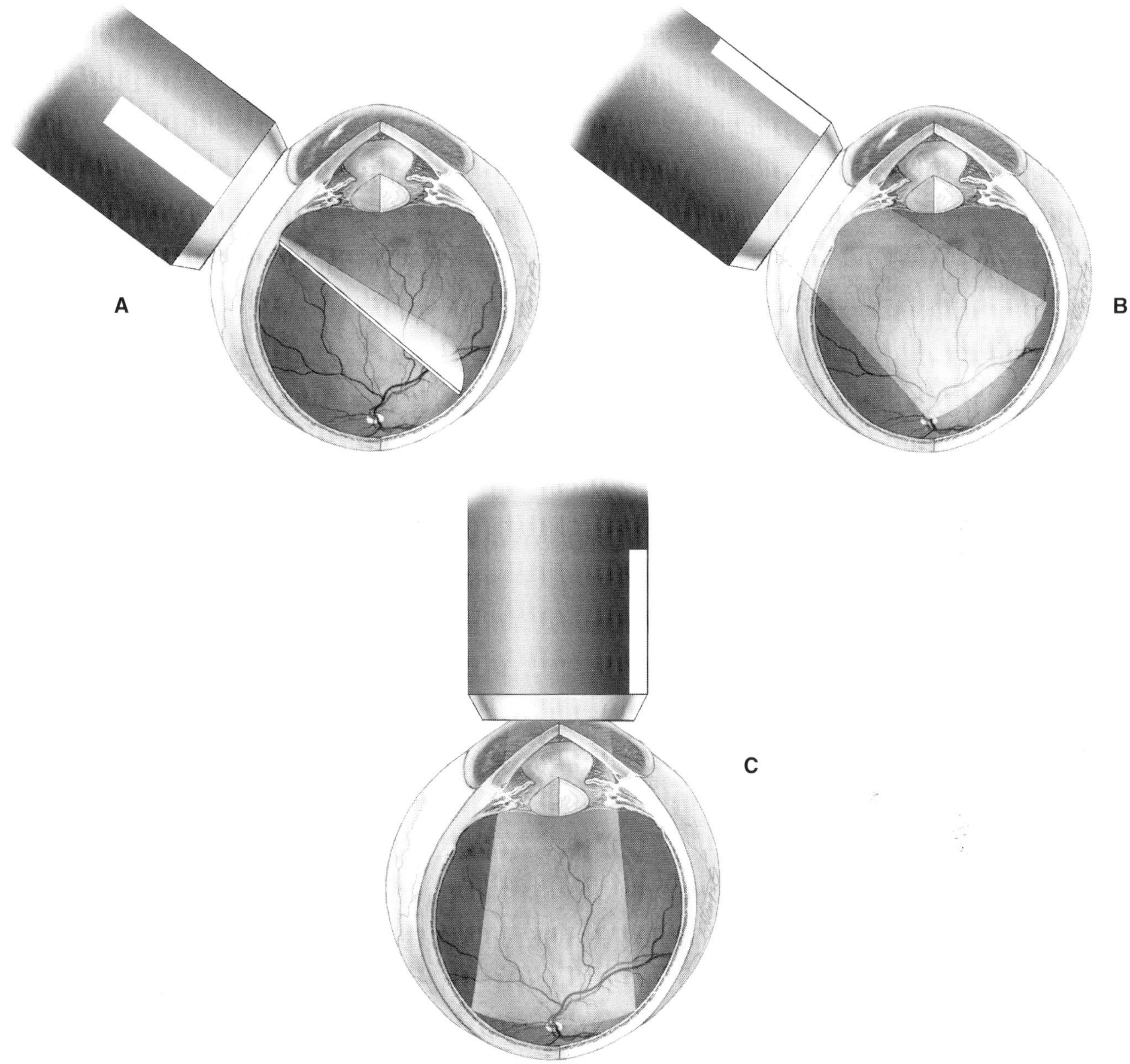

Figure 2-3 Three primary B-scan probe orientations. Transverse **(A)**, longitudinal **(B)**, and axial **(C)** scans.

Transverse and longitudinal scans are used most commonly because the probe is placed on the conjunctiva peripheral to the cornea. Thus, the sound beam bypasses the lens, allowing better sound beam penetration. Both transverse and longitudinal scans are performed with the patient's gaze directed away from the probe, toward the meridian being examined. This allows a wide surface of globe on which to place and shift the probe. In an axial scan, the patient fixates in primary gaze and the probe is placed on the center of the cornea, thereby displaying lens and optic nerve in the center of the echogram (Figure 2-3).

In the B-scan examination, the optic nerve is used as an anatomic reference for the posterior fundus. For the sake of clarification, the optic nerve is echographically considered to be the center of the posterior fundus rather than the macula (the true anatomic center). Furthermore, it serves as a reference point for the three primary B-scan probe positions (transverse, longitudinal, and axial) (Figure 2-4).

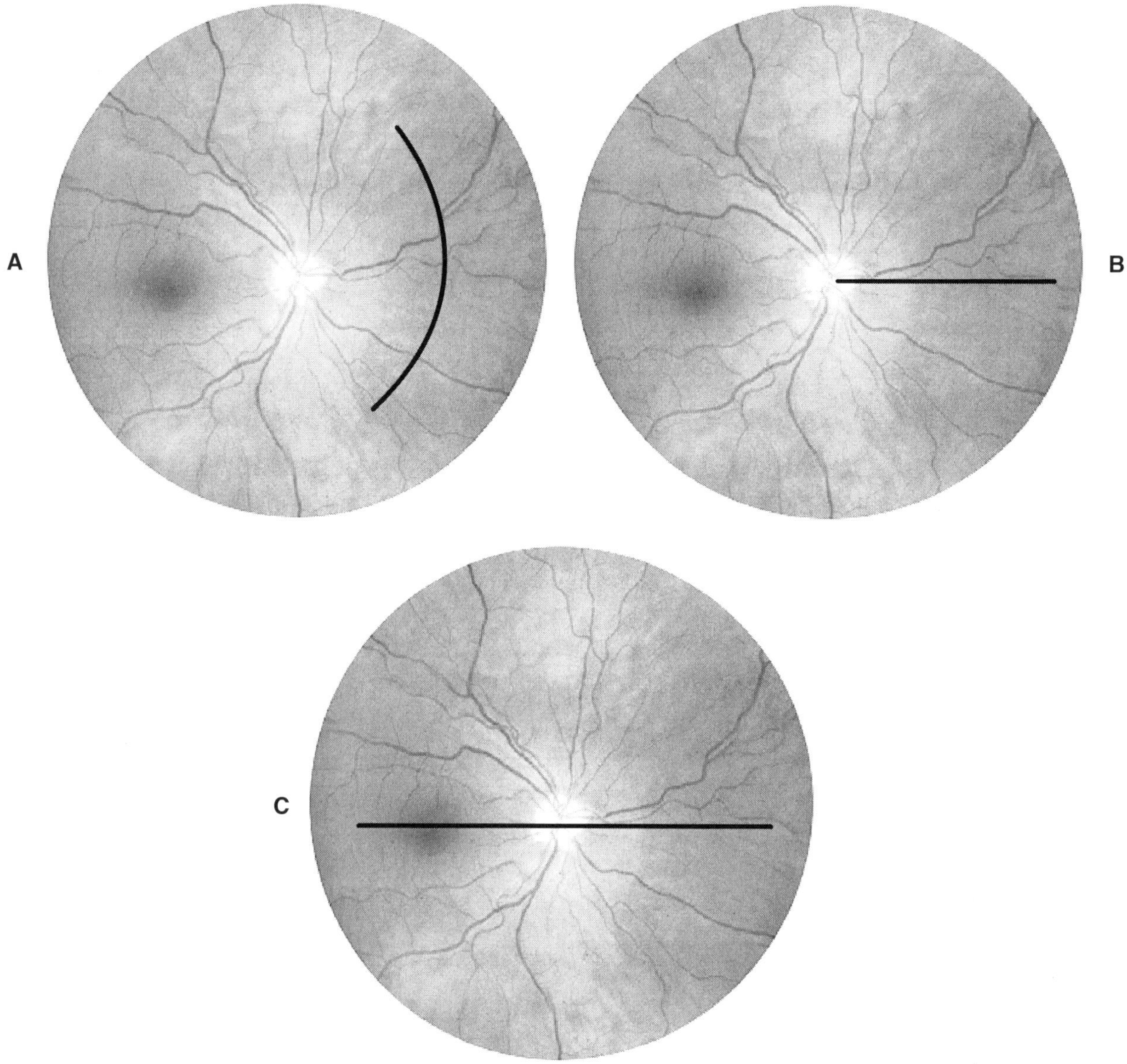

Figure 2-4 Optic nerve in center of posterior fundus serves as a reference point for the three primary B-scan probe orientations. Transverse **(A)**, longitudinal **(B)**, and axial **(C)** scans. Lines correspond to movement of the sound beam on the fundus for each probe position.

Transverse Scans

The probe, in a transverse scan, is placed on the globe so that the back-and-forth movement of the transducer occurs parallel (i.e., tangential) to the limbus. This causes the sound beam to move back and forth across the opposite fundus, producing a circumferential slice through several meridians of the globe. This orientation is appropriate for showing the lateral (i.e., circumferential) extent of a lesion (e.g., extending from 2- to 4-o'clock meridians, from 11:30- to 1:30-o'clock meridians, and so forth) (Figure 2-5; see also Figures 2-3, *A*, and 2-4, *A*).

The designation of the transverse scan is determined by the meridian that lies in the middle of the scanning section. For example, if the probe is held horizontally with its face centered on the 6-o'clock meridian, the middle of the echogram displays the 12-o'clock meridian of the fundus; this probe position is called a transverse scan of the 12-o'clock meridian. If the probe is placed in a vertical orientation at the 3-o'clock limbus, the sound beam sweeps across the 9-o'clock meridian of the fundus; this is called a transverse scan of the 9-o'clock meridian.

By convention, horizontal transverse scans (i.e., transverse scans of the 12- or 6-o'clock meridians) are performed with the marker oriented toward the patient's nose. Therefore, the upper part of the echogram always represents the nasal portion of the globe. On the other hand,

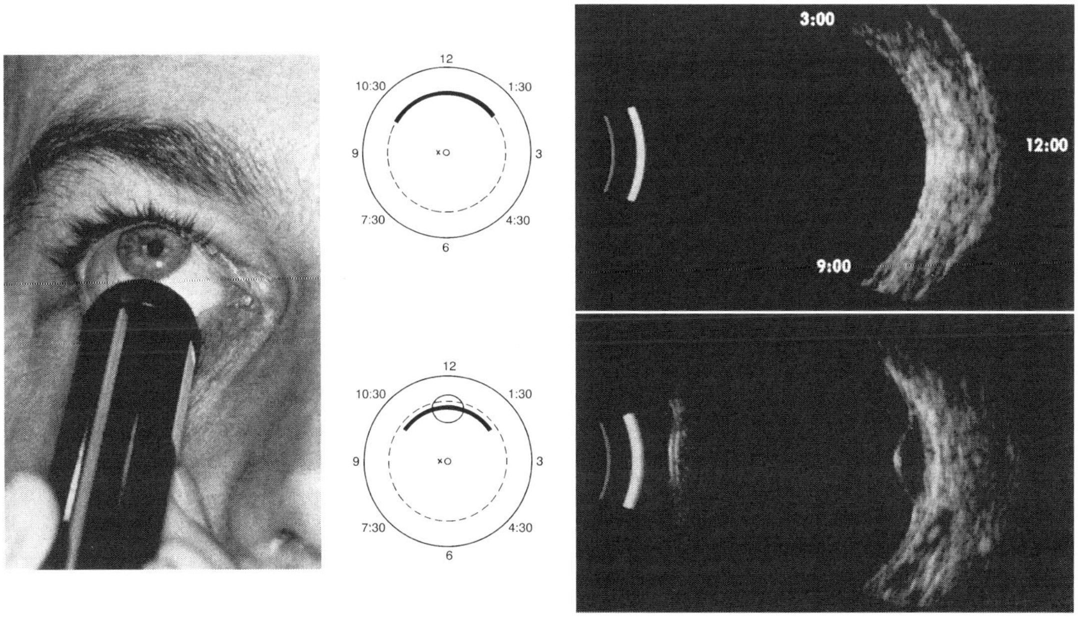

Figure 2-5 Technique for transverse B-scan approach. A horizontal transverse scan is demonstrated in this example. *Left*, The patient fixates superiorly, and the sound beam sweeps across the 12-o'clock meridian near the equator. *Top*, Normal globe. *Bottom*, Elevated lesion extending from 11:30- to 12:30-o'clock meridians. Note that the probe marker is oriented nasally. (From Green RL, Byrne SF: Diagnostic ophthalmic ultrasound, in Ryan SJ [ed]: *Retina*. ed 3, St Louis, Mosby, 2001, p 232.)

TABLE 2-1
Orientation of B-Scan Probe Marker

Probe Position	Direction of Marker
Transverse and Axial Scans	
Horizontal	Nasal
Vertical	Superior
Oblique	Superior
Longitudinal Scans	Toward center of cornea and meridian being examined

vertical transverse scans (i.e., transverse scans of the 3- or 9-o'clock meridians) are performed with the marker directed superiorly so the top of the echogram represents the upper portion of the globe. Oblique transverse scans (e.g., transverse scans of the 1:30-, 4:30-, 7:30-, or 10:30-o'clock meridians) are performed with the marker directed upward (Table 2-1 and Figure 2-6).

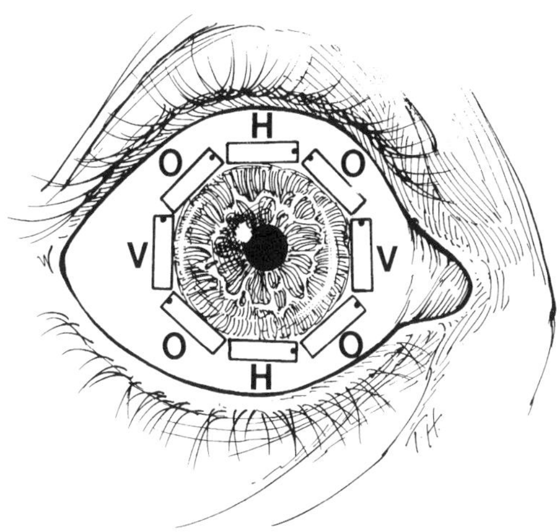

Figure 2-6 Probe marker orientation for various transverse B-scan approaches. *H*, Horizontal probe positions; *O*, oblique probe positions; *V*, vertical probe positions. Note that the marker is always oriented above the horizontal for vertical and oblique scans.

Longitudinal Scans

For longitudinal scanning the probe face is rotated 90 degrees from the position used for the transverse scan. This means that the back and forth movement of the transducer is oriented perpendicular (rather than parallel) to the limbus. The sound beam then sweeps *along* the single meridian located opposite the probe rather than *across* the meridian, in contrast to the transverse scan. In this way, the longitudinal scan shows the anterior-posterior extent of a lesion rather than the lateral extent (Figure 2-7; see also Figures 2-3, *B*, and 2-4, *B*). Another way to think of this orientation is as a radial section (like the spoke of a wheel) where the sound beam sweeps from the optic disc out toward the periphery along a given meridian.

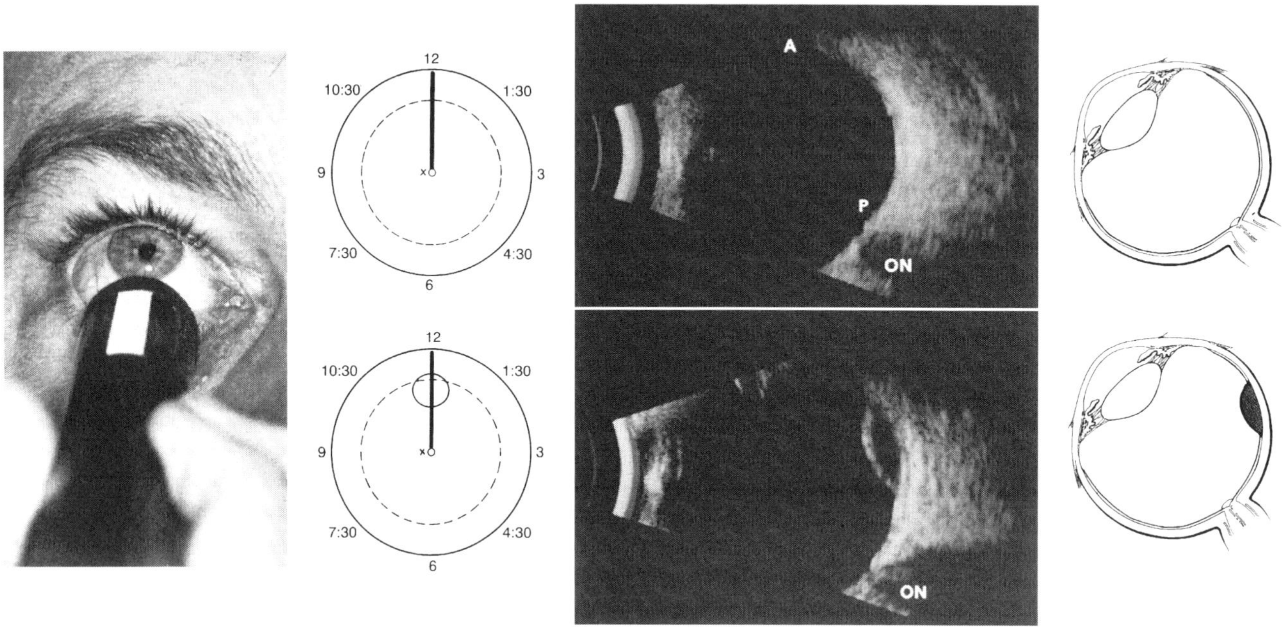

Figure 2-7 Technique for longitudinal B-scan approach. A longitudinal scan of the 12-o'clock meridian is demonstrated in this example. *Left*, The patient fixates superiorly and the sound beam sweeps along the 12-o'clock meridian. *Top*, Normal globe. *Bottom*, Elevated lesion. Note that the probe marker is oriented toward the cornea as well as the 12-o'clock meridian. *ON*, Optic nerve; *P*, posterior aspect of globe; *A*, anterior aspect of globe. (From Green RL, Byrne SF: Diagnostic ophthalmic ultrasound, in Ryan SJ [ed]: *Retina*. ed 3, St Louis, Mosby, 2001, p 233.)

In longitudinal scans, the marker is always directed toward the center of the cornea and the meridian being examined (Figure 2-8; see also Table 2-1). This produces an echogram that displays a section or slice through the globe along a given meridian. The optic disc and posterior aspect of the globe along the meridian are displayed on the lower portion of the screen. The peripheral aspect of the globe along the meridian is displayed on the upper aspect of the screen. The designation of the longitudinal scan is simply that meridian which is being examined. For example, if the probe is placed on the 6-o'clock meridian, the sound beam sweeps along the 12-o'clock meridian; this is designated as a longitudinal scan of the 12-o'clock meridian.

With the probe placed for the longitudinal scan orientation, it is possible to shift the probe on the globe either closer to the limbus or into the fornix. This provides either a more posterior or a more anterior view of the meridian being examined. With the probe placed so that it slightly overlaps the limbus, the sound beam sweeps through more of the posterior aspect of the eye, thus allowing better evaluation of the peripapillary region. Conversely, when the probe is placed close to the fornix, the sound beam extends more peripherally to better display the peripheral fundus and often the posterior ciliary body. It is of note that as the probe is shifted closer to the fornix, the optic nerve may move inferiorly off the screen display (Figure 2-9).

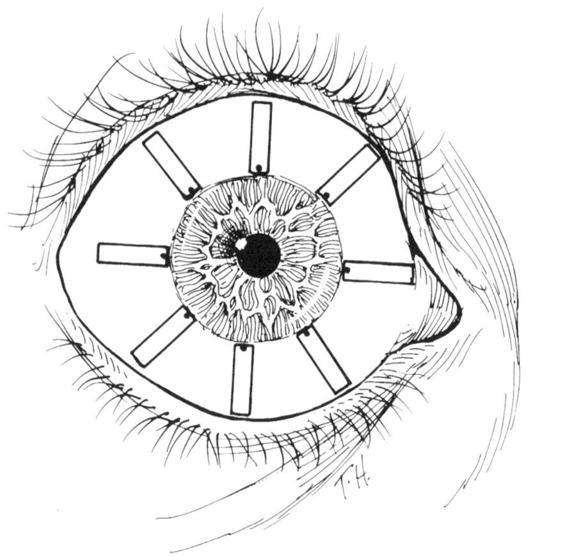

Figure 2-8 Probe marker orientation for various longitudinal B-scan approaches. Note that the probe marker is always oriented toward the center of the cornea as well as the meridian being scanned.

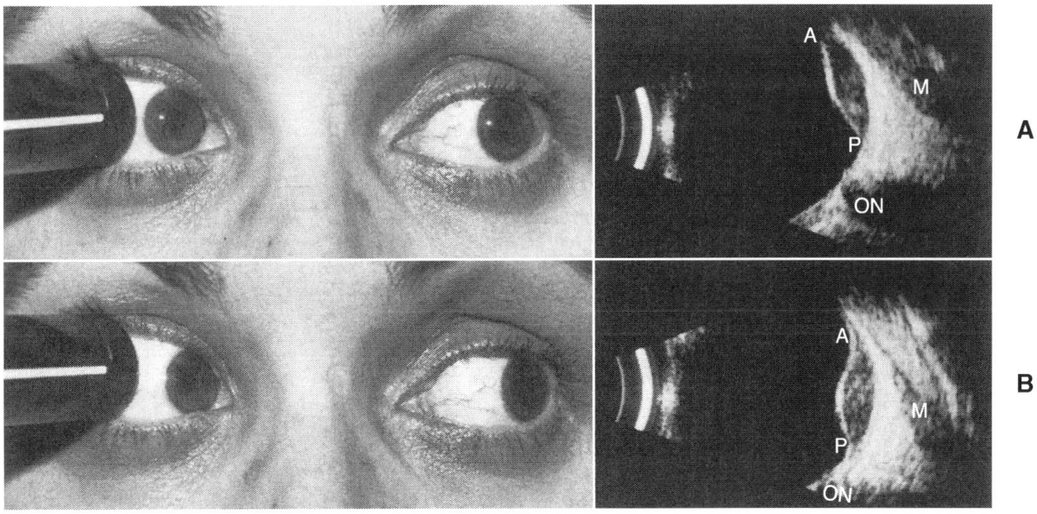

Figure 2-9 Anterior and posterior longitudinal B-scan probe positions. **A,** Posterior longitudinal scan of 3-o'clock meridian. Probe is placed near limbus with sound beam directed along posterior aspect of 3-o'clock meridian. Echogram shows dome-shaped lesion nasal to the optic nerve *(ON)*. Note that the posterior border *(P)* is well shown, but the anterior border *(A)* is not well imaged in this view. *M,* Medial rectus muscle. **B,** Anterior longitudinal scan of 3-o'clock meridian. Probe is shifted toward fornix to direct sound beam more anteriorly along the 3-o'clock meridian. The anterior margin of the lesion is now well demonstrated.

The use of a longitudinal probe orientation greatly facilitates three-dimensional thinking and promotes a better understanding of B-scan findings. It is often the best probe orientation for demonstrating the insertion of membranes into the optic disc. In many cases the axial approach, due to sound attenuation from the lens and from the angle of incidence, does not clearly demonstrate the relationship of membranes to the optic nerve. Therefore, the longitudinal approach should always be used to determine if a membrane inserts into the optic disc (see Figure 3-24). The longitudinal approach is useful also for demonstrating the peripheral insertions of a membrane.

Axial Scans

The axial orientation is the third type of B-scan probe position. The axial scan is performed with the patient fixating in primary gaze and with the probe face centered on the cornea. The sound beam is then directed through the center of the lens, sweeping along two opposing meridians, intersected by the optic nerve (Figure 2-10; see also Figures 2-3, *C*, and 2-4, *C*). As mentioned previously, this scan is the easiest to understand because it displays the lens and optic nerve in the center of the echogram, thus simplifying orientation while assessing the disease process. Unfortunately, however, sound attenuation and refraction from the lens often hinder resolution of the posterior portion of the globe, thus limiting the usefulness of axial scans. This position can be helpful in some situations, however, for documenting lesions and membranes in relation to the lens and optic nerve. It can also be useful for evaluating the macular region (see "Evaluation of the Macula" later in this chapter).

When a horizontal axial scan is performed, the marker is oriented toward the patient's nose, which places the macular region just below the optic disc in the echogram. A vertical axial scan is obtained with the marker in the superior position. In oblique axial scans (e.g., the sound beam is sweeping from the 1:30 to 7:30 or 10:30 to 4:30 meridians), the marker is oriented toward the upper of the two meridians being scanned (Figure 2-11; see also Table 2-1).

Para-Axial Scans

Para-axial scans often facilitate the evaluation of the peripapillary region. These scans are very similar to axial scans in that the probe is centered on the cornea with the sound beam directed through the lens. The sound beam, however, is slightly shifted so that the fundus adjacent to the optic nerve is imaged. In order to obtain a para-axial scan, an axial view is first displayed. The probe is then tilted slightly so that the sound beam passes through the fundus just next to the optic disc. If the probe is oriented vertically and the sound beam is shifted slightly right or left of the optic nerve, the nasal or temporal peripapillary region will be evaluated (see p 29). On the other hand, if the probe is oriented horizontally and the sound beam is shifted slightly above or below the optic nerve, the superior or inferior peripapillary region can be imaged. Finally, an oblique orientation can image the peripapillary region in other quadrants adjacent to the optic nerve

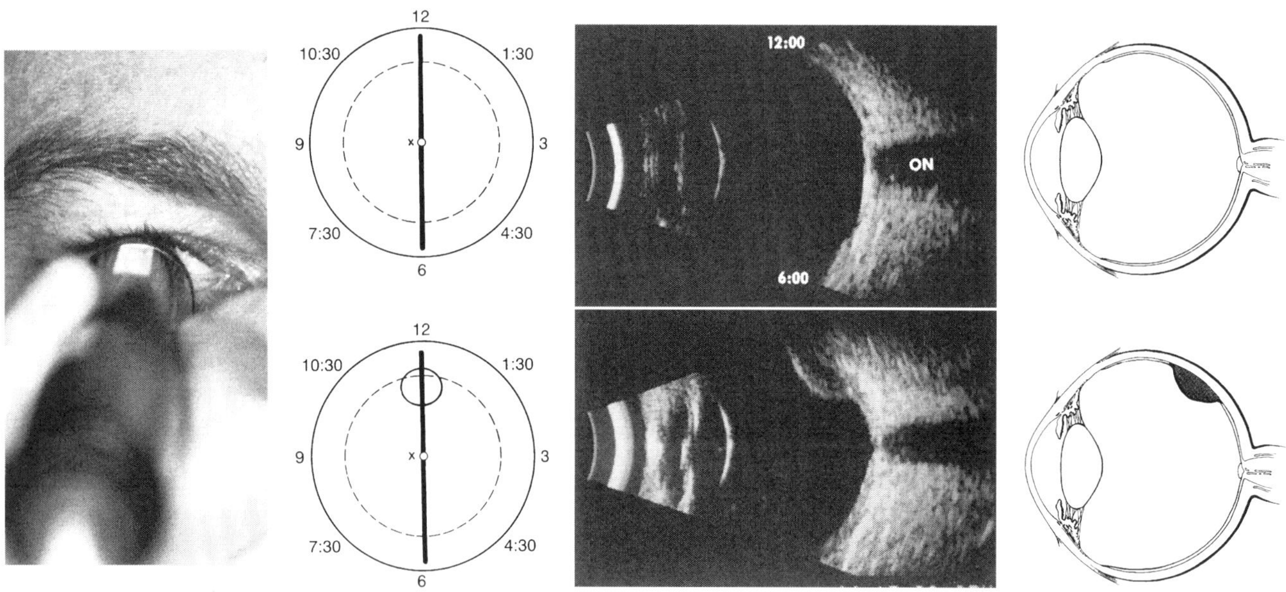

Figure 2-10 Technique for vertical axial B-scan. *Left*, Patient fixates in primary gaze, and probe is centered on cornea. *Top*, Normal globe. *Bottom*, Elevated lesion. *ON*, Optic nerve. Note that probe marker is directed toward the 12-o'clock meridian. (From Green RL, Byrne SF: Diagnostic ophthalmic ultrasound, in Ryan SJ [ed]: *Retina*. ed 3, St Louis, Mosby, 2001, p 234.)

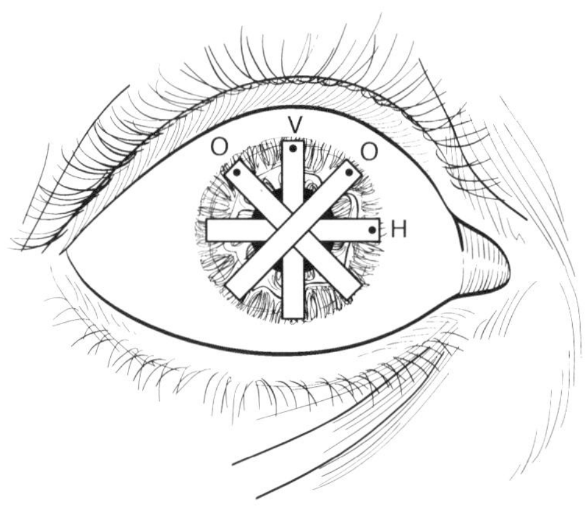

Figure 2-11 Probe marker orientation for various axial B-scan approaches. *O*, Oblique scans; *V*, vertical axial scan; *H*, horizontal axial scan. Note that the marker is directed upwards for vertical and oblique axial scans and nasally for horizontal axial scans.

(e.g., superotemporally or inferotemporally). The probe marker is oriented in exactly the same manner as for axial scans (see Table 2-1).

BASIC SCREENING EXAMINATION

The basic screening examination is performed to detect lesions in eyes with opaque ocular media. This examination can be performed with either B- or A-scan, although most examiners prefer to use B-scan. A systematic technique for screening the globe is used.

Basic B-Scan Screening Examination Technique

Transverse scans of the four major quadrants are performed initially at a high gain setting. The superior portion of the globe is first scanned with the patient's gaze directed superiorly. The probe is oriented horizontally with its face placed next to the inferior limbus and centered on the 6-o'clock meridian (horizontal transverse scan of the 12-o'clock meridian). Remember that the marker is directed nasally for this probe position. With the probe first positioned near the limbus, the superior, posterior fundus is examined initially. The probe is then shifted toward the lower fornix, thus screening progressively more peripheral aspects of the superior globe (Figure 2-12). As the probe is shifted, the echogram is continuously monitored to detect abnormal echoes. This maneuver thus examines the superior half of the globe. The nasal portion of the eye is next examined by having the patient look medially and by placing the probe in a vertical orientation, with the probe face centered near the temporal limbus (transverse scan of the 3-o'clock meridian [right eye] or 9-o'clock meridian [left eye]). Again the probe is shifted from limbus to fornix, thereby scanning the entire nasal half of the globe. Similar maneuvers are then performed for the inferior and temporal quadrants (see Appendix B).

It is also suggested that the eye be screened using longitudinal scans, along at least the four major meridians. These scans may help detect lesions located in the peripapillary region (including the macula) as well as in the far periphery of the globe.

Once the posterior segment has been thoroughly screened with transverse and longitudinal approaches, the

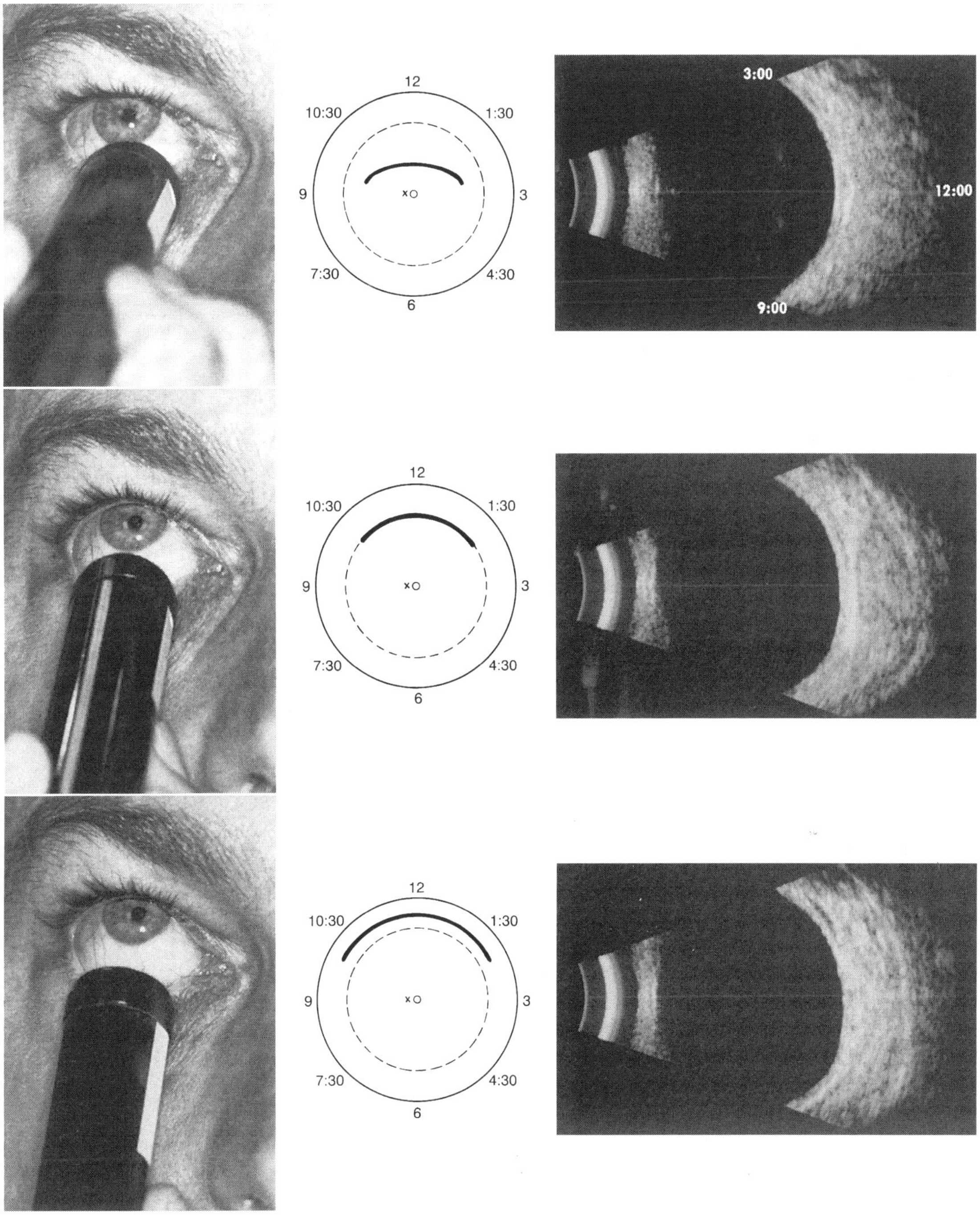

Figure 2-12 Technique for B-scan screening. In this example, the superior aspect of the globe is examined. Horizontal transverse approach is used to examine globe from posteriorly to anteriorly. Note that the probe marker is oriented nasally. (From Green RL, Byrne SF: Diagnostic ophthalmic ultrasound, in Ryan SJ [ed]: *Retina.* ed 3, St Louis, Mosby, 2001, p 236.)

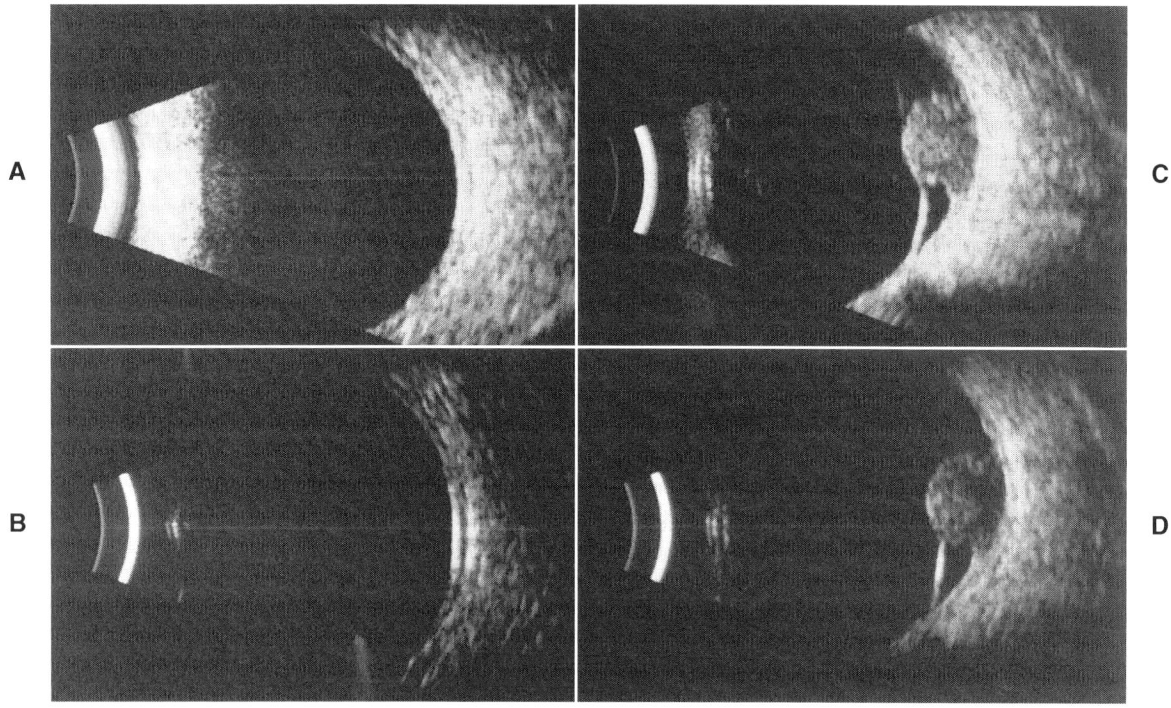

Figure 2-13 Transverse scans of normal globe (**A** and **B**) and choroidal tumor (**C** and **D**). **A** and **C**, High gain setting. **B** and **D**, Reduced gain setting. Note extremely bright echoes produced from normal retina and sclera when the sound beam is directed perpendicularly. Such artifacts can be mistaken for a foreign body or other very highly reflective lesion. (From Green RL, Byrne SF: Diagnostic ophthalmic ultrasound, in Ryan SJ [ed]: *Retina*. ed 3, St Louis, Mosby, 2001, p 237.)

globe is evaluated with both vertical and horizontal axial scans. For both of these positions, the patient fixates in primary gaze with the contralateral eye, and the probe is centered on the cornea of the examined eye.

The B-scan screening procedure is performed at both high and low gain settings. The high settings are used to detect vitreous opacities and gross fundus lesions, whereas the lower settings (which improve resolution) are helpful for detecting relatively flat fundus elevations and for better showing the topography of large lesions (Figure 2-13).

During the screening examination, the optic disc should also be evaluated to detect any abnormalities (see p 431).

Basic A-Scan Screening Examination Technique

Although A-scan is rarely used to screen the eye for abnormalities, the maneuver of shifting the probe along the surface of the eye is a necessary technique for the A-scan evaluation of intraocular lesions. For this technique, the patient's gaze is always directed away from the probe, toward the meridian to be examined. The probe is placed on the globe at the limbus opposite to the meridian and it is slowly shifted into the fornix as the screen is continuously monitored (Figure 2-14). This maneuver is generally first performed at the Tissue Sensitivity gain setting (see Figure 1-12) although reduced gain levels can also be used (Figure 2-15).

SPECIAL EXAMINATION TECHNIQUES

Special examination techniques (i.e., topographic, quantitative and kinetic echography) have been devised by Ossoinig[6-8] to provide a means of differentiating lesions through the analysis of specific acoustic characteristics (Box 2-1).

When one is initially learning this method, it is suggested that topographic techniques be performed first, followed by quantitative and then kinetic echography. However, once sufficient experience has been gained, the various techniques may be combined for greater efficiency.

Topographic Echography: Shape, Location, and Extension

As soon as a lesion is detected, topographic echography is performed to determine its location, general classification, and configuration (Figures 2-16 and 2-17). B-scan is ideally suited for the initial topographic evaluation because the moving, focused sound beam provides a two-dimensional display. It is also important, however, to appreciate a lesion's topography with A-scan in order to carry out quantitative and kinetic techniques. It is essential that scanning techniques be systematically performed with both B- and A-scan if reliable results are to be achieved (see Appendix C).

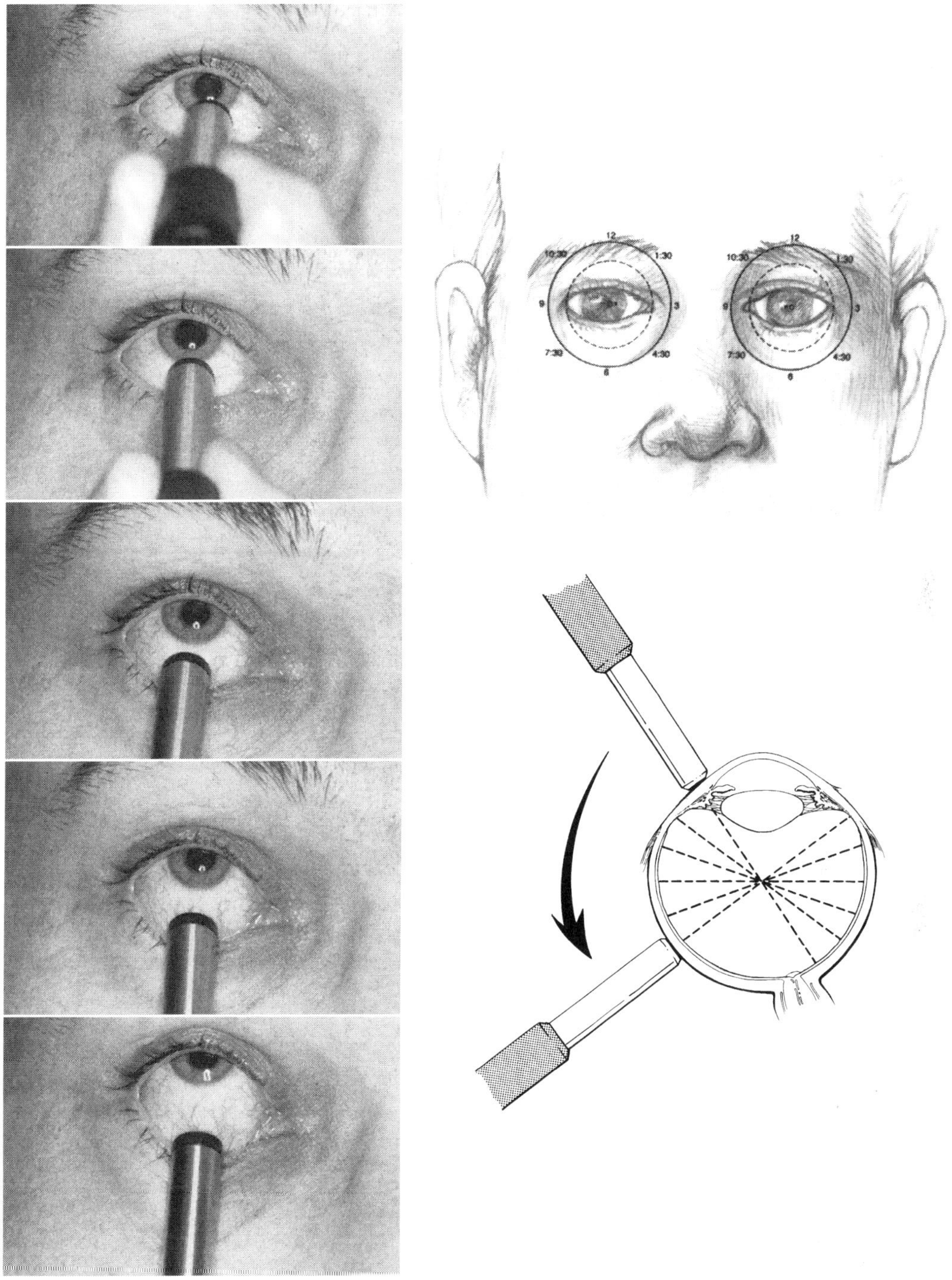

Figure 2-14 Technique for A-scan screening. In this example, the 12-o'clock meridian is examined. The patient fixates superiorly, and the probe is shifted from limbus to fornix along the 6-o'clock meridian (thereby examining the 12-o'clock meridian). This limbus-to-fornix shifting is performed in eight meridians to screen the entire posterior segment. (From Green RL, Byrne SF: Diagnostic ophthalmic ultrasound, in Ryan SJ [ed]: *Retina*. ed 3, St Louis, Mosby, 2001, p 229.)

A

B

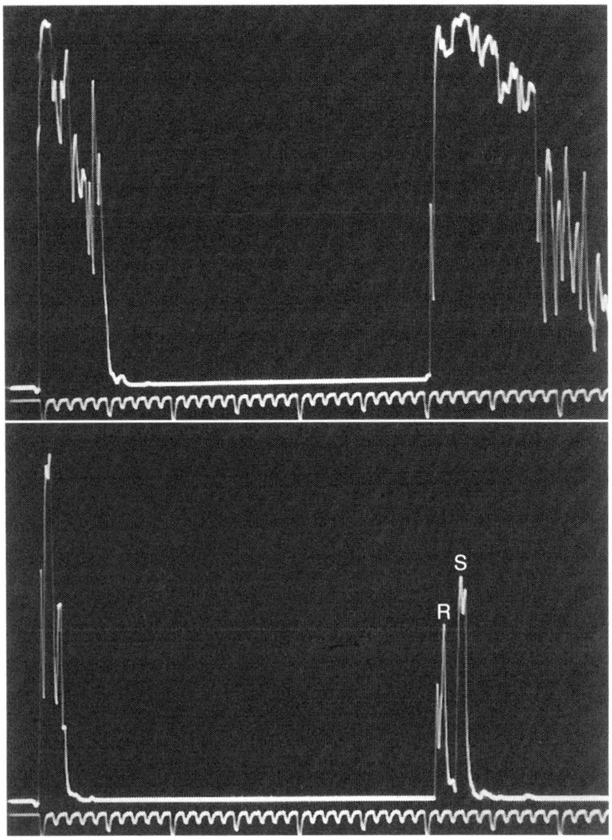

Figure 2-15 Normal A-scan echograms at Tissue Sensitivity **(A)** and reduced gain **(B)**. *R*, Retinochoroid layer; *S*, sclera. (From Green RL, Byrne SF: Diagnostic ophthalmic ultrasound, in Ryan SJ [ed]: *Retina*. ed 3, St Louis, Mosby, 2001, p 230.)

BOX 2-1

Differential Diagnosis of Intraocular Lesions*

Topographic
Location
Extension
Shape

Quantitative
Reflectivity
Internal structure
Sound attenuation

Kinetic
Aftermovement
Vascularity
Convection motion

*When an intraocular lesion is detected, these properties are assessed for differentiation.

Topographic B-Scan Evaluation

Once a lesion is detected, topographic evaluation of the lesion is then performed. The lesion is first assessed with the appropriate transverse B-scan approach where the probe is placed on the globe exactly opposite the lesion. For example, if a lesion is detected in the superior temporal quadrant of the right eye, a transverse scan of the 10:30 meridian is performed (probe is placed at 4:30, and marker is oriented supranasally). The probe is then shifted from limbus to fornix, thereby sweeping the sound beam through the lesion from posterior to anterior. This displays the gross shape and dimensions of the lesion as well as its lateral extent (i.e., the meridians that are affected by the lesion). The longitudinal approach is then applied, with the sound beam oriented radially, perpendicular to the transverse view. For a lesion located at the 10:30 position in the right eye, the probe face is placed on the 4:30 meridian with the marker directed toward the center of the cornea. The lesion's anterior-posterior extent (between the optic disc and ora along the 10:30 meridian) is assessed and its shape and gross dimensions are re-evaluated.

The lesion may also be displayed in axial orientation to document its position in relationship to the normal anatomic landmarks of the lens and optic nerve. This is accomplished by placing the probe on the cornea with the marker directed so that the sound beam slices through the lesion and optic nerve simultaneously (see Table 2-1). For a lesion located at the 10:30 position, the probe face is placed on the cornea and is rotated so that it is aligned along the 10:30 to 4:30 meridians. When the probe marker is oriented toward the uppermost of the two meridians being scanned (toward the 10:30 meridian in this example), the lesion is displayed above the optic nerve in the echogram (Figure 2-18). By compiling data obtained with these various scanning approaches, a three-dimensional concept of the lesion may be developed and its topography adequately documented.

Topographic B-scanning is also used to show the configuration and shape of a membrane. For example, a funnel-shaped retinal detachment (RD) typically displays a triangular or T-shaped configuration when an axial scan is performed. In these cases, the transverse scan provides a cross-section of the funnel and thus displays a circular or oval configuration. By combining the transverse with the axial approach, a three-dimensional image of a funnel-shaped retinal detachment can be formed. This topographic evaluation can then determine if the detachment is open or closed (Figure 2-19).

Topographic A-Scan Evaluation

Once the involved meridians have been generally determined with B-scan, A-scan is then applied. Lesion topography is always evaluated at the Tissue Sensitivity gain setting. The probe is first placed at the limbus of the meridian located opposite the center of the lesion. It is then shifted

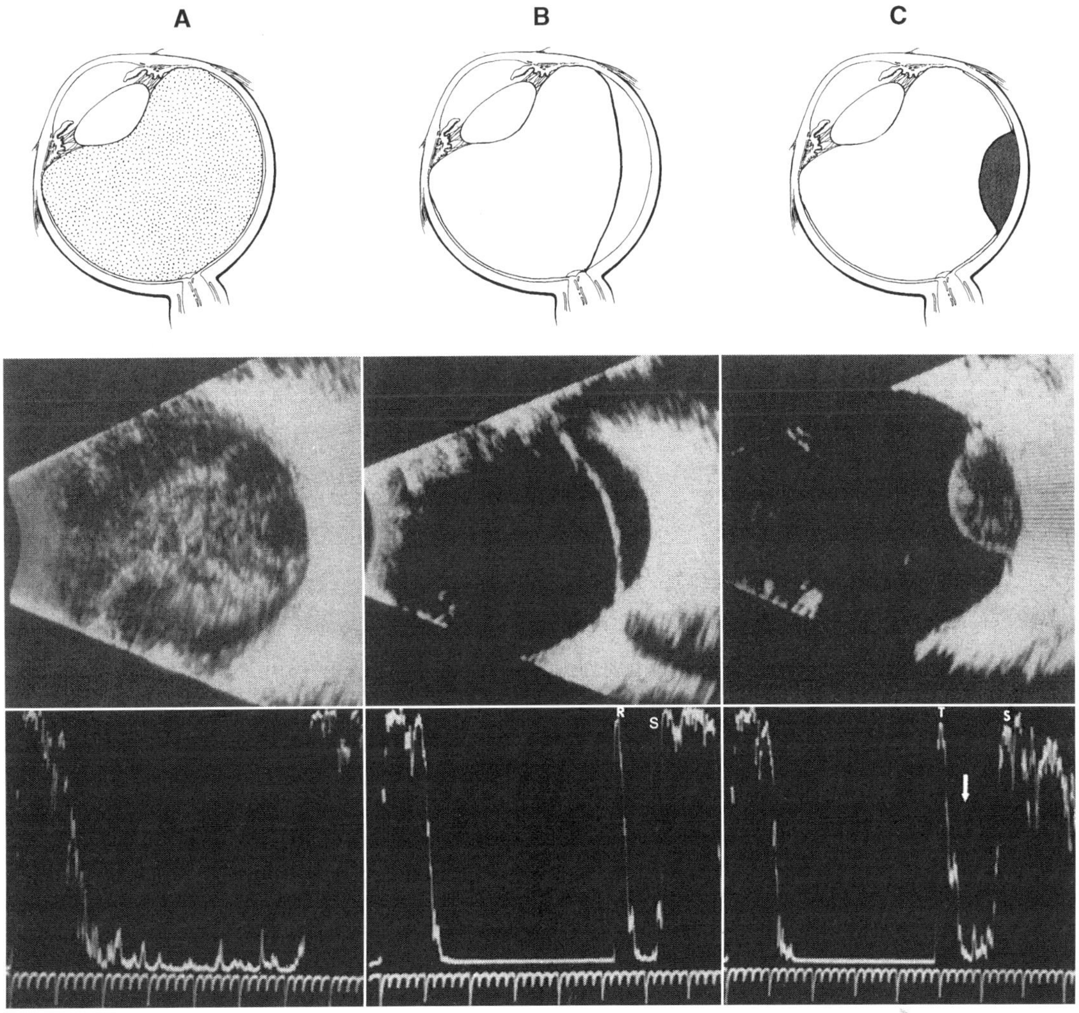

Figure 2-16 B- and A-scan echograms of the three major types of abnormal echo sources. **A,** Pointlike (e.g., fresh vitreous hemorrhage); **B,** membranelike (e.g., retinal detachment); **C,** masslike lesion (e.g., choroidal melanoma). *R,* Retina; *S,* sclera; *T,* tumor surface; *arrow,* internal tumor spikes. (From Green RL, Byrne SF: Diagnostic ophthalmic ultrasound, in Ryan SJ [ed]: *Retina.* ed 3, St Louis, Mosby, 2001, p 231.)

A

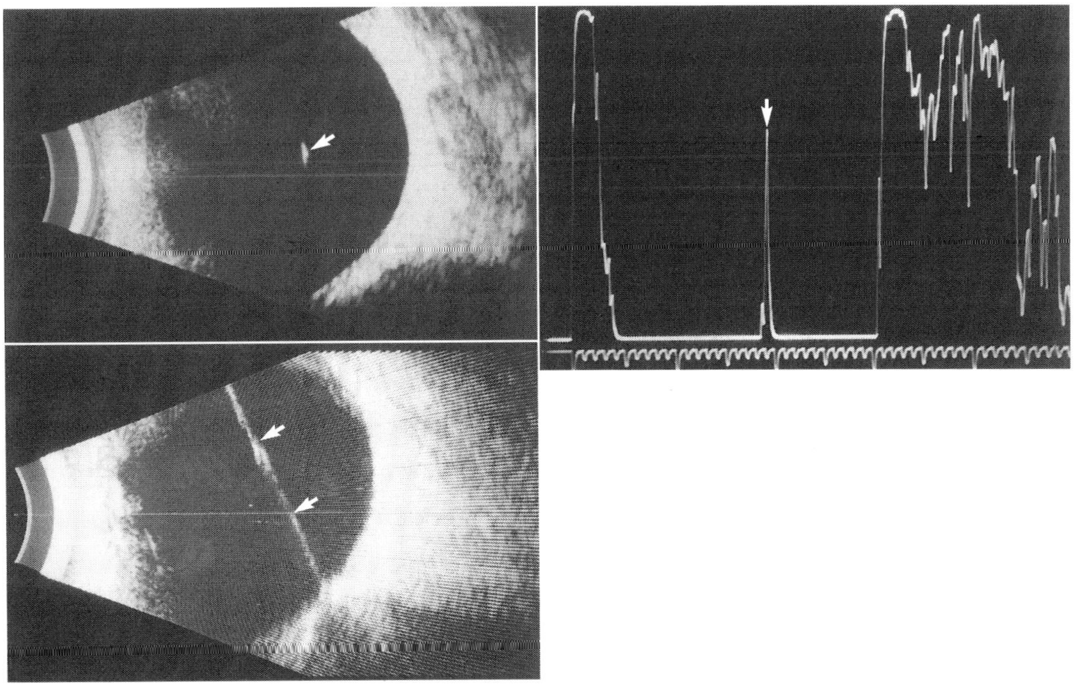

C

B

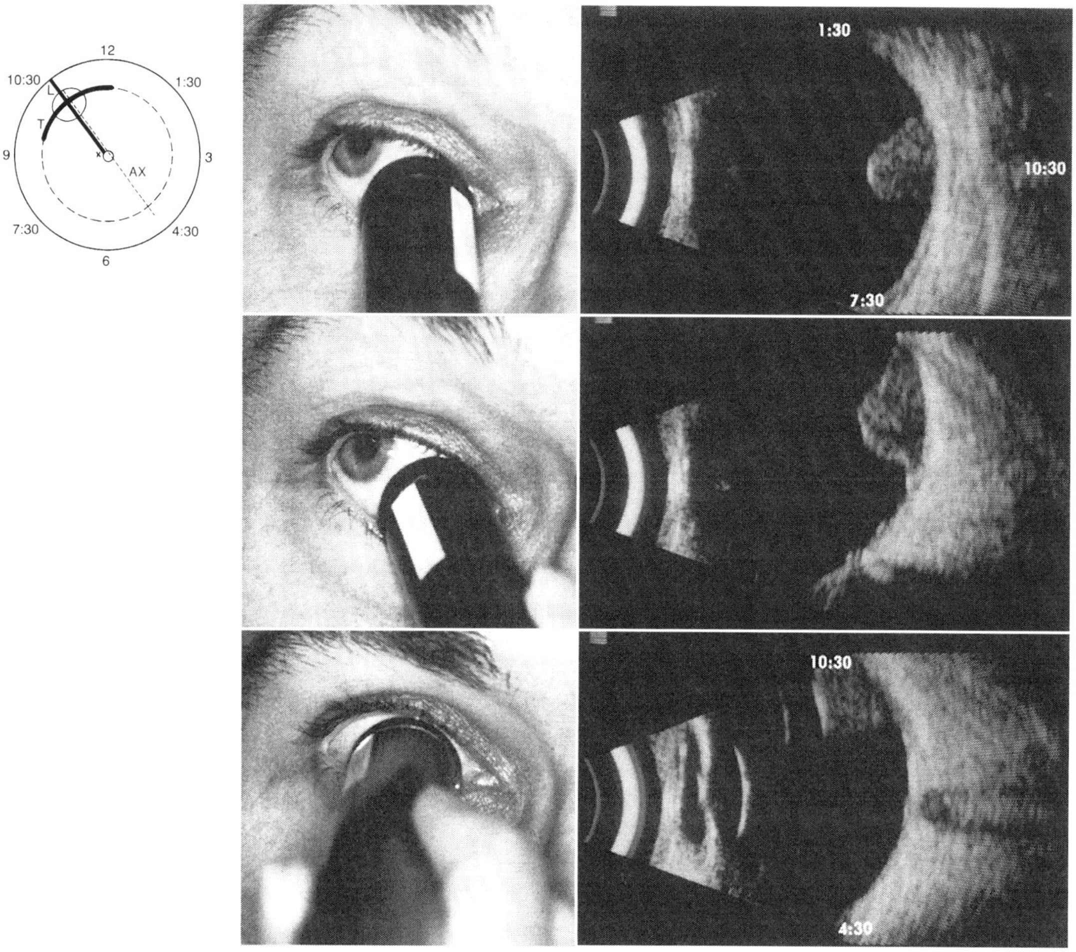

Figure 2-18 Topographic evaluation of tumor at 10:30 position with schematic drawing on *upper left* to illustrate sound beam orientation. *Top,* Transverse scan showing lateral extent of tumor. *Center,* Longitudinal scan showing radial extent of tumor. *Bottom,* Axial scan showing relationship of tumor to anatomic landmarks of lens and optic nerve. (From Green RL, Byrne SF: Diagnostic ophthalmic ultrasound, in Ryan SJ [ed]: *Retina.* ed 3, St Louis, Mosby, 2001, p 237.)

between limbus and fornix to assess the lesion anteroposteriorly (see p 24). Next, the probe is shifted from side-to-side (parallel to the limbus) to allow evaluation of the lesion laterally. Another helpful A-scan technique is to examine the lesion from different sound beam directions (i.e., with the probe placed in positions that are 90 degrees apart). These various A-scan maneuvers help to classify a lesion into a general category (pointlike, bandlike, membranelike, or masslike) and to evaluate its exact location and extent (see Figures 2-16 and 2-17).

Evaluation of the Macula

Because of the importance of the macular region, it is essential that this area be evaluated carefully to detect any abnormality. Several approaches are available for assessment of the macula. It is important to be familiar with these various alternatives because the optimal approach may vary from one eye to another.

There are four basic B-scan probe positions that allow perpendicular sound beam exposure to the macula. These include the horizontal axial, vertical transverse, longitudinal, and vertical macula approaches. A description of how to perform the first three of these approaches has been given earlier in this chapter. The fourth approach, vertical macula, is a type of para-axial scan previously described on p 21. This view is obtained by first displaying a vertical axial scan and by then directing the sound beam slightly temporal to the optic nerve (Figure 2-20). When evaluating a lesion in the macular area, it is helpful to display it from as many different probe orientations as possible in order to document its extent, configuration, and size (Figure 2-21).

In some cases, a nontraditional longitudinal probe approach is also used to assess the macula. This is accomplished by performing a longitudinal examination of the nasal meridian (i.e., 3:00 OD or 9:00 OS). The patient fixates in either primary gaze or only slightly nasally with the

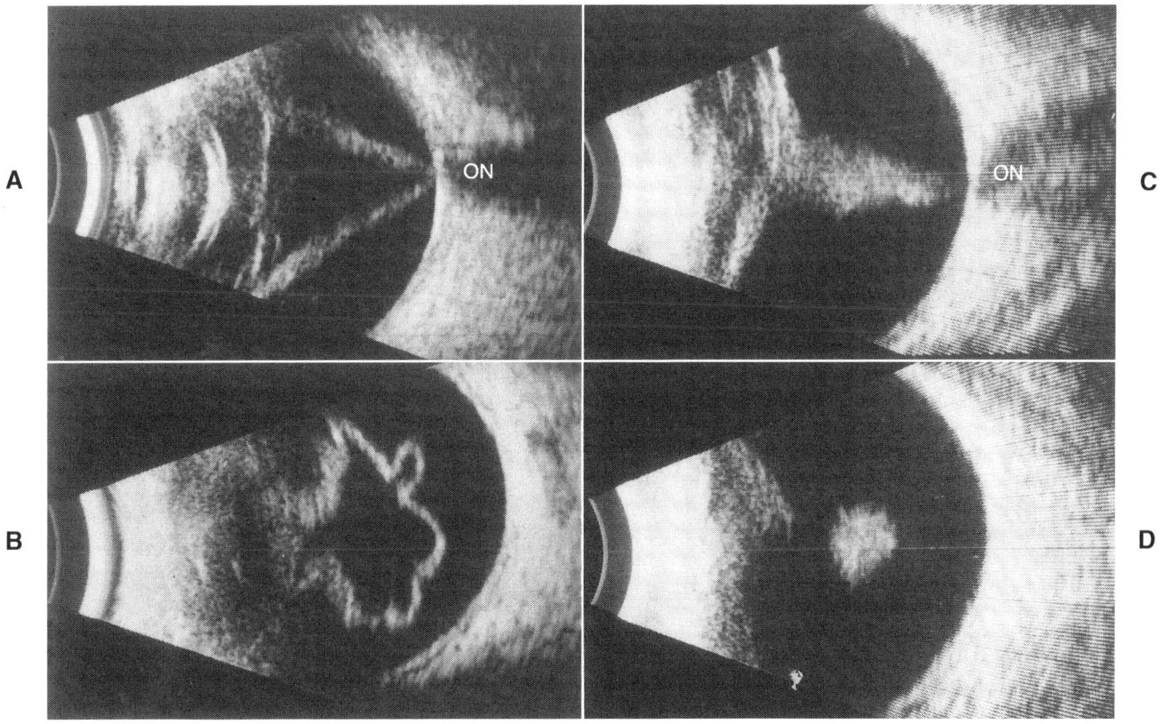

Figure 2-19 Three-dimensional conceptualization of funnel-shaped retinal detachments (RDs) using axial and transverse B-scan approaches. Open, triangular RD (**A** and **B**), and closed, T-shaped RD (**C** and **D**). **A,** Axial scan shows triangular shape of RD inserting into optic nerve *(ON)*. **B,** Transverse scan showing cross-section of open, funnel-shaped detachment. **C,** Axial scan shows T-shape of RD inserting into optic nerve *(ON)*. **D,** Transverse scan showing cross-section of closed, funnel-shaped detachment.

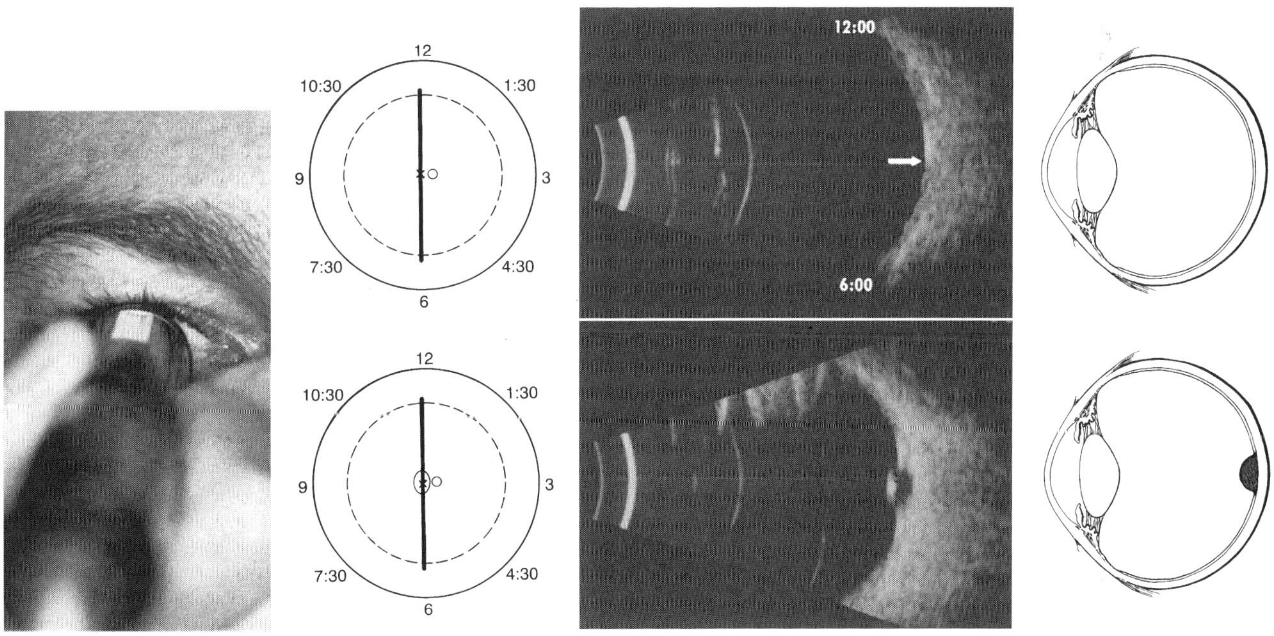

Figure 2-20 Technique for performing vertical scan through macula (vertical macula scan). *Left,* Patient fixates in primary gaze with probe centered on cornea. Note that the probe marker is directed superiorly. Sound beam is directed just temporal to optic disc. *Top,* Scan of normal macula *(arrow)*. *Bottom,* Elevated lesion at macula. (From Green RL, Byrne SF: Diagnostic ophthalmic ultrasound, in Ryan SJ [ed]: *Retina.* ed 3, St Louis, Mosby, 2001, p 238.)

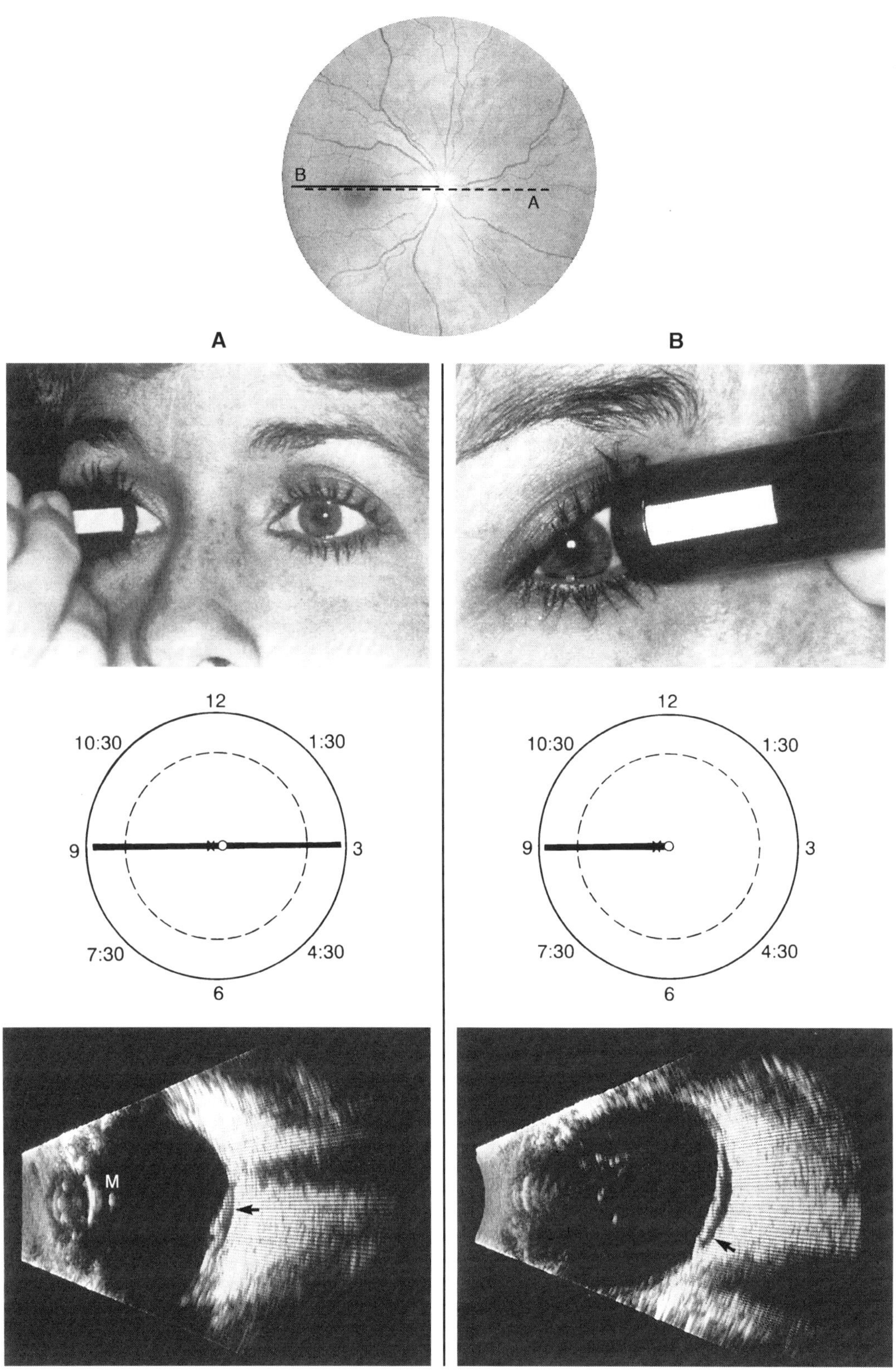

Figure 2-21 Four B-scan probe positions for evaluation of macula. Fundus photographs *(top)* indicate sound beam orientation. Photographs, schematic drawings, and echograms are of right eye. **A,** Horizontal axial scan. Patient fixates in primary gaze, probe is centered on cornea, and marker is oriented nasally. Sound beam sweeps across 3- and 9-o'clock meridians, intersected by the optic nerve. Echogram shows RD extending temporally from optic nerve. *M,* Multiple signal; *arrow,* macula. **B,** Longitudinal scan of 9-o'clock meridian. Patient fixates temporally, probe is placed nasally, and marker is directed toward center of cornea and 9-o'clock meridian. Echogram shows RD extending from optic nerve temporally to equator. *Arrow,* Macula.

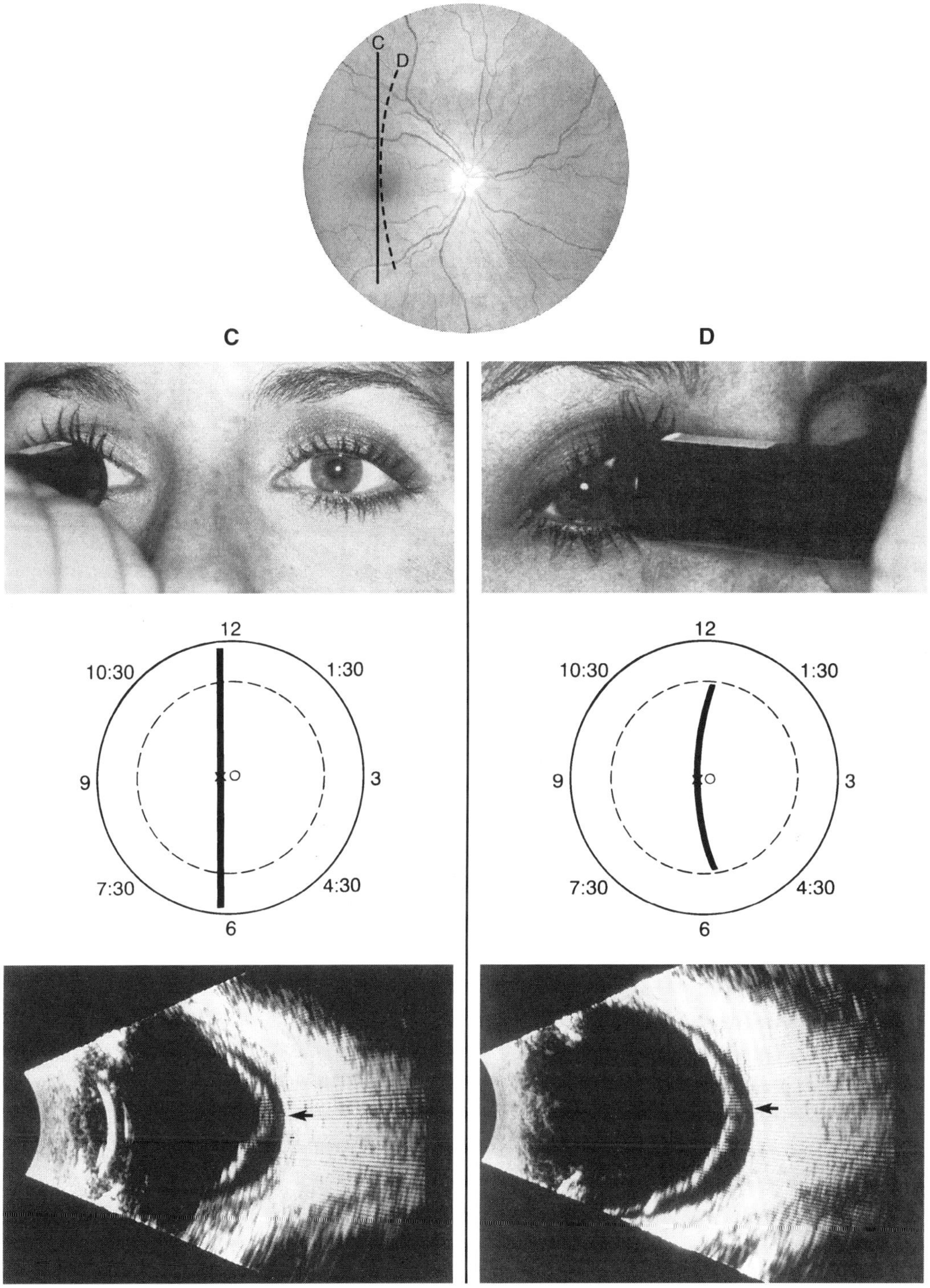

Figure 2-21 cont'd **C,** Vertical macula scan. Patient fixates in primary gaze, probe is centered on cornea, and marker is directed superiorly. Sound beam sweeps vertically through macula. Echogram shows RD extending from superior to inferior through macula *(arrow)*. **D,** Vertical transverse scan. Patient fixates temporally, probe is placed nasally near limbus, and marker is directed superiorly. Sound beam sweeps vertically through macula. Echogram shows RD extending from superior to inferior and involving macula *(arrow)*. Note that the lens is not present in this transverse scan as compared with the vertical macula view.

probe placed so that it slightly overlaps the temporal limbus. Using this technique, the macular region is located at the lower aspect of the echogram, inferior to the optic nerve[5] (see Figure 3-50, *B*). This examination technique is referred to as a reverse macula approach.

A-scan evaluation of the macula is performed by placing the probe either on the center of the cornea or at the nasal limbus. If the eye is phakic and the corneal approach is employed, care should be taken to direct the sound beam through the center of the lens to avoid refraction from the edges of the curved lens. Quantitation, however, should be performed with the sound beam bypassing the lens to avoid sound attenuation. Also, if there is a dense cataract or the eye is pseudophakic, it may be best to avoid the cornea and place the probe at the nasal limbus (Figure 2-22).

Quantitative Echography: Reflectivity, Internal Structure, and Sound Attenuation

Once the topographic findings have been ascertained, quantitative echography is performed to determine the reflectivity, internal structure, and sound attenuation of the lesion. In the globe, two types of quantitative echography have been described to evaluate reflectivity.[6-8]

Quantitative Echography Type I

REFLECTIVITY

Quantitative echography type I is used to estimate the reflectivity of all detected lesions. Reflectivity is evaluated by observing the spike height on A-scan and the signal brightness on B-scan. Before evaluating reflectivity, the sound beam must always be directed perpendicular to the lesion being assessed. There are several different types of intraoc-

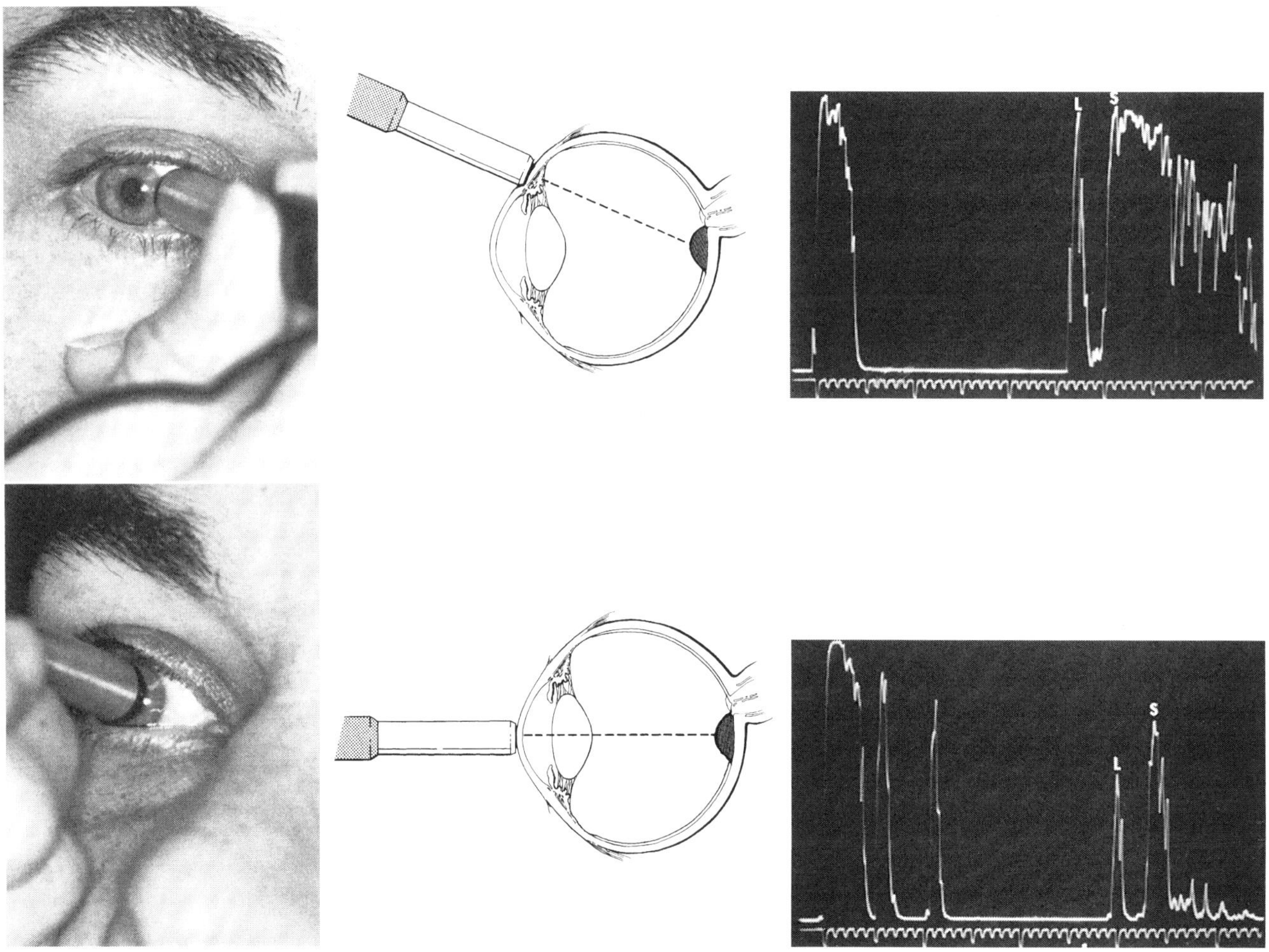

Figure 2-22 A-scan probe positions for evaluating lesion at the macula. *Top*, Using Tissue Sensitivity, probe is placed near limbus with sound beam bypassing lens to assess quantitative properties of lesion. *L*, Lesion surface; *S*, sclera. *Bottom*, Using reduced gain, probe is placed on cornea with sound beam directed through center of lens to measure height of lesion. (From Green RL, Byrne SF: Diagnostic ophthalmic ultrasound, in Ryan SJ [ed]: *Retina*. ed 3, St Louis, Mosby, 2001, p 238.)

ular lesions that can be assessed with quantitative echography. These include membranes and bands, opacities, foreign bodies, and tumors. The reflectivity of membranes, bands, and opacities is related to their configuration, size, thickness, and density. The reflectivity of a tumor, however, correlates with its histologic architecture, such as the character of cellular substance; the number, size, and distribution of cell aggregates; and the presence of large interfaces (e.g., blood vessels, connective tissue septa, calcification, and so forth).

On A-scan, using the Tissue Sensitivity gain setting, reflectivity is determined by estimating the height (i.e., amplitude) of a lesion's spikes in relation to the vitreous baseline (0%) and the top of the initial spike (100%) (Figures 2-23 and 2-24 and Table 2-2). On B-scan, the assessment of signal brightness is only a gross estimation and is not as precise as is determining spike height on A-scan. In order to assess the significance of a lesion's signal brightness on B-scan, the signal must be compared with that of either the normal highly reflective (echo-dense) sclera or the very low reflective (echolucent) vitreous cavity. A lesion's internal reflectivity, in comparison to these known tissues, is assessed in different degrees of echo density. Therefore, the most useful quantitative information obtained with B-scan is from those lesions that are extremely echo-dense and those that are echolucent (see Figure 4-44). Caution must be exercised in judging reflectivity from a B-scan echogram because it does not provide a standardized gain setting, as does the standardized A-scan (i.e., Tissue Sensitivity). Furthermore, the signal display characteristics of B-scan, such as gray scale, dynamic range, lines of resolution, and so forth, may vary from one instrument to another.

The technique of determining a lesion's reflectivity, especially with A-scan, is of great value in differentiating many types of intraocular lesions, such as membranes and intraocular tumors. For a mass lesion, the determination of reflectivity is necessary in order to evaluate its internal structure and degree of sound attenuation.

TABLE 2-2

Reflectivity Categories*

Category	Spike Height (%)
Extremely low	0-5
Low	5-40
Medium	40-60
Medium-high	60-80
High	80-100

*The reflectivity of a lesion is classified into a particular category depending on the height of the lesion spikes compared with the initial spike in the echogram. This quantitative technique is performed with standardized A-scan using the Tissue Sensitivity setting.

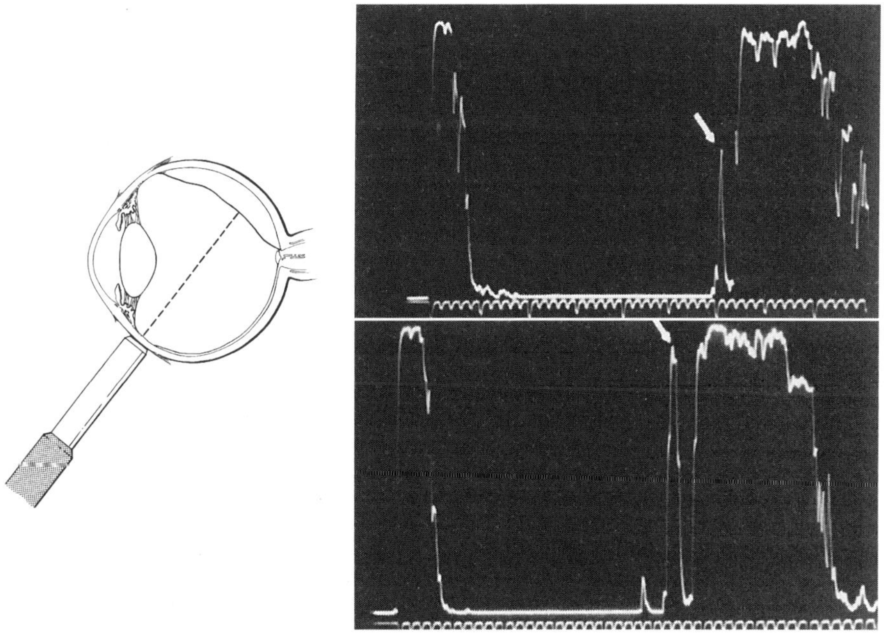

Figure 2-23 Quantitative echography type I to estimate lesion reflectivity with A-scan. Drawing shows sound beam directed perpendicular to a membrane. Echograms at Tissue Sensitivity from PVD *(top)* and RD *(bottom)*. PVD produces 50% high spike, whereas RD produces 100% high spike *(arrows)*. Most PVDs produce spike height of less than 100%, whereas only extremely dense PVDs and RD produce a spike of 100% height. (From Green RL, Byrne SF: Diagnostic ophthalmic ultrasound, in Ryan SJ [ed]: *Retina*. ed 3, St Louis, Mosby, 2001, p 240.)

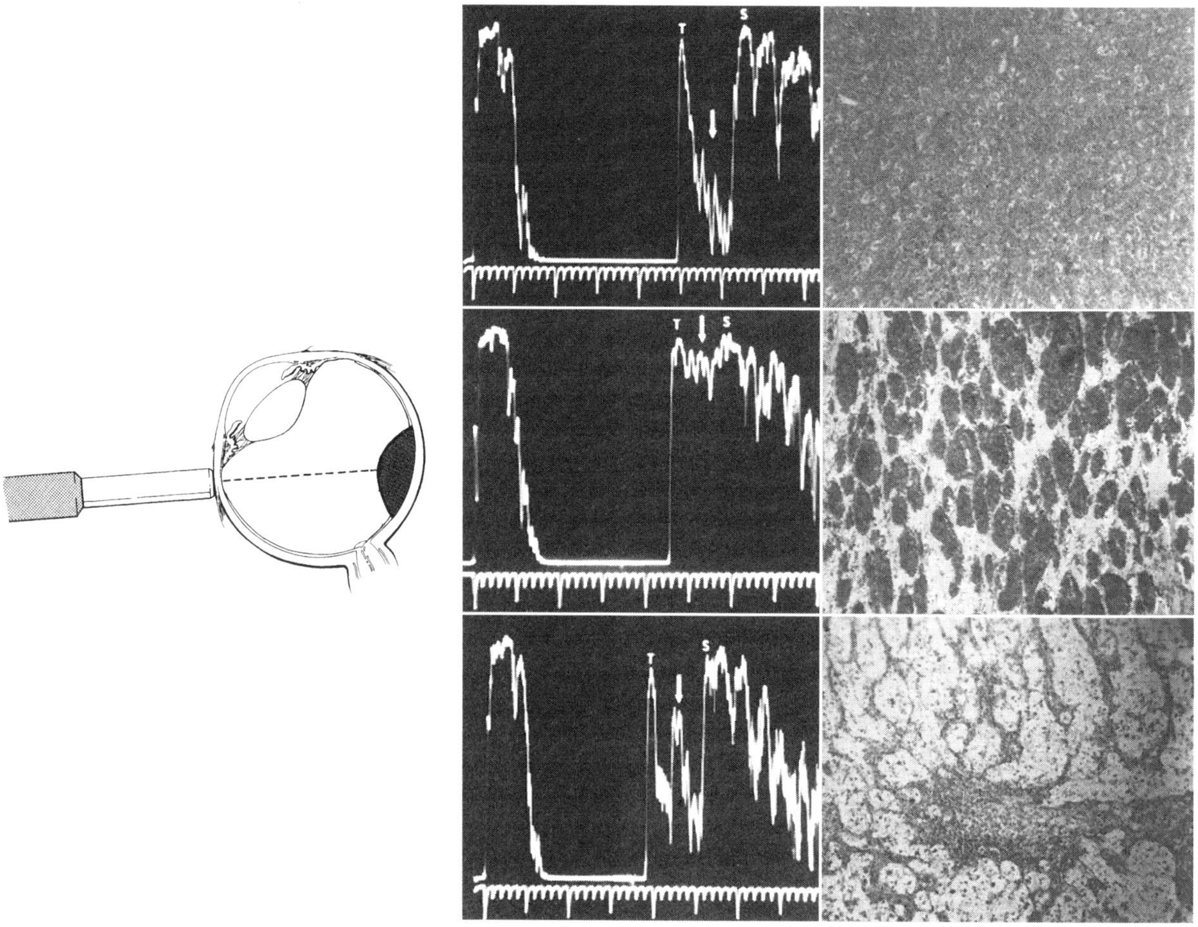

Figure 2-24 Typical tumor echograms taken at Tissue Sensitivity with histopathological correlation. Schematic drawing shows A-scan sound beam directed perpendicular to tumor surface. *Top*, Choroidal melanoma. Homogeneous cellular histology produces regular internal structure and low reflectivity. *Center*, Choroidal hemangioma. Multiple, small vascular spaces produce regular internal structure and high reflectivity. *Bottom*, Metastatic carcinoma. Irregular arrangement of tumor cells and variable size of interfaces produces irregular internal structure (i.e., variable reflectivity). *Arrows*, Internal tumor spikes; *T*, tumor surface; *S*, sclera. (From Green RL, Byrne SF: Diagnostic ophthalmic ultrasound, in Ryan SJ [ed]: *Retina*. ed 3, St Louis, Mosby, 2001, p 240.)

INTERNAL STRUCTURE

Internal structure refers to degrees of variation in histologic architecture within a masslike lesion. This feature is evaluated by noting differences in height and length of the A-scan spikes and, to a limited extent, differences in echo density on B-scan echograms. Such variations can occur within a single echogram or within different echograms obtained from the same lesion. Regular internal structure, indicating homogeneous architecture, is represented by little or no variation in the height and length of spikes on A-scan and a uniform appearance of echoes on B-scan. Conversely, irregular internal structure, indicating heterogeneous architecture, is represented by marked differences in echo appearance (see Figure 2-24). In some cases, slight variations can be present and the lesion will be classified as moderately irregular.

SOUND ATTENUATION

Sound attenuation occurs when the sound energy is scattered, reflected, or absorbed by a given medium. It may be more pronounced when the examination is performed through closed (especially swollen) lids, extremely dense opacities and membranes, or a medium that produces extremely high reflectivity (e.g., bone, calcium, or foreign material). Sound attenuation may be evaluated on both B- and A-scan and is indicated by a progressive decrease in the strength of echoes, either within or posterior to a lesion. On A-scan, this spike decrease, called angle kappa,[7,8] is determined by drawing an imaginary line through the peaks of the lesion spikes and estimating the angle that is then formed with the vitreous baseline. The steeper the angle, the greater is the sound attenuation. On B-scan, sound attenuation is indicated by a decrease in the brightness of the echoes (see Figures 5-4 and 5-7).

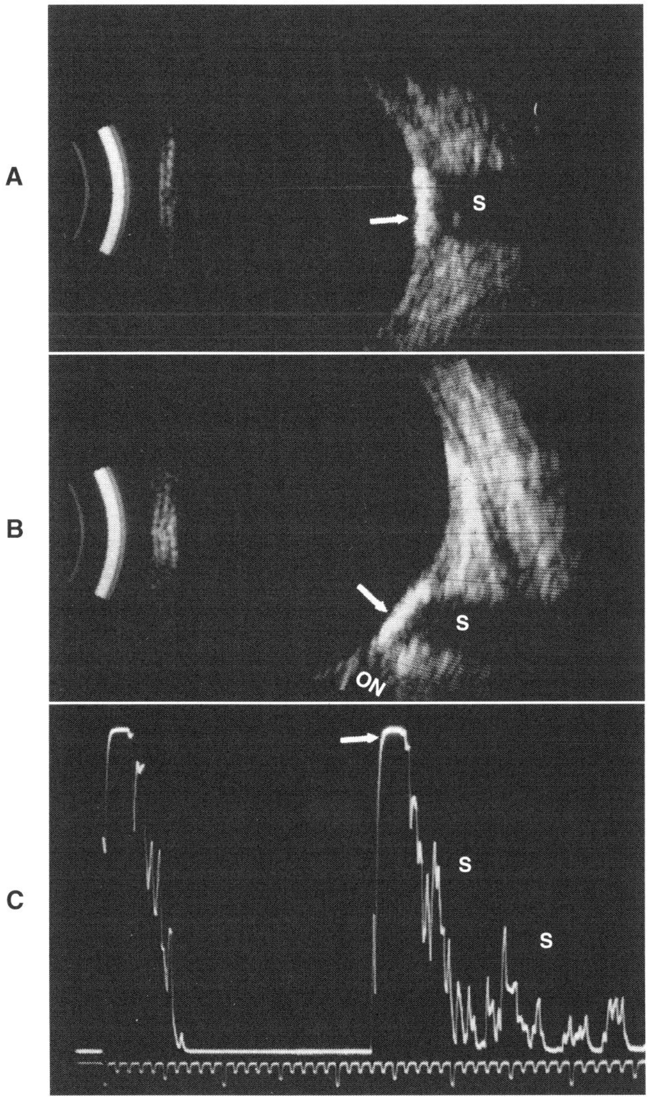

Figure 2-25 Strong sound attenuation produced by choroidal osteoma. Transverse **(A)** and longitudinal **(B)** B-scans through macula show a thick, plaquelike lesion *(arrow)* producing marked shadowing *(S)* of the scleral and orbital echoes. *ON,* Optic nerve. A-scan echogram **(C)** shows a very highly reflective, broad spike from the lesion with marked decrease in height of orbital spikes secondary to sound attenuation *(S)*. (From Green RL, Byrne SF: Diagnostic ophthalmic ultrasound, in Ryan SJ [ed]: *Retina.* ed 3, St Louis, Mosby, p 241.)

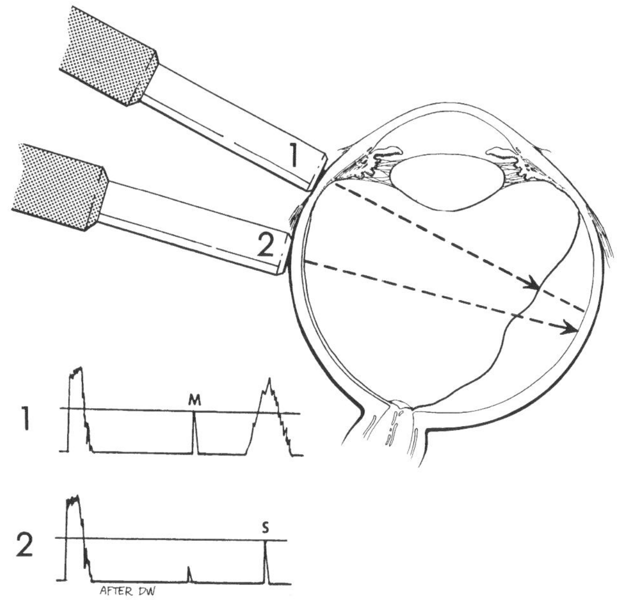

Figure 2-26 Quantitative echography type II to differentiate dense PVD from RD. Horizontal line is placed across the middle of the screen. *Probe position 1,* Sound beam directed perpendicular to membrane *(M)*. *Probe position 2,* Sound beam directed perpendicular to sclera *(S)*. The decibel level is decreased until the spike from these surfaces touches but does not surpass the horizontal line in the middle of the screen. The difference in the decibel setting required to display the membrane and sclera at this specific spike level may help differentiate retina from vitreous membrane (6 to 15 db = retina; >20 db = vitreous membrane). (From Green RL, Byrne SF: Diagnostic ophthalmic ultrasound, in Ryan SJ [ed]: *Retina.* ed 3, St Louis, Mosby, 2001, p 241.)

Various substances, such as bone, calcium, and most foreign bodies, typically produce strong sound attenuation. This results in decreasing signal strength or an actual void posterior to the lesion that is referred to as shadowing (Figure 2-25 and see p 466). However, when a dense echo source is extremely small, sound attenuation may be subtle or altogether absent (see Figure 4-31).

Quantitative Echography Type II

Quantitative type II echography is an A-scan method for the differentiation of a retinal detachment from a dense vitreous membrane (e.g., posterior vitreous detachment).[8] It can be applied when a membranelike lesion produces a 100% high spike at the Tissue Sensitivity gain setting during quantitative type I assessment, and the other acoustic characteristics are equivocal.

Quantitative echography type II allows precise measurement of a membrane's reflectivity in decibels as compared with reflectivity of the sclera in the same eye (Figure 2-26). However, because this technique is time consuming and has certain limitations (i.e., is more difficult if the lids are markedly swollen, if the eye has been severely injured, or the patient has recently undergone eye surgery), it is normally reserved for those situations where the other special examination techniques are unsuccessful in differentiating the lesion.

Kinetic Echography: Mobility, Vascularity, and Convection Movement

One of the unique abilities of conventional ultrasound instruments is the nearly instantaneous display of echoes. Therefore, any movement of or within a lesion is accurately depicted in the echogram (i.e., in real-time). Kinetic echography is used to dynamically assess the motion of or within a lesion. Three types of motion (i.e., aftermovement, vascularity, and convection movement) can be detected with the appropriate instrumentation.

Aftermovement, indicative of mobility, is determined by observing motion of the lesion echoes following cessation of eye or body movement. For example, a nonsolid lesion (e.g., vitreous membrane or retinal detachment) displays aftermovement, whereas a solid lesion (e.g., tumor) does not. Vascularity (fast spontaneous motion of echoes on the screen) represents blood flow within vessels. Convection movement (slow spontaneous movement of echoes on the screen) occurs due to convection currents of fine particles (e.g., cholesterol debris) within a large cavity (e.g., vitreous cavity or large orbital cyst).

Lesion Mobility (Aftermovement)

B-scan is used to assess the gross mobility of vitreous opacities and membranes. Aftermovement is evaluated before, during, and immediately following an eye movement. With the patient fixating a target, the lesion is imaged on the screen. The patient is then instructed to shift their gaze a short distance away from and then quickly back to the target in the same plane as the moving sound beam. Meanwhile, the echogram is continually monitored to evaluate any movement of lesion echoes.

One of the strengths of A-scan is the detection of subtle motion of a lesion. Spike aftermovement may be classified as horizontal or vertical. Horizontal spike motion is a lateral movement of the spike along the baseline, corresponding to lateral motion of the lesion. This type of motion is seen also on B-scan (Figure 2-27). Vertical spike motion, which is quite subtle, is a change in spike height caused by minimal change in position of the lesion relative to the sound beam. This slight aftermovement may not be appreciable with the B-scan (Figure 2-28).

A

B

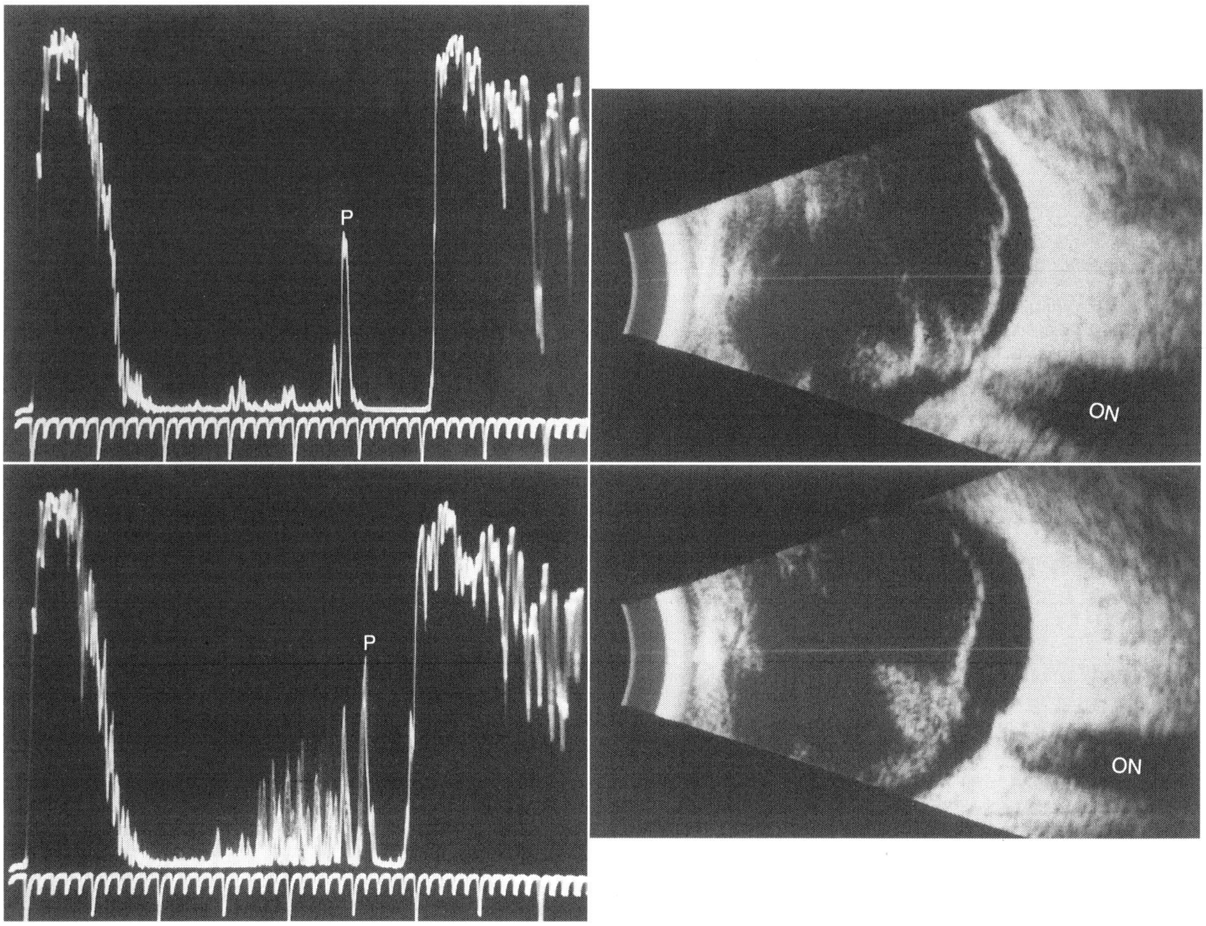

C

D

Figure 2-27 A-scan and B-scan demonstration of membrane mobility (aftermovement). **A** and **B,** A-scan echograms show vitreous hemorrhage and PVD *(P)* before **(A)** and immediately following **(B)** eye movement, using same probe position. Note change in position of PVD and blurred appearance of spikes in **B** compared with **A.** This changed appearance indicates that the PVD has moved closer to the surface of the retina and that there is continuing movement of the opacified vitreous gel. **C** and **D,** Longitudinal B-scans at reduced gain setting show PVD before **(C)** and immediately following **(D)** eye movement. PVD appears to insert into optic nerve *(ON)* in **C,** but **D** shows that the PVD is actually detached from the optic nerve.

A

B

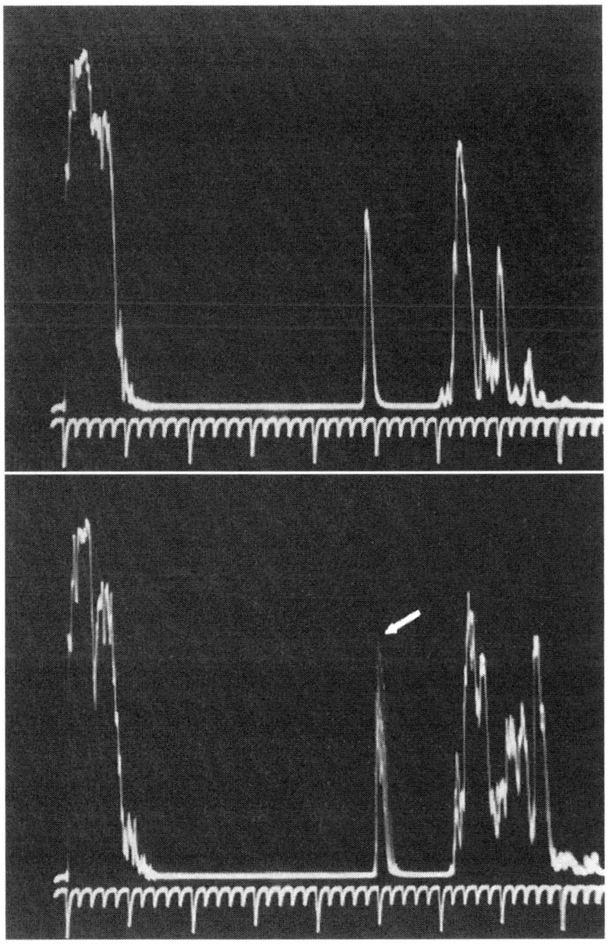

Figure 2-28 Aftermovement of RD shown with A-scan (reduced gain setting). RD before **(A)** and immediately following **(B)** eye movement. **A,** RD in focus before eye movement. **B,** Slight blurring of retinal spike *(arrow)* after eye movement indicates slight vertical aftermovement. (From Green RL, Byrne SF: Diagnostic ophthalmic ultrasound, in Ryan SJ [ed]: *Retina*. ed 3, St Louis, Mosby, 2001, p 242.)

Vascularity (Fast Spontaneous Motion)

Vascularity is a characteristic that is assessed in tumors. Fast spontaneous motion (i.e., low-amplitude, continuous flickering of the internal lesion spikes) is best detected with standardized A-scan, but in many cases may be appreciated also with B-scan. Vascularity is assessed with the probe held stationary and the eye steadily fixating on a target (Figure 2-29).

Convection Movement (Slow Spontaneous Motion)

Convection movement is a characteristic type of motion that can be observed in eyes with longstanding intraocular hemorrhage or in certain types of orbital cystic lesions containing cholesterol debris. This type of movement occurs because of convection currents that cause a continuous, slow movement of blood and/or cholesterol debris within the eye or large orbital cysts. Within the eye, the most common situation where this type of convection movement is seen is when hemorrhage, cholesterol debris, or both, accumulate

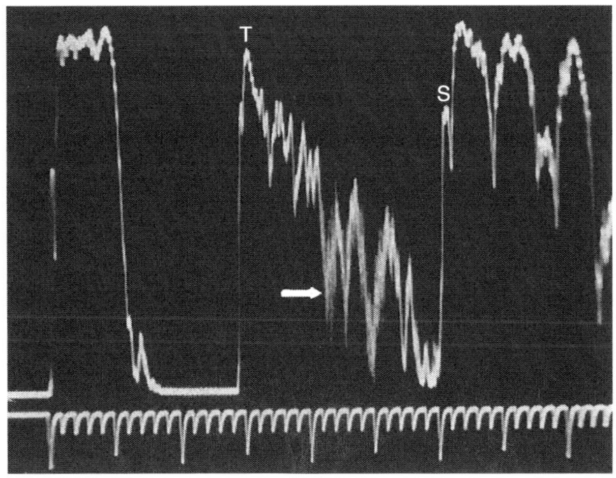

Figure 2-29 A-scan echogram of large melanoma shows internal vascularity (spontaneous motion). Vascularity is indicated by marked blurring of internal tumor spikes *(arrow)*. *T*, Tumor surface; *S*, sclera.

beneath a tight funnel-shaped retinal detachment. Coat's disease is a specific type of disorder that is typically associated with subretinal cholesterol (see p 187). In the orbit, the most common lesion associated with convection movement is the hematic cyst (cholesterol granuloma) (see p 340). The characteristic ultrasound finding for convection movement is a slow, up and down motion of spikes on A-scan and a slow, circular motion of pointlike echoes on B-scan. This type of movement is best assessed with the probe held stationary and the eye steadily fixating on a target.

ANTERIOR SEGMENT EVALUATION: IMMERSION TECHNIQUE

Contact scanning is not well suited for the anterior segment evaluation because the probe is unable to display echoes from the first few millimeters in front of the probe face (see Figure 1-13). As a result, immersion techniques have been developed to allow a fluid separation between the probe face and front of the eye. Although the same instruments used for contact scanning can be readily employed for immersion assessment of the anterior segment, newer higher frequency B-scan probes have been developed that allow better resolution of anterior segment structures and lesions. A-scan can also be used with the immersion technique to evaluate the reflectivity and size of anterior segment lesions and to measure the axial eye length (see Chapter 10).

In order to perform an immersion scan, some type of fluid bath must be used for the examination. Various types of scleral shells (see Appendix D) have been developed for use with contact instrumentation. These shells are placed between the eyelids and are filled with methylcellulose. The probes are then placed into or on the top of the shell (Figure 2-30, *A* and *D*). An alternative to the scleral shells is a balloonlike device created with a detached finger from a latex surgical glove. The finger is filled with water and the

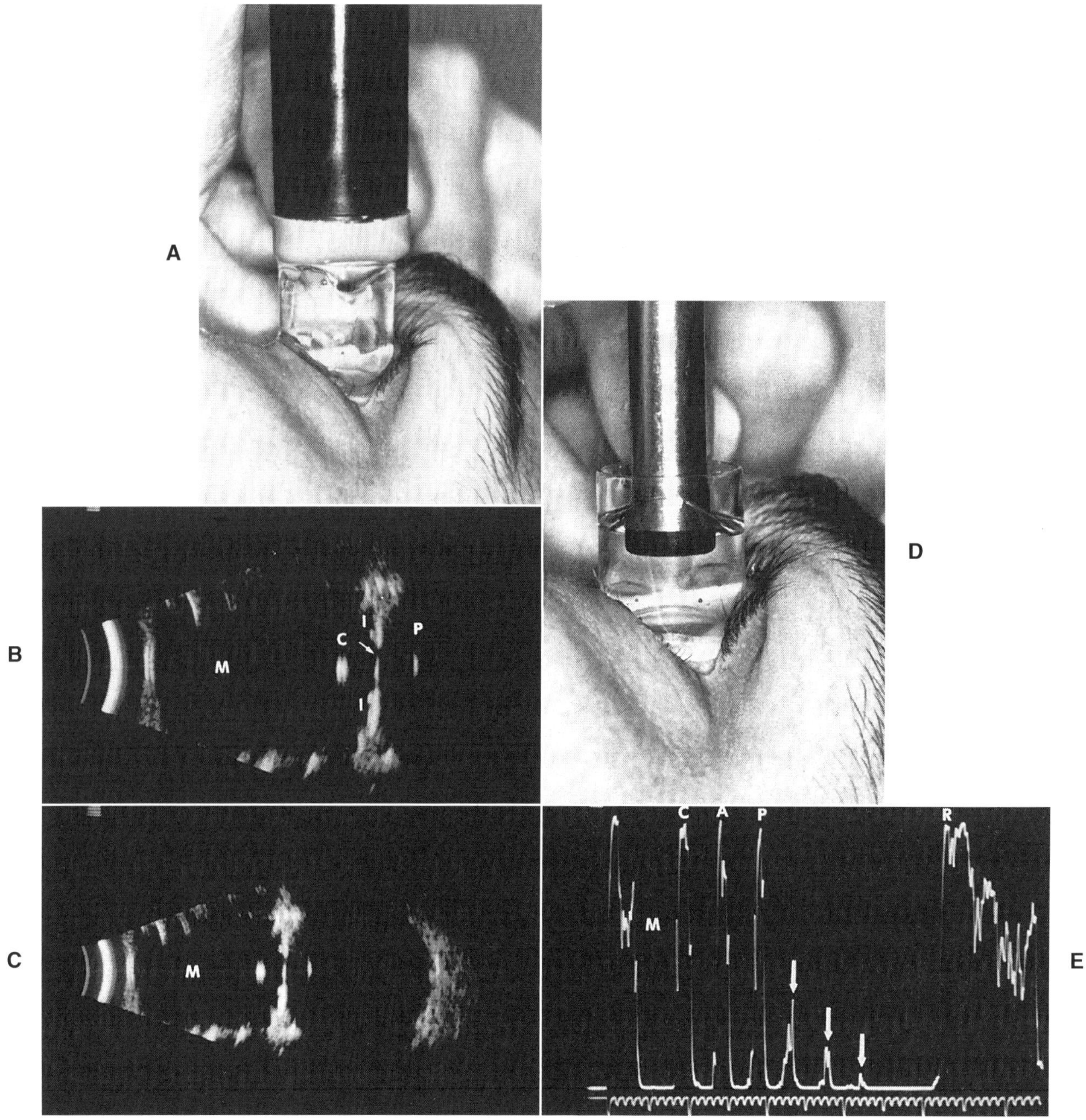

Figure 2-30 Immersion technique for anterior segment evaluation. **A,** B-scan probe is placed on top of small scleral shell filled with methylcellulose. **B,** B-scan echogram using globe screen expansion (posterior ocular wall not shown). *M,* Methylcellulose within shell; *C,* double line from anterior and posterior corneal surfaces; *I,* iris; *short arrow,* anterior lens capsule (pupil is dilated); *P,* posterior lens capsule. **C,** B-scan echogram using orbital screen expansion shows the entire eye. **D,** A-scan probe within fluid-filled scleral shell. **E,** A-scan echogram at Tissue Sensitivity gain setting. *Arrows,* Multiple signals along vitreous baseline; *R,* retina. (From Green RL, Byrne SF: Diagnostic ophthalmic ultrasound, in Ryan SJ [ed]: *Retina.* ed 3, St Louis, Mosby, 2001, p 243.)

A

B

C

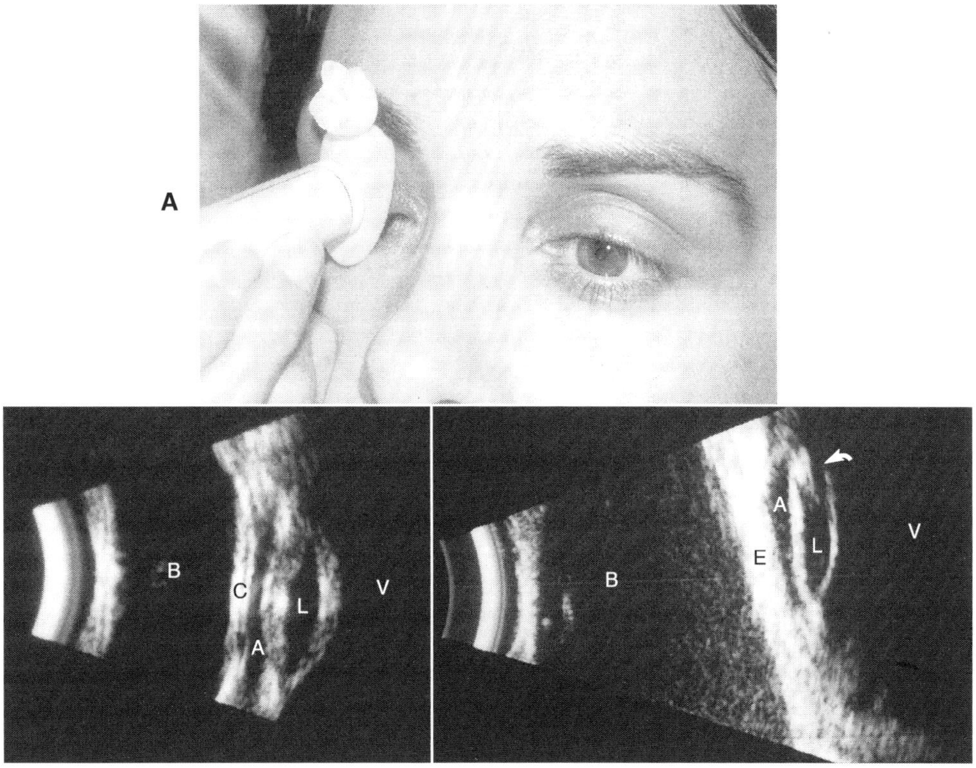

Figure 2-31 B-scan immersion examination of anterior segment using balloonlike device. **A,** Balloonlike device (created from latex glove tip) is placed directly over closed lid with probe on its surface. **B,** Echogram of anterior segment obtained with balloon directly on cornea. This was an examination of an eye with a dense cataractous lens. *B,* Balloon; *C,* cornea; *A,* anterior chamber; *L,* dense cataractous lens. Note echolucent lens nucleus surrounded by dense cortical lens material. *V,* Vitreous cavity. **C,** Echogram of anterior segment obtained with balloon placed on closed eyelid *(E).* This was an examination of a child with a history of corneoscleral laceration. *Curved arrow,* Rupture of peripheral aspect of posterior lens capsule.

open end is closed with suture material or dental floss. This balloonlike device can be placed over the closed eyelid or on the surface of the eye. The probe (with methylcellulose on its tip) is placed directly on the device (Figure 2-31, *A*).

B-Scan Immersion Techniques

Using the B-scan probe with an immersion scleral shell (see Figure 2-30, *A*), three different B-scan probe orientations (axial, longitudinal and transverse) can be used for the anterior segment examination. The axial scan is performed with the patient fixating in primary gaze and the sound beam directed through the center of the cornea. This allows for the display of the cornea, anterior chamber, iris, lens, and retrolental space along the visual axis (see Figure 2-30, *B* and *C;* see also Figure 2-32, *B*). The longitudinal approach is performed with the probe in exactly the same position as for the axial scan. However, instead of moving the probe, the patient's gaze is shifted so as to allow peripheral structures to be centered beneath the probe. Such scans provide a radial section through peripheral aspects of the cornea, iris, lens, and ciliary body and can demonstrate the posterior extent of anterior segment lesions (see Figures 3-62, *A* and *D,* and 5-82). The transverse approach is then performed with the patient's gaze in the same position as for the longitudinal scan. The probe, however, is rotated by 90 degrees so that the sound beam oscillates parallel (tangential) to the limbus. The transverse view provides a circumferential section of anterior segment structures and the lateral extent of anterior segment lesions (see Figures 3-62, *B* and *E,* and 5-79, *C*). For the various B-scan probe positions, the marker is generally orientated in the same manner as for contact scans of the posterior segment (see Table 2-1 and Figures 2-6, 2-8, and 2-11).

In recent years, instruments have been developed that allow the use of higher frequency B-scan probes to better demonstrate anterior segment structures and lesions. Although these higher frequencies provide better resolution, their depth of sound beam penetration is limited. One of these instruments is the I[3] SYSTEM-ABD (Innovative Imaging, Inc, Sacramento, California). This instrument uses a 20 MHz probe that can be used with an immersion

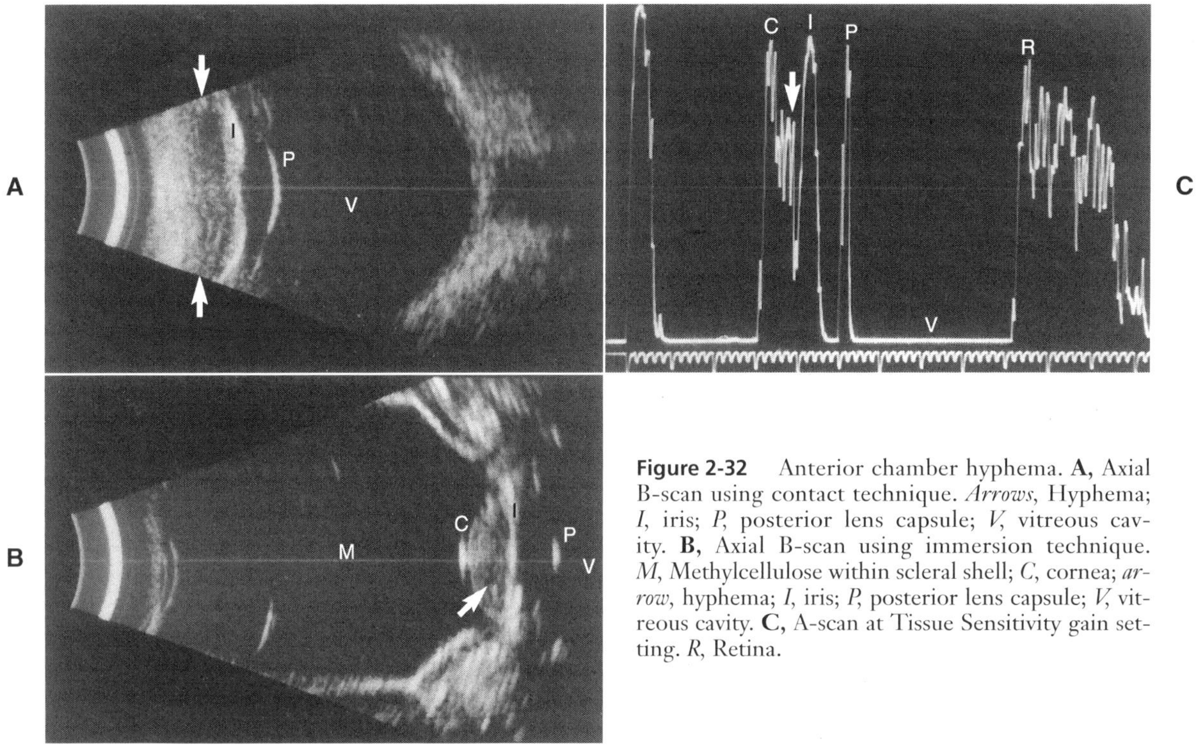

Figure 2-32 Anterior chamber hyphema. **A,** Axial B-scan using contact technique. *Arrows,* Hyphema; *I,* iris; *P,* posterior lens capsule; *V,* vitreous cavity. **B,** Axial B-scan using immersion technique. *M,* Methylcellulose within scleral shell; *C,* cornea; *arrow,* hyphema; *I,* iris; *P,* posterior lens capsule; *V,* vitreous cavity. **C,** A-scan at Tissue Sensitivity gain setting. *R,* Retina.

shell or a small water-filled balloon (latex tonometer cover) over the probe tip. This cover eliminates the need for a scleral shell immersion system, allows the probe to be used in a contact manner, and provides an easy method for imaging structures and lesions of the anterior segment (Figure 2-33; see also Figure 5-85).

The UBM[9,10] currently provides the highest resolution for the anterior segment examination. This technique utilizes frequencies in the range of 50 to 100 MHz and an immersion water bath system. The instrument and examination techniques as well as anatomy and lesions of the anterior segment are described in Chapter 8.

A-Scan Immersion Techniques

The immersion A-scan examination is initially performed with the patient fixating in primary gaze and the probe immersed into the methylcellulose. Spikes from the central aspect of the cornea, anterior chamber, iris, and lens are displayed (see Figure 2-30, *E;* see also Figure 2-32, *C*). Peripheral aspects of the anterior segment and lesions can be best demonstrated by having the patient shift their gaze so as to center the area of interest beneath the probe (see Figure 3-62, *C* and *F*).

EVALUATION OF THE LENS

The lens may be evaluated using either contact or immersion ultrasound techniques. B-scan is the primary modality for imaging the lens, although A-scan may provide measurements of lens thickness and, in some cases, is useful for evaluating internal reflectivity.

The contact B-scan technique primarily images the posterior aspect of the lens, including the posterior capsule (see Figure 2-32, *A*). Using this method, the lens is generally best evaluated with an axial approach (see p 21), although longitudinal (see p 19) and transverse (see p 18) probe positions are sometimes helpful. To obtain an adequate longitudinal view of the normal lens, an instrument with a wide scanning angle must generally be used, although instruments with less wide angles can display the lens if it is swollen. To show the normal lens with the transverse approach, a very anterior scan must be obtained. It is generally best to place the probe temporally with the patient fixating nasally. This transverse view is most effective for demonstrating a swollen lens and/or detecting an intralenticular foreign body (Figure 2-34).

The immersion B-scan technique is used to image the anterior lens capsule and the relationship of the lens to other anterior segment structures (i.e., cornea, anterior chamber, iris, and ciliary body). With this technique, the lens is best assessed with either an axial or a longitudinal approach. The axial approach can usually display both the anterior and posterior lens capsules with a traditional 10 MHz B-scan transducer. When higher resolution B-scan instruments are employed, the depth of penetration may not always allow display of the posterior capsule. The longitudinal approach is most beneficial when there is

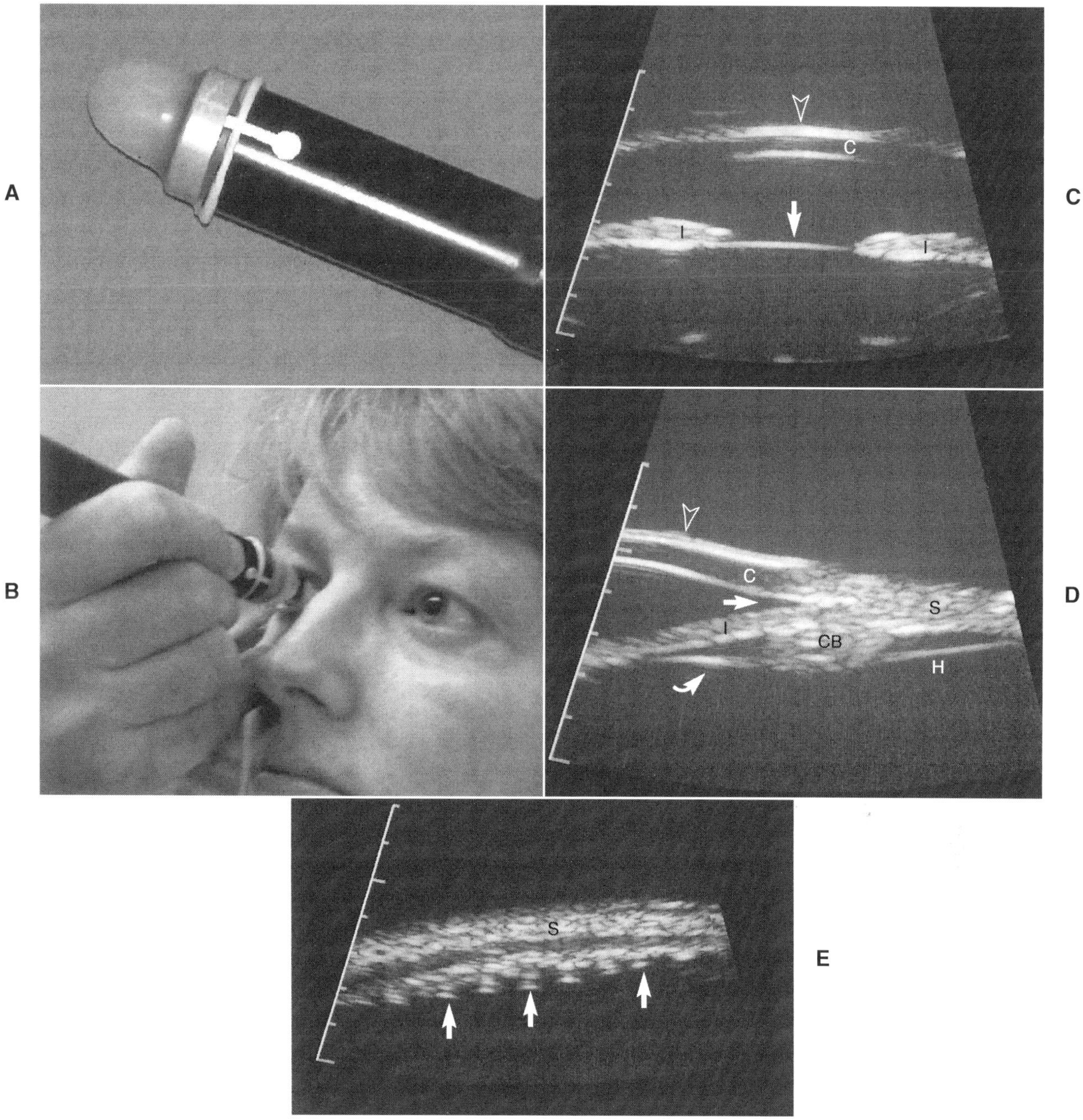

Figure 2-33 Immersion examination of anterior segment using high resolution B-scan (20 MHz) probe with balloonlike tip. **A,** High resolution I^3 B-scan probe with water-filled latex tonometer tip attached. **B,** High resolution probe with tip placed directly on cornea. **C,** Axial scan. *Open arrow,* Thin membrane representing probe balloon tip on cornea *(C); I,* iris; *straight white arrow,* anterior lens capsule. **D,** Longitudinal scan. *Straight white arrow,* Anterior chamber angle; *CB,* ciliary body; *curved white arrow,* Anterior lens capsule; *H,* surface of anterior hyaloid; *S,* sclera. **E,** Transverse scan through ciliary body. *Straight white arrows,* Ciliary processes. (Courtesy Cynthia Kendall, BMET, RDMS, Sacramento, California.)

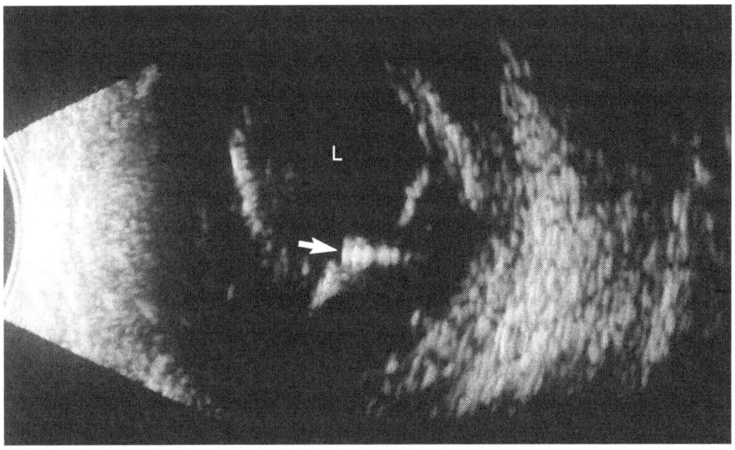

Figure 2-34 Glass foreign body within swollen, cataractous lens. Vertical transverse B-scan through lens at low gain setting. Foreign body *(arrow)* is located at inferior pole of the lens *(L)*. Note short comet tail artifact extending from foreign body.

significant pathology involving the lens, iris or ciliary body (see p 77). The display of zonular attachments to the lens requires the use of very high-resolution instruments such as the ultrasound biomicroscope (see p 223).

A-scan assessment of the lens (i.e., thickness and internal reflectivity) can be performed with either the contact or the immersion technique (see Figure 10-1). It should be noted, though, that to display both the anterior and posterior lens spikes with the contact method, the anterior chamber must be of normal or greater than normal depth.

The normal lens appears as a very well outlined, oval, echolucent structure on B-scan and exhibits very low internal reflectivity on A-scan. The anterior and posterior lens capsules produce distinct echoes on both B- and A-scan (see Figure 1-11). An axial B-scan view typically displays the center of the posterior capsule as a short, echo-dense crescent and peripheral aspects of the posterior capsule are not usually demonstrated (see Figures 1-13 and 4-2, *A*). A contact, longitudinal view, on the other hand, often shows the more complete, continuous nature of the posterior capsule (see Figure 4-6, *B*). The anterior capsule, which is best displayed with the immersion technique, appears as a smooth, slightly convex line. It often cannot be differentiated from the iris when using a traditional 10 MHz transducer unless the pupil is dilated (see Figures 2-30, *B*, and 4-2, *A*). On the other hand, dilatation of the pupil is not required to demonstrate the anterior lens capsule with high-resolution instruments (see Figure 2-33, *C*). In the normal lens, the nucleus generally cannot be differentiated from the cortex. Also, the normal lens can produce artifacts such as multiple signals (see Figures 1-11 and 2-21, *A*) and Baum's bumps (see p 467).

A wide variety of pathological conditions involving the lens can be demonstrated with ultrasound (Box 2-2). Cataracts, however, must usually be of moderate density for detection by echography. The cataractous lens exhibits varying degrees of echo density on B-scan (see Figure 4-2, *B*) and internal spikes of differing amplitude on A-scan (see Figures 10-11 and 10-12). In a dense nuclear cataract, B-scan can often differentiate the lens nucleus from the surrounding cortex (see Figure 7-3). Posterior subcapsular cataracts are best shown with an anterior transverse B-scan approach where the sound beam passes through the posterior capsule. The subcapsular cataractous changes appear as an echo-dense, roundish, plaque-like opacity in the echogram (Figure 2-35). In some cases, irregularities of the posterior lens capsule can be demonstrated. One example of this abnormal shape is posterior lenticonus (Figure 2-36).

Ultrasound can also be used to evaluate intraocular lenses. The appearance of an intraocular lens, with both conventional and high resolution instrumentation, is described elsewhere (see pp 109, 233, and 255).

BOX 2-2

Ultrasound Evaluation of the Lens

- Cataractous lens
- Intralenticular foreign body
- Posterior lenticonus
- Subluxation/dislocation of lens (see Figure 4-3)
- Dislocated lens nucleus (see Figure 4-40)
- Liquefaction of lens (see Figure 7-3)
- Measurement of lens thickness (see p 252)
- Retained lens material (see p 106)
- Retrolenticular (cyclitic) membrane (see Figure 3-63)
- Rupture of anterior or posterior lens capsule (see Figure 4-5)
- Shrunken (reabsorbed) lens (see Figure 4-15)
- Swollen (intumescent) lens (see Figure 5-78)
- Thin lens (PHPV) (see Figure 5-100)

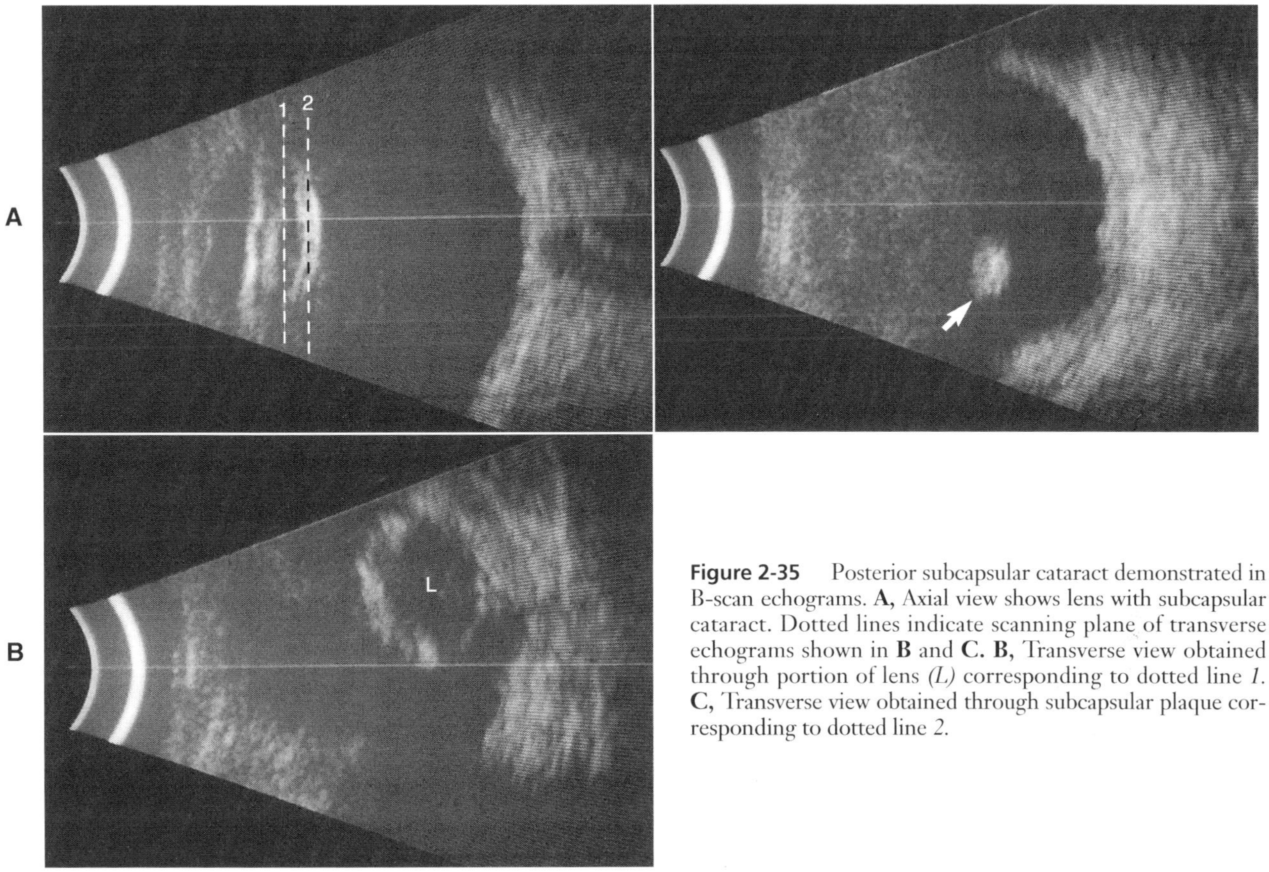

Figure 2-35 Posterior subcapsular cataract demonstrated in B-scan echograms. **A,** Axial view shows lens with subcapsular cataract. Dotted lines indicate scanning plane of transverse echograms shown in **B** and **C. B,** Transverse view obtained through portion of lens *(L)* corresponding to dotted line *1*. **C,** Transverse view obtained through subcapsular plaque corresponding to dotted line *2*.

EVALUATION OF THE PUPIL

Pupillary reaction may be evaluated with B-scan as the patient fixates in primary gaze. An extremely anterior transverse approach normally allows display of the iris and pupil. Pupillary response can be observed on the screen when a light is directed either toward the examined or the contralateral eye (Figure 2-37).

PEDIATRIC EXAMINATION

The echographic examination of small children can be extremely challenging. This is due primarily to inadequate cooperation and the frequent necessity to examine through closed eyelids. To perform a satisfactory examination, in some cases it is necessary to evaluate children under anesthesia. This evaluation can be carried out in the operating room under general anesthesia or in an outpatient setting under local sedation. This later situation should only be undertaken, however, if adequately trained personnel and appropriate devices are available to monitor the child both during and following the procedure. An additional echographic examination with the child awake may be helpful in some cases to assess the kinetic properties of certain lesions and structures that cannot be evaluated while the child was sedated.

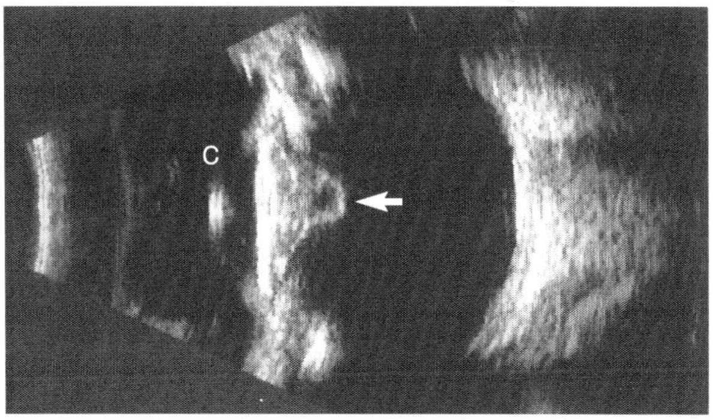

Figure 2-36 Posterior lenticonus. Immersion axial B-scan shows characteristic protrusion of posterior lens capsule *(arrow)*. *C*, Cornea. (Courtesy Dr. Cecelio Velasco-Barona, Mexico City, Mexico.)

An adequate examination can be performed on most children without sedation although various degrees of restraint may be necessary. Newborns and children up to 6 months of age can often be held by a parent with an assistant gently securing the head to prevent movement. Older children, however, often require immobilization of arms and legs that cannot be achieved without some type of external wrapping (Figure 2-38).

A

B

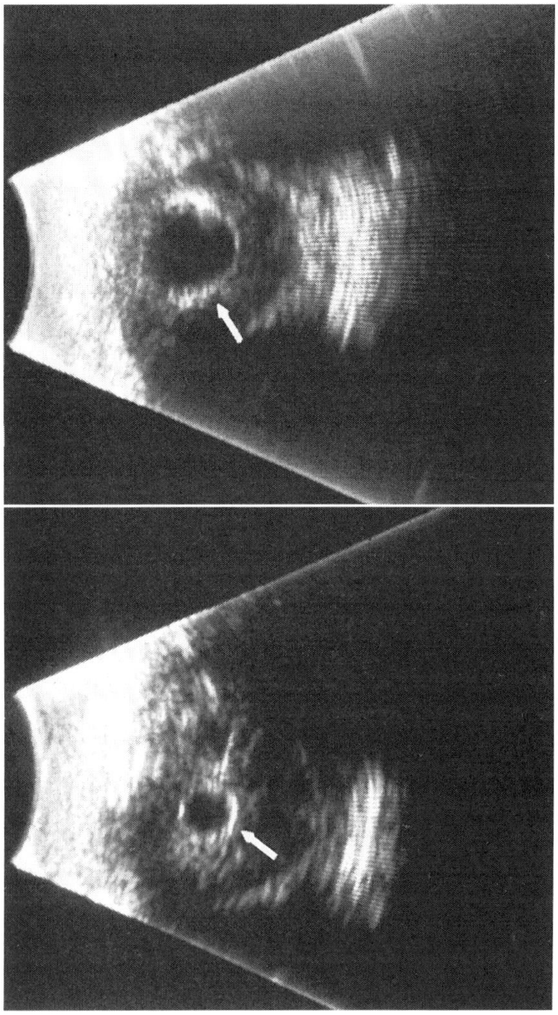

Figure 2-37 Evaluation of the pupil. The pupil can usually be imaged with the B-scan by using a very anterior transverse approach. The real-time features of the B-scan allow the examiner to monitor the pupillary light response on the screen. **A,** Dilated pupil *(arrow)*. **B,** Constricted pupil. (From Green RL, Byrne SF: Diagnostic ophthalmic ultrasound, in Ryan SJ [ed]: *Retina*. ed 3, St Louis, Mosby, 2001, p 261.)

As mentioned, it is often necessary to perform the examination through closed eyelids, especially if the child is awake. This limits the ability to accurately localize lesions and sometimes prevents adequate assessment of certain portions of the eye. Nevertheless, if a systematic approach is undertaken, in most cases, a satisfactory examination can be performed.

Evaluation of the anterior segment using an immersion technique is usually not possible when a child is awake. It has been shown, however, that the small finger-tip balloon technique used with conventional instrumentation (see Figure 2-31) or the 20 MHz probe with the latex tonometer cover (see Figure 2-33) can sometimes be beneficial in these patients.

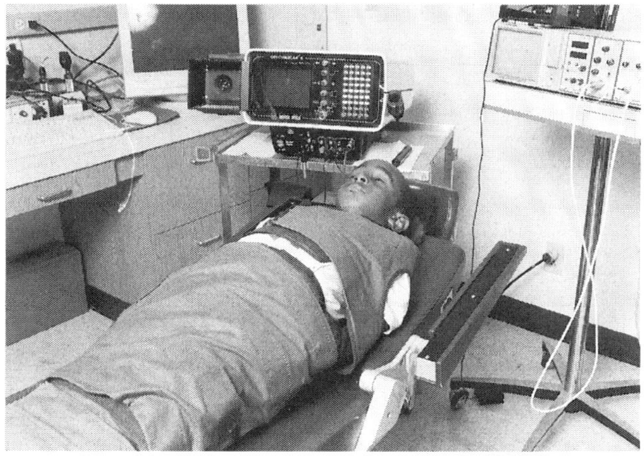

Figure 2-38 Young child in restraining device for ultrasound examination.

DOCUMENTATION OF FINDINGS

Adequate documentation of significant findings observed during an ultrasound examination is essential. Documentation serves to provide an accurate record of the examination and facilitates comparison at follow-up visits. Echograms are typically labeled with the specific area of the eye examined and for B-scan, the probe orientation (i.e., transverse, longitudinal or axial) is also recorded. For posterior segment lesions, the area of the eye examined is generally opposite to where the probe is placed (see Appendix E). For anterior segment lesions using an immersion technique, the area of the eye evaluated is directly adjacent to where the probe is placed. It should be mentioned, however, that pictorial documentation of all echographic findings may not always be possible due to the kinetic nature of the findings, the presence of artifacts, or poor patient compliance.

REFERENCES

1. Byrne SF: Standardized echography of the eye and orbit, in Naidich TB, Quencer R (eds): *Clinical Neurosonography*. Berlin, Springer-Verlag, 1987, p 252.
2. Byrne SF: Standardized echography. I. A-scan examination procedures. *Int Ophthalmol Clin* 1979;19(4):267.
3. Collaborative Ocular Melanoma Study Group: The procedures of echography (ultrasound) for the Collaborative Ocular Melanoma Study (COMS). COMS Report No. 12, part I. *J Ophthalmic Nurs Technol* 1999;18:143.
4. Collaborative Ocular Melanoma Study Group: The procedures of echography (ultrasound) for the Collaborative Ocular Melanoma Study (COMS). COMS Report No. 12, part II. *J Ophthalmic Nurs Technol* 1999;18:219.
5. Dugel PU, Smiddy WE, Byrne SF, et al: Macular hole syndromes. Echographic findings with clinical correlation. *Ophthalmology* 1994;101:815.
6. Ossoinig KC: *Standardized Ophthalmic Echography of the Eye, Orbit and Periorbital Region. A Comprehensive Slide Set and Study Guide*, ed 3, Iowa City, Goodfellow, 1985.
7. Ossoinig KC: Standardized echography: Basic principles, clinical applications, and results. *Int Ophthalmol Clin* 1979;19(4):127.
8. Ossoinig KC: Quantitative echography—the basis of tissue differentiation. *J Clin Ultrasound* 1974;2:33.
9. Pavlin CJ, Harasiewicz K, Sherar MD, et al: Clinical use of ultrasound biomicroscopy. *Ophthalmology* 1991;98:287.
10. Pavlin CJ, Foster FS: *Ultrasound Biomicroscopy of the Eye*. New York, Springer-Verlag, 1995.

3

William D. Bates

Vitreoretinal Disease

The accurate characterization of vitreoretinal disorders is important in the management of eyes with opaque ocular media.[54,57] The posterior segment must be evaluated systematically so that significant abnormalities are not overlooked. The evaluation should include an assessment of the vitreous body, posterior hyaloid, subvitreal space, retina, choroid, sclera, and optic disc. When indicated, the anterior segment may also be evaluated[47] (see p 77 and Chapters 2, 4, and 8).

VITREOUS BODY

The vitreous cavity should be assessed for the presence of opacities, bands, and membranes. Vitreous opacities produce dots or short lines on B-scan and vertical deflections from the baseline on A-scan. Opacities may originate from liquefied vitreous (syneresis) or clumps of cells, including calcium soaps (asteroid hyalosis), blood cells (hemorrhage), or inflammatory (uveitis) or infectious material (endophthalmitis).

Normal Vitreous

In the young person, the clear, jellylike vitreous body generally produces no echoes. However, scattered vitreous opacities of very low reflectivity may be detected in the aging eye. In addition, there may be a mobile posterior vitreous detachment (PVD) that manifests as a fine, thin line on B-scan and as a very low reflective spike on A-scan (Figure 3-1).

Asteroid Hyalosis

The ultrasound findings in this condition are usually quite typical, making the diagnosis straightforward. Calcium soaps produce bright, pointlike echo sources on B-scan that may be diffuse or focal. An area of clear vitreous is normally present between the posterior boundary of the opacities and the posterior hyaloid (Figure 3-2). This appearance may be confused with a PVD, especially when the hyaloid remains adherent to the retinal surface (Figure 3-3). On A-scan, asteroid hyalosis produces spikes of medium to high reflectivity that move with the vitreous gel.

Vitreous Hemorrhage

Vitreous hemorrhage, which is second only to cataract as a cause of opaque media, may be produced by or associated with a number of conditions. The most common of these are diabetic retinopathy, trauma, age-related macular degeneration (AMD), venous occlusion, and retinal tear. Echography is a useful adjunct to the clinical examination in establishing the density and location of the hemorrhage and may assist in determining the etiology of a clinically unexplained hemorrhage.

In fresh, mild hemorrhage, dots and short lines are displayed on B-scan, and a chain of low amplitude spikes is noted on A-scan. The more dense the hemorrhage, the greater the number of opacities and the higher their reflectivity.

If organization of the blood occurs, larger interfaces are formed, resulting in membranous surfaces on B-scan and even higher reflectivity on A-scan. Gravity may cause the blood to layer inferiorly, resulting in highly reflective pseudomembranes that can be confused with retinal detachment (RD) (Figure 3-4). However, these pseudomembranes can often be differentiated from RD with B-scan by noting a thinning of the membrane as it extends superiorly. This thinned membrane then appears to terminate within the vitreous gel (Figure 3-5) rather than inserting into the fundus as is characteristic of a partial RD. Also, a PVD commonly occurs in association with vitreous hemorrhage.

In some cases, hemorrhage may be confined to syneretic cavities within the vitreous body. In this situation, the blood is very homogeneous and does not form membranous surfaces and clumplike opacities, as occurs when it diffusely infiltrates the vitreous gel. The blood within these pockets appears very low reflective on A-scan and diffusely homogeneous on B-scan, similar to the hemorrhage in a vitrectomized eye (see Figure 4-45, *C* and *D*). It is important to appreciate that when both the solid vitreous gel and diffuse, homogeneous blood are present, the solid gel may appear echolucent on B-scan and can thus mimic cystic cavities (Figure 3-6).

A

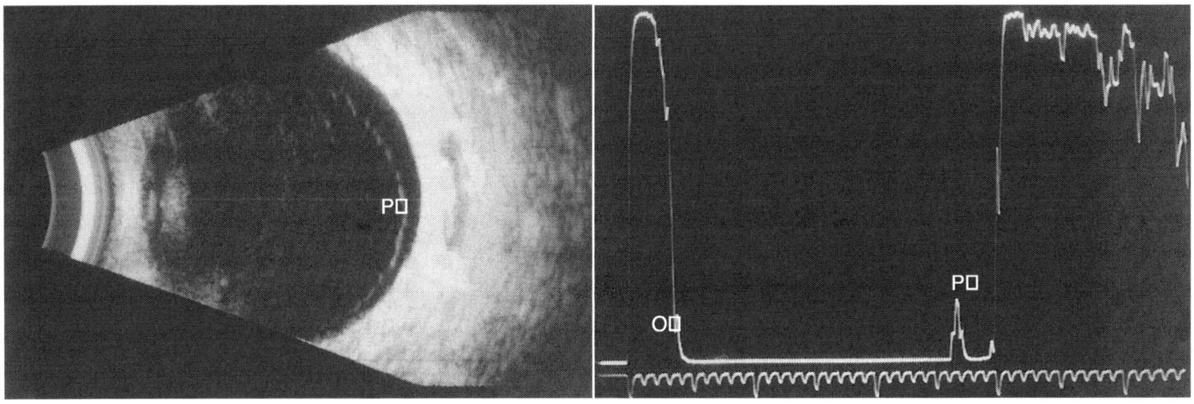

B

Figure 3-1 A PVD in the normal, aging eye. The PVD appears as a fine, thin line *(P)* on B-scan **(A)** and a low reflective spike on A-scan **(B).**

C

B

D

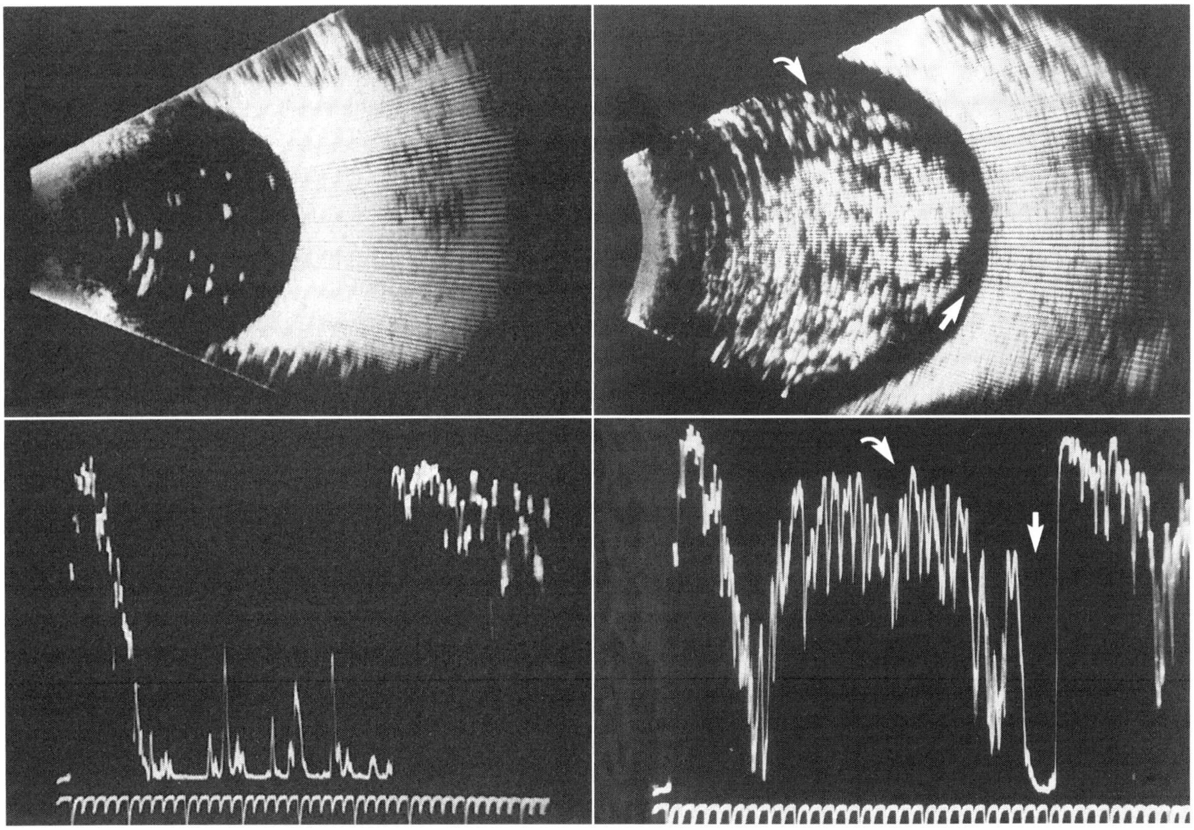

Figure 3-2 Asteroid hyalosis. Opacities can be mild (**A** and **B**) or extremely dense (**C** and **D**). Note the echolucent vitreous gel *(straight arrows)* located between asteroid opacities *(curved arrows)* and retina in **C** and **D.** This appearance can simulate a PVD. (**A** and **B** from Green RL, Byrne SF: Diagnostic ophthalmic ultrasound, in Ryan SJ [ed]: *Retina.* ed 3, St Louis, Mosby, 2001, p 245.)

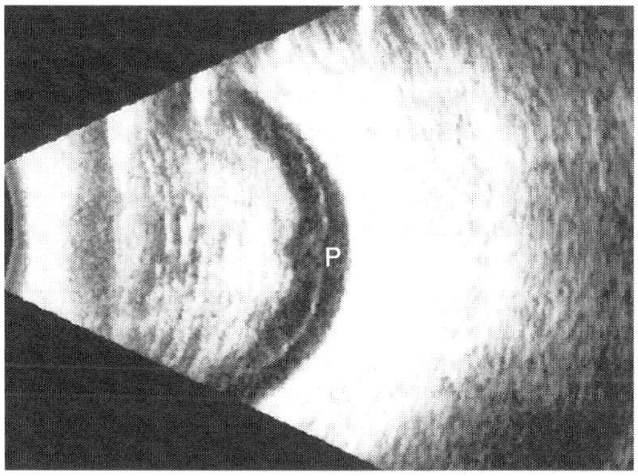

Figure 3-3 Dense asteroid hyalosis with PVD. Transverse B-scan demonstrates an area of clear vitreous between the posterior boundary of the dense opacities and the detached posterior hyaloid *(P)*.

A

B

C

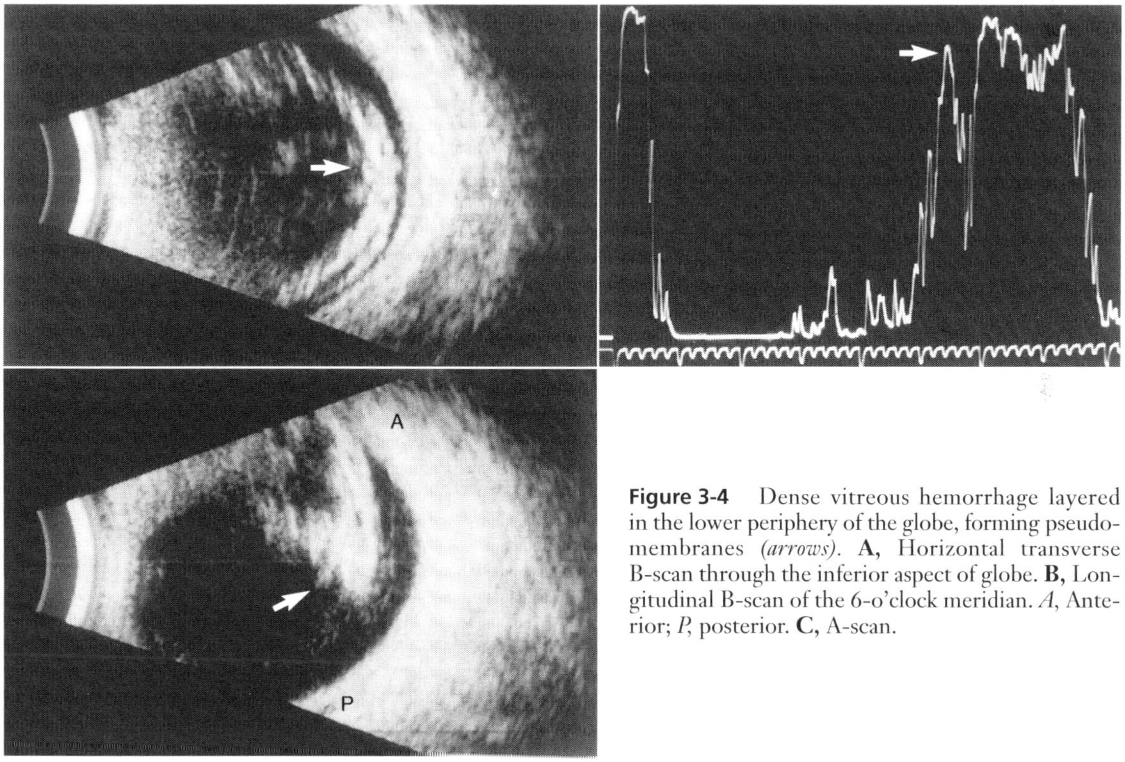

Figure 3-4 Dense vitreous hemorrhage layered in the lower periphery of the globe, forming pseudomembranes *(arrows)*. **A,** Horizontal transverse B-scan through the inferior aspect of globe. **B,** Longitudinal B-scan of the 6-o'clock meridian. *A,* Anterior; *P,* posterior. **C,** A-scan.

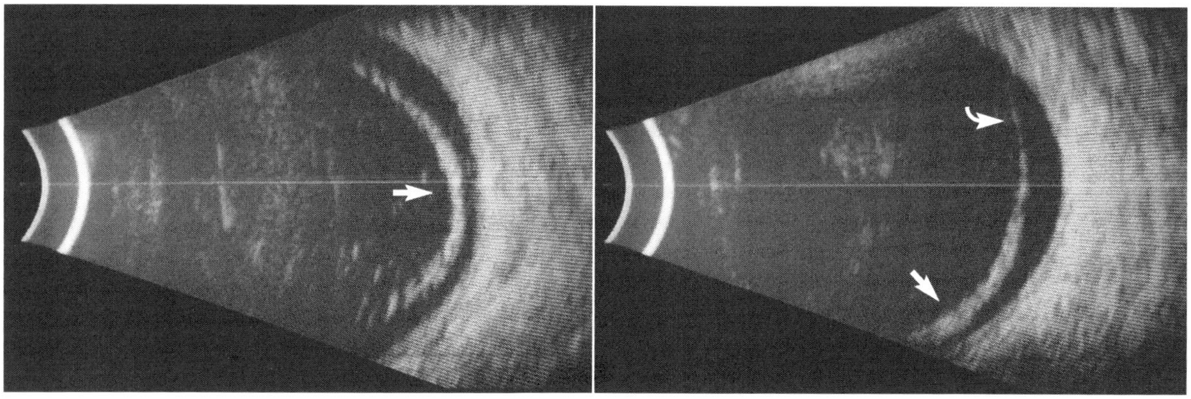

Figure 3-5 Technique for differentiation of layered blood from RD. **A,** Transverse B-scan through the inferior aspect of the globe in an eye with vitreous hemorrhage shows dense pseudomembrane produced by layered blood. *Straight arrow* indicates the 6-o'clock meridian. **B,** Transverse B-scan through 4:30 meridian shows thinning of pseudomembrane as it extends superiorly, appearing to terminate within the vitreous gel *(curved arrow)*. The 6-o'clock meridian is indicated by *straight arrow*.

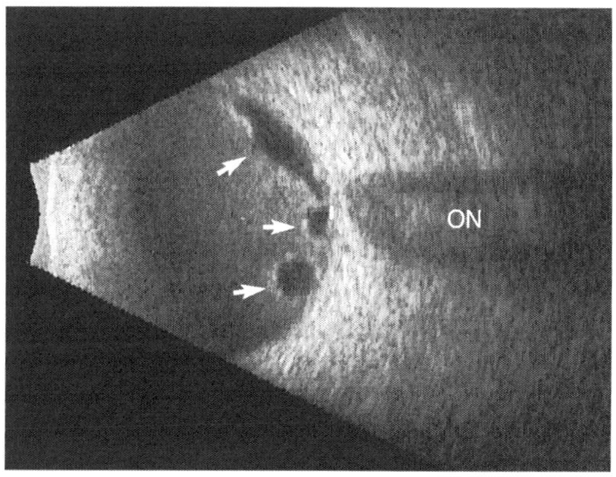

Figure 3-6 Vitreous hemorrhage and solid vitreous gel. Para-axial B-scan view demonstrates echolucent sections of solid vitreous gel *(arrows)* outlined by diffuse hemorrhage in the vitreous cavity. *ON*, Optic nerve.

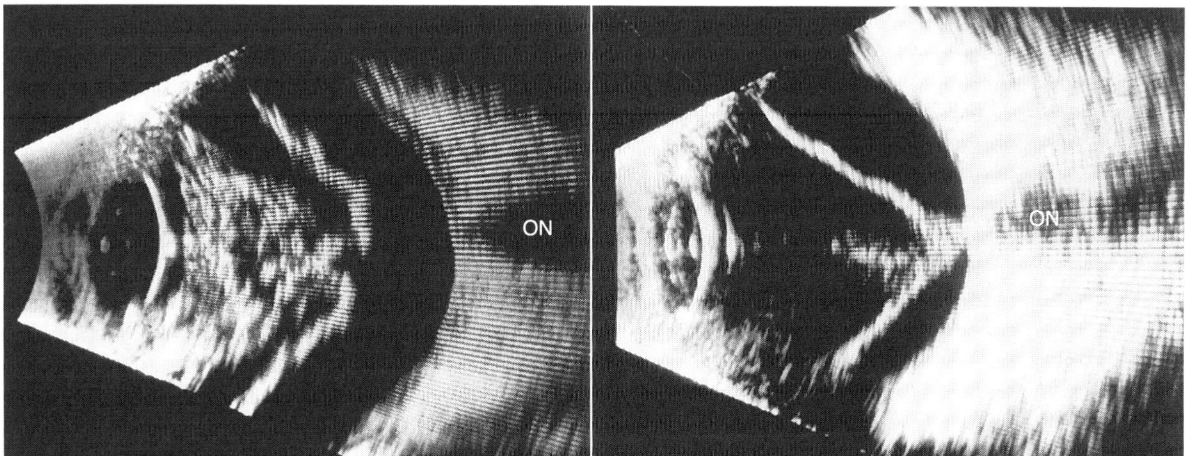

Figure 3-7 Axial B-scan views of two eyes with PVDs. **A,** Extensive PVD with complete separation of posterior hyaloid from optic nerve *(ON)*. **B,** Extensive PVD with persistent attachment of posterior hyaloid to optic nerve *(ON)*. Since this membrane may topographically simulate RD, quantitation and kinetic techniques should be used for differentiation.

A

B

C

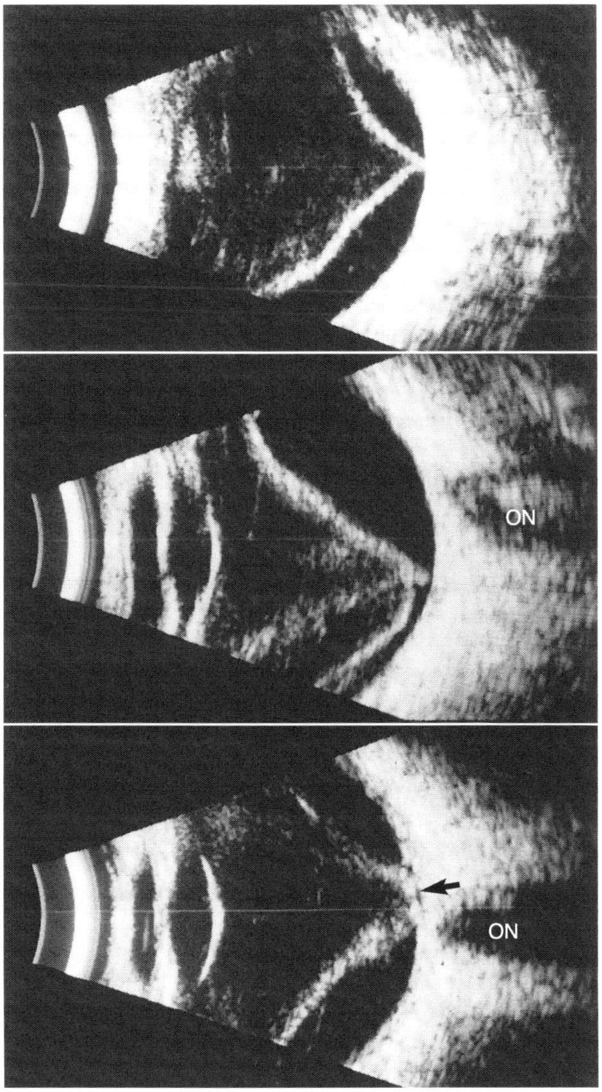

Figure 3-8 B-scans from different eyes showing PVDs with varied attachments to the retina. **A,** Horizontal transverse view near equator of eye shows area of vitreoretinal adherence. **B,** Horizontal axial scan shows PVD inserting into fundus temporal to macula. *ON,* Optic nerve. **C,** Vertical axial scan shows PVD inserting just superior to optic nerve, causing mild tractional detachment of retina *(arrow).*

Posterior Vitreous Detachment (PVD)

A PVD may occur in the normal aging eye, or it may be associated with vitreous hemorrhage or inflammation. The PVD may be focal or extensive. The posterior hyaloid may separate completely from the posterior pole, or it may remain attached to the optic disc, producing a funnel-shaped configuration (Figure 3-7). Vitreoretinal adhesions may occur at areas of retinal neovascularization (e.g., branch vein occlusion or diabetes) (Figure 3-8). In addition, vitreoretinal adhesions may be detected in areas other than the optic disc, often in association with a retinal tear or at impact site following penetrating trauma (see Chapter 4).

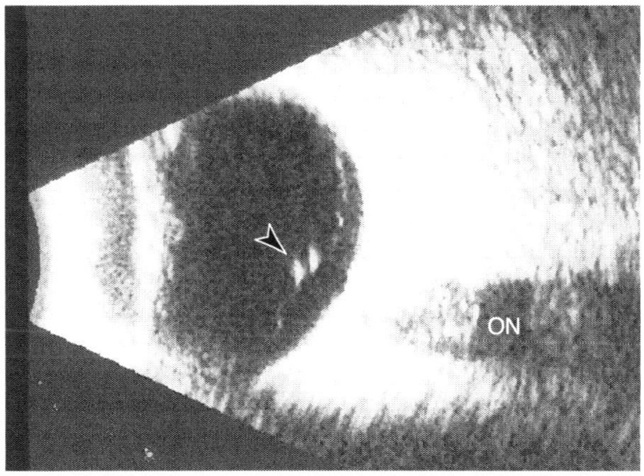

Figure 3-9 PVD with Weiss ring. Longitudinal B-scan demonstrates two closely spaced echo-dense opacities *(open arrow)* on surface of detached posterior hyaloid overlying optic nerve head. *ON,* Optic nerve.

On B-scan, in a normal eye, a PVD usually appears smooth and thin. When blood or inflammatory debris is layered on the surface of a PVD, the B-scan may show a thick line, especially posteriorly and inferiorly. Kinetic echography typically shows a very fluid, undulating aftermovement of the PVD. This characteristic fluid movement is helpful in differentiating a PVD from retinal and choroidal detachments, both of which are usually less mobile than a PVD.

Another B-scan finding in the normal eye where the vitreous is completely separated from the optic nerve is the presence of a Weiss ring.[26] The Weiss ring represents tissue that normally surrounds the optic nerve head and provides a firm attachment of the vitreous to the posterior pole. When the vitreous detaches from the optic nerve, this ring of tissue also separates and often appears on B-scan as two closely spaced opacities at the level of the PVD. This ring can usually be seen overlying the optic disc (Figure 3-9) but may be located elsewhere if the vitreous body has collapsed.

On A-scan, the reflectivity of a PVD can vary from extremely low, as in the normal eye, to extremely high, as is often the case in eyes with dense hemorrhage. Kinetic evaluation typically shows marked horizontal and vertical spike aftermovement (Table 3-1; also see Figure 2-27).

There are situations in which the acoustic behavior of a PVD is similar to that of an RD. Although differentiating between the two may be quite challenging, several techniques have been developed to facilitate this distinction (see "Retinal Detachment vs. Posterior Vitreous Detachment," on p 56).

Subvitreal Hemorrhage

Hemorrhage may occur in the subvitreal (subhyaloid) space in association with vitreous hemorrhage. Subvitreal

A

B

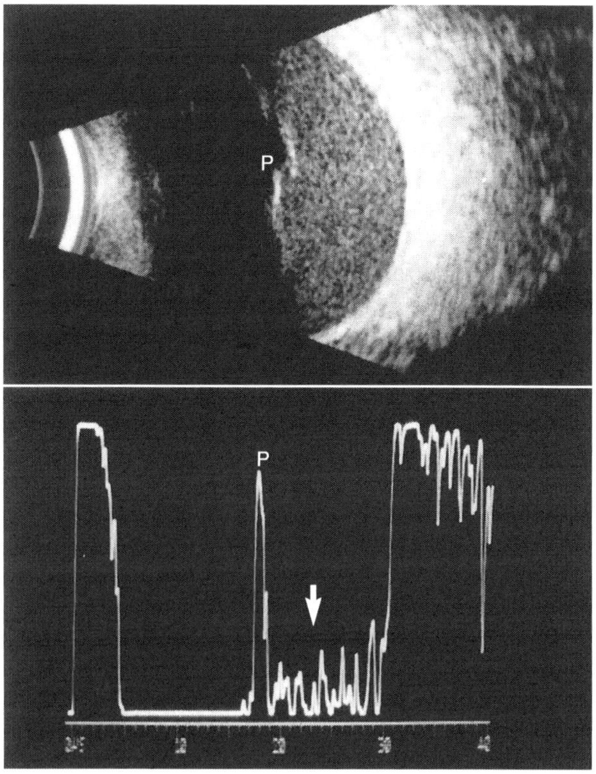

Figure 3-10 Subvitreal hemorrhage. **A,** Transverse B-scan echogram shows extensive PVD *(P)* and dense subvitreal hemorrhage. **B,** A-scan shows medium-high reflective spike from PVD *(P)* and low reflective spikes from the subvitreal fluid blood *(arrow)*.

A

B

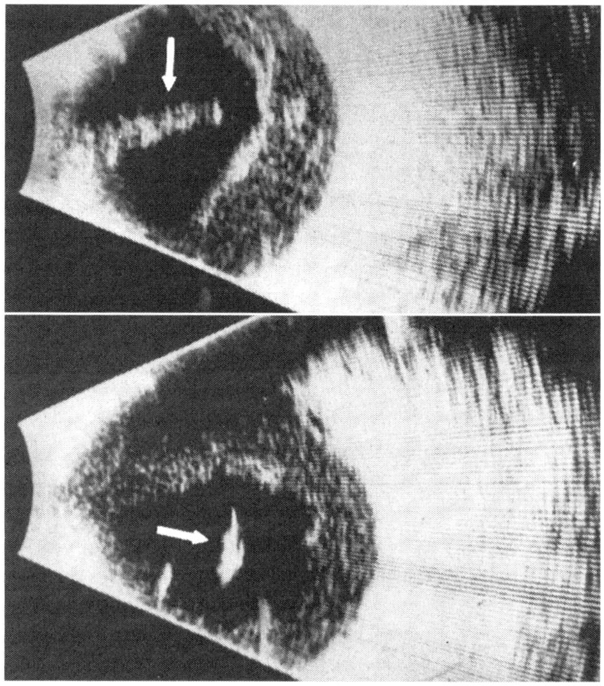

Figure 3-11 PVD with subvitreal hemorrhage and blood in Cloquet's canal *(arrows)*. **A,** Section along length of canal also shows PVD and dense subvitreal hemorrhage. The canal is surrounded by relatively clear vitreous gel. **B,** Cross-section of canal also shows PVD and subvitreal hemorrhage. (From Green RL, Byrne SF: Diagnostic ophthalmic ultrasound, in Ryan SJ [ed]: *Retina*. ed 3, St Louis, Mosby, 2001, p 247.)

TABLE 3-1

Differentiation of Posterior Vitreous Detachment (PVD), Retinal Detachment (RD), and Choroidal Detachment (CD)

Technique	PVD	RD	CD
Topographic	Smooth, open funnel with or without disc or fundus insertion; inserts at ora or ciliary body	Smooth or folded, open or closed funnel with disc insertion; may have associated cysts; inserts at ora	Smooth, dome or flat; no disc insertion; inserts at ora or ciliary body
Quantitative	Variable spike height; $<$100% high at ora superiorly	Steeply rising 100% high spike, including at ora superiorly	Steeply rising, thick, double-peaked 100% high spike
Kinetic (aftermovement)	Marked to moderate	Moderate to none	Mild to none

hemorrhage can be seen, however, even when there is no hemorrhage in the vitreous gel. On echography, a high gain setting is often needed to detect a mild subhyaloid hemorrhage (Figure 3-10). Subvitreal blood typically does not clot; therefore, it remains low reflective and mobile, even in longstanding cases. This is in contrast to the higher reflectivity of pseudomembranes and clumplike accumulations of blood that often form within the vitreous gel. Occasionally, subvitreal blood may extend anteriorly through Cloquet's canal (Figure 3-11).

Posterior Hyphema

The cellular component of blood in the subvitreal space may settle and layer, similar to a hyphema in the anterior chamber.[43] The surface of this layered blood may appear as

A

B

C

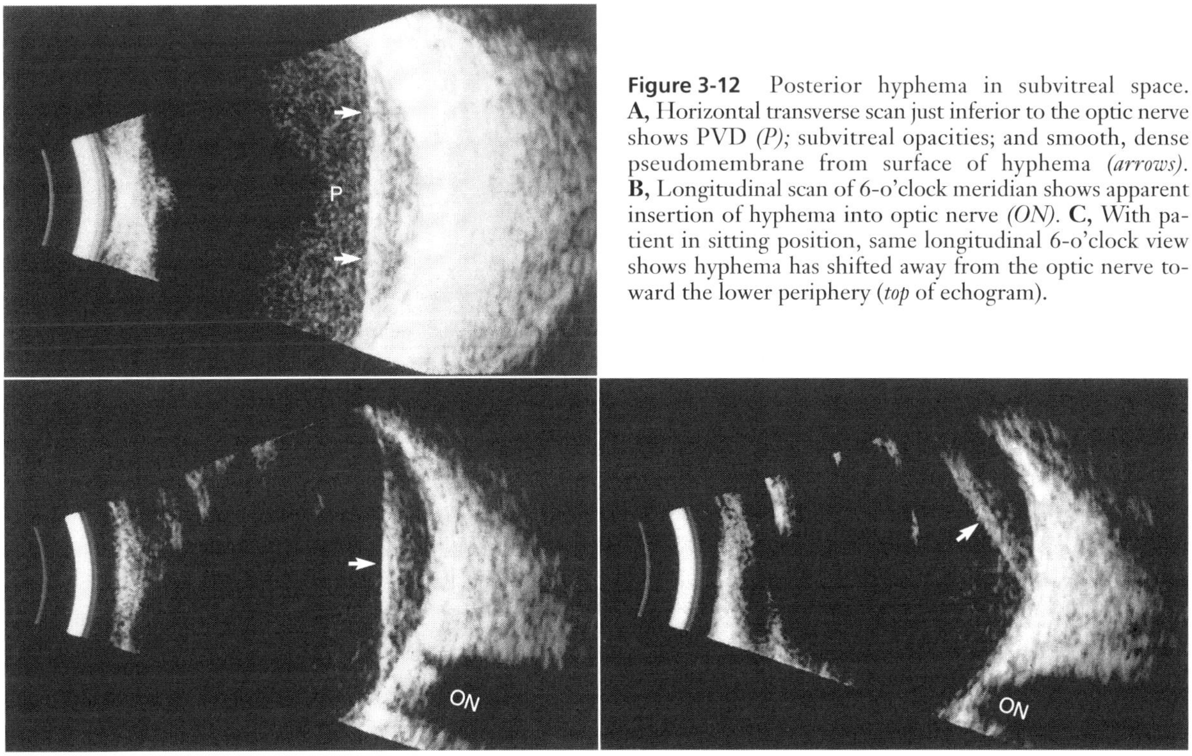

Figure 3-12 Posterior hyphema in subvitreal space. **A,** Horizontal transverse scan just inferior to the optic nerve shows PVD *(P)*; subvitreal opacities; and smooth, dense pseudomembrane from surface of hyphema *(arrows)*. **B,** Longitudinal scan of 6-o'clock meridian shows apparent insertion of hyphema into optic nerve *(ON)*. **C,** With patient in sitting position, same longitudinal 6-o'clock view shows hyphema has shifted away from the optic nerve toward the lower periphery (*top* of echogram).

a dense, smooth membrane on B-scan and as a highly reflective spike on A-scan, thus simulating a shallow RD. However, if the patient moves the eye back and forth, the hyphema normally slides across the fundus surface (Figure 3-12). If the patient sits upright or turns his or her head, the hyphema will shift its position.

When attempting to diagnose a hyphema in this way, it is important to use the same probe position before and after the head or body is moved. Use of this technique is recommended, even when the diagnosis of hyphema is obvious, to exclude underlying retinochoroid layer thickening or a shallow RD. Hyphemas can also be demonstrated in the presence of subretinal or suprachoroidal hemorrhage (see p 56 and Figure 5-70).

Vitreous Inflammation (Endophthalmitis/Uveitis)

See Chapter 6 for a review of vitreous inflammation (endophthalmitis/uveitis).

Vitreous Cysts

Vitreous cysts may be congenital or may be related to a disease process.[60] The congenital cysts are remnants of the hyaloid system. They are usually free floating, but in some cases remain attached to the surface of the optic disc. On B-scan they appear well outlined and either lobulated or round (Figure 3-13).

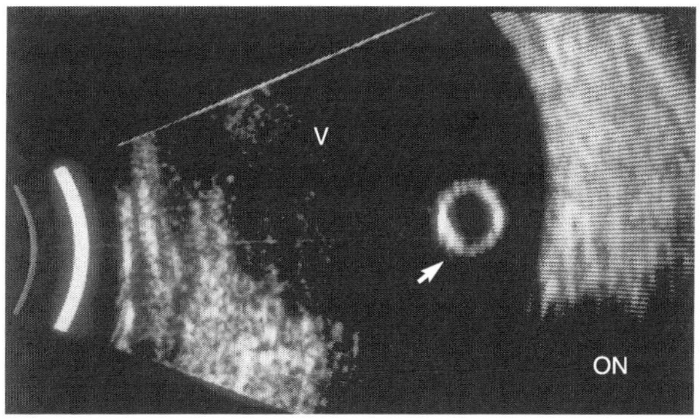

Figure 3-13 Congenital vitreous cyst. Longitudinal B-scan displays a large, round, echolucent lesion *(arrow)* that was freely floating in vitreous cavity *(V)*. *ON*, Optic nerve.

Cystic lesions of the vitreous can be associated with intraocular cysticercosis (see p 203) and have been described in eyes with medulloepithelioma (see p 187), as well as retinoblastoma (see p 180).

RETINA

One of the most important roles of echography is to evaluate the status of the retina in the presence of opaque media.

Retinal tears, RD, retinoschisis, and many other disorders can be accurately characterized.

Retinal Tears

A retinal tear is a type of retinal break that is readily detected with ultrasound and, therefore, should always be considered when screening an eye with opaque media. Focal retinal tears, a common cause of unexplained vitreous hemorrhage, are located most often in the superior peripheral fundus. The examiner should first search for a PVD and then for specific areas where the vitreous remains attached to the retinal surface. A retinal tear appears as a small, focal, echo-dense membrane extending from the surface of the fundus to which the posterior hyaloid is attached (Figure 3-14). Kinetic echography is important in confirming the area of vitreoretinal adherence and the presence of a retinal tear.

Other lesions that can simulate a retinal tear echographically include stalklike areas of neovascularization, as in diabetic retinopathy or branch vein occlusion, as well as small traction RDs. A focal accumulation of blood at an area of vitreoretinal adherence may also mimic a small retinal tear. In these situations, consideration of the history, location, and kinetic behavior of the lesion will generally allow differentiation from a true retinal tear. In addition, the presence of a shallow, focal RD surrounding the tear may be helpful in securing the diagnosis (Figure 3-15). It should also be noted that the echographic findings for treated and untreated retinal tears are similar.

Ultrasound has been incorporated into the treatment of retinal tears in some eyes with vitreous hemorrhage.[12,36] In these cases, B-scan is used instead of ophthalmoscopy to localize the tear and to monitor it during cryotherapy (Figure 3-16).

In most cases of extensive, rhegmatogenous RD, small tears usually cannot be detected with ultrasound. On the other hand, retinal folds can sometimes simulate small tears. One study has shown, however, that a retinal tear is usually located within 2 clock hours of the area of greatest retinal elevation.[6] Echography may thus indirectly aid in the localization of a tear by determining where the detachment is most elevated.

Giant retinal tears are often difficult to diagnose because they produce varied and unusual echographic findings[20,32] and because they are most often present in severely injured eyes. Whenever the insertion of a membrane appears to be unusual, the possibility of a giant tear should be considered (Figure 3-17). In some cases the detached retina may be folded over on itself, giving the false impression of two separate membranes (Figure 3-18). In addition, because of the large tear, the detached retina may show greater mobility than normal.

Another type of retinal break that may be encountered is a peripheral retinal dialysis. A retinal dialysis is a disinsertion of the retina from the ora serrata. Although these breaks can occur spontaneously, they are most often seen following blunt trauma. The most common locations for peripheral retinal dialyses include the supranasal and inferotemporal quadrants. These types of retinal breaks usually are associated with shallow rather than bullous RDs (see Figure 4-6).

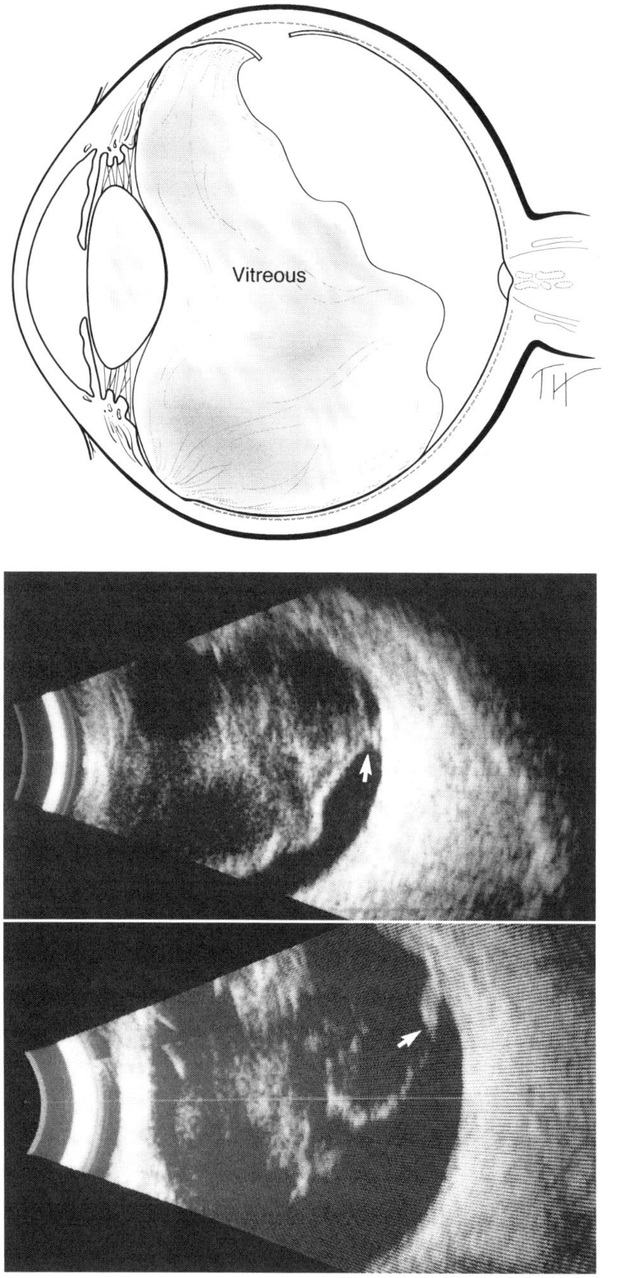

Figure 3-14 Peripheral retinal tears. **A,** Schematic drawing shows peripheral retinal tear with the posterior hyaloid remaining attached to its surface. Longitudinal B-scan echograms (**B** and **C**) from two different patients show adherence of posterior hyaloid to peripheral retinal tears *(arrows)*. Both eyes contain dense vitreous hemorrhage.

A 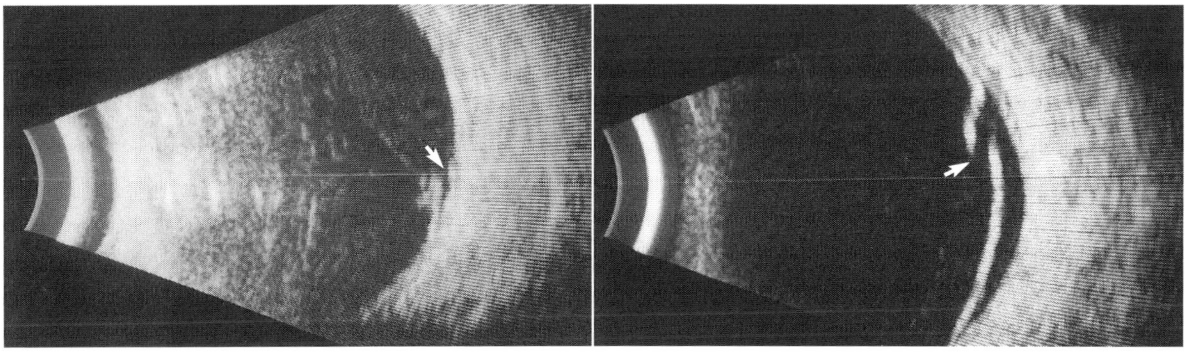 B

Figure 3-15 Peripheral retinal tear with shallow RD. Transverse B-scan echograms from two different patients show retinal tears *(arrows)* and associated RD. Detachment in **A** is more localized than detachment in **B.**

A 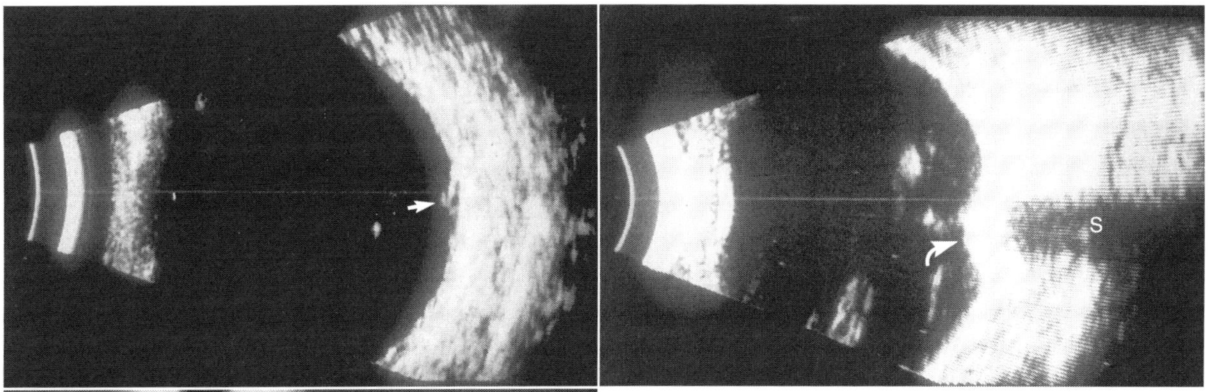 C

B 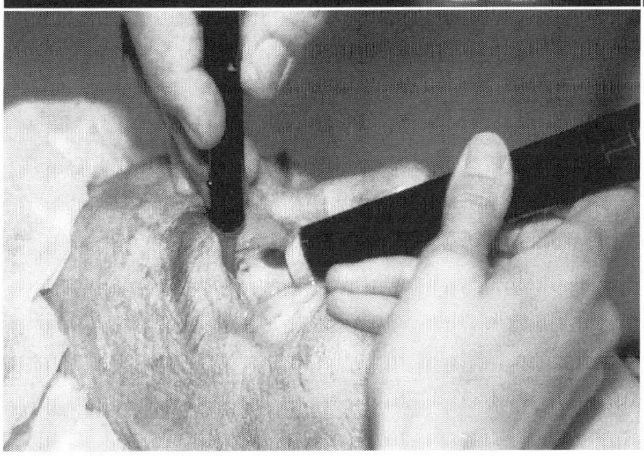

Figure 3-16 Ultrasound localization of retinal tear during cryotherapy. **A,** Transverse B-scan at reduced gain shows small peripheral tear in superior aspect of globe *(straight arrow)*. **B,** Photograph shows ultrasound guided localization of tear during cryotherapy. **C,** Transverse B-scan shows indentation of globe wall by cryoprobe *(arrow)* and shadowing *(S)* of orbital tissue. (**C** from DiBernardo C, Blodi B, Byrne SF: Echographic evaluation of retinal tears in patients with spontaneous vitreous hemorrhage. *Arch Ophthalmol* 1992;110:513.)

A

B

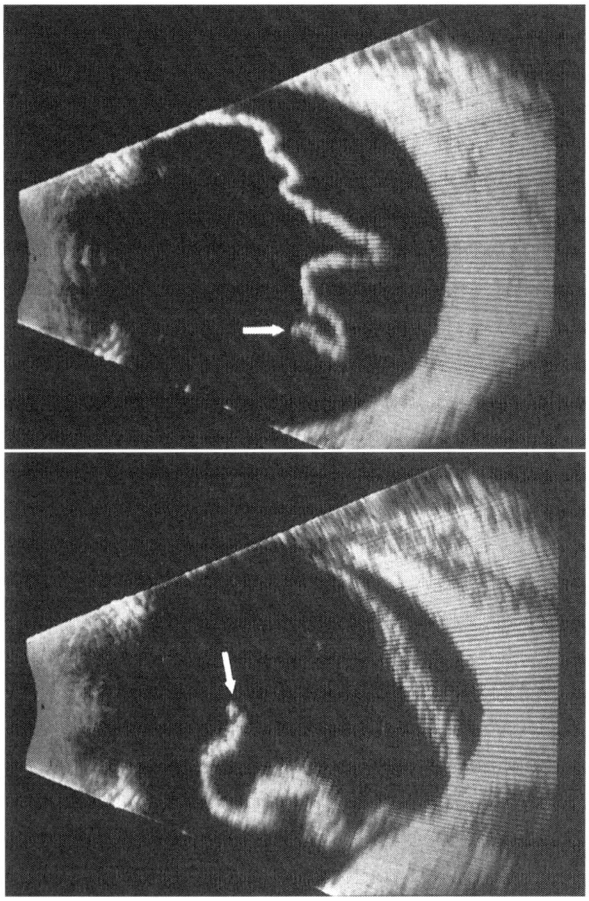

Figure 3-17 Giant retinal tear. Transverse **(A)** and longitudinal **(B)** views show extensive, folded RD with marked retraction of the retina and obvious disinsertion from the periphery *(arrows)*. (From Green RL, Byrne SF: Diagnostic ophthalmic ultrasound, in Ryan SJ [ed]: *Retina*. ed 3, St Louis, Mosby, 2001, p 249.)

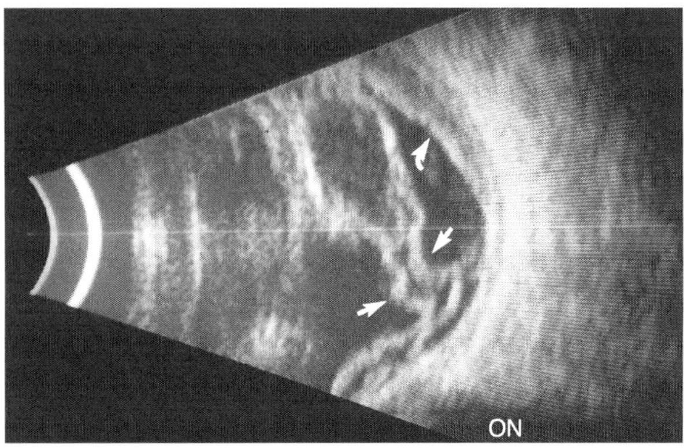

Figure 3-18 Giant retinal tear. Longitudinal B-scan demonstrates detached retina due to giant retinal tear. Note that retinal leaves are folded upon each other *(straight arrows)*, thus creating the impression of two separate membranes. *ON*, Optic nerve; *curved arrow*, shallow peripheral choroidal detachment.

Retinal Detachment (RD)

RD can have a number of etiologies, including tear (i.e., rhegmatogenous), exudate (e.g., uveal effusion, inflammation, central serous retinopathy, and intraocular tumors), hemorrhage (e.g., disciform lesions, trauma, and melanomas), and traction (e.g., diabetic retinopathy and trauma). The ultrasound findings differ somewhat according to the cause of the detachment.

The echographic features of RD are typically quite characteristic (see Table 3-1), thus making the differentiation from other membranes relatively straightforward. An RD (except those secondary to traction) generally appears as a bright, continuous, somewhat folded membrane on B-scan and as a highly reflective spike on A-scan[37] (Figure 3-19). There are certain situations, however, in which the retinal spike may be less than 100% high (e.g., atrophy, severe folding, or disruption of the retina).

In assessing an RD, it is always important to identify its insertions. An extensive or total RD can usually be shown to insert into the optic disc posteriorly and the ora serrata in the periphery. When the retina is only partially detached, it may not extend to the optic disc or the ora serrata but may appear to insert into the fundus in areas where it remains attached. Unusual situations in which the insertions may be atypical include peripheral retinal dialysis (see Figure 4-6), giant retinal tear (see p 52), and very rarely, complete avulsion of the retina from the optic disc due to severe trauma.

Peripheral rhegmatogenous RDs typically extend posteriorly as they extend laterally. This may not be true, however, following vitrectomy and 360-degree peripheral panretinal photocoagulation.[30] In this case, the photocoagulation creates retinal adhesions that prevent posterior extension of a peripheral rhegmatogenous detachment. This can lead to an unusual annular configuration of the detached retina that can simulate a choroidal detachment (see p 77 and Figure 7-8).

RD typically exhibits a tethered, restricted aftermovement that contrasts with the highly mobile, undulating movement of a PVD. However, certain factors can affect the mobility of the retina. For example, fresh, bullous detachments and those with large tears may be very mobile, whereas longstanding detachments with proliferative vitreoretinopathy (PVR) may be quite stiff. Additionally, exudative detachments show greater shifting of the subretinal fluid than do rhegmatogenous detachments. It should also be noted that atrophic retina, as may occur in endophthalmitis, may exhibit marked mobility, similar to that of a PVD.

An RD with underlying hemorrhage shows echoes in the subretinal space (Figure 3-20). The detection of mild hemorrhage generally necessitates the use of a high gain setting. As in subvitreal hemorrhage, subretinal blood typically does not clot and may produce a posterior hyphema (see p 50 and Figure 3-21). This is in contrast to suprachoroidal blood, which often produces solid clots (see p 106).

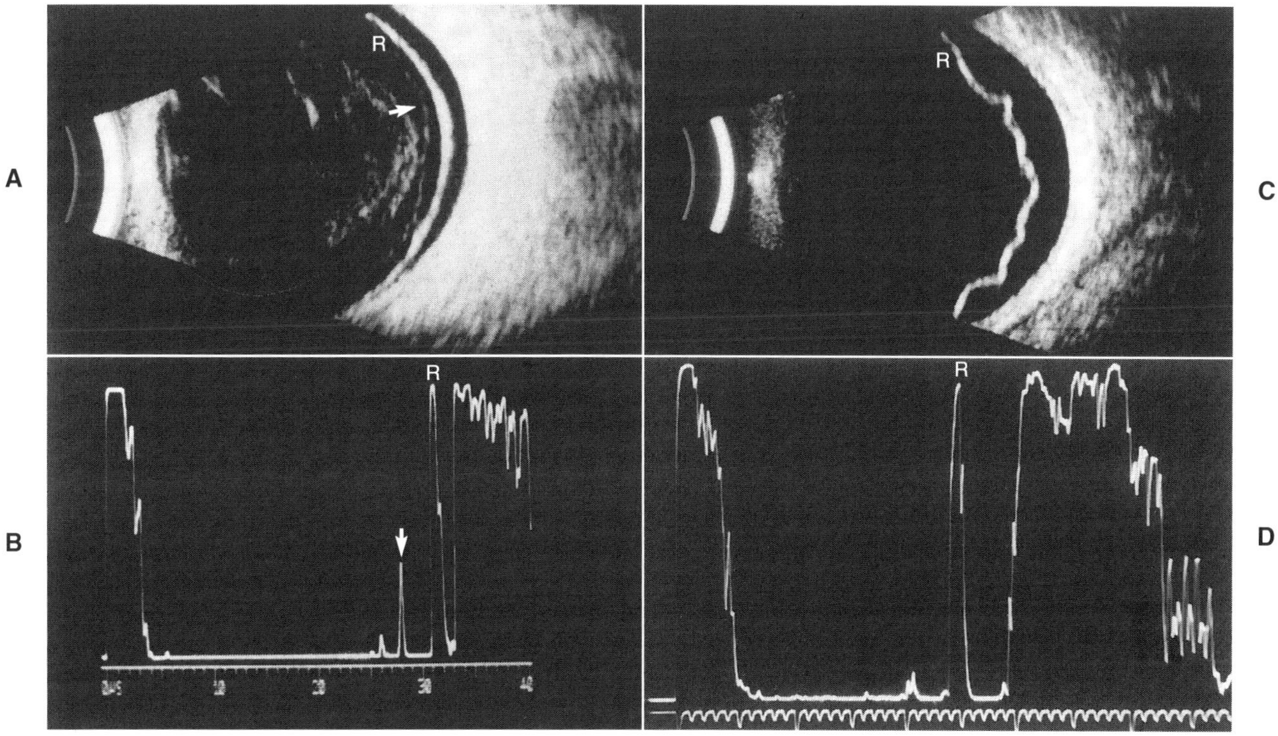

Figure 3-19 Smooth (**A** and **B**) and folded (**C** and **D**) RDs *(R)*. A-scans show characteristic 100% high, single-peaked spike at Tissue Sensitivity. Note mild vitreous opacities and PVD in **A** and **B** *(arrows)*. In **A** and **C**, note that the smooth surface of the fundus underlying the detached retina represents the inner surface of the retinal pigment epithelium. This surface is highly reflective on A-scan, similar to the retina.

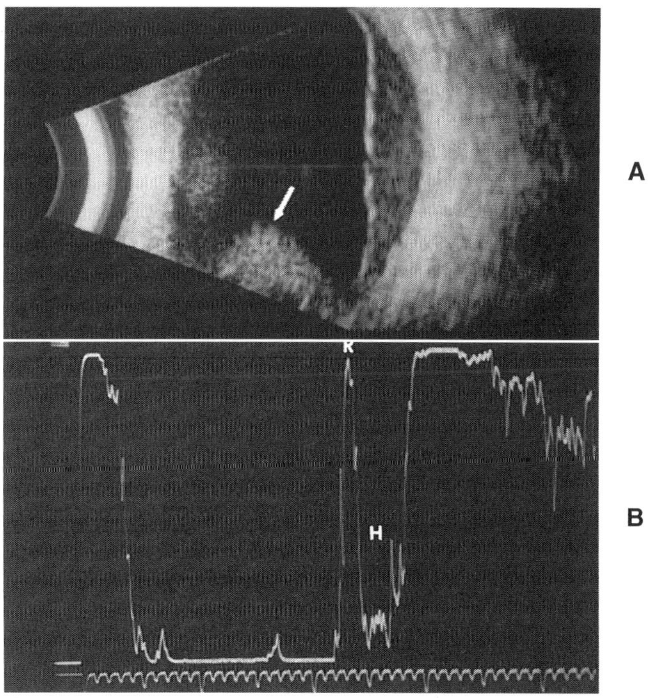

Figure 3-20 Hemorrhagic RD in an eye with choroidal melanoma. **A,** B-scan echogram shows mildly folded RD with dense subretinal hemorrhage (*arrow*, edge of melanoma). **B,** A-scan shows 100% high spike from retina *(R)* and low reflective echoes from subretinal hemorrhage *(H)*. (From Green RL, Byrne SF: Diagnostic ophthalmic ultrasound, in Ryan SJ [ed]: *Retina*. ed 3, St Louis, Mosby, 2001, p 250.)

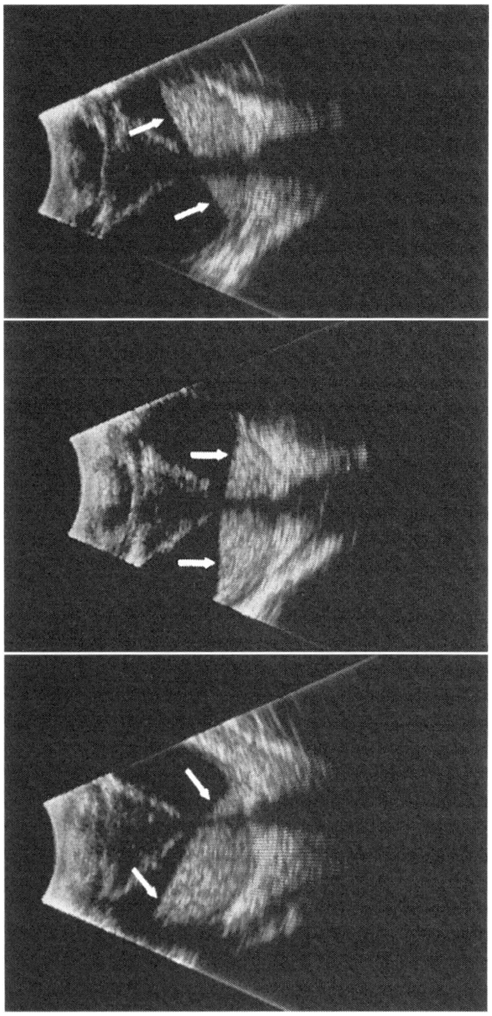

Figure 3-21 Posterior hyphema in subretinal space. Horizontal axial B-scan echograms from same patient with head turned toward nasal side **(A)**, with head straight **(B)**, and with head turned toward temporal side **(C)**. Echograms show shifting of hyphema *(arrows)* as head is moved from side to side. Note that the funnel-shaped RD appears echolucent when surrounded by dense opacities. (From Green RL, Byrne SF: Diagnostic ophthalmic ultrasound, in Ryan SJ [ed]: *Retina*. ed 3, St Louis, Mosby, 2001, p 248.)

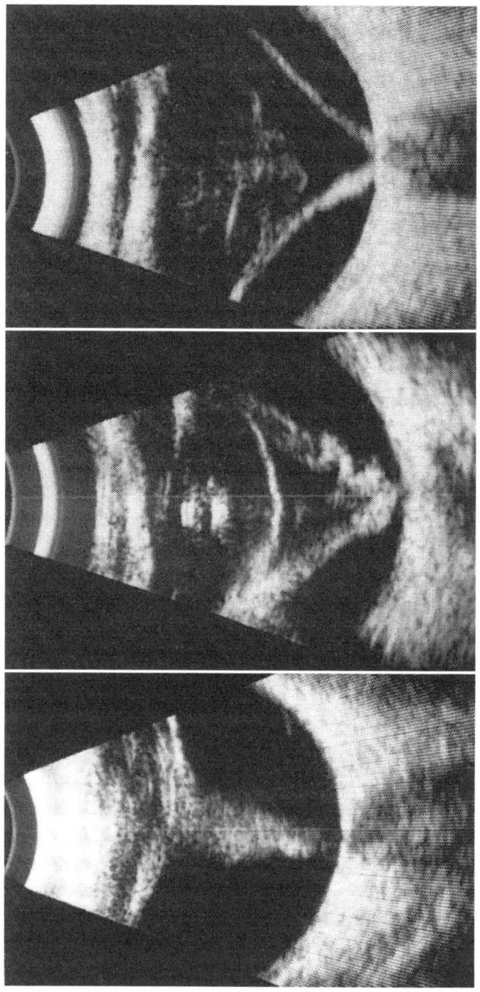

Figure 3-22 Axial B-scan echograms showing funnel-shaped RDs. **A,** Open funnel shape and mild PVD. **B,** Triangular shape with bridging membrane indicating PVR. **C,** T-shape *(closed funnel)* indicating PVR. (From Green RL, Byrne SF: Diagnostic ophthalmic ultrasound, in Ryan SJ [ed]: *Retina*. ed 3, St Louis, Mosby, 2001, p 250.)

The configuration of an RD may vary from shallow, flat, and smooth to bullous and highly folded. In addition, an extensive RD often takes the form of a funnel-shaped membrane. The funnel-shaped detachment may be open or closed (see Figure 2-19) and may be concave, triangular, or T-shaped. Detachments that are triangular or T-shaped, or that have fixed retinal folds, indicate PVR[19] (Figures 3-22 and 3-23). As mentioned in Chapter 2 (see p 21), an axial B-scan view may not always demonstrate the insertion of an RD into the optic nerve. Therefore, a longitudinal approach should always be used to assess the relationship of a membrane to the optic nerve (Figure 3-24). Shallow, extensive detachment of the retina is often secondary to a peripheral retinal dialysis. The possible presence of a peripheral retinal dialysis should be considered when examining an eye with a diffuse, shallow RD (see Figure 4-6).

Longstanding RDs may also develop retinal cysts and become partially calcified. Cholesterol debris may accumulate in the subretinal space (see p 37 and Figure 3-25).

Retinal Detachment vs. Posterior Vitreous Detachment

In some situations, the mobility of a PVD or an RD may be atypical, thus hindering differentiation of these two membranes. An incomplete PVD that is still attached to the op-

A 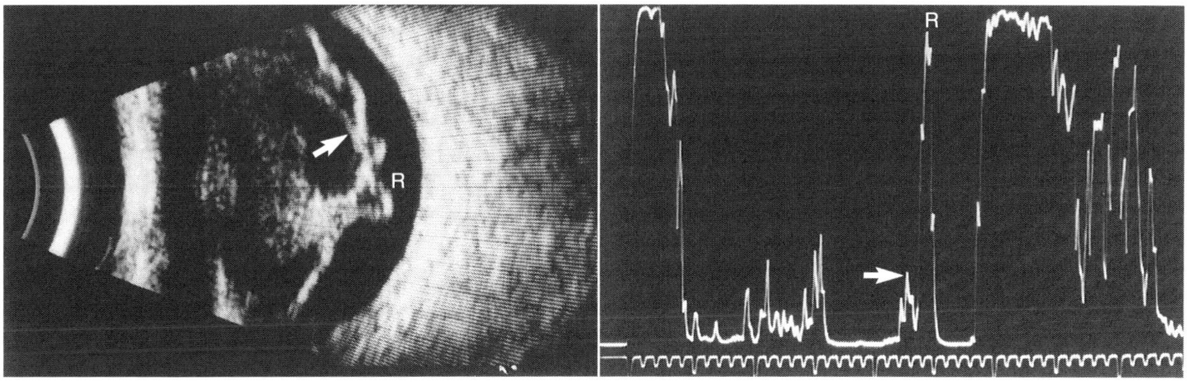 B

Figure 3-23 RD with fixed folds (PVR). **A,** Transverse B-scan echogram shows vitreous opacities and PVD *(arrow)* attached to extensive, folded RD *(R)*. **B,** A-scan shows low chain of spikes from vitreous opacities and 100% high spike from RD *(R)*. Note low reflective spike at left base of RD *(arrow)* corresponding to PVD that is adherent to the RD.

A C B D
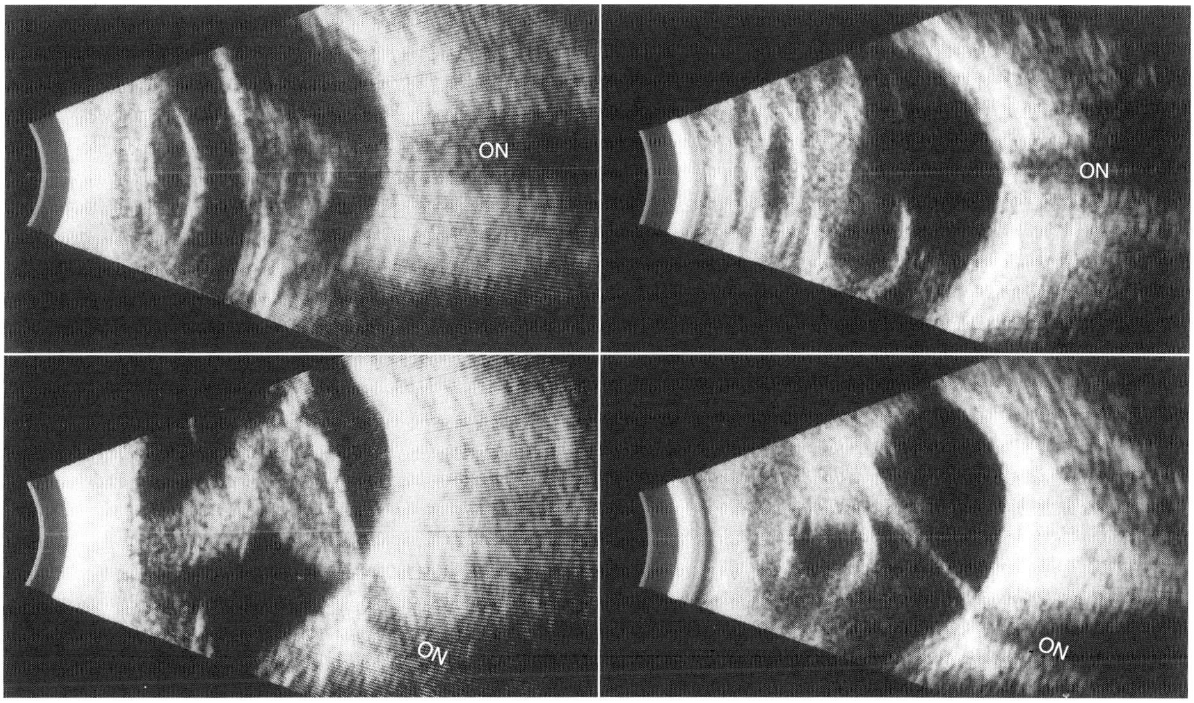

Figure 3-24 Axial vs. longitudinal B-scan approach for displaying posterior insertion of funnel-shaped RDs. Axial B-scan echograms from two different eyes with RD (**A** and **C**) do not demonstrate their insertion into the optic nerve *(ON)*. Longitudinal scans (**B** and **D**) from these same patients, however, clearly show the insertion of the detachments into the optic nerve.

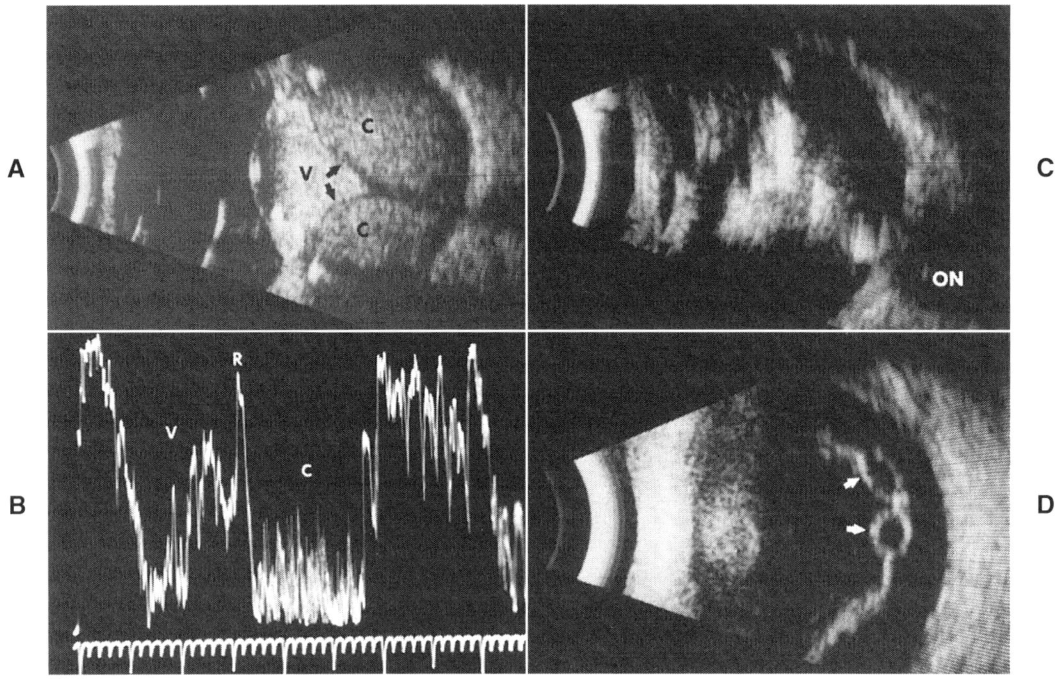

Figure 3-25 Various findings in three different longstanding RDs. **A,** Immersion B-scan echogram from aphakic eye shows closed funnel-shaped RD with dense vitreous hemorrhage *(V)* anteriorly and dense subretinal cholesterol *(C)* posteriorly. Note that funnel-shaped RD appears echolucent *(black arrows)* when surrounded on both sides by dense opacities. **B,** Corresponding A-scan echogram shows dense vitreous hemorrhage anteriorly *(V)* and the highly reflective RD *(R)*. Medium reflective, blurred spikes are displayed from the moving subretinal cholesterol *(C)* debris. **C,** Longitudinal B-scan shows calcified, funnel-shaped RD inserting into optic nerve *(ON)*. **D,** Transverse B-scan shows extensive RD with two retinal cysts *(arrows)*. (From Green RL, Byrne SF: Diagnostic ophthalmic ultrasound, in Ryan SJ [ed]: *Retina*. ed 3, St Louis, Mosby, 2001, p 251.)

tic disc may be less mobile than normal (e.g., trauma, diabetic retinopathy, or uveitis) and, therefore, may be confused with a funnel-shaped RD. Conversely, a detached retina can sometimes be more mobile than normal (e.g., endophthalmitis), thus simulating a PVD. In these situations, the echographic findings that are traditionally used (see Table 3-1) may be insufficient for differentiation, therefore necessitating the use of additional techniques.

In these atypical cases, the posterior insertion of the membrane in question should be reassessed with B-scan. It may be possible to rule out an RD merely by noting that the membrane inserts into the peripapillary region rather than into the optic disc (see Figure 3-7). Furthermore, the detection of a second membrane, located either anterior or posterior to the membrane in question, may be helpful in differentiating a PVD from an RD. If the etiology of the second membrane can be established, then the diagnosis of the membrane in question may often be clarified (Figure 3-26).

In extremely difficult cases, an A-scan technique has proved useful for differentiating PVD from RD.[18] This technique is based on the finding that the reflectivity of PVD and that of RD differ in the periphery. Whereas an RD remains highly reflective, a PVD often becomes less reflective as it inserts into the peripheral fundus[45] (Figures 3-27 and 3-28). The exception to this rule is in the inferior periphery, where the posterior hyaloid tends to remain higher reflective, similar to retina. B-scan can also be used in some instances to demonstrate the difference in reflectivity between a PVD and an RD in the periphery.

Traction Retinal Detachment

Vitreous membranes or bands that adhere to the fundus may exert traction on the retina. Traction is typically seen in diabetic retinopathy or trauma (see p 97) but can also occur in other conditions. Some of these include endophthalmitis (see p 191), uveitis, toxocariasis (see p 203), retinopathy of prematurity (see p 184), and persistent hyperplastic primary vitreous (see p 185).

Diabetic Retinopathy

Echography effectively demonstrates the nature and extent of abnormalities in patients with diabetic vitreous hemor-

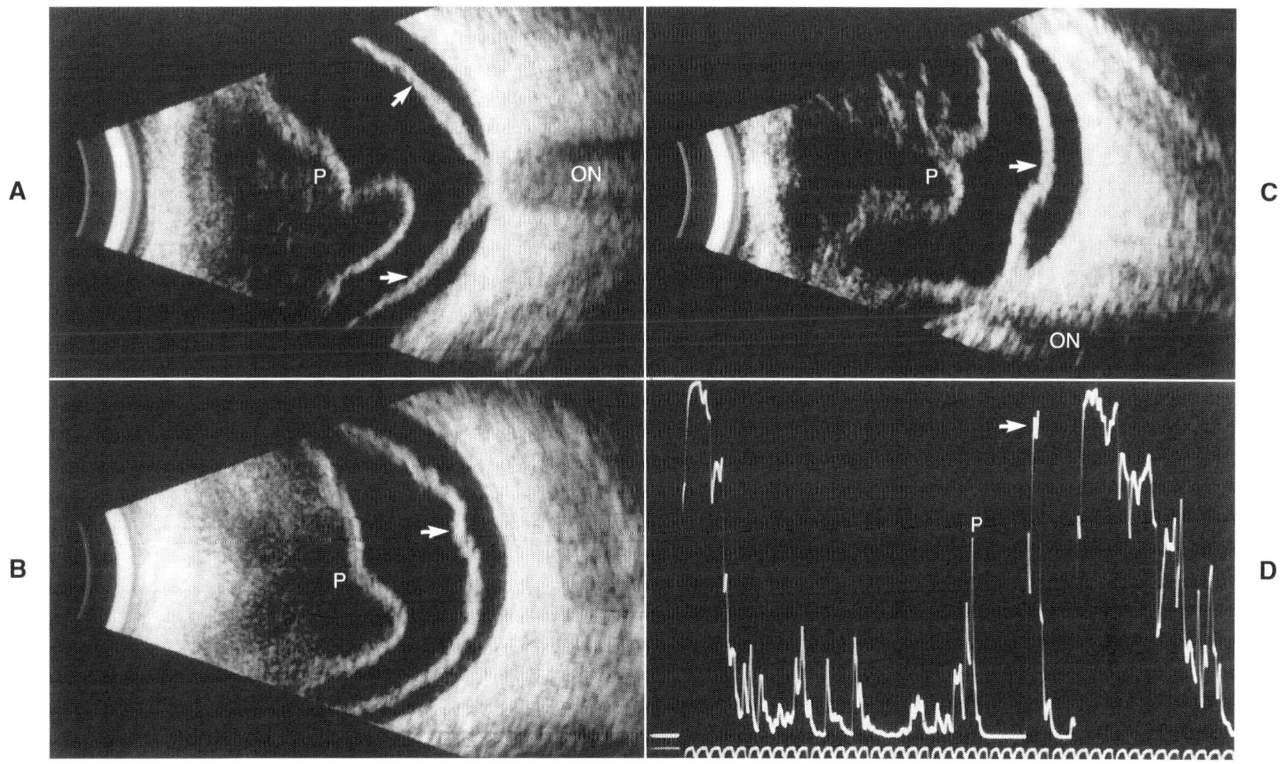

Figure 3-26 PVD and RD. It can sometimes be helpful to confirm that a membrane represents detached retina by identifying another membrane to be a PVD. A dense PVD *(P)* and RD *(arrows)* are shown in axial **(A)**, transverse **(B)**, and longitudinal **(C)** B-scan echograms. Note insertion of RD into optic nerve *(ON)* in **A** and **C. D,** A-scan shows medium reflective PVD and highly reflective RD.

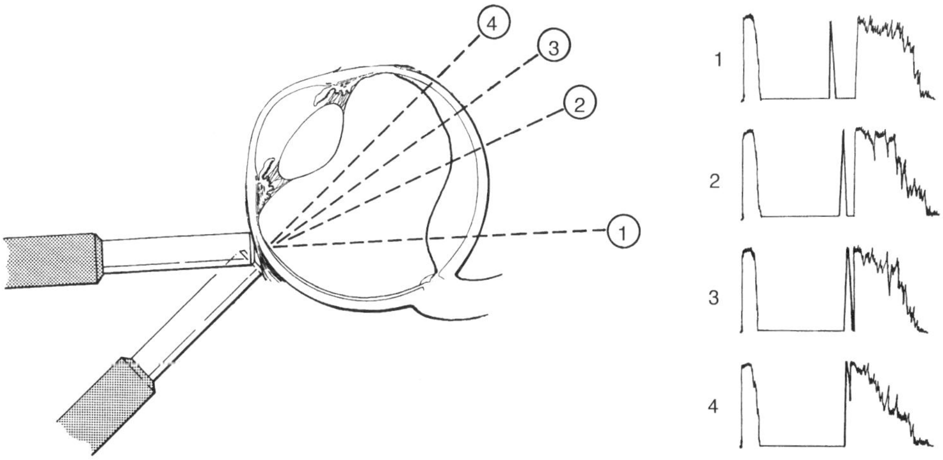

Figure 3-27 A-scan technique for differentiating dense PVD from RD in the superior portion of the globe. A 100% high spike is first displayed from the membrane posteriorly *(1)*. The probe is then shifted so as to trace the membrane to its insertion in the periphery (*2*, *3*, and *4*). Typically, a PVD becomes low reflective in the periphery, whereas retina remains highly reflective, as in this example. (From Green RL, Byrne SF: Diagnostic ophthalmic ultrasound, in Ryan SJ [ed]: Retina. ed 3, St Louis, Mosby, 2001, p 251.)

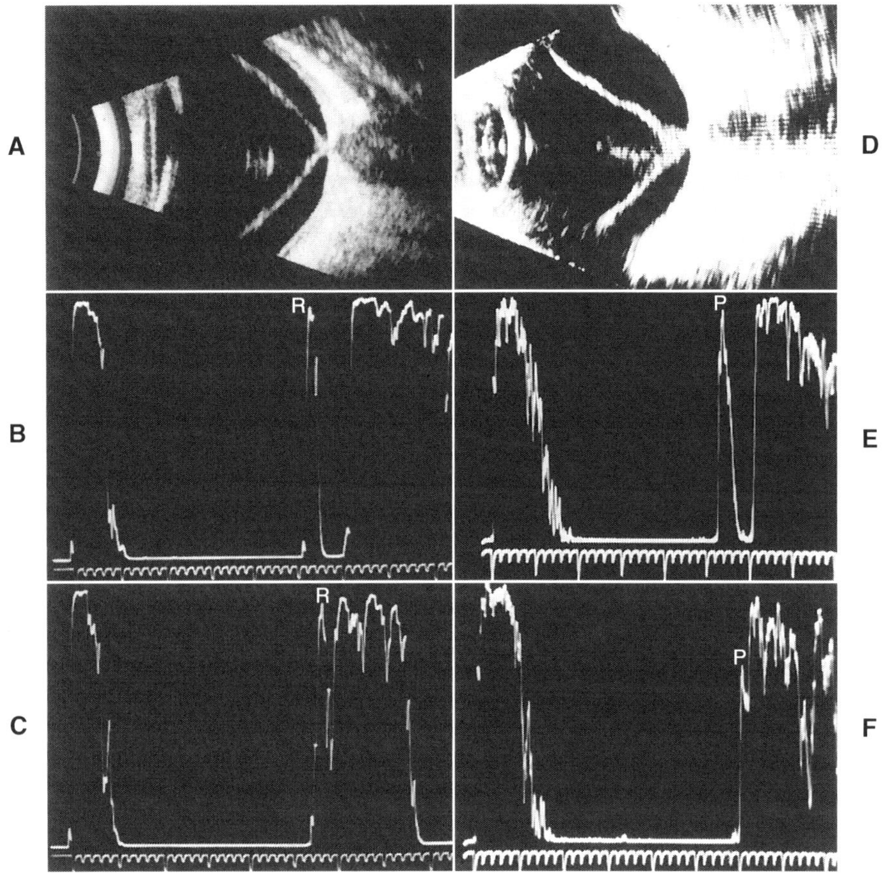

Figure 3-28 Funnel-shaped RD (**A** to **C**) and dense PVD (**D** to **F**). This example shows that evaluating the reflectivity of a membrane in the periphery can be helpful in differentiating retina from vitreous. Note the similar appearance of the RD *(R)* and PVD *(P)* on B-scan (**A** and **D**). Also, both membranes are highly reflective posteriorly (**B** and **E**). In the periphery, however, the retina **(C)** remains highly reflective, whereas the PVD **(F)** decreases in reflectivity.

rhage.[41] It is also used to monitor the progression of the disease. In previtrectomy evaluations, echography helps determine the timing of surgery and the optimal placement of instruments, as well as the visual prognosis.

Vitreous hemorrhage commonly occurs secondary to diabetic retinopathy. In these eyes, the blood may be located within the vitreous gel and/or the subvitreal space. Posterior hyphemas, which typically occur in the subvitreal space, can simulate RD (see Figure 3-12).

In the early stages of diabetic retinopathy, PVDs are typically shallow. They often begin in the temporal periphery and then extend posteriorly; the nasal posterior hyaloid tends to detach as the disease progresses. Vitreoretinal adhesions often occur in areas of proliferative preretinal membranes and stalks, which are usually located in the region of the optic nerve (Figure 3-29) or along the vascular arcades. Mild retinal elevation (i.e., very shallow, focal traction RD) or frank traction RD may be observed at the sites of adherence (Figure 3-30).

Splitting of the posterior cortical vitreous (posterior vitreoschisis)[9,50,51] may be present in eyes with proliferative diabetic retinopathy and vitreous hemorrhage. Such splitting produces schisis cavities that often contain fluid blood. The inner wall of the schisis cavity may be echographically confused with a PVD if the posterior hyaloid remains attached to the retinal surface (Figure 3-31). Serial examinations may clarify the situation, however, by showing detachment of the true posterior hyaloid. It is of interest that posterior vitreoschisis can also be seen in other conditions such as trauma and posterior uveitis (see Figure 6-5).

Using the B-scan examination techniques described in Chapter 2, the location of the PVD and retinal traction can be mapped out. Moreover, detachment or thickening of the macula (macular edema, see p 68) can usually be detected.

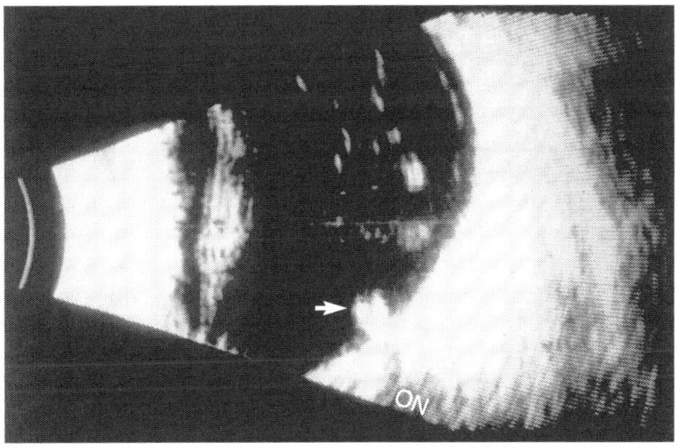

Figure 3-29 Proliferative, stalklike membrane in diabetic retinopathy. Longitudinal B-scan shows short, echo-dense membrane extending from optic disc. *ON*, Optic nerve. (Courtesy Dr. Barbara Blodi, Madison, Wisconsin, and Kathleen Meyer, RDMS, ROUB, Ann Arbor, Michigan.)

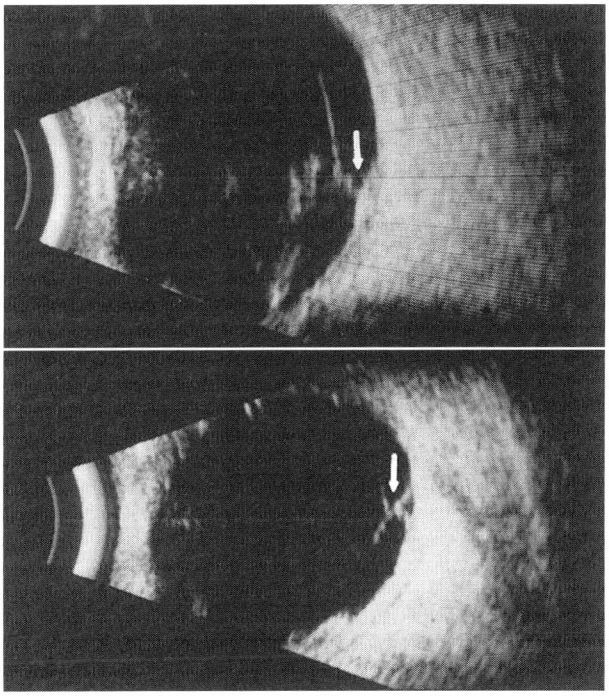

Figure 3-30 Diabetic retinal traction in the eyes of two different patients. **A,** Transverse B-scan echogram shows extensive PVD with vitreoretinal adherence producing slight elevation of retina *(arrow)*. **B,** Longitudinal B-scan shows PVD producing a frank, focal RD *(arrow)*. (From Green RL, Byrne SF: Diagnostic ophthalmic ultrasound, in Ryan SJ [ed]: *Retina.* ed 3, St Louis, Mosby, 2001, p 253.)

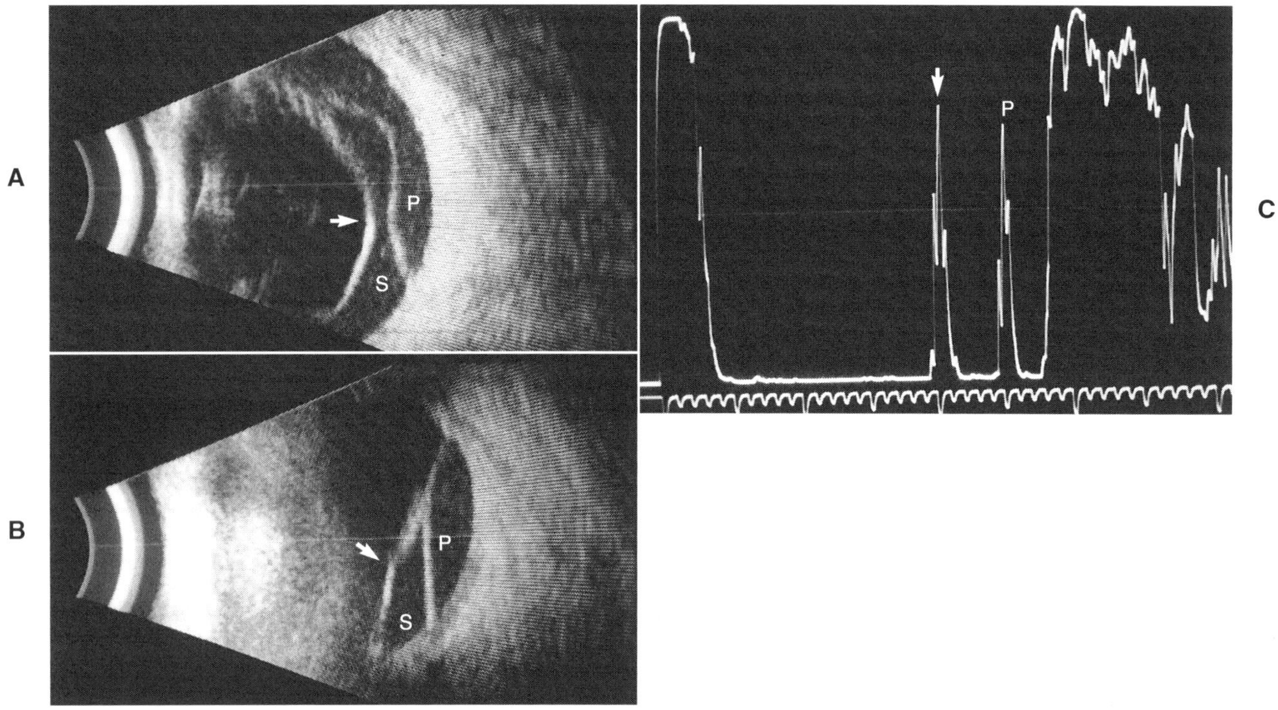

Figure 3-31 Posterior vitreoschisis in diabetic retinopathy. Transverse **(A)** and longitudinal **(B)** B-scans show splitting of posterior cortical vitreous that has produced schisis cavities *(S)*. The inner wall of the cavity *(arrows)* has a similar appearance to the detached posterior hyaloid *(P)* and may actually simulate a PVD in eyes in which the posterior hyaloid remains attached. Note hemorrhage present both in schisis cavity and subhyaloid space. **C,** A-scan displays spikes of medium reflectivity corresponding to the inner wall of the schisis cavity *(arrow)* and the posterior hyaloid *(P)*. (From Chu TG, Lopez PF, Cano MR, et al: Posterior vitreoschisis—An echographic finding in proliferative diabetic retinopathy. *Ophthalmology* 1996;103:317-318.)

In diabetic retinopathy, traction RDs are found most commonly in the peripapillary region and along the vascular arcades. Traction may present as mild elevation of the retina, a shallow or highly elevated detachment, or in extreme cases, an extensive or complete funnel-shaped detachment. These detachments must be examined using different probe positions to accurately delineate their appearance and extent.

The most common configurations of traction detachments are tentlike and tabletop (i.e., plateau). A tentlike detachment is produced by a pointlike vitreoretinal adherence, whereas a table-top detachment is the result of a broader vitreoretinal adherence, thus the table-top detachment is usually more extensive (Figure 3-32). In some cases, although a traction detachment may appear to be tentlike from one sound beam direction, it may actually be table-top. This can be determined by examining the lesion with a combination of transverse and longitudinal approaches (see Chapter 2).

A third type of traction RD that may occur in diabetic retinopathy is peripheral traction secondary to anterior hyaloidal fibrovascular proliferation. These peripheral detachments typically occur following vitrectomy in phakic eyes and are characterized by a ringlike or annular configuration[28] (Figures 3-33 and 3-34).

In some cases the posterior hyaloid may form a bridge between closely spaced, tentlike traction detachments (i.e., hammock appearance). This bridging membrane can be confused with a table-top traction RD. When occurring over the macula, this hammock-shaped membrane may be confused with a macular RD. A bridging membrane should be suspected when a vertical scan through the macula (see p 28) demonstrates a smooth membrane extending between the temporal arcades (Figure 3-35). It should be stressed, however, that whenever examining the macular region, a combination of transverse, longitudinal, and axial scans should be used (see Chapter 2).

The peripapillary region is a common location for diabetic traction RDs (Figure 3-36). Particular attention should always be given to the peripapillary region when examining patients with diabetic retinopathy.

Complex patterns of traction RD, secondary to posterior vitreoschisis (see p 60), can be caused by traction exerted by the inner wall of the schisis cavity and the posterior hyaloid (see Figure 3-37).

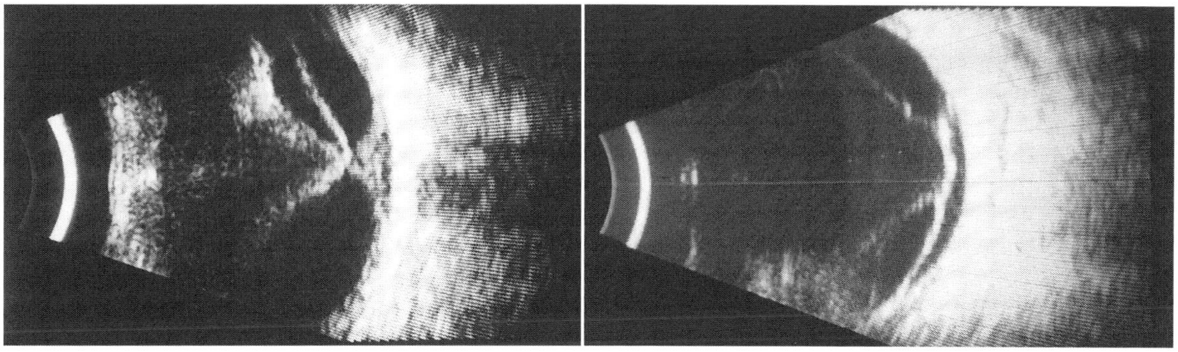

Figure 3-32 Diabetic traction RD. **A,** Small area of vitreoretinal adherence produces tentlike detachment. **B,** Broad area of vitreoretinal adherence in another patient produces tabletop detachment. (**A** from Green RL, Byrne SF: Diagnostic ophthalmic ultrasound, in Ryan SJ [ed]: *Retina*. ed 3, St Louis, Mosby, 2001, p 254.)

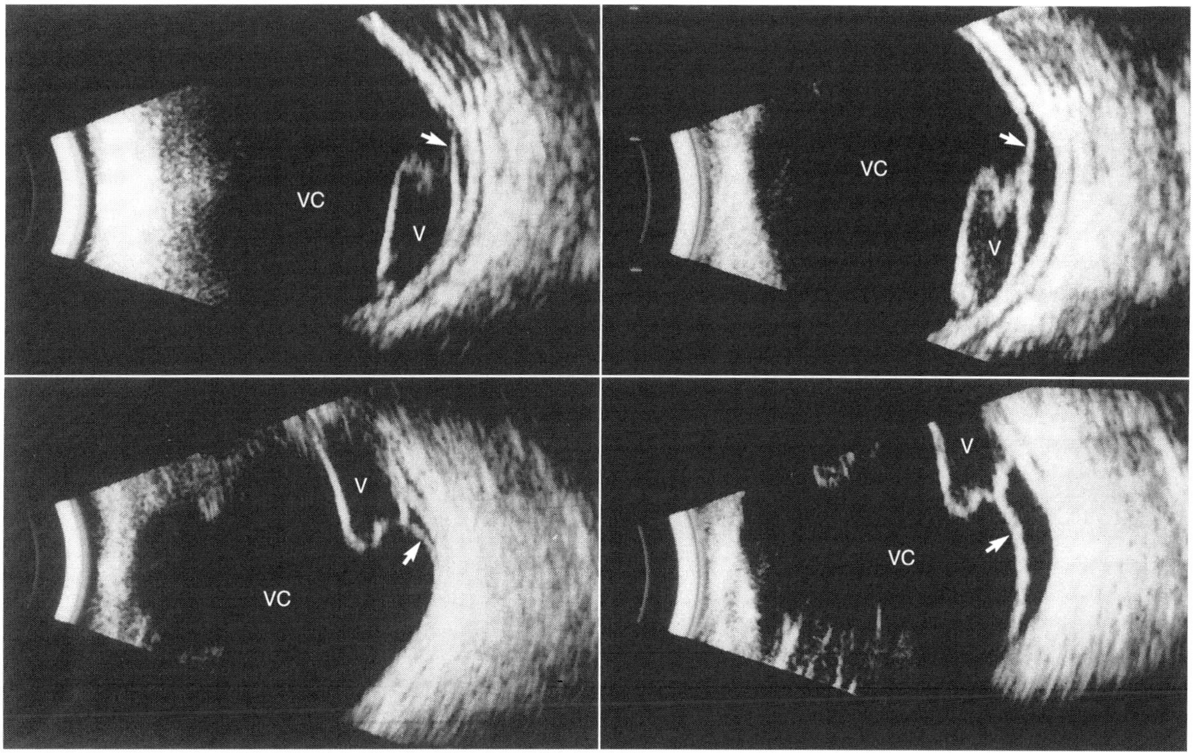

Figure 3-33 B-scans showing peripheral traction RD. Initial examination (**A,** transverse; **B,** longitudinal) shows shallow, peripheral traction RD *(arrows)*. *V,* Residual peripheral vitreous skirt; *VC,* vitreous cavity. Follow-up examination with corresponding transverse **(C)** and longitudinal **(D)** views shows increasing elevation and extent of traction RD.

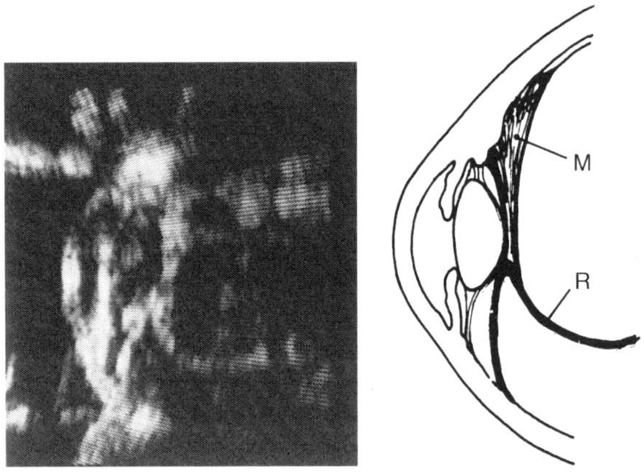

Figure 3-34 Retrolenticular traction in diabetic patient following vitrectomy (immersion technique). *M*, Retrolenticular membrane; *R*, retina. (From Green RL, Byrne SF: Diagnostic ophthalmic ultrasound, in Ryan SJ [ed]: *Retina.* ed 3, St Louis, Mosby, 2001, p 254.)

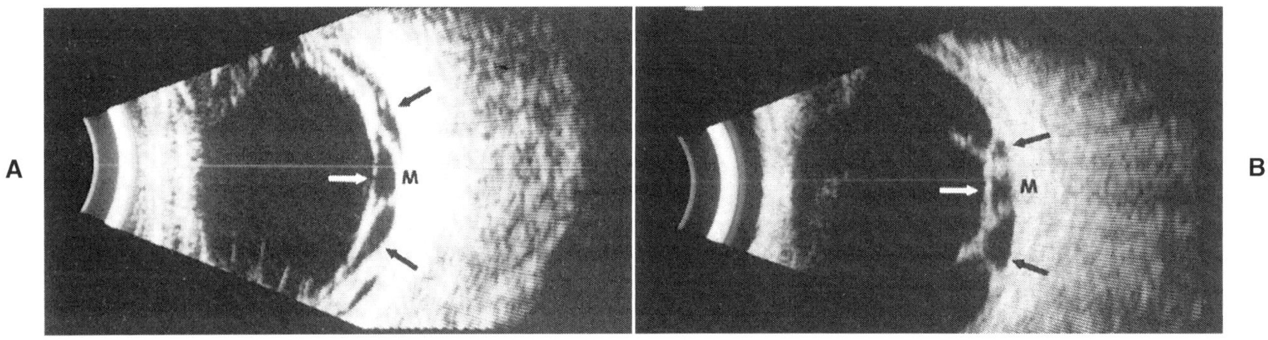

Figure 3-35 Traction RDs with bridging membrane in diabetic patients. Vertical transverse sections through macula show bridging membrane *(white arrows)* overlying the macula *(M)*. This bridging membrane is posterior hyaloid, which extends from one traction detachment to another. In these two cases, detachments are located at the superior and inferior temporal vascular arcades *(black arrows)*. The hammock-shaped appearance of these bridging membranes may be confused with a simple tabletop traction RD. (From Green RL, Byrne SF: Diagnostic ophthalmic ultrasound, in Ryan SJ [ed]: *Retina.* ed 3, St Louis, Mosby, 2001, p 254.)

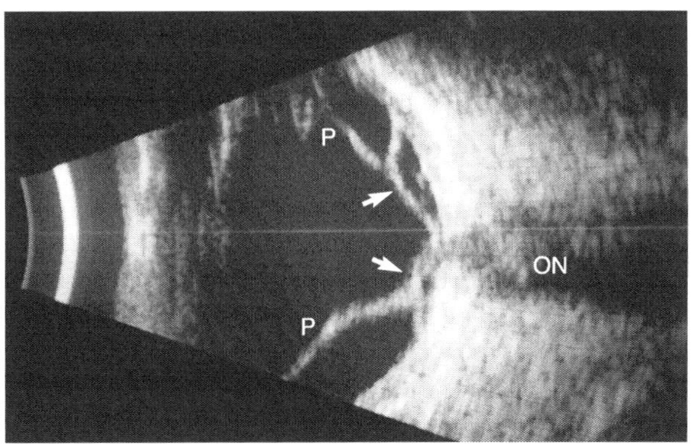

Figure 3-36 Peripapillary traction RD in a patient with diabetic retinopathy. Para-axial B-scan view demonstrates traction RDs *(arrows)* on either side of optic nerve *(ON)*. Note that vitreous is detached in the periphery but remains attached to the retina in the peripapillary region. *P*, Posterior hyaloid.

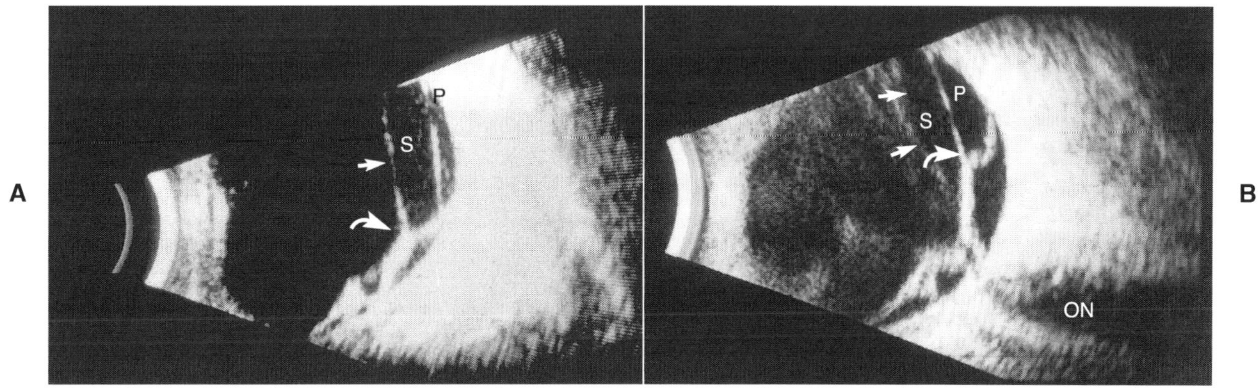

Figure 3-37 Complex traction RDs secondary to posterior vitreoschisis. Longitudinal B-scan echograms from two different patients with diabetic retinopathy show traction detachment produced by inner wall of schisis cavity **(A)** and posterior hyaloid **(B)**. *P,* Detached posterior hyaloid; *S,* schisis cavity; *straight arrows,* inner wall of schisis cavity; *curved arrows,* membranous attachment producing traction; *ON,* optic nerve.

BOX 3-1

Pitfalls in Diagnosing Retinal Detachment

Lesions Simulating Retinal Detachment

PVD with attachment to optic nerve (see p 49)
Vitreous hemorrhage with layered blood inferiorly (see p 45)
Posterior hyphema (see p 50)
Bridging vitreous membrane (e.g., diabetic retinopathy) (see p 62)
Vitreoschisis (see p 60)
Premacular hemorrhage (e.g., Terson's syndrome) (see p 73)
Peripheral vitreous skirt following vitrectomy (see p 109)
Vitreous track from penetrating injury (see p 95)
Vitreous incarceration secondary to penetrating injury (see p 90)
Blood in Cloquet's canal (see Figure 3-11)
Persistent hyaloid vessels in PHPV (see p 185)
360 degree peripheral choroidal detachments (see p 75 and 216)
Resolving choroidal detachments (see p 75)
Kissing choroidal detachments (see p 74)
Solid choroidal mass with subretinal hemorrhage (see p 118)
Retinoschisis (see p 66)
Scleral buckle with silicone band (see Figure 4-44)
Detachment of retinal pigment epithelium (see p 70)

Retinal Detachment Simulating Other Lesions

Atrophic RD (see p 54)
T-shaped RD in phakic or pseudophakic eyes (see p 56)
Tightly closed funnel-shaped RD with dense subretinal opacities (see Figures 3-21 and 3-25, *A* and *B*)
Peripheral annular RD after vitrectomy and panretinal photocoagulation (see p 54)
Giant retinal tear (see p 52)
Avulsion of retina from optic nerve (see p 54)

A thorough echographic examination should be carried out just prior to vitrectomy surgery.* Echography may often demonstrate the best area to insert the vitrectomy instruments and the safest regions to break through the posterior hyaloid. The findings also allow the surgeon to anticipate areas of vitreoretinal adherence and traction. Finally, a thorough examination may provide a reasonable assessment of the expected visual prognosis.

After vitrectomy, the examiner needs to be aware of the echographic appearance of residual vitreous gel and the characteristics of hemorrhage in the vitrectomized eye (see p 109).

Pitfalls in the Differentiation of Retinal Detachment

Although the diagnosis of an RD is generally straightforward (see p 54), a number of other lesions can simulate RD, and certain types of RDs can be quite challenging to diagnose. The examiner must be aware of both situations to avoid a misdiagnosis (Box 3-1).

*References 5, 10, 11, 44, 48, 57.

A

B

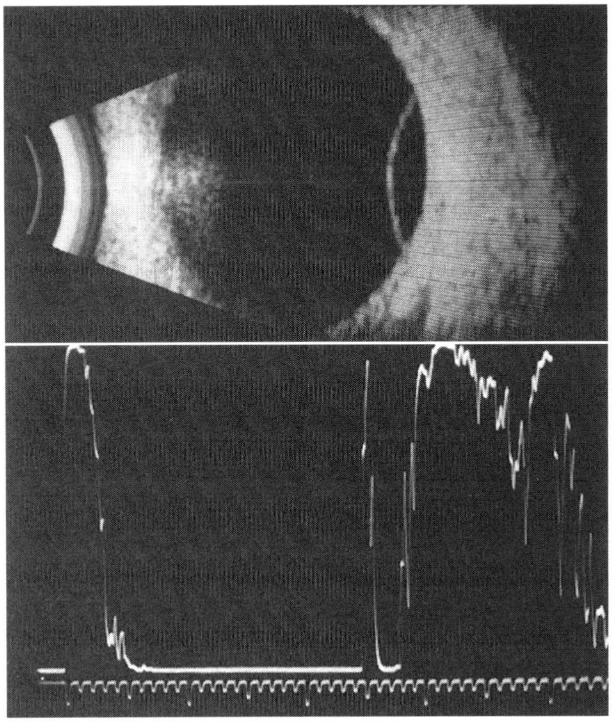

Figure 3-38 Retinoschisis. **A,** Transverse B-scan echogram shows moderately elevated, thin, smooth, dome-shaped membrane located in the inferotemporal periphery. **B,** Very thin 100% high spike is shown on A-scan. (From Green RL, Byrne SF: Diagnostic ophthalmic ultrasound, in Ryan SJ [ed]: *Retina.* ed 3, St Louis, Mosby, 2001, p 256.)

Retinoschisis

Retinoschisis, most often involving the inferotemporal peripheral fundus, is usually bilateral. On B-scan, retinoschisis appears as a smooth, thin, sharply demarcated, dome-shaped, non-mobile membrane. On A-scan, retinoschisis produces a 100% high, single-peaked spike, which may demonstrate slight vertical aftermovement (Figure 3-38).

Retinoschisis differs from RD in its more focal, smooth, and thin character and its lack of mobility. Although a choroidal detachment is also dome-shaped and is located in the periphery, it is thicker than retinoschisis and, on careful inspection, may show a double-peaked spike. Because retinoschisis is often bilateral, examination of the fellow eye may be helpful in establishing the diagnosis.

The use of scleral indentation in conjunction with B-scan[7] can differentiate retinoschisis from localized rhegmatogenous RD. After the membrane is localized with B-scan, scleral depression is simultaneously performed over the affected area. If the membrane in question represents an RD, the space between the sclera and the retina flattens as the subretinal fluid is forced through the break into the vitreous cavity (Figure 3-39). Conversely, if the membrane represents retinoschisis, the space between the sclera and the inner wall of the retinoschisis narrows but does not completely flatten (Figure 3-40).

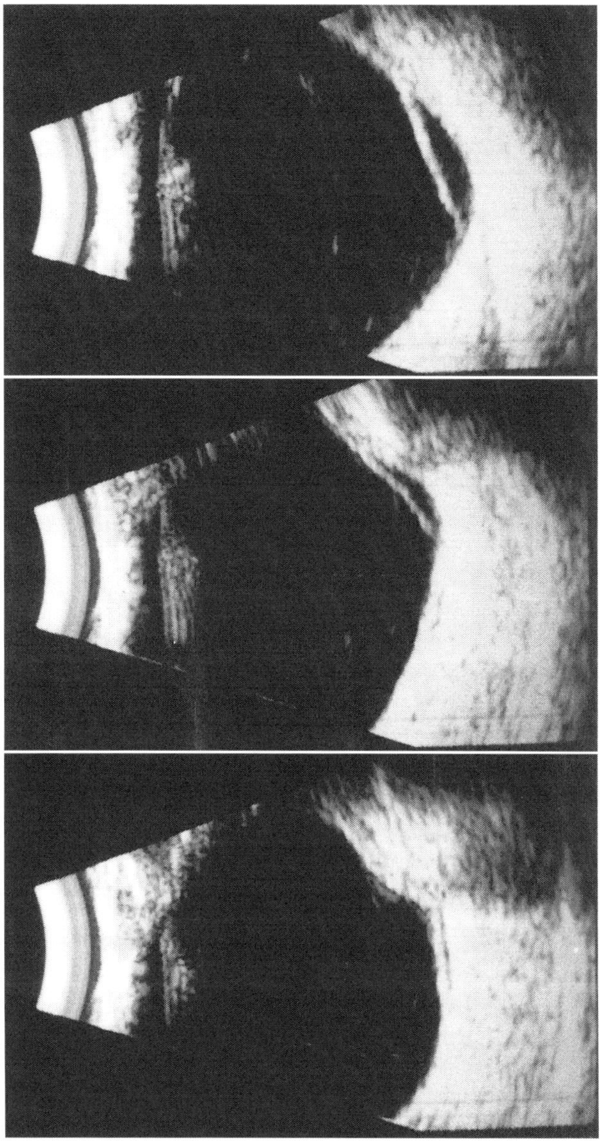

A

B

C

Figure 3-39 Scleral indentation for differentiating retinoschisis from peripheral RD. Example of peripheral RD. Longitudinal B-scan echograms show localized inferotemporal RD prior to depression **(A),** shallowing of subretinal space with slight depression **(B),** and complete flattening of subretinal space with full depression **(C).**

RETINAL PIGMENT EPITHELIUM

The retinal pigment epithelium (RPE) cannot generally be echographically differentiated from the overlying retina or underlying choroid. The inner surface of the RPE becomes exposed and echographically apparent when the overlying retina detaches. In this situation, the inner surface of the RPE appears smooth and echo-dense on B-scan and highly reflective on A-scan (see Figure 3-19).

The outer surface of the RPE and the sub-RPE space can be demonstrated echographically in the presence of an RPE detachment. These detachments are usually due to macular degeneration, most commonly AMD. RPE detachments may be focal (either serous, see p 70 and Figure

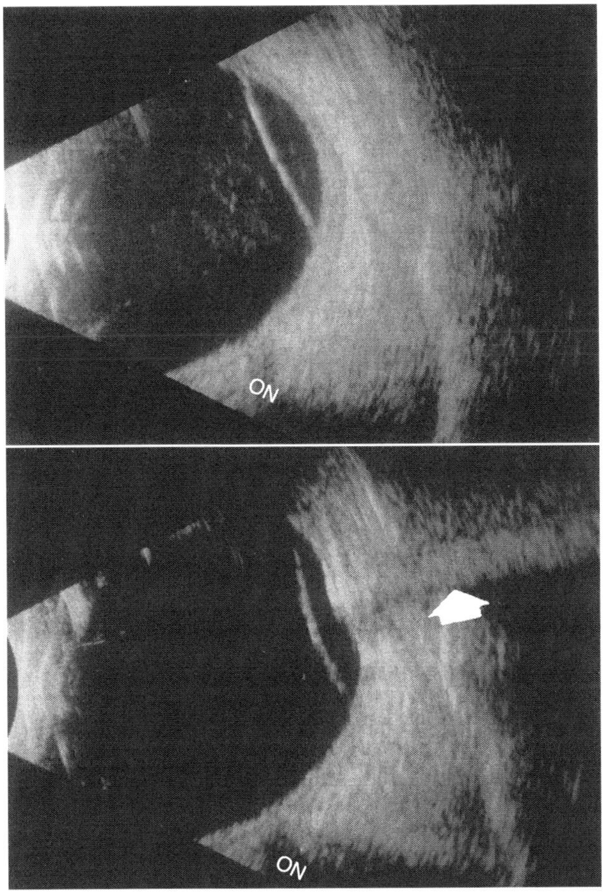

Figure 3-40 Scleral indentation for differentiating retinoschisis from peripheral RD. Longitudinal B-scan echograms show retinoschisis cavity in temporal periphery prior to depression **(A)** and with full depression **(B).** Note that schisis cavity shallows but does not collapse with full depression. *ON,* Optic nerve; *arrow,* chain of multiple signals produced by depressor tip. (From Boldt HC, Brown DM, McGeorge AJ: Echographic diagnosis of degenerative retinoschisis facilitated by scleral indentation [letter]. *Am J Ophthalmol* 1994;118:124.)

3-41, or hemorrhagic, see p 161) or massive, secondary to diffuse, dense sub-RPE hemorrhage (see Figure 5-65). In addition, certain intraocular tumors can occur beneath the pigment epithelium (see Figure 5-54).

MACULA

Macular edema, AMD, macular holes, and other disorders affecting the macula can be evaluated with ultrasound (Box 3-2). The macular region should always be assessed during an echographic screening examination of the eye. Techniques for examining the macular region have been described previously in Chapter 2 (see p 28).

Macular Edema

Macular edema is caused by leakage of fluid into the retina in the macular region. Causes of this disorder include apha-

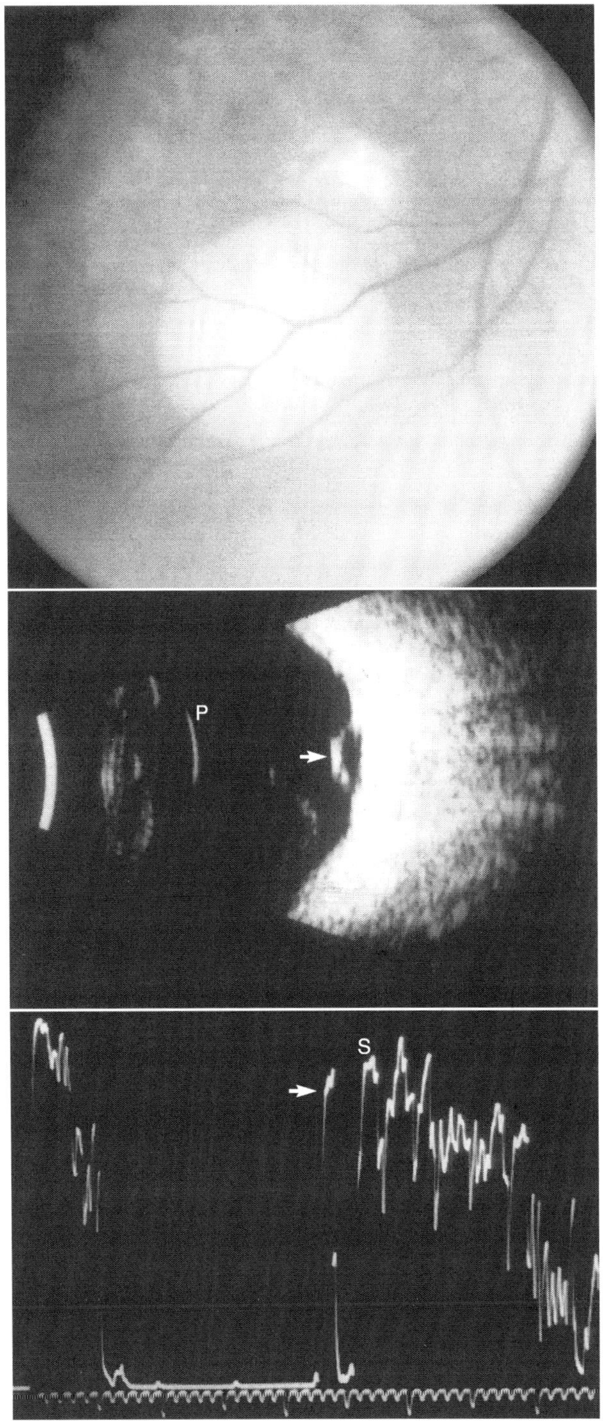

Figure 3-41 Serous detachment of the RPE in AMD. **A,** Fundus photograph demonstrates well circumscribed, nonpigmented lesion at inferior edge of macular region. **B,** Vertical macula B-scan shows smooth, dome-shaped, blisterlike, echolucent lesion *(arrow). P,* Posterior lens capsule. **C,** A-scan demonstrates very low internal reflectivity of lesion. *S,* Sclera.

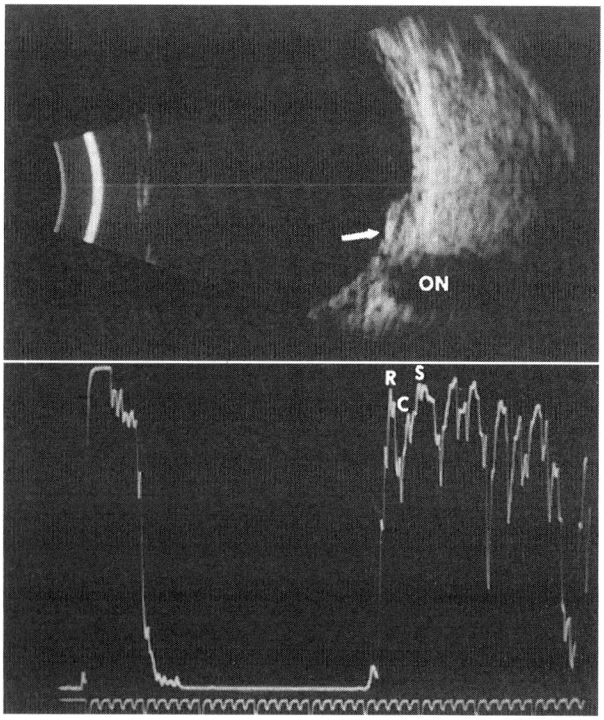

Figure 3-42 Macular edema. **A,** Longitudinal B-scan through the macula shows moderately elevated dome-shaped lesion *(arrow)* just temporal to the optic nerve *(ON)*. **B,** Lesion exhibits high internal reflectivity on A-scan. *R,* Retina; *C,* choroid; *S,* sclera. (From Green RL, Byrne SF: Diagnostic ophthalmic ultrasound, in Ryan SJ [ed]: *Retina.* ed 3, St Louis, Mosby, 2001, p 256.)

> **BOX 3-2**
> ## Macular Lesions
> Macular edema
> Age-related macular degeneration (AMD)
> RPE detachment
> Macular hole
> RD of the macula
> Hypotony maculopathy (see p 72)
> Premacular hemorrhage
> Staphyloma involving the macula

kic/pseudophakic cystoid macular edema (CME), diabetic retinopathy, uveitis, and retinal vein occlusions.

Macular edema is characterized echographically by an elevated, usually dome-shaped, lesion just temporal to the optic nerve. In many cases, these lesions are only very mildly elevated and show a somewhat irregular surface contour. Their small size usually precludes an accurate assessment of their internal reflectivity. When moderately elevated, however, they generally exhibit medium to high internal reflectivity on A-scan (Figure 3-42) and may show small cystic spaces on B-scan (Figure 3-43).

The echographic differential diagnosis of macular edema includes AMD, epiretinal membranes, macular holes (see p 71), inflammatory lesions of the retina (e.g., tuberculous granuloma [see p 205] and toxoplasmosis [see p 205]), as well as small tumors involving the macular region. These tumors include choroidal hemangioma (see p 147), metastatic carcinoma (see p 143), choroidal nevus (see p 151), and choroidal melanoma (see p 115).

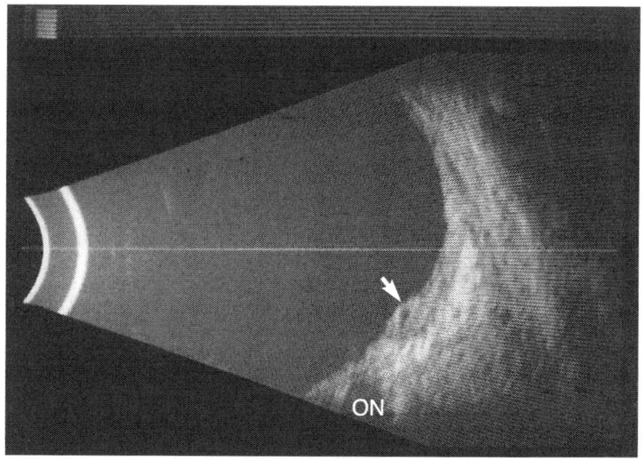

Figure 3-43 Cystoid macular edema. Longitudinal B-scan echogram demonstrates mildly elevated dome-shaped lesion *(arrow)* temporal to optic nerve *(ON)*. Note small cystic space within lesion.

Age-Related Macular Degeneration (AMD)

AMD is a chronic, degenerative disease, primarily involving the choriocapillaris, Bruch's membrane, and RPE in the macular region. Occasionally, however, this lesion can occur in an eccentric location. Other causes of macular degeneration that can simulate AMD, both clinically and echographically, include presumed ocular histoplasmosis (POH) and myopic degeneration.

There are two primary forms of AMD: wet and dry. The dry form produces degeneration and atrophy of the RPE and overlying retina. Although this disorder may be associated with slight thickening of the tissues in the macular region, ultrasound generally provides little assistance in its detection and evaluation. In longstanding cases, however, ultrasound can frequently detect small foci of calcification underlying the flat or minimally elevated retina (probably at the level of Bruch's membrane) (Figure 3-44).

In the wet form of AMD, choroidal neovascularization produces sub-RPE and subretinal exudate and/or hemorrhage. In the more chronic stages of this form of the disease, fibrosis, scarring, and calcification can occur. Clinically, the wet form of AMD is referred to as *senile disciform macular degeneration.* The ultrasound features of senile disciform macular degeneration vary according to the stage of the disease and the extent of exudate and/or hemorrhage present.

A disciform lesion generally appears as a mildly to moderately elevated, dome-shaped, heterogeneous lesion on B-scan and as two or three highly reflective spikes on A-scan[8] (Figure 3-45). The internal structure of these le-

A 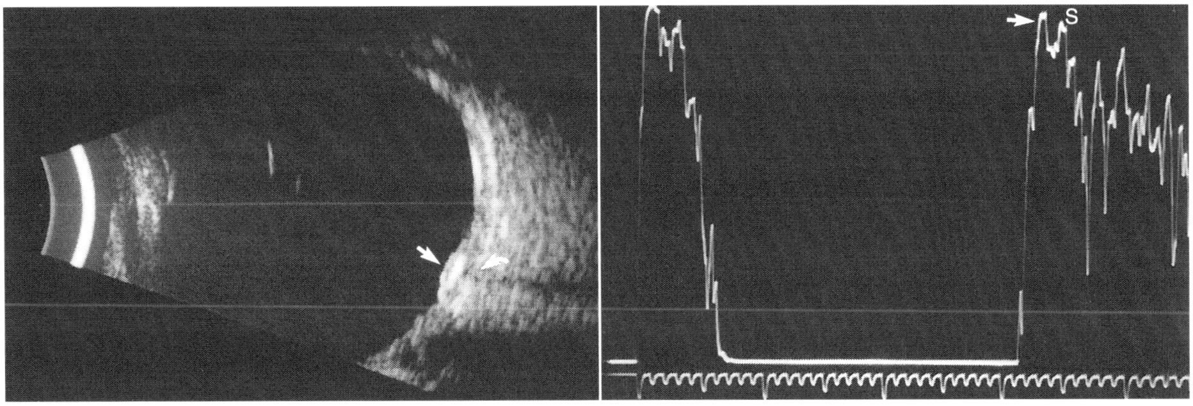 B

Figure 3-44 Dry form of AMD with calcification. **A,** Longitudinal B-scan through the macula shows a mildly elevated lesion containing echo-dense signal corresponding to calcific degeneration *(straight arrow)*. Note shadowing produced by the calcium *(curved arrow)*. **B,** A-scan demonstrates very high reflectivity of calcified lesion *(arrow)*. *S,* Sclera.

A 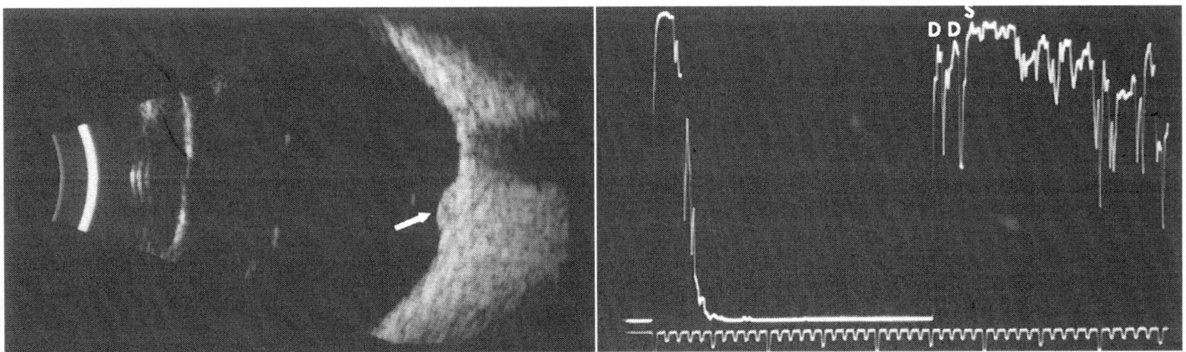 C

B 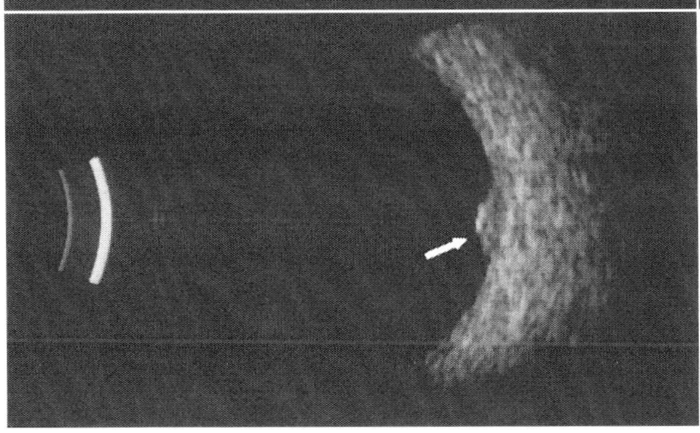

Figure 3-45 Disciform macular lesion. Horizontal axial **(A)** and vertical transverse **(B)** B-scan echograms show mildly elevated lesion in the macular region *(arrows)*. **C,** A-scan displays the two highly reflective spikes *(D)* that are suggestive of a disciform lesion. *S,* Sclera. (From Green RL, Byrne SF: Diagnostic ophthalmic ultrasound, in Ryan SJ [ed]: *Retina.* ed 3, St. Louis, Mosby, 2001, p 282.)

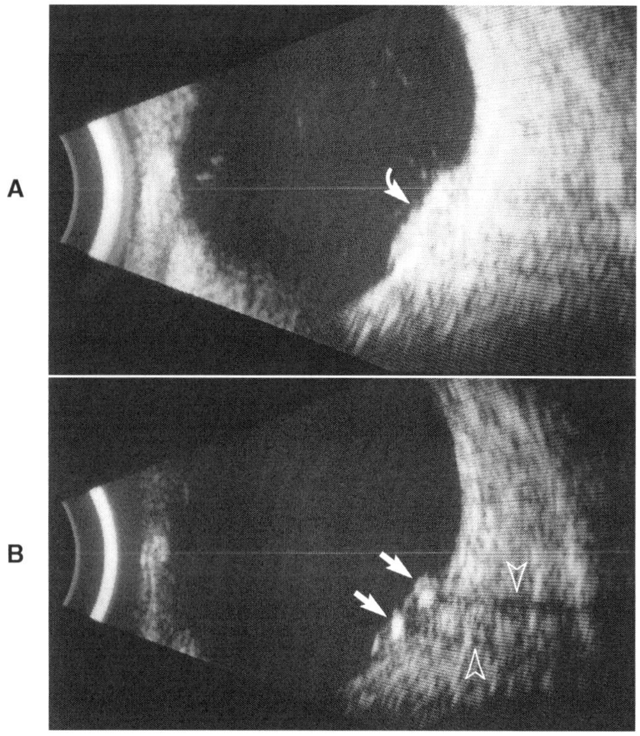

Figure 3-46 Longstanding disciform lesion with calcification. **A,** Longitudinal B-scan through macula at high gain shows moderately elevated lesion *(curved arrow)*. **B,** Same longitudinal B-scan view as in **A** at reduced gain shows two echo-dense nodules *(closed arrows)* representing foci of calcification within lesion. *Open arrows* indicate thin lines of shadowing produced by calcium.

sions can vary, depending on the degree and the extent of exudate and hemorrhage in the sub-RPE and/or subretinal spaces. Lesions that are only mildly elevated may demonstrate somewhat irregular surface contour. Because these findings are only suggestive of, rather than specific for, a disciform lesion, the diagnosis can be substantiated echographically only by observing a decrease in elevation with serial examinations. Another helpful sign is the presence of calcification that can occur in longstanding cases (Figure 3-46).

The echographic differential diagnosis of a disciform lesion includes metastatic carcinoma to the choroid, choroidal hemangioma, choroidal nevus, and macular edema. These lesions may all be highly reflective and, therefore, can be difficult to differentiate from disciform lesions. As previously mentioned, demonstrating a regression in size over time may be the only way to establish the diagnosis of a disciform lesion with echography. Furthermore, it should be noted that a mildly elevated disciform lesion can be difficult to differentiate from a small choroidal melanoma. Serial examinations may be helpful because choroidal melanomas typically show growth, whereas disciform lesions usually regress.

As previously mentioned, disciform lesions can be associated with sub-RPE and subretinal hemorrhage. When the hemorrhage is substantial, the echographic features of the lesion differ significantly from those described earlier and need to be differentiated from intraocular tumors. These hemorrhagic disciform lesions and their differential diagnoses are described in Chapter 5 (see p 160).

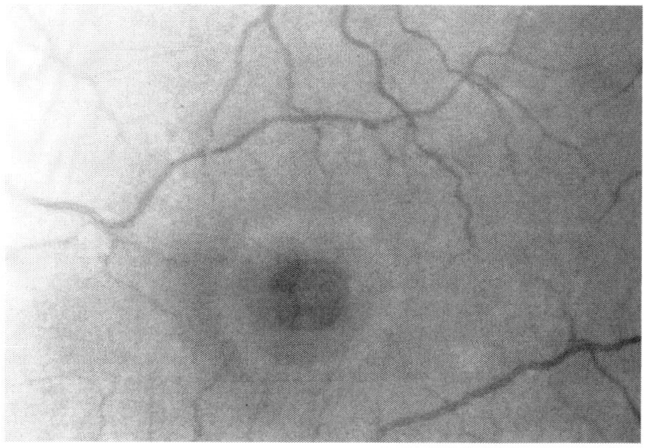

Figure 3-47 Fundus photograph showing full-thickness macular hole. (Courtesy Dr. Mark Johnson, Ann Arbor, Michigan.)

Another manifestation of AMD is the presence of serous RPE detachments. These lesions may occur in combination with, or instead of, the disciform lesion previously described. Clinically, RPE detachments appear as sharply demarcated, mildly elevated lesions, either in the macular region or in an eccentric location. These smooth, dome-shaped lesions appear blisterlike and echolucent on B-scan and very low reflective on A-scan (see Figure 3-41).

These blisterlike RPE detachments are often hemorrhagic and, as such, may masquerade as choroidal melanomas clinically. The echographic appearance of these lesions is described in Chapter 5 (see p 161 and Figure 5-68).

Macular Holes

Macular holes (Figure 3-47) can lead to significant central visual loss. The cause of macular hole formation is controversial, but the most widely accepted theory is that macular holes are a result of vitreous traction in the macular region.[21,35] Various stages of macular holes have been identified, ranging from impending holes to full-thickness holes. Until recently, there has been no effective treatment for this condition. Vitreoretinal procedures have now been developed, however, for the treatment of full-thickness macular holes.[52]

Ultrasound and ocular coherence tomography (OCT) are the two methods currently available for imaging the vitreoretinal relationship in the macular region.[29] OCT has been shown to provide high-resolution images of vitreous traction on the macula and full-thickness macular holes (Figure 3-48). The primary limitation of OCT is its inability to provide a broad perspective of the vitreous body and its relationship to the macula. Echography, on the other hand, can, in most cases, evaluate the overall status of the

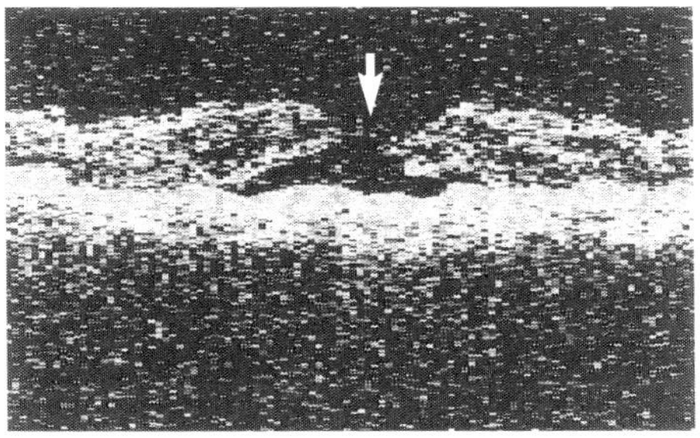

Figure 3-48 OCT showing full-thickness macular hole *(arrow)*. (Courtesy Dr. Gregg Kokame, Honolulu, Hawaii.)

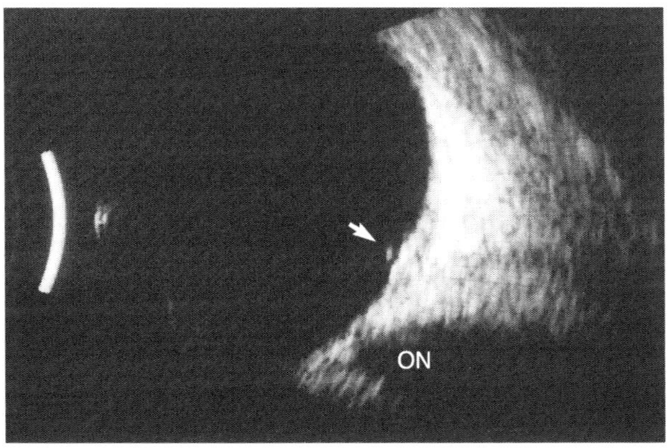

Figure 3-49 Full-thickness macular hole. Longitudinal B-scan at reduced gain demonstrates mild elevation in macular region with slight central depression corresponding to macular hole. Small opacity directly over depression *(arrow)* represents retinal operculum. *ON*, Optic nerve.

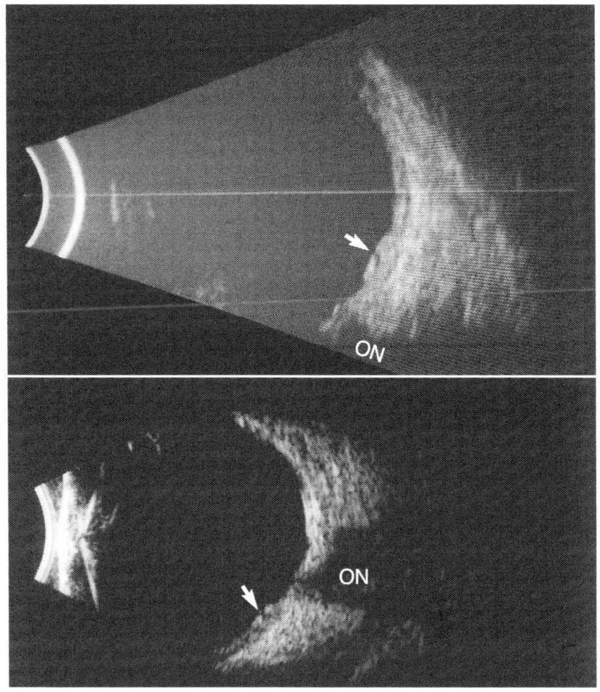

A

B

Figure 3-50 Two cases of full thickness macular holes resolved with B-scan. **A,** Longitudinal B-scan at reduced gain demonstrates elevated lesion in macular region with imaging of actual macular hole *(arrow)*. *ON*, Optic nerve. **B,** Reverse longitudinal B-scan of another case at reduced gain also displays macular hole *(arrow)*. (**B** courtesy Dr. Gregg Kokame, Honolulu, Hawaii.)

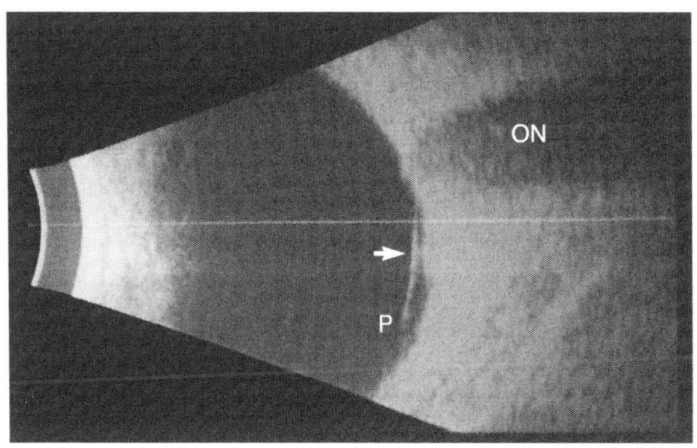

Figure 3-51 Relationship of PVD to macular hole (same case as in Figure 3-48). Para-axial B-scan at high gain displays shallow detachment of posterior hyaloid *(P)* overlying macular hole represented by mild elevation in macular region *(arrow)*. *ON*, Optic nerve. (Courtesy Dr. Gregg Kokame, Honolulu, Hawaii.)

vitreous in relation to the macula and can provide additional information to that given by OCT. Echography can also assess kinetic properties of the vitreous that can help clarify vitreoretinal attachments in the peripapillary region and macula.[13,16,17]

With macular holes, the echographic findings are very subtle. Several studies have shown, however, that these findings correlate well with the various stages of macular hole development.[13,34,58,59] Ultrasound demonstrates the relationship of the vitreous to the macula, as well as changes in the topography of the macular region.

As previously described, there are specific methods for examining the macular region (see p 28). It is suggested that the macula be examined with several different probe orientations to most accurately define the vitreomacular relationships.[34,38] A recent report emphasizes the importance of directing the sound beam perpendicular to the macular region. These investigators found that placing the probe on the cornea with the sound beam directed through the lens (horizontal axial and vertical macula scans) were the optimal probe positions for imaging the posterior hyaloid in the macula.[34]

In a fully developed macular hole, ultrasound typically shows an elevation in the macular region with a central depression corresponding to the hole (Figure 3-49). In some cases, B-scan can resolve the full thickness macular hole (Figure 3-50). A shallow PVD can often be demonstrated directly over the macular region, either still adherent to (stage 3) or completely separated from (stage 4) the optic disc (Figure 3-51).[13,59] In both instances, ultrasound often

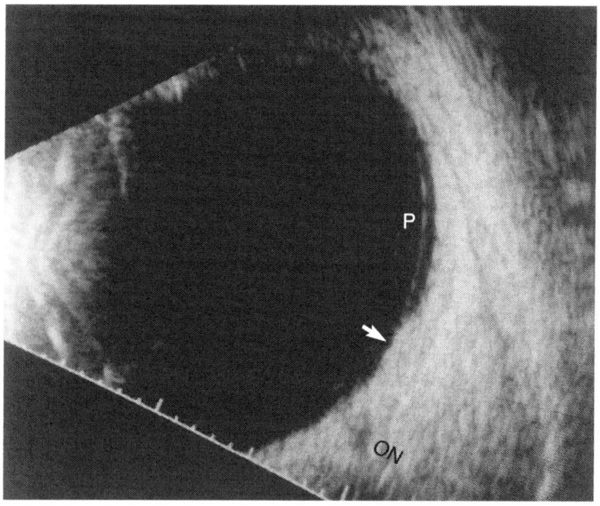

Figure 3-52 Stage 2 macular hole. Longitudinal B-scan shows shallow, partial detachment of the posterior hyaloid *(P)* adherent to surface of elevated macula *(arrow)*. *ON*, Optic nerve. (Courtesy Dr. Mark Johnson, Ann Arbor, Michigan.)

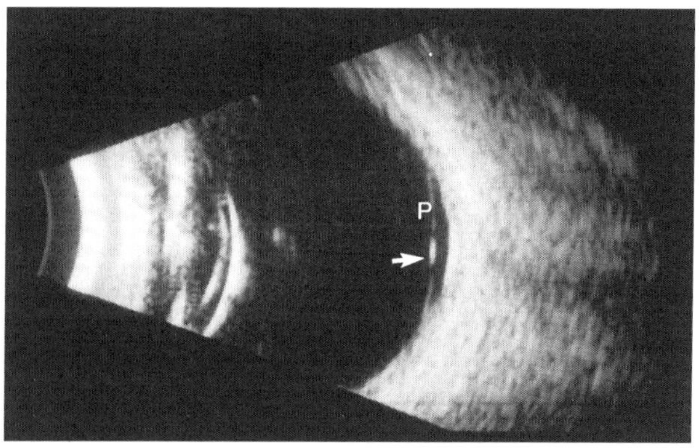

Figure 3-53 Pseudo-operculum. Vertical macula B-scan shows small echo-dense opacity *(arrow)* on surface of detached posterior hyaloid *(P)* overlying macula. Note absence of macular elevation.

identifies a small opacity on the posterior surface of the hyaloid directly over the macula. This opacity has been shown to correspond to an operculum attached to the posterior hyaloid (see Figure 3-49). In addition to the retinal operculum, ultrasound may identify opacities corresponding to the Weiss ring[26] (see Figure 3-9) when the vitreous is completely detached from the optic disc (see p 49). Rarely, the Weiss ring may be present (indicating detachment from the optic nerve) even though the vitreous is still attached in the macular region.[39,40]

In early stages of macular hole development (stages 1 and 2), ultrasound often reveals partial detachment of the posterior hyaloid, with persistent attachment to the macula. A slight elevation of the macula may be apparent, suggesting vitreous traction on the developing hole (Figure 3-52).[34]

Ultrasound may be a useful adjunct to biomicroscopy in the detection of a PVD in the fellow eyes of patients with a known macular hole. It has been shown that the presence of a PVD in the fellow eye significantly lowers the risk for hole formation. Biomicroscopy can only determine if a PVD is present when a pseudo-operculum is detected overlying the macula.[58] A pseudo-operculum is thought to represent a focal condensation of the vitreous cortex suspended on the detached hyaloid in front of the macula.[22,25] In eyes in which a pseudo-operculum cannot be seen with biomicroscopy, ultrasound may be the only means of demonstrating the presence of a shallow PVD overlying the macula (Figure 3-53).

Retinal Detachment of the Macula

Retinal detachment involving the macula can be secondary to traction (e.g., diabetic retinopathy), exudate (e.g., central serous retinopathy), hemorrhage (e.g., AMD), and tears or holes. They can also occur in association with optic pits (see Figure 16-29). The determination of whether an RD involves the macular region is essential in the management and prognosis of the disorder; therefore, precise echographic localization is essential (see p 28). When the ocular media are opaque, ultrasound can help determine the extent and cause of a macular RD. Ultrasound can even be useful in clear ocular media, especially in a large staphylomatous eye in which a shallow detachment of the macula may not be clinically apparent (see p 73).

As discussed in the section on diabetic retinopathy, bridging membranes overlying the macular region can simulate tractional detachment of the macula (see p 62). In addition, certain conditions can exhibit traction retinal folds through the macula. These include retinopathy of prematurity (see p 184) and toxocariasis (see p 203).

Hypotony Maculopathy

In chronic hypotony, diffuse thickening of the retinochoroid layer in the macular region results from thickening and shrinkage of the posterior sclera. This may lead to significant irreversible visual loss if the pressure is not restored to normal (see Figure 7-11).

The thickened retinochoroid layer and thickening of the posterior sclera can be demonstrated on B-scan examination. Focal detachment of the retina, RPE, and/or choroid at the macula can occasionally be detected (see Figure 7-10). This disorder is described in more detail in Chapter 7 on p 216.

Premacular Hemorrhage

Certain disorders produce hemorrhage in the premacular region. This premacular hemorrhage, located either in the subhyaloid space or beneath the internal limiting membrane, may be associated with a vitreous hemorrhage that precludes visualization of the posterior pole. Disorders that may cause premacular hemorrhage include Terson's syndrome,[61] hypertensive retinopathy, retinal artery micro-

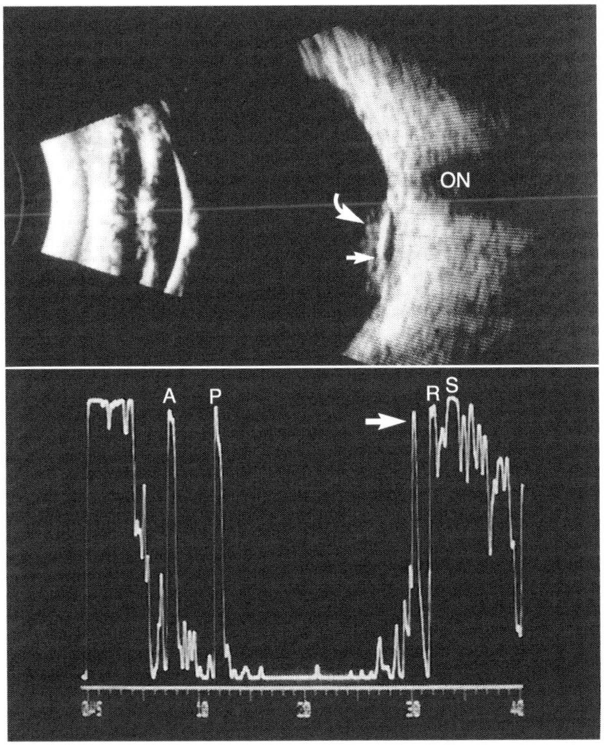

Figure 3-54 Premacular hemorrhage due to Terson's syndrome. Echograms show shallow retina-like membrane resulting from dense preretinal hemorrhage. **A,** Horizontal axial B-scan at reduced gain shows shallow, smooth, echo-dense, dome-shaped membrane *(straight arrow)* overlying macula and inserting into optic nerve *(ON)*. Note mild hemorrhage in posterior vitreous overlying membrane *(curved arrow)*. **B,** A-scan obtained with probe on cornea shows high reflectivity of membrane *(arrow)* compared to retina *(R)* and sclera *(S)*. *A,* Anterior lens capsule; *P,* posterior lens capsule. (**A** courtesy Dr. Barbara Blodi, Madison, Wisconsin, and Kathleen Meyer, RDMS, ROUB, Ann Arbor, Michigan.)

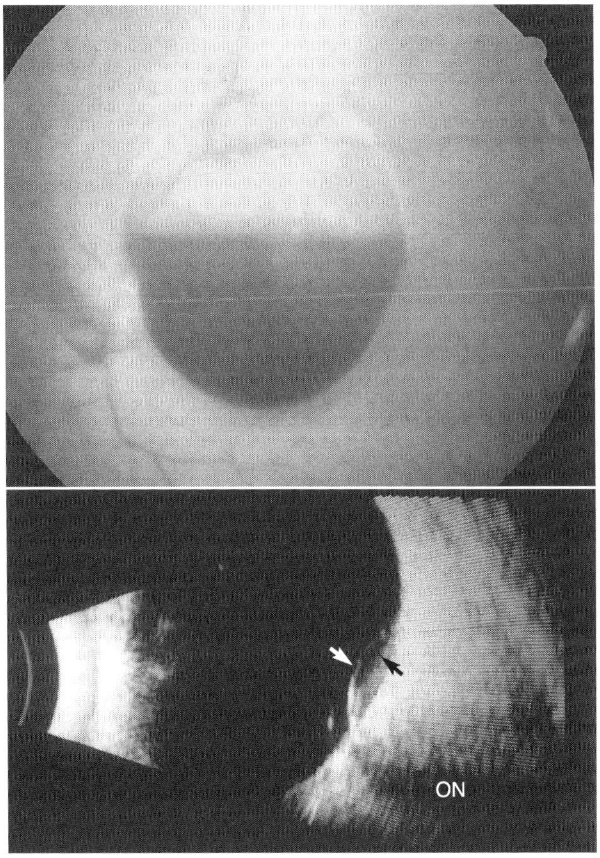

Figure 3-55 Premacular hemorrhage. **A,** Fundus photograph shows layering of premacular hemorrhage. **B,** Longitudinal B-scan through macula demonstrates smooth, dome-shaped membrane overlying macula *(white arrow)* and layering of submembranous blood *(black arrow)*. *ON,* Optic nerve. (Courtesy Dr. Barbara Blodi, Madison, Wisconsin, and Kathleen Meyer, RDMS, ROUB, Ann Arbor, Michigan.)

aneurysm, leukemia, shaken-baby syndrome, and Valsalva maculopathy.

On ultrasound, premacular hemorrhage appears as a dome-shaped, smooth, mildly elevated, nonmobile membrane overlying the macula.[46] This membrane, which represents the posterior hyaloid or internal limiting membrane, is usually highly reflective due to the submembranous blood adherent to its posterior surface (Figures 3-54 and 3-55). Consequently, it may mimic a localized detachment of the macula. Differentiation from RD can usually be made by considering the history and other clinical findings. Serial echographic examinations will also often show resolution of the hemorrhage and flattening of the overlying membrane.

Staphyloma Involving the Macula

Staphylomas involving the macular region are most commonly associated with elongated, highly myopic globes, or they may be secondary to congenital disorders and colobomas that involve the macula. Ultrasound can easily demonstrate the bowing out of the posterior scleral wall (see Figure 10-25). As previously mentioned, shallow RDs in the macular area in the presence of a posterior staphyloma can sometimes be appreciated better with ultrasound than with ophthalmoscopy (Figure 3-56).

The echographic localization of a posterior staphyloma is very important in obtaining accurate axial eye length measurements for intraocular lens calculations (see Chapter 10).

Trauma Involving the Macula

Trauma can cause several different types of macular lesions, including Berlin's edema (commotio retinae, see p 90), choroidal ruptures (see Figure 4-7), and traction detachments (see p 58), as well as intraretinal and preretinal hemorrhage (see above).

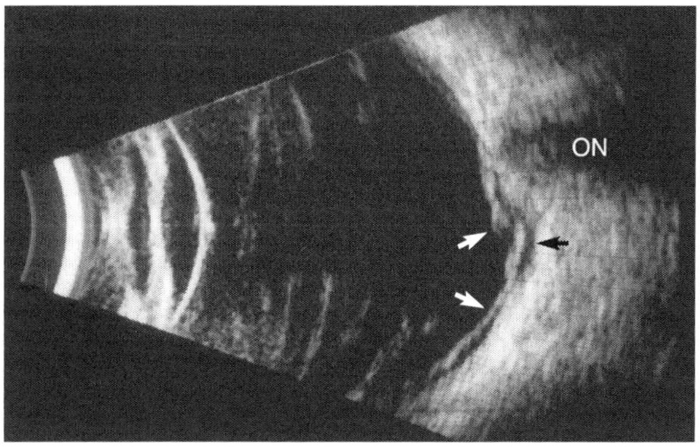

Figure 3-56 Staphyloma of macula with shallow RD. Horizontal axial B-scan shows staphyloma temporal to the optic nerve *(ON)* involving macula. *White arrows*, shallow RD involving macula; *black arrow*, macula.

CHOROID

Although the choroid and suprachoroidal space can be examined indirectly with ophthalmoscopy and fluorescein angiography, ultrasound has greatly enhanced the examination of this region of the eye. In the normal eye, ultrasound is generally unable to differentiate the thin layer of choroid from the overlying retina and underlying sclera. This complex of surfaces (i.e., posterior ocular coats) appears as an echo-dense band on B-scan and as a small group of highly reflective spikes on A-scan. However, when the choroid and/or suprachoroidal space are expanded by fluid or infiltration, ultrasound is then able to image this region to provide topographic, quantitative, and kinetic information not obtainable by other means.

Choroidal Thickening

Choroidal thickening, either focal or diffuse, may be associated with many conditions. The causes of choroidal thickening include edema, inflammatory infiltration, tumor, and idiopathic choroidal folds.

Choroidal Edema

Choroidal edema can be produced by inflammation, vascular congestion, and hypotony. In the presence of choroidal edema, the posterior ocular coats appear thicker than normal, and in some cases, the retinochoroid layer is distinguishable from the sclera. In this situation, two bands can be identified on B-scan: one representing the retinochoroid layer, the other the sclera. On A-scan, the group of highly reflective spikes representing the posterior ocular coats is thicker and the individual spikes are more distinct (see Figure 7-10). In most cases, the retina cannot be distinguished from the edematous choroid unless the retina is detached.

Choroidal Inflammation

Choroidal thickening can also be produced by diffuse inflammatory infiltration, such as Vogt-Koyanagi-Harada syndrome (see p 200), sympathetic ophthalmia (see p 201), and lymphoid hyperplasia of the uvea (see p 153). In these conditions, the homogeneous nature of the choroidal inflammatory infiltration contrasts with the highly reflective retinal and scleral borders, facilitating detection with ultrasound. On B-scan the thickened choroid appears as an echolucent band, whereas on A-scan, the infiltration exhibits low to medium internal reflectivity. The ability of ultrasound to image the choroid in these conditions has greatly enhanced their detection and diagnosis. In addition, ultrasound is often more reliable than CT scan and MRI in differentiating choroidal from scleral thickening (see Figures 5-55 and 6-8).

Choroidal Tumors

Choroidal thickening may also be caused by either primary or metastatic tumors (see Chapter 5). Mildly elevated, diffuse choroidal tumors may be difficult to differentiate echographically and, therefore, can be confused with choroidal thickening of other etiologies. These choroidal tumors include diffuse melanomas, metastatic carcinomas, lymphomas, and diffuse hemangiomas (as in Sturge-Weber syndrome) (see Figures 5-46 and 5-47).

Choroidal Folds

Choroidal folds can produce diffuse thickening of the posterior choroid. This thickening appears related to diffuse thickening of the posterior sclera; together, these produce distinct echographic findings (see p 80).

Choroidal Detachment

Choroidal detachment occurs when serous fluid, blood, or inflammatory debris accumulates in the suprachoroidal space. Choroidal detachments usually occur in peripheral aspects of the eye, but they may extend to the posterior pole. Peripheral choroidal detachments usually also involve the ciliary body (ciliochoroidal detachments). Choroidal detachments may be shallow or bullous in nature. They can be associated with a number of conditions and can develop following surgery or trauma[49] (Box 3-3).

The characteristic echographic features of choroidal detachments generally facilitate differentiation from other conditions (see Table 3-1).

A choroidal detachment typically presents as a smooth, thick, dome-shaped membrane on B-scan and as a thick, steeply rising, 100% high spike on A-scan (Figure 3-57). On careful inspection at low gain, a double-peaked spike may be observed. The kinetic evaluation typically shows little or no aftermovement with either A- or B-scan. Choroidal detachments that extend for 360 degrees produce a typical scalloped appearance when scanned with a transverse approach (Figure 3-58, *A*). Highly elevated de-

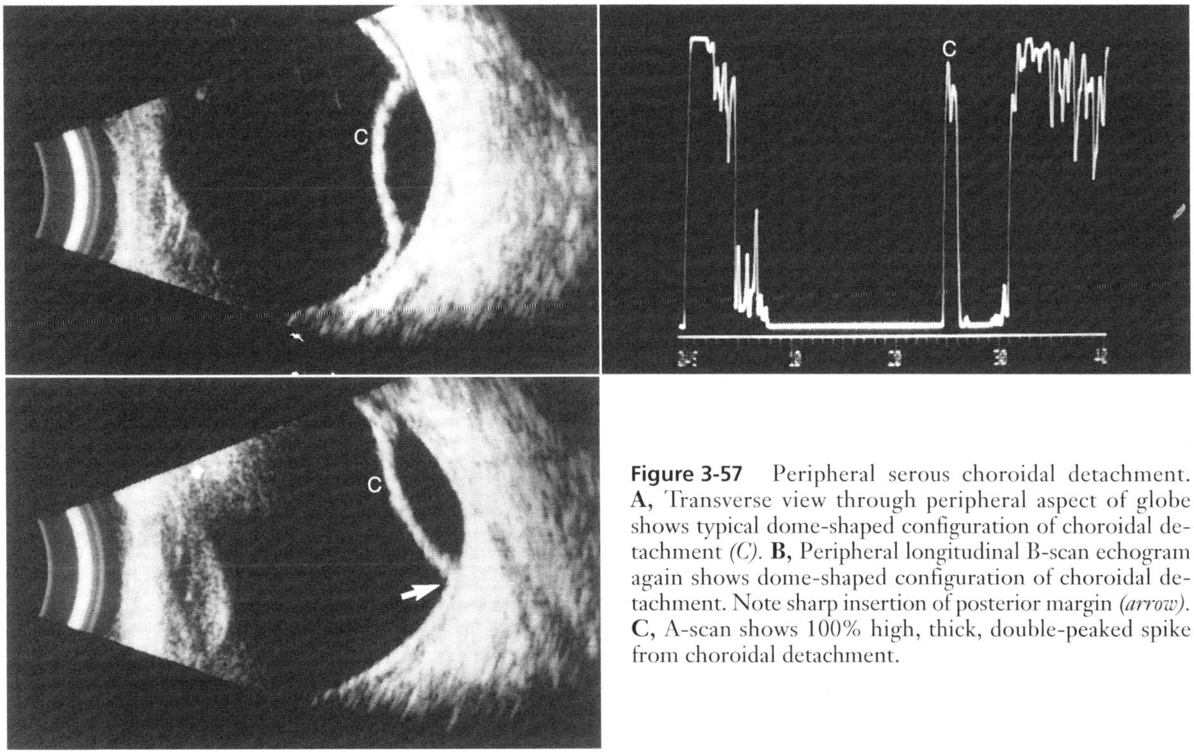

Figure 3-57 Peripheral serous choroidal detachment. **A,** Transverse view through peripheral aspect of globe shows typical dome-shaped configuration of choroidal detachment *(C)*. **B,** Peripheral longitudinal B-scan echogram again shows dome-shaped configuration of choroidal detachment. Note sharp insertion of posterior margin *(arrow)*. **C,** A-scan shows 100% high, thick, double-peaked spike from choroidal detachment.

BOX 3-3

Causes of Choroidal (Ciliochoroidal) Detachment

- Idiopathic
  - Uveal effusion syndrome (see p 82)
  - Nanophthalmos (see p 82)
- Inflammatory
  - Uveitis (infectious or noninfectious, see p 194)
  - Scleritis (see p 195)
- Hypotony (see p 214)
- Intraocular surgery (see pp 109 and 216)
- Trauma
- Intraocular tumor (see p 144)
- Arteriovenous fistula (see p 355)
- Renal disease
- Toxic reactions to systemic medications (see p 216)

tachments are more likely to extend to the posterior pole and may insert adjacent to but not directly into the optic disc (Figure 3-58, *B* and *C*).

In some cases of 360 degree, highly elevated choroidal detachments, apposition of the temporal and nasal detachments may occur in the central aspect of the vitreous cavity (kissing or appositional choroidal detachments) (Figure 3-58, *B* and *C*). When the detachment is sufficiently elevated, a thin band stretching from the inner aspect of the detached choroid to the sclera may be noted. This band is postulated to represent a vortex vein or a ciliary blood vessel and/or nerve (Figures 3-58, *C* and 3-59).

Choroidal detachments very often extend anteriorly to involve the ciliary body and, in such cases, are more appropriately referred to as ciliochoroidal detachments. Shallow peripheral choroidal detachments typically appear flat and smooth on B-scan, as opposed to the scalloped appearance described earlier. When an annular ciliochoroidal detachment extends a full 360 degrees, it can be easily confused with a shallow, peripheral RD. It should be noted, however, that it is very rare for a nontractional RD to be so extensive and yet confined only to the periphery[30] (see p 54).

The accumulation of hemorrhage and/or cellular debris in the suprachoroidal space produces echoes in this region (Figure 3-60). Dense hemorrhage may produce solid clots that can be detected and monitored with ultrasound (see p 106). A focal (especially hemorrhagic) choroidal detachment may initially simulate a melanoma, but it can usually be differentiated by noting mobility of the fluid suprachoroidal blood and/or by changes observed with follow-up examinations (see p 106 and Figure 5-71). It is also of interest that choroidal detachments can be associated with uveal tumors (see Chapter 5 and Figure 5-43), as well as venous congestion (see p 355).

Choroidal detachments can usually be differentiated from RDs. However, when choroidal detachments decrease

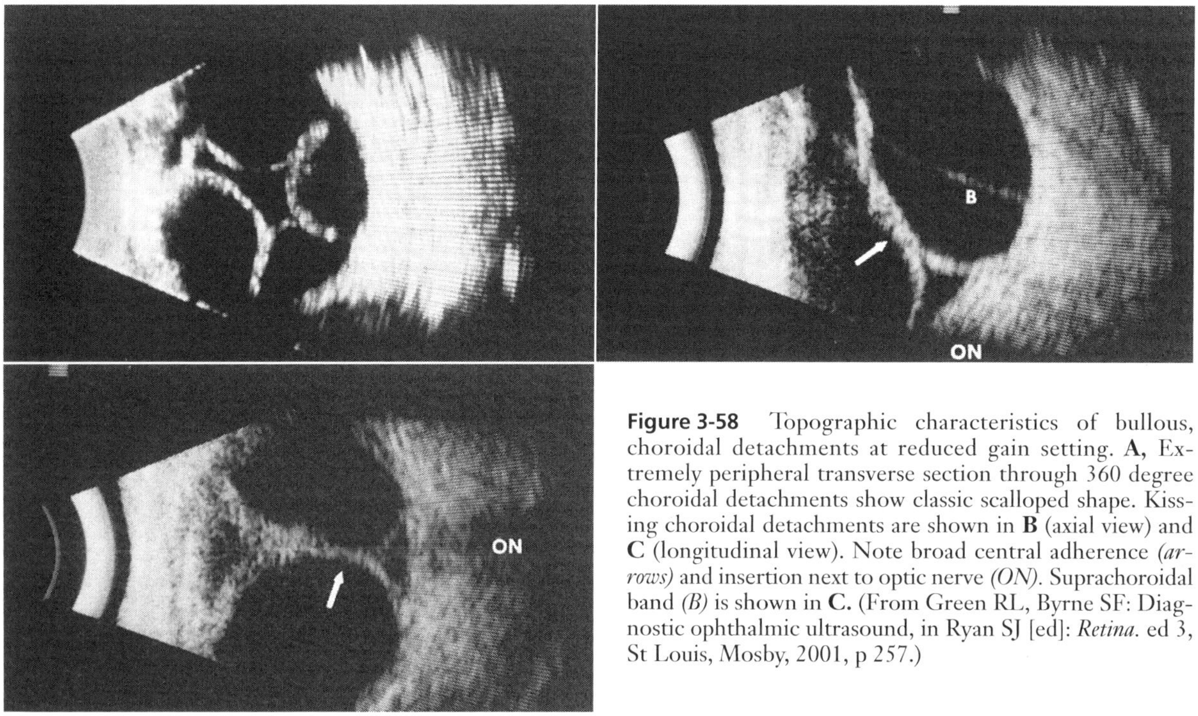

Figure 3-58 Topographic characteristics of bullous, choroidal detachments at reduced gain setting. **A,** Extremely peripheral transverse section through 360 degree choroidal detachments show classic scalloped shape. Kissing choroidal detachments are shown in **B** (axial view) and **C** (longitudinal view). Note broad central adherence *(arrows)* and insertion next to optic nerve *(ON)*. Suprachoroidal band *(B)* is shown in **C.** (From Green RL, Byrne SF: Diagnostic ophthalmic ultrasound, in Ryan SJ [ed]: *Retina.* ed 3, St Louis, Mosby, 2001, p 257.)

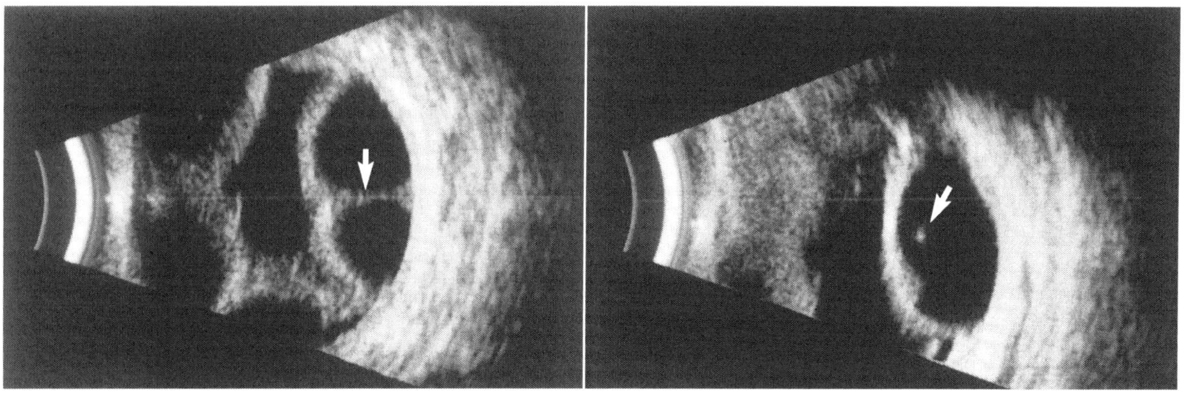

Figure 3-59 Bullous choroidal detachments with band in suprachoroidal space. **A,** Peripheral transverse section through choroidal detachments shows typical scalloped appearance and suprachoroidal band *(arrow)*. **B,** Longitudinal view displays cross-section of band *(arrow)*.

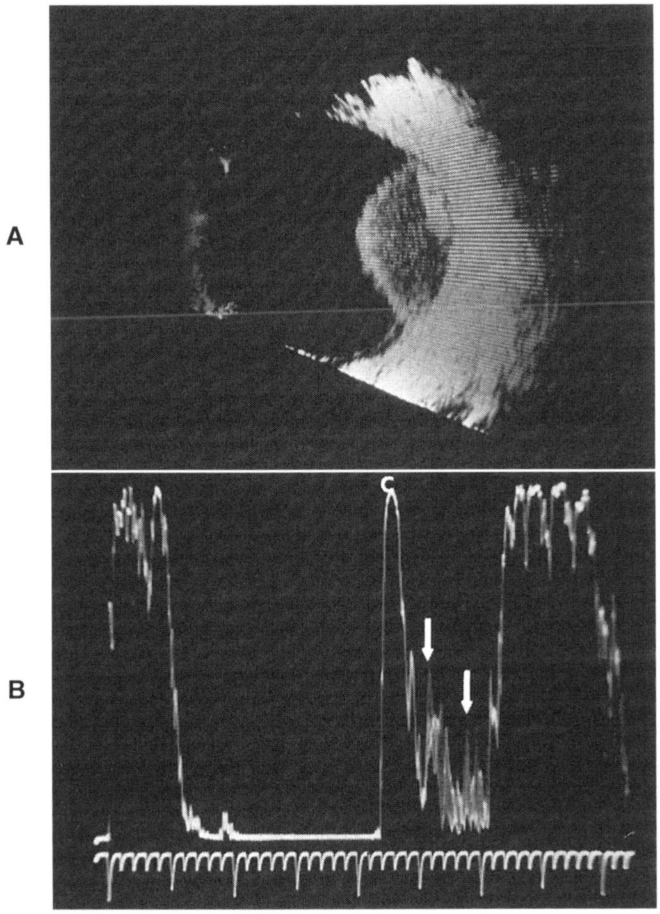

Figure 3-60 Hemorrhagic choroidal detachment. **A,** Transverse B-scan echogram demonstrates moderately elevated, thick, dome-shaped membrane with dense suprachoroidal hemorrhage. **B,** A-scan shows thick, 100% high choroidal spike *(C)* and blurred, low-to-medium reflective spikes *(arrows)* from the mobile suprachoroidal blood. (From Green RL, Byrne SF: Diagnostic ophthalmic ultrasound, in Ryan SJ [ed]: *Retina.* ed 3, St Louis, Mosby, 2001, p 258.)

in elevation, they may exhibit more pronounced aftermovement and a more folded appearance, similar to that of an RD.

CILIARY BODY

The ciliary body can be difficult to assess using conventional ultrasound because of its extreme anterior location and its irregular surface contour. Abnormalities of the ciliary body that can be detected with ultrasound include thickening due to edema or infiltration, detachment, or tumors (see p 173). In addition, cyclitic membranes and in some cases, cyclodialysis clefts can be demonstrated.

The contact method of ultrasound can assess the more posterior aspects of the ciliary body (i.e., pars plana) and sometimes the anterior ciliary body (i.e., pars plicata), especially nasally. Whenever an abnormality is suspected, comparison with the same region of the contralateral eye is recommended. Ciliochoroidal detachments can be demonstrated with both B- and A-scan (Figure 3-61). The contact technique can also show posterior ciliary body tumors or peripheral choroidal tumors that extend into the pars plana (see p 173).

An immersion technique is often more effective for evaluating the ciliary body[31,42] (see p 37 and Chapter 8). Detachments of the ciliary body (Figure 3-62), cyclitic membranes (Figure 3-63), and in some cases, cyclodialysis clefts are best shown using this technique. These findings are shown even better with the newer high resolution B-scan instrumentation (Figure 3-64; see also Figure 8-19). The position of intraocular lenses and their haptics can also be shown with this equipment[47,53] (see Figure 8-18).

SCLERA

Many disorders affect the sclera. However, clinical evaluation of the sclera, especially posteriorly, is often difficult because the sclera cannot be directly visualized. As a result, scleral disorders often go undetected or misdiagnosed. The imaging capabilities of ultrasound make it an ideal tool to assist in the evaluation of the sclera and its various disorders (Box 3-4).

Examination Techniques for the Sclera

Examination of the sclera is best achieved using B-scan. Certain probe positions can facilitate the assessment of scleral topography and thickness, as well as the relationship of the sclera to other ocular and orbital structures. Immersion techniques can be helpful for evaluating the anterior sclera, especially with the use of high resolution B-scan (see Chapter 8). A-scan can be used as well to evaluate the quantitative features of thickened sclera.

A relatively high gain setting is used initially to image the sclera with B-scan. Once the sclera is displayed, the gain is reduced to better distinguish the scleral borders from the surrounding tissues. The posterior sclera is best evaluated with a combination of axial, para-axial, and longitudinal probe positions, whereas transverse and longitudinal approaches are primarily used for the peripheral sclera (see Chapter 2).

Normal Sclera

The appearance of normal sclera varies with the size of the globe being examined. Scleral thickness increases as eye size decreases (i.e., hyperopia) and decreases as eye size increases (i.e., myopia). In all cases, however, the normal sclera is thickest posteriorly, measuring approximately 1.0 mm in an eye of average size. In the anterior aspects of the globe, the sclera thins, measuring 0.6 mm at the equator

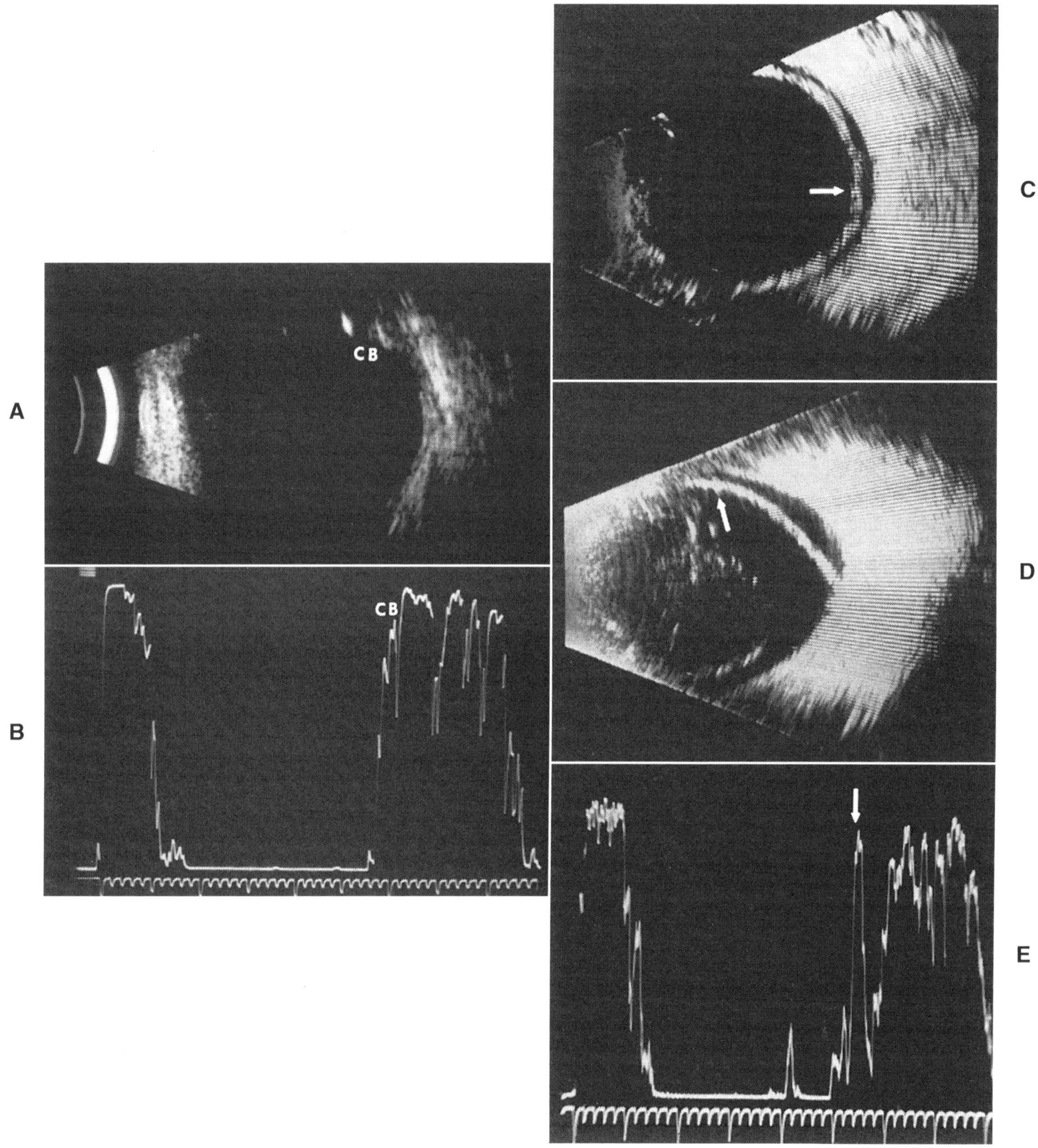

Figure 3-61 Normal ciliary body and ciliochoroidal detachment (contact technique). Normal ciliary body *(CB)* is shown in **A** and **B** and ciliochoroidal detachment *(arrows)* is shown in **C** to **E. A,** Peripheral longitudinal B-scan of normal ciliary body shows slight elevation. **B,** A-scan shows thick, irregular spike from coarse surface of normal ciliary body. Extremely peripheral transverse **(C)** and longitudinal **(D)** B-scans show detachment of ciliary body and peripheral choroid. **E,** A-scan demonstrates 100% high spike from detachment. (**C** to **E** from Green RL, Byrne SF: Diagnostic ophthalmic ultrasound, in Ryan SJ [ed]: *Retina.* ed 3, St Louis, Mosby, 2001, p 259.)

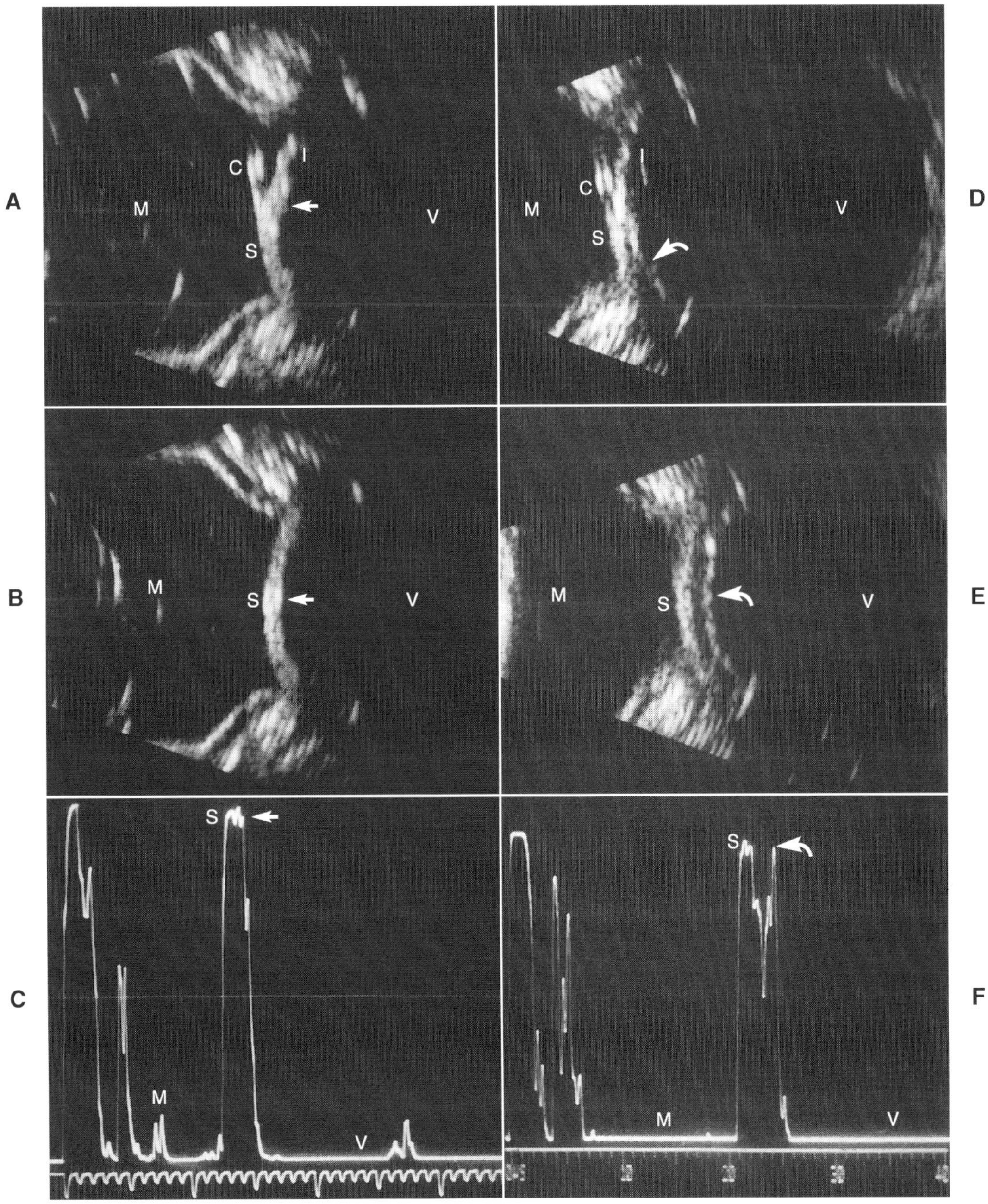

Figure 3-62 Normal and ciliary body detachment (immersion technique). Normal ciliary body *(straight arrows)* is shown in **A** to **C** and ciliary body detachment *(curved arrows)* is shown in **D** to **F**. **A** and **D**, Longitudinal B-scans. **B** and **E**, Transverse B-scans. **C** and **F**, A-scan echograms. *C*, Cornea; *I*, iris; *M*, methylcellulose within scleral shell; *S*, sclera; *V*, vitreous cavity.

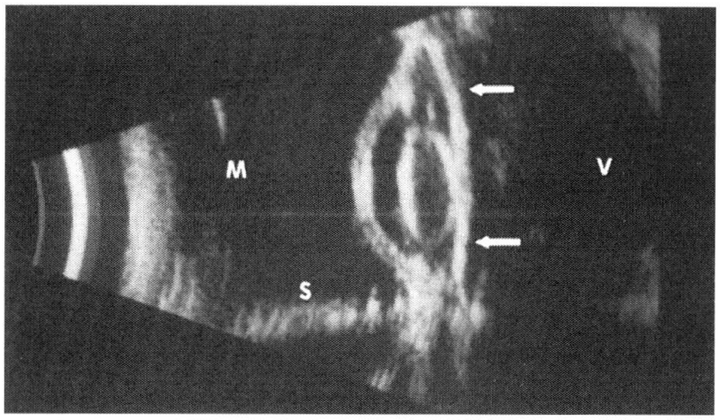

Figure 3-63 Cyclitic membrane. Immersion B-scan shows shallow anterior chamber, cataractous lens, and dense cyclitic membrane *(arrows)*. Membrane inserts into the ciliary body at edges of echogram. *M*, Methylcellulose within scleral shell; *S*, side of scleral shell; *V*, vitreous cavity. (From Green RL, Byrne SF: Diagnostic ophthalmic ultrasound, in Ryan SJ [ed]: *Retina*. ed 3, St Louis, Mosby, 2001, p 260.)

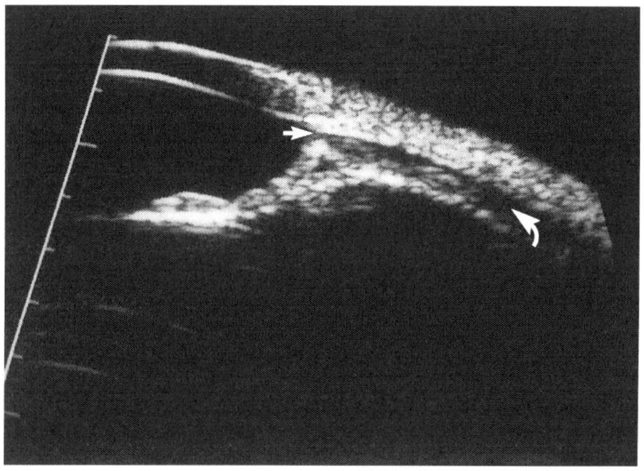

Figure 3-64 Cyclodialysis cleft. High resolution B-scan (20 MHz) (longitudinal view) is through peripheral aspect of anterior chamber and ciliary body. *Arrow* indicates cyclodialysis cleft between the anterior chamber and supraciliary space *(curved arrow)* created by the detachment of the ciliary body. (Courtesy Rhonda Waldron, MMSc, COMT, Atlanta, Georgia.)

and only 0.3 mm directly beneath the insertions of the rectus muscles.[55]

Echographically, the outer scleral surface can be distinguished from the adjacent highly reflective Tenon's capsule by reducing the gain. The relationship of the sclera to the optic nerve is best evaluated using axial and/or longitudinal scans. However, the inner scleral surface may be difficult to distinguish from the adjacent retinochoroid layer unless there is thickening or infiltration of the choroid and/or retina. Consequently, the very thin retinochoroid layer may have to be included in the assessment of scleral thickness (Figure 3-65).

As previously mentioned, the peripheral sclera is best assessed using both transverse and longitudinal scans. Because transverse scans are used for screening the globe (see p 22), overall scleral thickness is usually evaluated with this probe orientation. To confirm the presence of scleral abnormalities, however, longitudinal scans should also be utilized. The extraocular muscle insertions are important landmarks that can aid in the evaluation of peripheral scleral thickness because the insertion of the muscle highlights the outer surface of the sclera (see Chapter 15).

BOX 3-4

Disorders of the Sclera

- Thickening of sclera
  - Hyperopia
  - Choroidal folds
  - Nanophthalmos
  - Uveal effusion syndrome
  - Anterior ischemic optic neuropathy (AION)
  - Scleritis
  - Hypotony
- Thinning of sclera
  - Myopia
  - Staphyloma
  - Necrotizing scleritis
  - Plaque radiotherapy
- Scleral rupture (see pp 90 and 95)
- Scleral infolding (see p 97)
- Scleral calcification (see pp 114, 148, and 151)
- Scleral tumor (see p 155)

Disorders of the Sclera

In most cases, scleral abnormalities include thickening, thinning, deformity, or infiltration. These findings may be either diffuse or focal.

Thickening of the Sclera

HYPEROPIA

Hyperopia is generally associated with a shorter than normal eye and thicker than normal sclera (Figure 3-66). Although thickened sclera in the hyperopic globe is a normal finding, these eyes, as well as those of normal size with atypically thickened sclera, are predisposed to certain disorders, including choroidal folds, uveal effusion syndrome, and anterior ischemic optic neuropathy (AION).

CHOROIDAL FOLDS (CHORIORETINAL FOLDS)

Although choroidal folds represent folding or wrinkling of the choroid and retina, the underlying cause appears to be scleral thickening.[22] A number of conditions cause secondary choroidal folds, including indentation of the sclera by a retrobulbar mass, a foreign body, or a scleral buckle. In these conditions, it is postulated that the folds are due to thickening and indentation of the sclera. Scleritis may also cause thickening of the sclera and secondary choroidal

A 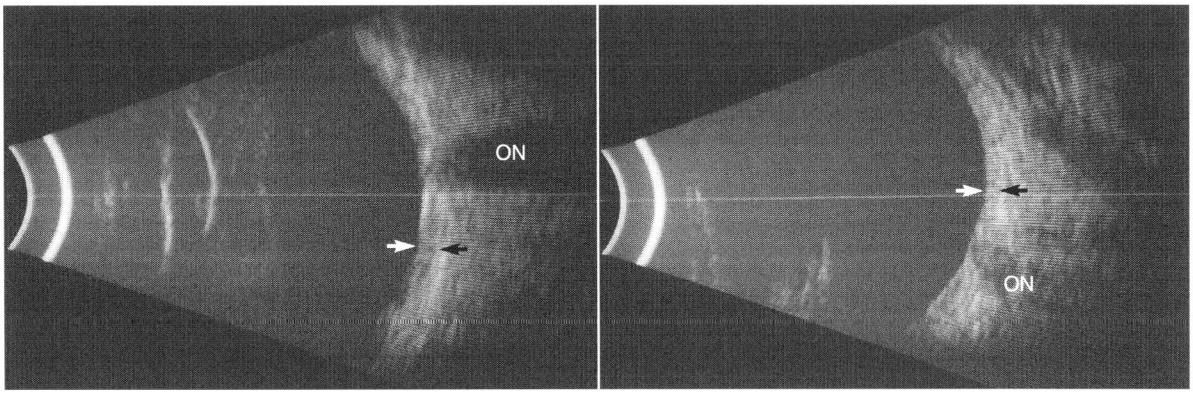 B

Figure 3-65 B-scan imaging of sclera in eye of normal size. Horizontal axial **(A)** and longitudinal **(B)** scans show band corresponding to normal sclera combined with thin retinochoroid layer *(arrows)*. *ON*, Optic nerve.

A 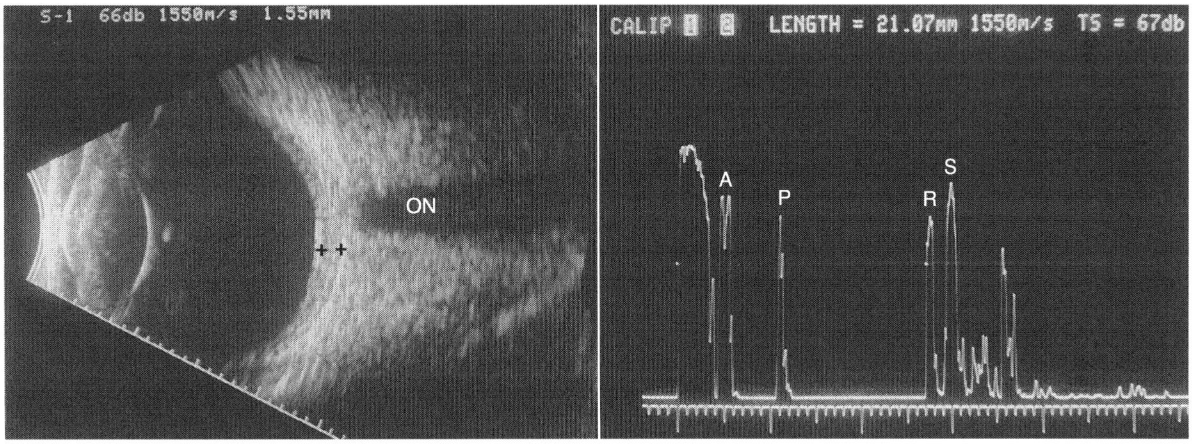 B

Figure 3-66 Short hyperopic globe with thick sclera. **A,** Horizontal axial B-scan demonstrates the thick nature of posterior sclera. Thickness of sclera temporal to optic nerve *(ON)* measures 1.56 mm. **B,** Contact A-scan measurement of axial length = 21.07 mm. *A*, Anterior lens capsule; *P*, posterior lens capsule; *R*, retina; *S*, sclera.

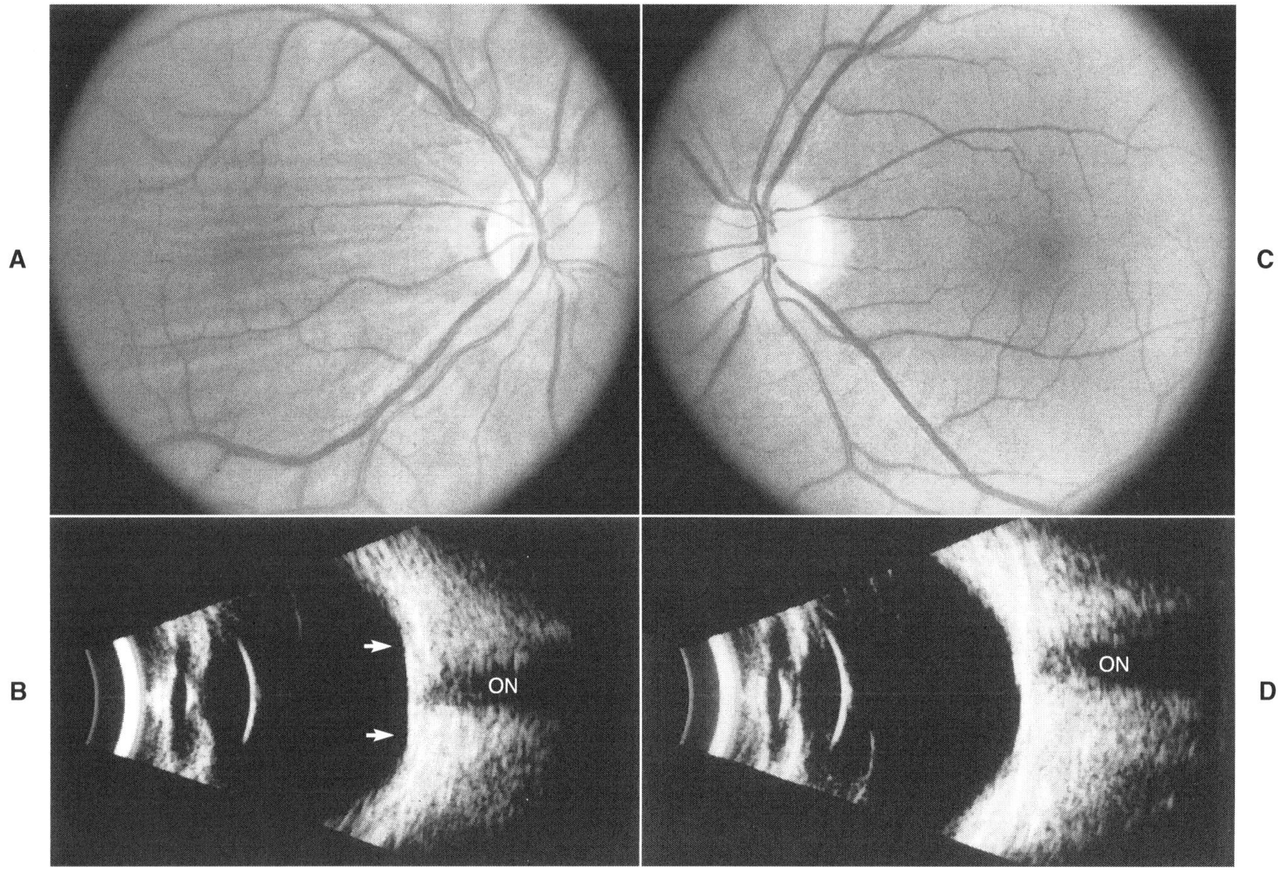

Figure 3-67 Choroidal folds associated with flattening of posterior ocular wall. **A,** Fundus photograph shows choroidal folds radiating horizontally from the optic disc. **B,** Corresponding horizontal axial B-scan echogram shows typical flattening of posterior ocular wall *(arrows)*. *ON,* Optic nerve. **C,** Fundus photograph of normal fellow eye. **D,** Corresponding horizontal axial B-scan echogram of fellow eye shows normal concave appearance of posterior ocular wall.

folds (see p 195). Choroidal folds have also been associated with choroidal tumors (e.g., melanoma and metastatic carcinoma) and infiltrative disorders such as VKH (see p 200). Hypotony caused by uveitis or trauma, or occurring as a result of glaucoma surgery, may also cause choroidal folds because of shrinkage of the globe and subsequent scleral thickening. However, the majority of choroidal folds are idiopathic. They are often found as an incidental finding, usually in patients who are hyperopic.

The most striking echographic feature of idiopathic choroidal folds is flattening of the posterior ocular wall caused by diffuse thickening of the posterior sclera and retinochoroid layer (Figure 3-67). These eyes frequently have a shorter than normal axial length (see p 244), and there may be echographic evidence of increased fluid surrounding the retrobulbar optic nerve[2] (see p 419).

NANOPHTHALMOS

This bilateral condition is characterized by diffuse, marked thickening of the sclera and very short axial eye lengths. Scleral thickness in these eyes has been reported to be at least 2 mm[1] and axial eye lengths can range from 14.0 to 20.5 mm.[33] Other findings include a shallow anterior chamber and diffuse thickening of the retinochoroid layer. Although the lens in these very short eyes is of normal size, it occupies a proportionately greater than normal volume (Figure 3-68). Nanophthalmic eyes are predisposed to angle closure glaucoma (see p 214), as well as to postoperative or spontaneous serous ciliochoroidal and retinal detachments (i.e., uveal effusion syndrome).

UVEAL EFFUSION SYNDROME

Uveal effusion syndrome, which produces spontaneous, serous ciliochoroidal and retinal detachments, appears to be caused by diffuse thickening of the sclera. It is hypothesized that the thickened sclera leads to obstruction of the vortex veins and subsequent accumulation of proteinaceous fluid in the suprachoroidal and, in some cases, the subretinal space.[22] In addition to demonstrating the ciliochoroidal and retinal detachments, ultrasound can show thickening of the sclera and retinochoroid layer (Figure 3-69). These eyes are usually shorter than normal and may be very short

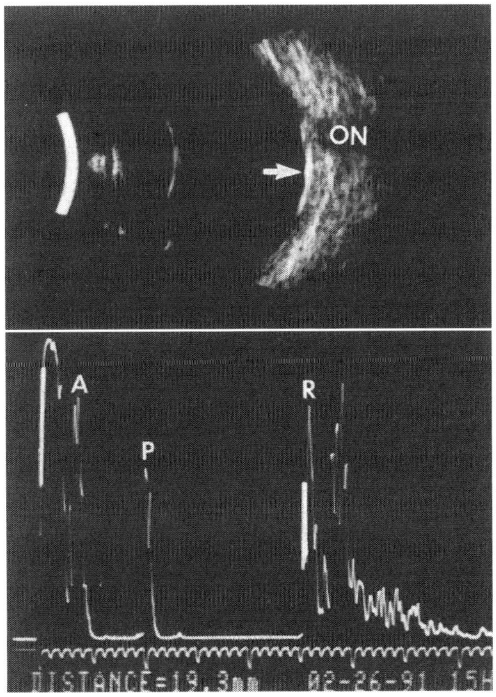

A

B

Figure 3-68 Nanophthalmos. **A,** Horizontal axial B-scan at reduced gain shows thickening of posterior retinochoroid layer and sclera *(arrow)*. *ON*, Optic nerve. **B,** A-scan at reduced gain shows contact axial length measurement of 19.3 mm. *A*, Anterior lens capsule; *P*, posterior lens capsule; *R*, retina.

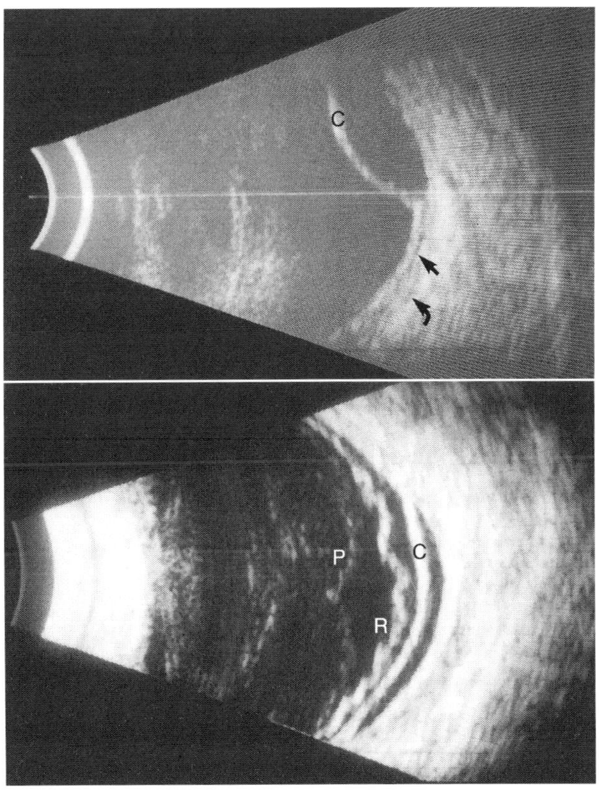

A

B

Figure 3-69 Choroidal detachment **(A)** and choroidal and retinal detachment **(B)** in uveal effusion syndrome. **A,** Anterior longitudinal B-scan displays peripheral dome-shaped, serous choroidal detachment *(C)* as well as diffuse thickening of retinochoroid layer *(black straight arrow)* and sclera *(black curved arrow)*. **B,** Anterior transverse B-scan shows shallow choroidal detachment *(C)*, RD *(R)*, and PVD *(P)*.

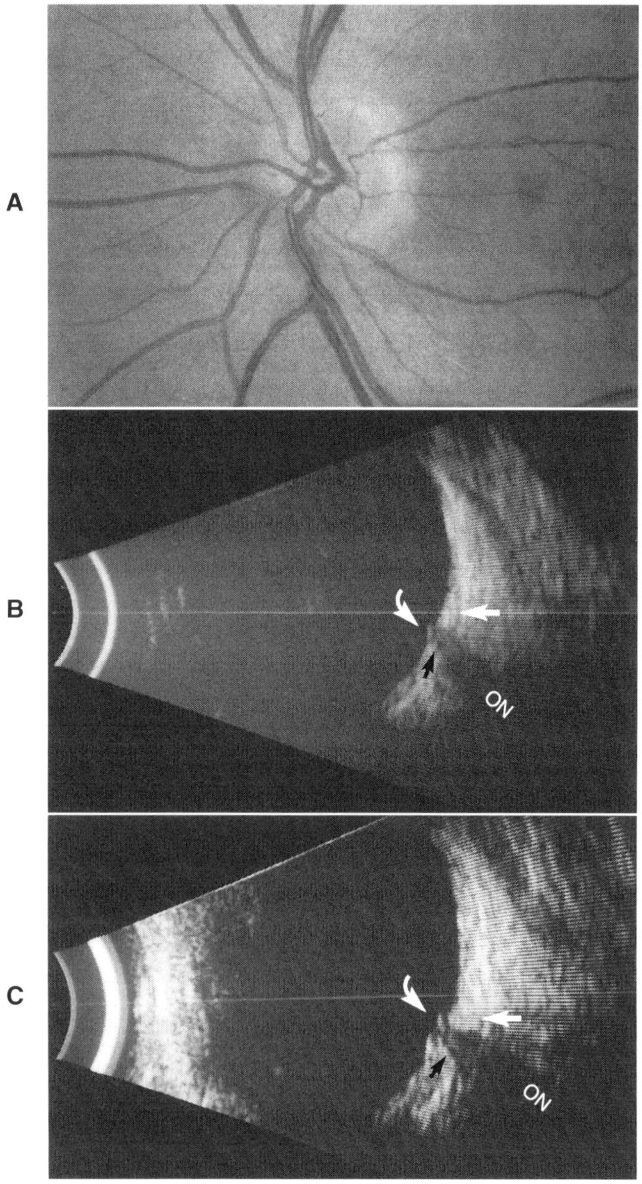

Figure 3-70 Crowded optic disc. **A,** Fundus photograph shows blurring of the disc margins (pseudopapilledema) due to crowded optic disc. Longitudinal B-scans from two different patients show eye of average length **(B)** and short hyperopic eye **(C).** Note mild elevation of optic disc *(curved white arrows)*, long scleral optic canals *(black straight arrows)*, and thickened posterior sclera *(straight white arrows)*.

as occurs in nanophthalmos (see p 82).[56] In some cases, ultrasound can detect increased subarachnoid fluid around the optic nerve (see p 419 in Chapter 16). These patients may also present with secondary angle closure glaucoma (see p 214).

ANTERIOR ISCHEMIC OPTIC NEUROPATHY

Anterior ischemic optic neuropathy (AION) may be caused, in part, by thickening of the posterior sclera. The thickened sclera in these patients produces long, narrow scleral canals and the clinical finding of a crowded disc[15,23] (see p 434). These findings may be implicated in the pathogenesis of AION.[3,14] Ultrasound in these eyes demonstrates thickened sclera and long scleral canals (Figure 3-70). The axial length measurement is usually normal or moderately short.[15] These findings are similar to those of patients with idiopathic chorioretinal folds that can sometimes be clinically identified in eyes with AION.

SCLERITIS

Ultrasound can be used to evaluate both anterior and posterior scleritis and is, in fact, the best imaging modality for diagnosing posterior scleritis.[4,23,27] The scleral thickening in posterior scleritis can vary from mild to marked and can be either diffuse or localized (i.e., nodular; see p 196). Along with the thickened sclera, there is generally thickening of the choroid, as well as edema or inflammatory infiltration in sub-Tenon's space. Scleritis is discussed in detail in Chapter 6 (see p 195).

HYPOTONY

Longstanding hypotony following glaucoma surgery or secondary to uveitis, ruptured globe or a cyclodialysis cleft usually leads to shrinkage of the globe and diffuse thickening of the sclera. This condition is also often associated with diffuse thickening of the retinochoroid layer, and choroidal detachments may develop. Hypotony maculopathy can also occur (see p 72).[22] The ultrasound findings for hypotony are described in detail in Chapter 7 on p 216.

Thinning of the Sclera

MYOPIA

Large myopic globes have thinner than normal sclera. Because it is much more difficult to distinguish the sclera from the adjacent ocular coats using ultrasound, it is often necessary to include the retina and choroid when evaluating the scleral thickness. As in eyes of normal axial length, the sclera tends to be thinner in the periphery than posteriorly in the myopic eye.

STAPHYLOMA

Focal or localized thinning of the sclera can produce a staphyloma. These lesions may be congenital, or they may develop following chronic inflammation or intraocular surgery. Anterior staphylomas can be confused with intraocular tumors, whereas posterior staphylomas can complicate the biometry examination (see p 263). Large, broad staphylomas in the posterior pole are often associated with high axial myopia. However, staphylomas may be eccentric, located near the equator. When these eccentric staphylomas are large, they have been observed to be associated with significant corneal astigmatism.[24]

NECROTIZING SCLERITIS

Thinning of the sclera can develop secondary to necrotizing scleritis. When the scleral thinning presents anteriorly, the underlying choroid may sometimes be visible through the thin sclera, thus producing a dark or pigmented appearance that may clinically simulate a tumor. In these situations, ultrasound can be used to identify the thin sclera and exclude the presence of an intraocular tumor (see p 196 and Figure 6-12).

PLAQUE RADIOTHERAPY (BRACHYTHERAPY)

Radioactive plaques are often used to treat choroidal melanomas. Thinning of the sclera can occur following this treatment.

Scleral Deformity

The normal shape of the globe can be altered in a number of ways, including flattening and indentation by external sources, folds secondary to hypotony (see pp 82 and 214), ruptures and perforations due to trauma (see Chapter 4), longstanding degeneration as in phthisis bulbi (see p 114), and changes in contour due to choroidal tumors.

Indentation or flattening of the globe may present on clinical examination with choroidal folds and elevation of the fundus. Ultrasound can usually identify the cause of the scleral abnormality. Possible causes include pressure from an orbital mass (see p 297), a foreign body (see Figure 17-14), a scleral buckle (see p 109), or a bleb secondary to a glaucoma drainage device (see p 219). In addition, collapse of the sclera due to sudden or chronic hypotony can produce scleral infolding (see p 97).

Scleral Calcification

There are a number of disorders associated with calcification of the sclera. These include idiopathic sclerochoroidal calcification (see p 148), Cogan's plaques (see p 151), and phthisis bulbi (see p 114).

Scleral Tumors

See p 155 in Chapter 5 for a review of scleral tumors.

REFERENCES

1. Anand R, Tasman WS: Nonrhegmatogenous retinal detachment, in Ryan SJ (ed): *Retina.* ed 3, vol 3. St Louis, 2000, Mosby, p 2089.
2. Atta HA, Byrne SF: The findings of standardized echography for choroidal folds. *Arch Ophthalmol* 1988;106:1234.
3. Beck RW, Savino PJ, Repka MX, et al: Optic disc structure in anterior ischemic optic neuropathy. *Ophthalmology* 1944;91:1337.
4. Benson WE, Shields JA, Tasman W, et al: Posterior scleritis. A cause of diagnostic confusion. *Arch Ophthalmol* 1979;97:1482.
5. Bigar F, Bosshard C, Klüti R, et al: Combined A- and B-scan echography. Preoperative evaluation of vitrectomy patients. *Mod Probl Ophthalmol* 1977;18:2.
6. Blumenkranz MS, Byrne SF: Standardized echography (ultrasonography) for the detection and characterization of retinal detachment. *Ophthalmology* 1982;89:821.
7. Boldt HC, Brown DM, McGeorge AJ: Echographic diagnosis of degenerative retinoschisis facilitated by scleral indentation [letter]. *Am J Ophthalmol* 1994;118:123.
8. Byrne SF: Differential diagnosis of disciform lesions using standardized echography, in Hillman JS, Lemay MM (eds): *Ophthalmic Ultrasonography.* Dordrecht, Dr W Junk, 1983, p l49.
9. Chu TG, Lopez PF, Cano MR, et al: Posterior vitreoschisis. An echographic finding in proliferative diabetic retinopathy. *Ophthalmology* 1996;103:315.
10. Coleman DJ, Franzen LA: Vitreous surgery: preoperative evaluation and prognostic value of ultrasonic display of vitreous hemorrhage. *Arch Ophthalmol* 1974;92:375.
11. Coleman DJ: Preoperative evaluation of the vitreous with ultrasound, in McPherson A (ed): *New and Controversial Aspects of Vitreoretinal Surgery.* St Louis, Mosby, 1977, p 95.
12. DiBernardo C, Blodi BA, Byrne SF: Echographic evaluation of retinal tears in patients with spontaneous vitreous hemorrhage. *Arch Ophthalmol* 1992;110:511.
13. Dugel PU, Smiddy WE, Byrne SF, et al: Macular hole syndromes. Echographic findings with clinical correlation. *Ophthalmology* 1994;101:815.
14. Feit RH, Tomsak RL, Ellenberger C Jr: Structural factors in the pathogenesis of ischemic optic neuropathy. *Am J Ophthalmol* 1984;98:105.
15. Feldon SE, Sadun AA, DuBois LG, et al: Echographic features pre- and post-optic nerve sheath fenestration for progressive aion. *Invest Ophthalmol Vis Sci* 1991;32:951.
16. Fisher YL, Slakter JS, Friedman RA, et al: Kinetic ultrasound evaluation of the posterior vitreoretinal interface. *Ophthalmology* 1991; 98:1135.
17. Fisher YL, Slakter JS, Yannuzzi LA, et al: A prospective natural history study and kinetic ultrasound evaluation of idiopathic macular holes. *Ophthalmology* 1994;101:5.
18. Freyler H, Egerer I: Echography and histological studies in various eye conditions. *Arch Ophthalmol* 1977;95:1387.
19. Fuller DG, Laqua H, Machemer R: Ultrasonographic diagnosis of massive periretinal proliferation in eyes with opaque media (triangular retinal detachment). *Am J Ophthalmol* 1977;83:460.
20. Fuller DG, Hutton WL: *Presurgical Evaluation of Eyes With Opaque Media.* New York, Grune & Stratton, 1982, p 109.
21. Gass JDM: Idiopathic senile macular hole: its early stages and pathogenesis. *Arch Ophthalmol* 1988;106:629.
22. Gass JDM: *Stereoscopic Atlas of Macular Diseases.* ed 4, vol 2. St Louis, Mosby, 1997.
23. Green RL: Echographic diagnosis of posterior scleritis, in Ossoinig KC (ed): *Ophthalmic Echography.* Dordrecht, Dr W Junk, 1987, p 515.
24. Green RL: Personal communication. March 2001.
25. Green RL, Byrne SF: Diagnostic ophthalmic ultrasound, in Ryan SJ (ed): *Retina.* ed 2, vol 1. St Louis, Mosby, 1989, p 191.
26. Green WR, Sebag J: Vitreoretinal interface, in Ryan SJ (ed): *Retina.* ed 3, vol 3. St Louis, Mosby, 2000, p 1895.
27. Guthoff RF, Singh G: Posterior scleritis—the role of ultrasonography in the follow-up of the disease, in Hillman JS, LeMay MM (eds): *Ophthalmic Ultrasonography.* Dordrecht, Dr W Junk, 1984, p 169.
28. Han DP, Lewandowski M, Mieler WF: Echographic diagnosis of anterior hyaloidal fibrovascular proliferation. *Arch Ophthalmol* 1991;109:842.
29. Haouchine B, Massin P, Gaudric A: Foveal pseudocyst as the first step in macular hole formation—prospective study by optical coherence tomography. *Ophthalmology* 2001;108:15.
30. Hudson HL, Chong LP, Frambach DA, et al: Encircling panretinal laser photocoagulation may prevent macular detachment after vitrectomy for proliferative diabetic retinopathy. *Int Ophthalmology* 1994;18:101.
31. Iijima Y, Asanagi K: A new B-scan ultrasonographic technique for observing ciliary body detachment. *Am J Ophthalmol* 1983;95:498.
32. Jalkh AE, Jabbour N, Avila MP, et al: Ultrasonographic findings in eyes with giant retinal tears and opaque media. *Retina* 1983;3:154.
33. Jin JC, Anderson DR: Laser and unsutured sclerotomy in nanophthalmos. *Am J Ophthalmol* 1990;109:576.
34. Johnson MW, Van Newkirk MR, Meyer KA: Perifoveal vitreous detachment is the primary pathogenic event in idiopathic macular hole formation. *Arch Ophthalmol* 2001;119:215.
35. Johnson RN, Gass JDM: Idiopathic macular holes: observations, stages of formation, and implications for surgical intervention. *Ophthalmology* 1988;95:917.
36. Kelley LM, Walker JP, Wing GL, et al: Ultrasound-guided cryotherapy for retinal tears in patients with vitreous hemorrhage. *Ophthalmic Surg Lasers* 1997;28:565.
37. Kerman BM, Coleman DJ: B-scan ultrasonography of retinal detachments. *Ann Ophthalmol* 1978;10:903.
38. Kokame GT: Ultrasound of macular holes [letter]. *Ophthalmology* 1995;102:366.

39. Kokame GT: Clinical correlation of ultrasonographic findings in macular holes. *Am J Ophthalmol* 1995;119:441.
40. Kokame GT: Macular traction associated with a premacular circular dehiscence of the detached posterior vitreous cortex. *Vitreotech* 2000;5:4.
41. McLeod D, Restori M: Ultrasonic examination in severe diabetic eye disease. *Br J Ophthalmol* 1979;63:533.
42. Ormerod LD, Baerveldt G, Green RL: Cyclodialysis clefts: natural history, assessment, and management, in Weinstein GW (ed): *Open-Angle Glaucoma.* New York, Churchill Livingstone, 1986, p 201.
43. Ossoinig KC: Echographic detection and classification of posterior hyphemas. *Ophthalmologica* 1984;189:2.
44. Ossoinig KC, Frazier SL, Watzke RC, et al: Combined A-scan and B-scan echography as a diagnostic aid for vitreoretinal surgery, in McPherson A (ed): *New and Controversial Aspects of Vitreoretinal Surgery.* St Louis, Mosby, 1977, p 106.
45. Ossoinig KC, Islas G, Tamayo GE, et al: Detached retina versus dense fibrovascular membrane: standardized A-scan and B- scan criteria, in Ossoinig KC (ed): *Ophthalmic Echography.* Dordrecht, Germany, Dr W Junk, 1987, p 275.
46. Ossoinig KC, Reshef DS, Weingeist TA, et al: Echographic findings in Terson's syndrome, in Ossoinig KC (ed): *Ophthalmic Echography.* Dordrecht, Dr W Junk, 1987, p 247.
47. Pavlin CJ, Foster FS: *Ultrasound Biomicroscopy of the Eye.* New York, Springer-Verlag, 1995.
48. Purnell EW, Frank KE, Cappaert WE: Preoperative ultrasonographic evaluation of vitrectomy candidates with diabetic retinopathy, in McPherson A (ed): *New and Controversial Aspects of Vitreoretinal Surgery.* St Louis, Mosby, 1977, p 84.
49. Sabti K, Lindley SK, Mansour M, et al: Uveal effusion after cataract surgery: an echographic study. *Ophthalmology* 2001;108:100.
50. Schwartz SD, Alexander R, Hiscott P, et al: Recognition of vitreoschisis in proliferative diabetic retinopathy. A useful landmark in vitrectomy for diabetic traction retinal detachment. *Ophthalmology* 1996;103:323.
51. Seabag J: Diabetic vitreopathy [editorial]. *Ophthalmology* 1996; 103:205.
52. Sjaarda RN, Thompson JT: Macular hole, in Ryan SJ (ed): *Retina.* ed 3, vol 3. St Louis, Mosby, 2001, p 2547.
53. Sorenson AL, Holladay JT, Kim T, et al: Ultrasonographic measurement of induced myopia associated with capsular bag distention syndrome. *Ophthalmology* 2000;107:902.
54. Till P, Ossoinig KC: Ten-year study on clinical echography in intraocular disease. *Bibl Ophthalmol* 1975;83:49.
55. Torczinski E: Sclera, in Duane TD, Jaeger EA (eds): *Biomedical Foundations of Ophthalmology.* vol 1. Philadelphia, JB Lippincott, 1988, p 3.
56. Uyama M, Takahashi K, Kozaki J, et al: Uveal effusion syndrome. Clinical features, surgical treatment, and pathophysiology. *Ophthalmology* 2000;107:441.
57. van Heuven WAJ, Ossoinig KC: Ultrasonography before vitrectomy, in *Symposium on Retinal Diseases.* St Louis, Mosby, 1977, p 11.
58. Van Newkirk MR, Gass JDM, Callanan D, et al: Follow-up and ultrasonographic examination of patients with macular pseudo-operculum. *Am J Ophthalmol* 1994;117:13.
59. Van Newkirk MR, Johnson MW, Hughes JR, et al: B-scan ultrasonographic findings in the stages of idiopathic macular hole. *Trans Am Ophthalmol Soc* 2000;98:163.
60. Yanoff M, Fine BS: *Ocular Pathology.* ed 4, London, Mosby-Wolfe, 1996, p 444.
61. Weingeist TA, Goldman EJ, Folk JC, et al: Terson's syndrome. Clinicopathologic correlations. *Ophthalmology* 1986;93:1435.

4

William D. Bates

Trauma and Postsurgical Findings

One of the most difficult clinical examinations for the ophthalmologist is that of the traumatized globe. The patient may be unable or unwilling to open the lids because of severe pain. Opacification of the anterior chamber, lens, or vitreous cavity may further hinder the clinical examination. In these cases, ultrasound can provide valuable information that may be unobtainable by other means.*

In a severely injured eye, marked lid swelling and patient discomfort often necessitate examination through closed lids. Nevertheless, with a systematic approach, sufficient information can usually be obtained to allow a reasonable assessment of the extent of intraocular injuries. Whenever possible, open wounds should be repaired prior to the echographic examination. In those few cases, however, in which the intraocular contents must be assessed before initial wound closure, it is possible to perform an examination without further injuring the globe. This can be achieved by placing the probe gently on the closed lids, using copious amounts of sterile methylcellulose. With this method, virtually no pressure need be exerted to obtain useful echograms. When examining through closed lids, however, relatively high gain settings must be used to help overcome the effects of sound attenuation by the lids. For anterior segment examinations through the lids, a soft stand-off technique may be used (see p 39).

Because examination of the traumatized eye may be limited and because only a brief examination may be possible, it is important that the echographer be aware of the various types of pathologic changes that are most likely to occur with different types of injuries. The three main categories of intraocular trauma are blunt injuries, penetrating injuries, and surgical complications.

In addition to ocular trauma, this chapter will also address typical echographic findings in the post-surgical eye.

BLUNT TRAUMA

Blunt trauma to the eye can produce marked, sudden distortion of the globe, resulting in more severe damage than may be clinically apparent. Blunt trauma injuries include those caused by blows from fists or elbows, inflating airbags, tennis balls or racquetballs, and paint balls. Specific injuries to both the anterior and posterior segments of the eye should be considered (Box 4-1).

Anterior Segment

Ultrasound can be used to assess the anterior segment in the presence of corneal opacification or anterior chamber hyphema. If a hyphema is present, ultrasound can demonstrate both the presence of the clot and the depth of the anterior chamber. The status of the lens may also be readily assessed by ultrasound (Figure 4-1).

If the trauma is such that traditional immersion techniques using a scleral shell cannot be used, the anterior segment can be examined through closed lids (see p 39). One of the newer high resolution B-scan probes utilizes a soft, water-filled, balloon-like tip that can be very useful in these circumstances (see p 37 and Figure 2-33).

Blunt trauma can also affect the lens. Although mild cataractous changes may not be obvious with ultrasound, moderately dense cataracts can usually be detected. On B-scan, a cataractous lens exhibits varying degrees of echo density, whereas the normal lens is echolucent (Figure 4-2). Subluxation or dislocation of the lens may also be easily detected. A subluxated lens may lie in the anterior chamber, or it may be displaced laterally or posteriorly (Figure 4-3). A dislocated lens can usually be detected floating within the vitreous cavity; or sometimes it can be observed sliding along the surface of the retina (see Figure 5-77). Vitreous membranes or strands are occasionally attached to the dislocated lens (Figure 4-4).

Severe blunt trauma can also result in rupture of the lens capsule, either anteriorly or posteriorly. Echographic detection of a lens rupture is useful for determining the best surgical approach for cataract extraction (Figure 4-5).

Blunt trauma to the anterior segment may cause dehiscence of a corneal or limbal surgical wound. These cases are often associated with anterior chamber hyphemas.

*References 6, 7, 11, 12, 16, 18, 21, 23, 26.

BOX 4-1

Sequelae of Blunt Trauma

Anterior Segment

- Hyphema
- Cataract
- (Sub)luxation of lens or IOL
- Lens capsule rupture
- Corneoscleral rupture
- Cyclodialysis cleft

Posterior Segment

- Vitreous hemorrhage
- Posterior vitreous detachment
- Retinal tear
- Retinal dialysis
- Retinal detachment
- Edema of retinochoroid layer
- Hemorrhagic choroidal detachment
- Posterior scleral rupture
- Avulsion of optic nerve

A B

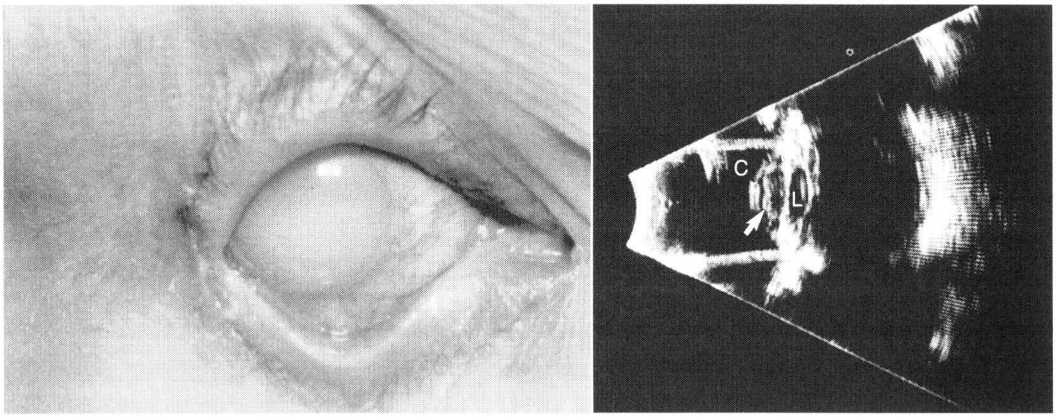

Figure 4-1 Anterior chamber hyphema. **A,** External photograph showing diffuse corneal blood staining. **B,** Immersion axial B-scan shows anterior chamber hyphema *(arrow)*. *C,* Cornea; *I,* iris; *L,* lens. (From Green RL, Byrne SF: Diagnostic ophthalmic ultrasound, in Ryan SJ [ed]: *Retina.* ed 3, St Louis, Mosby, 2001, p 263.)

A B

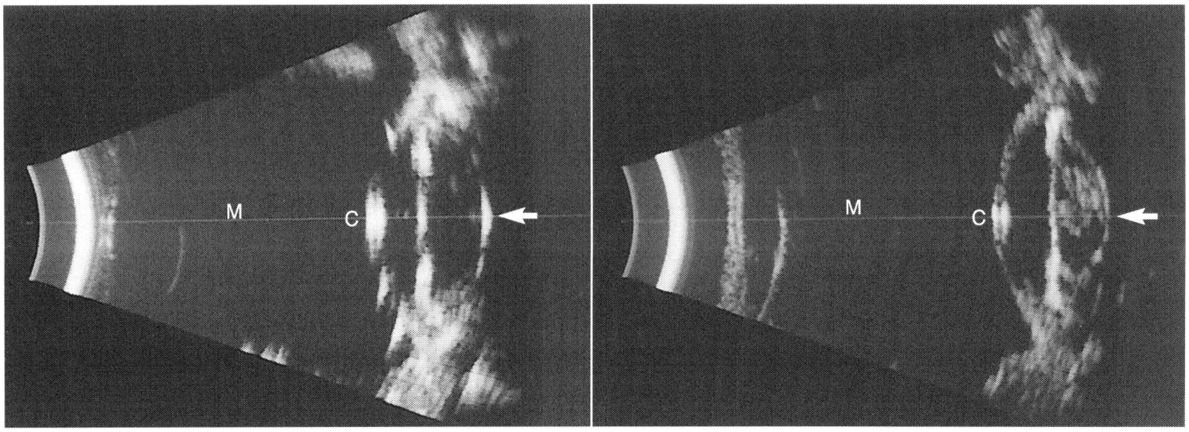

Figure 4-2 Normal lens and traumatic cataract due to blunt trauma. Immersion axial B-scans are at reduced gain setting. **A,** Normal lens *(arrow)* with typical echolucent appearance. *C,* Cornea; *M,* methylcellulose within scleral shell. **B,** Cataractous lens.

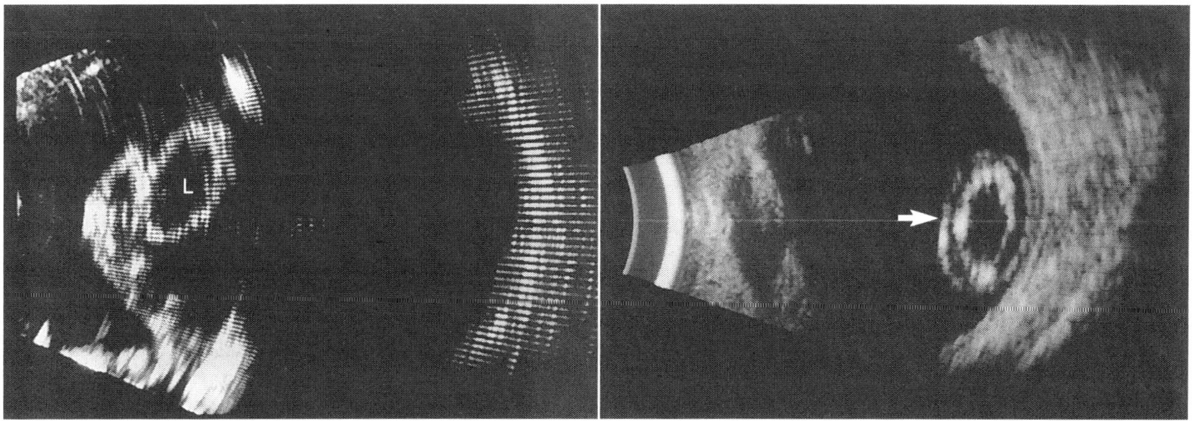

Figure 4-3 Subluxated and dislocated lenses following blunt trauma. **A,** Immersion B-scan echogram shows subluxated lens *(L)*. **B,** Contact B-scan shows cataractous, dislocated lens *(arrow)* lying on surface of retina.

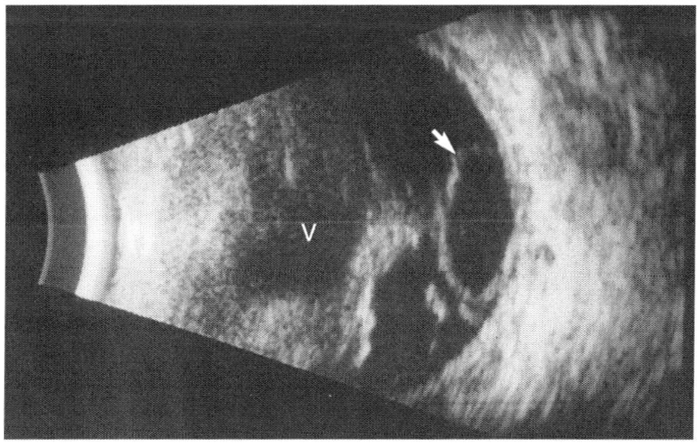

Figure 4-4 Dislocated lens following blunt trauma injury. Transverse B-scan shows oval-shaped lens *(arrow)* on surface of retina. Vitreous opacities and membranes are attached to lens. *V,* Vitreous cavity.

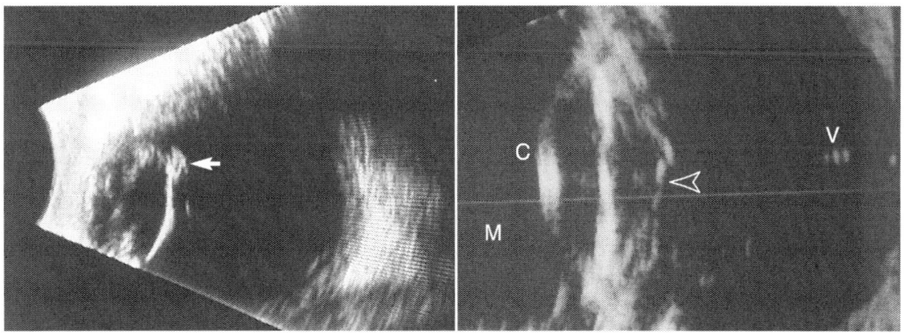

Figure 4-5 Two examples of ruptured lenses from severe blunt trauma. **A,** Para-axial B-scan shows extrusion of lens material through small rupture at periphery of posterior lens capsule *(arrow)*. **B,** Immersion axial B-scan shows irregular contour of posterior lens capsule *(open arrow)* due to lens rupture. *C,* Cornea; *M,* methylcellulose within scleral shell; *V,* vitreous cavity. (From Green RL, Byrne SF: Diagnostic ophthalmic ultrasound, in Ryan SJ [ed]: *Retina.* ed 3, St Louis, Mosby, 2001, p 263.)

Ultrasound is useful for determining the status of the anterior chamber and the crystalline lens or intraocular lens (IOL) implant. Ultrasound is often needed to determine whether the lens has been extruded from the eye.

A cyclodialysis cleft following blunt trauma to the anterior segment may sometimes occur. This can lead to persistent hypotony and should be considered whenever there is hypotony of unknown etiology. Clinically, these clefts may be difficult to detect if the anterior chamber is shallow and/or the cornea is opacified. High resolution B-scan instrumentation is usually necessary to image these lesions (see Figures 3-64 and 8-19).

Posterior Segment

Vitreoretinal Injuries

A wide variety of posterior segment abnormalities can occur secondary to blunt trauma. These include vitreous hemorrhage, posterior vitreous detachment (PVD), peripheral retinal tears, subretinal hemorrhage, and macular holes. The typical echographic findings for these posterior segment abnormalities have already been described in Chapter 3. When the ocular media are opaque, the eye should be carefully evaluated to detect the presence of any of these conditions.

Additional findings that should be considered in patients with blunt ocular trauma include peripheral retinal dialysis, Berlin's edema (commotio retinae), and choroidal rupture. A retinal dialysis, a disinsertion of the peripheral retina from the ora serrata, is best detected with B-scan using a longitudinal approach (Figure 4-6). Although a retinal dialysis may be located in any quadrant, common locations are supranasally and inferotemporally.[8] When a retinal detachment (RD) results from a peripheral retinal dialysis, it is usually shallow rather than bullous, and, when longstanding, it may develop multiple intraretinal cysts.[8]

Berlin's edema is often associated with acute visual loss. On ultrasound, this condition appears as diffuse thickening of the retinochoroid layer, usually in the posterior pole (Figure 4-7).

A choroidal rupture consists of a tear in the retinal pigment epithelium (RPE), Bruch's membrane, and choroid. Acutely, a choroidal rupture may be associated with Berlin's edema, intraretinal, or subretinal hemorrhage and generally cannot be differentiated from these conditions with ultrasound. However, once the hemorrhage and/or edema have partially resolved, the choroidal rupture can in some cases be imaged echographically (see Figure 4-7).

Posterior Scleral Rupture

Severe blunt trauma can result in rupture of the posterior sclera. These eyes usually present clinically with marked hemorrhagic chemosis as well as vitreous hemorrhage.[17] In most cases, these ruptures are occult with no external signs of rupture, and the intraocular pressure may be normal. On ultrasound, the sclera in the area of the rupture may show an irregular contour, thickening, and decreased reflectivity.[15] An actual split in the scleral fibers may, however, not be detectable.

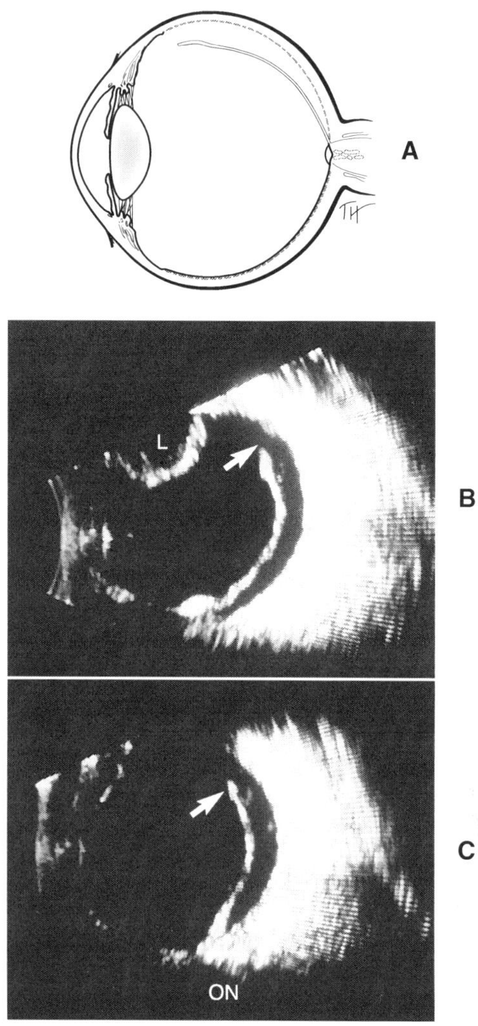

Figure 4-6 Peripheral retinal dialysis following blunt trauma. **A,** Schematic drawing showing retinal dialysis. **B,** Anterior longitudinal B-scan shows RD with peripheral dialysis *(arrow). L,* Lens. **C,** Posterior longitudinal view shows the peripheral dialysis and RD inserting into the optic nerve *(ON).* (From Green RL, Byrne SF: Diagnostic ophthalmic ultrasound, in Ryan SJ [ed]: *Retina.* ed 3, St Louis, Mosby, 2001, p 264.)

Other findings associated with scleral rupture include (1) vitreous incarceration associated with vitreous hemorrhage and PVD, (2) thickening or detachment of the surrounding retina and/or choroid, and (3) hemorrhage in the immediate episcleral space (Figure 4-8).[15] Additionally, the incarcerated vitreous may produce traction folds or bands extending across the vitreous cavity toward the site of incarceration. Retinal incarceration can also occur. In one case, nearly the entire retina was extruded through a large scleral defect into the orbit (Figure 4-9).

A

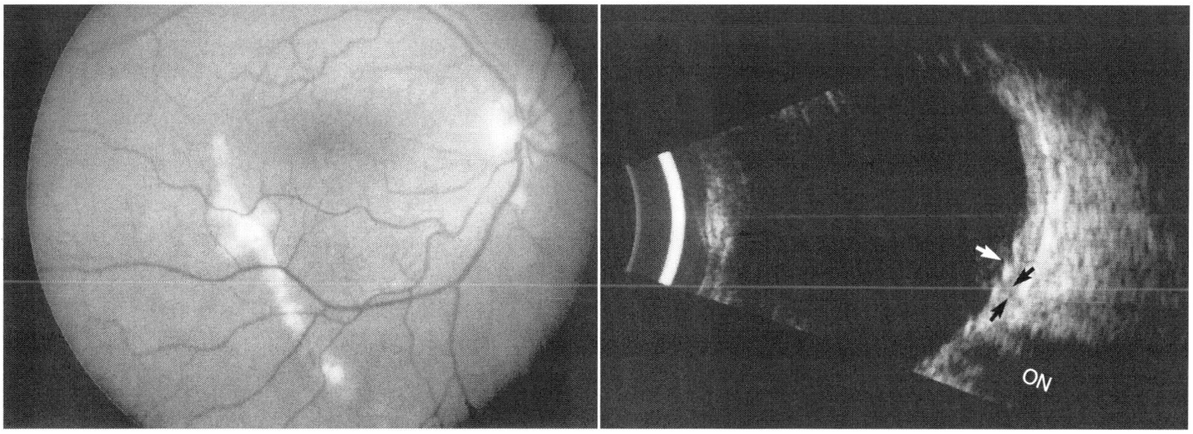

B

Figure 4-7 Choroidal rupture following blunt trauma. **A,** Fundus photograph demonstrates choroidal rupture at temporal edge of macular region. **B,** Longitudinal B-scan shows thin echolucent line representing choroidal rupture *(black arrows)* and associated irregular thickening of retinochoroid layer in macular region *(white arrow)*. *ON*, Optic nerve.

A

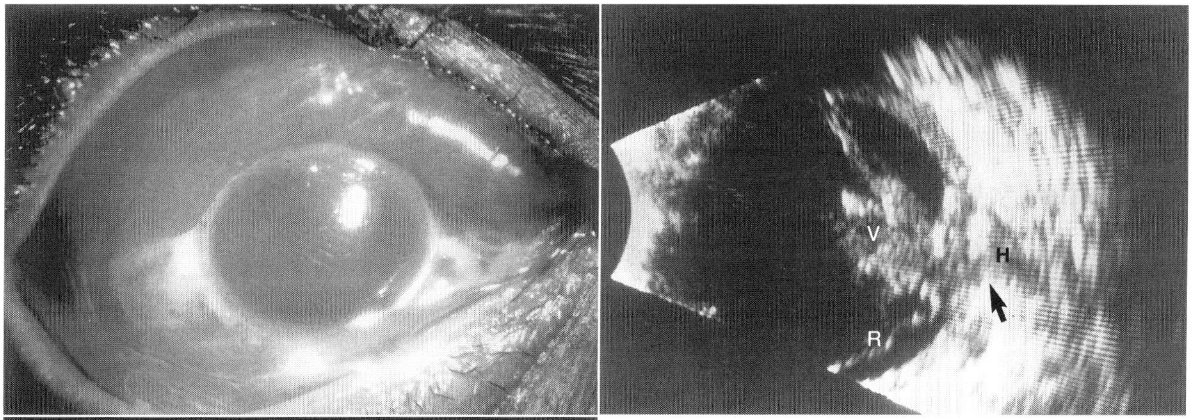

C

B

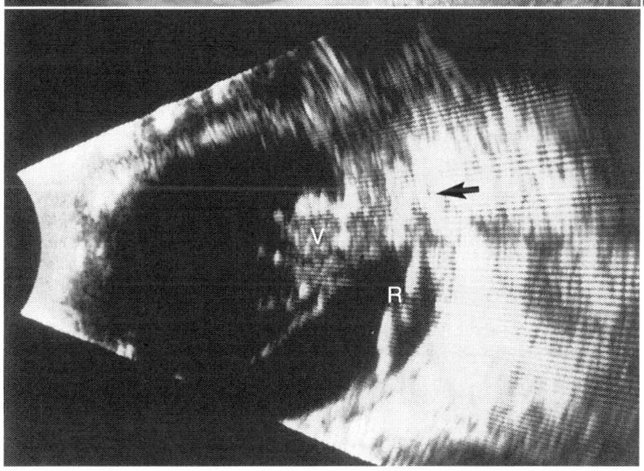

Figure 4-8 Scleral rupture following blunt trauma. **A,** External photograph showing anterior chamber hyphema and hemorrhagic chemosis. **B,** Longitudinal B-scan displays vitreous hemorrhage *(V)*, incarceration of vitreous into scleral rupture *(arrow)*, and inferior RD *(R)*. **C,** Transverse B-scan view through area of scleral rupture shows vitreous incarcerated into scleral wound and RD *(R)*. *H*, Orbital hemorrhage.

A

B

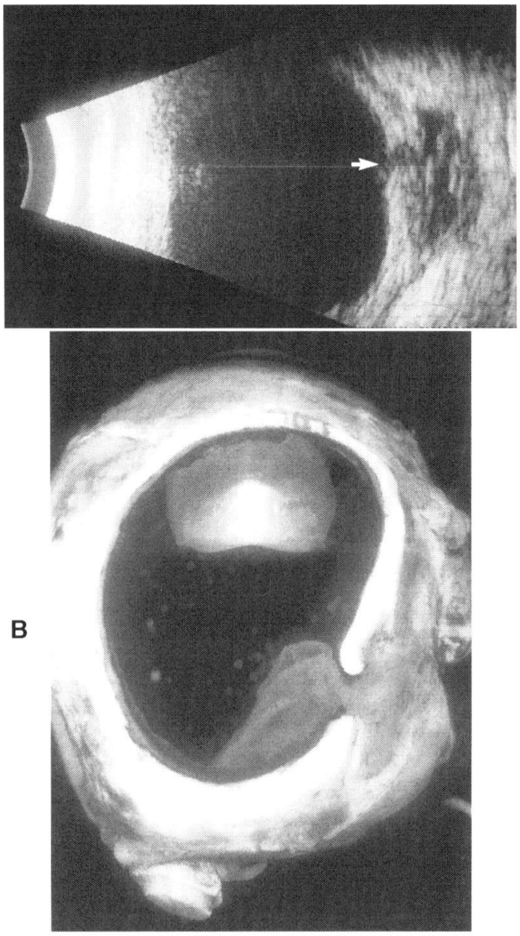

Figure 4-9 Large posterior scleral rupture following severe blunt trauma. **A,** Transverse B-scan shows large defect in posterior sclera *(arrow)* and adjacent extraocular cavity containing extruded retina. **B,** Gross pathology specimen demonstrates scleral rupture and extruded retinal tissue.

Hemorrhagic Choroidal Detachment

Hemorrhagic choroidal detachments commonly occur following a posterior scleral rupture. Moreover, experience has shown that the presence of a hemorrhagic choroidal detachment indicates that there has been a rupture of the globe.

Traumatic hemorrhagic choroidal detachments may be localized or quite extensive, even reaching the edge of the optic disc. Focal detachments are mildly dome-shaped, whereas those that are more extensive have a relatively flat configuration similar to those seen in penetrating injuries (see p 97). The exception to this rule is in aphakic eyes in which blunt trauma caused a corneal or limbal wound rupture or in pseudophakic eyes in which the IOL was extruded through a wound dehiscence. In these cases, the hemorrhagic choroidal detachments may be highly elevated and dome-shaped and may adhere centrally (kissing or appositional choroidal detachments) (see the section, "Expulsive Hemorrhage," on p 104). The presence of choroidal detachments can alter the timing of surgical intervention as well as the surgical approach.[3,4,16,25]

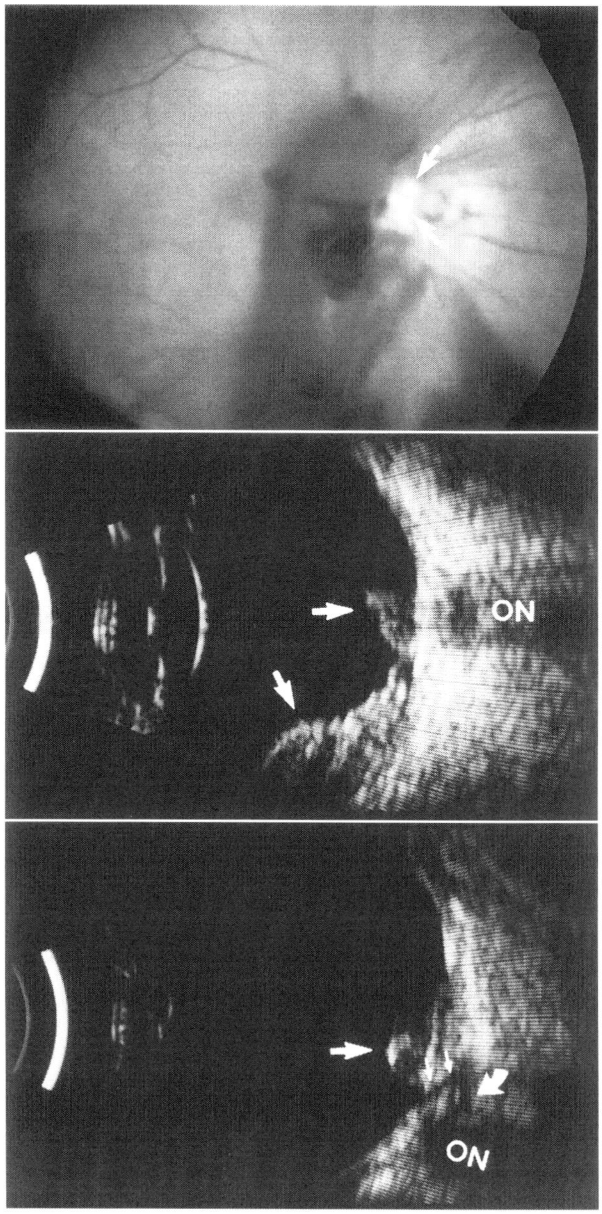

A

B

C

Figure 4-10 Acute avulsion of the left optic nerve following severe blunt trauma. Patient experienced immediate total loss of vision. **A,** Fundus photograph of left eye shows vitreous hemorrhage overlying optic disc and area of bare sclera *(arrows)* at edge of optic disc (not shown). **B,** Axial B-scan echogram shows vitreous hemorrhage emanating from optic disc and extending inferiorly *(arrows)*. *ON,* Optic nerve. **C,** Longitudinal B-scan along temporal fundus shows vitreous hemorrhage *(large straight arrow)*, thin scleral rupture at edge of optic disc *(small arrow)*, and small area of orbital hemorrhage *(curved arrow)*.

Avulsion of the Optic Nerve

Avulsion of the optic nerve is a rare sequela of blunt trauma. B-scan may show an actual break in the sclera near the optic disc (Figure 4-10). There can also be enlargement of the retrobulbar optic nerve (see p 429). In longstanding cases, proliferative membranes develop at the optic disc, and the

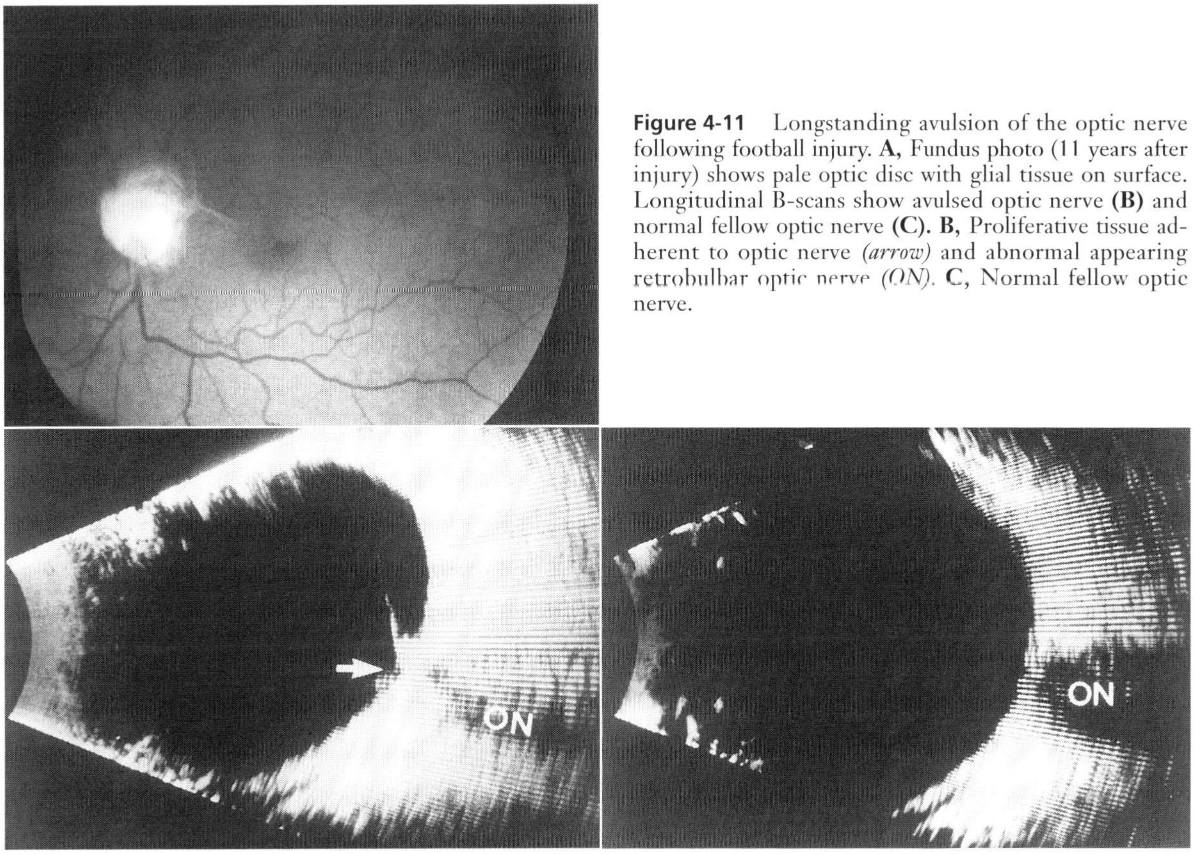

Figure 4-11 Longstanding avulsion of the optic nerve following football injury. **A,** Fundus photo (11 years after injury) shows pale optic disc with glial tissue on surface. Longitudinal B-scans show avulsed optic nerve **(B)** and normal fellow optic nerve **(C)**. **B,** Proliferative tissue adherent to optic nerve *(arrow)* and abnormal appearing retrobulbar optic nerve *(ON)*. **C,** Normal fellow optic nerve.

insertion of the optic nerve into the globe may appear atypical[10,13] (Figure 4-11).

PENETRATING TRAUMA

Penetrating ocular injuries can cause marked disruption and distortion of normal anatomical structures. Nevertheless, a systematic ultrasound examination will often yield useful information (Box 4-2).

Anterior Segment

Marked disruption of the anterior segment can occur following a penetrating injury. This can produce hyphema, iridodialysis, and disruption of the lens. Ultrasound can demonstrate many of these lesions and is ideal for determining the status of the anterior chamber, iris, and lens. Lens abnormalities that can be shown include cataractous changes (see Figure 4-2), subluxation/dislocation (Figure 4-12), lens capsule rupture (Figures 4-13 and 4-14), and reabsorption of lens material (Figure 4-15). Dislocation of an IOL can be determined as well (Figure 4-16). Cyclitic membranes may also be demonstrated posterior to the

BOX 4-2

Sequelae of Acute Penetrating Trauma

Anterior Segment

- Hyphema
- Shallow anterior chamber
- Iridodialysis
- Cataract
- (Sub)luxation of lens or IOL
- Lens capsule rupture
- Cyclitic membrane
- Ciliary body detachment

Posterior Segment

- Vitreous hemorrhage
- Posterior vitreous detachment
- Hemorrhagic track through the vitreous
- Incarceration of vitreous and/or retina
- Retinal detachment
- Posterior scleral rupture
- Hemorrhagic choroidal detachment
- Scleral fold

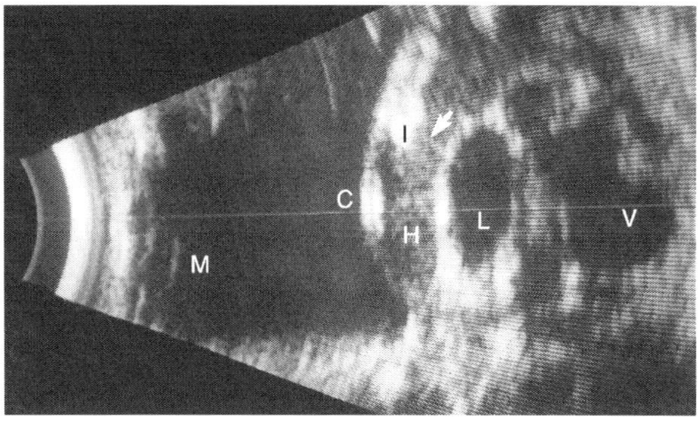

Figure 4-12 Hyphema, iridodialysis, and subluxation of lens following penetrating injury. Immersion axial B-scan echogram. *C*, Cornea; *H*, anterior chamber hyphema; *I*, iris; *L*, lens; *M*, methylcellulose within scleral shell; *V*, vitreous hemorrhage; *arrow*, iridodialysis.

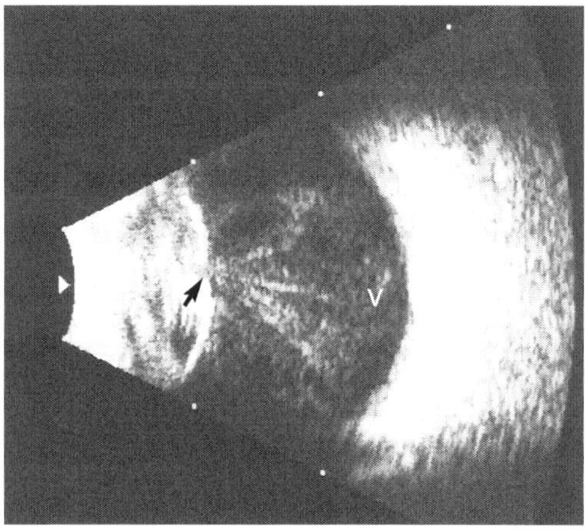

Figure 4-13 Posterior lens capsule rupture secondary to penetrating injury. Para-axial B-scan demonstrates rupture of posterior capsule *(arrow)* with incarceration of anterior vitreous. Note vitreous traction bands extending toward site of incarceration. *V*, Vitreous cavity.

A

C

B

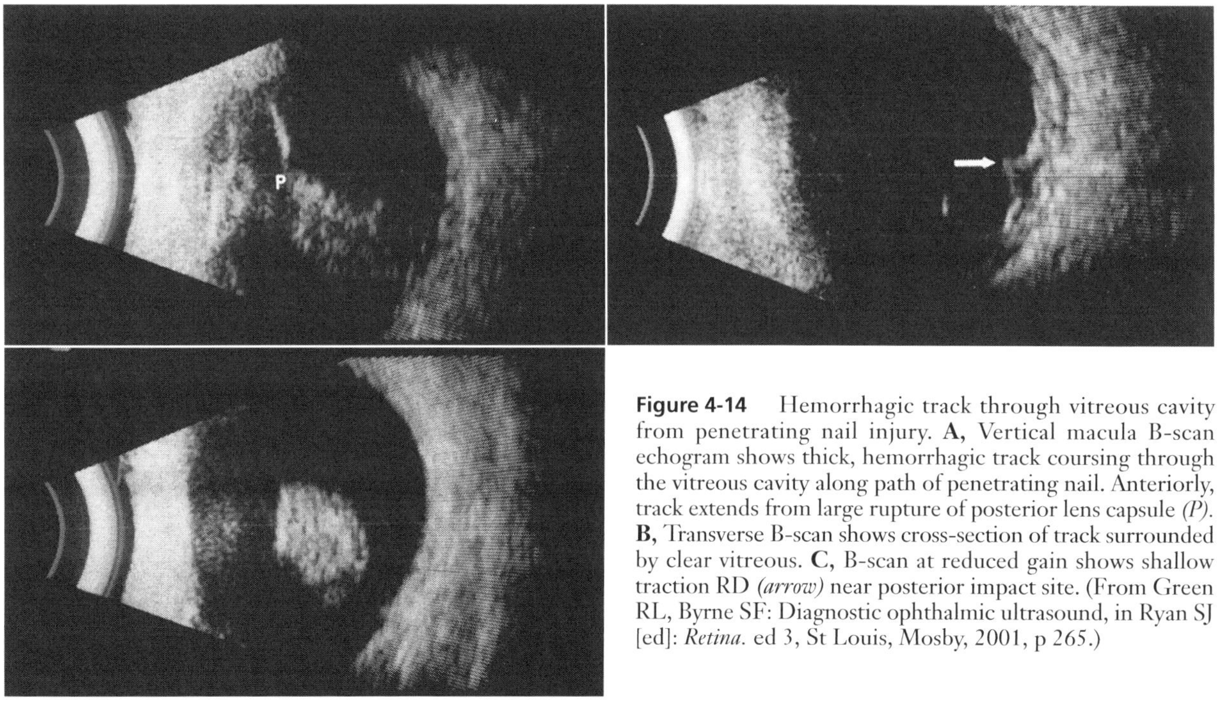

Figure 4-14 Hemorrhagic track through vitreous cavity from penetrating nail injury. **A,** Vertical macula B-scan echogram shows thick, hemorrhagic track coursing through the vitreous cavity along path of penetrating nail. Anteriorly, track extends from large rupture of posterior lens capsule *(P)*. **B,** Transverse B-scan shows cross-section of track surrounded by clear vitreous. **C,** B-scan at reduced gain shows shallow traction RD *(arrow)* near posterior impact site. (From Green RL, Byrne SF: Diagnostic ophthalmic ultrasound, in Ryan SJ [ed]: *Retina*. ed 3, St Louis, Mosby, 2001, p 265.)

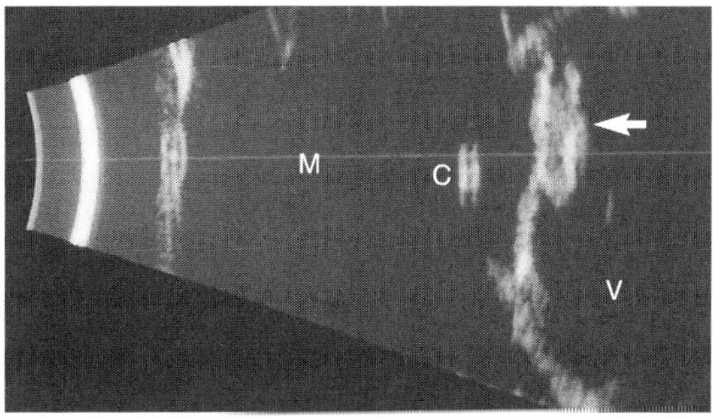

Figure 4-15 Marked disruption of lens following penetrating injury. Immersion axial B-scan echogram demonstrates residual lens material *(arrow)*. *C*, Cornea; *M*, methylcellulose within scleral shell; *V*, vitreous cavity.

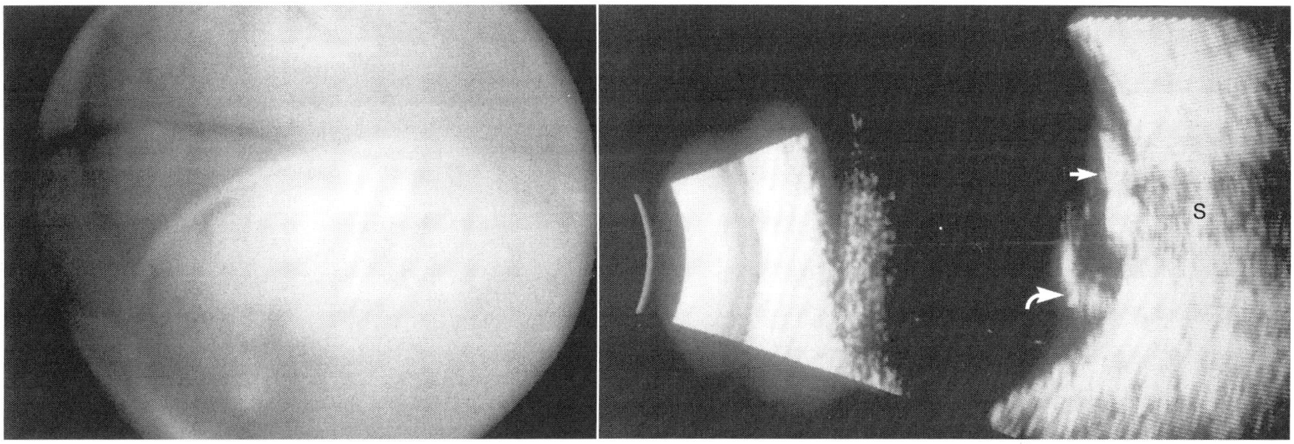

Figure 4-16 Dislocated IOL. **A,** Fundus photograph shows dislocated IOL on posterior retina. **B,** Transverse B-scan displays echodense dislocated lens *(straight arrow)* on posterior retinal surface. *S*, Shadowing from IOL; *curved arrow*, lens haptic. (Courtesy Dr. Barbara Blodi, Madison, Wisconsin, and Kathleen Meyer, RDMS, ROUB, Ann Arbor, Michigan.)

crystalline lens (see Figure 3-63), an IOL, or the iris (in aphakic eyes).

Ciliary body or ciliochoroidal detachments, either secondary to hypotony or the result of traction from cyclitic membranes, may be present (see Figure 3-61). Epithelial downgrowth is a rare complication of penetrating trauma. In this condition, a sheet of epithelial cells extends onto the surface of anterior segment structures. Occasionally, this downgrowth proliferates to form a cyst or solid mass that can be demonstrated by ultrasound (see p 177).

Posterior Segment

Vitreoretinal Injuries/Posterior Scleral Rupture

Penetrating injuries to the posterior segment frequently produce vitreous hemorrhage (see p 45). When a penetrating injury is caused by a sharp object (e.g., needle, nail, screwdriver, or pencil) or a projectile-type of foreign body, a hemorrhagic track through the vitreous cavity is usually present. The track appears as a bandlike structure that occurs along the path of the foreign object. The track may terminate in the vitreous or at an impact site in the fundus. In some cases, the track may lead to an intraocular foreign body (Figure 4-17), a posterior exit wound (posterior scleral rupture) (Figure 4-18), or a foreign body outside of the globe (Figure 4-19; see also Figure 17-9). Thickening or detachment of the retina and/or choroid is typically present near an impact site (see Figures 4-14 and 4-18).

Unless the sound beam is properly aligned with the track, it may not be displayed in its entirety and, therefore, may not be appreciated. Whenever there has been a penetrating injury, a careful search should be made for a hemorrhagic track. It is usually beneficial to know the location of the anterior entrance wound and the direction from which the foreign body entered the eye to determine its

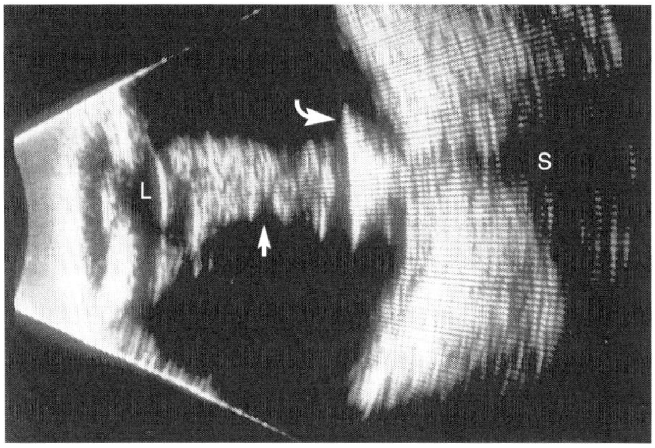

Figure 4-17 Hemorrhagic track produced by intraocular foreign body. Para-axial B-scan shows thick hemorrhagic track *(straight arrow)* extending from region of lens *(L)* and terminating at foreign body *(curved arrow)* located in front of posterior retina. Note foreign body shadow *(S)*, which simulates optic nerve.

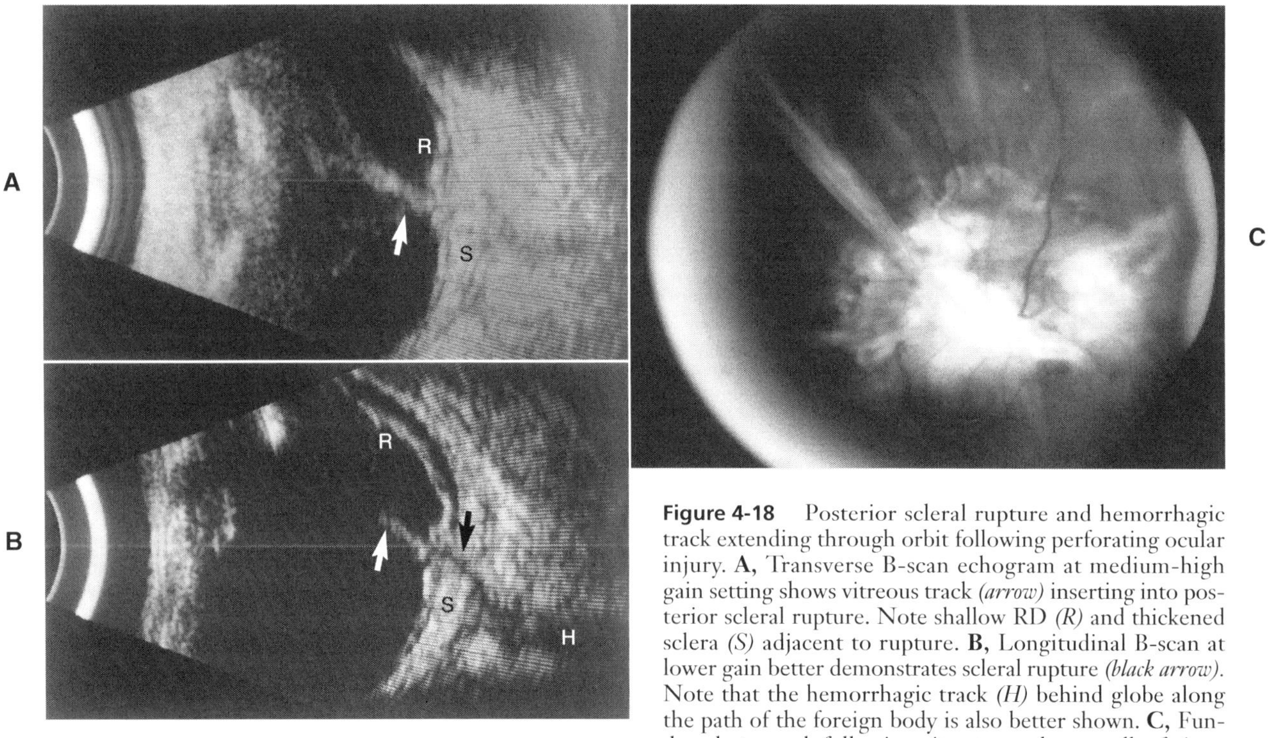

Figure 4-18 Posterior scleral rupture and hemorrhagic track extending through orbit following perforating ocular injury. **A,** Transverse B-scan echogram at medium-high gain setting shows vitreous track *(arrow)* inserting into posterior scleral rupture. Note shallow RD *(R)* and thickened sclera *(S)* adjacent to rupture. **B,** Longitudinal B-scan at lower gain better demonstrates scleral rupture *(black arrow)*. Note that the hemorrhagic track *(H)* behind globe along the path of the foreign body is also better shown. **C,** Fundus photograph following vitrectomy shows stalk of vitreous still attached to fundus in area of impact site.

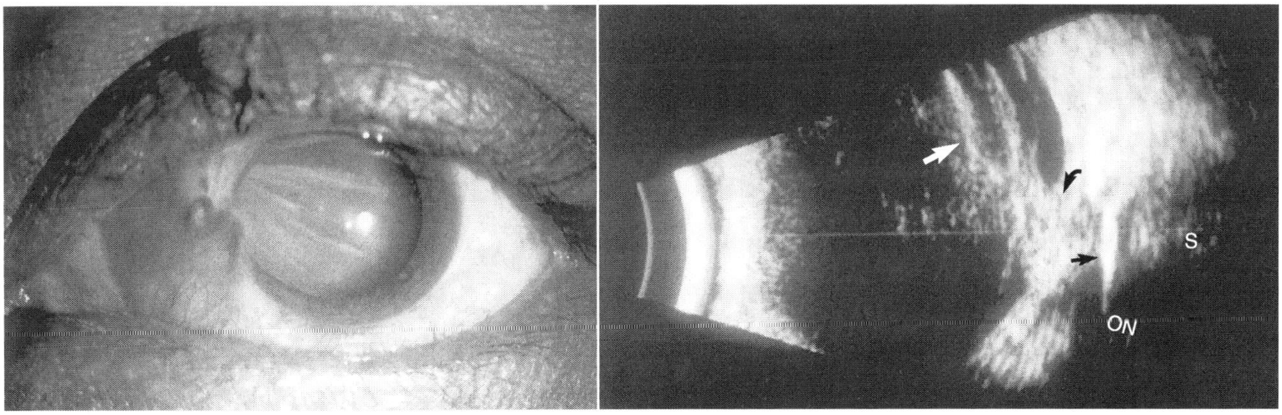

Figure 4-19 Perforating foreign body injury demonstrating vitreous incarceration. **A,** External photograph showing repaired corneoscleral wound and opacified anterior vitreous. **B,** Longitudinal B-scan demonstrates vitreous incarceration into posterior exit wound *(curved black arrow)* located adjacent to optic nerve *(ON)*. Note vitreous traction bands *(white arrow)* extending toward exit site. *Straight black arrow,* Extraocular foreign body; *S,* shadowing produced by foreign body.

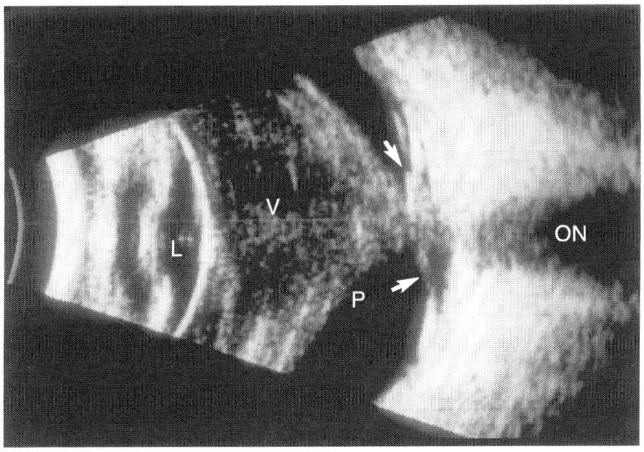

Figure 4-20 Traction RD following perforating foreign body injury (same case as in Figure 4-19). Axial B-scan echogram shows traction RD *(arrows)* adjacent to optic nerve *(ON)* produced by vitreous incarceration anteriorly. *L,* Lens; *P,* posterior hyaloid; *V,* vitreous hemorrhage.

path within the globe. This information can help determine proper probe positioning.

Ultrasound can often show vitreous incarceration at the site of a penetrating injury. When, however, there has been a perforating injury (both entrance and exit wounds), incarceration may be observed at both wound sites. As has been described for ruptured globes secondary to blunt trauma (see Blunt Trauma on p 87), the vitreous incarceration, regardless of location, usually forms traction bands that can be easily demonstrated echographically (see Figure 4-19). Once the origin of such traction bands has been determined, the opposite side of the globe should be evaluated to rule out traction RD.

Traumatic Retinal Detachment

Anterior penetrating injuries that lead to significant vitreous loss often result in traction on the posterior retina. Traction RDs can occur immediately following the injury, or they may develop subsequently (Figure 4-20). Frequent echographic follow-up is therefore very useful for detecting the onset of traction RD in eyes with vitreous incarceration.[18]

Rhegmatogenous RDs may develop at the site of penetration, and RDs with subretinal blood are a common finding following penetrating injury (see p 54).[18] Incarceration of the retina into a scleral wound can sometimes be demonstrated as well (Figure 4-21).

Hemorrhagic Choroidal Detachment

Hemorrhagic choroidal detachments can occur after a penetrating or perforating injury. In fact, the majority of globes with a scleral laceration develop an associated hemorrhagic choroidal detachment.

As described for scleral ruptures secondary to blunt trauma, hemorrhagic choroidal detachments occurring after penetrating trauma are usually only mildly to moderately elevated and have a slightly dome-shaped or flat configuration (Figure 4-22). They may be localized to the area of rupture, or they can be quite diffuse, extending posterior to the equator.

Scleral Folds

Sudden decompression of the globe, from a penetrating injury or a perforated corneal ulcer, may result in a collapse of the scleral wall. This collapse can produce scleral infolding that may be easily detected with echography.[19] Scleral folds are typically dome-shaped on B-scan, and the apex of the dome may be very highly reflective. In

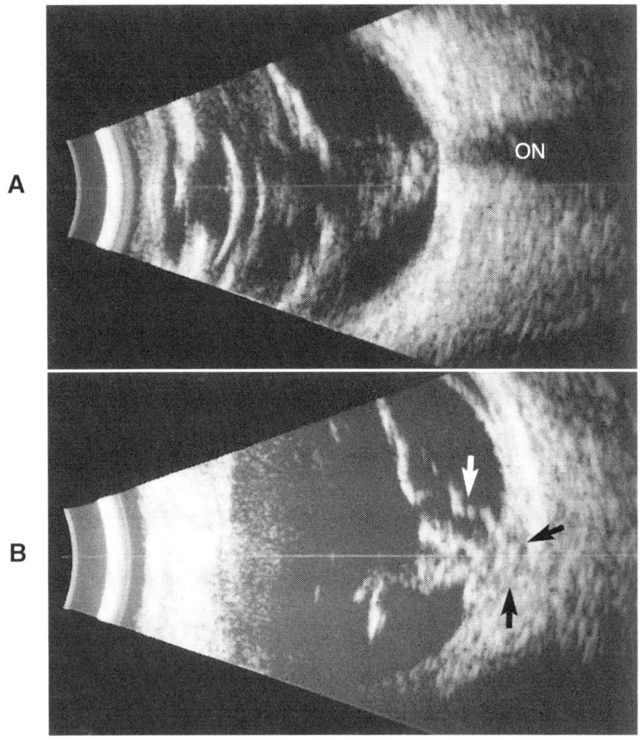

Figure 4-21 Retinal incarceration following penetrating injury (knife wound). **A,** Axial B-scan shows funnel-shaped RD inserting into optic nerve *(ON)*. **B,** Transverse B-scan view through inferior aspect of eye shows incarceration of retina *(white arrow)* into sclera *(black arrows)*.

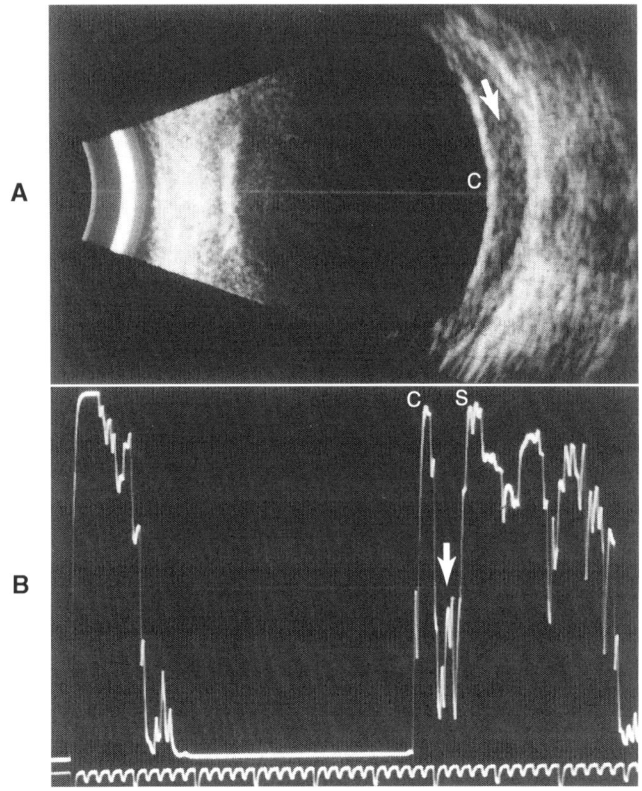

Figure 4-22 Shallow hemorrhagic choroidal detachment following penetrating injury. **A,** Peripheral transverse B-scan at reduced gain shows smooth, concave appearance of choroidal detachment *(C)* and opacities in suprachoroidal space *(arrow)*. **B,** Corresponding A-scan displays spikes beneath choroid *(arrow)* due to suprachoroidal hemorrhage. *S,* Sclera.

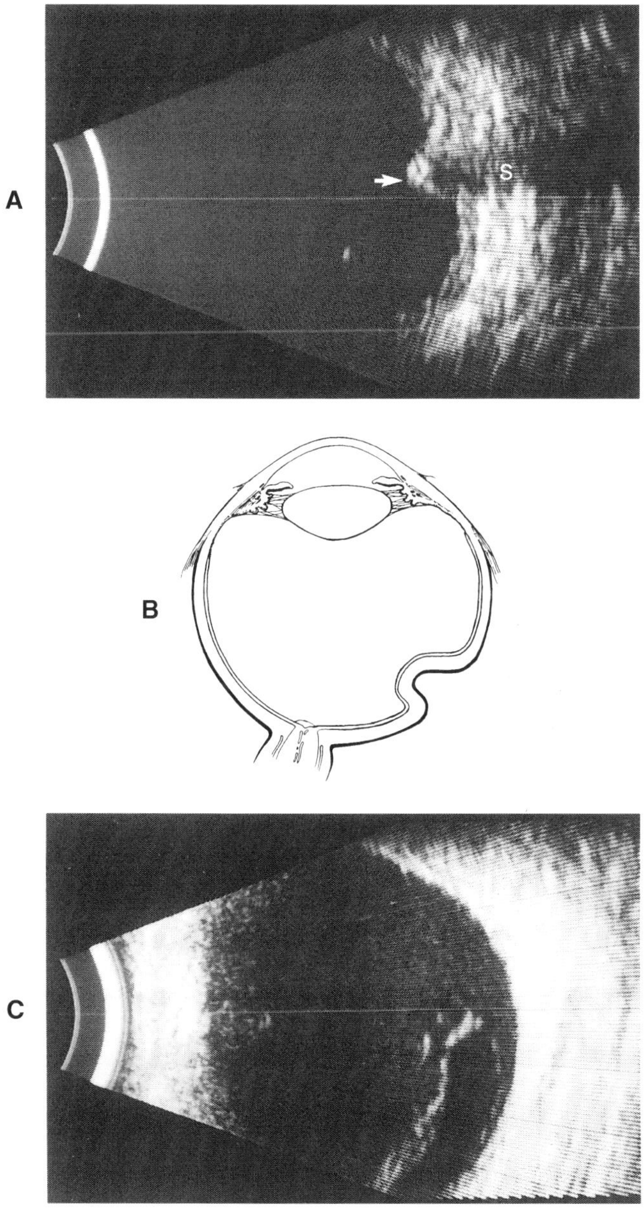

Figure 4-23 Scleral fold in patient with ruptured cataract wound (open eye at time of examination). **A,** Scleral infolding produces localized convex-shaped appearance *(arrow)*. The irregularly shaped sclera is highly reflective and produces shadowing *(S)*. This appearance may simulate an intraocular foreign body. **B,** Schematic drawing showing scleral fold. **C,** Same area of globe 3 days after wound repair shows resolution of fold. (**A** and **C** from Green RL, Byrne SF: Diagnostic ophthalmic ultrasound, in Ryan SJ [ed]: *Retina*. ed 3, St Louis, Mosby, 2001, p 262.)

addition, the folded sclera may produce shadowing of posterior orbital tissues (Figure 4-23; also see p 466). Scleral folds can be mistaken for choroidal detachments, foreign bodies, or scleral buckles. The presence of a scleral fold should be anticipated in an eye with very low intraocular pressure, (either from sudden decompression or secondary to severe inflammation).

BOX 4-3

Foreign Bodies Following Penetrating Trauma

Intraocular Foreign Bodies

Metallic
Spherical
Glass
Organic material
Air bubbles

Orbital foreign bodies (see p 439)

Foreign Bodies

Intraocular Foreign Bodies

Various types of intraocular foreign bodies are, in most instances, readily detectable with echography (Box 4-3).* Even when a foreign body has been previously localized by means of computed tomography (CT), ultrasound examination should be performed for more precise localization and for determination of the extent of intraocular damage. Moreover, if a foreign body is located next to the scleral wall, CT scanning may be unable to indicate whether it lies just within or just outside of the globe.

METALLIC FOREIGN BODIES

Although no two foreign bodies are exactly alike, the echographic findings for metallic foreign bodies (or other very hard substances) are generally similar. On B-scan, these foreign bodies produce a very echo-dense signal that persists at low gain settings. In addition, there is usually marked shadowing of the ocular and orbital structures just posterior to the foreign body (Figure 4-24). As mentioned previously (see p 95), the echographic detection of a foreign body can be facilitated if it has produced a hemorrhagic track within the eye (see Figure 4-17).

The examiner should be aware of two situations in which an intraocular foreign body may be overlooked during the ultrasound examination. First, shadowing from a foreign body located posteriorly can be confused with the optic nerve void, causing the foreign body to go undetected. To avoid this situation, it is important always to identify the optic nerve in relationship to the foreign body. Second, small foreign bodies (less than 0.5 mm in diameter or thin pieces of wire) may not produce obvious shadowing even though they can be quite echo-dense. In this case, other imaging studies may be important to help confirm the presence of a foreign body.

Metallic foreign bodies produce very high reflectivity on A-scan, regardless of the sound beam direction. In these cases, examination with the A-scan, using oblique sound beam incidence, can be helpful in confirming the presence of a foreign body.

*References 1, 2, 16, 22, 24, 27.

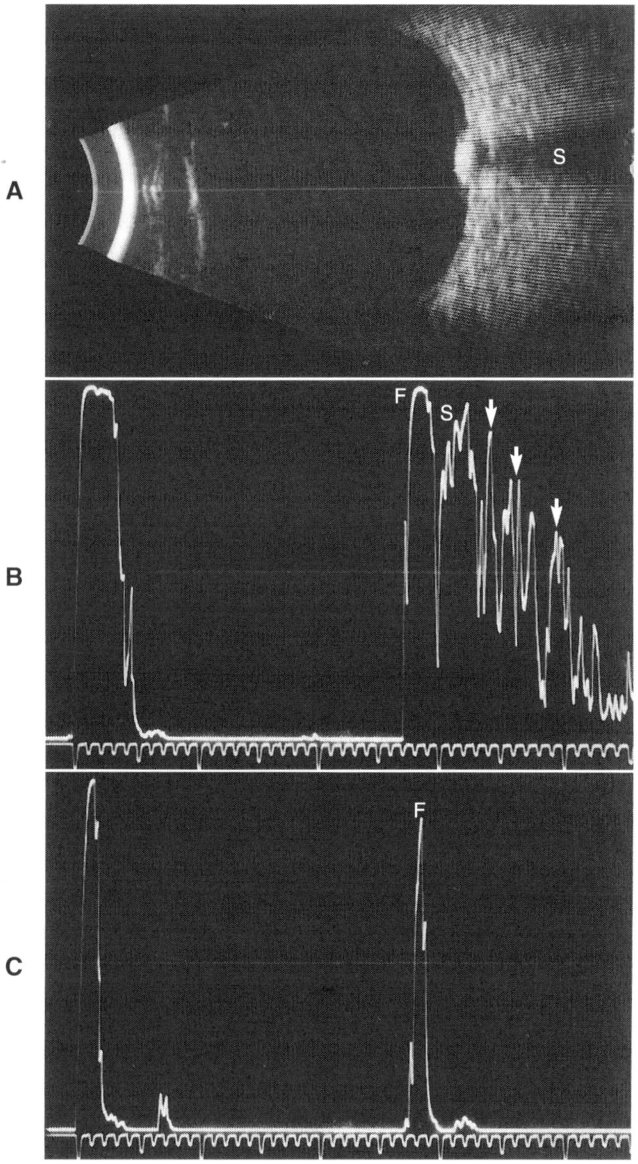

Figure 4-24 Metallic intraocular foreign body several years following injury. **A,** B-scan echogram shows foreign body on surface of retina and marked shadowing *(S)*. **B,** A-scan at Tissue Sensitivity shows thick, very highly reflective spike from foreign body *(F)* and decreased spike height of sclera *(S)* and orbital tissue *(arrows)* as a result of sound attenuation. **C,** Foreign body spike persists at a very low gain setting. (From Green RL, Byrne SF: Diagnostic ophthalmic ultrasound, in Ryan SJ [ed]: *Retina.* ed 3, St Louis, Mosby, 2001, p 267.)

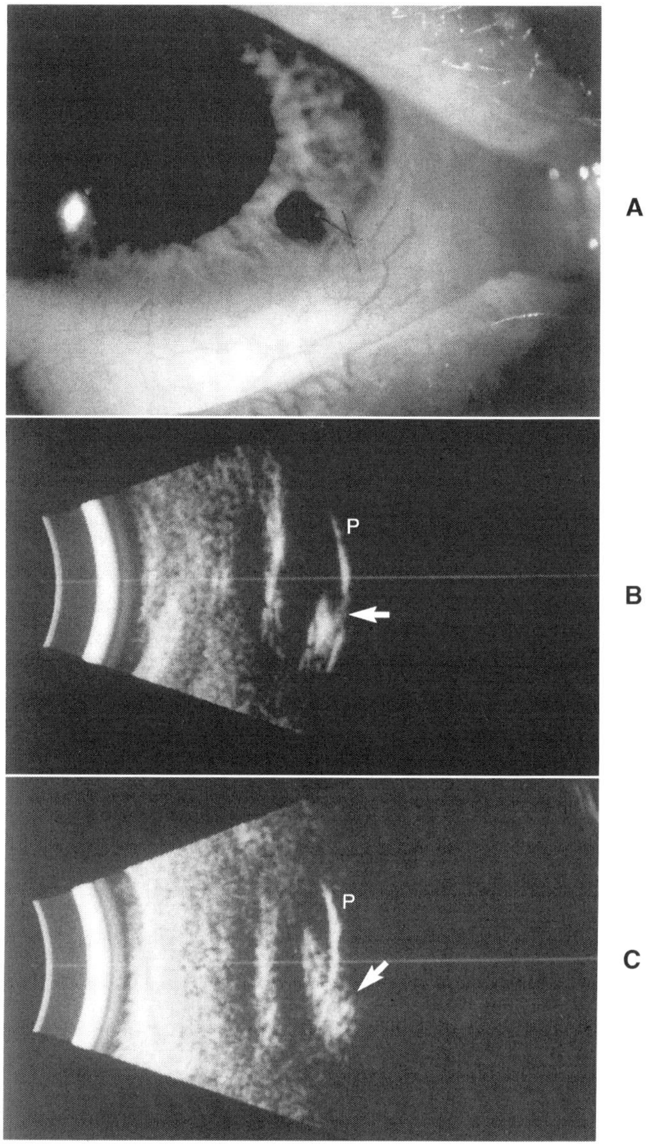

Figure 4-25 Intralenticular foreign body. **A,** External photograph showing perforation of iris. **B,** Vertical axial B-scan echogram at reduced gain shows small, echo-dense lesion *(arrow)* within lens. *P,* Posterior lens capsule. **C,** Horizontal axial B-scan shows long section of sliverlike foreign body protruding through posterior lens capsule.

Foreign bodies in the anterior segment, especially those in the lens, can often be detected with a contact technique (Figure 4-25; see also Figure 2-34). However, if the foreign body is small and is situated adjacent to the lens capsule, in the plane of the iris, or in the pars plicata, an immersion technique (see p 37) may be necessary for detection and localization. This technique, however, should be used only if the entrance wound has been sutured or has healed. Examination through the lids with a soft stand-off technique (see p 40) may also be necessary if the standard immersion method cannot be performed.

SPHERICAL FOREIGN BODIES

Spherical foreign bodies (e.g., BBs or gunshot pellets) produce unique and specific echographic signals.[22,27] When sound waves pass through a spherical, metallic for-

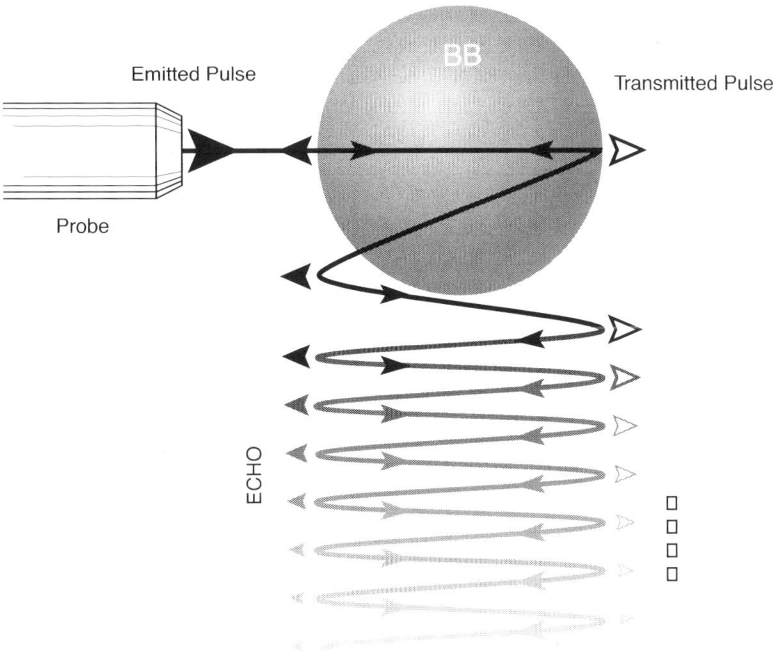

Figure 4-26 Schematic drawing shows reverberations from BB pellet. (Redrawn from Ossoinig KC: *Standardized Ophthalmic Echography of the Eye, Orbit and Periorbital Region. A Comprehensive Slide Set and Study Guide.* ed 3, Iowa City, Goodfellow, 1985, p 12.)

A

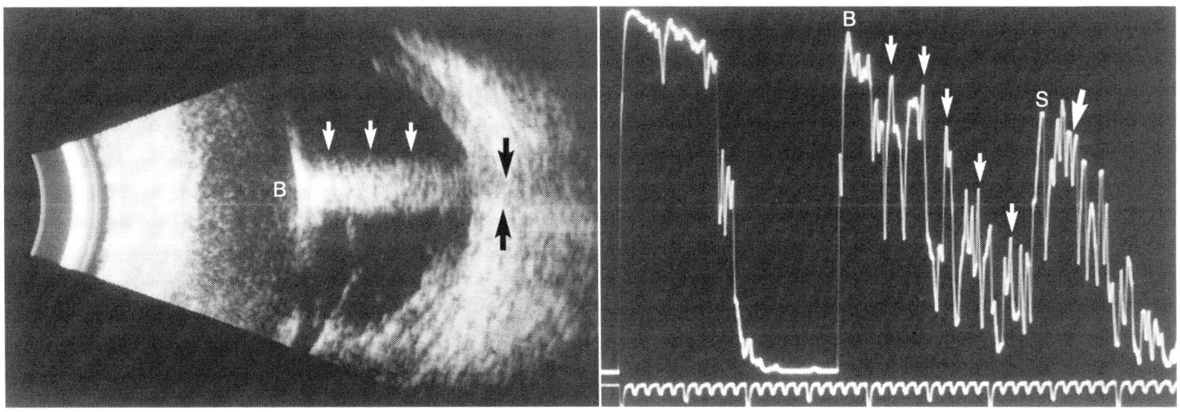

B

Figure 4-27 Intraocular BB. **A,** Transverse B-scan echogram shows BB *(B)* in center of vitreous cavity followed by characteristic chain of multiple signals (comet tail artifact) *(small white arrows)*. Note mild shadowing of sclera and orbital signals *(black arrows)*. **B,** Corresponding A-scan echogram. Note decreased height of sclera *(S)* and orbital spikes *(large arrow)* due to sound attenuation.

eign body, a portion of the sound wave reverberates within the object. Each time a reverberation occurs, some of the sound energy passes back to the transducer, producing a series of echo signals of decreasing amplitude that appear to the right of the foreign body echo (i.e., reduplication or multiple signals) (Figure 4-26). On B-scan, this chain of multiple signals is referred to as a comet tail artifact. As the sound beam strikes the foreign body, this chain of multiple signals appears instantly on the screen, thus allowing very easy detection and localization of this specific type of foreign body (Figures 4-27 and 4-28).

GLASS AND ORGANIC MATERIAL

Glass foreign bodies exhibit certain unique echographic characteristics. In most cases, glass enters the eye as a sliver. When the sound beam strikes the long, smooth surface of a glass sliver with an oblique incidence, most of the sound is reflected away from the probe, resulting in the display of only a weak echo. For this reason, a relatively large piece of glass may be completely missed or mistaken for a small foreign body. Only when the sound beam is directed perpendicular to the long, flat surface of the glass sliver is a very echo-dense signal displayed that accurately indicates the foreign body's density and size

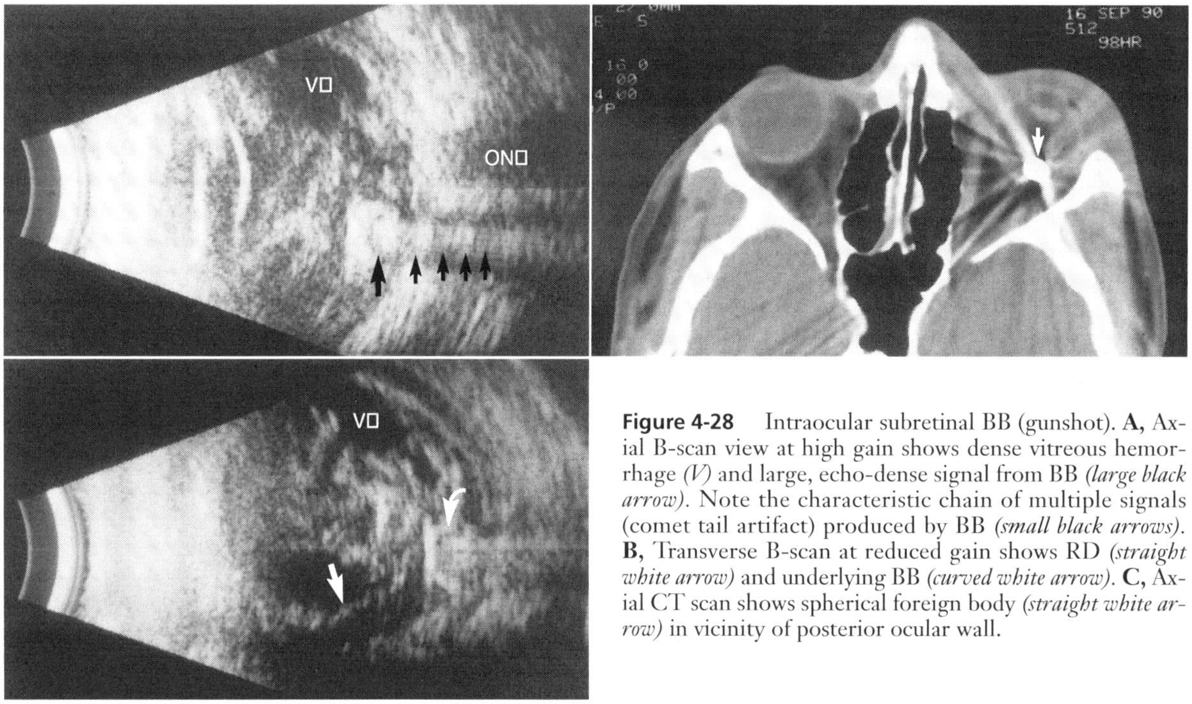

Figure 4-28 Intraocular subretinal BB (gunshot). **A,** Axial B-scan view at high gain shows dense vitreous hemorrhage *(V)* and large, echo-dense signal from BB *(large black arrow)*. Note the characteristic chain of multiple signals (comet tail artifact) produced by BB *(small black arrows)*. **B,** Transverse B-scan at reduced gain shows RD *(straight white arrow)* and underlying BB *(curved white arrow)*. **C,** Axial CT scan shows spherical foreign body *(straight white arrow)* in vicinity of posterior ocular wall.

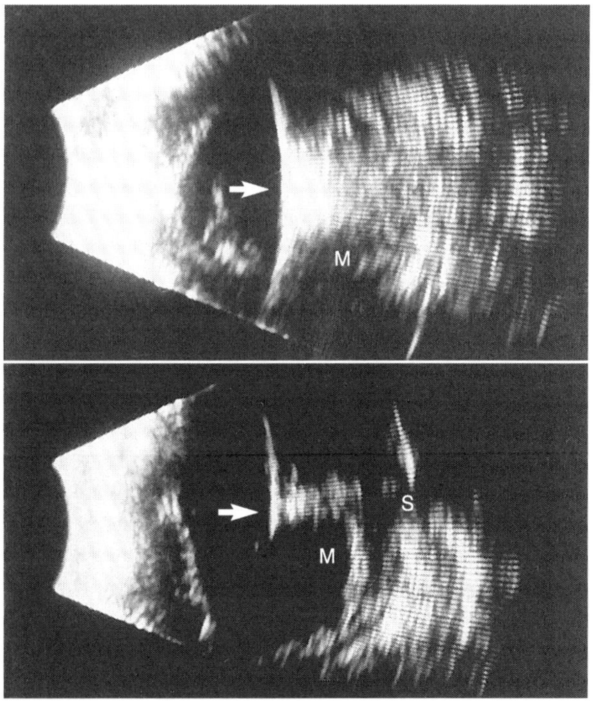

Figure 4-29 Intraocular glass splinter. **A,** Sound beam aligned with length of splinter *(arrow)*. **B,** Cross-section through splinter. Note multiple signals *(M)* produced by the glass foreign body and shadowing of sclera and orbital tissue *(S)*. (From Green RL, Byrne SF: Diagnostic ophthalmic ultrasound, in Ryan SJ [ed]: *Retina*. ed 3, St Louis, Mosby, 2001, p 268.)

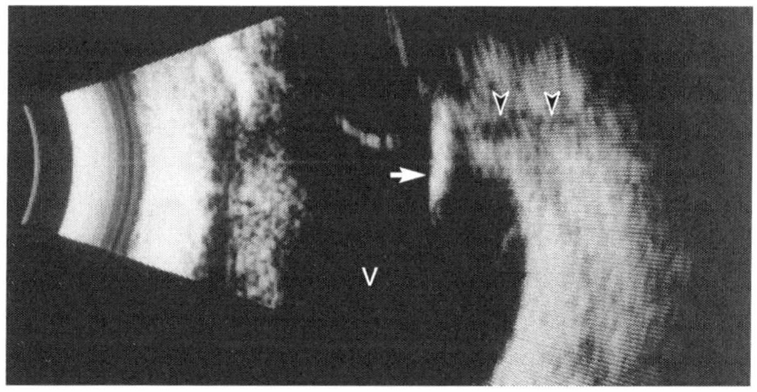

Figure 4-30 Intraocular thorn (from brambleberry bush). Longitudinal B-scan shows thorn as echo-dense line *(closed arrow)* in anterior aspect of vitreous cavity *(V)*. Open arrows indicate shadowing produced by thorn. (Courtesy Dr. Barbara Blodi, Madison, Wisconsin, and Kathleen Meyer, RDMS, ROUB, Ann Arbor, Michigan.)

(Figure 4-29). Therefore, when a glass foreign body is suspected, it is essential that a very thorough screening examination be performed to ensure accurate detection and localization.

Wood or other types of vegetable matter can produce various echographic findings, depending on their size and density (Figure 4-30). Initially, these foreign bodies may be highly reflective, but their reflectivity may decrease over time, thus making detection extremely difficult.

Penetrating ocular injuries may introduce eyelashes (cilia)

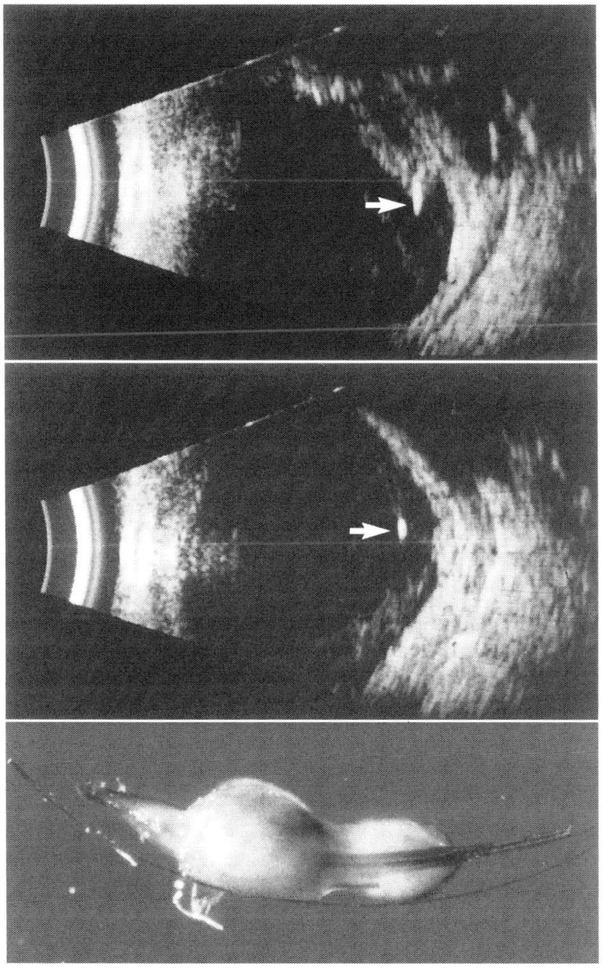

Figure 4-31 Intraocular cilia following penetrating injury. **A,** Anterior longitudinal B-scan echogram along 6-o'clock meridian shows thin, foreign body-like echo *(arrow)* corresponding to cilia. **B,** Transverse B-scan view shows cross-section of cilia. **C,** Photograph showing encapsulated cilia that was removed during vitrectomy.

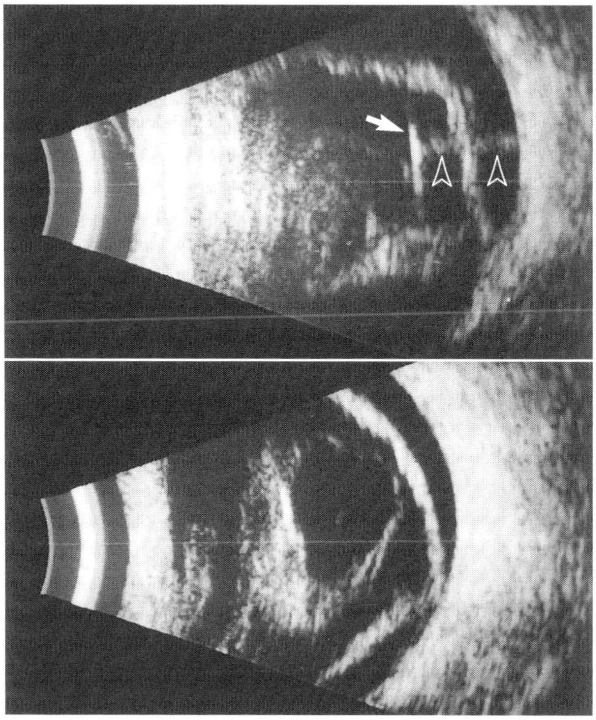

Figure 4-32 Intraocular air following penetrating injury. **A,** Transverse B-scan view through superior globe immediately following repair of penetrating injury shows highly reflective foreign bodylike signal *(arrow)* produced by intraocular air bubble. *Open arrows,* Multiple signals. **B,** Transverse B-scan echogram through same section of globe 2 days later shows complete resolution of bubble. (From Green RL, Byrne SF: Diagnostic ophthalmic ultrasound, in Ryan SJ [ed]: *Retina.* ed 3, St Louis, Mosby, 2001, p 269.)

into the eye. These foreign bodies typically show a thin, elongated shape on B-scan. They do not produce shadowing but appear relatively echo-dense (Figure 4-31). The possibility of an eyelash foreign body should always be considered when examining an eye following a penetrating injury.

AIR BUBBLES

Small air bubbles may enter the globe as a result of a penetrating ocular injury. These focal, point-like echo sources are extremely high reflective, resulting in echograms that are similar to those of true intraocular foreign bodies. Like spherical foreign bodies, they can produce multiple signals (Figure 4-32) as well as shadowing (Figure 4-33, *A*).

Certain findings may help to differentiate air bubbles from true foreign bodies. The first clue may be the display of more than one foreign bodylike echo when the history indicates that only one foreign body should be present (Figure 4-33, *B*). In addition, there are some differences between the acoustic properties of air bubbles and those of true intraocular foreign bodies. The majority of true foreign bodies are irregularly shaped; consequently, their echoes may differ slightly in appearance when examined from different sound beam directions. Moreover, true foreign bodies generally do not move, even when the patient's head or body position is changed. Conversely, air bubbles, because of their spherical and smooth nature, produce echoes of similar appearance when evaluated from different sound beam orientations. And since they are normally found in the vitreous cavity and are lighter than vitreous, they tend to move opposite to the direction of head tilt. If the diagnosis is uncertain, a follow-up examination, performed a day or two later, may be of great help because small air bubbles usually disappear within this time period (see Figure 4-32).

Orbital Foreign Bodies

See p 439 in Chapter 17 for a review of orbital foreign bodies.

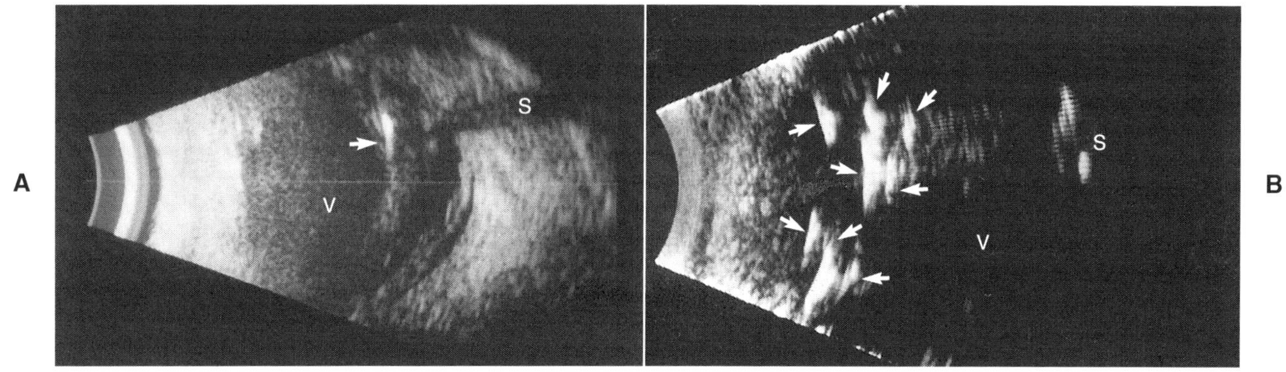

Figure 4-33 Two examples of intraocular air following recent penetrating injury. **A,** Single bright echo corresponding to intra-vitreal air bubble *(arrow)*. Note shadowing *(S)* produced by air bubble. *V,* Vitreous cavity. **B,** Axial B-scan echogram (through closed lids at reduced gain) shows numerous bright echo signals *(arrows)* from small air bubbles. These echoes moved freely as the patient shifted body position.

> **BOX 4-4**
> ### Surgical Trauma (Complications)
> Endophthalmitis/uveitis (see pp 191 and 194)
> Expulsive hemorrhage
> Retained lens material
> Dislocated IOL
> Macular edema (see p 67)
> Penetrating needle injuries of the eye
> Sympathetic ophthalmia (see p 201)
> Epithelial downgrowth and inclusion (implantation) cyst (see Figures 5-80 and 5-92)

SURGICAL TRAUMA (COMPLICATIONS)

Ultrasound is an important adjunct for evaluating some of the complications that follow intraocular surgery. Many of the possible findings (e.g., vitreous hemorrhage or RD) have already been described in Chapter 3. Other complications (Box 4-4) will be described in this chapter and elsewhere in the book.

Endophthalmitis/Uveitis

See Chapter 6 for a review of endophthalmitis and uveitis.

Expulsive Hemorrhage

One of the most devastating complications of intraocular surgery is an expulsive hemorrhage. In this condition, massive suprachoroidal hemorrhagic detachments can partially or totally fill the vitreous cavity. In some cases, a massive hemorrhagic choroidal detachment may involve only one or two quadrants of the eye (Figure 4-34). In more severe cases, however, 360 degree choroidal detachments may adhere in the central aspect of the vitreous cavity, producing an appositional (kissing) configuration.

On B-scan, these large, dome-shaped membranes can be seen to adhere to one another in the central portion of the eye. These detachments may extend to the posterior pole, inserting next to rather than into the optic disc (Figure 4-35).

Massive hemorrhagic choroidal detachments also can occur on a delayed basis following intraocular surgery in aphakic or pseudophakic eyes. These are most likely to occur following glaucoma procedures (see p 218) or corneal transplant surgery. Expulsive hemorrhagic choroidal detachments also may be observed following rupture of the globe, in either aphakic or pseudophakic eyes.

In some cases, the hemorrhagic choroidal detachments are so massive and the hemorrhage so dense that it may be extremely difficult to detect them with B-scan. The echographic findings in these cases are sometimes confused with very dense vitreous hemorrhage. A B-scan sign that is occasionally helpful in detecting hemorrhagic choroidal detachments is the presence of spontaneous motion from blood vessels on the surface of the choroidals. In some cases, reducing the gain level may allow better resolution of the closely adherent choroidal surfaces (Figure 4-36).

Echography can be used to follow the course of hemorrhagic choroidal detachments and to help determine whether intervention is indicated and, if so, when it should be undertaken.[3,4] Studies have shown that many of these detachments separate after a few weeks, although shallow detachments may persist for months.[3,4,25] It is of note that shallow RDs may occur at the posterior aspect of highly el-

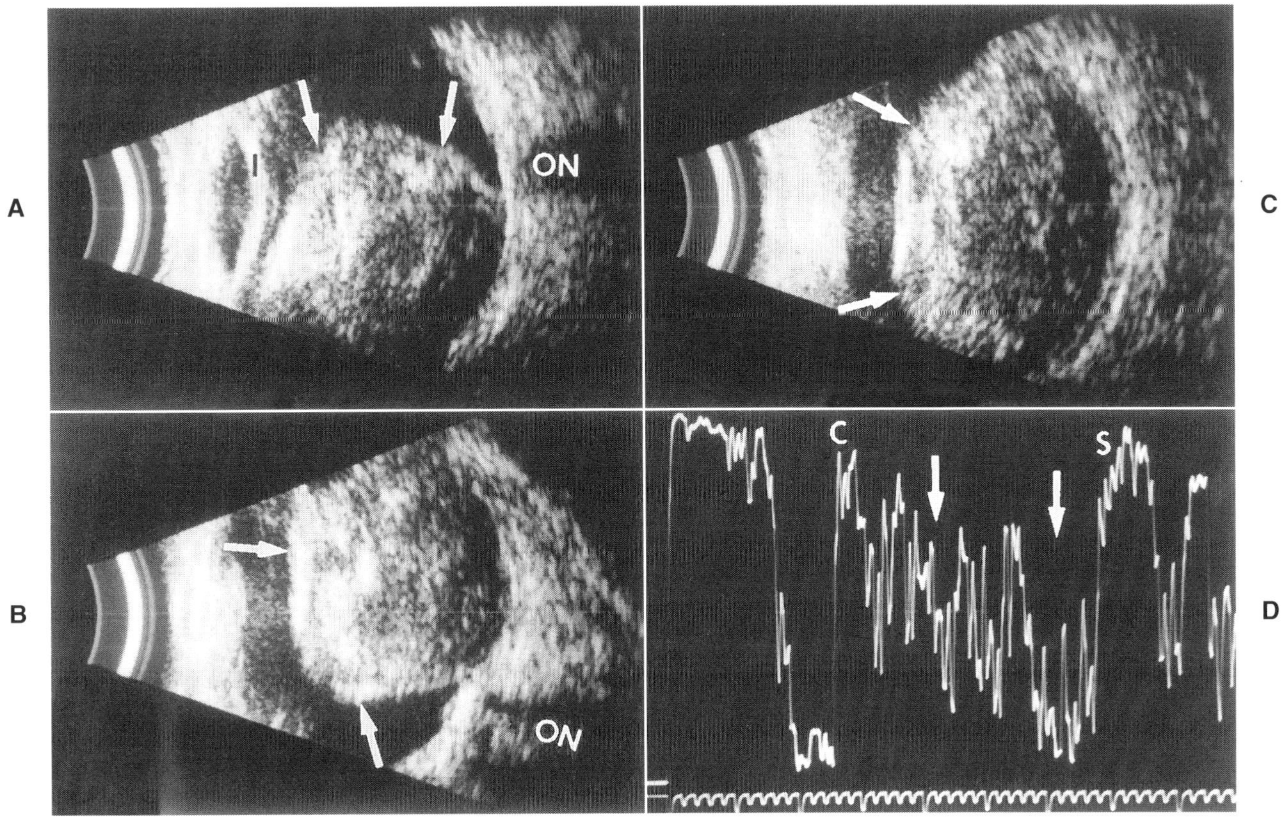

Figure 4-34 Large hemorrhagic choroidal detachment resulting from expulsive hemorrhage at the time of cataract surgery. **A,** Horizontal axial B-scan echogram shows highly elevated, hemorrhagic choroidal detachment *(arrows)* extending from temporal aspect of globe and overlying optic nerve *(ON)*. *I,* Iris. **B,** Longitudinal B-scan view along temporal meridian shows large hemorrhagic choroidal detachment. **C,** Transverse B-scan view through temporal periphery of eye shows large, dome-shaped choroidal detachment. **D,** A-scan of choroidal detachment *(C)* in area of greatest elevation from the sclera *(S)*. Note medium-high internal reflectivity and decreasing spike height (due to sound attenuation) produced by clotted blood in suprachoroidal space *(arrows)*.

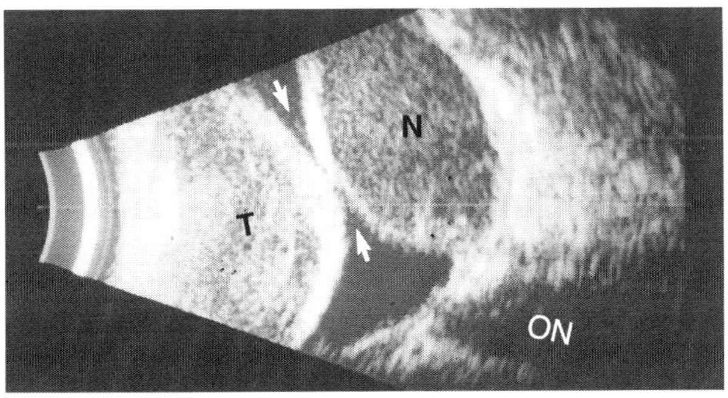

Figure 4-35 Appositional (kissing) hemorrhagic choroidal detachments. Longitudinal B-scan of 3-o'clock meridian in right eye demonstrates highly elevated nasal *(N)* and temporal *(T)* choroidal detachments adhering in central aspect of vitreous cavity *(arrows)*. *ON,* Optic nerve. Note dense hemorrhage in suprachoroidal space.

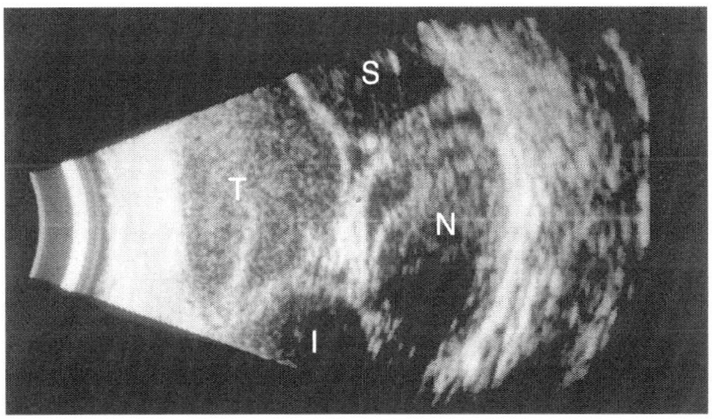

Figure 4-36 Appositional (kissing) hemorrhagic choroidal detachments. Peripheral transverse B-scan at reduced gain shows 360-degree massive choroidals with temporal *(T)*, superior *(S)*, nasal *(N)*, and inferior *(I)* detachments meeting in the central vitreous cavity and almost completely obliterating the vitreous space. This example shows that typical configuration in which the nasal and temporal detachments adhere to one another in the central aspect of the vitreous cavity.

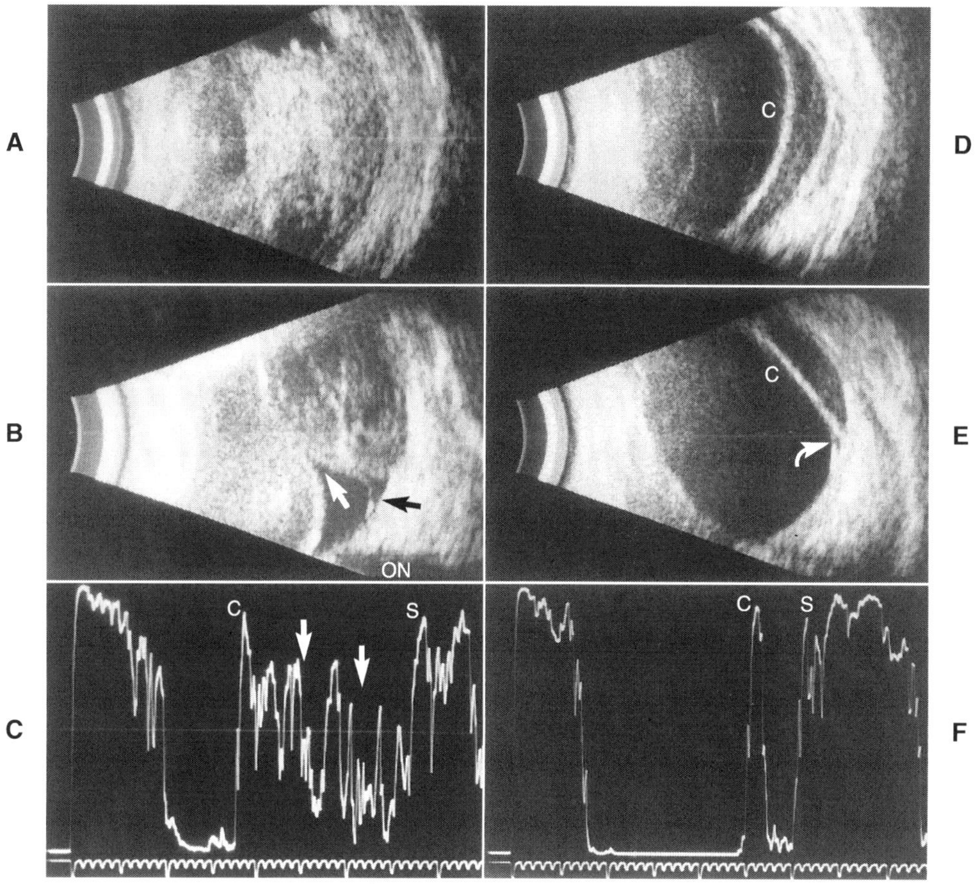

Figure 4-37 Massive appositional (kissing) hemorrhagic choroidal detachments immediately following expulsive hemorrhage (**A** to **C**) and at follow-up examination (**D** to **F**). **A,** Transverse B-scan. Note that surfaces of choroidal detachments cannot be identified because of their marked adherence centrally. **B,** Longitudinal B-scan view shows central adherence of choroidals *(white arrow).* Note sharp posterior insertion of choroidals near optic nerve *(ON)* and shallow RD *(black arrow).* **C,** A-scan of hemorrhagic choroidal *(C)* shows medium-high internal reflectivity *(arrows)* of clotted suprachoroidal blood. *S,* Sclera. **D,** Transverse B-scan corresponding to **A** shows marked reduction and concave appearance of choroidal detachment. **E,** Longitudinal B-scan corresponding to **B** also shows marked decrease in choroidal detachment. Note that very shallow RD is still present at posterior edge of choroidal detachment *(curved white arrow).* **F,** A-scan corresponding to **C** shows decreased elevation of detachment and very low reflectivity of fluid blood in suprachoroidal space.

evated hemorrhagic choroidal detachments. In some cases, these detachments may be caused by the mass effect of the choroidal detachments. As the choroidals resolve, these RDs tend to decrease and/or resolve (Figure 4-37).

In most cases of large, hemorrhagic choroidal detachments, highly reflective solid blood clots are initially present in the suprachoroidal space. Over time, however, these clots diminish in size and become lower reflective (Figure 4-38).

The echographic documentation of clot appearance and size may be useful in determining the optimal timing for drainage. Also, as these choroidal detachments decrease in size, RDs may become echographically apparent. Delayed hemorrhagic choroidal detachments often flatten out completely, with residual retinal traction only in the periphery. This is in contrast to surgical or traumatic expulsive hemorrhages, in which RDs are often present after the choroidal detachments have begun to resolve.[3,4]

Retained Lens Material

When rupture of the posterior capsule occurs during cataract surgery, cortical lens material, lens nucleus fragments, or the entire lens nucleus may fall back into the vitreous gel. The cortical material and nuclear fragments typically appear echographically as irregularly shaped, medium to high reflective opacities of varying size in the vitreous cavity (Figure 4-39). The lens nucleus is usually oval in shape. Inflammatory vitreous opacities and/or membranes are normally associated with retained lens material (Figure 4-40). A dislocated lens nucleus may adhere to the retina, and, thus,

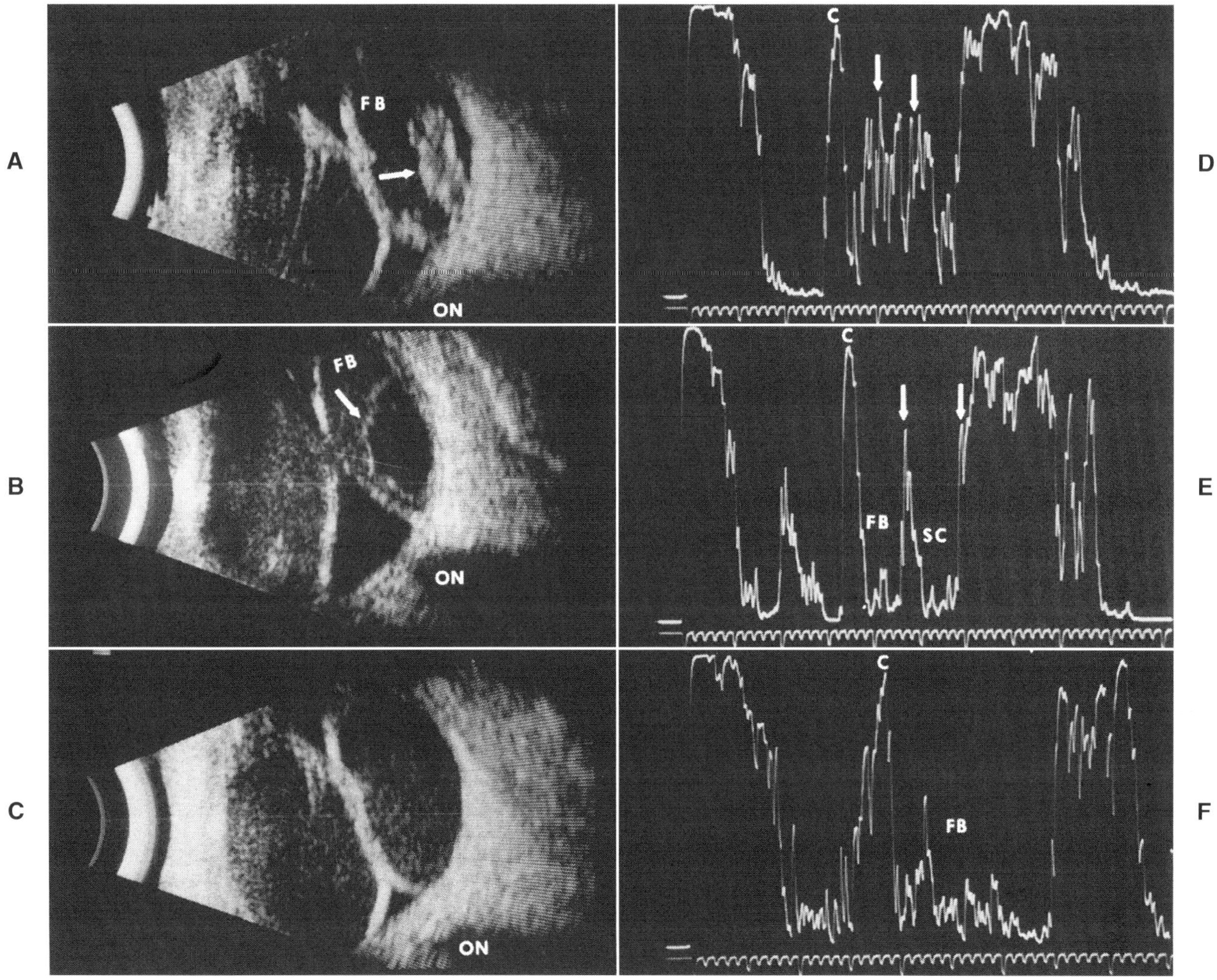

Figure 4-38 Massive appositional (kissing) hemorrhagic choroidal detachments demonstrating clot lysis. Longitudinal B-scan and corresponding A-scan echograms are from three different patients showing various stages of clot lysis. **A,** B-scan 2 days after hemorrhage shows large, dense, solid clot *(arrow)* surrounded by fluid blood *(FB)* in suprachoroidal space. *ON,* Optic nerve. **B,** B-scan of second patient 7 days after hemorrhage also shows solid clot surrounded by fluid blood in the suprachoroidal space. Note that this older clot appears echolucent, whereas the fresher clot in **A** is more echo-dense. **C,** B-scan from third patient obtained 2 weeks after choroidal hemorrhage shows complete resolution of solid clot, with fluid blood completely filling suprachoroidal space. **D,** A-scan corresponding to **A** shows choroidal detachment *(C)* and medium-high reflectivity of suprachoroidal solid clot *(arrows).* **E,** A-scan corresponding to **B** shows low reflectivity of both fluid blood *(FB)* and solid clot *(SC). Arrows,* Borders of SC. **F,** A-scan corresponding to **C** shows low reflectivity of fluid blood. (From Green RL, Byrne SF: Diagnostic ophthalmic ultrasound, in Ryan SJ [ed]: *Retina.* ed 3, St Louis, Mosby, 2001, p 271.)

A

B

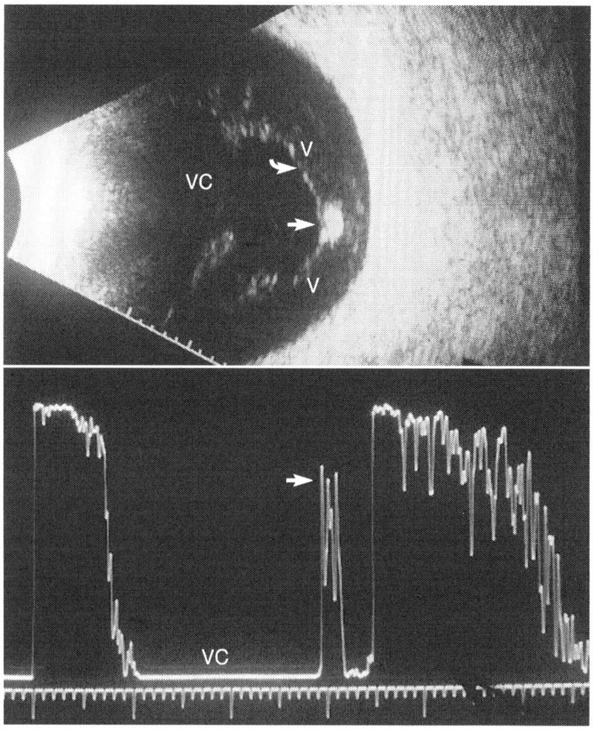

Figure 4-39 Retained lens fragments following cataract surgery and anterior vitrectomy. **A,** Transverse B-scan displays relatively large, echo-dense, irregularly shaped lens fragment *(straight arrow)* within residual vitreous gel *(V)*. Curved arrow, inner surface of remaining vitreous skirt. *VC,* Vitrectomy cavity created by removal of anterior vitreous gel. **B,** Lens fragment produces medium-high reflective, multi-peaked spike on A-scan.

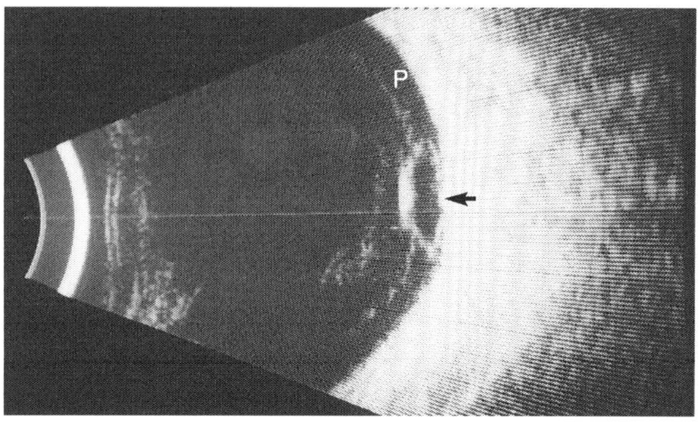

Figure 4-40 Dislocated lens nucleus following cataract surgery. Transverse B-scan shows oval-shaped echolucent lens nucleus on surface of retina *(arrow)*. Note attachment of posterior hyaloid *(P)* to nucleus.

unlike a dislocated intact lens (see Figure 5-77), it may not move during kinetic echography.

Dislocated Intraocular Lens

An IOL may sometimes dislocate posteriorly, and in these cases, it appears as a large, foreign body–like structure within the vitreous cavity (see Figure 4-16).

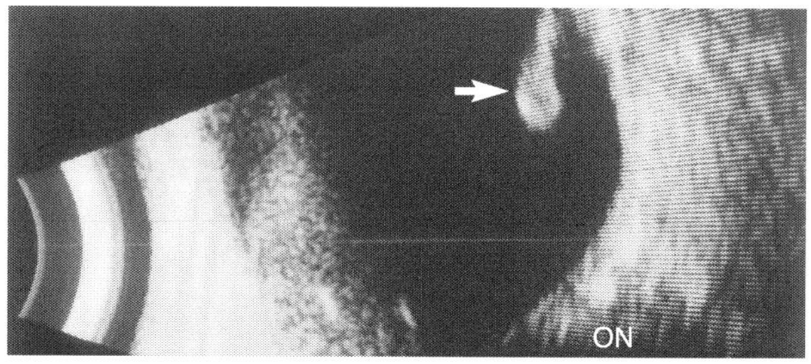

Figure 4-41 Inadvertent injection of steroid into the vitreous cavity. Longitudinal B-Scan shows echo-dense, well-circumscribed appearance of Depo-Medrol *(arrow)*. *ON,* Optic nerve.

Macular Edema

See p 67 in Chapter 3 for a review of macular edema.

Penetrating Needle Injuries of the Eye

Inadvertent penetration of the eye can occur during retrobulbar or sub-Tenon's injections. A variety of echographic findings may be present following this event.[9,14] In some cases, because of the sharp needles used, only minimal findings, such as mild vitreous hemorrhage and localized PVD, may be observed. In other cases, however, vitreous incarceration, retinal and choroidal detachments, and scleral thickening may be detected. The inadvertent injection of steroids into the vitreous cavity has also been shown with echography (Figure 4-41).

Sympathetic Ophthalmia

See Chapter 6 for a review of sympathetic ophthalmia.

Epithelial Downgrowth and Inclusion (Implantation) Cyst

Epithelial downgrowth or implantation of epithelial cells may occur following intraocular surgery or penetrating trauma. This can result in the formation of masslike lesions (see p 177) or the development of epithelial inclusion cysts involving the iris or ciliary body (see p 170).

POSTSURGICAL FINDINGS

Certain echographic findings may be present after intraocular surgery. These findings are due to changes in the anatomy of the globe as a result of the surgical procedure and to various types of implants or devices that may be inserted in or around the eye (Box 4-5). Familiarity with these findings and the related artifacts that may occur is necessary to avoid misdiagnosis. In addition, the ultrasound examination may help to clarify a vague or inadequate clinical history.

BOX 4-5

Postsurgical Findings

IOL
Scleral buckle
Vitreous skirt/vitreous hemorrhage
Intraocular gas/air
Perfluorocarbon
Intraocular silicone
Glaucoma-filtering implant devices (shunts) (see p 218)
Ganciclovir implant (see Figure 6-23)

Intraocular Lens Implants

IOLs can create strong artifacts that may complicate the echographic examination of the posterior segment. The smooth, highly reflective surface of the lens implant produces numerous multiple signals that can hinder visualization of the vitreous cavity and posterior fundus when an axial A- or B-scan approach is used (Figure 4-42). To evaluate the posterior segment of these eyes reliably, the probe must be placed peripheral to the limbus.

Scleral Buckle

Scleral buckling procedures produce indentation of the ocular wall. Reflectivity of the buckle varies, depending on the type of scleral buckle used. A solid silicone buckle produces a very highly reflective surface that is indistinguishable from the sclera. The interior of the silicone buckle, however, is echolucent on B-scan and low reflective on A-scan. A scleral sponge, on the other hand, produces highly reflective surface signals, and the sponge material is echo-dense and highly reflective. Both types of buckle produce strong sound attenuation and orbital shadowing (Figures 4-43 and 4-44). A silicone encircling band indents the globe only minimally and extends around the globe circumferentially. These thin bands usually cause only mild sound attenuation. Longitudinal views are usually the best means of demonstrating the presence of an RD extending posteriorly from the buckle margin (see Figure 6-14).

Vitreous Skirt/Vitreous Hemorrhage

Residual vitreous gel may remain in the periphery of the eye following a vitrectomy. This remnant of the vitreous body (i.e., vitreous skirt) can easily be missed on an ultrasound examination if the far periphery of the eye is not adequately evaluated. In addition, if the residual vitreous gel is detected but is not correctly identified, it can be confused with a peripheral RD.

The unique topography of a vitreous skirt usually facilitates its recognition. A transverse B-scan section through the far periphery of the globe typically shows the circumferential configuration of the vitreous skirt. A longitudinal B-scan section, on the other hand, shows that the gel remains attached at the vitreous base, with its posterior surface moving freely in the vitreous cavity (Figure 4-45, *A* and *B*). The internal reflectivity of the remaining vitreous gel is very low, appearing echolucent on B-scan.

In a vitrectomized eye, a diffuse hemorrhage in the vitreous cavity usually produces very weak echoes because the blood remains in a liquefied state and does not become clumped as it does in the vitreous gel. Therefore, when examining a vitrectomized eye, it is important to use high gain settings to assess the vitreous cavity for the presence of hemorrhage (Figure 4-45, *C* and *D*).

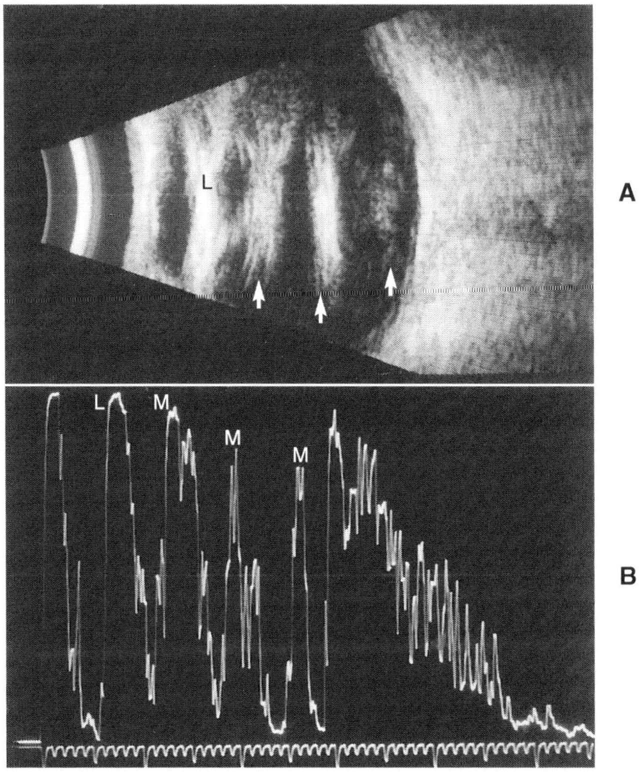

Figure 4-42 IOL producing multiple signals. **A,** Axial B-scan echogram shows bright anterior echo from an IOL implant *(L)*. Note multiple signals *(arrows)* produced by reverberations between the lens implant and probe face. **B,** A-scan shows highly reflective spike from IOL implant *(L)* and spikes of decreasing height from the multiple signals *(M)*. (From Green RL, Byrne SF: Diagnostic ophthalmic ultrasound, in Ryan SJ [ed]: *Retina.* ed 3, St Louis, Mosby, 2001, p 300.)

Intraocular Gas/Air

Large gas or air bubbles located in the vitreous cavity may hinder or prevent echographic examination of the posterior segment. This occurs because gas or air strongly reflects the sound waves and thus precludes imaging of any structures located posterior to the bubble (shadowing). Multiple signals, produced by reverberations between the probe and bubble, are also typically present. In some cases, the bubble may be small enough to allow a

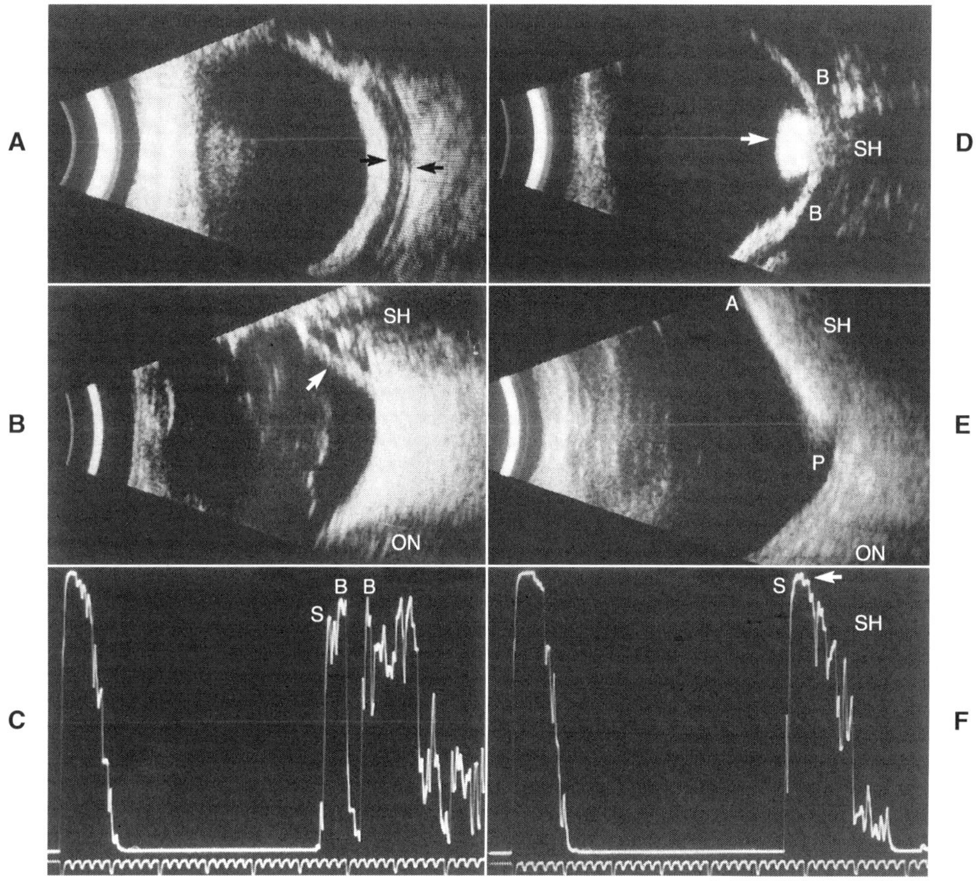

Figure 4-43 Circumferential solid scleral buckle (**A** to **C**) and radial scleral sponge (**D** to **F**). **A,** Peripheral transverse B-scan echogram shows echolucent area corresponding to scleral buckle as it surrounds the globe *(black arrows).* **B,** Anterior longitudinal B-scan view shows cross section of buckle *(white arrow)* near the equator. The buckle is indenting the globe and produces shadowing *(SH)* of the orbital tissue. *ON,* Optic nerve. **C,** Corresponding A-scan shows low internal reflectivity of solid silicone buckle. *B,* Buckle surfaces; *S,* sclera. **D,** Peripheral transverse B-scan at very low gain shows cross-section of radial sponge that is markedly indenting globe *(white arrow).* The solid scleral buckle *(B)* lies adjacent to the sponge. *SH,* Shadowing. **E,** Longitudinal B-scan demonstrates the anterior *(A)* and posterior *(P)* extent of the echo-dense sponge. **F,** Corresponding A-scan shows highly reflective sponge *(arrow)* adjacent to sclera *(S).*

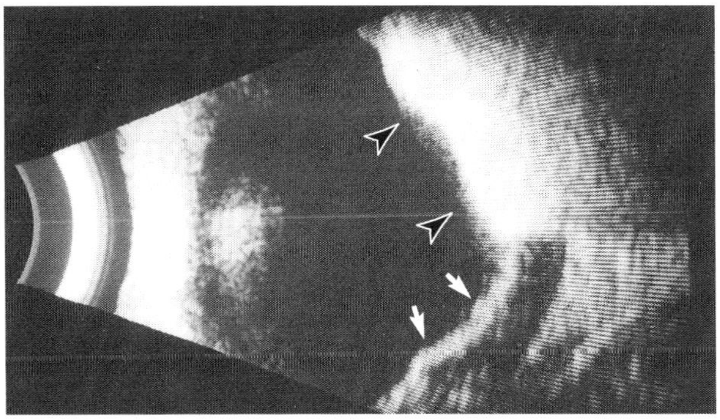

Figure 4-44 Circumferential scleral sponge and solid scleral buckle. Transverse B-scan at equator shows sponge *(open arrows)* adjacent to solid buckle *(closed arrows)*.

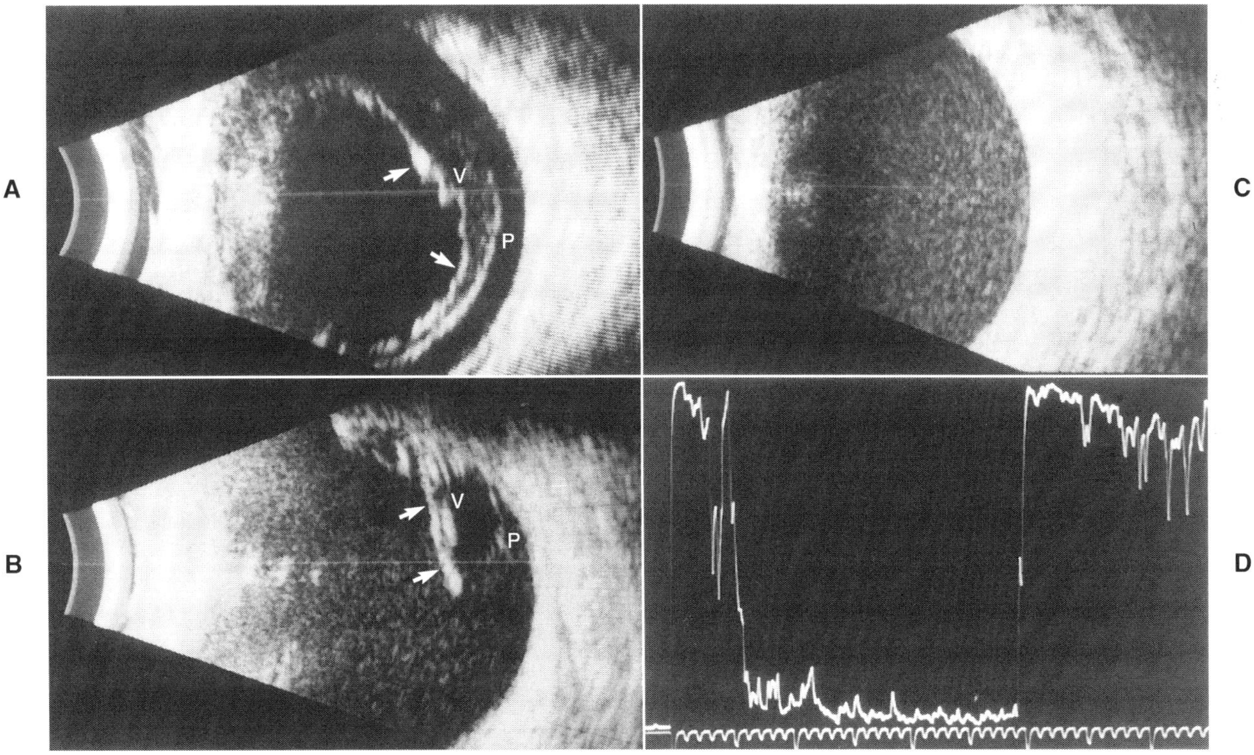

Figure 4-45 Recurrent hemorrhage and residual vitreous gel following vitrectomy for diabetic retinopathy. **A,** Peripheral transverse B-scan shows core of remaining vitreous gel (vitreous skirt). *P,* Detached posterior hyaloid; *V,* vitreous gel; *arrows,* inner surface of peripheral vitreous skirt. **B,** Anterior longitudinal B-scan echogram shows cross-section of vitreous skirt attached to vitreous base. Note diffuse vitreous opacities from recurrent vitreous hemorrhage detected at this high gain setting. **C** and **D** are from a different patient. **C,** Transverse B-scan at a very high gain shows diffuse opacities from the fluid blood within the vitreous cavity. **D,** Corresponding A-scan (also at very high gain setting) shows a chain of low reflective spikes corresponding to the fluid vitreous blood.

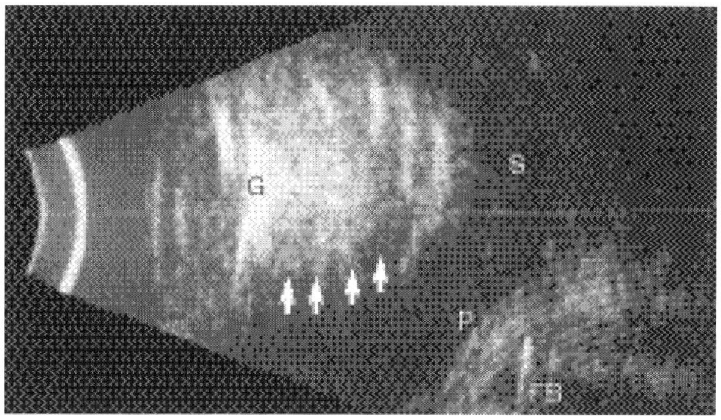

Figure 4-46 Intraocular gas bubble *(G)* after vitrectomy. The gas bubble is producing multiple signals *(arrows)* as well as total shadowing and obscuration of the adjacent ocular and orbital tissues *(S)*. The sound beam, however, partially bypasses the large anterior bubble and penetrates a small portion of the posterior globe *(P)*. An orbital foreign body *(FB)* is located just posterior to the globe inferiorly. (From Green RL, Byrne SF: Diagnostic ophthalmic ultrasound, in Ryan SJ [ed]: *Retina*. ed 3, St Louis, Mosby, 2001, p 300.)

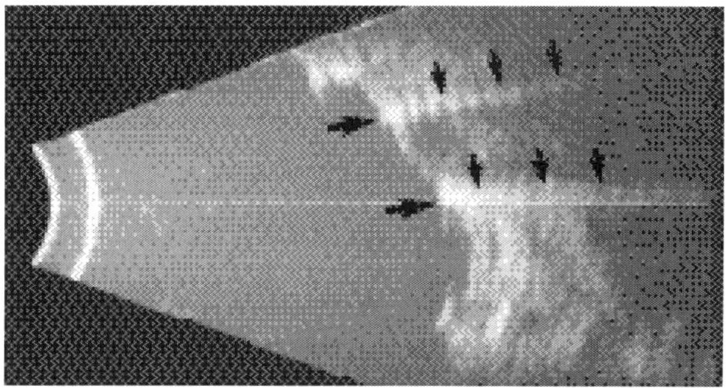

Figure 4-47 Retained intraocular perfluorocarbon bubble following vitrectomy surgery. B-scan shows two chains of multiple signals *(small arrows)* emanating from bubbles on surface of retina *(large arrows)*.

portion of the fundus to be imaged. However, it is often necessary to have the patient either sit upright or tilt their head so as to move the bubble away from the central axis of the eye. This frequently allows at least the posterior aspect of the vitreous cavity, fundus, and optic disc to be evaluated (Figure 4-46). A follow-up examination is often helpful in these eyes since gas and air bubbles dissipate over time. Mirror-image artifacts[29] may occasionally be encountered in these eyes.

Perfluorocarbon

Residual perfluorocarbon bubbles may remain in the eye following vitrectomy surgery. These bubbles have a tendency to adhere to the surface of the fundus. On B-scan, they appear as small, bright echoes followed by a prominent chain of multiple signals[20] (Figure 4-47).

Intraocular Silicone

The sound velocity of silicone oil is much slower than that of normal ocular tissue and the majority of intraocular lesions (see Table 10-2).[5,28] Consequently, echograms of silicone-filled eyes typically appear much larger than normal. Silicone may also produce significant sound attenuation, thus hindering reliable evaluation of the posterior segment (Figure 4-48). Although techniques for detecting RDs in eyes with silicone oil have been reported,[28] experience indicates that ultrasound is generally not reliable for detecting detachments in these eyes. See p 265 for a discussion of silicone oil and the measurement of axial eye length.

Glaucoma-Filtering Implant Devices (Shunts)

See p 218 in Chapter 7 for a review of glaucoma-filtering shunts.

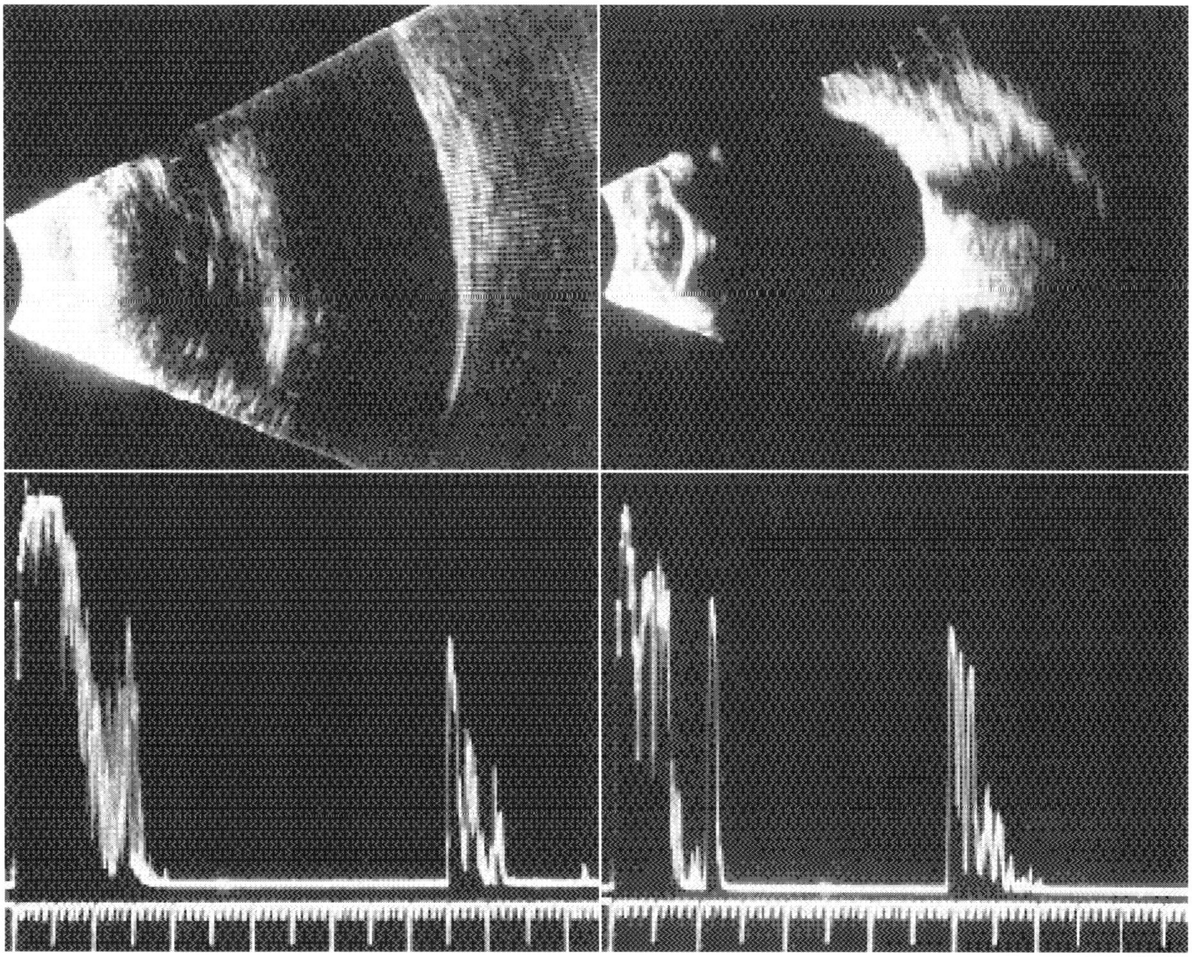

Figure 4-48 A- and B-scan echograms of globe filled with silicone oil (**A** and **B**) and normal fellow eye (**C** and **D**) at same screen expansion. Silicone oil produces marked sound attenuation, preventing resolution of the posterior ocular wall and orbital contents. The sound velocity in the silicone oil is significantly slower than that of aqueous and vitreous, which causes echograms to appear larger than normal. (From Green RL, Byrne SF: Diagnostic ophthalmic ultrasound, in Ryan SJ [ed]: *Retina.* ed 3, St Louis, Mosby, 2001, p 301.)

A

B

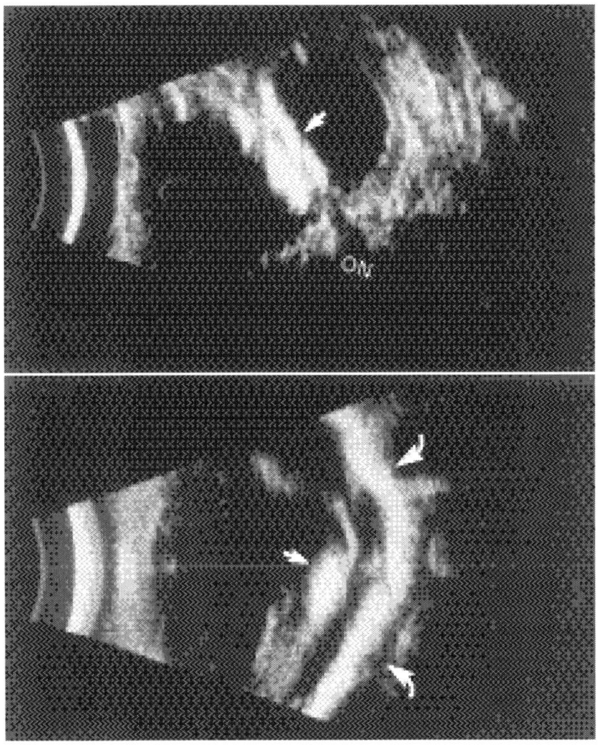

Figure 4-49 Phthisis bulbi. B-scan echograms at reduced gain from two patients show decreased size of globes and intraocular calcification. **A,** Longitudinal B-scan shows total, closed funnel-shaped RD *(arrow)* inserting into optic nerve *(ON)*. Note very echo-dense appearance of retina as a result of extensive calcification. **B,** Transverse B-scan shows extensive calcification of ocular wall *(curved arrows)* and partial calcification of retina *(straight arrow)*.

Ganciclovir Implant

See Figure 6-23 for an example of a ganciclovir implant.

Phthisis Bulbi

Many conditions can result in severe degeneration of the globe. Phthisis bulbi is characterized by marked irregular shrinkage of the eye. One of the main features of this disorder is extensive calcification of the posterior ocular coats. These eyes also often have a total, funnel-shaped RD that may be partially calcified (Figure 4-49). The subretinal space is typically filled with dense opacities, representing either hemorrhage or cholesterol debris (see Figure 3-25, *A* and *B*). In phthisis bulbi, the globe may be so shrunken and calcified that the normal ocular structures cannot be recognized. In such cases, it may be impossible to completely rule out the presence of an intraocular tumor.

REFERENCES

1. Awschalom L, Meyers SM: Ultrasonography of vitreal foreign bodies in eyes obtained at autopsy. *Arch Ophthalmol* 1982;100:979.
2. Bronson NR: Techniques of ultrasonic localization and extraction of intraocular and extraocular foreign bodies. *Am J Ophthalmol* 1965;60:596.
3. Chu TG, Cano MR, Green RL, et al: Massive suprachoroidal hemorrhage with central retinal apposition. A clinical and echographic study. *Arch Ophthalmol* 1991;109:1575.
4. Chu TG, Green RL: Suprachoroidal hemorrhage. *Surv Ophthalmol* 1999;43:471.
5. Clemens S, Kroll P, Rochels R: Ultrasonic findings after treatment of retinal detachment by intravitreal silicone instillation. *Am J Ophthalmol* 1984;98:369.
6. Coleman DJ, Lizzi FL, Jack RL: *Ultrasonography of the Eye and Orbit.* Philadelphia, Lea & Febiger, 1977, p 248.
7. Diamond JG, Kaefring S, Ossoinig KC: Echography in vitrectomy, in White D, Brown RE (eds): *Ultrasound in Medicine.* New York, Plenum Press, 1977, 3A:971.
8. Dugel PU, Ober RR: Posterior segment manifestations of closed-globe contusion injury ultrasound, in Ryan SJ (ed): *Retina.* ed 3, vol 3. St Louis, 2001, Mosby, p 2391.
9. Duker JS, Belmont JB, Benson WE, et al: Inadvertent globe perforation during retrobulbar and peribulbar anesthesia. *Ophthalmology* 1991;98:519.
10. Foster BS, Glenville AM, Lucarelli MJ: Optic nerve avulsion. *Arch Ophthalmol* 1997;115:823.
11. Fuller DG, Hutton WL: *Presurgical Evaluation of Eyes With Opaque Media.* New York, Grune & Stratton, 1982, p 168.
12. Green RL, Byrne SF: Diagnostic ophthalmic ultrasound, in Ryan SJ (ed): *Retina.* St Louis, Mosby, 1989, p 234.
13. Green RL, Byrne SF: Diagnostic ophthalmic ultrasound, in Ryan SJ (ed): *Retina.* St Louis, Mosby, 1989, p 191.
14. Hay A, Flynn HW Jr, Hoffman JI, et al: Needle penetration of the globe during retrobulbar and peribulbar injections. *Ophthalmology* 1991;98:1017.
15. Hughes JR, Byrne SF: Detection of posterior ruptures in opaque media, in Ossoinig KC (ed): *Ophthalmic Echography.* Dordrecht, Dr W Junk, 1987, p 333.
16. Keenum DG, Boldt HC, Byrne SF: Modern diagnostic techniques in the evaluation of ocular trauma. *Ophthalmol Clin North Am* 1995;8:589.
17. Liggett PE, Mani N, Green RE, et al: Management of traumatic rupture of the globe in aphakic patients. *Retina* 1990;10(suppl 1):59.
18. Liggett PE, Gauderman WJ, Moreira CM, et al: Pars plana vitrectomy for acute retinal detachment in penetrating ocular injuries. *Arch Ophthalmol* 1990;108:1724.
19. Loewenstein A, McKinnon S, DiBernardo C: Echographic diagnosis of scleral folds in hypotony. *Am J Ophthalmol* 1997;124:260.
20. Nemeth J, Suveges I: Echographic signs of perfluorodecalin [letter to the editor]. *Am J Ophthalmol* 1993;115:679
21. Ossoinig KC: Standardized echography: Basic principles, clinical applications and results. *Int Ophthalmol Clin* 1979;19:127.
22. Ossoinig KC, Bigar F, Kaefring SL, et al: Echographic detection and localization of BB shots in the eye and orbit. *Bibl Ophthalmol* 1975;83:109.
23. Ossoinig KC, Frazier SL, Watzke RC, et al: Combined A-scan and B-scan echography as a diagnostic aid for vitreoretinal surgery, in McPherson A (ed): *New and Controversial Aspects of Vitreoretinal Surgery.* St Louis, Mosby, 1977, p 106.
24. Ossoinig KC, Seher K: Ultrasonic diagnosis of intraocular foreign bodies, in Gitter KA, Keeney AH, Sarin LK, et al (eds). *Ophthalmic Ultrasound.* St Louis, Mosby, 1969, p 311.
25. Reynolds MG, Haimovici R, Flynn HW, et al: Suprachoroidal hemorrhage. Clinical features and results of secondary surgical management. *Ophthalmology* 1993;100:460.
26. Rubsamen PE, Cousins SW, Winward KE, et al: Diagnostic ultrasound and pars plana vitrectomy in penetrating ocular trauma. *Ophthalmology* 1994;101:809.
27. Sawada A, Frazier SL, Ossoinig KC: The role of ultrasound in the management of ocular foreign bodies, in White D, Brown RE (eds): *Ultrasound in Medicine.* New York, Plenum Press, 1977, 3A:1003.
28. Shugar JK, de Juan E Jr, McCuen BW II, et al: Ultrasonic examination of the silicone-filled eye. Theoretical and practical considerations. *Graefes Arch Clin Exp Ophthalmol* 1986;224:361.
29. Whitacre MM: B-scan ultrasonography of eyes containing intravitreal gas. *Am J Ophthalmol* 1991;112:272.

William D. Bates

5 Intraocular Tumors

Ultrasound has become increasingly important in the evaluation of eyes with intraocular tumors.* Aside from its obvious benefits for eyes with opaque ocular media, it has now become the most useful, noninvasive adjunct to the clinical examination for the differentiation of intraocular tumors in the presence of clear ocular media. In addition, ultrasound can provide accurate measurements of tumor size and is therefore valuable for the assessment of growth or regression. Both anterior segment and posterior segment tumors can be evaluated. Standardized Echography,[34,60,61] three-dimensional B-scan imaging[81] (see Chapter 9), spectrum analysis,[20,21,47] ultrasound biomicroscopy (UBM)[72] (see Chapter 8), and color Doppler imaging (CDI) (see Chapter 14) are useful for evaluating intraocular tumors.

DETECTION OF LESIONS

An intraocular tumor must be of a minimum thickness (i.e., elevation) before it can be resolved by ultrasound. In most cases, a lesion arising within the choroid must be more elevated than the surrounding retinochoroid layer to be detected. Experience has shown[60] that a lesion usually must be elevated by approximately 0.75 mm before it can be distinguished from surrounding tissue. Lesions involving the ciliary body normally need to have an even greater elevation to be detected because of the irregular nature of the normal ciliary body and its anterior location. It should be noted, however, that very small ciliary body lesions can be detected with the new high resolution B-scan instrumentation (see pp 39 and 173 and also Chapter 8).

Although a choroidal lesion may be large enough to be detected by ultrasound, effective quantitation may require even more elevation. This height is usually 2 mm or greater, but the size required for differentiation in many cases depends on the location and internal reflectivity of the lesion. In general, anterior segment lesions need to be thicker than choroidal lesions to be differentiated. Additionally, low reflective lesions require less elevation than do highly reflective lesions to be diagnosed with echography.

In determining whether an elevated fundus lesion is a tumor, it is important to assess whether it is solid or nonsolid (e.g., serous or hemorrhagic detachment of the choroid, retina, or pigment epithelium). This is accomplished by observing the lesion's surface to detect the presence of aftermovement (see p 36). Another indication that the lesion may not be solid is the lack of internal echoes when an extremely high gain setting is used. It should be pointed out, however, that these criteria may be difficult to evaluate when a lesion is only mildly elevated. Consequently, the determination of whether a slightly elevated lesion is solid or nonsolid cannot always be made.

OCULAR MELANOMA

The evaluation and measurement of ocular melanomas is one of the most important functions of ophthalmic ultrasound.[16,17,52] Ultrasound has proved to be a useful diagnostic imaging modality for determining the presence of a melanoma in opaque ocular media,[51] but it also offers a reliable, independent diagnosis in clear ocular media. In several large studies, it has been shown that Standardized Echography, in particular, is highly accurate for the diagnosis of ocular melanoma.[28,56,59,98] Echography has proved to be useful also for the detection of extraocular tumor growth, and it is a reliable method of obtaining accurate measurements of tumor dimensions.[56]

Typical Acoustic Properties of Ocular Melanoma

Specific criteria are used to diagnose an ocular melanoma with Standardized Echography.[60-62] The cardinal features include (1) solid consistency, (2) collar button (i.e., mushroom) shape, (3) low to medium internal reflectivity, (4) regular internal structure, and (5) internal blood flow (i.e., vascularity) (Figure 5-1). Additional factors, including the presence of sound attenuation, the extent of associated exudative retinal detachment, and the status of the adjacent scleral/orbital interface are also important considerations.

Echographically, most melanomas are dome shaped, but some may be lobulated or have an irregular surface contour (Figure 5-2). The classic configuration of a melanoma, however, is the collar button shape. In addition, melanomas may have a diffuse configuration with a relatively flat but irregular surface. The collar button shape, indicating that

*References 7, 17, 58, 62-64, 67.

A

B

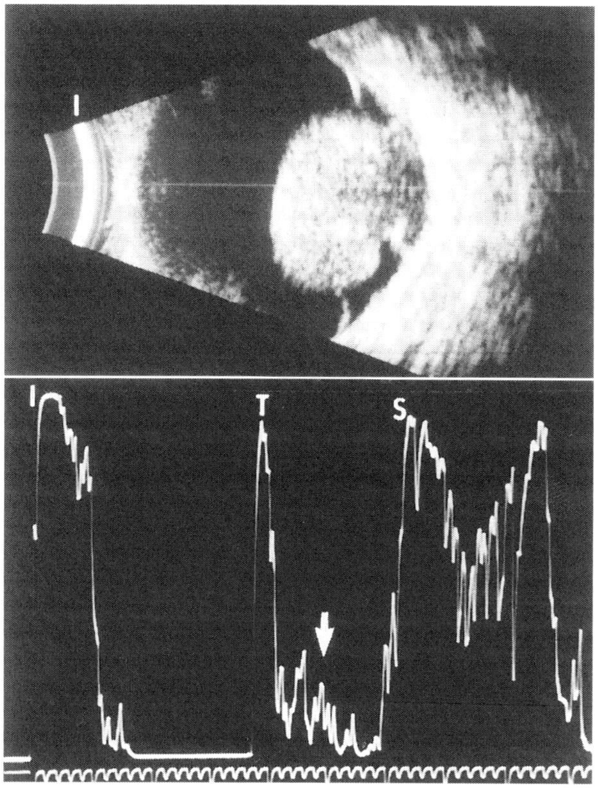

Figure 5-1 Choroidal melanoma. **A,** Transverse B-scan echogram shows typical collar button (i.e., mushroom) configuration. *I,* Initial line corresponding to probe face. **B,** A-scan echogram shows low to medium internal reflectivity that is typical of choroidal melanoma. *I,* Initial spike corresponding to probe tip; *T,* tumor surface; *arrow,* internal tumor spikes; *S,* sclera.

A

B

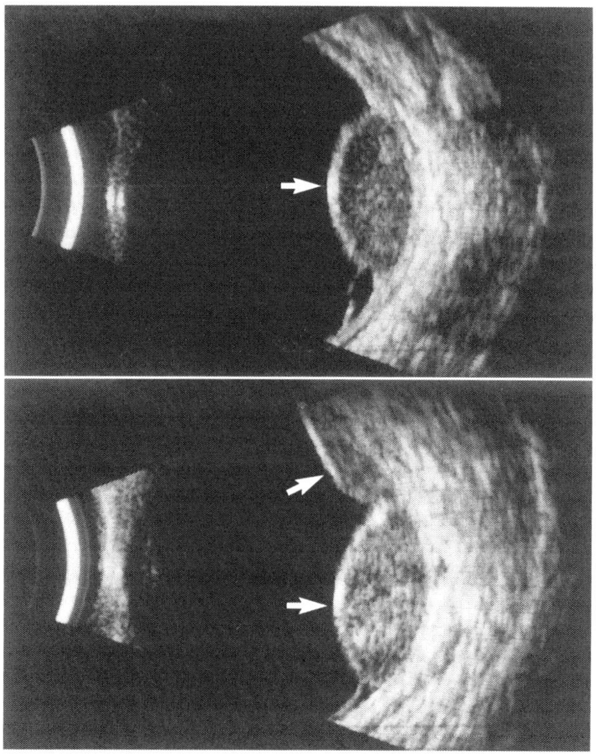

Figure 5-2 Choroidal melanomas. Transverse B-scans demonstrate dome **(A)** and lobulated **(B)** configurations. *Arrows,* Tumor.

the tumor has broken through Bruch's membrane, gives the tumor a distinct, nearly pathognomonic appearance on B-scan. The break usually occurs near the center of the tumor, but it sometimes occurs in an eccentric area of the lesion. The collar button shape is most often noted in larger tumors, but it can be present in smaller lesions as well (Figure 5-3). This finding is usually easy to detect, although in some cases, it is discovered only through careful topographic evaluation. It should be noted that rarely the collar button shape can be seen in tumors other than melanoma (see p 144).

The internal reflectivity of an ocular melanoma is an important criterion for diagnosis. Because of their cellular, homogeneous histologic architecture, these tumors typically demonstrate low to medium reflectivity. For the same reason, their internal structure is, in most cases, quite regular[42,44,62] (see Figures 2-24 and 5-1).

Internal blood flow (i.e., vascularity) is another important acoustic property that can be observed in nearly all ocular melanomas. Vascularity, on A-scan, is indicated by the presence of a fast, spontaneous, low-amplitude flickering motion occurring within the internal tumor spikes (see Figure 2-29). Internal blood flow can also be detected with B-scan,[34] as well as with CDI (see p 373).

Other Findings in Ocular Melanoma

There are several other findings that may be encountered in the ultrasound examination of an ocular melanoma. These include sound attenuation, choroidal excavation, posterior scleral bowing, and retinal detachment, as well as vitreous and subretinal hemorrhage. In addition, certain melanomas may exhibit an atypical irregular internal structure, cystic spaces, signs of inflammation, and/or calcification.

Sound Attenuation

Large ocular melanomas often produce significant internal sound attenuation.[32,53] As previously described (see p 34), sound attenuation, represented by a decrease in echo strength, occurring from left to right in the echogram, results in the display of lower reflectivity at the base of the tumor. On B-scan, this decreased reflectivity at the tumor base has been described by some authors as acoustic hollowing.[18,43] The lower reflectivity on A-scan and acoustic hollowing on B-scan at the base of a large melanoma may also be due in part to the more homogeneous nature of the tumor in this region (Figure 5-4). Occasionally, melanomas produce very strong sound attenuation that causes decreased reflectivity of the orbital echoes behind the tumor (i.e., shadowing).

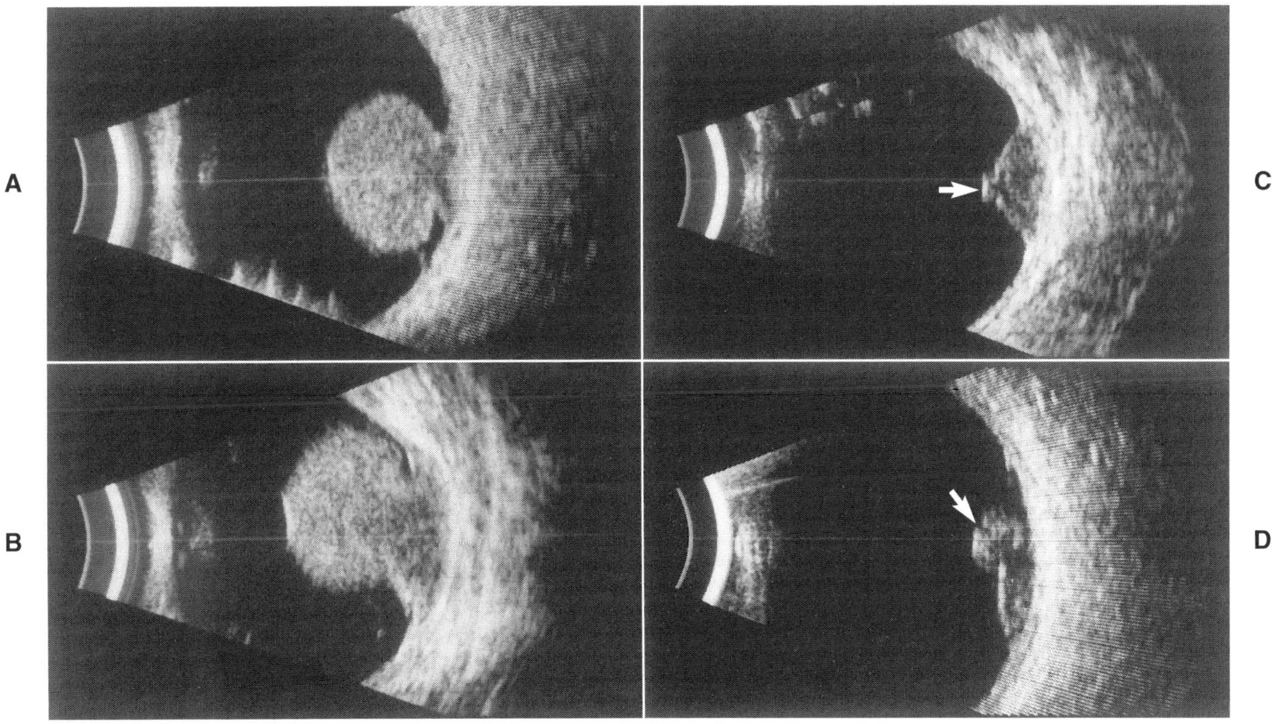

Figure 5-3 Four different collar button–shaped choroidal melanomas (transverse B-scan echograms). **A,** Large collar button, centered over the tumor base. **B,** Large collar button, located eccentrically. **C,** Very small collar button *(arrow)*, centered over the tumor base. **D,** Small collar button *(arrow)*, located eccentrically.

A

B

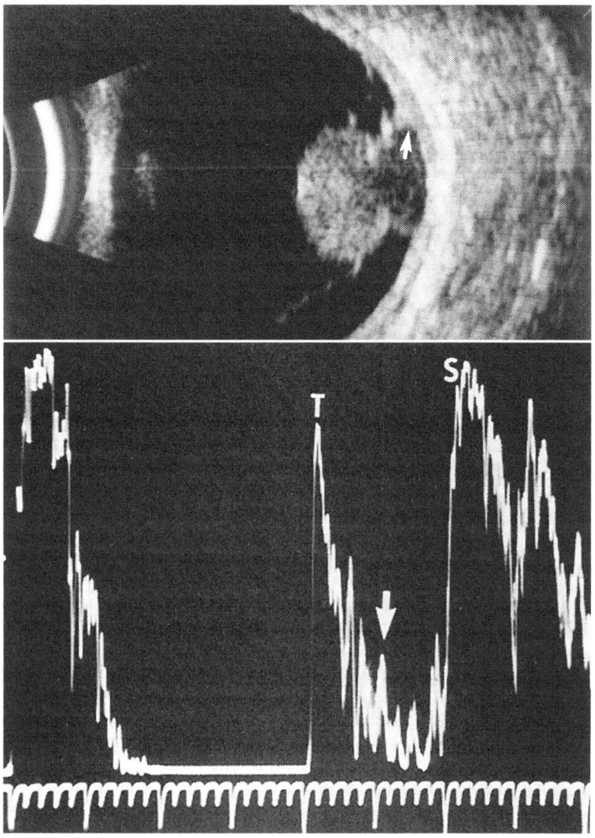

Figure 5-4 Collar button–shaped melanoma demonstrating strong internal sound attenuation and "choroidal excavation." **A,** Transverse B-scan echogram shows echolucent area at base of tumor produced by sound attenuation. This echolucency (acoustic hollowing) can also be due, in part, to a more homogeneous cellular architecture at the base of the tumor. *Arrow,* apparent choroidal excavation due to curving of tumor base at its margin. **B,** A-scan echogram shows moderately steep angle kappa, indicative of internal sound attenuation and/or a change in the cellular architecture at the tumor base. *T,* Tumor surface; *arrow,* internal tumor spikes; *S,* sclera.

Choroidal Excavation

A B-scan finding that has been described in melanomas is choroidal excavation.[16,18] This B-scan characteristic, noted at the tumor base, is thought to be caused by homogeneous tumor infiltration of the normal choroid (see Figure 5-4). The normal choroid, however, is of microscopic thickness, and therefore, tumor infiltration does not adequately explain this phenomenon. Another explanation is that the finding of choroidal excavation is merely an illusion created by the curved appearance of the tumor base at its margins. It should also be noted that choroidal excavation has been demonstrated in a variety of other choroidal lesions and is therefore not specific for melanoma.[28]

Posterior Scleral Bowing

Another finding that has recently been described in melanomas occurring in younger individuals is scleral bowing posterior to the tumor.[9] This bowing is caused by increased concavity of the sclera underlying the tumor (Figure 5-5) and can be associated with scleral infiltration (see p 131). Posterior scleral bowing can be confused with choroidal excavation but can be differentiated by noting the increased concavity of the sclera. It should also be noted that posterior scleral bowing is not specific for choroidal melanoma and has been reported in other tumors occurring in younger individuals (see p 154).

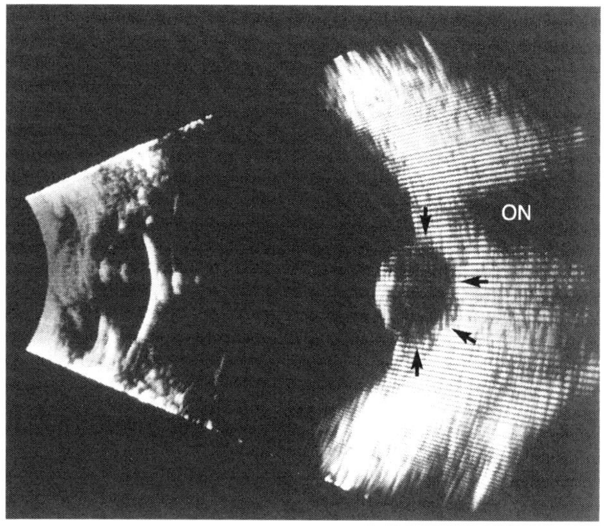

Figure 5-5 Scleral bowing. Axial B-scan showing dome-shaped melanoma adjacent to optic nerve *(ON)* with bowing of sclera posterior to the tumor *(arrows).*

Retinal Detachment

Serous retinal detachments are commonly associated with choroidal melanomas. These exudative detachments often extend from the margins of the tumor and are also frequently present in the lower periphery of the globe, away from the tumor mass. In rare cases, the retina may be detached over the apex of the tumor (see p 123).

Hemorrhage

Vitreous hemorrhage and/or subretinal hemorrhage may occur secondary to an ocular melanoma (Figure 5-6). When such hemorrhage is extremely dense, it can mask an underlying tumor. Therefore, whenever a dense hemorrhage is present, the eye should be carefully screened to rule out a solid mass. If a lesion of questionable solidity is found, serial examinations may be necessary to rule out a melanoma.

Irregular Internal Structure

Some melanomas have been shown to exhibit atypical features such as irregular structure and higher internal reflectivity.[32] These features are most commonly noted in very large melanomas that contain hemorrhage and

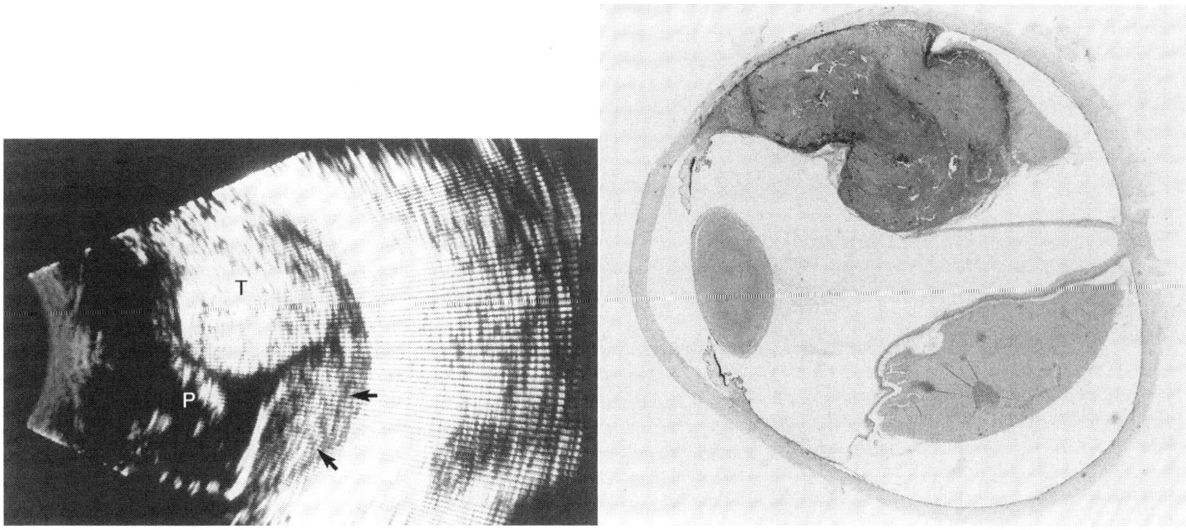

Figure 5-6 Large collar button–shaped melanoma with vitreal and subretinal hemorrhage. **A,** Transverse B-scan echogram shows posterior vitreous detachment *(P)*, tumor *(T)*, and subretinal hemorrhage *(black arrows)*. **B,** Photograph of gross pathologic specimen shows large choroidal melanoma (mixed cell type) and subretinal hemorrhage.

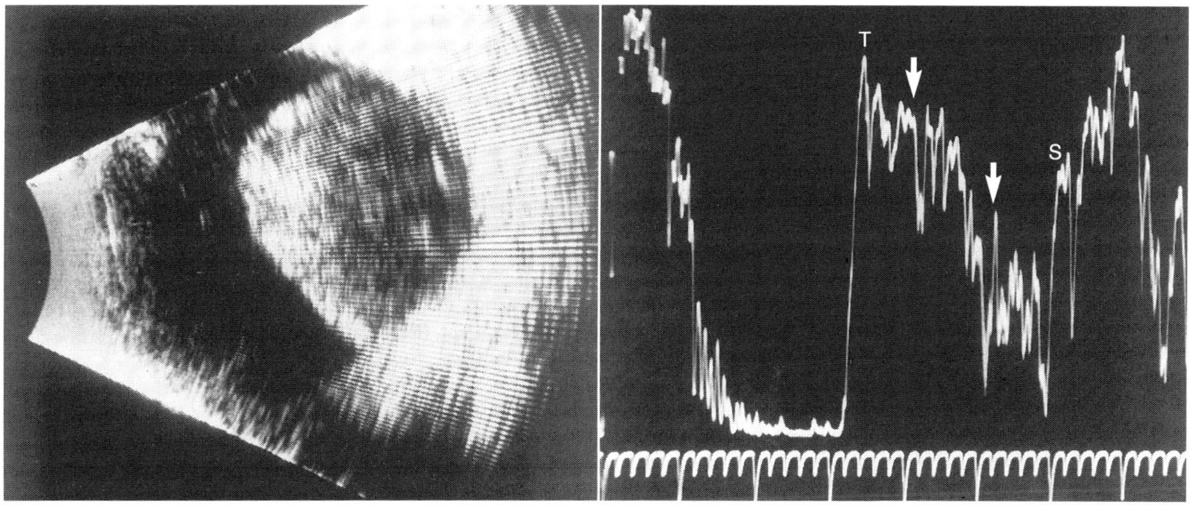

Figure 5-7 Large ciliochoroidal melanoma with irregular internal structure. **A,** Transverse B-scan shows large dome-shaped melanoma with relatively echolucent base due to sound attenuation. **B,** A-scan shows somewhat irregular internal structure, although there is a moderately steep angle kappa. *T,* Tumor surface; *arrows,* internal tumor spikes; *S,* sclera. Note the higher internal reflectivity within the anterior portion of the tumor.

necrosis, as well as dilated blood vessels, especially in more anterior portions of the lesion. This can result in a higher, more irregular internal reflectivity in these portions of the tumor. Additionally, these lesions may produce moderate sound attenuation (Figure 5-7).[53,62] A-scan echograms may also be more irregular when a tumor has broken through Bruch's membrane and shows a collar button appearance on B-scan. In these cases, spikes may be produced by both the tumor surface and the edges of Bruch's membrane, resulting in an irregular internal structure on A-scan. However, with slight movement of the probe, directing the sound beam completely through the break, the A-scan pattern often becomes lower reflective and more regular (Figure 5-8). Lesions with a very bumpy

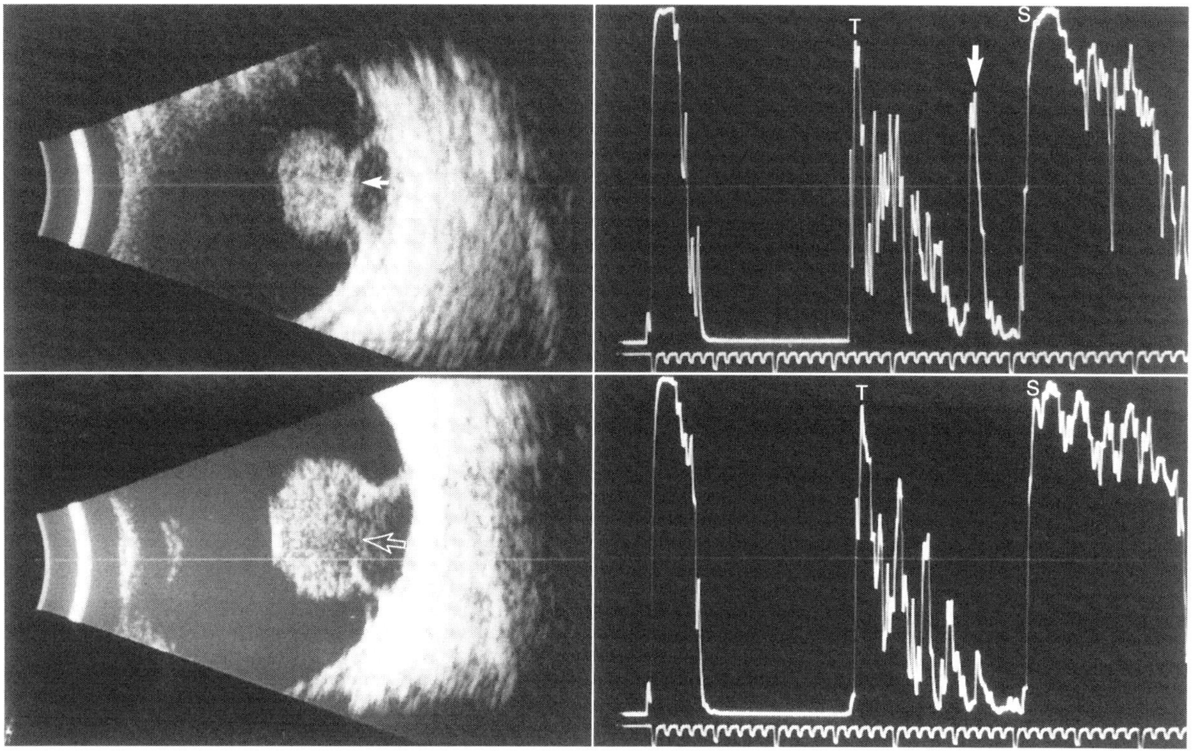

Figure 5-8 Collar button–shaped melanoma with irregular internal structure due to rupture in Bruch's membrane. **A,** Transverse B-scan echogram through periphery of tumor in area where Bruch's membrane is intact *(closed arrow)*. **B,** Transverse B-scan view through center of tumor shows break in Bruch's membrane *(open arrow)*. **C,** A-scan corresponding to B-scan in **A** displays irregular internal structure owing to a highly reflective spike produced by Bruch's membrane *(arrow)*. *T,* Tumor surface; *S,* sclera. **D,** A-scan corresponding to B-scan in **B** shows more regular internal structure as sound beam passes through break in Bruch's membrane.

surface contour also may produce a slightly irregular pattern on A-scan examination.

Cystic Spaces

B-scan may demonstrate tiny cystlike spaces within ocular melanomas. This finding is not specific for melanoma, however, and may occur in other types of intraocular tumors. On the other hand, very large cystic cavities are more characteristic of ciliochoroidal melanomas[50] (see p 173).

Inflammation

Scleritis, sub-Tenon's edema or inflammatory infiltration, and orbital inflammation can sometimes be detected echographically in association with ocular melanomas.[3,89] In two such cases, the inflammation resolved and the size of the choroidal melanoma decreased following treatment with corticosteroids (Figure 5-9). The etiology of this inflammatory reaction was not entirely clear. Neither case showed any histopathologic evidence of scleral or extrascleral invasion, although one tumor showed partial necrosis. In a report of three similar cases, histopathology demonstrated microscopic extraocular extension in one case.[107] Another report described three cases of choroidal melanoma with clinical signs of inflammation that underwent partial spontaneous regression.[89] One of these tumors was found to be highly necrotic on histopathologic examination. A more recent histopathologic study from the Armed Forces Institute of Pathology (AFIP)[55] reported on the association of scleritis and episcleritis with choroidal and ciliary body melanoma. This investigation showed that scleritis and episcleritis were significantly associated with tumor necrosis. It is important to note that the echographic findings of scleritis and episcleritis can mimic extraocular extension. Follow-up examination is, therefore, essential whenever there is a question of inflammation vs. extraocular extension (see p 131).

Calcification

Another rare finding in ocular melanoma is the presence of calcification. Calcium usually appears as a solitary focus on the surface of the tumor, in most cases, underlying an area of localized retinal detachment (Figure 5-10). One case

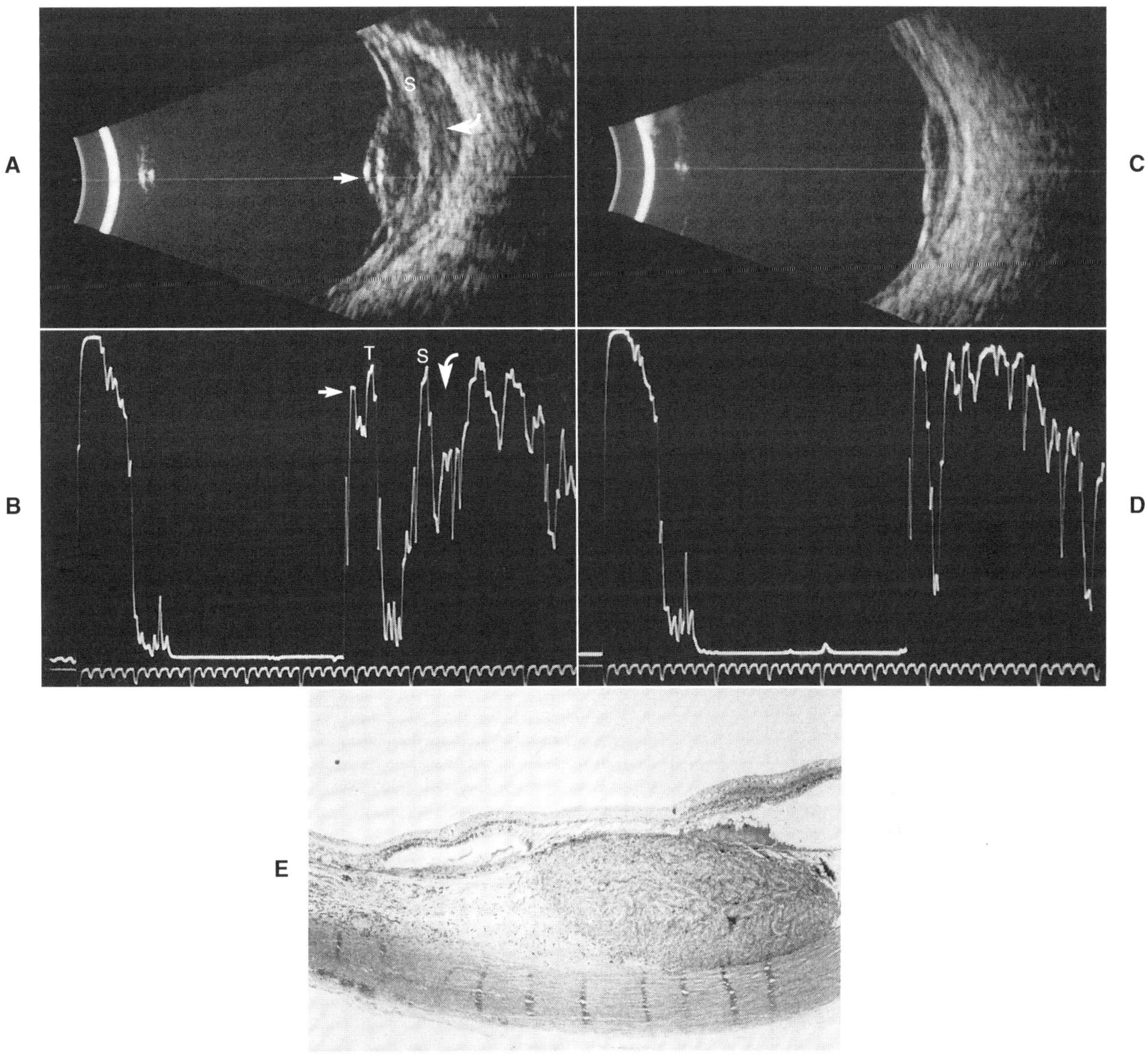

Figure 5-9 Choroidal melanoma with associated scleritis and orbital inflammation. Echograms show initial evaluation (**A** and **B**) and following corticosteroid therapy (**C** and **D**). **A,** Transverse B-scan demonstrates dome-shaped intraocular mass with shallow overlying serous retinal detachment *(straight arrow)* and diffuse sub-Tenon's lesion adjacent to intraocular tumor *(curved arrow)*. *S,* Sclera. **B,** Corresponding A-scan shows low reflectivity of choroidal mass as well as shallow retinal detachment and medium reflectivity of lesion posterior to sclera. *T,* Tumor surface; *S,* sclera. **C** and **D** show significant decrease in elevation of intraocular tumor and nearly complete resolution of orbital mass. Note retinal detachment is no longer present. **E,** Histopathology shows partially necrotic melanoma (mixed cell type) without evidence of extrascleral extension.

A

B

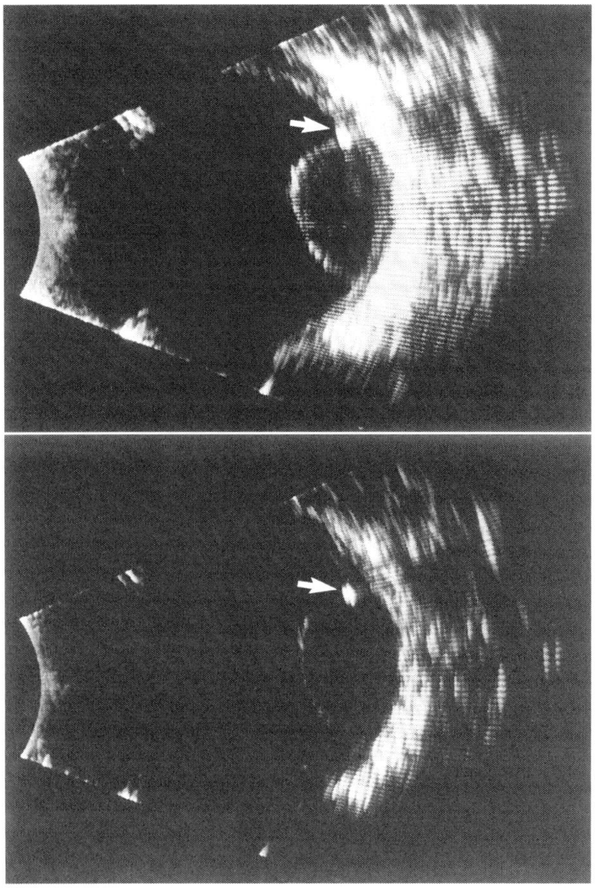

Figure 5-10 Dome-shaped melanoma showing calcified nodule *(arrow)* on peripheral surface of tumor. Transverse B-scan echograms are at medium gain **(A)** and low gain setting **(B).**

A

B

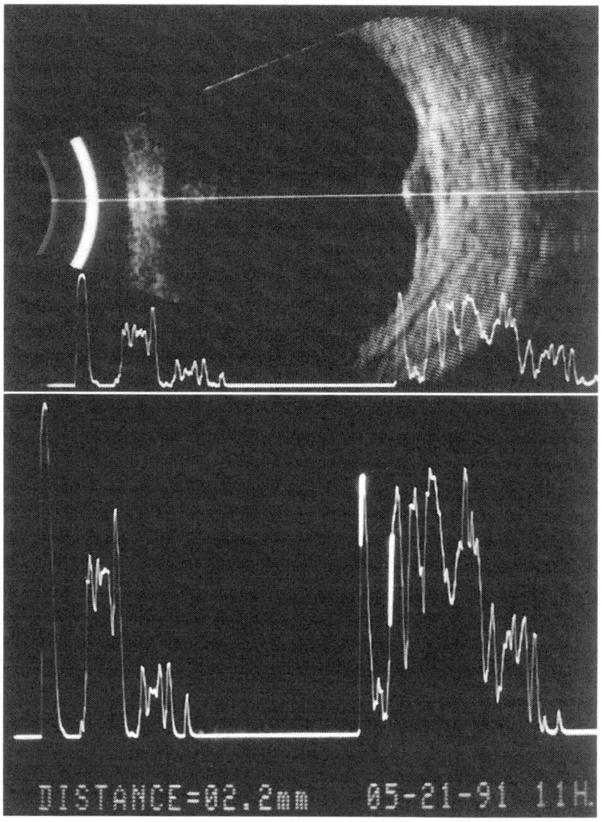

Figure 5-11 Measurement of tumor elevation using simultaneous vector A-scan. **A,** Transverse B-scan with vector A-scan through center of dome-shaped tumor. **B,** Vector A-scan displayed without B-scan shows cursors positioned on tumor surface and inner sclera. Height of tumor = 2.2 mm.

report describes a large plaque of calcified bone within a choroidal melanoma.[10]

Spectrum Analysis of Ocular Melanoma

Coleman and associates have developed a technique using spectrum analysis for tissue characterization of intraocular tumors.[19,47,48] This technique uses computer analysis of certain ultrasound parameters to provide acoustic signatures of intraocular tumors. Spectrum analysis has been successful in differentiating ocular melanoma from other intraocular tumors and has shown the potential to identify different cell types of melanoma (e.g., spindle B and mixed epithelioid).[20] More recently, this technique has been used to demonstrate microcirculatory patterns in uveal melanomas. It has been shown that the histologic presence of microvascular networks in ocular melanoma is associated with increased mortality.[91] The microcirculatory networks appear to provide a specific acoustic signature with spectrum analysis. This method may prove beneficial for the prognosis and management of patients with ocular melanoma.

Tumor Biometry

One of the more important functions of echography in the evaluation of melanomas is the measurement of tumor dimensions.[56] Accurate measurements are important for planning tumor management (e.g., observation vs. treatment and radiation dosimetry) and for monitoring tumor growth or regression.

Tumor Height Measurements

The measurement of apical tumor height (i.e., maximum elevation) should first be performed using B-scan. With some B-scan instruments, measurements can be obtained directly from the screen using electronic cursors; in others, it may be necessary to measure a photograph of the echogram (see Appendix F). The measurement of tumor height can also be performed in some instruments by using a vector A-scan placed on the B-scan echogram (Figure 5-11).

For B-scan measurements, either a transverse or a longitudinal view can be employed; but ideally, measurements should be obtained using both views. There are situations, however, in which one approach may be more reliable than the other, depending on the location and shape of the lesion. Peripheral lesions are frequently better assessed with a longitudinal view. With a transverse scan through a peripheral tumor, the sound beam may be unknowingly directed obliquely, resulting in a falsely high tumor elevation. Furthermore, it should be stressed that it is not possible to obtain an accurate height measurement of a tumor located in the periphery using the vector A-scan technique.

For most tumors, the initial step in obtaining an apical height measurement with B-scan is to examine the tumor with a transverse probe position. Using a medium gain setting, the tumor is centered in the echogram and the probe is angled back and forth, thus sweeping the acoustic section across the lesion. As this maneuver is carried out, the echogram is monitored in an attempt to direct the sound beam perpendicular to both the apex of the tumor and the inner sclera at the tumor base. The inner sclera can be identified as the first distinct line at the base of the tumor that is continuous with the surrounding fundus (Figure 5-12). Once optimal display of both the apex and the inner sclera has been achieved, the apical height of the tumor can be measured from the B-scan echogram. A similar maneuver, using a longitudinal scan, is then performed to obtain a second apical height measurement.

Axial and para-axial B-scan probe approaches (e.g., vertical macular scan, see p 28) are usually best suited for measuring lesions in the peripapillary region (see Figure 2-20). These approaches are not appropriate, however, for measuring more peripheral tumors.

Once a preliminary measurement of tumor elevation has been obtained with B-scan, this value is confirmed with standardized A-scan. The A-scan is first set at Tissue Sensitivity and the probe is placed on the area of the globe opposite the tumor. The probe is then shifted as needed to direct the sound beam toward the tumor apex. Localization of the tumor apex can be further accomplished by shifting the sound beam back and forth across the tumor. The sound beam should be shifted until it is simultaneously aligned perpendicular to both the surface of the tumor at its apex and the inner sclera. Perpendicularity is achieved once steeply rising spikes of maximum height are displayed from both surfaces (Figure 5-13).

When both the tumor surface spike and the scleral spike have been adequately displayed at Tissue Sensitivity, a measurement of the elevation is obtained. For further refinement of the measurement, the gain is reduced slightly (as the screen is continuously monitored) to display distinct peaks from both the tumor surface spike and the inner scleral spike. Measurements are obtained from the screen by means of electronic cursors positioned on the same phase or region of the tumor surface spike and the inner scleral spike (Figure 5-14). Some instruments lack electronic cursors and thus require that measurements be made from photographs using calipers and conversion tables[59] (see Appendix A).

The examiner should strive to obtain several consistent measurements from the best-quality echograms that can be obtained. There should be a close correlation between measurements obtained with B-scan and standardized A-scan techniques. The measurements obtained with these two methods should generally be within 0.2 to 0.3 mm for small tumors and 0.5 mm for large tumors. When greater differences are encountered, the quality of the echograms should be re-evaluated and those considered suboptimal repeated. The echograms should also be assessed to ensure that the correct surfaces were measured.

Correct identification of A-scan spikes originating from the tumor surface and the inner sclera is critical for accurate measurements. In cases in which the retina is attached to the apex of the tumor, the tumor surface spike includes both retina and tumor surface. This results in the tumor surface spike appearing relatively thick at Tissue Sensitivity and sometimes double peaked at reduced gain. In these cases, measurements should always be obtained from the retinal portion of the surface spike. Conversely, if B-scan examination shows that the retina is detached from the tumor apex, measurements should be taken from the actual tumor surface spike rather than from the retinal spike (Figure 5-15). In some tumors, it may be impossible to display the surface spike at 100% height. This can occur in tumors with a very convex surface configuration, steep elevation, or an irregular, bumpy surface. In such cases, the highest amplitude tumor surface spike that can be displayed should be used for the measurement.

The spike produced by the inner sclera may sometimes be difficult to identify correctly. The most common error in this regard is measuring to the outer sclera/Tenon's capsule interface and thus obtaining a falsely large measurement. This can occur because the outer sclera/Tenon's interface is often more highly reflective than the inner scleral surface; therefore, it is easier to display for measurement. This error can be avoided, however, by recognizing that the inner sclera produces the first distinct spike at the base of the tumor when using both Tissue Sensitivity and reduced gain (Figure 5-16). The use of a medium or slightly higher gain setting can facilitate identification of the inner scleral spike. In addition, A-scan measurements should always be correlated with those obtained from B-scan to help assure accurate readings (Figure 5-17).

It is important to point out that the steepness and height of the inner scleral spike may diminish due to scleral tumor infiltration or associated scleritis (Figure 5-18), or as a result of plaque radiotherapy (see p 137). In these

Text continued on p 129

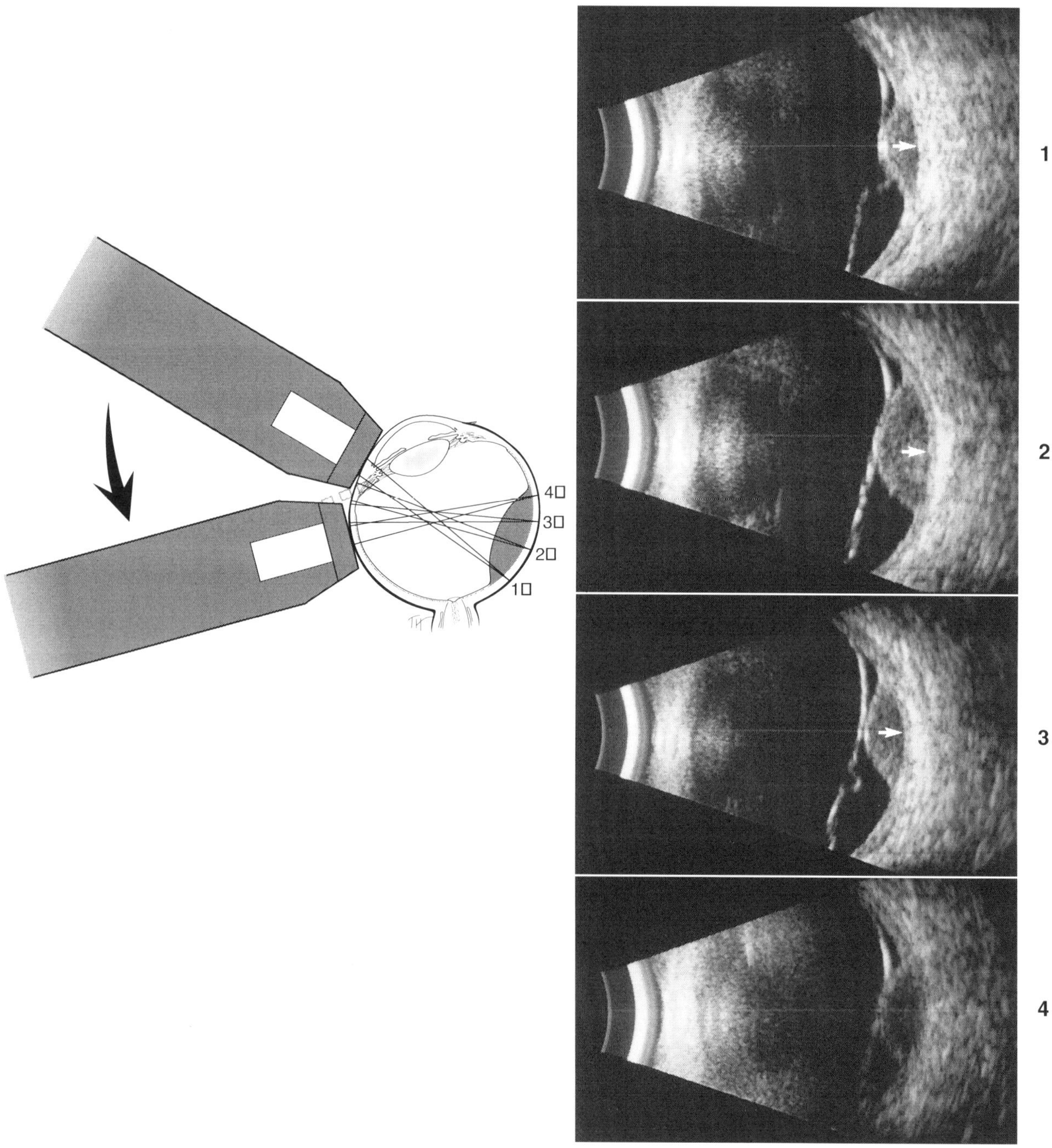

Figure 5-12 Dynamic B-scan technique to localize tumor apex (maximum elevation). Schematic drawing shows probe placement for transverse scanning. Probe is first placed near the limbus on the meridian opposite the tumor and is shifted toward the fornix. This provides multiple sections of the tumor from its posterior *(1)* to its anterior border *(4)*. The maximum tumor height is displayed with probe position 2. Note exudative retinal detachment overlying and adjacent to tumor. *Arrows*, Inner sclera.

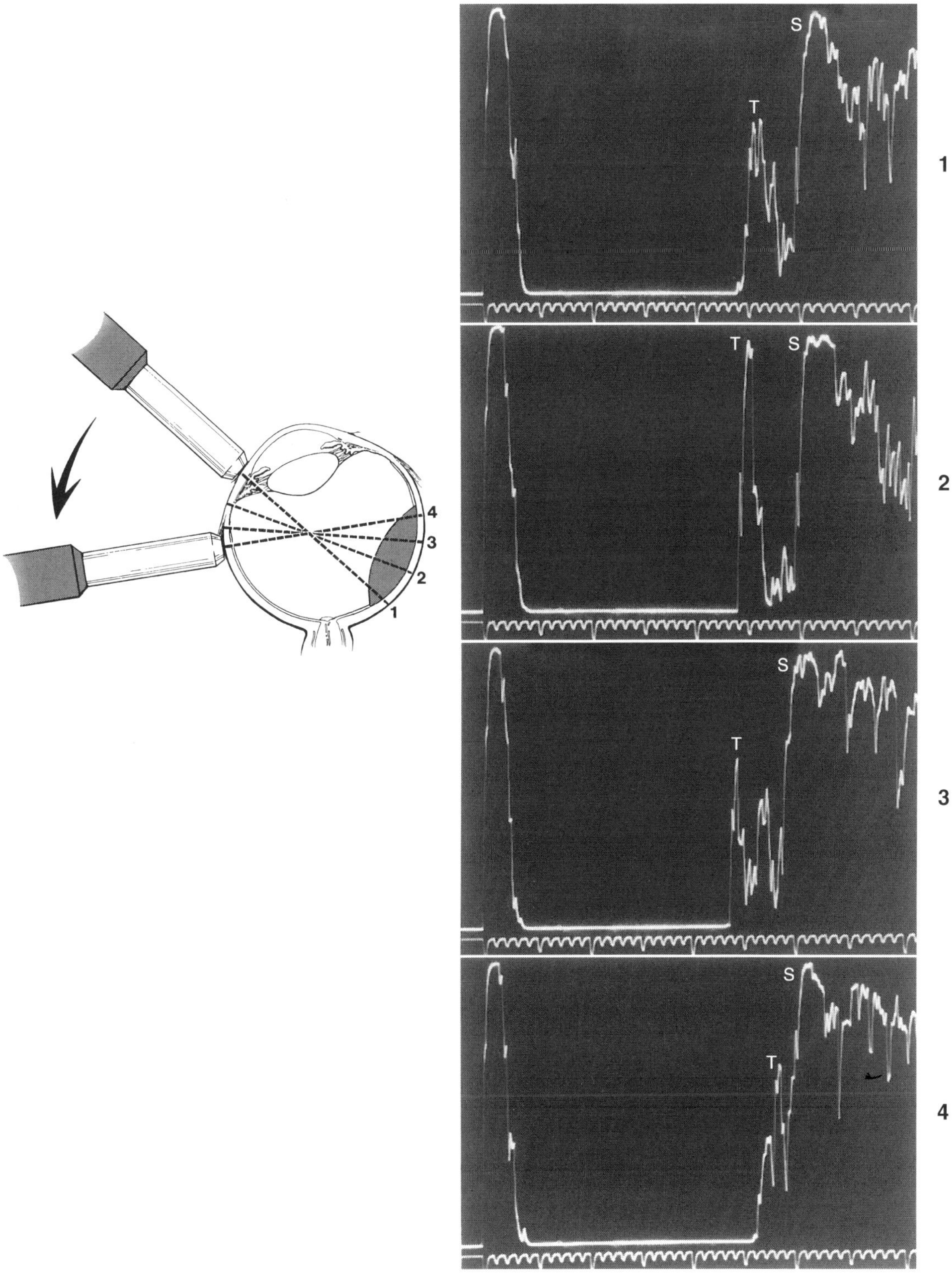

Figure 5-13 Dynamic A-scan technique to localize tumor apex (maximum elevation). Schematic drawing shows probe shifted from limbus to fornix. This displays the lesion from its posterior margin *(1)* to its anterior margin *(4)*. Note that maximum tumor height is displayed with probe position 2. In the corresponding echogram *(2)*, the steeply rising, high spikes from the retina and sclera indicate that the sound beam is directed perpendicular to these surfaces. *T,* Tumor surface; *S,* sclera.

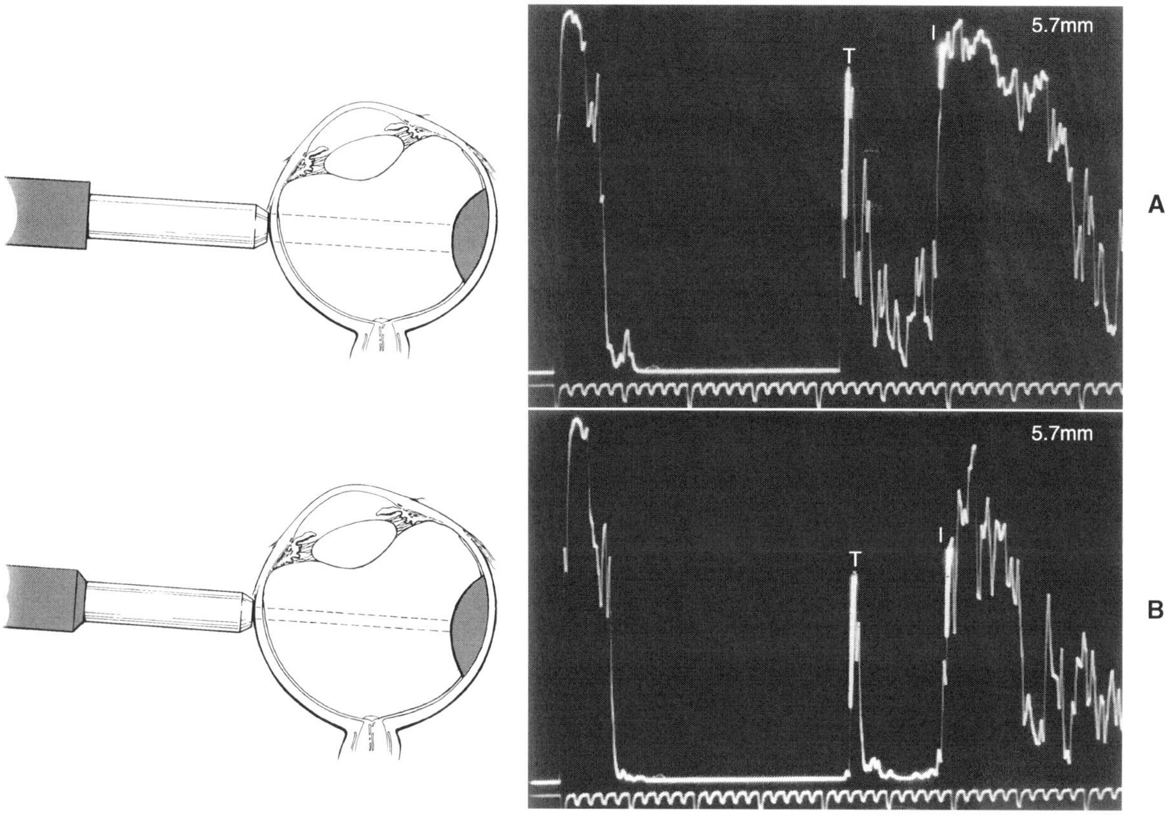

Figure 5-14 A-scan measurement of choroidal melanoma. **A,** A-scan echogram at Tissue Sensitivity gain setting to examine and measure tumor with relatively wide portion of sound beam. *T,* Tumor surface; *I,* inner sclera. Elevation = 5.7 mm. **B,** A-scan at reduced gain setting. At lower gain, the sound beam is effectively narrowed (only center of beam is used), thus improving axial resolution and providing more accurate measurements. Maximum elevation = 5.7 mm.

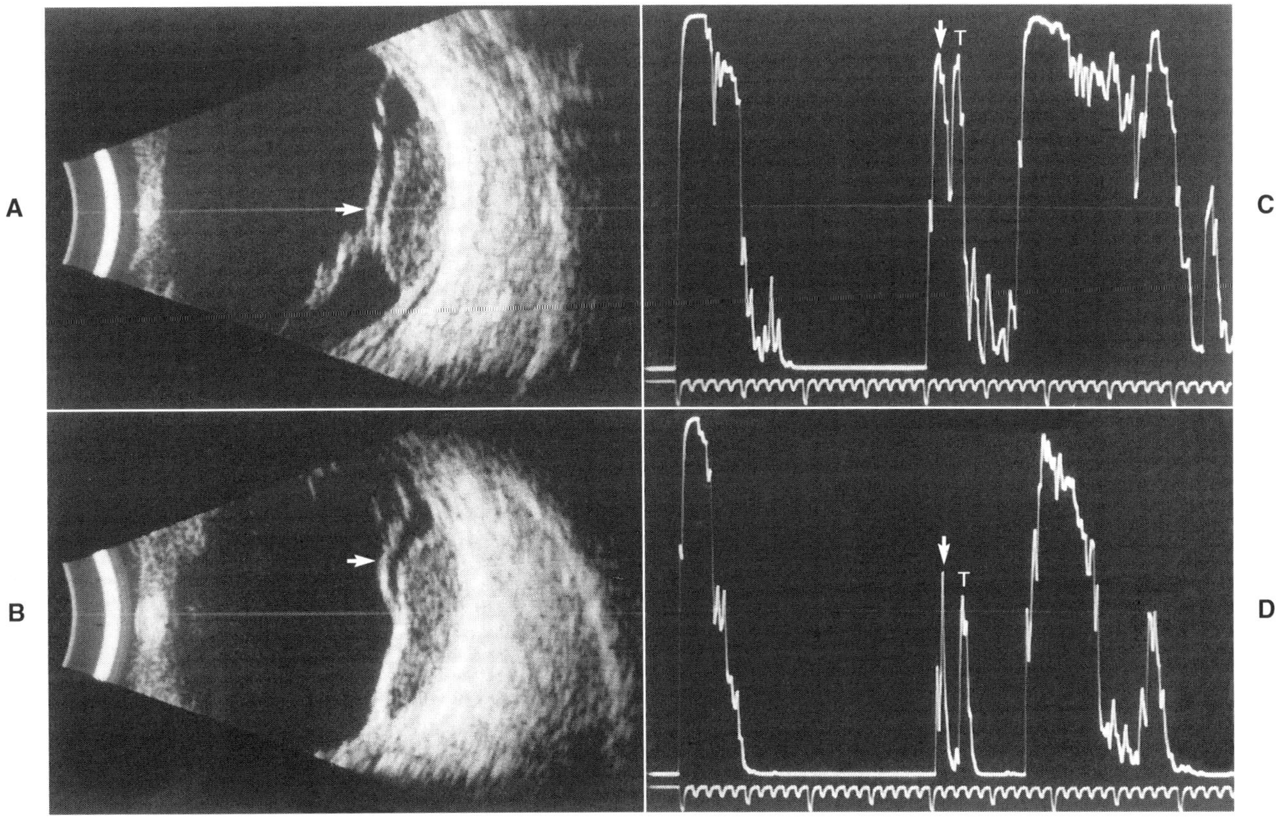

Figure 5-15 Choroidal melanoma with overlying retinal detachment. Measurement of tumor height must be obtained from actual tumor surface rather than from detached retina. Transverse **(A)** and longitudinal **(B)** B-scans show retinal detachment *(arrow)* overlying apex of tumor. A-scan views at Tissue Sensitivity **(C)** and reduced gain setting **(D)** show separate spikes from detached retina *(arrow)* and tumor surface *(T)*.

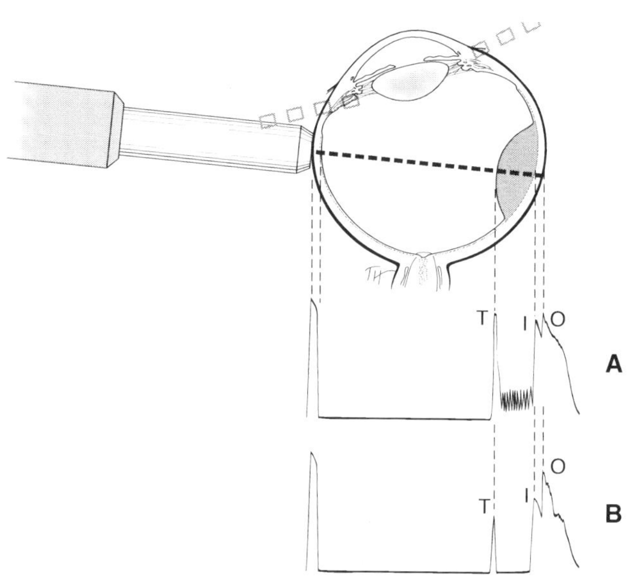

Figure 5-16 Schematic drawing showing A-scan technique for measuring tumor height. Probe is placed on globe opposite tumor with sound beam directed perpendicular to apex of tumor and sclera. Measurement is obtained at both Tissue Sensitivity **(A)** and moderately reduced gain **(B)**. To obtain an accurate measurement, the sound beam must be directed perpendicular to both the tumor surface *(T)* and the inner sclera *(I)*. Note that an erroneously large measurement can be obtained if the tumor is measured to the outer sclera *(O)*. This can be avoided by maintaining the display of the inner scleral spike as the gain is reduced for measurement.

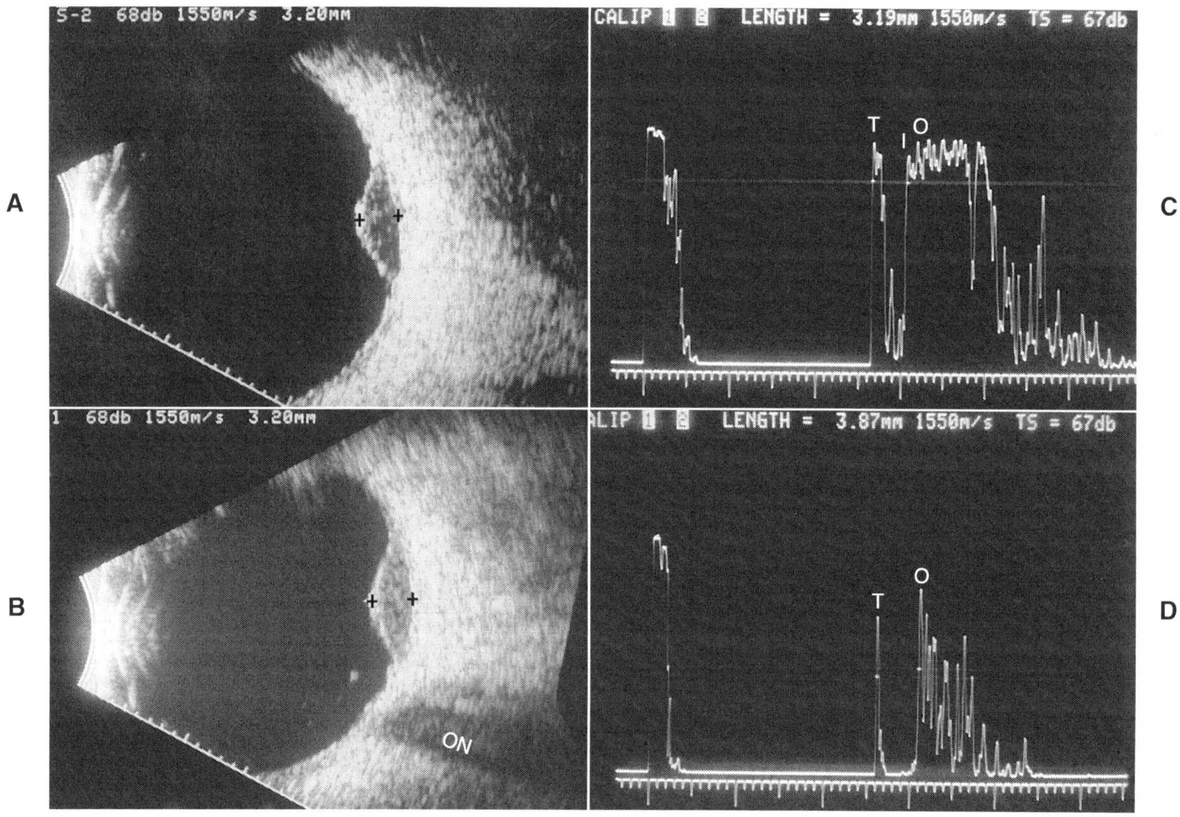

Figure 5-17 Erroneous measurement of intraocular tumor height. Apical height is first measured from transverse **(A)** and longitudinal **(B)** B-scans with electronic cursors *(black crosses)* placed on tumor surface and inner sclera. The apical height measures 3.20 mm. *ON*, Optic nerve. The tumor is then measured with A-scan, first at Tissue Sensitivity **(C)** and then at reduced gain **(D)**. **C,** With cursors placed on surface of tumor *(T)* and inner sclera *(I)*, apical height measures 3.19 mm. *O*, Outer scleral spike. **D,** At reduced gain, the weaker inner scleral spike is no longer displayed and an erroneous measurement (3.87 mm) is obtained to the outer scleral spike *(O)*. This error can be avoided by correctly identifying the inner scleral spike at the higher gain level (Tissue Sensitivity) and then maintaining its display as the gain is reduced. This example demonstrates the importance of always correlating A- and B-scan measurements.

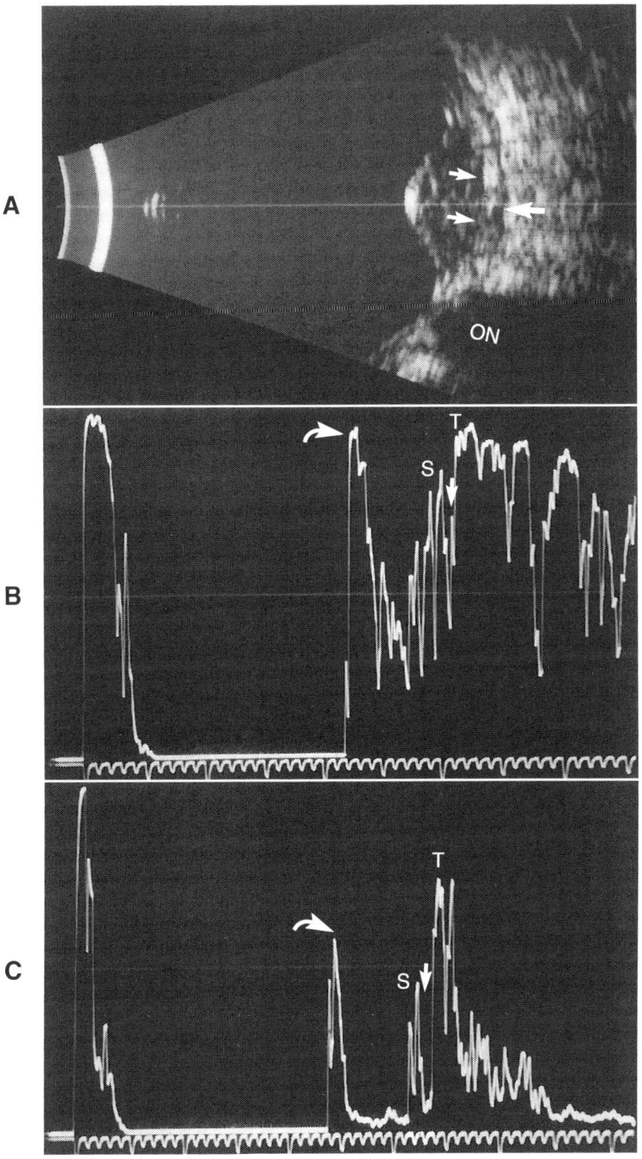

Figure 5-18 Choroidal melanoma with scleritis resulting in decreased reflectivity of sclera. **A,** Longitudinal B-scan view at reduced gain setting shows irregular, indistinct scleral surface *(small arrows)* and edema in sub-Tenon's space *(large arrow)* due to scleritis. *ON,* Optic nerve. **B,** A-scan echogram shows reduced height of scleral spike *(S)* due to inflammation. *Curved arrow,* Surface of tumor; *vertical arrow,* edema in sub-Tenon's space; *T,* Tenon's capsule. **C,** Corresponding A-scan at reduced gain again shows Tenon's capsule *(T)* to be more highly reflective than the inflamed sclera *(S)*. *Vertical arrow,* Inflammation in sub-Tenon's space.

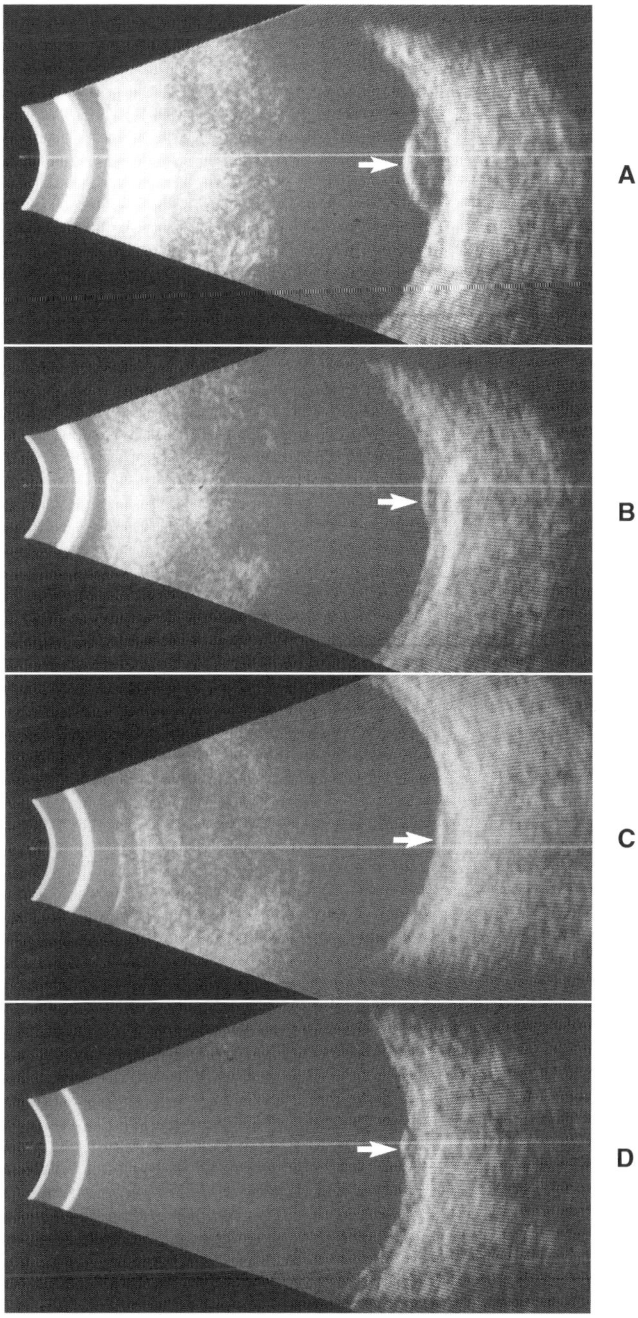

Figure 5-19 B-scan monitoring for growth of small choroidal melanoma treated with laser. Transverse B-scan echograms show tumor prior to laser therapy **(A)**, during ongoing treatment (**B** and **C**) and following treatment **(D)**. Note that tumor is almost completely flat in **C** after last laser treatment, but shows mild increase in height 3 months after completion of treatment **(D)**.

more difficult cases, identification of the scleral spike can be aided by correlating A- and B-scan echograms.

The A-scan measurement of small tumors (<1.5 mm) can be quite challenging. This is due to the difficulty of simultaneously directing the sound beam perpendicular to both the tumor apex and the inner sclera. It is therefore recommended that B-scan measurements be used to monitor the apical height of small tumors (Figure 5-19).

Tumor Base Measurements

Ultrasound can be utilized to measure the basal diameter of a tumor by examining it with both transverse and longitudinal approaches. The transverse approach measures the circumferential (lateral) diameter, whereas the longitudinal approach measures the radial (anteroposterior) diameter.

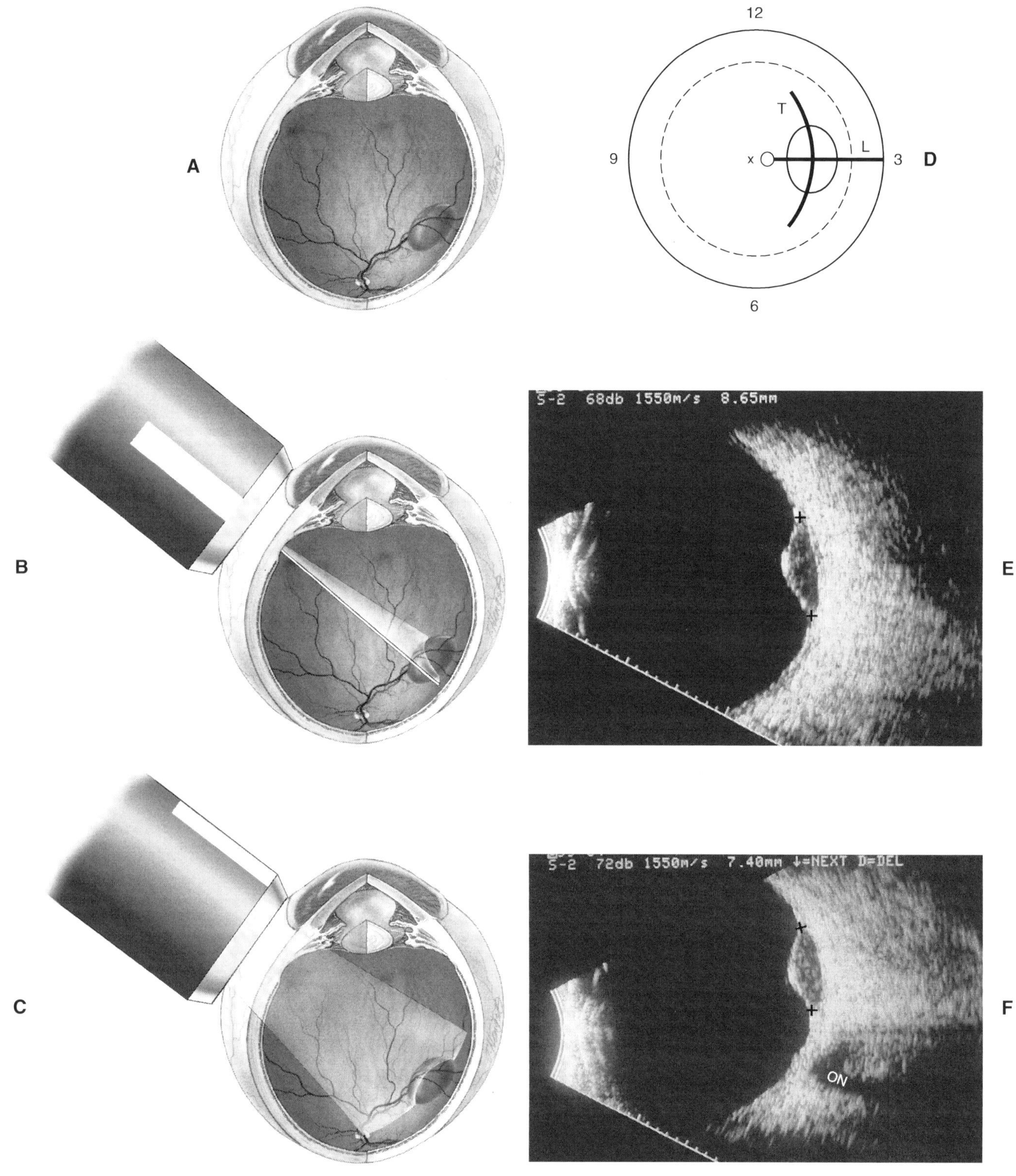

Figure 5-20 Basal diameter measurements of choroidal tumor using transverse and longitudinal B-scan approaches. Three-dimensional schematic drawings show choroidal tumor **(A)** with transverse **(B)** and longitudinal **(C)** sound beam approaches. Schematic drawing **(D)** shows path of sound beam through tumor for the transverse *(T)* and longitudinal *(L)* scans. Transverse **(E)** and longitudinal **(F)** echograms show dome-shaped tumor with correct placement of cursors at tumor margins. The transverse approach provides the lateral (i.e., circumferential) extent whereas the longitudinal approach displays the anteroposterior (i.e., radial) extent of the tumor. In this example, the tumor base measures 8.65 mm circumferentially and 7.40 mm radially. *ON*, Optic nerve.

A

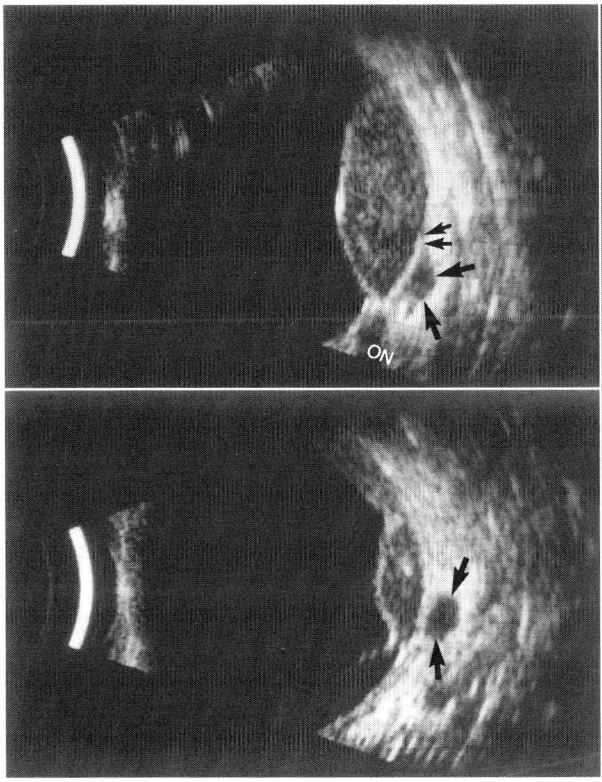

B

C

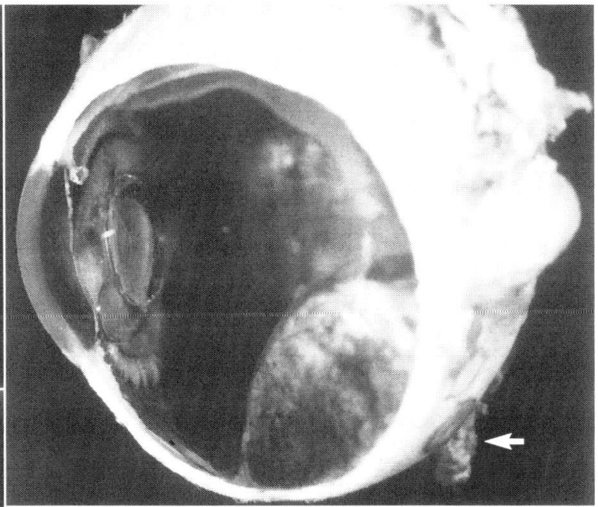

Figure 5-21 Choroidal melanoma with extrascleral extension. **A,** Longitudinal B-scan shows dome-shaped tumor with extrascleral nodule *(large arrows)* located near the optic nerve *(ON)*. Note communication of nodule with intraocular tumor through small vessel in sclera *(small arrows)*. **B,** Transverse B-scan obtained through posterior aspect of tumor also shows extrascleral tumor nodule *(arrows)*. **C,** Gross pathologic specimen shows choroidal melanoma (mixed cell tumor) with extrascleral extension *(arrow)*.

These measurements can be performed from the screen with electronic cursors or from photographs, using calipers (Figure 5-20; see also Appendix F).

In some cases, the longitudinal and transverse views may not demonstrate the largest basal diameter of the tumor. This can sometimes be appreciated, however, by simply rotating the probe while performing either a transverse or a longitudinal scan.

Measurements from B-scan are most accurate and useful when the tumor has very distinct margins that can be easily identified echographically. B-scan measurements are less reliable in areas of the tumor that have tapered, indistinct margins. In cases in which the tumor margins are clinically visible, B-scan measurements should be compared with the clinical estimate. If the tumor is to be plaqued, a general rule of thumb is that the greater of the clinical and echographic measurements should be used. Also, it should be realized that when a choroidal tumor extends into the ciliary body, the anterior border may not be clearly imaged (see p 174). As a result, measurement of the radial basal diameter for such tumors may be inaccurate.

Tumor Volume Measurements/ Three-Dimensional Imaging

As previously described (see p 122), traditional methods of measuring intraocular tumors utilize a combination of the one-dimensional (A-scan) and two-dimensional (B-scan) forms of ultrasound. This combination is used to evaluate tumor size and to establish whether growth or regression has occurred. The one measurement that eludes this method, however, is an accurate determination of tumor volume. Many investigators believe that an assessment of tumor volume is the most effective and reliable means of measuring and following choroidal melanomas. The development of new three-dimensional (3-D) ultrasound technology[81] now provides a more effective and reliable means of measuring tumor volume (see Chapter 9).

Extrascleral Extension

B-scan can be very useful in detecting extrascleral extension of an intraocular melanoma.[23,52,78,79] Extrascleral tumor extension typically appears as one or more nodules located near the sclera, adjacent to the base of the tumor (Figure 5-21). The thickness of the nodule must be approximately 1.5 mm before it can be reliably detected. When the lesion is of sufficient thickness, standardized A-scan can also be used to assess internal reflectivity (Figure 5-22) and blood flow within the nodule.

Small areas of suspected tumor extension may be identified, but in many cases, the small size precludes confident diagnosis at the initial examination. When a suspicious area is detected, follow-up examinations can be useful to look for an increase in size or changes in configuration that may in-

A
B
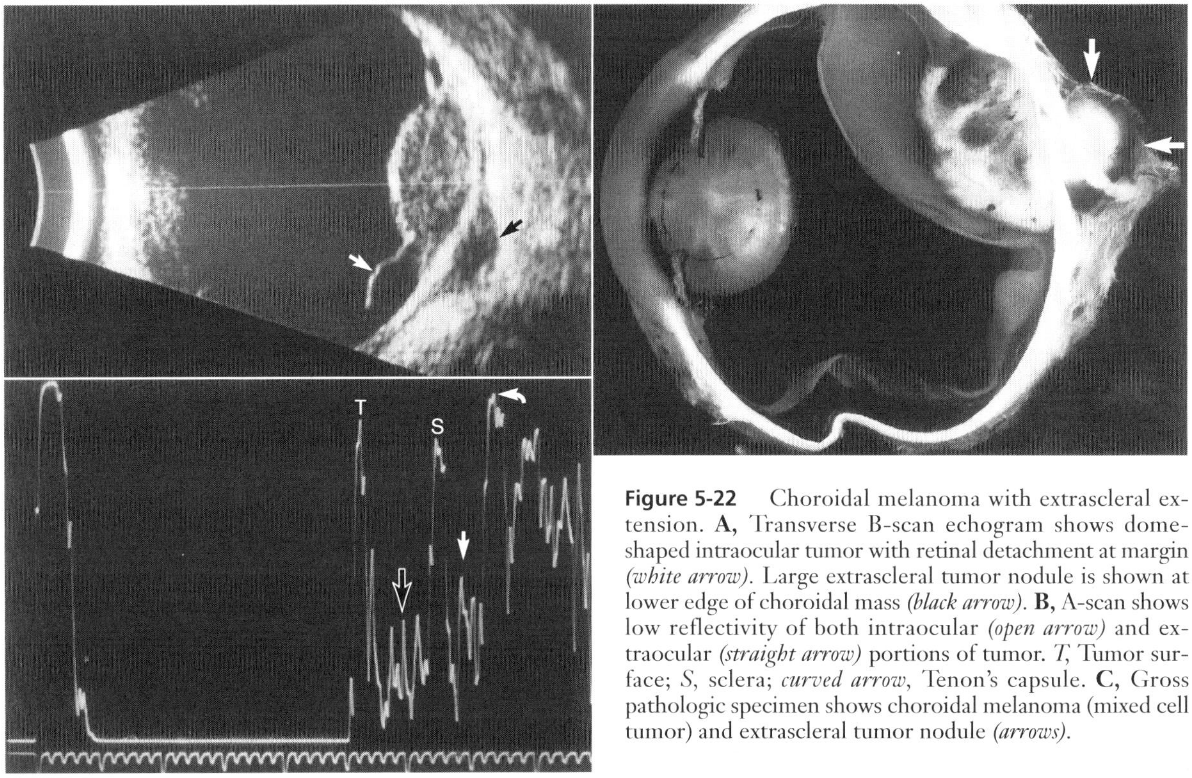

C

Figure 5-22 Choroidal melanoma with extrascleral extension. **A,** Transverse B-scan echogram shows dome-shaped intraocular tumor with retinal detachment at margin *(white arrow)*. Large extrascleral tumor nodule is shown at lower edge of choroidal mass *(black arrow)*. **B,** A-scan shows low reflectivity of both intraocular *(open arrow)* and extraocular *(straight arrow)* portions of tumor. *T,* Tumor surface; *S,* sclera; *curved arrow,* Tenon's capsule. **C,** Gross pathologic specimen shows choroidal melanoma (mixed cell tumor) and extrascleral tumor nodule *(arrows)*.

A
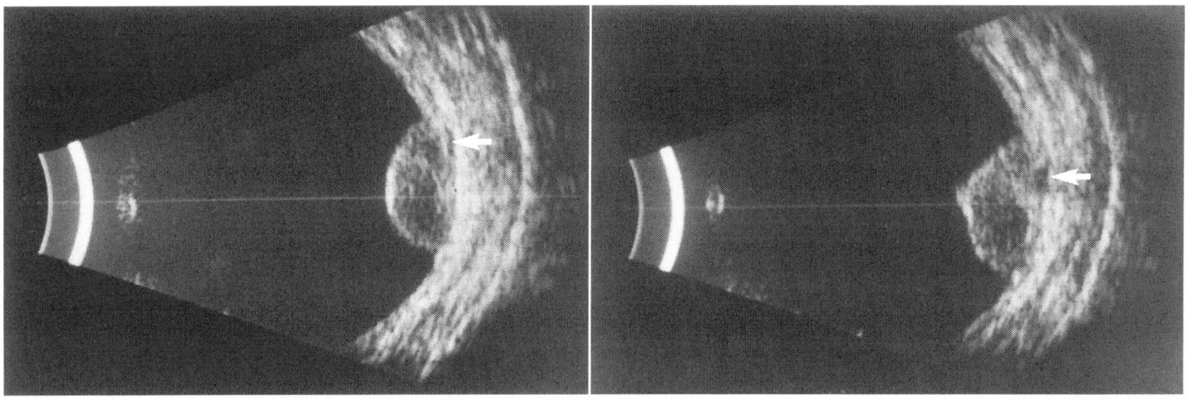
B

Figure 5-23 Choroidal melanoma with extrascleral extension. Transverse B-scan echograms show growth of suspicious area of extraocular extension. **A,** At initial examination, there is a small area of echolucency in the episcleral region adjacent to tumor *(arrow)*. **B,** At follow-up examination 1 year later, there is growth of both intraocular tumor and extraocular lesion *(arrow)*. Note that the extrascleral lesion now has a nodular appearance.

dicate true extraocular growth (Figure 5-23). It should also be emphasized that small choroidal melanomas can be associated with significant extraocular tumor growth (Figure 5-24). As a result, small tumors should be monitored with ultrasound, even when there is no clinically apparent change in the size of the intraocular lesion.

In some cases, scleral infiltration, with or without extraocular extension, can be demonstrated echographically (Figure 5-25). In addition, extension through the sclera within small blood vessels may sometimes be detected; and occasionally, the vessel may be shown to communicate with an extraocular nodule (see Figure 5-21). In one instance, the extension of a melanoma into the orbit by way of a vortex vein was observed[34] (Figure 5-26; see also Figure 9-3).

A

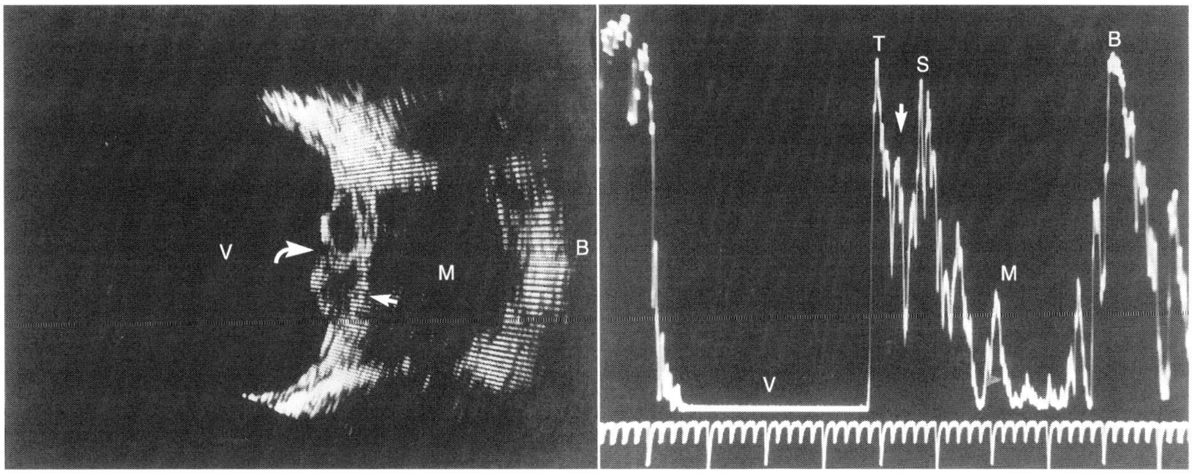

B

Figure 5-24 Small intraocular melanoma with large extrascleral tumor extension. **A,** Transverse B-scan echogram (at reduced gain setting) shows relatively small, lobulated intraocular melanoma *(curved arrow)* and large melanoma in orbit *(M)*. *V,* Vitreous cavity; *straight arrow,* sclera; *B,* orbital bone. **B,** A-scan shows small, medium reflective intraocular melanoma *(arrow)*, and large, low reflective portion in orbit. *T,* Tumor surface; *S,* sclera.

A

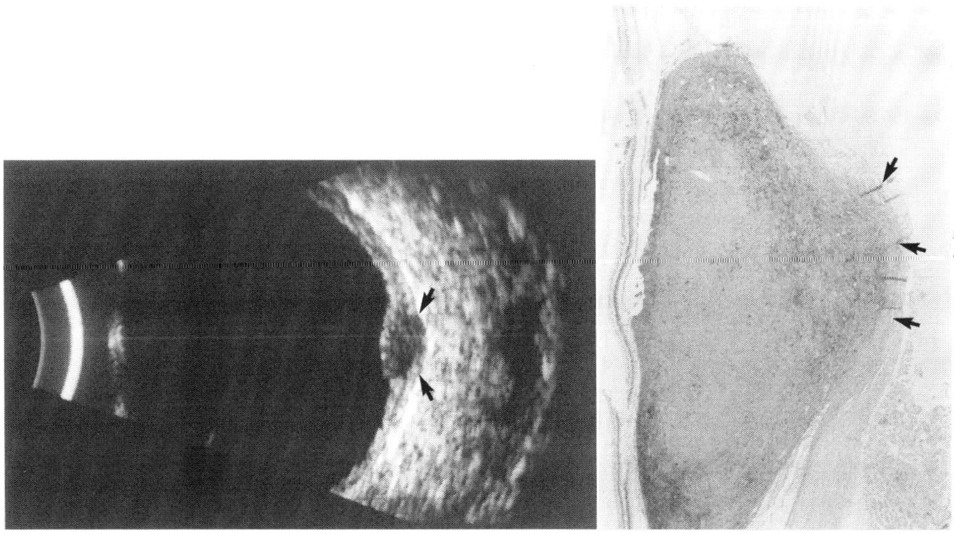

B

Figure 5-25 Small choroidal melanoma showing infiltration and bowing of posterior sclera. **A,** Transverse B-scan demonstrates dome-shaped tumor with diffuse infiltration and bowing of sclera *(arrows)*. **B,** Histopathologic specimen of the melanoma (spindle cell type) shows scleral infiltration *(arrows)* and bowing of sclera.

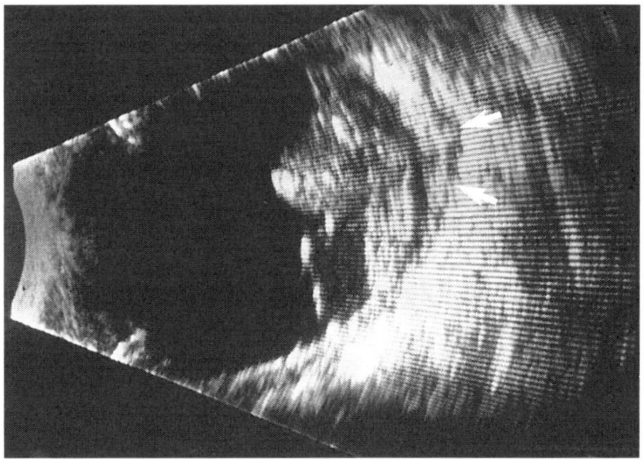

Figure 5-26 Large, irregularly shaped melanoma with extension into orbit via vortex vein *(arrow)*. (From Green RL, Byrne SF: Diagnostic ophthalmic ultrasound, in Ryan SJ [ed]: *Retina*. ed 3, St Louis, Mosby, 2001, p 274.)

A

B

C

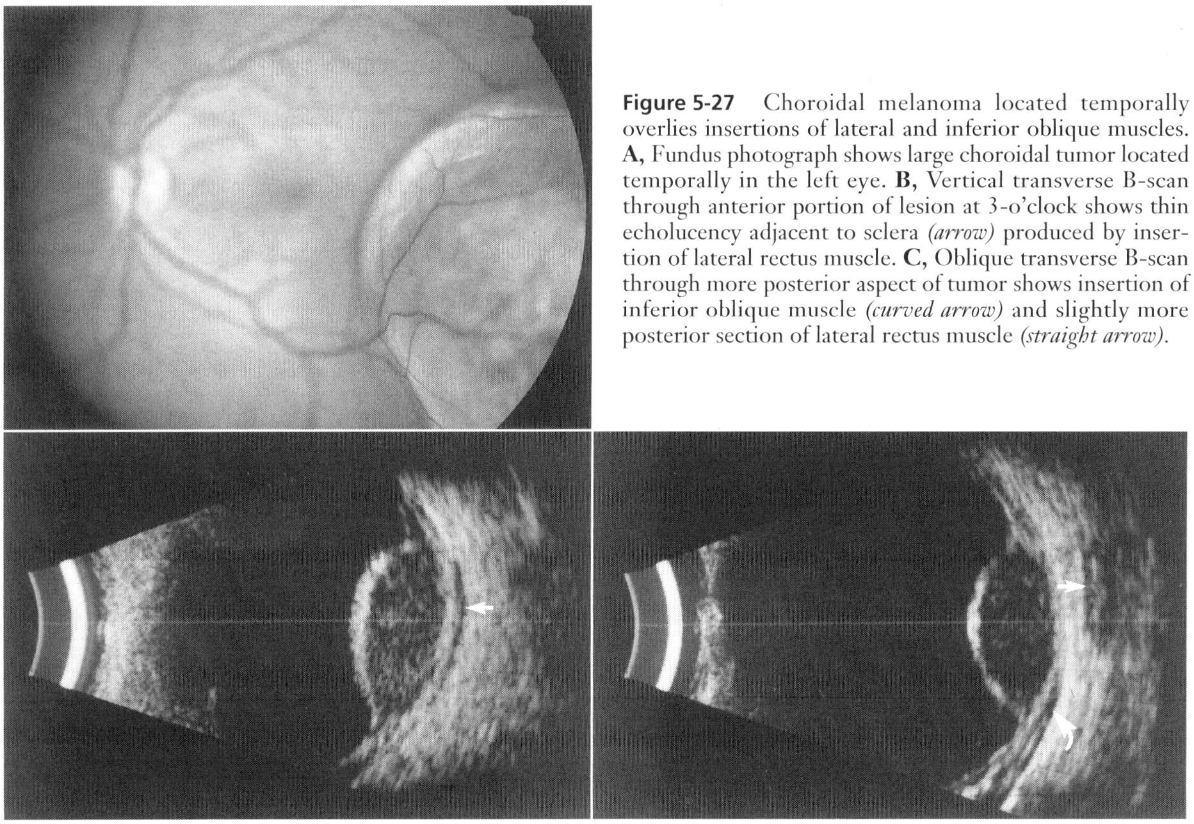

Figure 5-27 Choroidal melanoma located temporally overlies insertions of lateral and inferior oblique muscles. **A,** Fundus photograph shows large choroidal tumor located temporally in the left eye. **B,** Vertical transverse B-scan through anterior portion of lesion at 3-o'clock shows thin echolucency adjacent to sclera *(arrow)* produced by insertion of lateral rectus muscle. **C,** Oblique transverse B-scan through more posterior aspect of tumor shows insertion of inferior oblique muscle *(curved arrow)* and slightly more posterior section of lateral rectus muscle *(straight arrow)*.

Pseudoextrascleral Extension

Certain findings can simulate extraocular growth of a melanoma. These include congested blood vessels, extraocular muscles, and inflammation in sub-Tenon's space.[24,80] A dilated episcleral blood vessel adjacent to an intraocular tumor may be difficult to distinguish from extraocular extension but should not change in size on follow-up examination.

The insertion of an extraocular muscle, especially the inferior oblique, can be mistaken for extrascleral extension (Figure 5-27). This misinterpretation can usually be avoided, however, if the examiner is aware of the location and normal appearance of the extraocular muscles (see Chapter 15 and Figure 15-2). It should be pointed out, however, that the presence of a muscle adjacent to an intraocular tumor can mask small areas of extrascleral extension. If, in such cases, the pattern in the region of the extraocular muscle has a somewhat nodular or irregular configuration, then extraocular tumor extension should be strongly suspected (Figure 5-28).

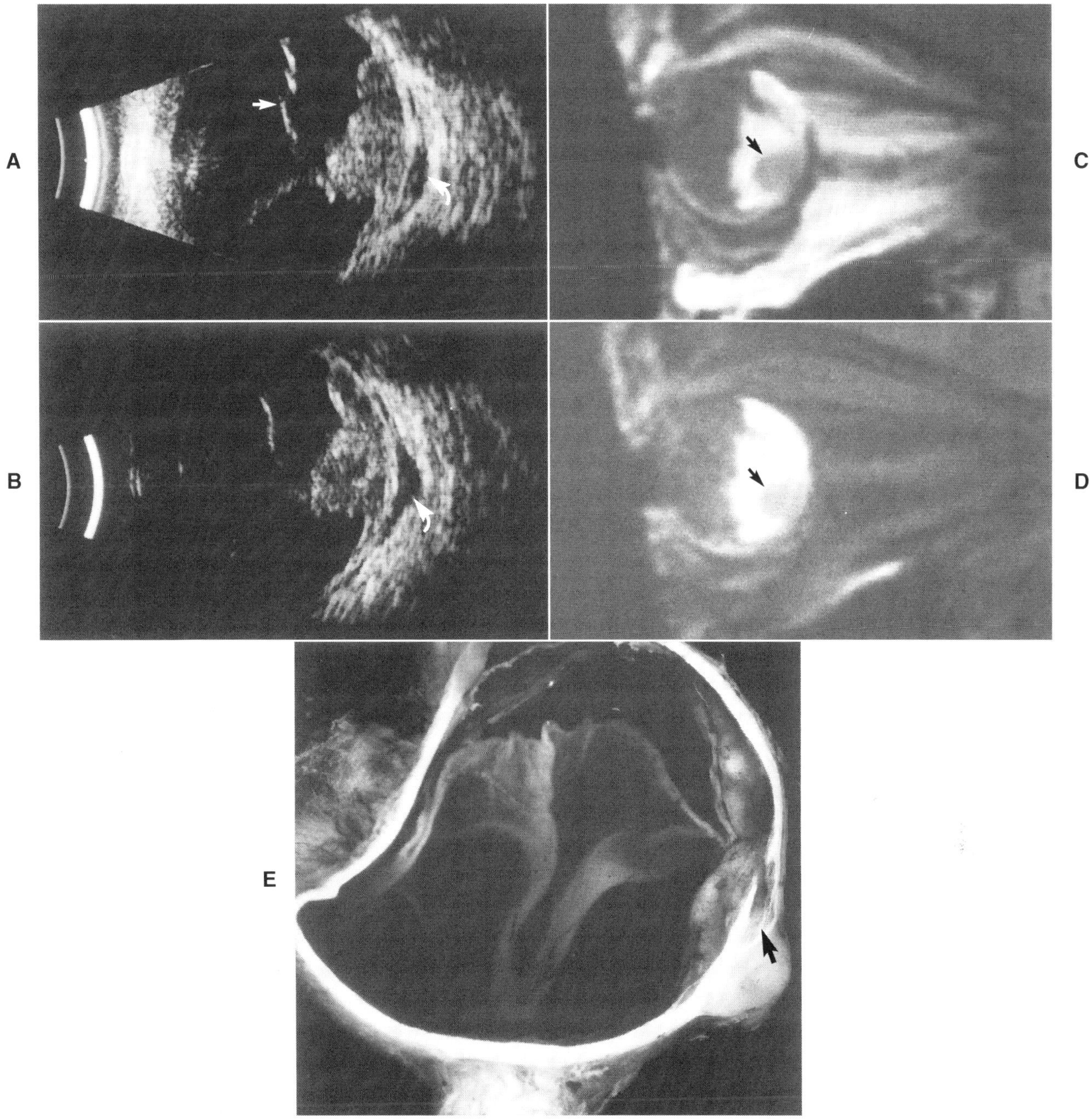

Figure 5-28 Choroidal melanoma with extrascleral extension. Patient with painful eye was referred for echography with suspected scleritis. Although view of the fundus was hazy, an amelanotic lesion was visible in the lower temporal periphery beneath a bullous retinal detachment. Echograms were typical for melanoma. In addition, there was an extraocular lesion in the region of the inferior oblique muscle adjacent to the tumor. On initial examination, it could not be determined whether this represented thickening of the muscle or actual extraocular tumor growth. **A,** Transverse B-scan echogram from initial examination shows large, irregularly shaped intraocular tumor with adjacent echolucent lesion in orbit *(curved arrow). Straight arrow,* RD. **B,** Transverse B-scan 4 weeks later shows increased thickness and slight change in shape of extraocular lesion *(curved arrow).* Definite extrascleral extension was diagnosed by echography at this visit. Sagittal MRI scans (**C** and **D**) obtained at time of second echography examination failed to disclose extrascleral portion of tumor. Intraocular tumor, *arrows.* **C,** T1-weighted scan. **D,** Scan with fat suppression. **E,** Gross pathologic specimen shows melanoma (mixed cell tumor) and extraocular tumor nodule *(arrow).*

Episcleral inflammation adjacent to a choroidal melanoma can also mimic extraocular extension. As mentioned earlier (see p 120), some choroidal melanomas have been associated with scleritis and episcleritis. In all of these cases, the inflammation resolved following corticosteroid therapy, thereby eliminating the echographic suspicion of extraocular extension. However, subsequent histopathologic examination of some of these eyes indicated the presence of microscopic extrascleral and/or scleral extension.[107] Changes involving the sclera, episclera, and extraocular muscle insertions following plaque radiotherapy can also mimic extraocular extension (see p 137).

Diffuse Melanoma

Diffuse melanomas can be difficult to diagnose, both clinically and echographically. Although these tumors are usually flat and diffuse, they may have a slightly irregular, bumpy surface with indistinct margins. When the tumor is sufficiently elevated, the internal reflectivity is typically low to medium (Figure 5-29). Internal vascularity is often difficult to assess because of the shallow nature of these tumors. Additionally, diffuse melanomas are associated with a high incidence of extrascleral extension.[25] The echographic differential diagnosis of diffuse melanoma includes metastatic carcinoma to the choroid (see p 143), diffuse choroidal

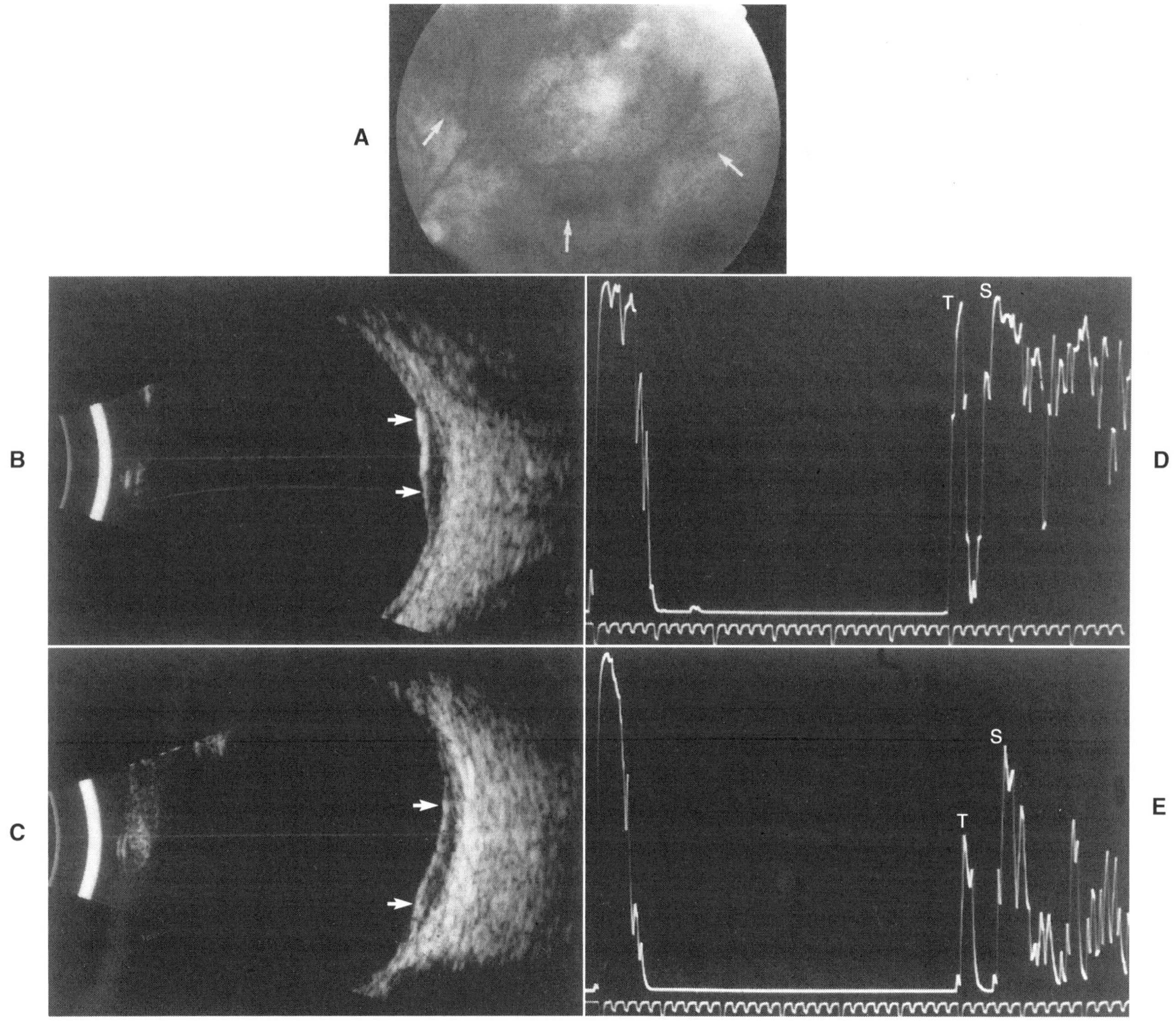

Figure 5-29 Diffuse choroidal melanoma. **A,** Fundus photograph shows extensive, pigmented choroidal melanoma *(arrows)*. **B,** Transverse B-scan echogram shows mildly elevated lesion with flat surface contour *(arrows)*. **C,** Longitudinal B-scan shows much larger base of tumor in this view *(arrows)*. **D,** A-scan at Tissue Sensitivity shows very low reflective, thin lesion. *T,* Tumor surface; S, sclera. **E,** A-scan at reduced gain setting.

nevus (see p 151), Vogt-Koyanagi-Harada syndrome[26] (see p 200), uveal lymphoid hyperplasia (see p 153), diffuse choroidal hemangioma (see p 147), and disciform lesion (see p 160).

Radiation Therapy

Radiation therapy, either by plaque or external beam, has become a common alternative modality for treating eyes with choroidal melanomas.[68,94] Echography is used to follow these tumors in order to assess the effectiveness of treatment and to ensure proper placement of radioactive plaques.[22,70,71]

Postradiation Findings

Typical echographic findings have been observed following radiation treatment of ocular melanoma. These lesions tend to become more irregular in structure and higher reflective as they decrease in size (Figure 5-30). Such changes in internal characteristics appear to be due largely to necrosis within the lesion.[79,80] Loss of internal vascularity is also usually noted following effective treatment. Although treated

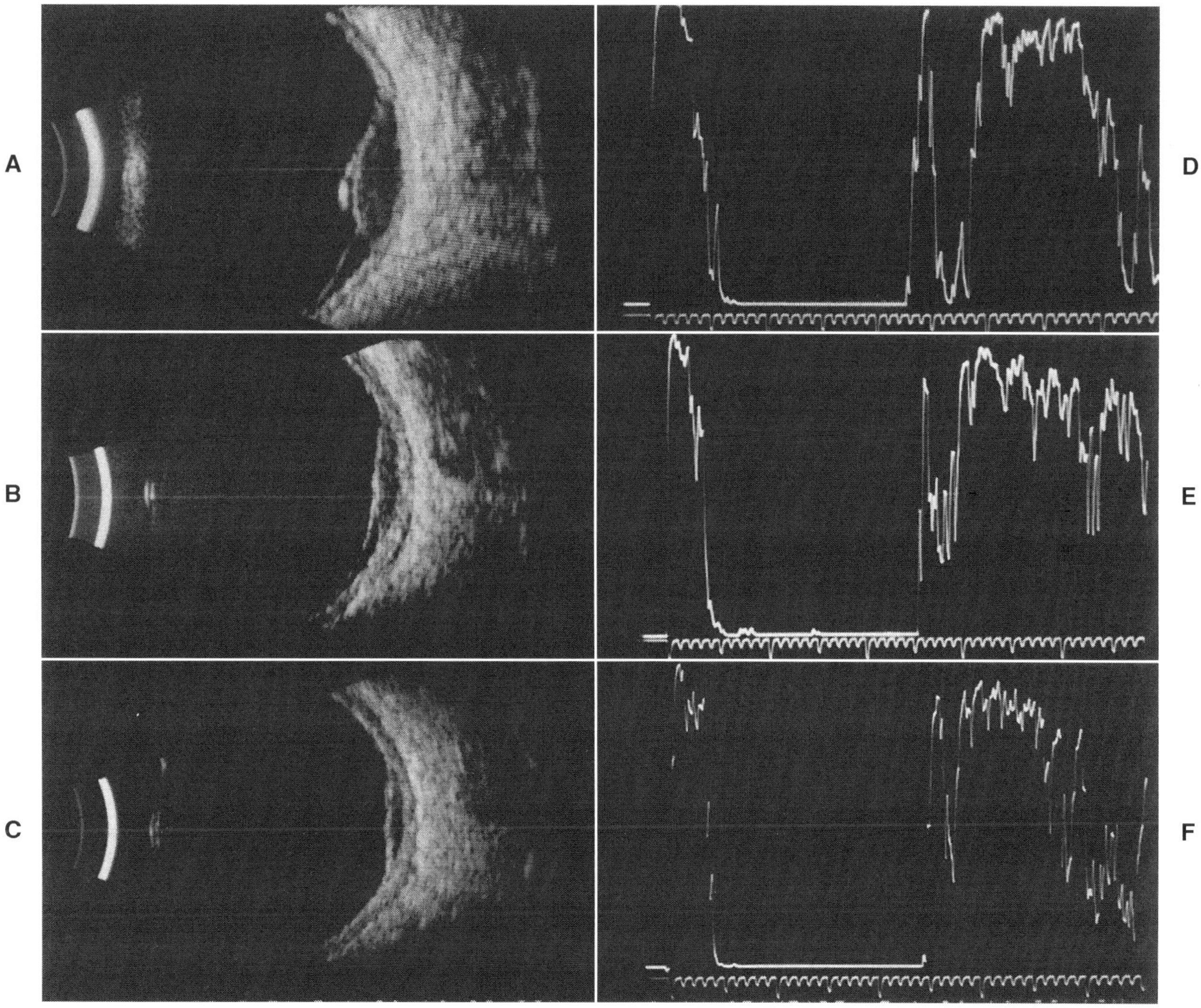

Figure 5-30 Dome-shaped choroidal melanoma before plaque radiotherapy (**A** and **D**), at 4 months (**B** and **E**), and at 8 months (**C** and **F**) after treatment. Transverse B-scan **(A)** shows shallow overlying retinal detachment and corresponding A-scan **(D)** shows low internal reflectivity. At 4 months, transverse B-scan **(B)** shows marked decrease in tumor elevation and flattened surface; corresponding A-scan **(E)** shows increased reflectivity and lower elevation. At 8 months, transverse B-scan **(C),** demonstrates further decrease in elevation and complete resolution of serous retinal detachment; corresponding A-scan **(F)** also shows decrease in tumor elevation. (From Green RL, Byrne SF: Diagnostic ophthalmic ultrasound, in Ryan SJ [ed]: *Retina.* ed 3, St Louis, Mosby, 2001, p 276.)

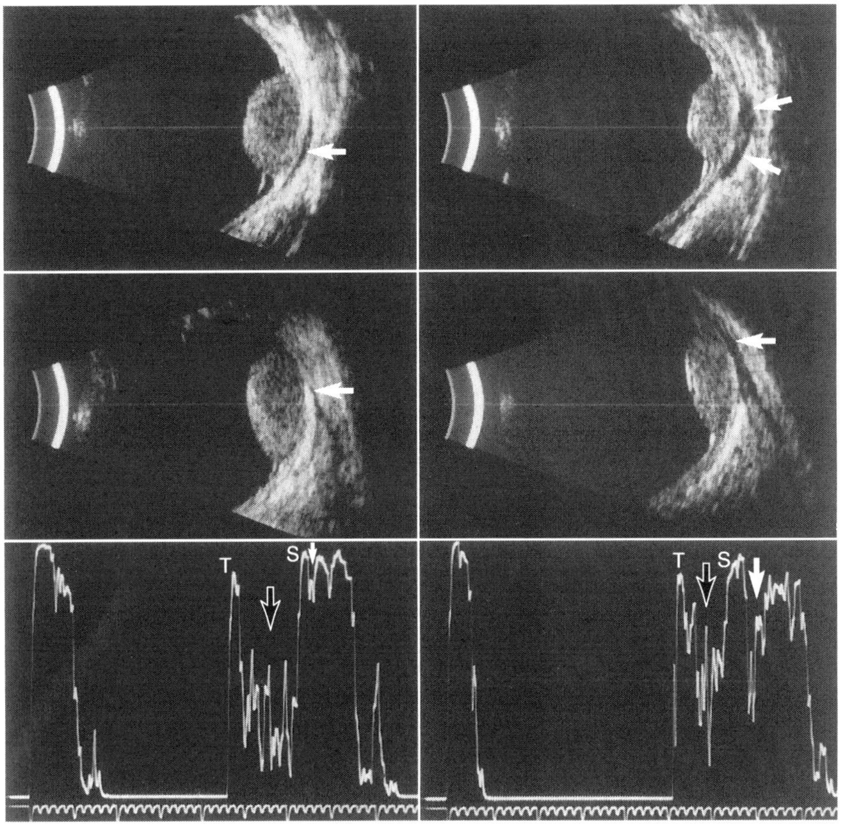

Figure 5-31 Dome-shaped choroidal melanoma overlying insertion of lateral rectus muscle before treatment (**A** to **C**) and 8 months after plaque radiation therapy (**D** to **F**). Transverse (**A**), longitudinal (**B**) B- scans and A-scan (**C**) show dome-shaped, medium-reflective melanoma adjacent to insertion of lateral rectus muscle *(closed arrows)*. *T*, Tumor surface; *open arrow*, internal tumor spikes; *S*, sclera. Corresponding echograms at follow-up examination after treatment (**D** to **F**) show decreased height of tumor, increased internal reflectivity and thickened insertion of muscle. Note how the thickened muscle can simulate extraocular tumor extension.

melanomas typically become smaller over time, some tumors may enlarge shortly after radiotherapy. In the majority of these cases, however, the tumors eventually decrease in size. This initial enlargement appears to be due to edema of the tumor after irradiation. Continued enlargement of the tumor may indicate true tumor growth.

Other possible associated findings include thickening of an adjacent extraocular muscle insertion (Figure 5-31) and decreased reflectivity of the sclera. In addition, inflammatory changes may appear in sub-Tenon's space behind the tumor in the area where the plaque had been placed. It is important to recognize these post-treatment changes because they may affect the appearance of the posterior scleral spike when measuring the tumor after treatment (Figure 5-32). As previously mentioned, changes in the sclera, episclera, and thickening of extraocular muscles can be mistaken for extraocular tumor growth. Consequently, such findings should be closely observed to ensure that there is no increase in size over time. Any enlargement on follow-up examination suggests the possibility of extraocular extension.

Although treated melanomas usually become gradually smaller, long-term follow up should be performed. This is because tumors can show signs of growth after significant regression (Figure 5-33).

Plaque and External Beam Localization Techniques

Ultrasound examination can be a useful adjunct to transillumination for verifying the position of a radioactive plaque adjacent to an ocular melanoma.* Ultrasound is especially useful for localization of a plaque behind a posterior tumor that lies close to the optic nerve, where transillumination may not adequately indicate the tumor margins. Echography can also be of value in cases in which the entire tumor base cannot be visualized with ophthalmoscopy (e.g., collar button tumors with overhang) (see Figure 5-34, *A* and *B*).

The technique for plaque localization incorporates the use of B-scan, either in the operating room under sterile

*References 22, 41, 68, 70, 71, 96, 103.

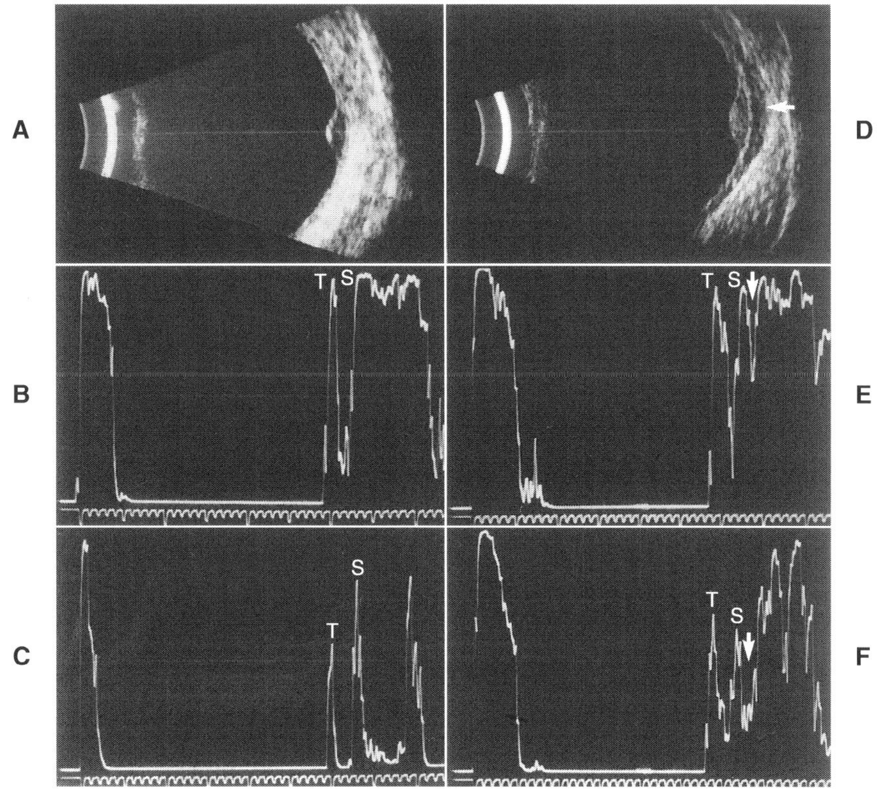

Figure 5-32 Small choroidal melanoma before treatment (**A** to **C**) and 6 months following radioactive plaque therapy (**D** to **F**) show diffuse episcleral inflammation after treatment. **A,** Transverse B-scan echogram shows dome-shaped tumor. **B,** A-scan at Tissue Sensitivity shows low internal reflectivity. *T,* tumor surface; *S,* sclera. **C,** A-scan at reduced gain shows maximum height of tumor. **D,** Extensive echolucent lesion in episcleral space *(arrow)* adjacent to tumor following treatment. **E,** A-scan echogram at Tissue Sensitivity shows mild increase in reflectivity of tumor and thin lesion in episcleral space *(arrow).* **F,** A-scan view at reduced gain shows maximum height of tumor and lesion in episcleral space. Note reduced height of scleral spike due to inflammation following therapy.

A B C

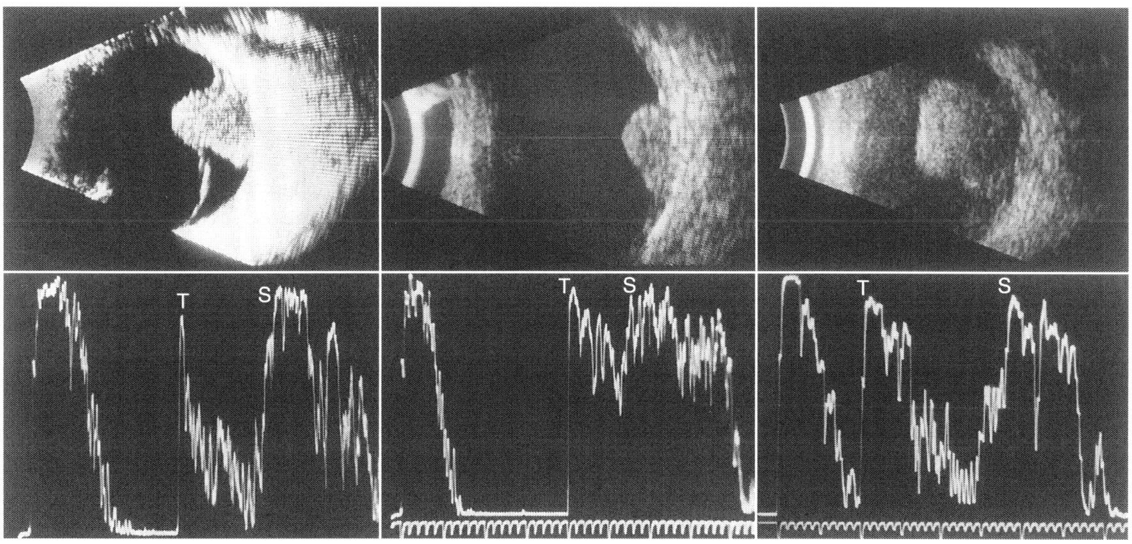

Figure 5-33 Choroidal melanoma at initial examination **(A),** at 1 year **(B)** and 3 years **(C)** after plaque radiation therapy. **A,** Large collar button–shaped tumor demonstrates low to medium reflectivity. *T,* Tumor surface; *S,* sclera. **B,** Tumor shows marked decrease in height as well as increase in internal reflectivity. The internal vascularity was also markedly diminished compared to the initial examination. **C,** Tumor is much larger, and reflectivity has decreased. Also, the internal vascularity had increased markedly compared to the first follow-up examination.

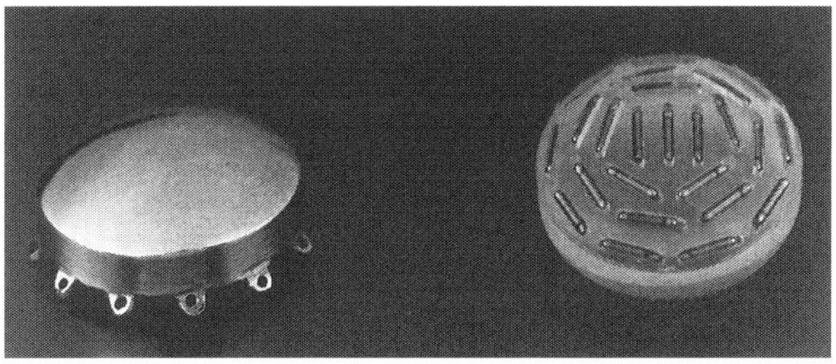

Figure 5-34 Gold shield *(left)* and I-125 plaque containing radioactive seeds *(right)*.

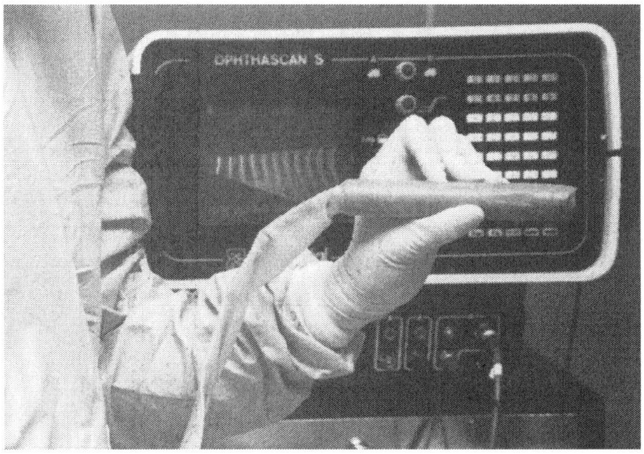

Figure 5-35 B-scan probe placed in sterile rubber sleeve. (Roper Hall, model 2606-P-6078, Kieler.)

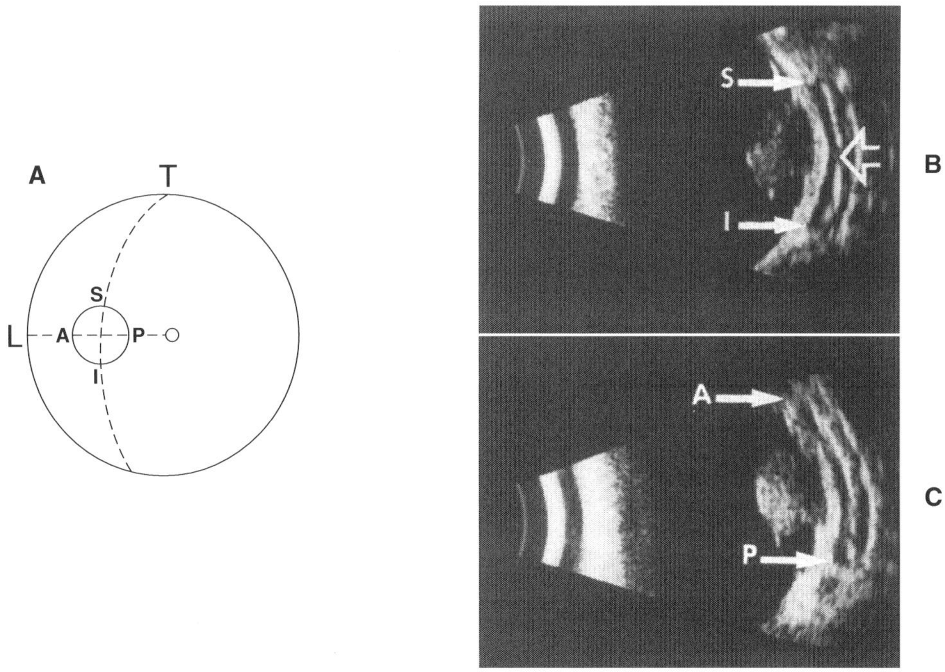

Figure 5-36 B-scan technique for localizing radioactive plaque behind choroidal melanoma. **A,** Schematic drawing shows tumor temporal to the optic disc and path of transverse *(T)* and longitudinal *(L)* scans through tumor. *S,* superior tumor margin; *P,* posterior tumor margin; *I,* inferior tumor margin; *A,* anterior tumor margin. **B,** Transverse B-scan echogram through choroidal melanoma and plaque *(open arrow)* shows superior *(S)* and inferior *(I)* margins of plaque. **C,** Longitudinal B-scan through tumor and plaque shows anterior *(A)* and posterior *(P)* margins of plaque. Note that plaque margins extend beyond tumor borders, indicating proper placement.

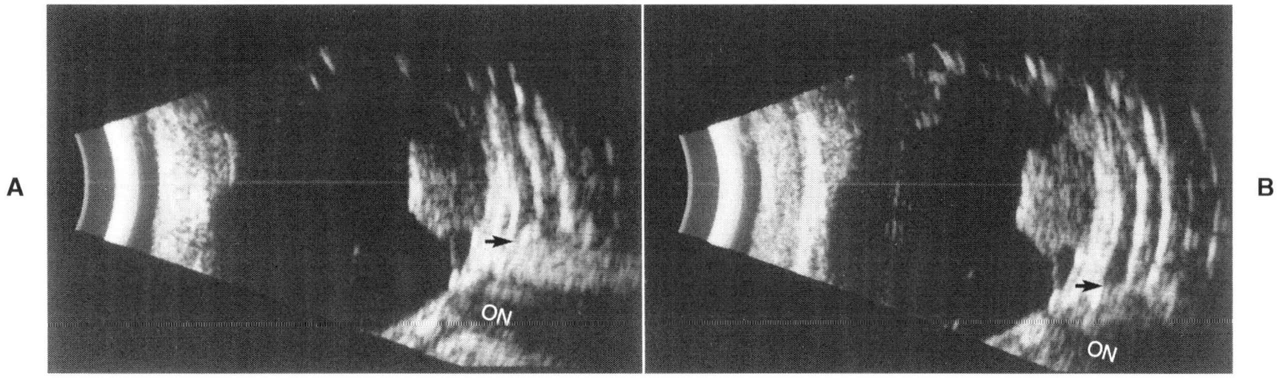

Figure 5-37 Longitudinal B-scan echograms demonstrate repositioning of I-125 plaque. **A,** Initial examination after plaque placement shows that the plaque does not properly extend beyond the posterior tumor margin *(arrow)*. *ON,* Optic nerve. **B,** Examination after repositioning of plaque shows that plaque is now correctly positioned.

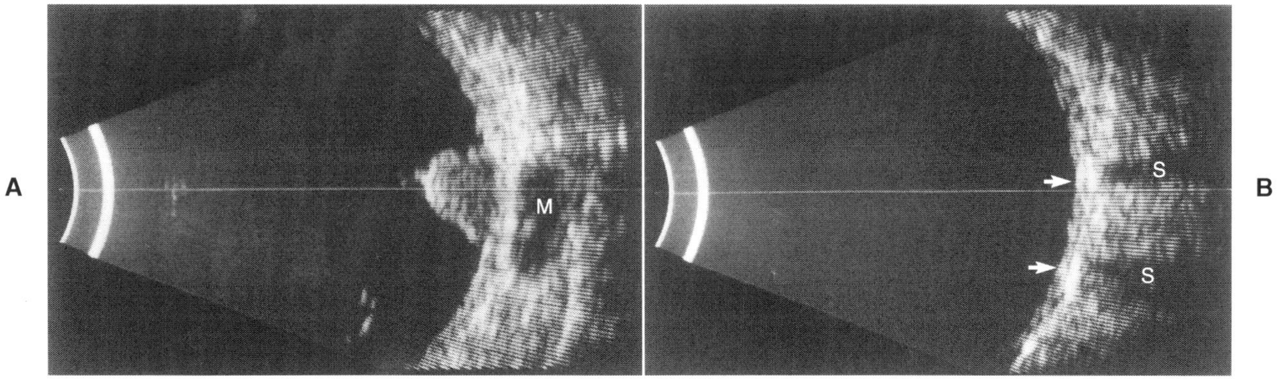

Figure 5-38 B-scan echograms of choroidal melanoma following external beam irradiation. **A,** Transverse view shows choroidal tumor adjacent to enlarged medial rectus muscle *(M)*. **B,** Transverse scan just adjacent to tumor shows two small, highly reflective echoes from tantalum rings *(arrows)* placed next to tumor prior to treatment. S, Shadowing from tantalum rings.

conditions or postoperatively, where strict sterility is unnecessary. The iodine-125 (I-125) plaques typically consist of a gold shield with a plastic insert containing the radioactive seeds[46] (Figure 5-34). On B-scan, these plaques produce a distinct, echolucent pattern in the orbit adjacent to the sclera, with marked shadowing of the orbital tissues.

When the plaque is to be localized under sterile conditions, the B-scan probe can be placed into a sterile rubber sleeve (Figure 5-35). Sterile methylcellulose is placed into the rubber sleeve before inserting the probe and is also applied to the surface of the globe just prior to the examination. The probe is then placed on the eye, opposite the tumor. The base of the tumor is imaged in both transverse and longitudinal orientations to display the relationship of the plaque to the tumor margins (Figure 5-36). If the plaque is shown to be improperly positioned or appears tilted, it can be moved and the echogram repeated to ensure that adequate coverage has been accomplished (Figure 5-37). As previously mentioned, this technique is more useful for tumors located posteriorly, near the optic nerve. Also, this method is most suitable for tumors that have very distinct, steeply rising margins, where the true edges of the tumor can be identified with ultrasound. Echography is less reliable for localizing the plaque behind tumors with sloping, indistinct borders (see Figure 5-29).

For external beam irradiation, tantalum rings are sutured to the globe to help localize the tumor for treatment. Echography can often demonstrate these rings adjacent to the tumor (Figure 5-38).

Ciliary Body and Iris Melanomas

See p 169 for a review of ciliary body and iris melanomas.

BOX 5-1

Pseudomelanomas*

Tumors	Nontumors
Metastatic carcinoma	Disciform lesion
Choroidal hemangioma	Hemorrhagic retinal pigment epithelium detachment (HRPED)
Calcific tumors (e.g., osteoma)	Choroidal hemorrhage (focal)
Nevus	Hemorrhage into retinal cyst/retinoschisis
Melanocytoma (magnocellular nevus)	Posterior nodular scleritis (see p 196)
Intraocular B-cell lymphoma (reticulum cell sarcoma)	Inflammatory lesions of choroid (e.g., VKH, sympathetic ophthalmia, see Chapter 6)
Uveal lymphoid hyperplasia	Bilateral diffuse uveal melanocytic proliferation (BDUMP)
Leukemia	Ampulla of vortex vein
Leiomyoma	Posterior coloboma
Uveal schwannoma (neurilemoma)	Dislocated lenses and lens nuclei
Neurofibroma	Intumescent lens
Hamartomas of the retina (capillary and combined)	Cyst
Scleral tumors	Epithelial downgrowth
Adenoma	
Medulloepithelioma (diktyoma)	

*These lesions can simulate an ocular melanoma clinically and/or echographically.

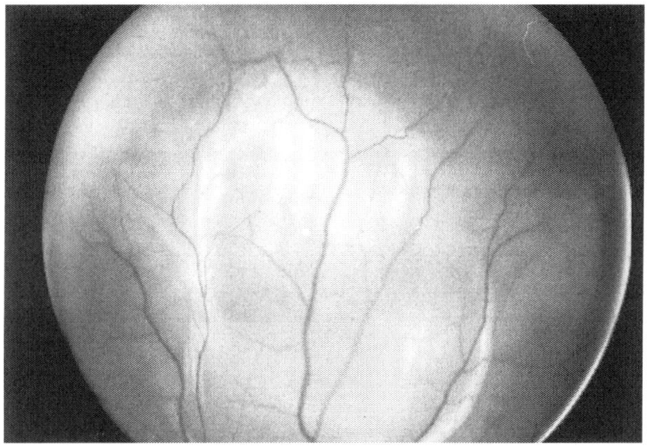

Figure 5-39 Fundus photograph showing metastatic carcinoma to choroid.

Differential Diagnosis of Ocular Melanoma

Many pigmented and nonpigmented lesions can clinically simulate a melanoma[28,58] (Box 5-1). The most common lesions include choroidal nevi, metastatic neoplasms, choroidal hemangiomas, disciform lesions, and choroidal hemorrhages (Table 5-1). There are, however, a large variety of less common conditions that also can simulate a melanoma, including posterior nodular scleritis, melanocytoma, and even dislocated lenses. Echography can be used to differentiate and diagnose many of these disorders. Whenever a suspicious lesion is detected, a systematic echographic examination should be performed using topographic, quantitative, and kinetic techniques (see Chapter 2).

OTHER TUMORS OF THE UVEA, RETINA, RETINAL PIGMENT EPITHELIUM, AND SCLERA

Metastatic Carcinoma

Metastatic carcinoma to the choroid presents clinically as a yellowish, mildly elevated, diffuse lesion with irregular borders (Figure 5-39) that may occur in one or both eyes.[87,88] These tumors are often located in the posterior aspect of the fundus and can be focal or multifocal. They are frequently associated with a serous retinal detachment.

Echographically, metastatic carcinomas are usually mildly to moderately elevated, although they can occasionally become quite elevated. These tumors typically have an irregular, bumpy surface contour, often with central excavation.[6,34] They are frequently diffuse and are sometimes

TABLE 5-1

Differential Diagnosis of Ocular Melanoma*

Lesion	Location	Shape	Reflectivity	Structure	Vascularity
Melanoma	Choroid/ciliary body	Dome/collar button	Low-medium	Regular	+
Metastatic carcinoma	Posterior choroid	Diffuse/irregular	Medium to high	Irregular	−
Choroidal hemangioma	Posterior choroid	Dome	High	Regular	−
Choroidal nevus	Choroid	Dome	High	Regular	−
Disciform lesion	Macula	Dome/irregular	High	Variable	−
Choroidal hemorrhage	Choroid	Dome	Variable	Variable	−

*This table lists the main echographic findings for the most common intraocular lesions that clinically simulate a melanoma.

A C B D

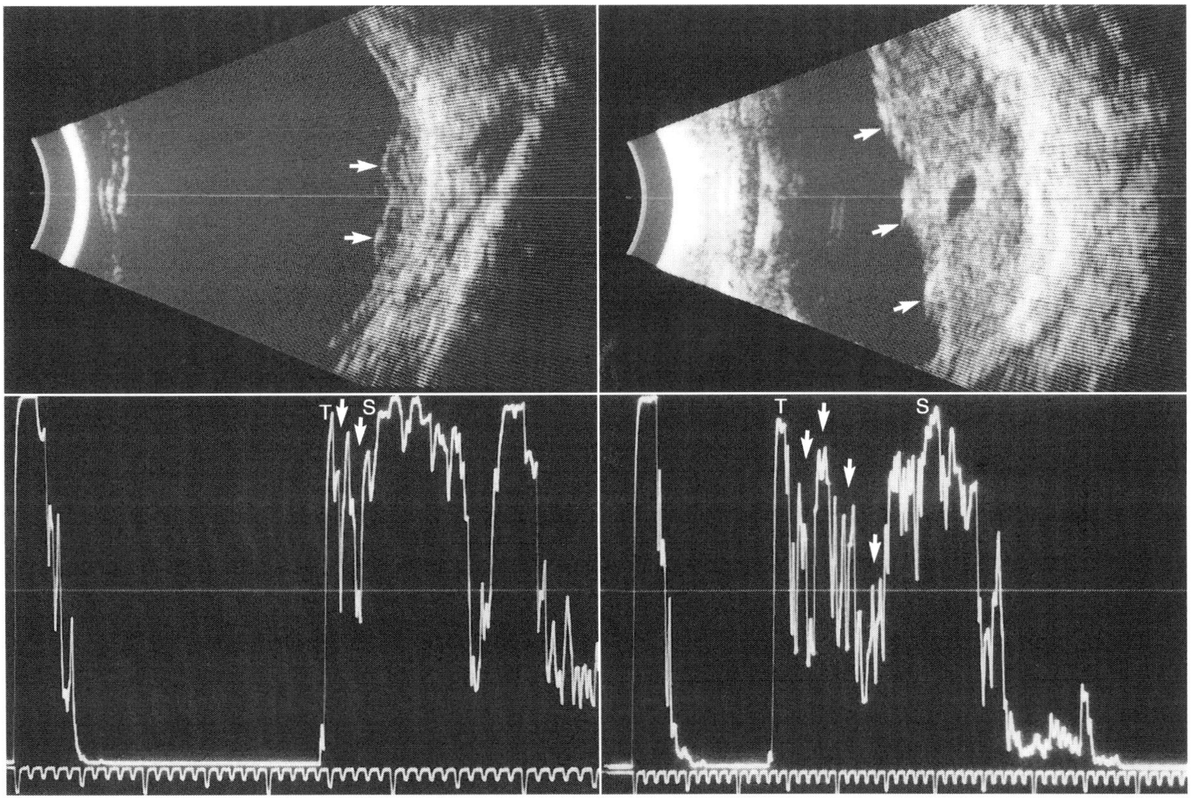

Figure 5-40 Two cases of metastatic carcinoma to the choroid. **A** and **B,** Mildly elevated tumor; **C** and **D,** highly elevated tumor. B-scans (**A** and **C**) show both lesions to have an irregular, bumpy or lobulated surface *(arrows)*. The A-scans (**B** and **D**) of both patients show relatively high reflectivity but also variability of the internal tumor spikes *(arrows)*, indicating irregular structure. *T,* Tumor surface; *S,* sclera. (From Green RL, Byrne SF: Diagnostic ophthalmic ultrasound, in Ryan SJ [ed]: *Retina.* ed 3, St Louis, Mosby, 2001, p 281.)

found by echography to be more extensive than is clinically appreciable. The internal reflectivity of metastatic carcinomas is generally medium to high, but the internal structure can be somewhat irregular (Figure 5-40). These findings result from the varied histologic architecture produced by the growth pattern of metastatic carcinomas to the choroid (see Figure 2-24). Additionally, internal vascularity is typically minimal or absent in these lesions. The serous retinal detachments associated with metastatic carcinomas tend to be more elevated and extensive than are those occurring with melanomas of similar size[87] (Figure 5-41). In some cases, metastatic tumors present with simultaneous intraocular and orbital lesions (Figure 5-42). Vitreous and subretinal hemorrhage is rarely associated with metastatic carcinoma.

Echographically, metastatic carcinomas to the choroid can be confused with diffuse choroidal melanomas (see

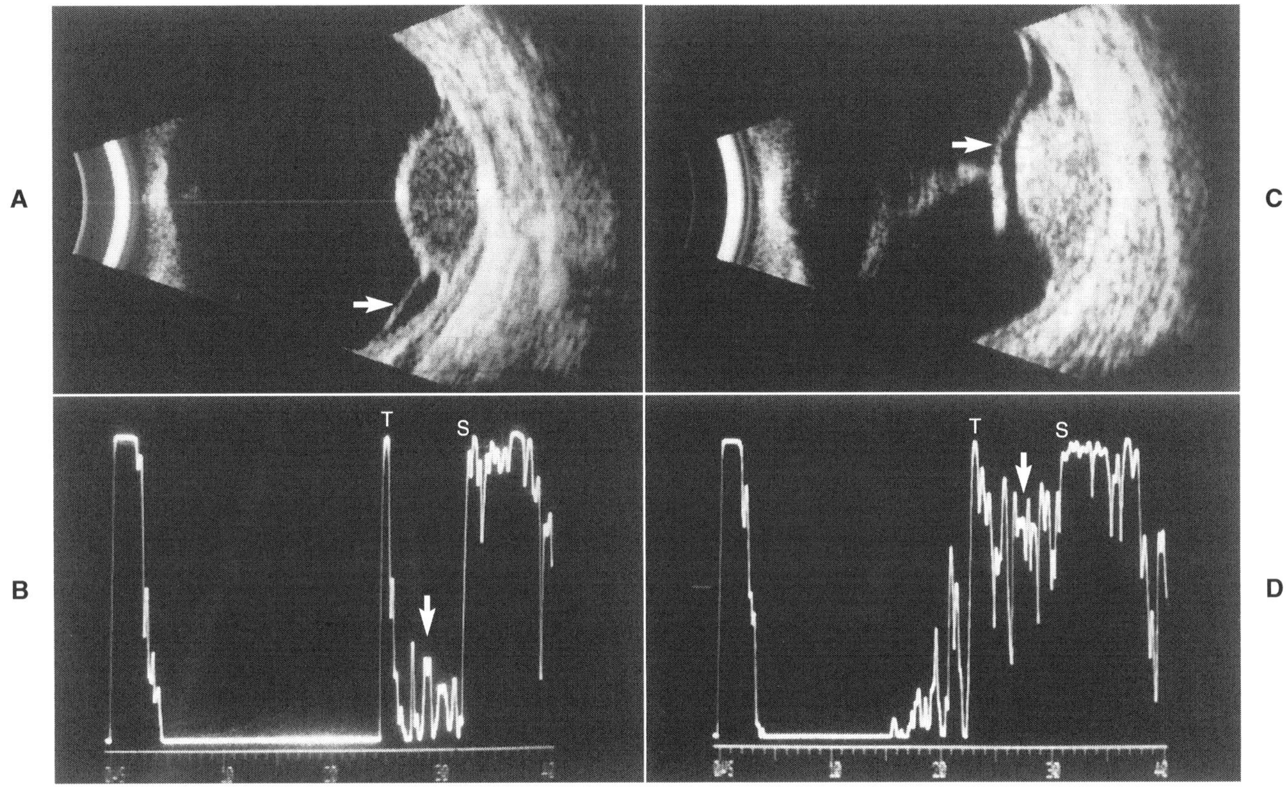

Figure 5-41 Choroidal melanoma (**A** and **B**) and metastatic carcinoma to the choroid (**C** and **D**) of similar size. B-scans (**A** and **C**) show dome-shaped tumors with associated retinal detachments *(arrows)*. Note that detachment is much more extensive in **C,** as is typical for metastatic tumors. A-scan of melanoma **(B)** is also much lower reflective than metastatic tumor **(D).** *T,* Tumor surface; *arrows,* internal tumor spikes; *S,* sclera.

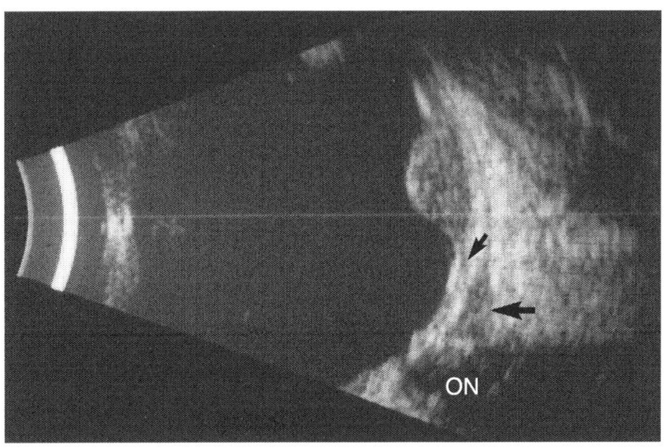

Figure 5-42 Metastatic carcinoma to choroid and orbit. Longitudinal B-scan shows dome-shaped intraocular mass and smaller extrascleral mass *(large arrow)* adjacent to optic nerve *(ON)*. Note possible communication between intraocular and extraocular lesions through scleral canal *(small arrow)*.

p 136), uveal lymphoid hyperplasia (see p 153), disciform lesions (see p 159), choroidal hemangiomas (see p 147), posterior nodular scleritis (see p 196), choroidal nevi (see p 151), and Vogt-Koyanagi-Harada syndrome (see p 200).

In some cases, metastatic choroidal tumors present with atypical findings. Some tumors may exhibit low internal reflectivity as well as internal vascularity and may be therefore confused echographically with choroidal melanomas. The most common type of metastatic tumor to produce these echographic findings is the small cell (oat cell) carcinoma of the lung.[101] Another unusual finding that may be observed is the presence of bullous choroidal detachments[93] (Figure 5-43). An additional rare finding in metastatic carcinoma to the choroid is a collar button shape.[102] One case

A

B

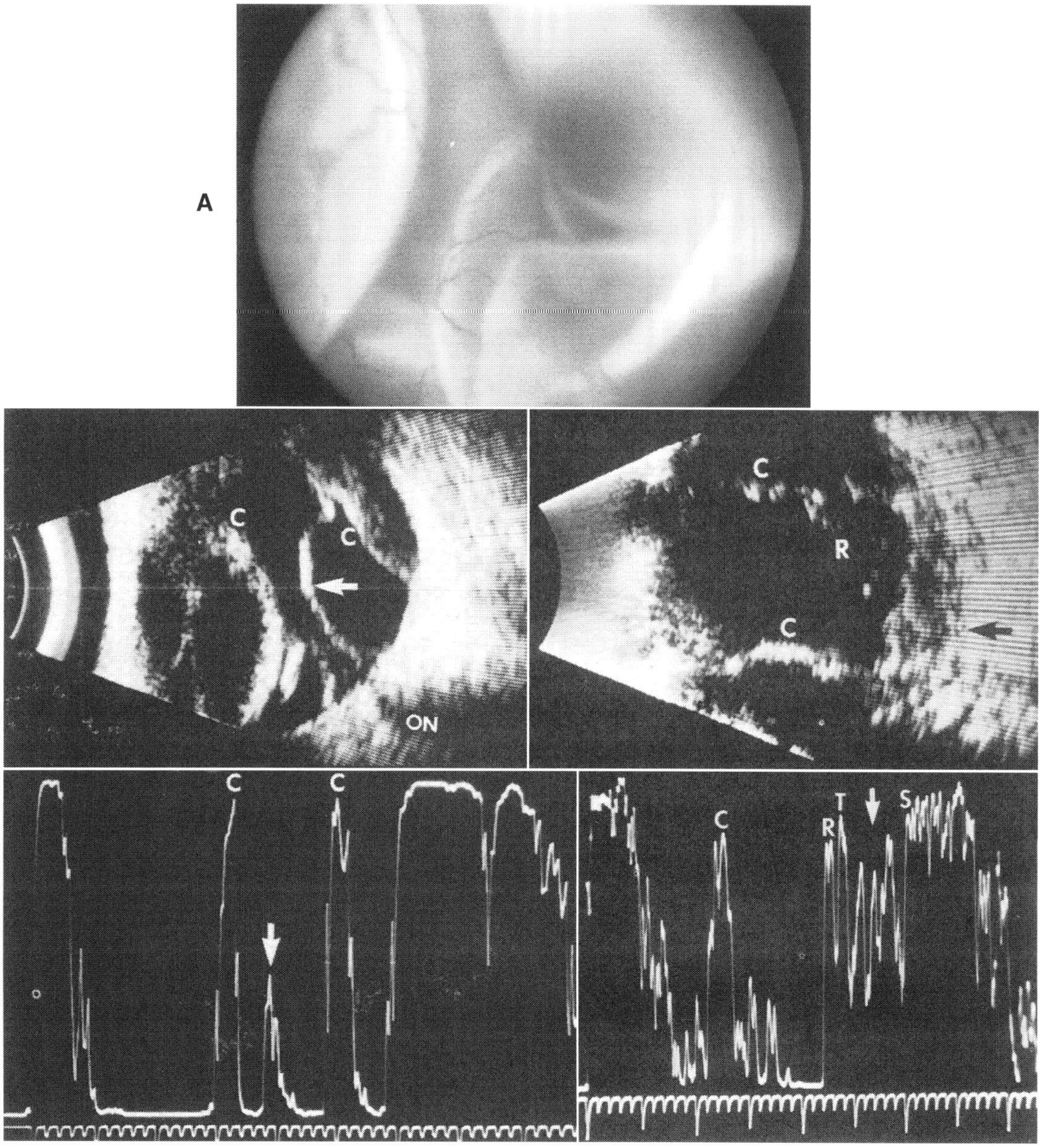

D

C

E

Figure 5-43 Metastatic carcinoma to the choroid with associated retinal and choroidal detachments. **A,** Fundus photograph shows bullous choroidal detachments. **B,** Longitudinal B-scan echogram of 3-o'clock meridian shows peripheral dome-shaped choroidal detachments *(C)* and funnel-shaped retinal detachment *(arrow)* inserting into optic nerve *(ON)*. **C,** Corresponding A-scan echogram shows thick, highly reflective, double-peaked spikes from choroidal detachments *(C)* and lower spike from retinal detachment *(arrow)* as a result of oblique sound beam incidence. **D,** Transverse B-scan through lower periphery of globe shows diffuse tumor mass *(arrow)* with irregular surface contour. Note peripheral choroidal detachments *(C)* and overlying retinal detachment *(R)*. **E,** A-scan shows irregular internal structure and high reflectivity of metastatic tumor *(arrow)*. *C,* Choroidal detachment; *R,* retinal detachment overlying tumor; *T,* tumor surface; *arrow,* internal tumor spikes; *S,* sclera. (From Sneed RS, Byrne SF, Meiler WF, et al: Choroidal detachments associated with malignant choroidal tumors. *Ophthalmology* 1991; 98:968.)

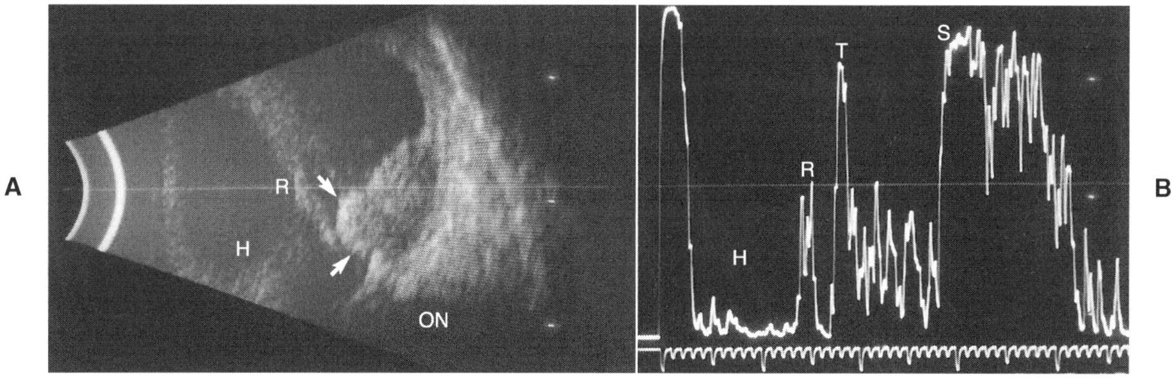

Figure 5-44 Metastatic carcinoma with collar button configuration. **A,** Longitudinal B-scan shows choroidal mass with eccentric collar button *(arrows)* located adjacent to optic nerve *(ON)*. Total, closed funnel-shaped retinal detachment *(R)* and subretinal hemorrhage *(H)* are also present. **B,** A-scan shows medium to low internal reflectivity of tumor. *T,* Tumor surface; *S,* sclera, *H,* hemorrhage in subretinal space; *R,* retina. Low height and double-peaked nature of retinal spike are due to closed funnel shape and oblique sound beam incidence. This eye was enucleated due to uncontrollable intraocular pressure. Histopathologic examination showed metastatic carcinoma from the lung and confirmed that the tumor had broken through Bruch's membrane. (From Read RW, Green RL, Rao NA: Metastatic adenocarcinoma with rupture through the Bruch membrane simulating a choroid melanoma. *Am J Ophthalmol* 2002;132:994.)

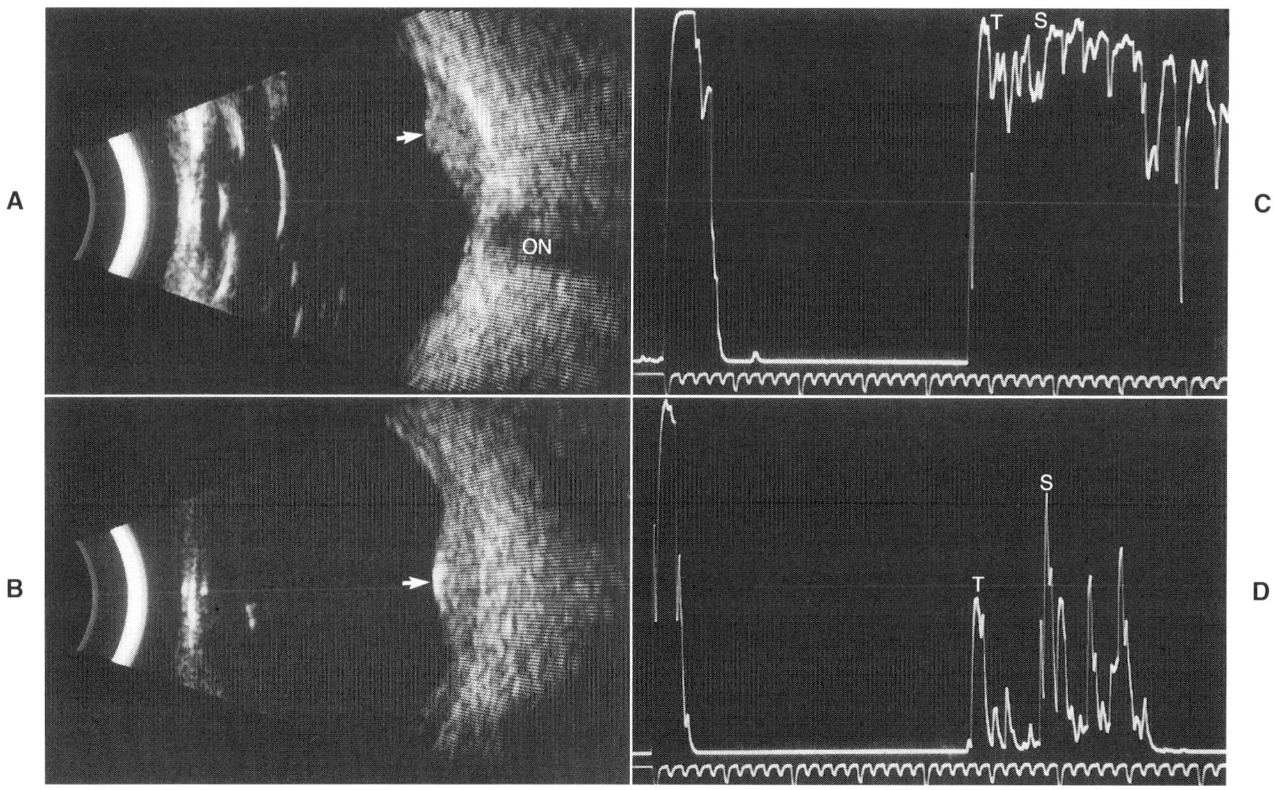

Figure 5-45 Choroidal hemangioma located adjacent to optic nerve. Axial **(A)** and transverse **(B)** B-scan echograms show dome-shaped lesion *(arrows)*. *ON,* Optic nerve. **C,** A-scan at Tissue Sensitivity shows regular internal structure and high reflectivity typical of a choroidal hemangioma. *T,* Tumor surface; *S,* sclera. **D,** A-scan of tumor at reduced gain.

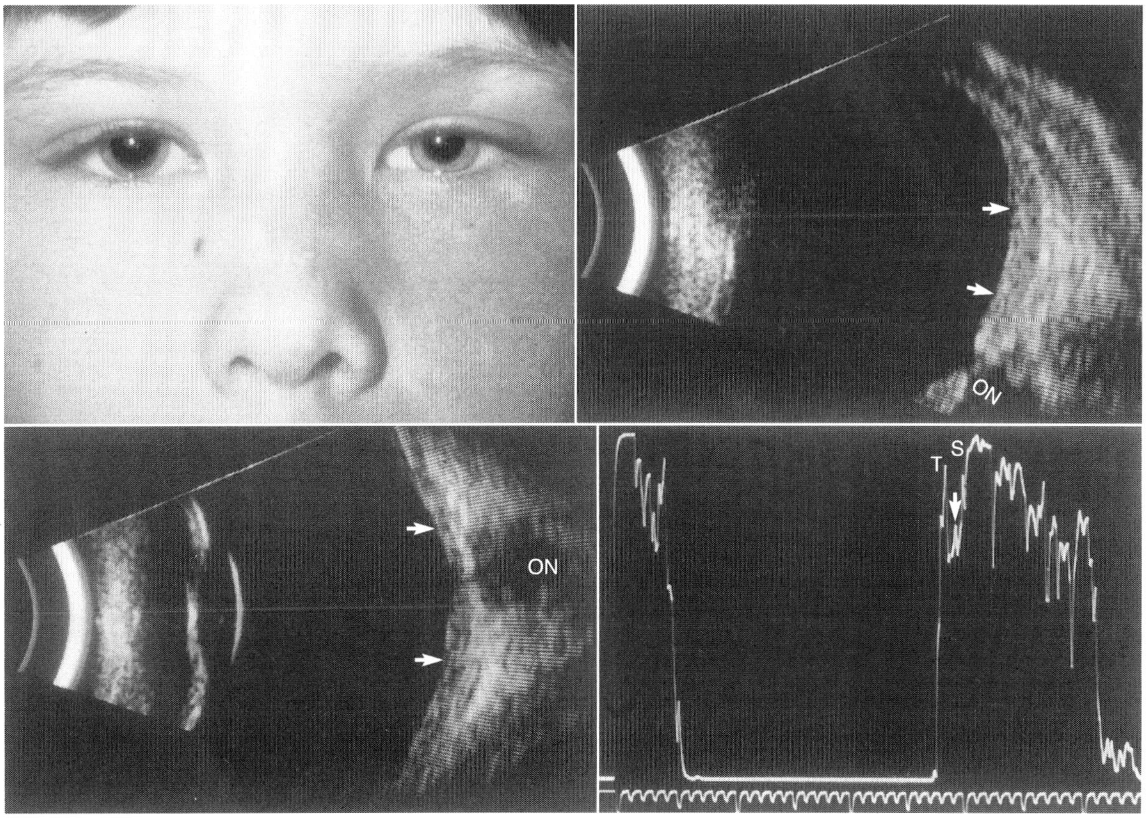

Figure 5-46 Diffuse choroidal hemangioma in child with Sturge-Weber syndrome. **A**, External photograph shows port wine stain typical of Sturge-Weber syndrome. **B**, Axial B-scan echogram shows diffuse, mildly elevated lesion *(arrows)* surrounding the optic nerve *(ON)*. **C**, Longitudinal B-scan shows diffuse lesion extending from ON to the periphery. **D**, A-scan shows mildly elevated lesion with medium-high internal reflectivity. *T*, Tumor surface; *arrow*, internal tumor spikes; *S*, sclera.

of metastatic carcinoma from lung presented with a collar button configuration and a massive subretinal hemorrhage. The internal structure of the tumor was slightly irregular and the reflectivity was medium to low (Figure 5-44). This patient developed severe secondary glaucoma.

Choroidal Hemangioma

This tumor often presents as an orange-red, mildly elevated lesion in the posterior fundus, temporal to the optic nerve.[29] These dome-shaped lesions typically exhibit high internal reflectivity and regular internal structure (Figure 5-45). Although hemangiomas are classified as vascular lesions, significant internal blood flow is usually not observed echographically. Serous retinal detachments can be present at the tumor margins and cystic degeneration of the overlying retina can occur. Calcification occasionally can be seen on the surface of a choroidal hemangioma.[105] Echographically, hemangiomas can be confused with other highly reflective lesions such as metastatic carcinomas, disciform lesions, choroidal nevi, and occasionally, posterior nodular scleritis.

Sturge-Weber syndrome is associated with a more diffuse type of choroidal hemangioma.[75] These tumors are often less elevated than the focal, dome-shaped lesions described earlier (Figure 5-46). In some cases, these hemangiomas are so diffuse that they can be mistaken for nonspecific retinochoroid layer thickening (see p 74). Therefore, in cases of Sturge-Weber syndrome, retinochoroid layer thickness should be carefully compared between the two eyes. Occasionally, these diffuse tumors can be moderately elevated and partially dome shaped. Serous retinal detachments may develop, and associated thickening of adjacent extraocular muscles may be present (Figure 5-47).

Choroidal Osteoma and other Calcific Lesions of the Eye

Certain intraocular tumors are associated with calcification. In addition, there are numerous other lesions that demonstrate signs of calcification on the ultrasound examination (Box 5-2).

A choroidal osteoma usually presents as a yellow-white to orange-red lesion in the peripapillary region, most com-

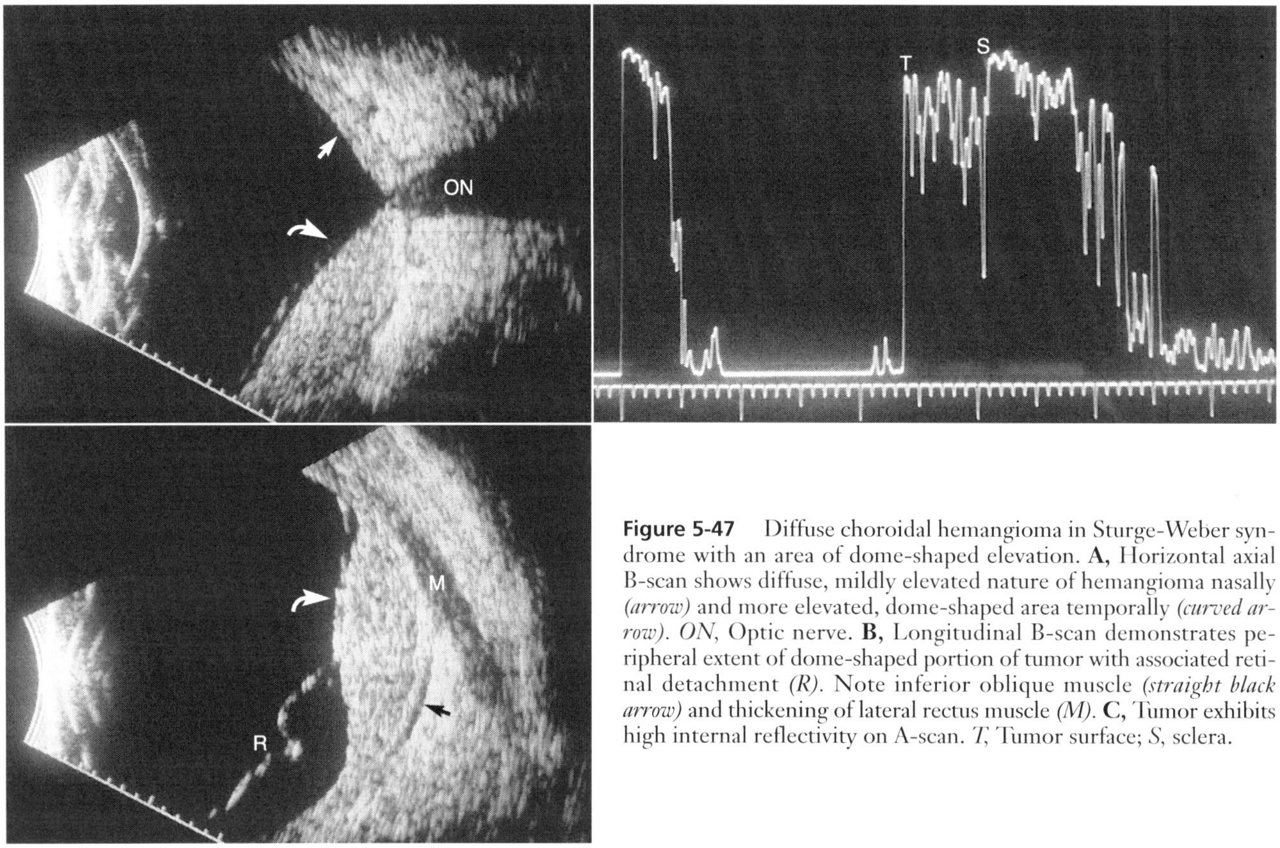

Figure 5-47 Diffuse choroidal hemangioma in Sturge-Weber syndrome with an area of dome-shaped elevation. **A,** Horizontal axial B-scan shows diffuse, mildly elevated nature of hemangioma nasally *(arrow)* and more elevated, dome-shaped area temporally *(curved arrow)*. *ON,* Optic nerve. **B,** Longitudinal B-scan demonstrates peripheral extent of dome-shaped portion of tumor with associated retinal detachment *(R)*. Note inferior oblique muscle *(straight black arrow)* and thickening of lateral rectus muscle *(M)*. **C,** Tumor exhibits high internal reflectivity on A-scan. *T,* Tumor surface; *S,* sclera.

BOX 5-2

Conditions Associated with Calcification

- Choroidal osteoma (see p 147)
- Sclerochoroidal calcification (see below)
- Retinoblastoma (see p 180)
- Retinal angioma (see p 155)
- Retinal astrocytic hamartoma (see p 155)
- Choroidal melanoma (see p 120)
- Choroidal hemangioma (see p 147)
- Optic nerve head drusen (see p 434)
- Disciform lesions (see p 68)
- Granuloma (e.g., toxocariasis) (see p 203)
- Cysticercosis (see p 203)
- Mature cataracts (see p 265)
- Trauma
- Calcification underlying longstanding retinal detachment
- Phthisis bulbi (see p 114)
- Cogan's plaques (see p 149)

monly in young women.[4] Osteomas are typically unilateral, focal, and only mildly elevated.[29] Because these lesions consist of bone, they produce extremely high internal reflectivity and marked shadowing of the scleral and orbital signals posterior to the lesion (see Figure 2-25). Although many osteomas have a relatively smooth, flat appearance, they occasionally show an irregular surface contour[29] (Figure 5-48).

Idiopathic sclerochoroidal calcification is a disorder that can simulate choroidal osteoma.[40,49,73,88] This condition, which is usually bilateral, is characterized by multiple, discrete, yellowish plaquelike lesions. They are typically found in the midperipheral fundus, often supratemporally. Echographically, these lesions are usually flat or only mildly elevated. They produce extremely high reflectivity and marked shadowing of the orbital tissues posterior to the lesion[76,92] (Figure 5-49). It has been shown that echography may detect bilateral lesions, although clinically they may only be visible in one eye.[40] Similar types of lesions have been described in patients with hyperparathyroidism and other metabolic disorders.[40]

Other intraocular tumors can also show signs of calcification. The tumor most often associated with calcification

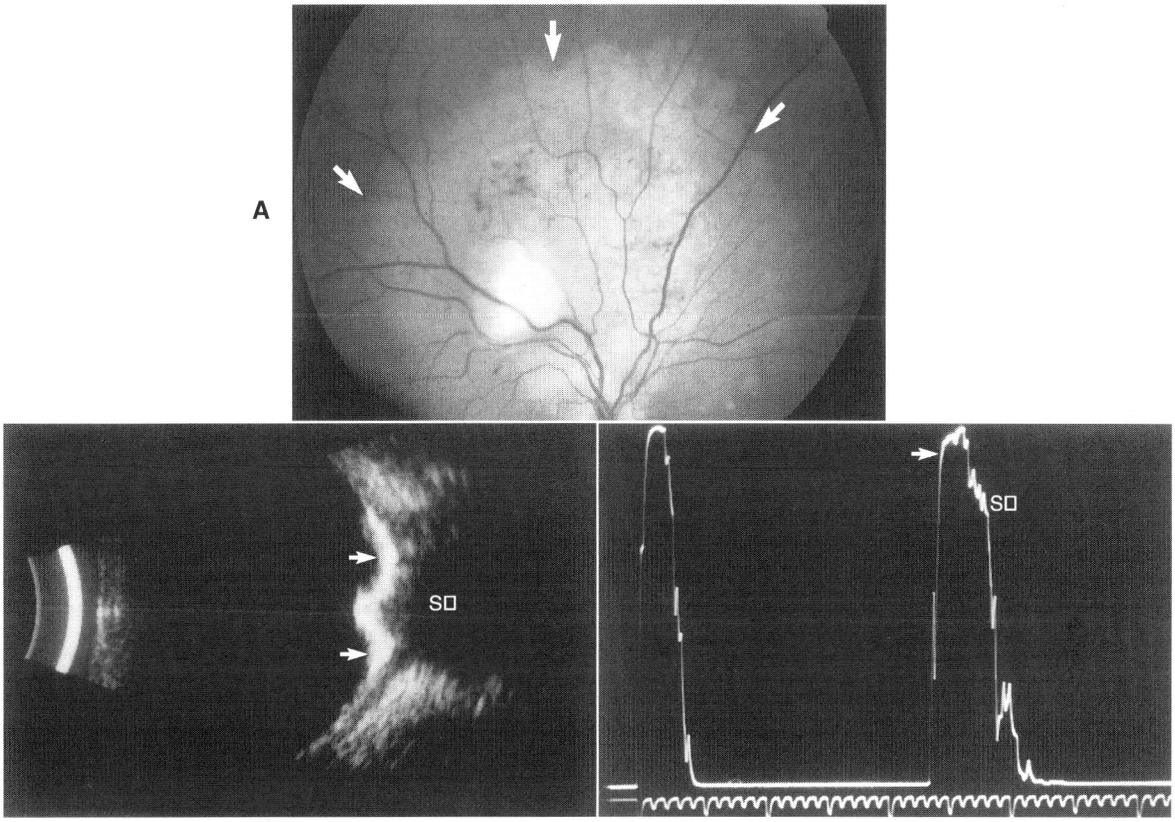

Figure 5-48 Choroidal osteoma. **A,** Fundus photograph shows extensive hypopigmented lesion superiorly *(arrows).* **B,** Transverse B-scan echogram shows very echo-dense lesion with irregular surface contour *(arrows).* Note wide area of shadowing *(S)* behind lesion. **C,** A-scan shows very high reflectivity of osteoma *(arrow).* Orbital spikes are absent because of very strong shadowing *(S).*

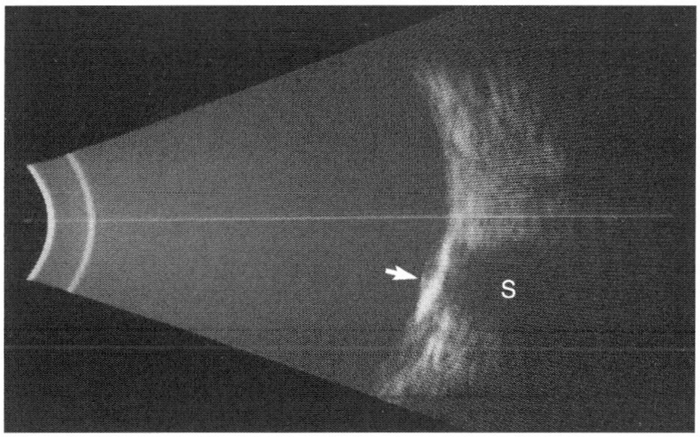

Figure 5-49 Idiopathic sclerocalcification. Transverse B-scan displays slightly irregular, echo-dense plaque at level of retinochoroid layer and sclera *(arrow). S,* Shadowing produced by calcified lesion.

is retinoblastoma (see p 180). Retinal angiomas and retinal astrocytic hamartomas (see p 155) are also known to demonstrate calcific deposits. Calcified nodules have also been observed in choroidal melanomas (see p 120 and Figure 5-10) and choroidal hemangiomas, usually on the tumor surface.

Nontumorous causes of calcification within the eye include optic nerve head drusen (see p 434), degenerative changes of the eye, and Cogan's plaques.[15] Examples of degenerative lesions associated with calcification include longstanding disciform lesions, granulomas from toxocariasis, cysticercosis, and lesions caused by trauma. Dense, mature cataracts can also demonstrate extensive calcification. Plaquelike calcification of the choroid and/or sclera may be seen in

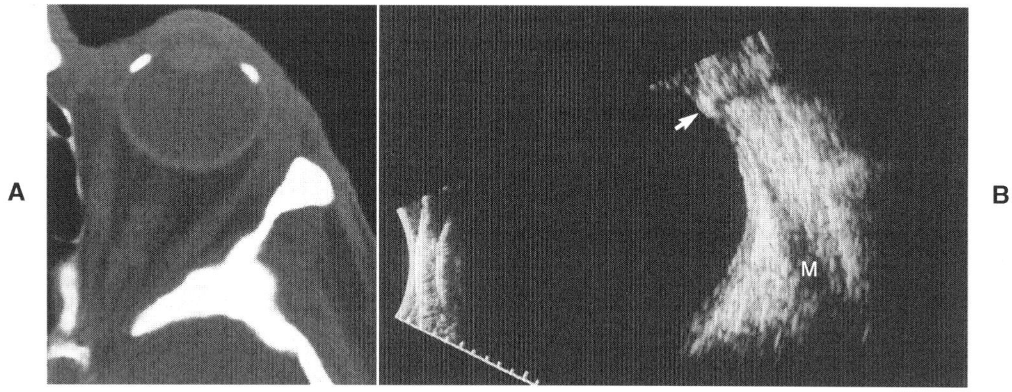

Figure 5-50 Cogan's plaque. **A,** Axial CT scan (bone window) shows plaquelike calcifications of nasal and temporal peripheral sclera. **B,** Anterior longitudinal B-scan demonstrates small, echo-dense lesion involving peripheral sclera *(arrow)*. *M,* Lateral rectus muscle.

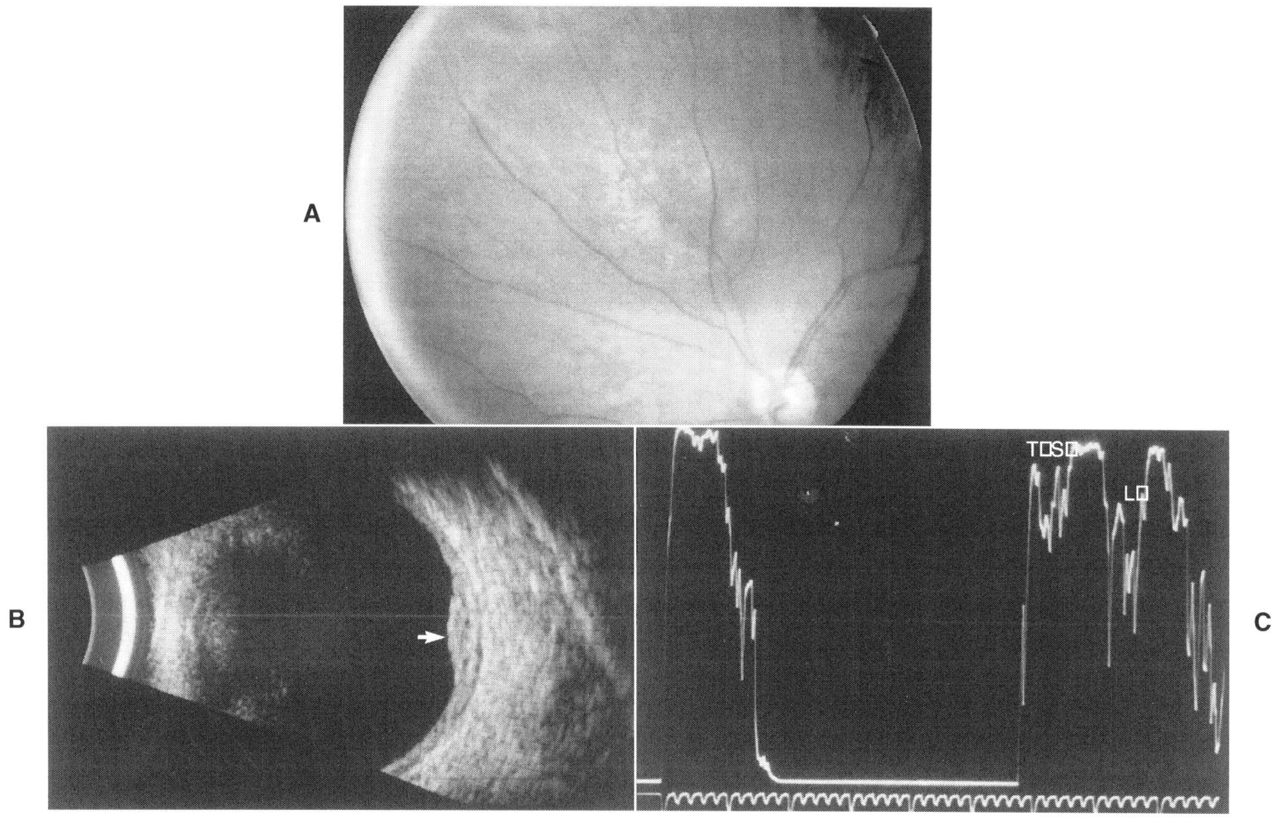

Figure 5-51 Choroidal nevus. **A,** Fundus photograph shows pigmented lesion. **B,** Transverse B-scan echogram shows mildly elevated lesion *(arrow)*. **C,** A-scan shows mild elevation and high internal reflectivity of lesion. *T,* Tumor surface; *S,* sclera.

eyes with longstanding retinal detachment. Finally, dense calcification of the posterior ocular coats and other structures including the detached retina and lens, occurs secondary to phthisis bulbi (see p 114).

Cogan's plaques are focal areas of scleral calcification that are located anterior to the insertion of the horizontal rectus muscles. They are frequently bilateral and are often detected during routine ultrasound screening examinations. These small lesions are nodular and echo dense (Figure 5-50).

Choroidal Nevus

Choroidal nevi are usually minimally elevated and, in many cases, are too flat even to be detected by echography. Although there is scant pathologic correlation with echographic findings, most elevated choroidal nevi appear to be highly reflective and nonvascular[66] (Figures 5-51 and 5-52). Their small size, however, often prevents effective differentiation, and therefore, echography frequently cannot distinguish nevi from small melanomas. As a result, suspected nevi should be observed closely to detect any changes in size or internal reflectivity. Nevi usually show little or no growth, whereas melanomas tend to increase in size. In addition, as small melanomas grow, their internal reflectivity tends to decrease. It should be noted, however, that choroidal nevi can develop subneovascular membranes with subretinal fluid, thus mimicking growth.[8]

Choroidal nevi also can be echographically confused with other highly reflective lesions, such as choroidal hemangiomas, metastatic carcinomas, and disciform lesions.

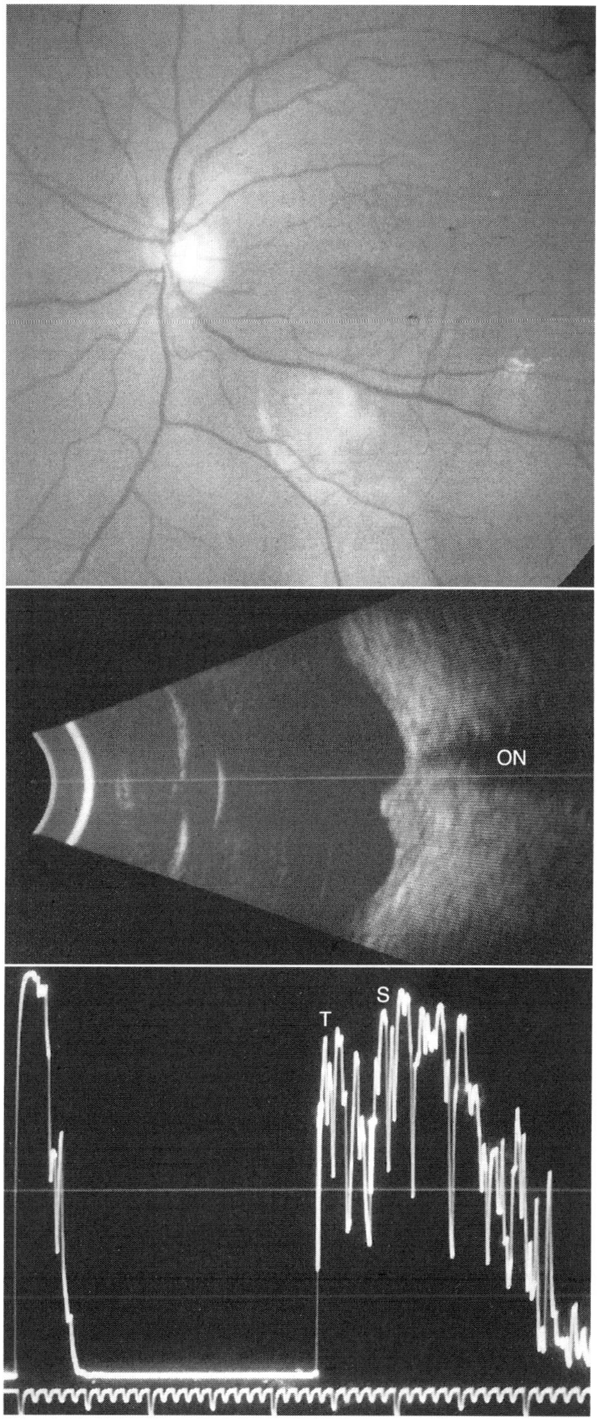

Figure 5-52 Choroidal nevus that was clinically suspicious for choroidal melanoma. **A,** Fundus photograph shows pigmented lesion inferotemporal to optic nerve. **B,** Oblique axial B-scan shows slightly irregular, dome-shaped mass adjacent to optic nerve *(ON)*. **C,** Lesion exhibits high internal reflectivity with slightly irregular internal structure on A-scan. *T,* Tumor surface; *S,* sclera. Needle biopsy confirmed benign nature of the tumor.

Melanocytoma (Magnocellular Nevus)

This darkly pigmented, benign tumor, most often situated at the optic nerve head, can be clinically confused with a melanoma. Melanocytomas are usually only mildly elevated and have a smooth, dome shape. They are typically highly reflective, with regular internal structure and no internal vascularity (Figure 5-53). These tumors sometimes involve the choroid or ciliary body (see p 177). Rarely melanocytomas undergo malignant transformation[88]; therefore, they should be monitored for growth.

Intraocular B-Cell Lymphoma (Reticulum Cell Sarcoma)

These lesions have a yellow-white appearance, are often bilateral, and may be associated with a diffuse cellular infiltration of the vitreous, presenting clinically as a uveitis.[12] The fundus lesions usually represent neoplastic infiltration in the sub-retinal pigment epithelium (sub-RPE) space. In most cases, they are only mildly elevated, with a bumpy, irregular surface contour. The few lesions examined have demonstrated irregular internal structure without evidence of internal vascularity (Figure 5-54). The echographic

A

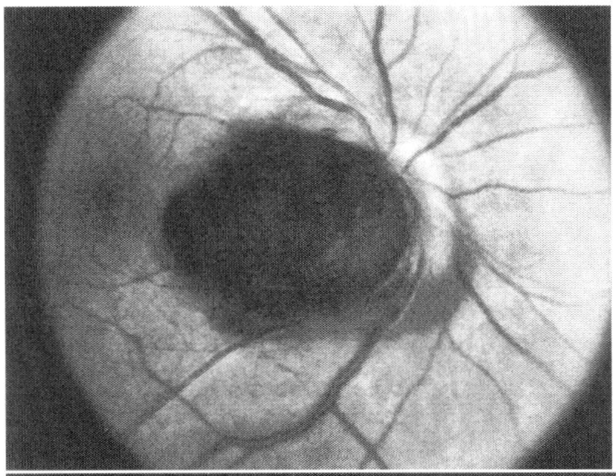

Figure 5-53 Melanocytoma. **A,** Fundus photograph shows darkly pigmented tumor overlying optic disc. **B,** Axial B-scan echogram shows mildly elevated lesion *(arrow)* overlying surface of optic nerve *(ON)*. **C,** A-scan shows regular internal structure and high reflectivity of lesion. *T,* Tumor surface; *O,* surface of optic disc.

B

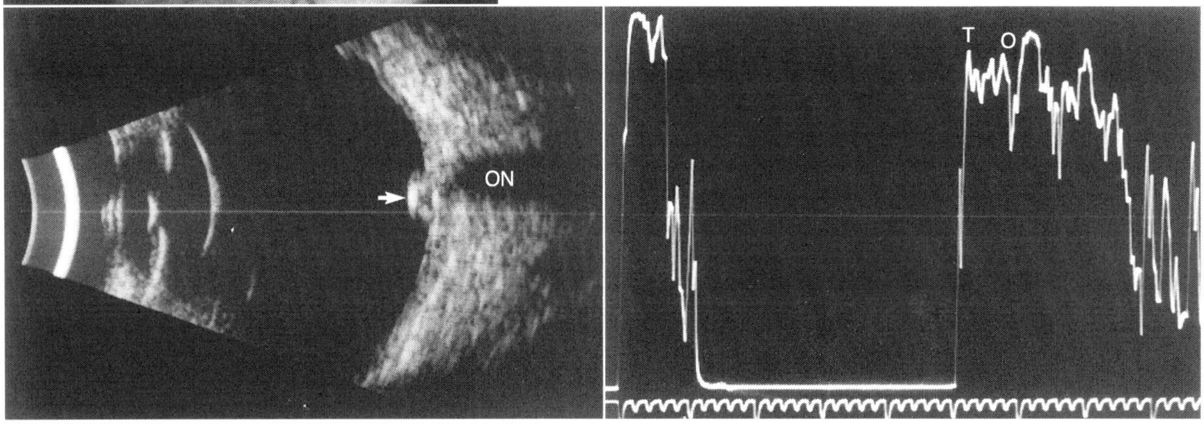

C

A

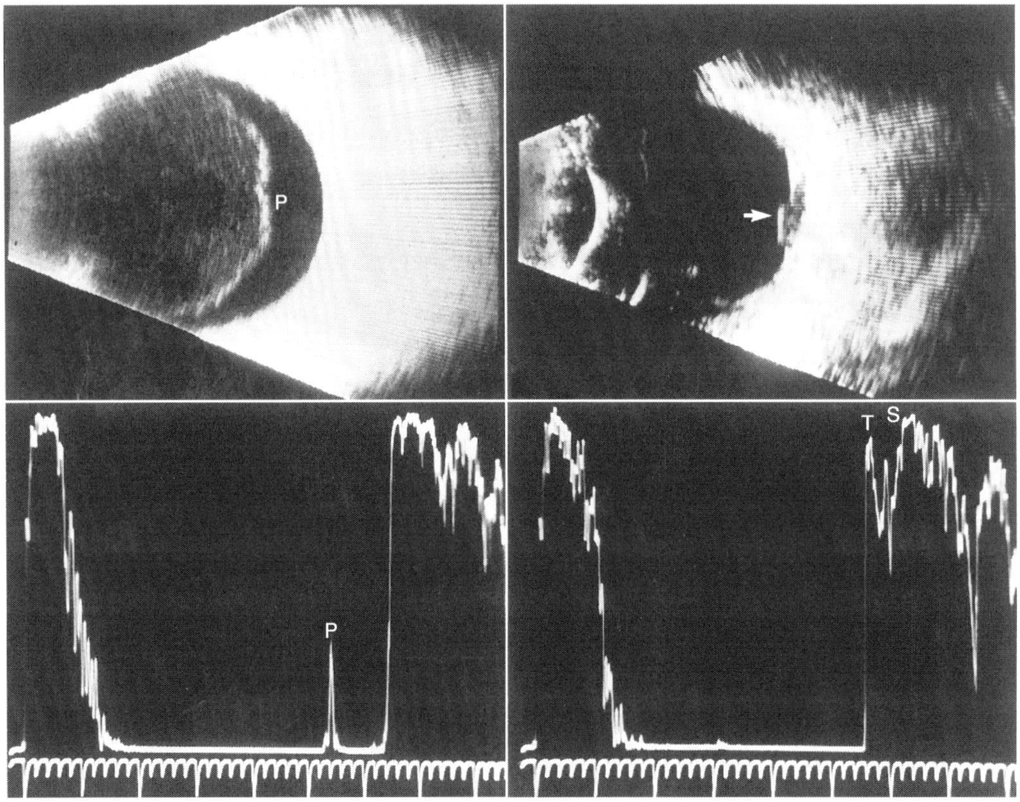

C

B

D

Figure 5-54 B-cell lymphoma (reticulum cell sarcoma). **A,** Transverse B-scan echogram shows opacification of vitreous and extensive PVD *(P)*. **B,** A-scan echogram shows low to medium reflectivity of PVD *(P)*. **C,** Vertical macula B-scan echogram shows mildly elevated lesion with irregular surface contour *(arrow)*. **D,** Corresponding A-scan shows high internal reflectivity of lesion. *T,* Tumor surface; *S,* sclera.

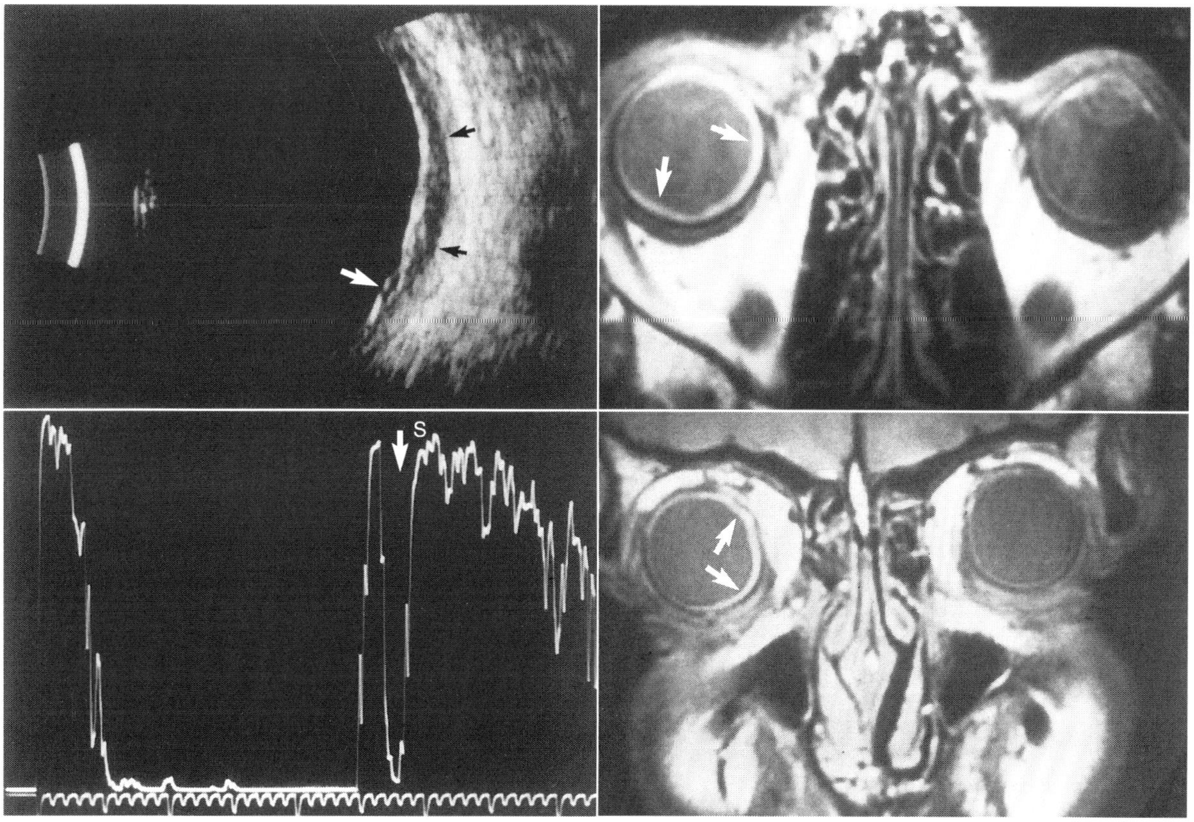

Figure 5-55 Uveal lymphoid hyperplasia involving the choroid of the right eye. **A,** Transverse B-scan echogram shows diffuse, echolucent thickening of choroid *(black arrows)* with focal, very shallow retinal detachment at inferior aspect of lesion *(white arrow)*. **B,** A-scan shows low reflective choroidal thickening *(arrow)*. *S,* Sclera. Axial **(C)** and coronal **(D)** MRI scans show diffuse thickening of ocular wall in the right eye *(arrows)*.

appearance of these tumors can be very similar to that of metastatic carcinoma to the choroid. Unlike metastatic carcinomas, however, B-cell lymphomas are not usually associated with extensive serous retinal detachments.[63]

Uveal Lymphoid Hyperplasia

Lymphoid hyperplasia is an uncommon, often unilateral, lymphoproliferative disorder that involves primarily the uveal tract. This condition has been referred to as inflammatory pseudotumor,[29,74] benign reactive lymphoid hyperplasia,[11,74] and more recently, uveal lymphoid infiltration.[36] Recent investigations have shown that most of these lesions are actually a type of low-grade lymphoma.[14]

Clinically, lymphoid hyperplasia presents as a diffuse or nodular amelanotic choroidal lesion.[11] One investigator has described the appearance as multifocal, creamy choroidal infiltrates.[45] Serous retinal detachments have also been reported. The uveal infiltration may involve the ciliary body, causing shallowing of the anterior chamber and, in some cases, secondary angle-closure glaucoma.[11] These patients may also present with salmon-colored conjunctival lesions. Iris lesions have also been described.

On ultrasound, uveal lymphoid hyperplasia appears as a diffuse lesion with a smooth or somewhat bumpy surface contour. This lesion exhibits low to medium internal reflectivity, and internal vascularity has been reported (Figure 5-55).[11] Extraocular nodules are frequently demonstrated in the peripapillary region (Figure 5-56). These nodules appear to extend through emissary canals from the intraocular lesion.[11,36] More extensive orbital lesions can also occur.

The primary differential diagnoses for uveal lymphoid hyperplasia, both clinically and echographically, include diffuse melanoma (see p 136), metastatic carcinoma (see p 142), posterior scleritis (see p 196), uveal effusion syndrome (see p 82), Vogt-Koyanagi-Harada syndrome (see p 200), sympathetic ophthalmia (see p 201), and leukemia (see p 154). The majority of these conditions can be differentiated by combining the clinical and echographic findings.[26] The most challenging diagnosis to exclude, however, is diffuse amelanotic melanoma. This difficulty arises from the fact that both disorders may exhibit low to medium reflective choroidal thickening, as well as extrascleral nodules. Differentiation can be made in some cases by noting a prompt response to steroid therapy, thus favoring the diagnosis of lymphoid hyperplasia. It is of interest, however,

A

C

B

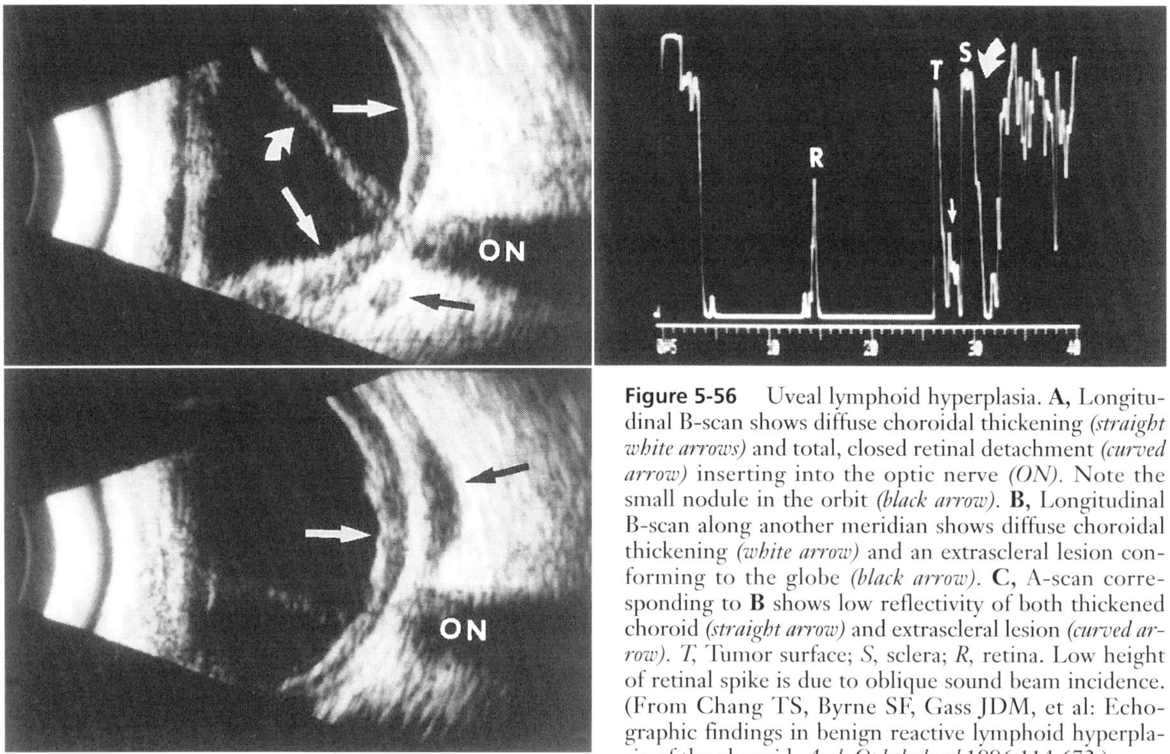

Figure 5-56 Uveal lymphoid hyperplasia. **A,** Longitudinal B-scan shows diffuse choroidal thickening *(straight white arrows)* and total, closed retinal detachment *(curved arrow)* inserting into the optic nerve *(ON)*. Note the small nodule in the orbit *(black arrow)*. **B,** Longitudinal B-scan along another meridian shows diffuse choroidal thickening *(white arrow)* and an extrascleral lesion conforming to the globe *(black arrow)*. **C,** A-scan corresponding to **B** shows low reflectivity of both thickened choroid *(straight arrow)* and extrascleral lesion *(curved arrow)*. *T,* Tumor surface; *S,* sclera; *R,* retina. Low height of retinal spike is due to oblique sound beam incidence. (From Chang TS, Byrne SF, Gass JDM, et al: Echographic findings in benign reactive lymphoid hyperplasia of the choroid. *Arch Ophthalmol* 1996;114:672.)

A

B

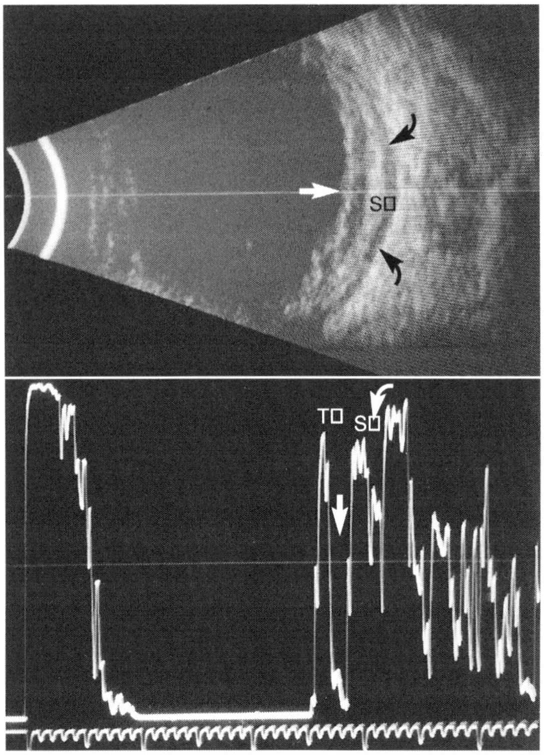

Figure 5-57 Diffuse leukemic infiltration of choroid. **A,** Transverse B-scan demonstrates diffuse thickening of choroid *(straight white arrow)* and sclera *(S)*. *Curved arrows* show diffuse infiltration of sub-Tenon's space. **B,** A-scan displays low internal reflectivity of thickened choroid *(straight arrow)* and widening of sub-Tenon's space *(curved arrow)*. *T,* Tumor surface; *S,* sclera.

that choroidal melanomas can be associated with inflammatory episcleral lesions, which also may respond to anti-inflammatory therapy (see p 120).

Leukemia

Leukemia can affect the eye by diffusely infiltrating the choroid. Echographically, leukemic infiltrates exhibit low to medium reflectivity, similar to other highly cellular choroidal lesions (Figure 5-57).

Leiomyoma

This rare tumor, occurring most often in young women, is typically located in the peripheral choroid and/or ciliary body.[83] Leiomyomas may be difficult to differentiate from melanomas both clinically and echographically.[83] The few tumors that have been examined showed a smooth, domed configuration and internal vascularity. They exhibited regular or slightly irregular internal structure and predominantly low to medium internal reflectivity (Figure 5-58). It is interesting, however, that leiomyomas are known to transilluminate very well.[83,88]

Uveal Schwannoma (Neurilemoma)

Schwannoma of the choroid is a benign tumor that arises from peripheral nerve sheaths.[29,85,88] These lesions may be amelanotic or pigmented and may simulate a choroidal melanoma both clinically and echographically.[88] A rare

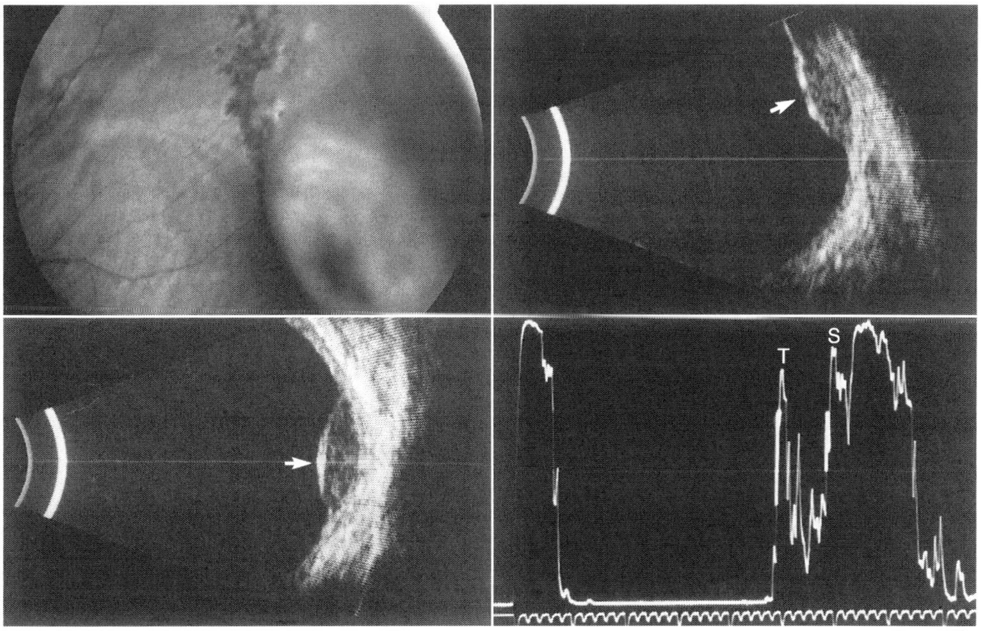

Figure 5-58 Leiomyoma in teenage girl. **A,** Fundus photograph shows elevated lesion in periphery of eye. The pigment clumping adjacent to the lesion is secondary to a previous retinal detachment. Transverse **(B)** and longitudinal **(C)** B-scan echograms show smooth, dome-shaped lesion in periphery *(arrows)*. A-scan **(D)** shows low to medium internal reflectivity with moderately irregular internal structure. *T,* Tumor surface; *S,* sclera. Histopathology confirmed the diagnosis of leiomyoma 12 years later, when the eye was enucleated due to significant growth of the lesion.

form of this tumor, occurring in younger individuals, is diffuse uveal melanocytic schwannoma, also referred to by one author[29] as diffuse choroidal melanocytic nevus. On B-scan, these lesions are diffuse and typically involve the posterior choroid. They exhibit regular internal structure and low internal reflectivity on A-scan. In addition, they demonstrate significant internal vascularity. An unusual echographic finding in these cases, similar to that seen in younger individuals with choroidal melanoma (see p 118), is thickening and bowing of the posterior sclera in the region of the tumor (Figure 5-59). Histopathology has demonstrated scleral infiltration in these tumors.[29]

Neurofibroma

Neurofibromas of the uveal tract are usually associated with neurofibromatosis. They appear as a diffuse, either pigmented or nonpigmented lesion, that may involve the entire uveal tract. Serous retinal detachments may also be present. The echographic features of these tumors include a diffuse lesion that demonstrates regular internal structure and low to medium internal reflectivity.

Hamartomas of the Retina (Capillary, Combined Retinal/Retinal Pigment Epithelium, Astrocytic)

Retinal hamartomas, usually located at the optic disc or in the peripheral fundus, are typically mildly elevated with a domed configuration. Peripheral capillary hemangiomas associated with von Hippel–Lindau syndrome are predominantly medium reflective (Figure 5-60) and show some degree of internal vascularity. Two cases of retinal astrocytic hamartoma have been seen, both of which were associated with tuberous sclerosis. The lesion in one patient was heavily calcified, exhibiting very high reflectivity and marked shadowing (Figure 5-61). The second patient had bilateral tumors, one of which showed medium internal reflectivity without calcification. The tumor in the other eye demonstrated a small focus of calcification but otherwise exhibited low reflectivity (Figure 5-62).

Scleral Tumors

Tumors primarily involving the sclera are extremely rare. These unusual lesions, however, can mimic choroidal melanoma both clinically and echographically. Two types of scleral tumors are scleral cysts and focal fibrosclerosis (scleral pseudotumor). Scleral cysts present as nonpigmented, well-circumscribed, dome-shaped fundus lesions. On B-scan, these very well-circumscribed lesions are dome shaped and echolucent. In addition, they appear to cause an outward bowing of the posterior scleral surface. On A-scan, these lesions produce low internal reflectivity. The histopathology of one case is shown in Figure 5-63.

The systemic disorder of multifocal fibrosclerosis (most commonly associated with retroperitoneal fibrosis) can produce focal lesions of the sclera.[35] These tumors may either be unilateral or bilateral and may occur as a solitary mass or

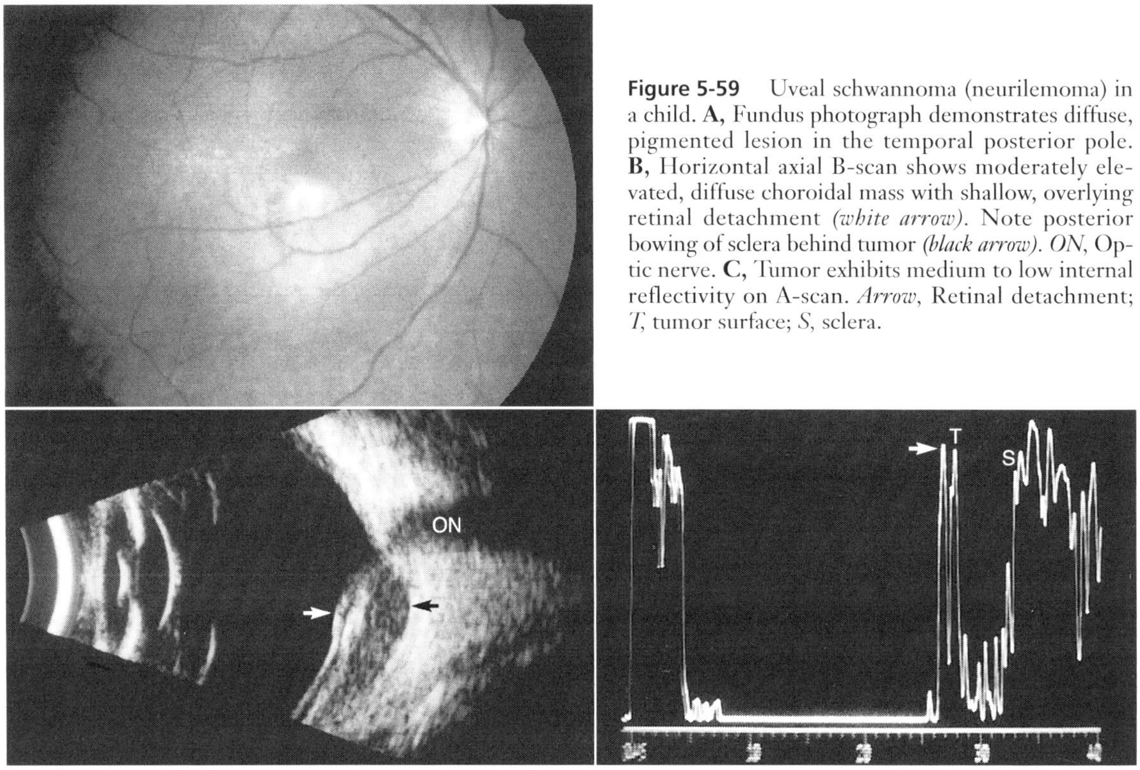

Figure 5-59 Uveal schwannoma (neurilemoma) in a child. **A,** Fundus photograph demonstrates diffuse, pigmented lesion in the temporal posterior pole. **B,** Horizontal axial B-scan shows moderately elevated, diffuse choroidal mass with shallow, overlying retinal detachment *(white arrow)*. Note posterior bowing of sclera behind tumor *(black arrow)*. *ON,* Optic nerve. **C,** Tumor exhibits medium to low internal reflectivity on A-scan. *Arrow,* Retinal detachment; *T,* tumor surface; *S,* sclera.

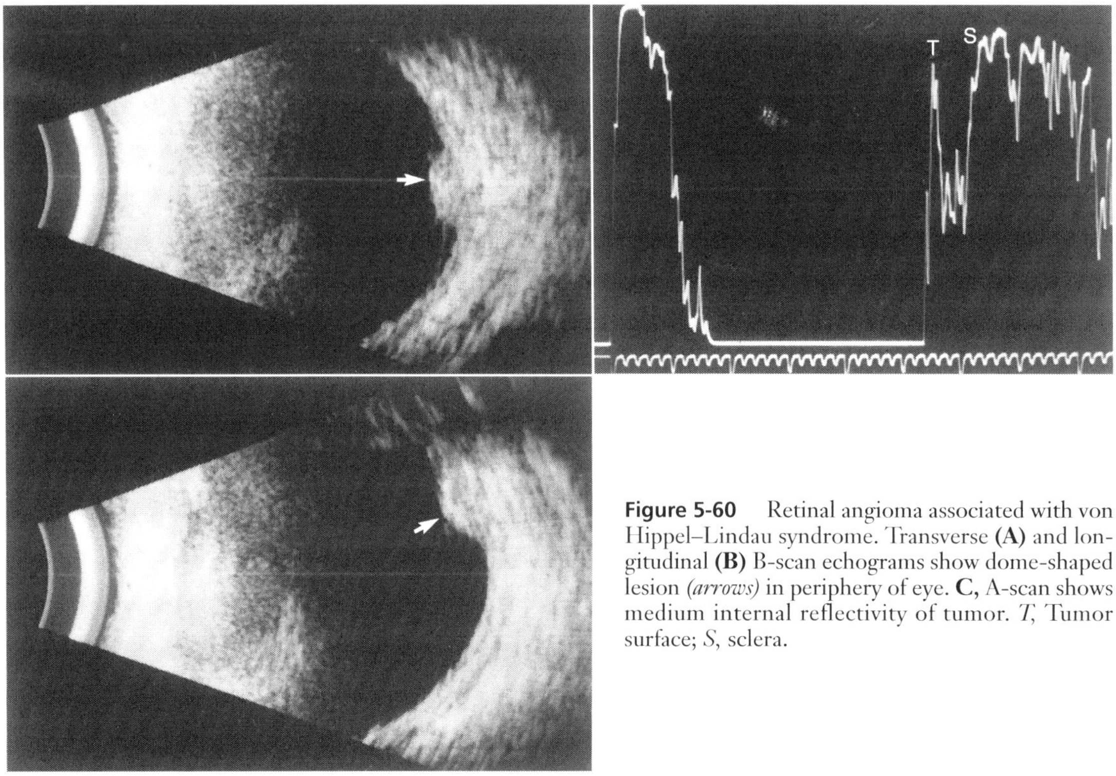

Figure 5-60 Retinal angioma associated with von Hippel–Lindau syndrome. Transverse **(A)** and longitudinal **(B)** B-scan echograms show dome-shaped lesion *(arrows)* in periphery of eye. **C,** A-scan shows medium internal reflectivity of tumor. *T,* Tumor surface; *S,* sclera.

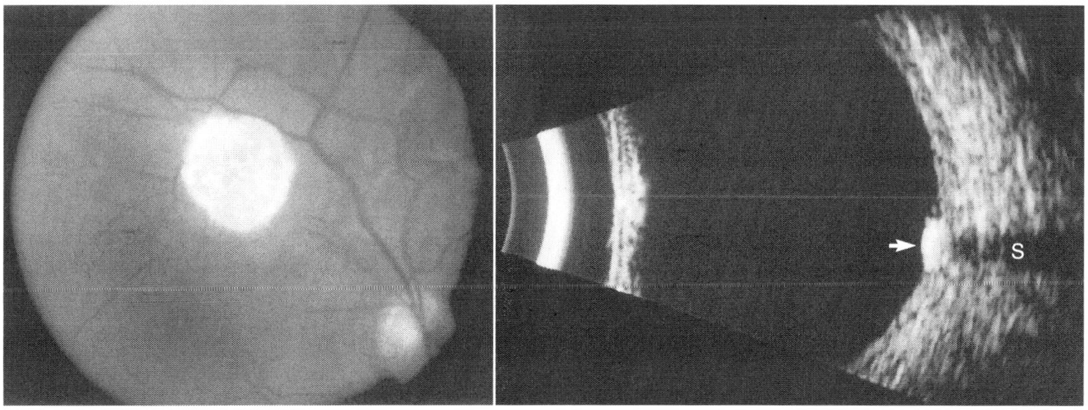

Figure 5-61 Astrocytic hamartoma. **A,** Fundus photograph shows well-outlined, nonpigmented lesion supratemporal to optic disc. **B,** Transverse B-scan demonstrates highly echodense, mildly elevated lesion. Marked shadowing *(S)* indicates calcified nature of lesion.

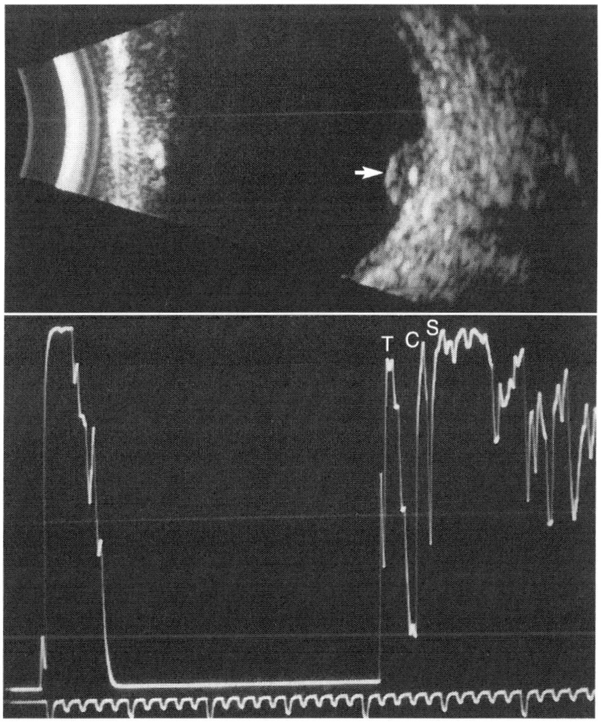

Figure 5-62 Astrocytic hamartoma. **A,** Transverse B-scan displays smooth, dome-shaped lesion *(arrow)*. Note echo-dense nodule at base of lesion representing small focus of calcification. **B,** A-scan shows low internal reflectivity of lesion and high reflectivity of calcified nodule *(C)*. *T,* Tumor surface; *S,* sclera.

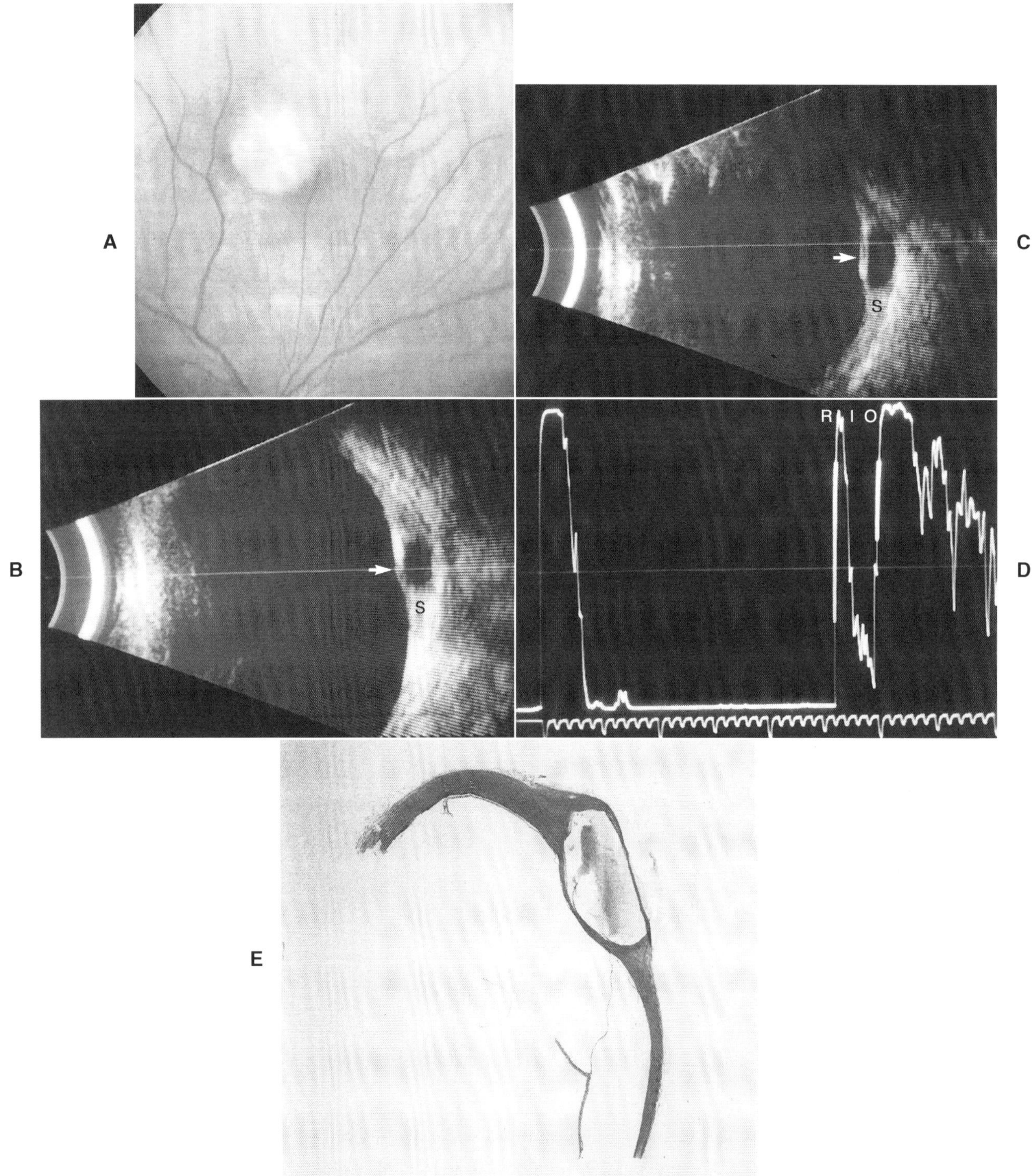

Figure 5-63 Intrascleral cyst. **A,** Fundus photograph demonstrates well-outlined, nonpigmented lesion superior to optic disc. Transverse **(B)** and longitudinal **(C)** B-scans at reduced gain display well-outlined, echolucent lesion within the sclera *(S)*. Internal echoes were present at higher gain settings. Note slight bowing of both the inner and outer scleral walls. *Arrow,* surface of retina. **D,** A-scan shows low internal reflectivity of lesion. *R,* Retina; *I,* inner scleral wall; *O,* outer scleral wall. **E,** Pathology shows epithelial-lined scleral cyst containing mucin.

as multiple lesions within one eye. Clinically, they appear as a nonpigmented, elevated fundus lesion, usually with a dome shape. In addition, outer scleral fibrous plaques have been identified adjacent to the intraocular lesion. On B-scan, this lesion appears as a solid, elevated, dome-shaped mass with a thick surface. The outer scleral surface appears to be slightly bowed outward, and the tapered lateral margins of the lesion can be shown to be contiguous with the episcleral space rather than with the choroid. This latter finding is important in helping to differentiate these primarily scleral lesions from choroidal masses which they can easily mimic. On A-scan, these lesions exhibit low internal reflectivity and regular internal structure (Figure 5-64). No internal vascularity has been identified. They have been shown to decrease in size with anti-inflammatory therapy. Although lesions with similar histopathology have been previously described as pseudotumors in the orbit, their occurrence in the sclera is extremely rare. In addition, several authors have reported cases of fibrosclerotic lesions involving both the uvea and the sclera.[54,77,99] Because these scleral lesions can mimic choroidal lesions, choroidal involvement in some of the reported cases may have actually represented primarily scleral involvement.[35]

OTHER LESIONS SIMULATING MELANOMA

Disciform Macular Degeneration (Disciform Lesion)

Disciform macular degeneration is the wet form of age-related macular degeneration (AMD). It is caused by choroidal neovascularization, producing sub-RPE and subretinal exudate and/or hemorrhage. In the more chronic stages of this form of the disease, fibrosis and scarring can occur, as can calcification.

Disciform lesions can usually be differentiated clinically from choroidal melanomas by the presence of drusen and exudate, and by their location in the macular region. The fellow eye may have similar changes of disciform macular degeneration. In some cases, however, these associated

A C B D

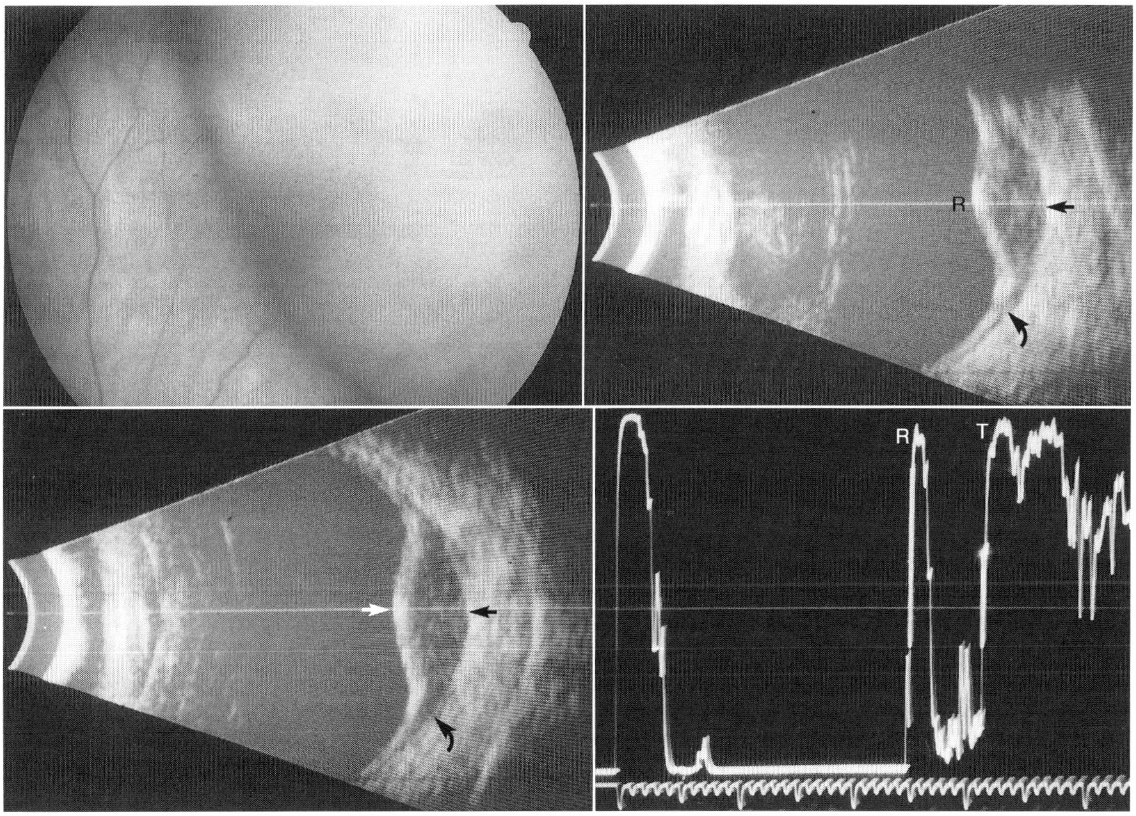

Figure 5-64 Scleral lesion secondary to multifocal fibrosclerosis. **A,** Fundus photograph shows well-outlined, elevated mass lesion. Transverse **(B)** and longitudinal **(C)** B-scan echograms show an elevated dome-shaped lesion with a thick inner surface representing indentation of the retina and choroid *(straight white arrow). Straight black arrows* show slight bowing of outer surface where lesion contacts Tenon's capsule. Note how lesion merges with the episclera *(curved arrows)* at its margins. **D,** Lesion exhibits low internal reflectivity on A-scan. *R,* Retinochoroid layer; *T,* Tenon's capsule.

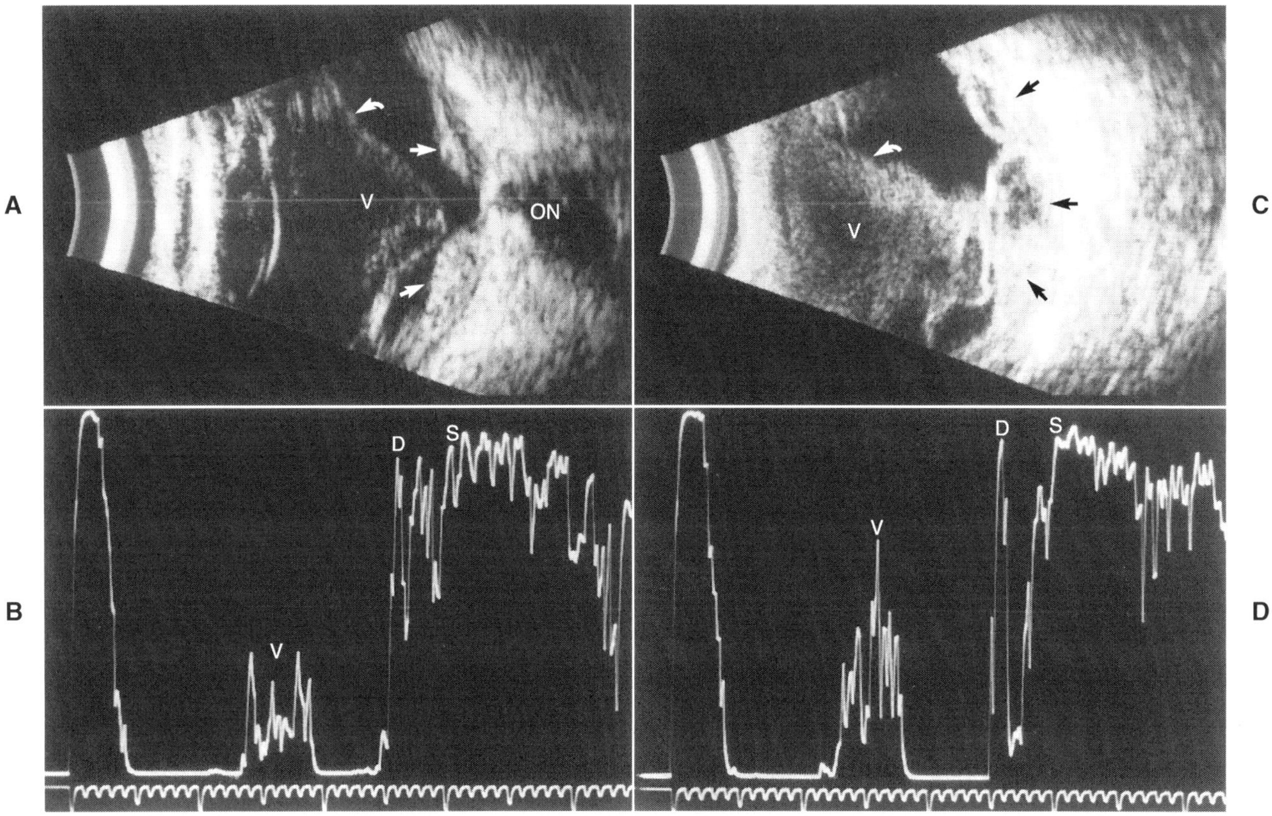

Figure 5-65 Large hemorrhagic disciform lesion. **A,** Horizontal axial B-scan echogram at reduced gain setting shows extensive peripapillary disciform lesion *(straight arrows)* surrounding optic nerve *(ON)* with greatest elevation at macula (just below optic nerve in echogram). *V,* Vitreous hemorrhage; *curved arrow,* PVD. **B,** Corresponding A-scan through macula shows typical high internal reflectivity of lesion. *V,* Vitreous hemorrhage; *D,* surface of disciform lesion; *S,* sclera. **C,** Transverse B-scan through inferotemporal quadrant shows peripheral extension of hemorrhagic lesion *(black arrows)*. *V,* Vitreous hemorrhage; *curved arrow,* PVD. **D,** Corresponding A-scan shows low internal reflectivity of lesion in this region.

findings may not be present, thus obscuring the clinical diagnosis. Disciform lesions can also occur in eccentric areas of the fundus. The clinical differentiation from a small melanoma in these circumstances may not be straightforward. Ultrasound may be of assistance in distinguishing these lesions. The echographic features of nonhemorrhagic disciform lesions are described in detail in Chapter 3 (see p 68).

Hemorrhagic Disciform Lesion

Hemorrhagic disciform lesions are primarily the result of hemorrhage and fibrovascular proliferation in the sub-RPE space. They may be associated with subretinal hemorrhage. The blood in the sub-RPE space may be partially clotted. The echographic features of hemorrhagic disciform lesions differ significantly from the nonhemorrhagic form described in Chapter 3 (see p 68). They may be quite well localized or diffuse and extensive, involving the entire posterior fundus and, in some cases, extending into the periphery.[6,100] These hemorrhagic lesions often begin in the macular region and progress inferotemporally. Hemorrhagic disciform lesions usually exhibit a bumpy, lobulated surface, and may have very indistinct margins. Their internal structure is often quite irregular with areas of both high and low internal reflectivity. This heterogeneous appearance is due to the presence of sub-RPE hemorrhage (clotted and unclotted), as well as to fibrovascular proliferation. These lesions do not show internal vascularity. The retinal detachments with subretinal hemorrhage that occur in these eyes are usually very shallow, although they can be quite extensive and elevated (Figure 5-65; see also Figure 7-7).

Plaquelike foci of calcification are observed in some hemorrhagic disciform lesions, presumably at the level of Bruch's membrane.[100] In addition, shallow suprachoroidal hemorrhages can underlie a disciform lesion (Figure 5-66). It has been observed that these patients are often on anticoagulant therapy at the time they develop the hemorrhagic disciform lesions.

Vitreous hemorrhage can be associated with hemorrhagic disciform lesions. In fact, disciform lesions have been

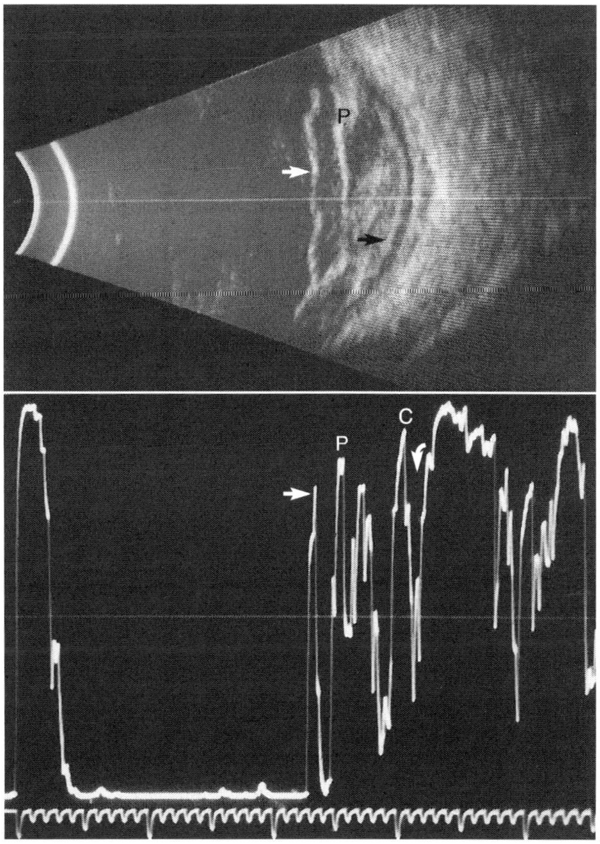

Figure 5-66 Hemorrhagic disciform lesion. **A,** Transverse B-scan demonstrates hemorrhage beneath retina *(white arrow)*, retinal pigment epithelium *(P)*, and choroid *(black arrow)*. **B,** A-scan shows highly irregular structure of lesion. *White arrow,* Retina; *P,* retinal pigment epithelium; *C,* choroid; *curved arrow,* suprachoroidal space.

shown to be one of the most common causes of dense vitreous hemorrhage in older patients.[33] When vitreous hemorrhage occurs in these eyes, the posterior hyaloid usually separates from the posterior fundus and the underlying lesion (see Figure 5-65).

The echographic differential diagnosis of a hemorrhagic disciform lesion includes large choroidal melanoma and metastatic carcinoma. Generally, choroidal melanomas are more regularly structured and demonstrate low to medium reflectivity, although very large tumors can demonstrate increased heterogeneity as a result of hemorrhage and necrosis within the tumor (see p 118). In addition, these tumors may be associated with vitreous hemorrhage, which can also occur secondary to a hemorrhagic disciform lesion. Distinguishing between these two entities can sometimes be difficult, but the detection of internal vascularity favors the diagnosis of melanoma. Otherwise, serial examinations can be performed for differentiation. Hemorrhagic disciform lesions tend to decrease in size (Figure 5-67), whereas melanomas remain the same or become more elevated. In rare instances, spontaneous regression of choroidal melanoma can occur[89] (see p 120).

Choroidal metastases may share some of the echographic features of hemorrhagic disciform lesions (e.g., irregular surface contour and medium to high internal reflectivity) but the clinical differentiation is usually not difficult. As a rule, metastatic carcinomas are only mildly elevated and it is rare for them to be associated with vitreous hemorrhage or extensive subretinal hemorrhage.

Hemorrhagic Retinal Pigment Epithelial Detachment

Hemorrhagic retinal pigment epithelial detachments (HRPED) and hemorrhagic disciform lesions comprise a clinical and histopathologic continuum.[100] The HRPED represents a limited sub-RPE hemorrhage resulting in a dark, smooth, dome-shaped lesion that can clinically simulate a choroidal melanoma. They may occur in the macular region or in eccentric locations, often in the temporal periphery. This limited hemorrhage is in contrast to the more extensive, diffuse hemorrhage that produces the more highly elevated, irregularly shaped disciform lesion.

Echographically, HRPED produces a smooth, domed configuration on B-scan, often with very sharp, distinct margins (Figure 5-68). This blister-like appearance is more suggestive of a pigment epithelial detachment than a solid tumor.[34] On A-scan, the reflectivity varies according to the size and consistency of the blood (clotted vs. liquefied) in

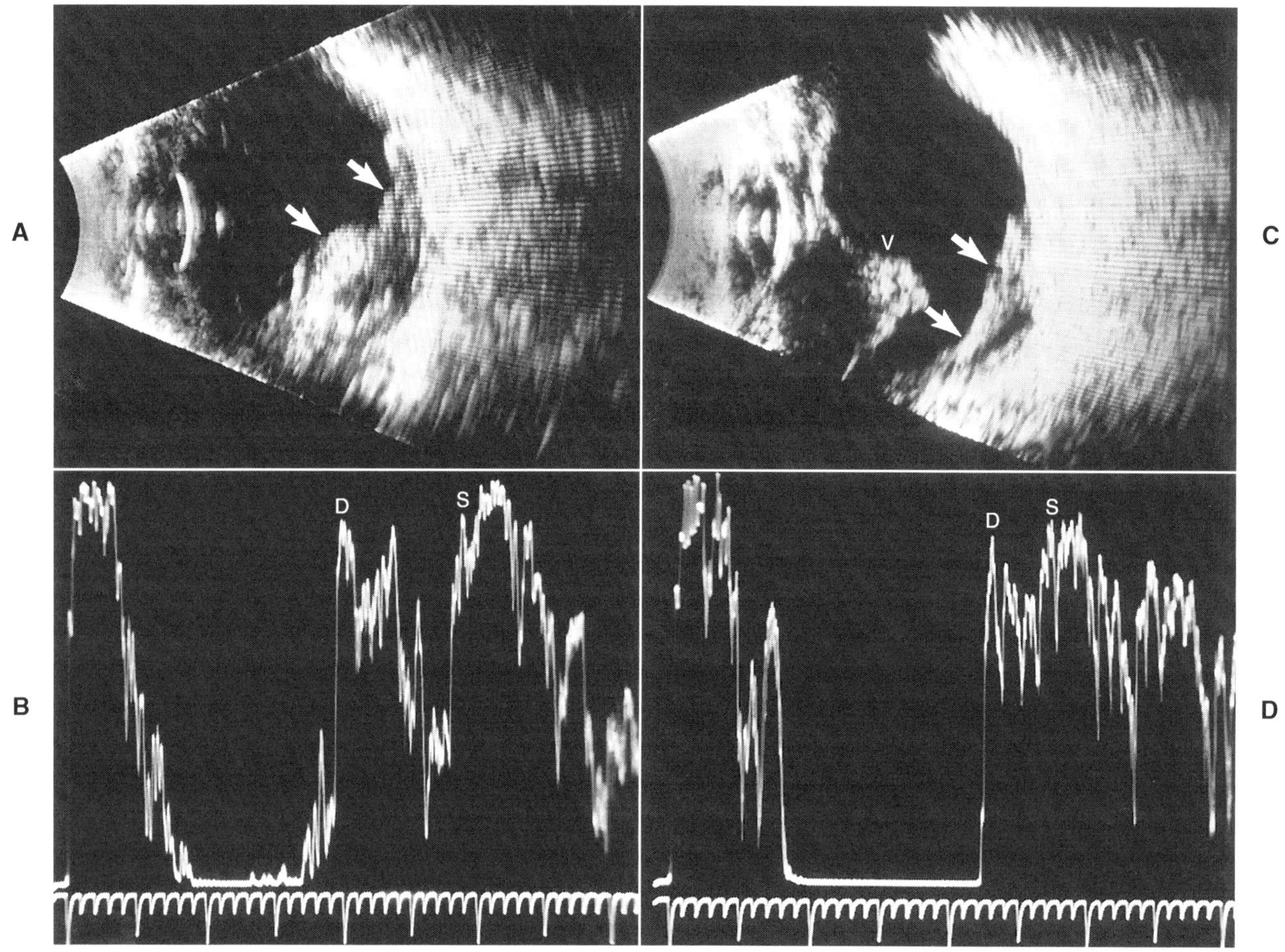

Figure 5-67 Large hemorrhagic disciform lesion (**A** and **B**) with follow-up examination 1 month later (**C** and **D**) showing regression. **A,** Vertical macula B-scan echogram shows a very irregular, bumpy surface *(arrows)*. **B,** A-scan shows irregular internal structure with areas of both high and low internal reflectivity. *D,* Lesion surface; *S,* sclera. Vertical macula B-scan **(C)** shows marked decrease in size of lesion. Also, note vitreous hemorrhage and PVD *(V)*. **D,** A-scan shows more regular internal structure and higher reflectivity. (From Green RL, Byrne SF: Diagnostic ophthalmic ultrasound, in Ryan SJ [ed]: *Retina.* ed 3, St Louis, Mosby, 2001, p 283.)

the sub-RPE space. These lesions do not demonstrate internal vascularity. Echographically, the diagnosis of HRPED is confirmed only when the lesion is observed to decrease on follow-up examination (Figure 5-69). However, in some cases HRPED may persist for weeks or months.

Choroidal Hemorrhage

Focal choroidal hemorrhages occurring after intraocular surgery or for other reasons[95] have been confused clinically with melanomas. Echographically these lesions have a domed configuration and can be mildly to highly elevated. The internal reflectivity and structure of choroidal hemorrhages can vary due to the consistency of the blood (i.e., clotted vs. liquefied) (see p 106 and Figure 4-38). When they initially develop, the suprachoroidal blood is usually clotted. As the blood liquefies, however, echography may show aftermovement of the surface spike and/or mobility of the blood echoes. In rare cases, a suprachoroidal hyphema may be present (Figure 5-70; see also p 51).

Whenever a patient presents with an intraocular mass postoperatively, the possibility of a choroidal hemorrhage should be considered. In these cases, a follow-up examination performed after 2 to 3 weeks typically shows a decrease in the size of the lesion, as well as a change in the internal reflectivity resulting from liquefaction of the blood (Figure 5-71).

Hemorrhage into Retinal Cyst/Retinoschisis

Two cases of hemorrhage into a large retinal cyst have been evaluated. In both patients, the initial clinical impression was that of a solid tumor. In one case, an oval-shaped cyst was associated with a shallow retinal detachment. The other lesion was round and was attached to the leaf of a funnel-shaped retinal detachment (Figure 5-72). In both cases,

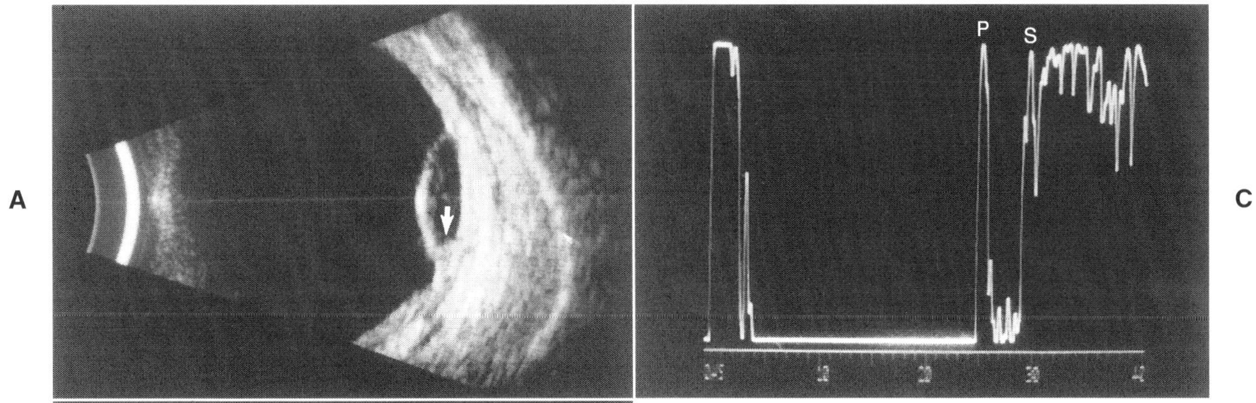

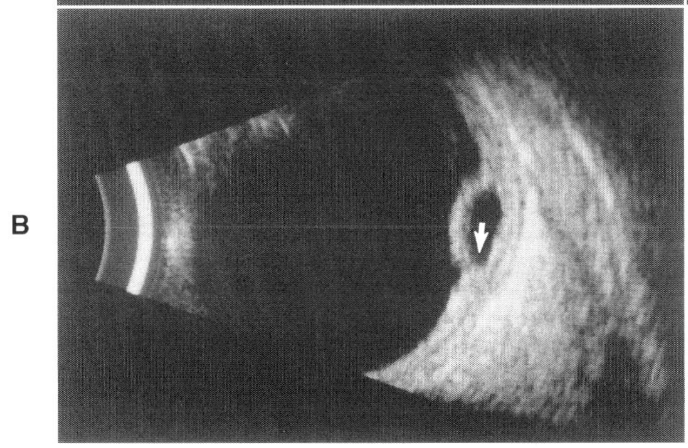

Figure 5-68 Hemorrhagic pigment epithelial detachment (HRPED). Transverse **(A)** and longitudinal **(B)** B-scan echograms show smooth dome-shaped peripheral lesion. Note steep insertions *(arrows)*, characteristic of RPE detachments. A-scan **(C)** shows a relatively thin, highly reflective surface spike *(P)* and very low internal reflectivity. *S*, Sclera.

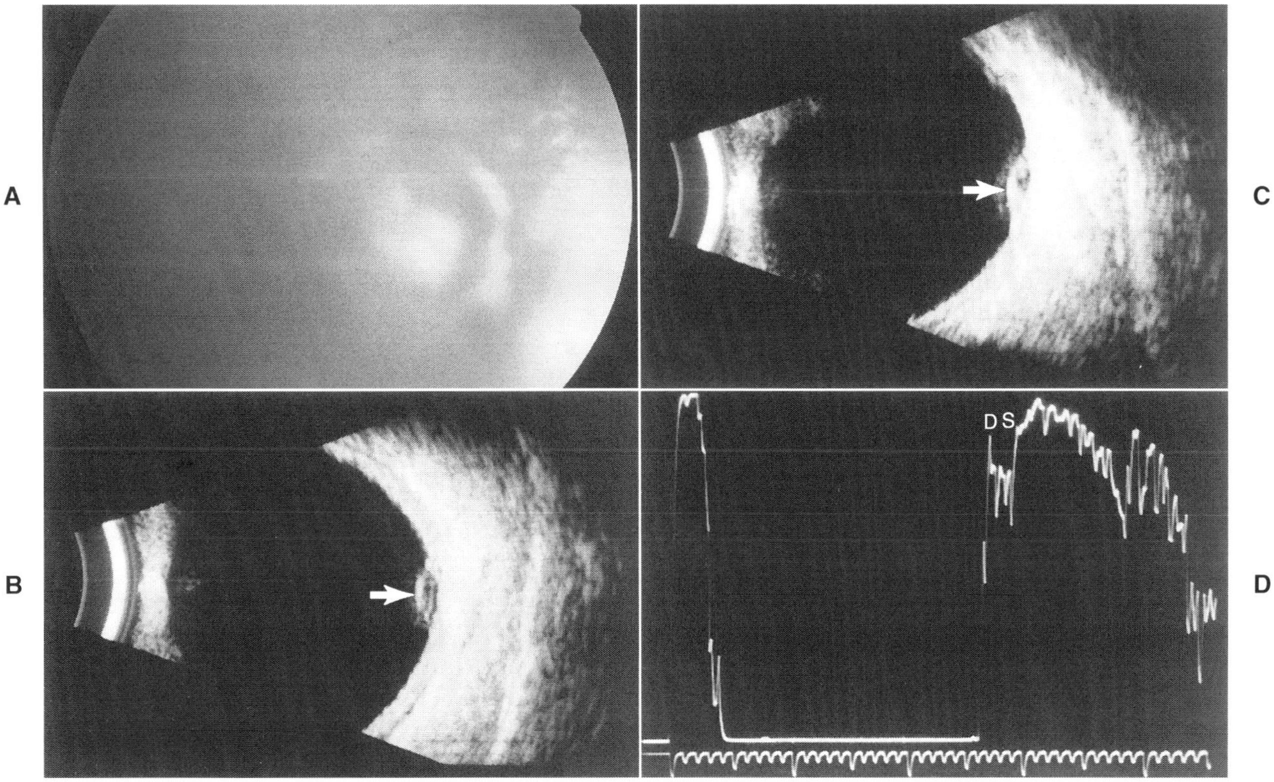

Figure 5-69 Peripheral eccentric HRPED at initial visit (**A** to **D**) and at follow-up examination 2 months later (**E** to **H**) showing regression. **A,** Fundus photograph at initial examination shows hazy vitreous with lesion temporal to the macula. Transverse **(B)** and longitudinal **(C)** B-scan echograms show smooth, dome-shaped lesion located in temporal aspect of peripheral fundus. Note mild opacities from vitreous hemorrhage overlying lesion in **C.** A-scan **(D)** shows high internal reflectivity of lesion. *D*, Surface of disciform lesion; *S*, sclera.

Continued

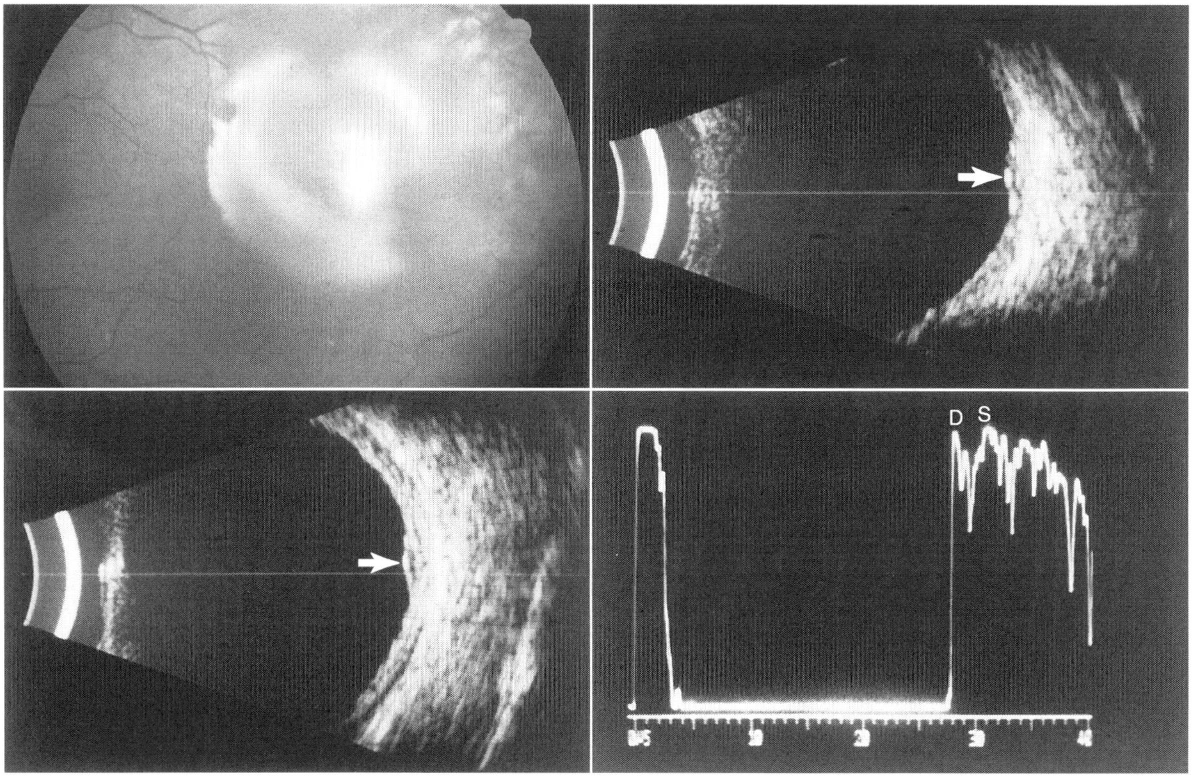

Figure 5-69, cont'd E, Fundus photograph at follow-up examination shows clearing vitreous hemorrhage with exudation surrounding slightly elevated choroidal lesion. Corresponding echograms in **F, G,** and **H** show lesion regression.

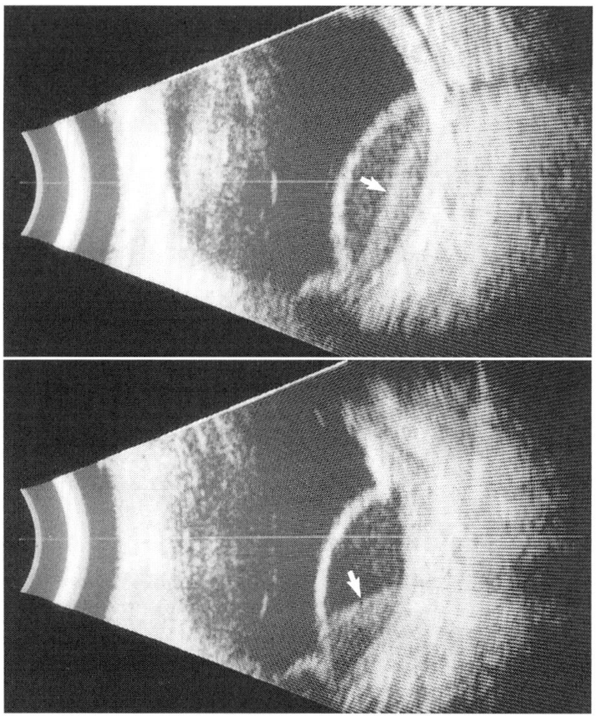

Figure 5-70 Hemorrhagic choroidal detachment with suprachoroidal hyphema. B-scan echograms using same probe position were obtained with patient in reclined **(A)** and upright **(B)** positions. Echograms demonstrate dome-shaped choroidal detachment with liquefied blood in the suprachoroidal space. Note shifting of hyphema *(arrows)* as body position is changed.

A C B D

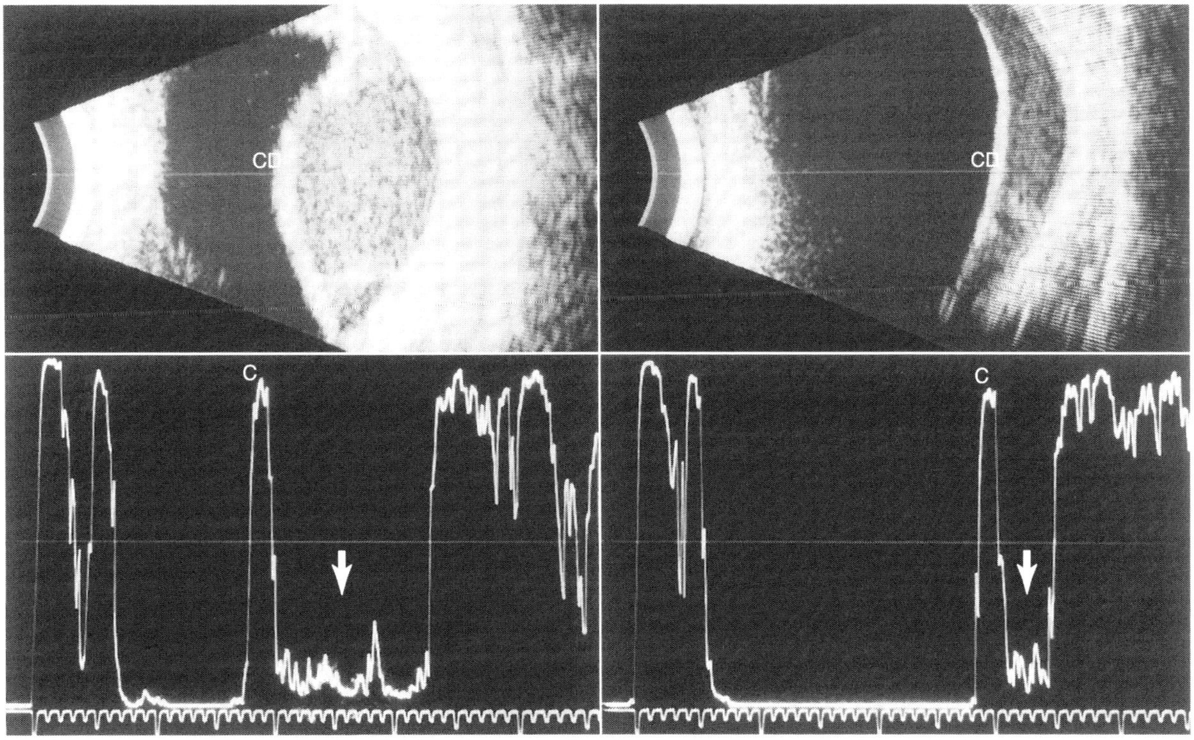

Figure 5-71 Large hemorrhagic choroidal detachment at initial presentation (**A** and **B**) and at follow-up examination 10 days later (**C** and **D**). **A,** Peripheral transverse B-scan echogram shows thick, smooth, detached choroid *(C)* with dense opacities in the suprachoroidal space. **B,** A-scan shows highly reflective, thick, spike from detached choroid *(C)* and low reflective spikes from fluid suprachoroidal blood *(arrow)*. **C,** B-scan corresponding to **A** shows significant decrease in elevation of the choroidal detachment. **D,** A-scan corresponding to **B** also shows decreased elevation.

A B

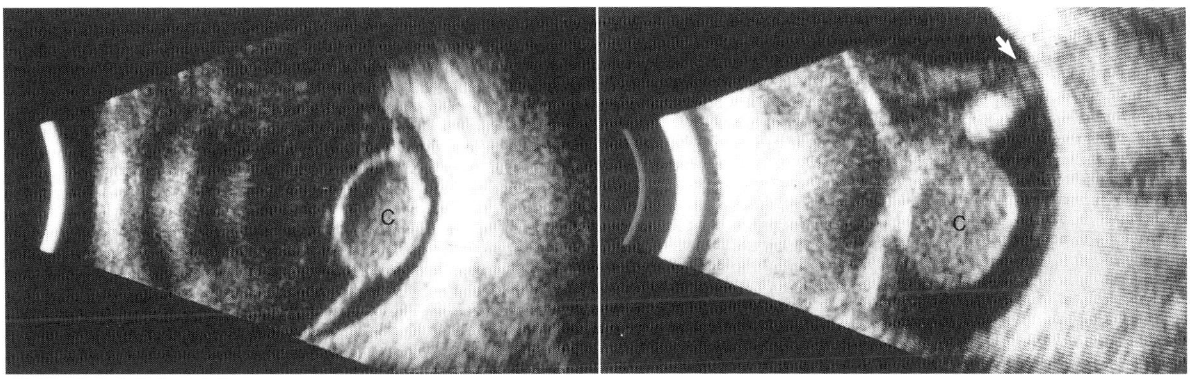

Figure 5-72 Two examples of hemorrhagic retinal cysts. **A,** Longitudinal B-scan demonstrates large retinal cyst *(C)* within shallow retinal detachment. Note layering of blood within cyst. **B,** Eccentric horizontal axial B-scan echogram shows large cyst *(C)* attached to temporal leaf of funnel shaped retinal detachment. *Arrow,* Insertion of retina into optic disc. Note dense opacities within retinal cyst.

A

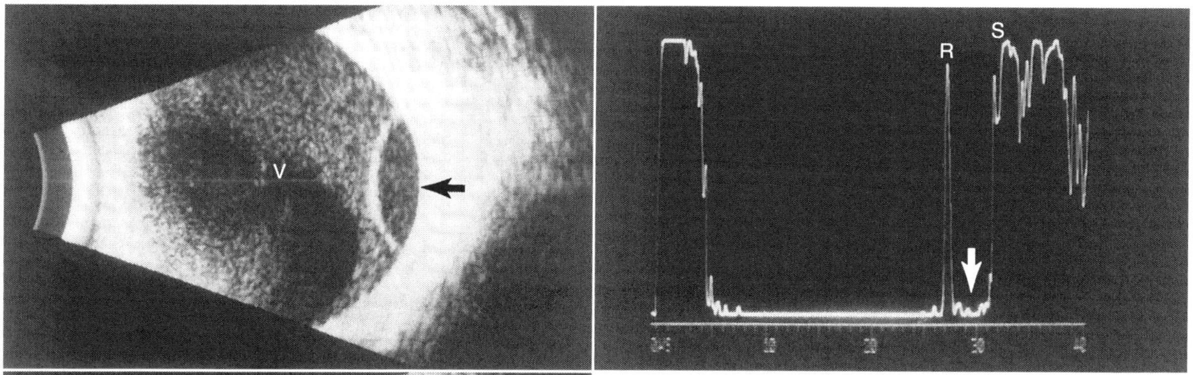

C

B

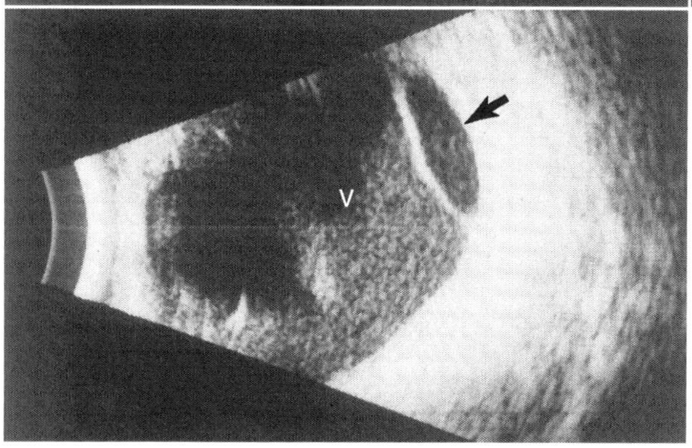

Figure 5-73 Retinoschisis with hemorrhage. Peripheral transverse **(A)** and longitudinal **(B)** B-scan echograms show smooth, dome-shaped membrane with moderately dense opacities within schisis cavity *(arrows)*. *V*, Vitreous hemorrhage. **C,** A-scan shows thin, highly reflective spike from surface of retinoschisis *(R)* and very low reflective spikes from hemorrhage in schisis cavity *(arrow)*. *S*, Sclera.

mobile, liquefied blood was identified within the cyst and aftermovement of the surface spike was observed. Hemorrhage into a peripheral retinoschisis (see p 66) can also be confused with an intraocular tumor (Figure 5-73).

Posterior Nodular Scleritis

See p 196 in Chapter 6 for a review of posterior nodular scleritis.

Bilateral Diffuse Uveal Melanocytic Proliferation (BDUMP)

Bilateral diffuse uveal melanocytic proliferation (BDUMP), an unusual paraneoplastic syndrome, is an ocular disorder that is associated with systemic carcinoma (e.g., small cell carcinoma of the lung and ovarian cancer).[2,30,31] This disorder is characterized by diffuse thickening of the uveal tract with multiple, slightly elevated, pigmented and nonpigmented melanocytic tumors. In addition, these eyes develop exudative retinal detachments and cataracts. The etiology of the ocular findings is unknown, and treatment (e.g., corticosteroids or irradiation) is ineffective.

Echographically, there is diffuse, mild, irregular thickening of the retinochoroid layer that is usually too minimal for any reliable assessment of internal reflectivity. Shallow exudative retinal detachments may be demonstrated. The echographic findings are generally nonspecific, although a diffuse, mildly elevated metastatic carcinoma of the choroid (see p 143) should be considered in the differential diagnosis.

Ampulla of Vortex Vein

Dilated vortex vein ampullae are darkish appearing, smoothly contoured, mildly elevated lesions. They are typically found where the vortex veins exit the globe, near the equator.[5,57] Echographically, these lesions demonstrate a dome shape, low to medium internal reflectivity, and no vascularity. These dilated veins are generally not present when the patient is fixating in primary gaze; they become apparent only when gaze is directed toward the involved vortex vein. Mild pressure exerted on the globe by the ultrasound probe may cause the lesion to collapse (Figure 5-74).

Posterior Coloboma

Colobomas of the posterior fundus associated with staphylomas of the sclera have been misinterpreted as an elevated lesion by ophthalmoscopy. It is possible for the sharp margin of a coloboma to be mistaken for the edge of a mass lesion. Alternatively, the edge of a coloboma may be mistaken for the apex of a tumor with the bottom of the staphyloma simulating the tumor base. B-scan can easily demonstrate the staphylomatous nature of the lesion, thus ruling out an intraocular tumor (Figure 5-75).

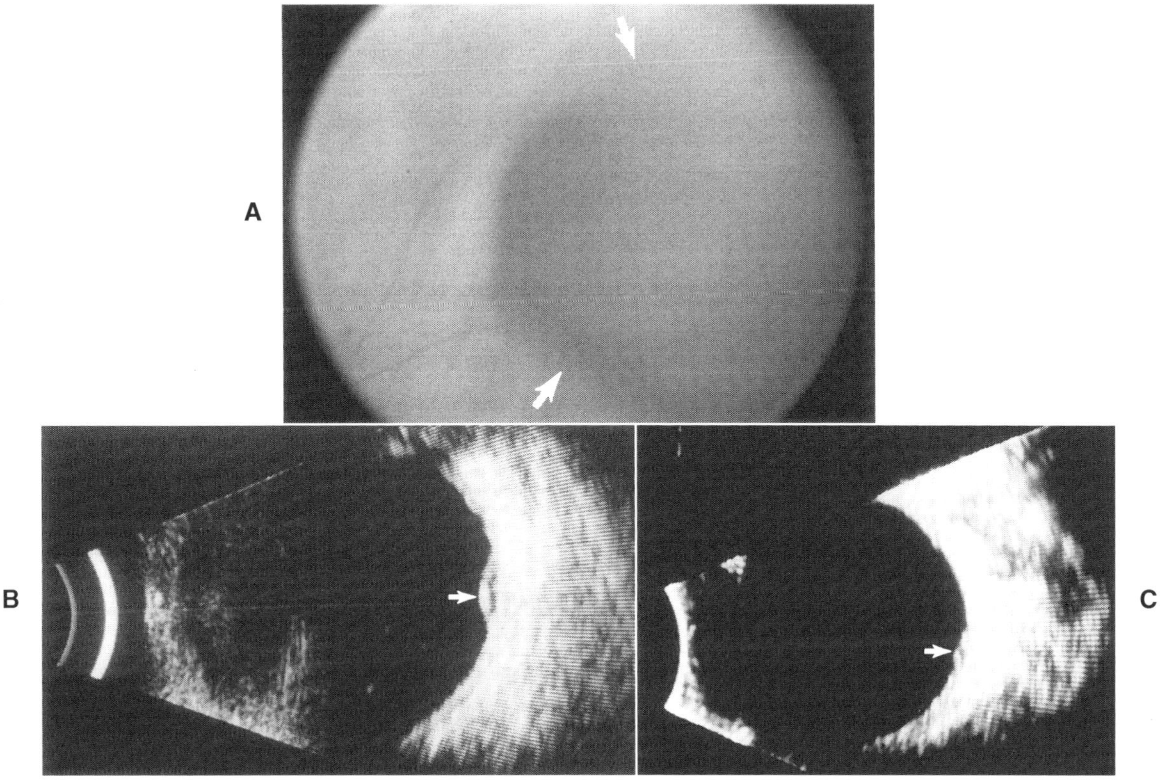

Figure 5-74 Ampulla of vortex vein. **A,** Fundus photograph shows dark, mildly elevated lesion *(arrows)* located in the supranasal aspect of the eye near the equator. **B,** Transverse B-scan echogram shows mildly elevated, dome-shaped lesion *(arrow)* as patient fixates supranasally, **C,** Transverse B-scan view through same region with slight pressure of probe against globe causes collapse and disappearance of lesion.

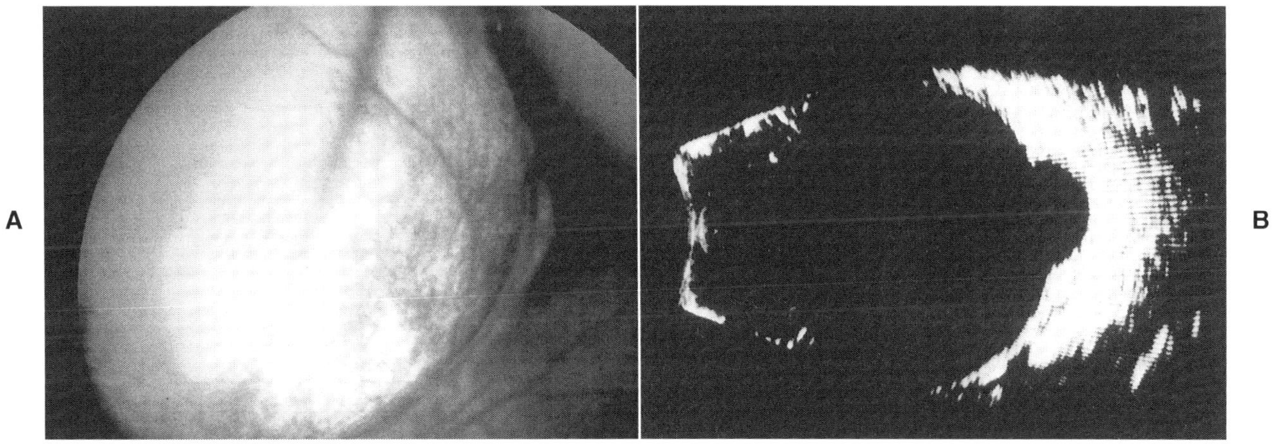

Figure 5-75 Posterior coloboma. **A,** Fundus photograph shows well-circumscribed posterior coloboma. **B,** Transverse B-scan demonstrates staphylomatous nature of the lesion.

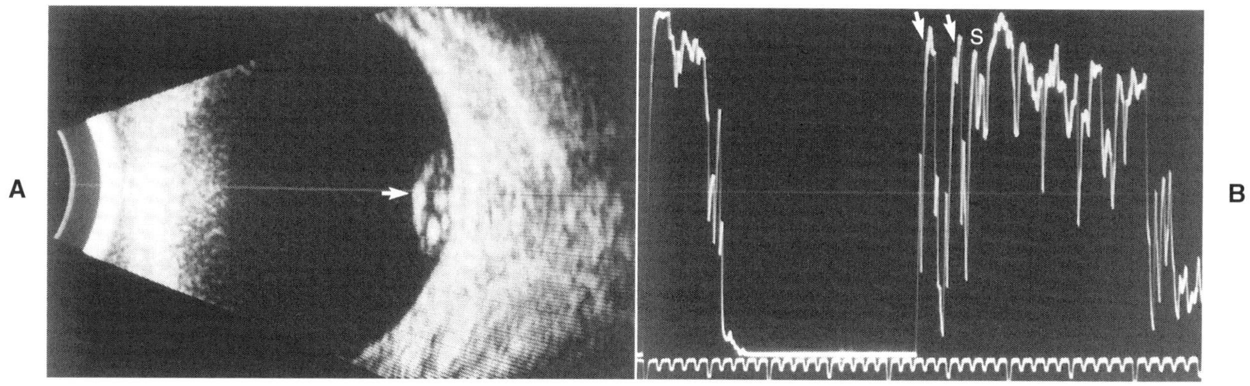

Figure 5-76 Dislocated lens nucleus. **A,** Transverse B-scan echogram through inferior aspect of globe shows oval-shaped lens nucleus lying on surface of the retina *(arrow)*. **B,** A-scan shows highly reflective spikes from the anterior and posterior surfaces of the nucleus. *S,* Sclera.

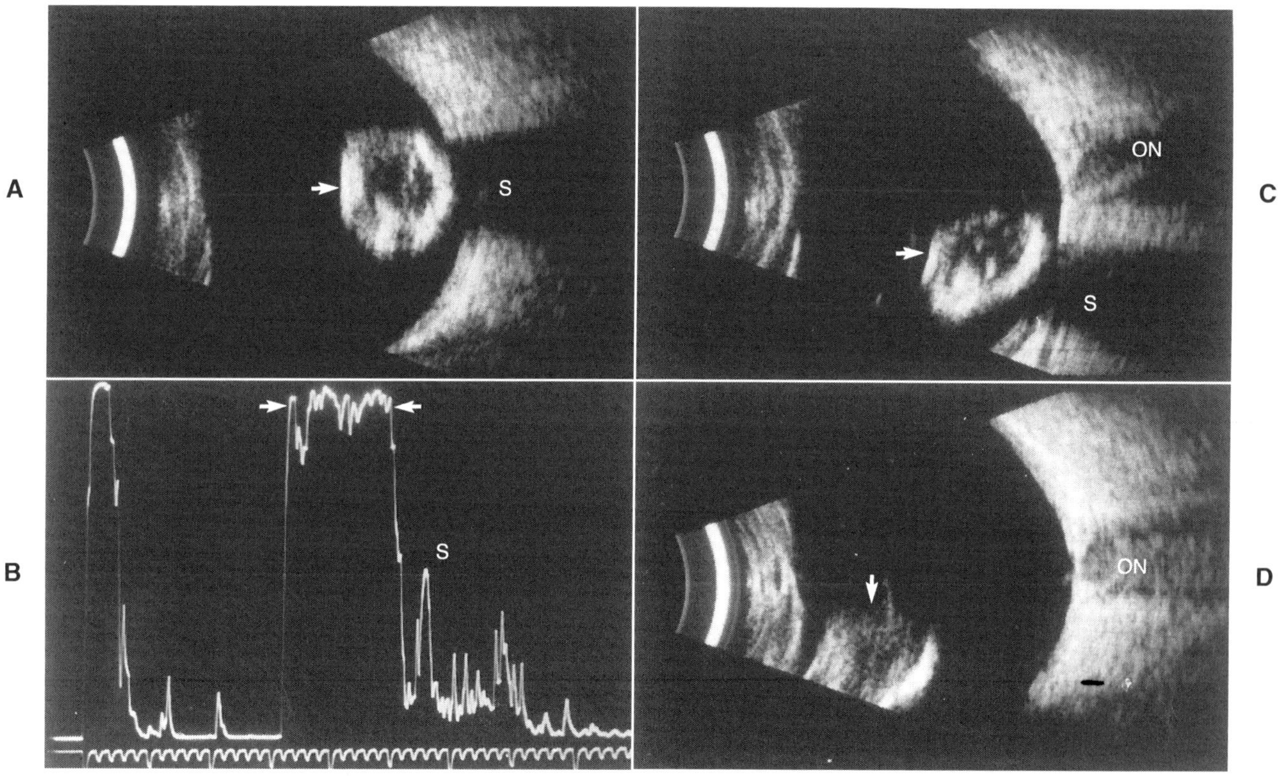

Figure 5-77 Dislocated, cataractous lens. **A,** Horizontal transverse B-scan echogram through inferior posterior globe (at reduced gain setting) shows round, swollen, partially calcified dislocated lens *(arrow)* lying near surface of retina. Note marked shadowing *(S)* of posterior ocular and orbital structures produced by the calcified lens. **B,** Corresponding A-scan view of the lens shows very high reflectivity *(arrows)*. *S,* Decreased spike height of orbital tissues due to strong sound attenuation. **C,** Vertical axial B-scan obtained with patient in normal reclined position shows dislocated lens *(arrow)* just inferior to optic nerve *(ON)*. **D,** Vertical axial B-scan obtained with patient in sitting position shows lens has moved more inferiorly and anteriorly *(arrow)*.

Dislocated Lens

Lenses and lens nuclei that dislocate into the posterior segment, usually following blunt trauma or during intraocular surgery (see p 106), have been confused with intraocular tumors clinically.[1] When the lens is adherent to the posterior fundus, it can simulate a tumor, but in most cases, these lesions are mobile and can be observed to move during eye movement.

Echographically, dislocated lenses and lens nuclei typically appear oval and their internal reflectivity varies, depending on the degree of cataract formation (Figure 5-76). With eye movement, B-scan may show mobility of the lens within the vitreous cavity or sliding of the lens along the retinal surface (Figure 5-77). Another common finding is the adherence of vitreous membranes or strands to the surface of the lens or lens nucleus (see Figure 4-40). A dislocated lens should always be considered in the differential diagnosis of an intraocular mass. In many cases, a tumor can be easily ruled out by noting that the lens is not located in its normal position.

Intumescent Lens

A swollen, cataractous lens located in its normal position may be mistaken for a peripheral tumor. This confusion results from the appearance of the lens when it is displayed in cross-section on a very anterior transverse scan. In this probe position, the lens may appear as a mass emanating from the ciliary body or peripheral choroid. This lesion usually can be identified as a lens, however, by performing an axial or longitudinal scan and noting that the lens is swollen and is located in its normal position (Figure 5-78).

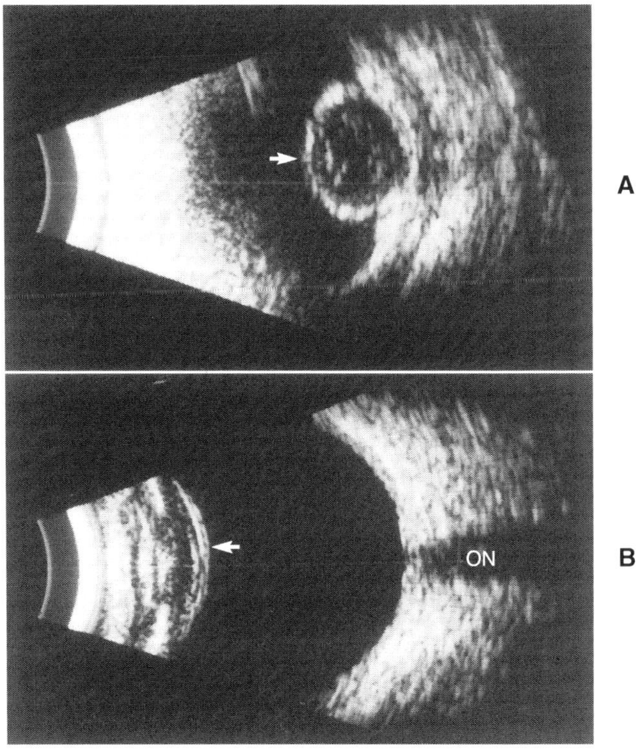

Figure 5-78 Intumescent, cataractous lens masquerading as intraocular tumor. **A,** Very anterior transverse B-scan echogram displays cross-section of swollen lens *(arrow)*. Note that in this view the lens appears very similar to a large ciliary body tumor. **B,** Axial B-scan of same eye shows cataractous lens in its normal position. *ON,* Optic nerve.

ANTERIOR SEGMENT TUMORS

Many of the different types of lesions (tumors, inflammatory lesions, and cysts) that can affect the posterior segment of the eye can also occur in the anterior segment (i.e., iris and ciliary body) (see Box 5-1).

Until recently, the only echographic method for evaluating the anterior segment was through the use of conventional contact B- and A-scan instrumentation. An immersion technique was adapted to allow imaging of anterior segment structures (see p 37). As a rule, iris lesions must be at least 1.0 mm thick and ciliary body lesions must be at least 1.5 mm for reliable detection with this method. Newer instrumentation, however, using higher frequency transducers, now provides greater resolution of both normal anatomic structures and lesions of the anterior segment. As a result, lesions of smaller size can be detected and more information can be obtained. A complete discussion and illustration of anterior segment pathology, with UBM, is provided in Chapter 8.

Because anterior segment lesions are relatively small, the use of the standardized A-scan for tissue differentiation is generally limited to the assessment of lesions that are greater than 2.0 mm in thickness. A-scan can evaluate the internal reflectivity of these lesions and can help determine whether they are vascularized. This acoustic information can be of value in differentiating certain lesions.

This section will address the use of conventional B- and A-scan instrumentation for the evaluation of anterior segment pathology. This technology is still the most widely available throughout the world and is routinely used in clinical settings. In most cases, conventional ultrasound is adequate for documenting the size and extent of anterior segment lesions and for monitoring their growth. Examples of anterior segment pathology, utilizing one of the new high resolution B-scan (20 MHz) probes (see p 39), will also be shown.

Iris Lesions

An iris lesion can present as either a pigmented or an amelanotic lesion on slit-lamp examination, or it can present as an elevation (bulging) of the iris. The main role for echography in these cases is to differentiate a solid from a cystic lesion, and to document its size and extent.

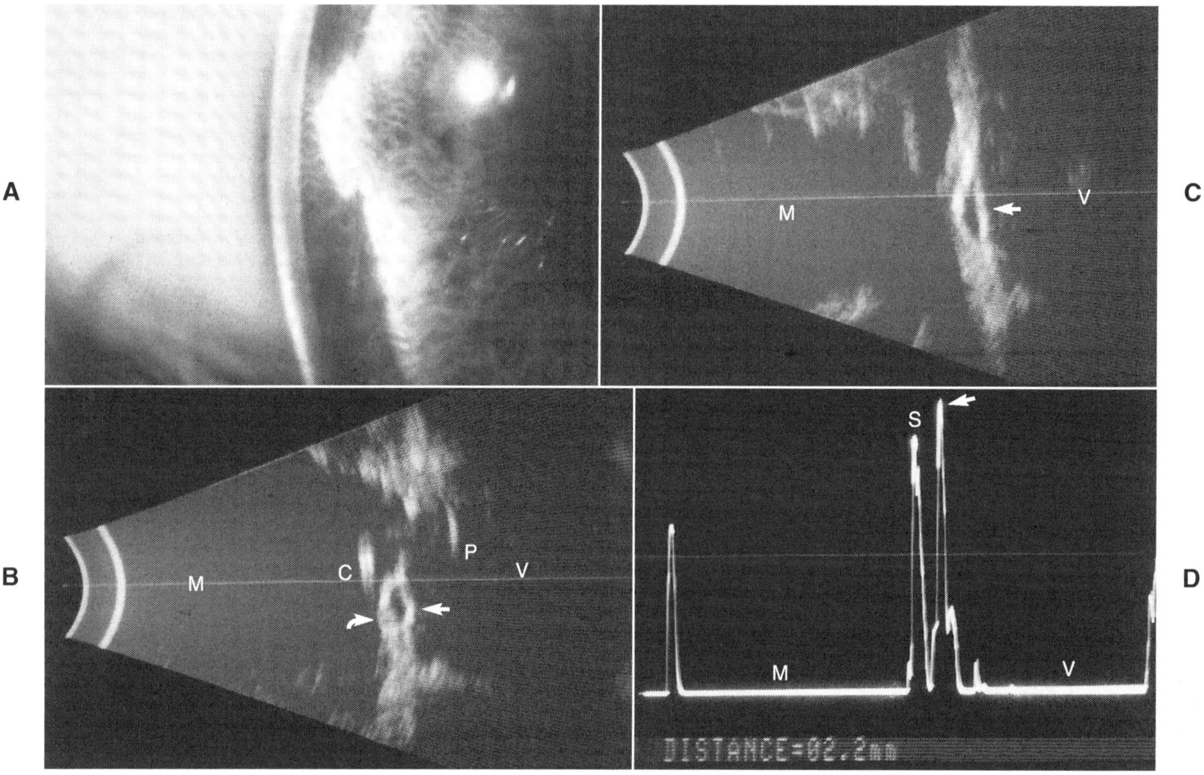

Figure 5-79 Posterior iris cyst (immersion technique). **A,** External photograph showing bulging of iris. **B,** Longitudinal B-scan echogram shows small, well-outlined, oval, echolucent lesion at posterior aspect of peripheral iris *(straight arrow)*. Lesion is bowed forward, causing narrowing of anterior chamber near angle *(curved arrow)*. *M,* Methylcellulose within scleral shell; *C,* cornea; *P,* posterior lens capsule; *V,* vitreous cavity. **C,** Transverse B-scan (with sound beam directed through limbus) shows the lateral extent of the lesion. **D,** Vector A-scan through lesion displays thickness of 2.2 mm. *S,* Sclera; *arrow,* posterior wall of cyst. (**A** courtesy Rosario Bate, CRA, Ottawa, Canada.)

Iris Cyst

Cystic lesions may be developmental or acquired. The most common developmental cysts are primary cysts of the iris pigment epithelium. These lesions usually present clinically as a bulging of the peripheral iris. Generally, they cannot be visualized with slit-lamp or ophthalmoscopic examination. Echographically, they are well circumscribed, round or oval, and echolucent. They are located in the peripheral iris at the junction of the anterior ciliary body (Figure 5-79). One study of 52 eyes[90] showed these cystic lesions to have a mean sagittal thickness of 1.6 mm. In this study, the sagittal thickness was defined as the distance from the anterior surface of the iris to the inner surface of the posterior cyst wall.

Acquired cysts, which occur most commonly following surgery or trauma, result from the implantation of surface epithelium. These lesions can be located on the anterior or the posterior iris, usually near the wound site. They are typically well outlined and echolucent, often with an irregular shape (Figure 5-80).

Iris Melanoma and Nevus

Iris melanomas can be either pigmented or amelanotic. They may be located at the pupil or may involve the iris near the angle. B-scan shows a solid lesion that may vary in shape (Figure 5-81). In addition, B-scan is useful for determining whether a peripheral iris melanoma extends posteriorly into the ciliary body (Figure 5-82). If the lesion is sufficiently thick, A-scan shows medium internal reflectivity and may demonstrate internal vascularity (Figure 5-83).

Clinically, iris nevi may appear very similar to iris melanomas. Criteria for differentiating these lesions with echography have not been established.

A

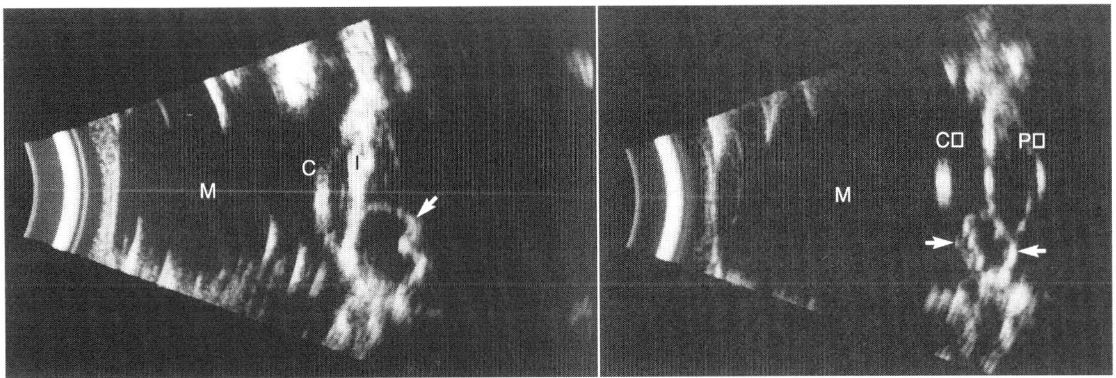

C

B

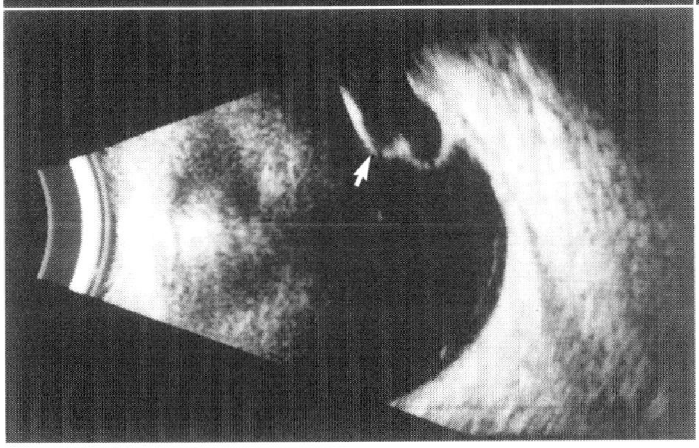

Figure 5-80 Two examples of epithelial implantation cysts following corneoscleral laceration. Immersion axial B-scan **(A)** and contact B-scan **(B)** show well-outlined, lobulated, echolucent lesion *(arrows)* located in ciliary body region. *M*, Methylcellulose within scleral shell; *C*, cornea; *I*, iris. **C,** Axial immersion B-scan from second patient shows irregularly shaped, echolucent lesion *(horizontal arrows)* in the angle of the anterior chamber. *P*, Posterior lens capsule.

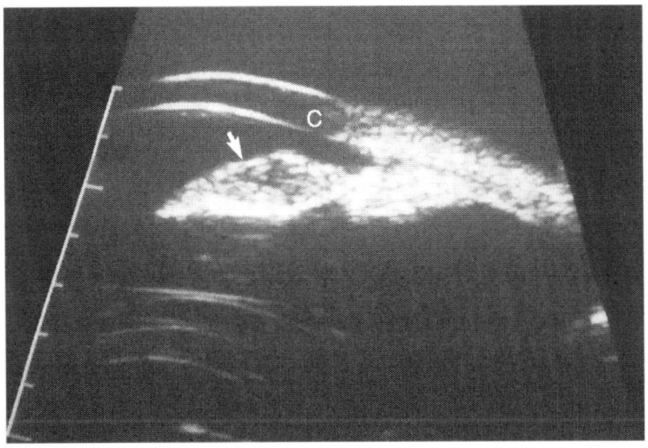

Figure 5-81 Iris melanoma examined with high resolution B-scan (20 MHz). *Arrow*, Dome-shaped iris mass; *C*, cornea. (Courtesy Rhonda Waldron, MMSc, COMT, Atlanta, Georgia.)

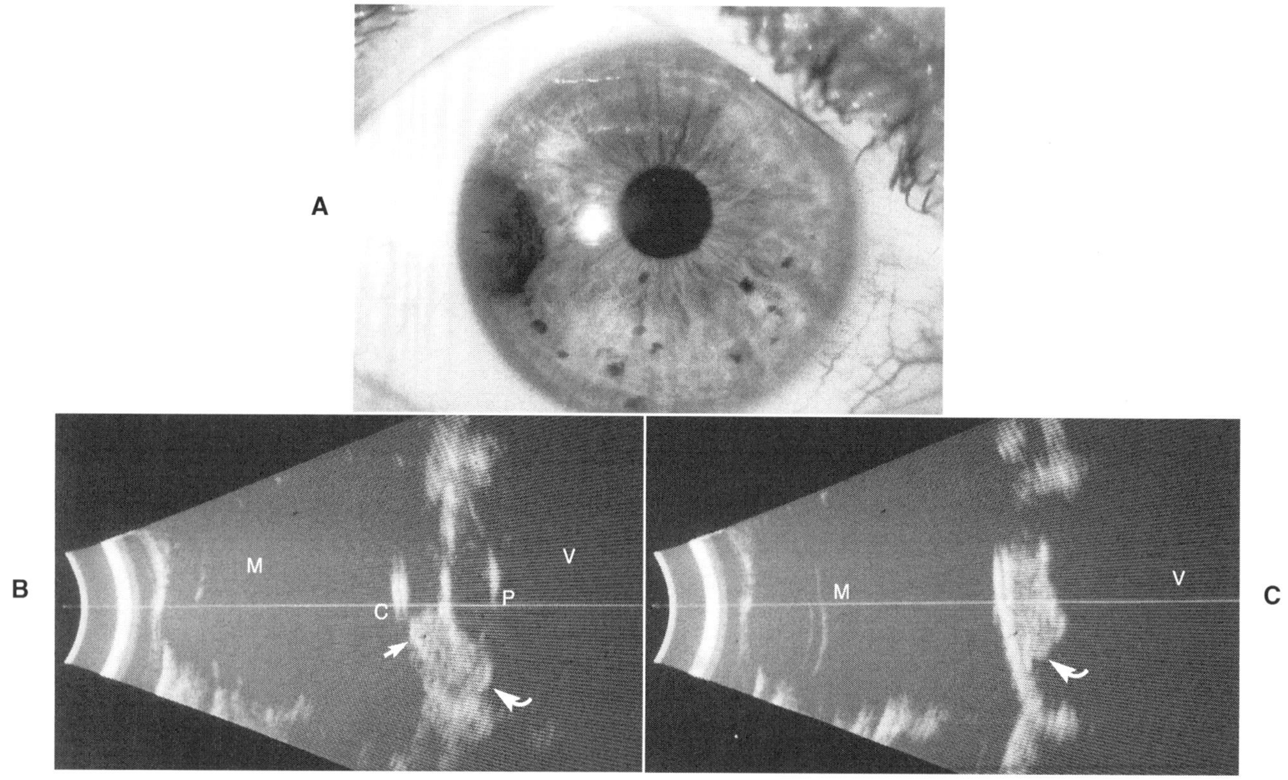

Figure 5-82 Peripheral iris melanoma with extension into ciliary body (immersion technique). **A,** External photograph shows pigmented tumor involving peripheral aspect of iris in right eye. **B,** Horizontal axial B-scan demonstrates irregularly shaped mass lesion extending from the anterior chamber *(straight arrow)* posteriorly into ciliary body *(curved arrow)*. Lesion is in contact with lens. *M,* Methylcellulose within scleral shell; *C,* cornea; *P,* posterior lens capsule; *V,* vitreous cavity. **C,** Longitudinal scan with posterior aspect of ciliary body mass centered beneath probe. Patient gaze is such that cornea and other anterior segment structures are not visible. This view clearly delineates the posterior tumor margin *(curved arrow)*.

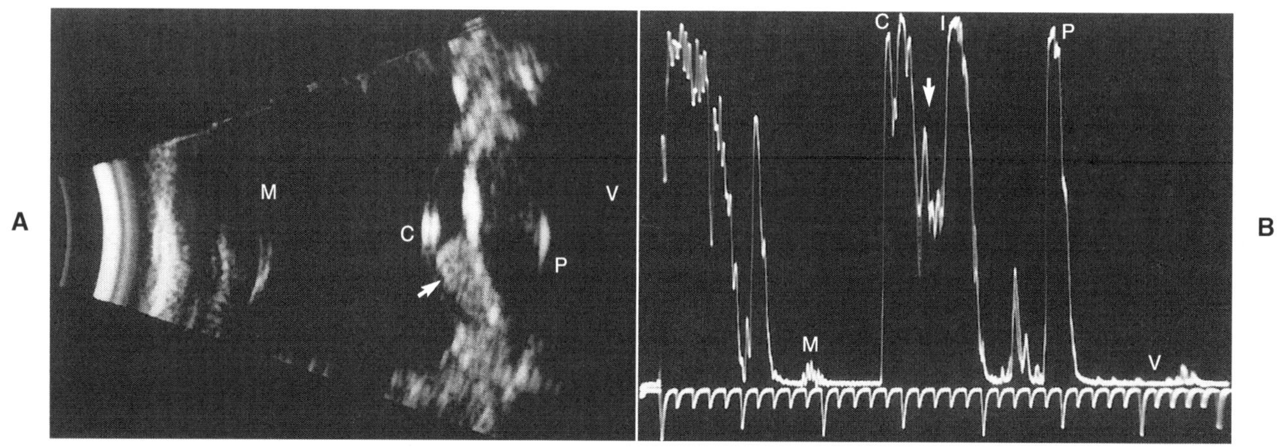

Figure 5-83 Iris melanoma (immersion technique). **A,** Vertical axial B-scan echogram shows iris mass filling inferior aspect of anterior chamber *(arrow)*, including the angle. *M,* Methylcellulose within scleral shell; *C,* cornea; *I,* iris; *P,* posterior lens capsule; *V,* vitreous cavity. **B,** A-scan shows medium internal reflectivity of lesion *(arrow)*.

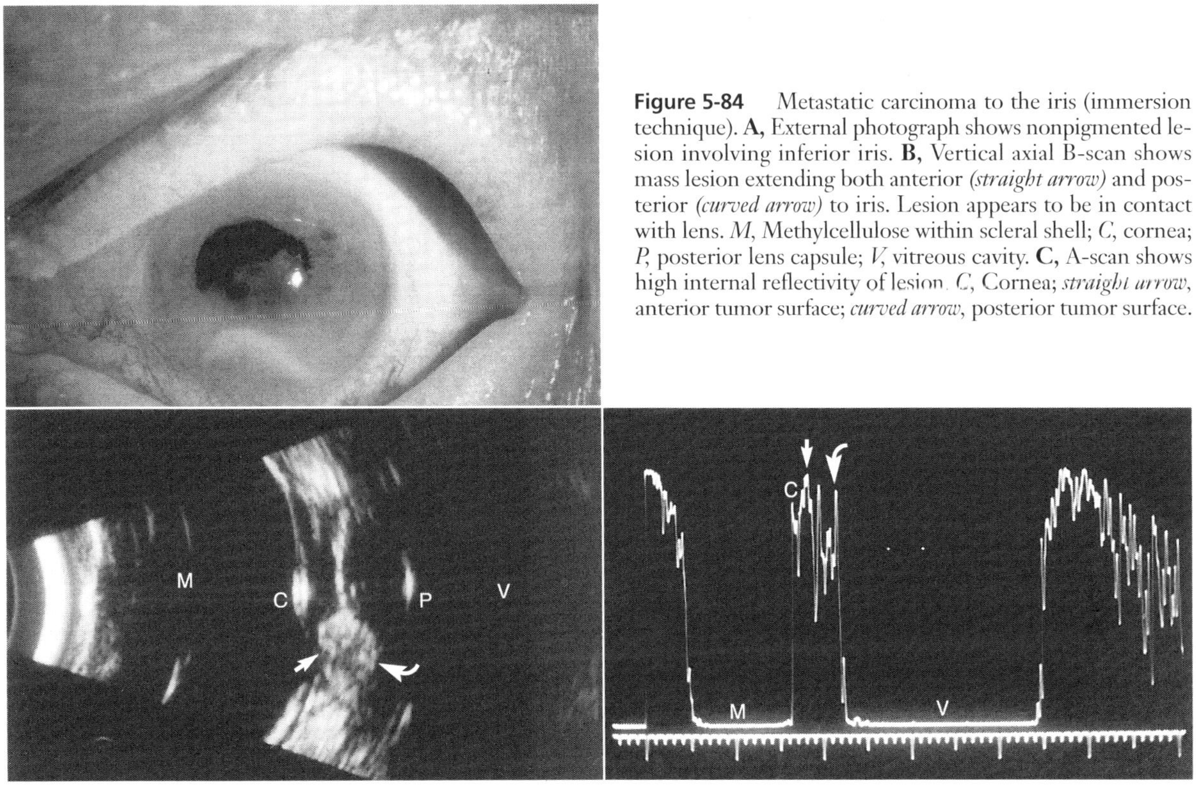

Figure 5-84 Metastatic carcinoma to the iris (immersion technique). **A,** External photograph shows nonpigmented lesion involving inferior iris. **B,** Vertical axial B-scan shows mass lesion extending both anterior *(straight arrow)* and posterior *(curved arrow)* to iris. Lesion appears to be in contact with lens. *M,* Methylcellulose within scleral shell; *C,* cornea; *P,* posterior lens capsule; *V,* vitreous cavity. **C,** A-scan shows high internal reflectivity of lesion. *C,* Cornea; *straight arrow,* anterior tumor surface; *curved arrow,* posterior tumor surface.

Iris Metastasis

Clinically, metastatic lesions appear as pink or yellow nodules involving the iris stroma.[88] B-scan shows a solid lesion with a somewhat irregular shape that may extend into the ciliary body. A-scan demonstrates an irregular internal structure with predominantly medium to high internal reflectivity (Figure 5-84). Vascularity is typically not detected.

Ciliary Body Lesions

Lesions of the ciliary body are often masked by their peripheral location and can sometimes become quite large before manifesting clinically. The immersion technique is often the best method for documenting the topography and measuring the thickness of a ciliary body tumor. Nevertheless, the contact method can sometimes be of value in assessing these lesions.

Ciliary Body Melanoma

Although ciliary body melanomas cannot be easily visualized ophthalmoscopically, they are frequently associated with clinical findings that may indicate the diagnosis.[88] These findings include dilated episcleral blood vessels, extrascleral extension, a dome-shaped mass behind the pupil, cataract and subluxation of lens, and extension into the iris and anterior chamber. These patients may also develop secondary glaucoma.

On B-scan, ciliary body melanomas exhibit a smooth, dome shape (Figure 5-85); larger lesions may develop a collar button shape (see Figure 5-6). They may be confined to the anterior ciliary body or may extend posteriorly into the pars plana and peripheral choroid. The contact method, using a longitudinal B-scan approach, is usually best suited for demonstrating the extent of peripheral choroidal involvement (Figure 5-86). B-scan may also show extension into the anterior chamber and impingement on the lens (Figure 5-87; see also Figure 5-86), and A-scan may demonstrate the characteristic low to medium internal reflectivity, as well as internal vascularity.

Another interesting echographic feature of some ciliary body melanomas is the presence of one or more cystic cavities (i.e., cavitary melanoma)[50] (Figure 5-88). In some cases, the cystic cavities occupy nearly the entire volume of the tumor and may simulate a benign cyst of the ciliary body. Two features of these melanomas that may help differentiate them from benign cysts are (1) a solid mass at the base of the lesion and (2) a thick wall surrounding the cavities within the tumor (Figure 5-89).

When large choroidal melanomas extend anteriorly, contact techniques may be unable to display the anterior border of the lesion. Immersion B-scan is then recommended to document the anterior extent of the lesion and the degree of ciliary body involvement (see Figure 5-87).

A B

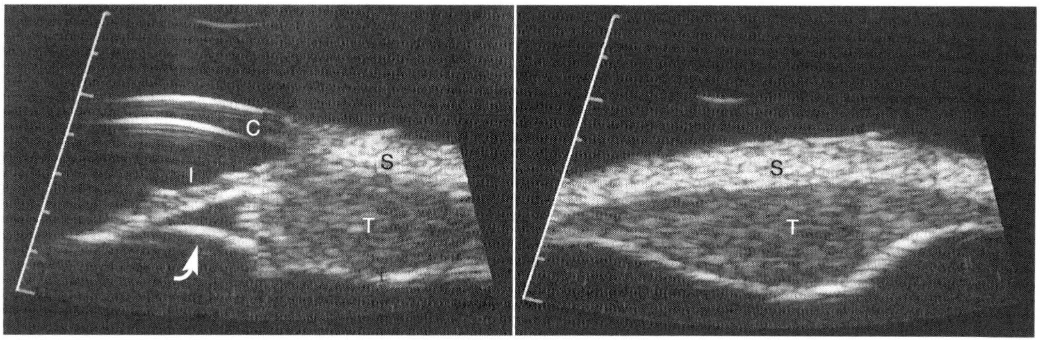

Figure 5-85 Ciliary body melanoma examined with high resolution B-scan (20 MHz). **A,** Longitudinal scan demonstrates well-outlined, oval tumor *(T)*. *C,* Cornea; *S,* sclera; *I,* iris; *curved arrow,* anterior lens surface. **B,** Transverse B-scan shows circumferential slice through tumor. (Courtesy Cynthia Kendall, BMET, RDMS, Sacramento, California.)

A C B D

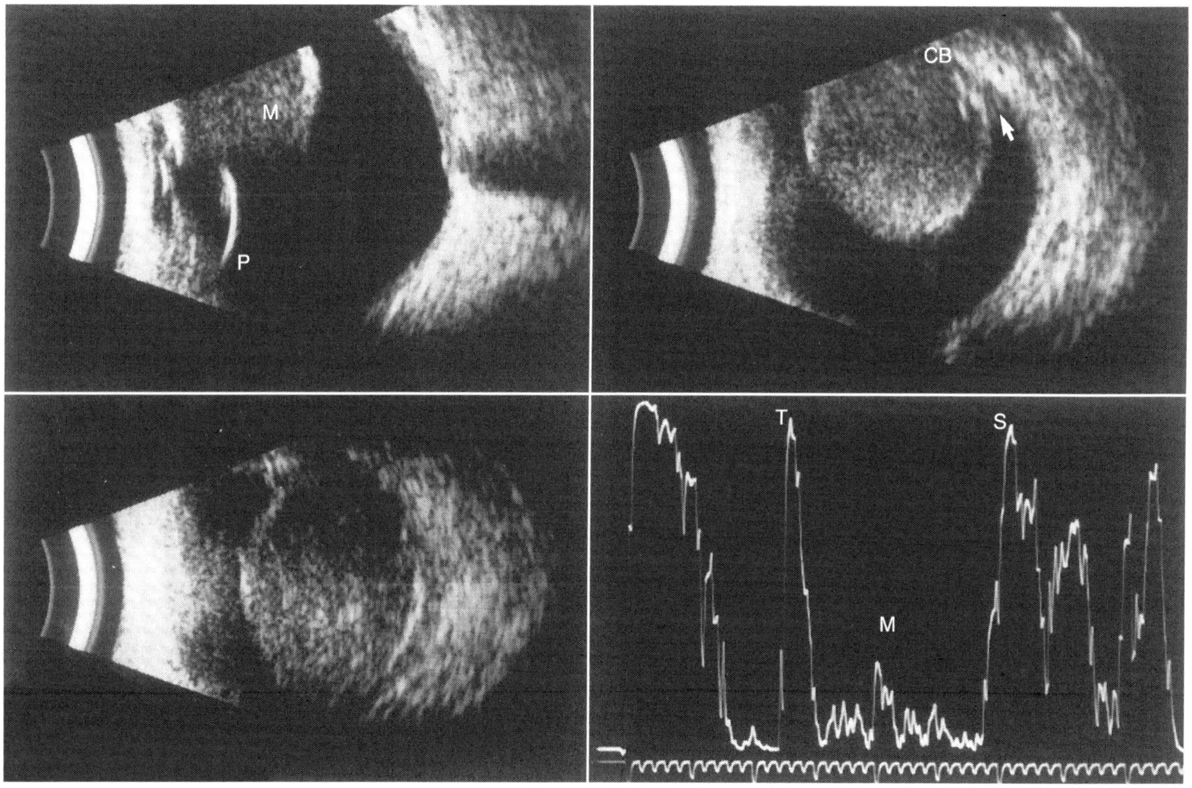

Figure 5-86 Large ciliary body melanoma displayed with contact technique. **A,** Oblique axial B-scan view shows large, peripheral melanoma *(M)* displacing lens inferiorly. *P,* Posterior lens capsule. **B,** Oblique transverse B-scan through superior aspect of ciliary body shows very large, dome-shaped tumor. Note that the tumor and sclera are not well shown because of difficulty in maintaining perpendicularity in the periphery of the globe. **C,** Anterior longitudinal B-scan shows extreme peripheral location of tumor. Note that in this view the entire radial extent of tumor cannot be displayed. *CB,* Ciliary body; *arrow,* posterior aspect of tumor. **D,** A-scan at Tissue Sensitivity shows very low reflectivity of melanoma *(M)*. *T,* Tumor surface; *S,* sclera.

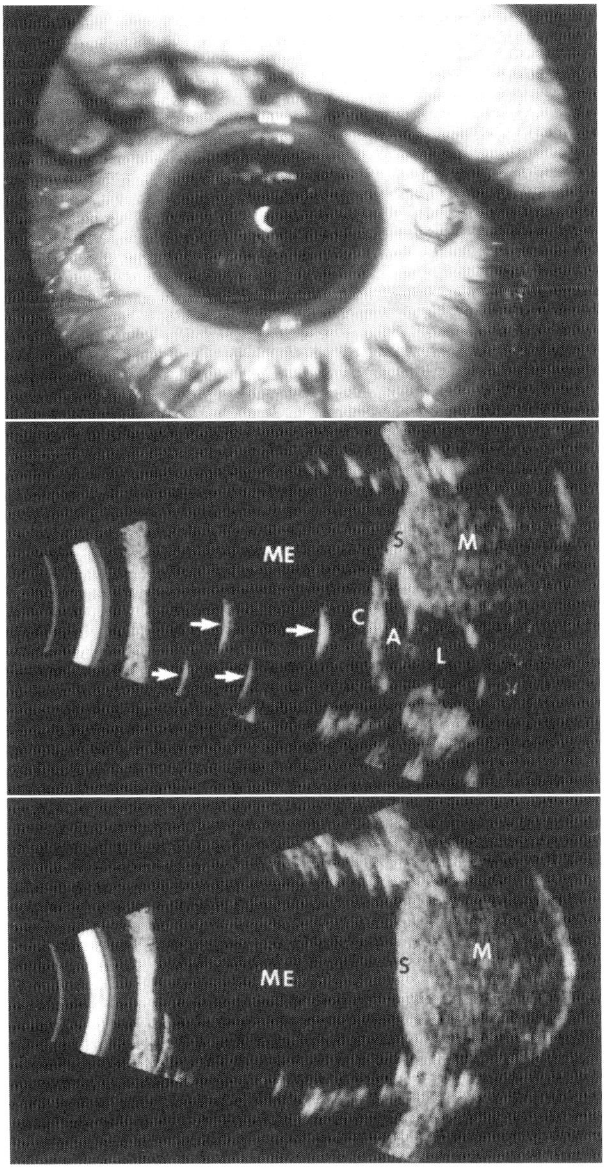

Figure 5-87 Large ciliochoroidal melanoma (immersion technique, same tumor as in Figure 5-86). **A,** Large ciliary body mass located supratemporally is visible through pupil on external photograph. **B,** Axial B-scan view shows large melanoma *(M)* displacing the lens *(L)*. *ME,* Methylcellulose within scleral shell; *arrows,* small air bubbles; *C,* cornea; *S,* sclera; *A,* anterior chamber. **C,** Transverse B-scan with tumor centered beneath probe (patient fixating inferonasally) shows melanoma *(M)*.

A C B D

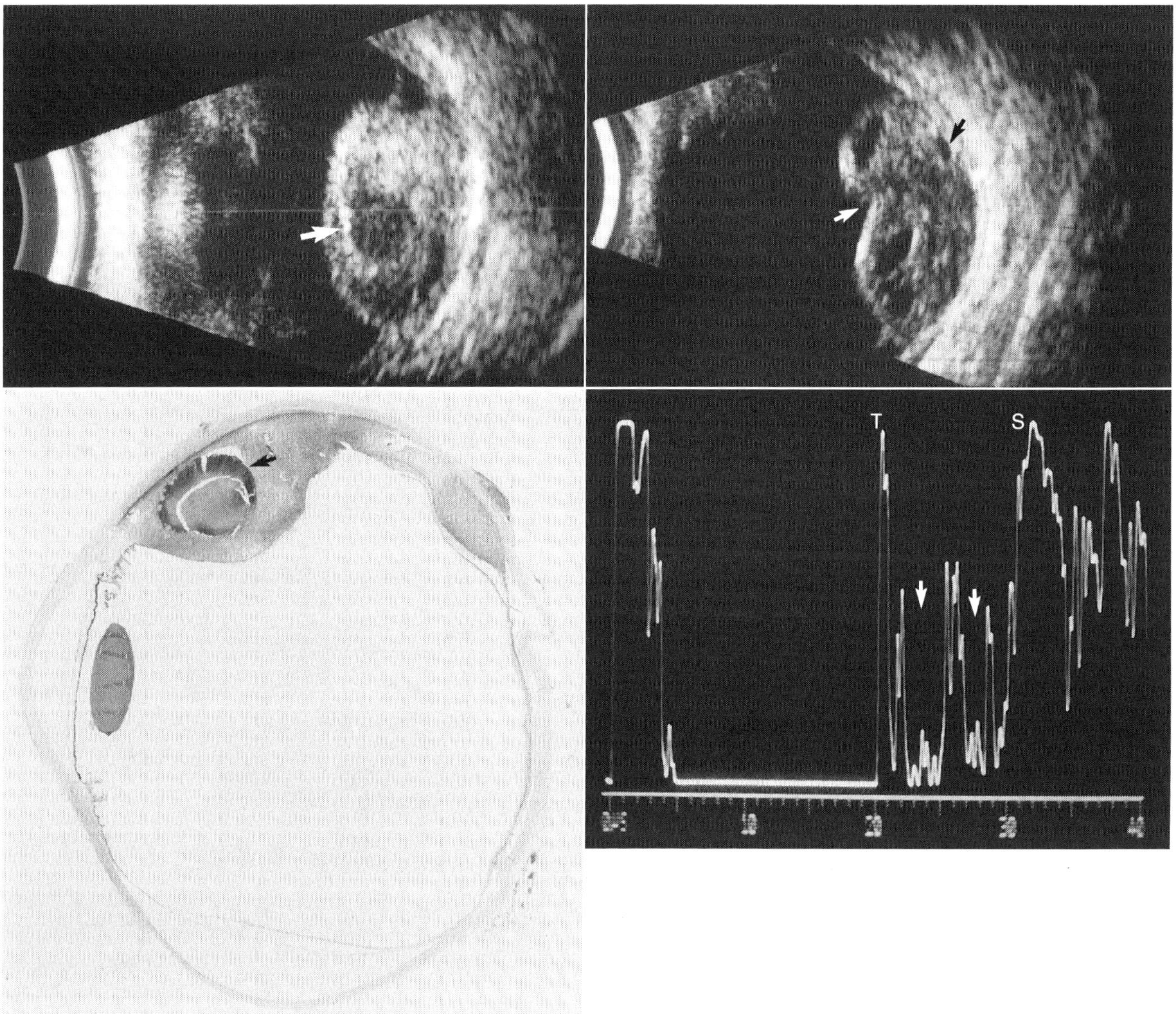

Figure 5-88 Two examples of ciliochoroidal melanoma with cystic degeneration (cavitary melanoma). **A,** Transverse B-scan demonstrates large dome-shaped tumor with area of cystic degeneration *(arrow)*. **B,** Gross pathologic specimen shows large ciliochoroidal melanoma (mixed cell tumor) with hemorrhagic degeneration *(arrow)*. **C,** Transverse B-scan of second case shows large mass with eccentric collar button *(arrows)* containing multiple cystic spaces. **D,** A-scan corresponding to **C** shows moderately irregular structure with areas of low reflectivity due to cystic cavities *(arrows)*. *T,* Tumor surface; *S,* sclera.

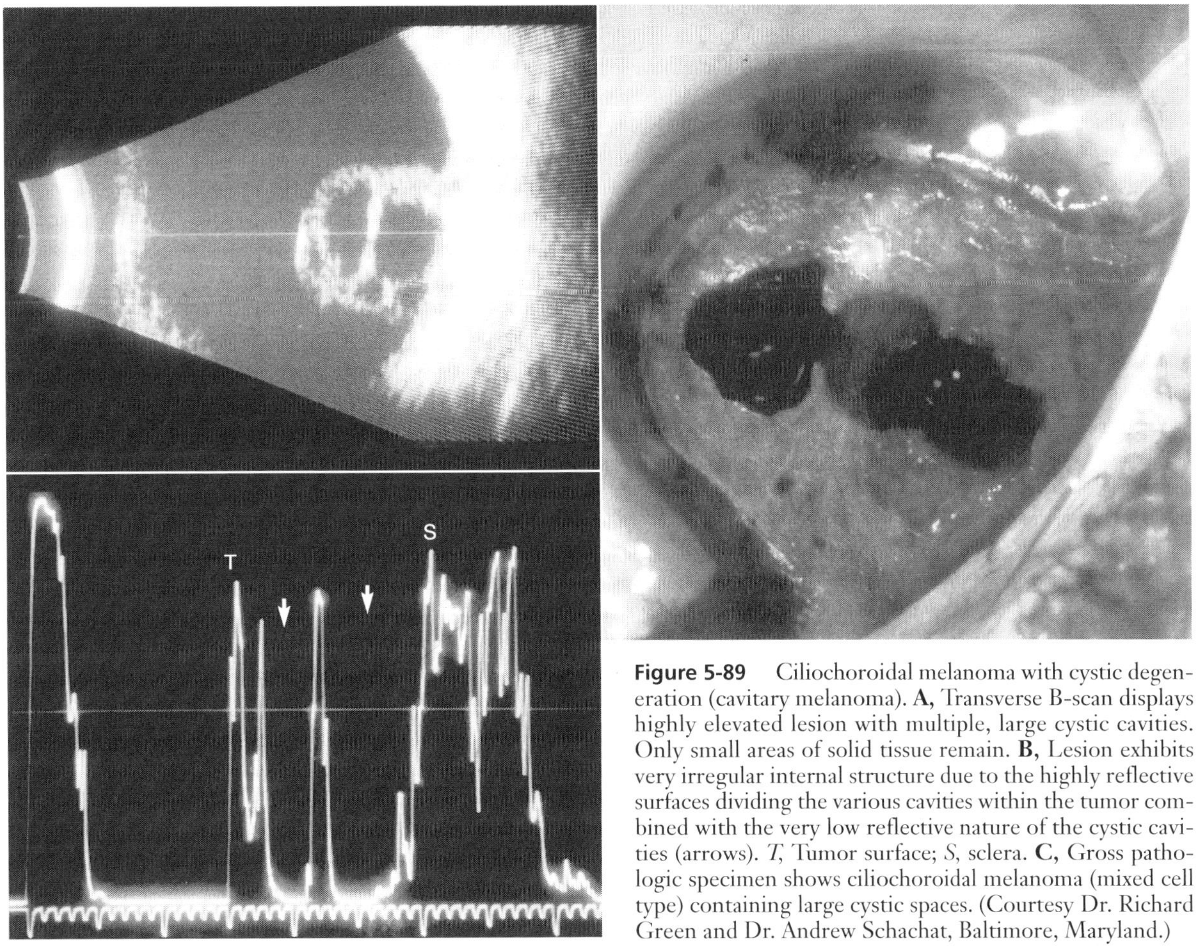

Figure 5-89 Ciliochoroidal melanoma with cystic degeneration (cavitary melanoma). **A,** Transverse B-scan displays highly elevated lesion with multiple, large cystic cavities. Only small areas of solid tissue remain. **B,** Lesion exhibits very irregular internal structure due to the highly reflective surfaces dividing the various cavities within the tumor combined with the very low reflective nature of the cystic cavities (arrows). *T,* Tumor surface; *S,* sclera. **C,** Gross pathologic specimen shows ciliochoroidal melanoma (mixed cell type) containing large cystic spaces. (Courtesy Dr. Richard Green and Dr. Andrew Schachat, Baltimore, Maryland.)

Other Lesions of the Ciliary Body

A number of other lesions can involve the ciliary body and may mimic a melanoma clinically. Some of these include melanocytoma, adenoma, leiomyoma, medulloepithelioma (see p 187), benign cysts, and epithelial downgrowth. On B-scan, most of these lesions are well outlined and dome shaped.

Melanocytomas and adenomas usually demonstrate regular internal structure and high internal reflectivity on A-scan (Figure 5-90). In contrast, leiomyomas exhibit low to medium internal reflectivity. These tumors are also highly vascularized (see p 154 and Figure 5-58).

Benign cysts involving the ciliary body are usually round or oval and appear echolucent on B-scan (Figure 5-91). As mentioned earlier, cavitary melanomas can simulate these lesions and must be considered in the differential diagnosis (see p 173 and Figure 5-89).

Epithelial downgrowth can present as a masslike lesion involving the ciliary body. This lesion may demonstrate an irregular shape on B-scan and high internal reflectivity on A-scan (Figure 5-92). Epithelial downgrowth should be suspected if there has been previous penetrating trauma or complicated intraocular surgery.

Conjunctival (limbal) dermoid tumors usually present in childhood. In many cases, they extend onto the cornea. These lesions can often be assessed with ultrasound using the immersion technique previously described for evaluation of the anterior segment (see p 37). Typically,

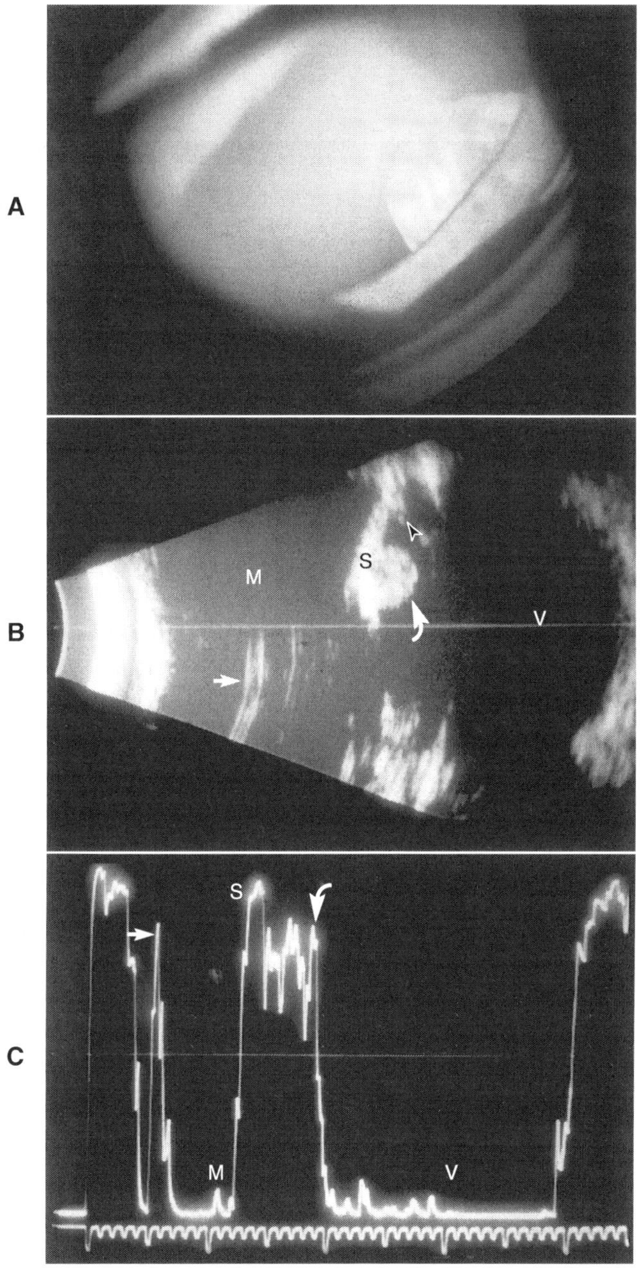

Figure 5-90 Adenoma of ciliary body (immersion technique). **A,** Photograph shows nonpigmented ciliary body mass behind iris. **B,** Longitudinal B-scan shows roundish ciliary body mass *(curved arrow)*. *M,* Methylcellulose within scleral shell; *straight arrow,* air bubble; *S,* sclera; *open arrow,* posterior extent of lesion along ciliary body; *V,* vitreous cavity. Patient gaze is such that cornea and iris are not visible. **C,** A-scan indicates high internal reflectivity of tumor. (**A** courtesy James Gilman, CRA; **B** and **C** courtesy Rhonda Waldron, MMSc, COMT, Atlanta, Georgia.)

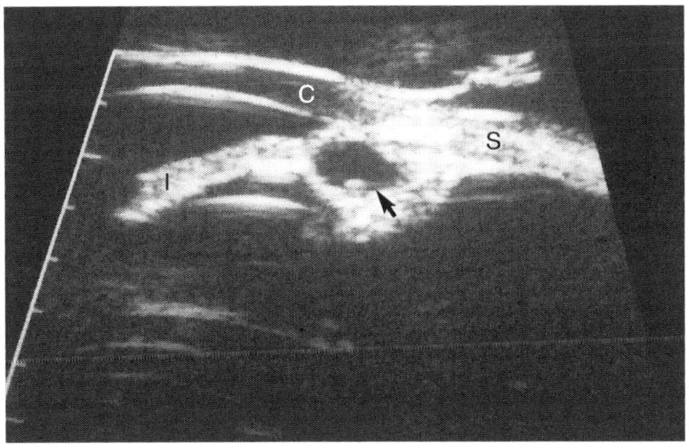

Figure 5-91 Ciliary body cyst examined with high resolution B-scan (MHz). Longitudinal scan. *Arrow,* Ciliary body cyst; *C,* cornea; *I,* iris; *S,* sclera. (Courtesy Rhonda Waldron, MMSc, COMT, Atlanta, Georgia.)

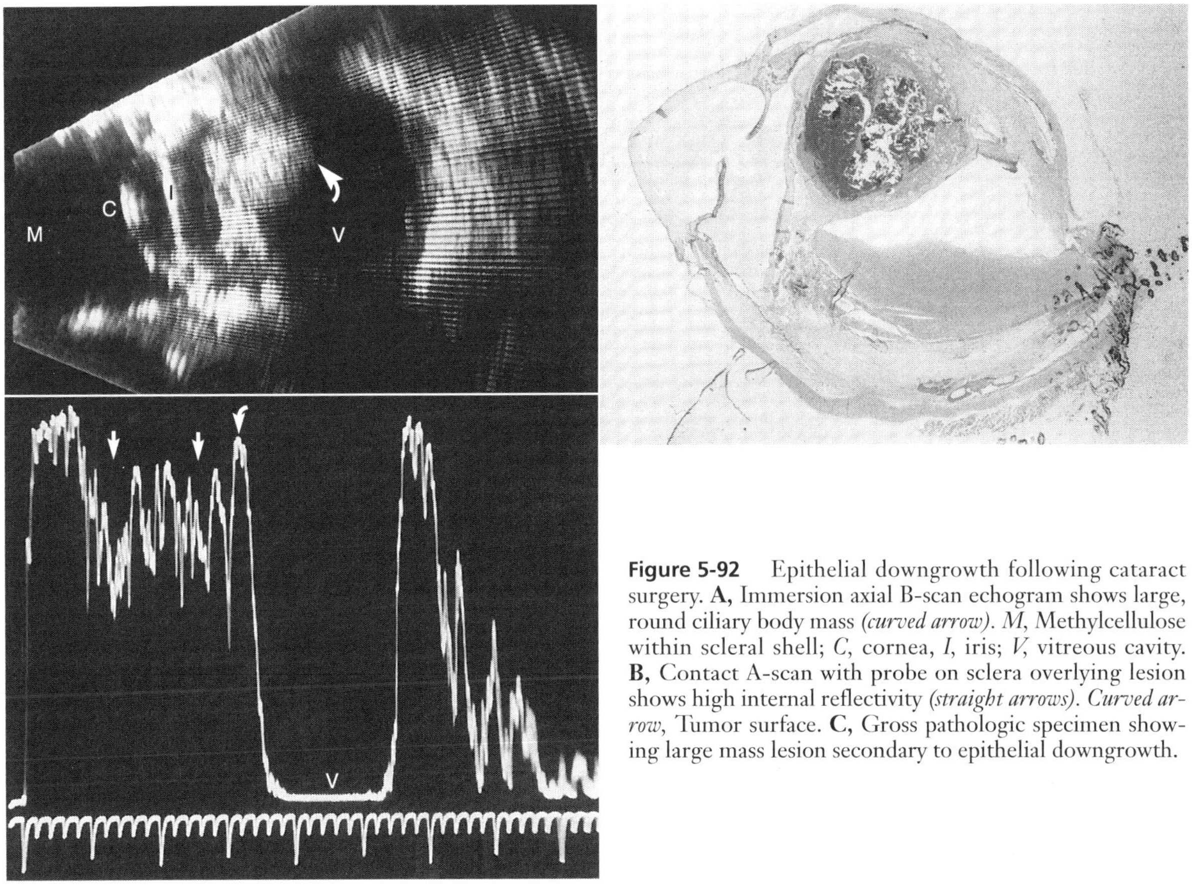

Figure 5-92 Epithelial downgrowth following cataract surgery. **A,** Immersion axial B-scan echogram shows large, round ciliary body mass *(curved arrow). M,* Methylcellulose within scleral shell; *C,* cornea, *I,* iris; *V,* vitreous cavity. **B,** Contact A-scan with probe on sclera overlying lesion shows high internal reflectivity *(straight arrows). Curved arrow,* Tumor surface. **C,** Gross pathologic specimen showing large mass lesion secondary to epithelial downgrowth.

A 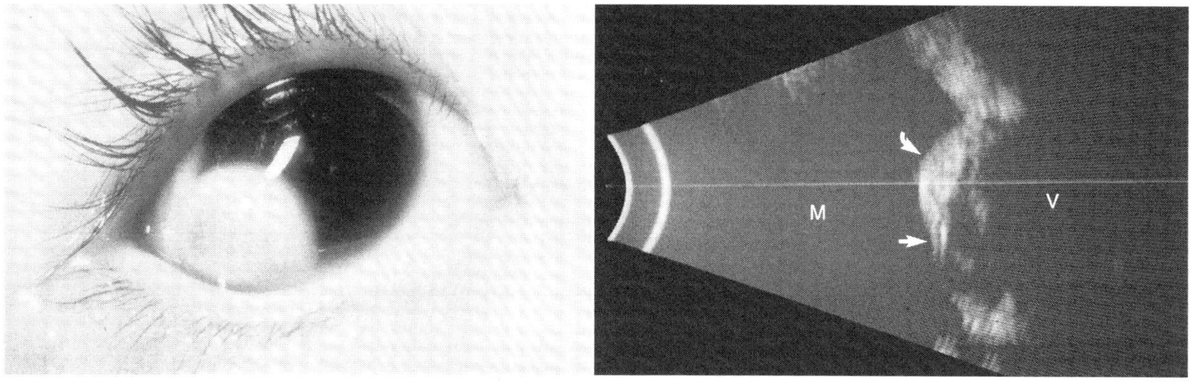 B

Figure 5-93 Limbal dermoid (immersion technique). **A,** External photograph from child shows limbal dermoid. **B,** Longitudinal B-scan shows dome-shaped mass *(curved arrow)* in perilimbal region with extension onto cornea *(straight arrow)*. Lesion is relatively echo-dense and cannot be differentiated from underlying sclera. *M,* Methylcellulose within scleral shell; *V,* vitreous cavity. (**A** courtesy Dr. Jonathon Dutton, Carey, North Carolina.)

ultrasound demonstrates a smooth, dome-shaped lesion on the surface of the globe at the limbus. They exhibit high internal reflectivity and often appear to infiltrate the underlying sclera (Figure 5-93).

RETINOBLASTOMA

Echography is useful for the detection and differentiation of intraocular tumors in children and is particularly valuable in the diagnosis of retinoblastoma.[58,65] Retinoblastomas can be unilateral or bilateral, focal or multifocal, and frequently have a creamy, yellow-white appearance. These tumors can grow either anteriorly from the inner surface of the retina toward the vitreous (endophytic) or posteriorly from the outer aspect of the retina toward the choroid (exophytic).[108] Retinoblastomas commonly contain calcium.

Echographically, retinoblastomas may have a smooth, dome shape, but more typically, they have a very irregular configuration. The internal reflectivity can vary according to the degree of calcification within the lesion. Noncalcified tumors demonstrate low to medium reflectivity, whereas calcium produces extremely high internal reflectivity. The calcium may be quite dense and located throughout the lesion, or it may be limited to a few small foci (Figure 5-94). When these deposits are numerous and/or large, shadowing of the adjacent sclera and orbit may occur (Figures 5-95 and 5-96). Because the demonstration of calcium is so important in diagnosing a retinoblastoma, these eyes should be examined very carefully. Internal vascularity may or may not be detected in these lesions. It should also be mentioned that these eyes are usually of normal size or larger.[97] Consequently, axial eye length measurements can often be helpful in differentiating a retinoblastoma from other causes of leukokoria that present with small globes (Table 5-2). It should also be mentioned that orbital inflammation can occur in association with retinoblastoma.[37,84]

In some cases, a retinoblastoma can present as a mildly elevated, diffuse lesion at the level of the retina, with a bumpy, irregular contour. These diffuse tumors, which usually occur in older children, may contain little or no calcium (Figure 5-97). In these eyes, tumor cells may accumulate in the anterior chamber as a pseudohypopyon or in the vitreous, simulating a vitritis.[84,97] They may also produce cysts within the vitreous cavity.[106] Because the clinical presentation can mimic an inflammatory disorder and because calcification may not be present on ultrasound, the diagnosis of retinoblastoma may not be readily apparent. Therefore, whenever a diffuse, bumpy, noncalcified lesion is detected in a child, the diagnosis of retinoblastoma should be considered.

Retinoblastomas can infiltrate the optic nerve or extend into the orbit. This may be difficult to detect with ultrasound because of shadowing from intraocular calcification. Consequently, computed tomography (CT) or magnetic

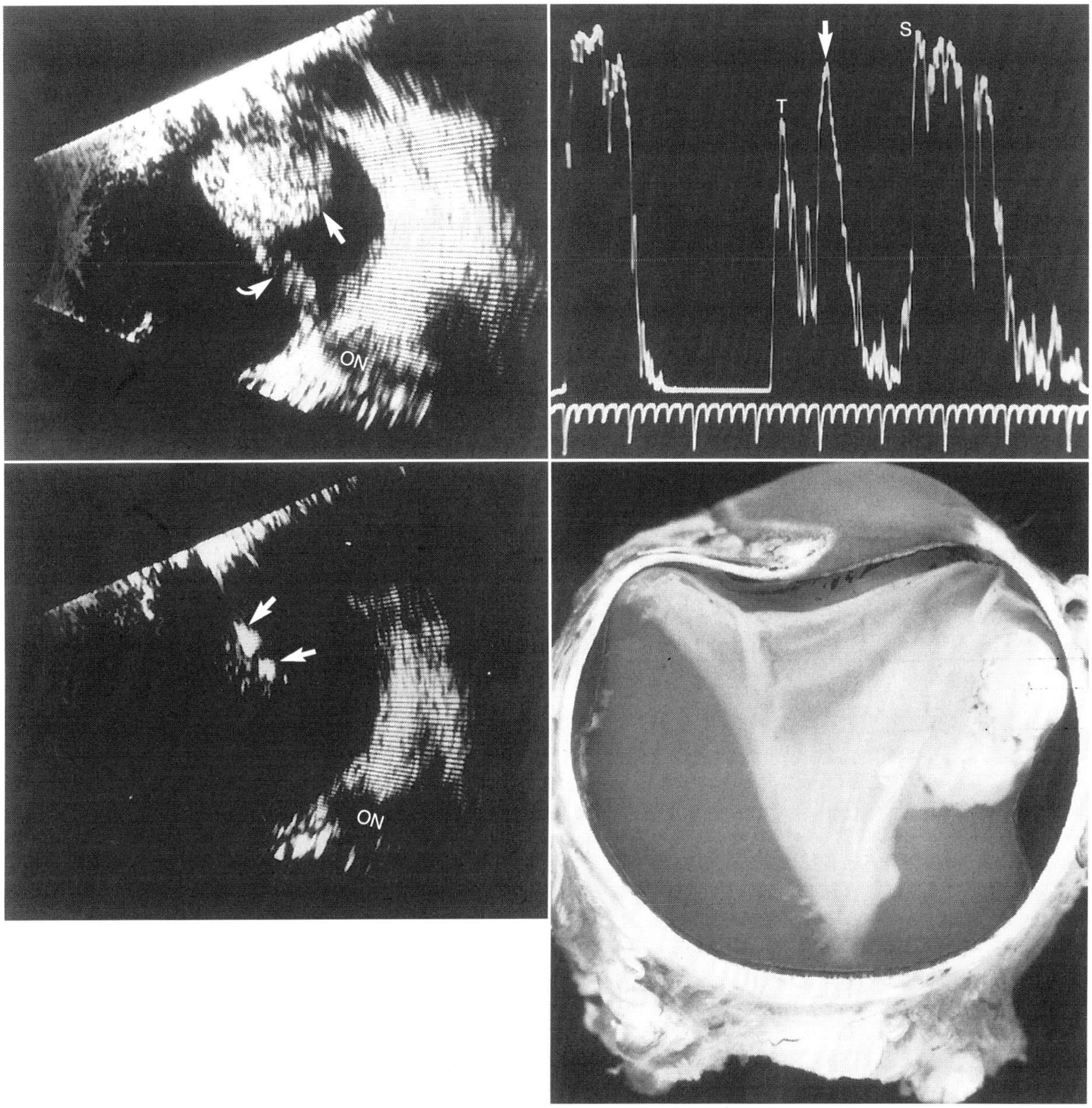

Figure 5-94 Large exophytic retinoblastoma showing only mild calcification. **A,** Longitudinal B-scan echogram displays large, roundish, echo-dense lesion *(straight arrow)* in peripheral aspect of eye. Retinal detachment *(curved arrow)* is noted extending from lesion to optic nerve *(ON)*. **B,** Same view as **A** (at reduced gain setting) shows persistent, echo-dense signals from calcium deposits within tumor *(arrows)*. **C,** A-scan through tumor shows highly reflective spike from focus of calcium *(arrow)*. *T,* Tumor surface; *S,* sclera. **D,** Gross pathologic specimen shows total retinal detachment with large exophytic tumor.

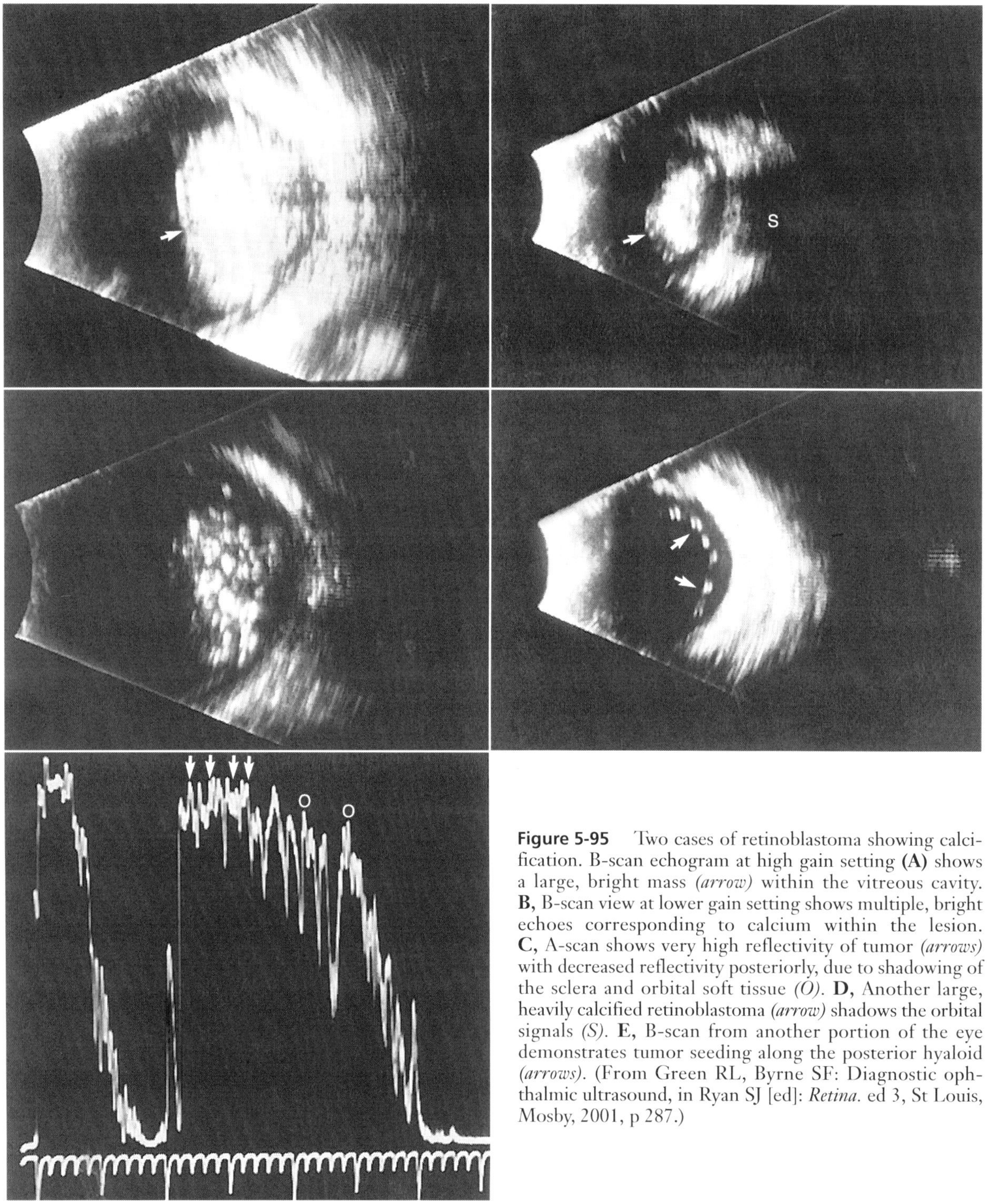

Figure 5-95 Two cases of retinoblastoma showing calcification. B-scan echogram at high gain setting **(A)** shows a large, bright mass *(arrow)* within the vitreous cavity. **B,** B-scan view at lower gain setting shows multiple, bright echoes corresponding to calcium within the lesion. **C,** A-scan shows very high reflectivity of tumor *(arrows)* with decreased reflectivity posteriorly, due to shadowing of the sclera and orbital soft tissue *(O)*. **D,** Another large, heavily calcified retinoblastoma *(arrow)* shadows the orbital signals *(S)*. **E,** B-scan from another portion of the eye demonstrates tumor seeding along the posterior hyaloid *(arrows)*. (From Green RL, Byrne SF: Diagnostic ophthalmic ultrasound, in Ryan SJ [ed]: *Retina.* ed 3, St Louis, Mosby, 2001, p 287.)

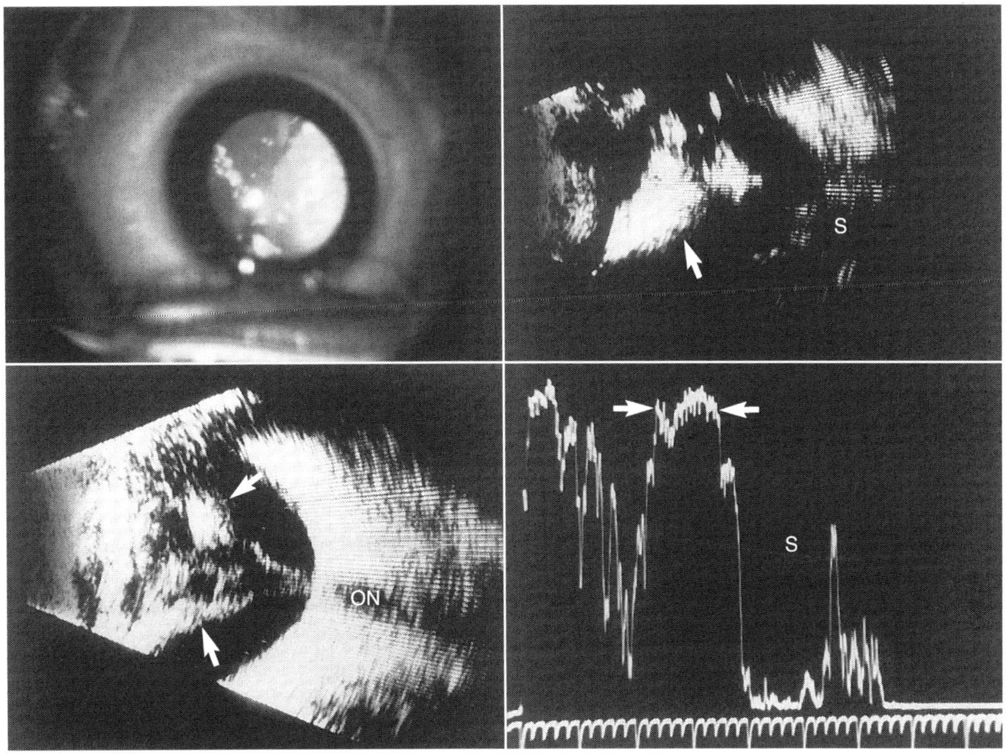

Figure 5-96 Highly calcified endophytic retinoblastoma. **A,** External photograph shows whitish mass posterior to lens. **B,** Axial B-scan echogram shows calcified retinoblastoma within funnel-shaped retinal detachment *(arrows)*. *ON,* Optic nerve. **C,** Transverse B-scan view at reduced gain setting shows large focus of calcium within tumor *(arrow)* and shadowing of orbital soft tissue *(S)*. **D,** A-scan shows very high reflectivity of calcified tumor *(arrows)*. *S,* Strong sound attenuation prevents display of orbital soft tissue.

TABLE 5-2

Conditions Associated with Leukokoria*

Condition	Main Echographic Finding	Axial Eye Length	Unilateral/Bilateral
Retinoblastoma	Calcified mass	Normal	Unilateral/bilateral
Retinopathy of prematurity (ROP) (stage V)	Total retinal detachment with retinal loops	Short	Bilateral
Persistent hyperplastic primary vitreous (PHPV)	Vitreous band from lens to optic nerve	Short	Unilateral
Coats' disease	Exudative retinal detachment	Normal	Unilateral
Toxocariasis	Peripheral glaucoma; retinal folds and posterior traction retinal detachment	Normal	Unilateral
Endophthalmitis	Vitreous opacities	Normal	Unilateral
Cysticercosis	Cyst with scolex	Normal	Unilateral
Medulloepithelioma (diktyoma)	Ciliary body mass with cystic cavities	Normal	Unilateral

*This table lists the main echographic findings for the most common conditions associated with leukokoria.

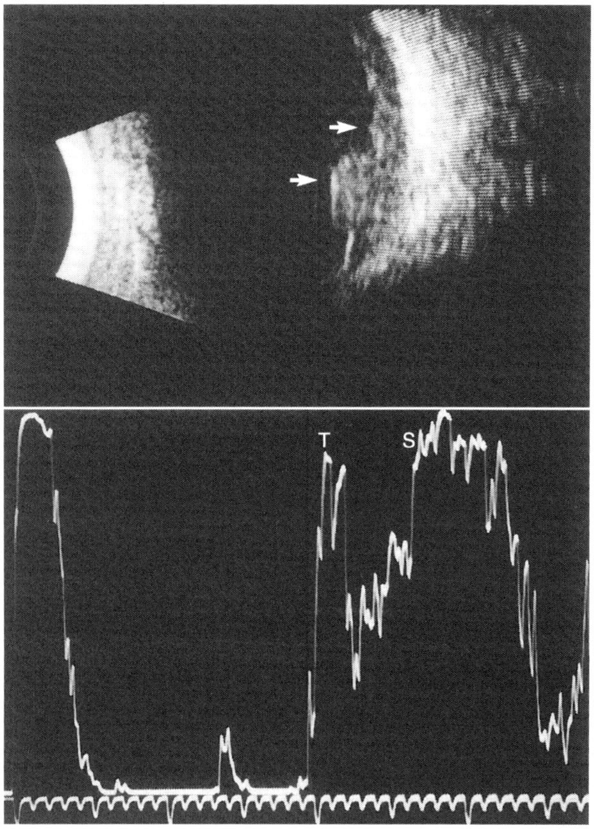

Figure 5-97 Diffuse, noncalcified retinoblastoma. **A,** B-scan echogram shows diffuse lesion with irregular, bumpy contour *(arrows)*. **B,** A-scan shows medium internal reflectivity with no evidence of calcium. *T,* Tumor surface; *S,* sclera. (From Green RL, Byrne SF: Diagnostic ophthalmic ultrasound, in Ryan SJ [ed]: *Retina.* ed 3, St Louis, Mosby, 2001, p 288.)

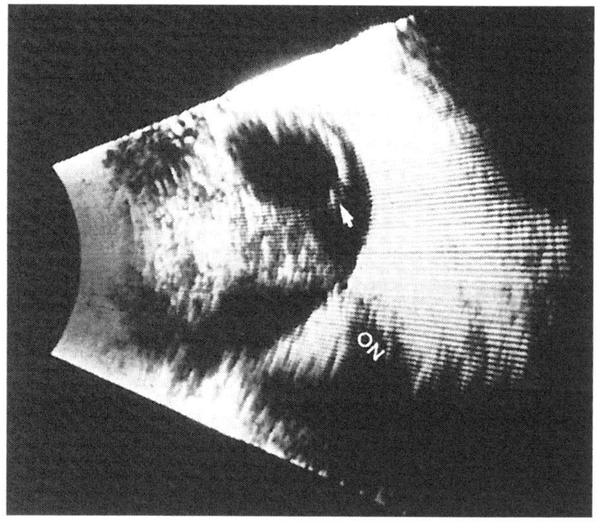

Figure 5-98 Stage V ROP. Longitudinal B-scan echogram of total funnel-shaped retinal detachment demonstrates large, peripheral retinal loop *(arrow)*. Note dense opacities within moderately open funnel. *ON,* Optic nerve. (From Pulido JS, Byrne SF, Clarkson JG, et al: Evaluation of eyes with advanced stage V of retinopathy of prematurity using standardized echography. *Ophthalmology* 1991;98:1100.)

resonance imaging (MRI) are better modalities for the detection of optic nerve or orbital involvement.

Echography is also important for monitoring the size of retinoblastomas that have been treated with radiation or alternative methods of therapy. In most instances, tumors that recur or continue to grow after treatment tend to exhibit low to medium internal reflectivity and usually do not show calcification.

Differential Diagnosis of Retinoblastoma

There are several intraocular conditions associated with leukokoria that must be considered in the differential diagnosis of retinoblastoma (see Table 5-2). The primary conditions are (1) retinopathy of prematurity (ROP), (2) persistent hyperplastic primary vitreous (PHPV), (3) Coats' disease, (4) toxocariasis, (5) cysticercosis, (6) medulloepithelioma, and (7) endophthalmitis (see p 191). Unlike retinoblastomas, these lesions do not usually contain calcium unless the eye has undergone chronic degeneration. The calcification that is detected in degenerative conditions typically occurs within the retina or choroid and therefore has a plaquelike configuration[34] (see Figure 4-49). This is in contrast to the clumplike calcification that is usually observed in retinoblastomas.

A number of rare or unusual conditions that were clinically suggestive of retinoblastoma have been evaluated. These included a large, collar button–shaped melanoma in a 6-year-old child and a rhabdomyosarcoma of the ciliary body, also in a 6-year-old child. Other unusual lesions that have been evaluated with echography include combined hamartoma of the retinal pigment epithelium and neurofibroma of the choroid (see p 155). It should also be mentioned that astrocytomas of the retina can also be calcified (see p 155) and thus may simulate retinoblastoma.

OTHER LESIONS ASSOCIATED WITH LEUKOKORIA

Retinopathy of Prematurity

Retinopathy of prematurity (ROP) is typically a bilateral condition that affects mainly the vitreous and peripheral retina.[69] In advanced cases (i.e., stage V), the retina is extensively detached, often in a funnel-like configuration. The peripheral retina frequently has a loop or troughlike appearance as a result of traction by dense retrolental membranes. Echography can show the presence of these peripheral loops, as well as the extent and configuration of the retinal detachment (Figure 5-98).[13,34,73,82] It should be mentioned that these retinal loops can appear echographi-

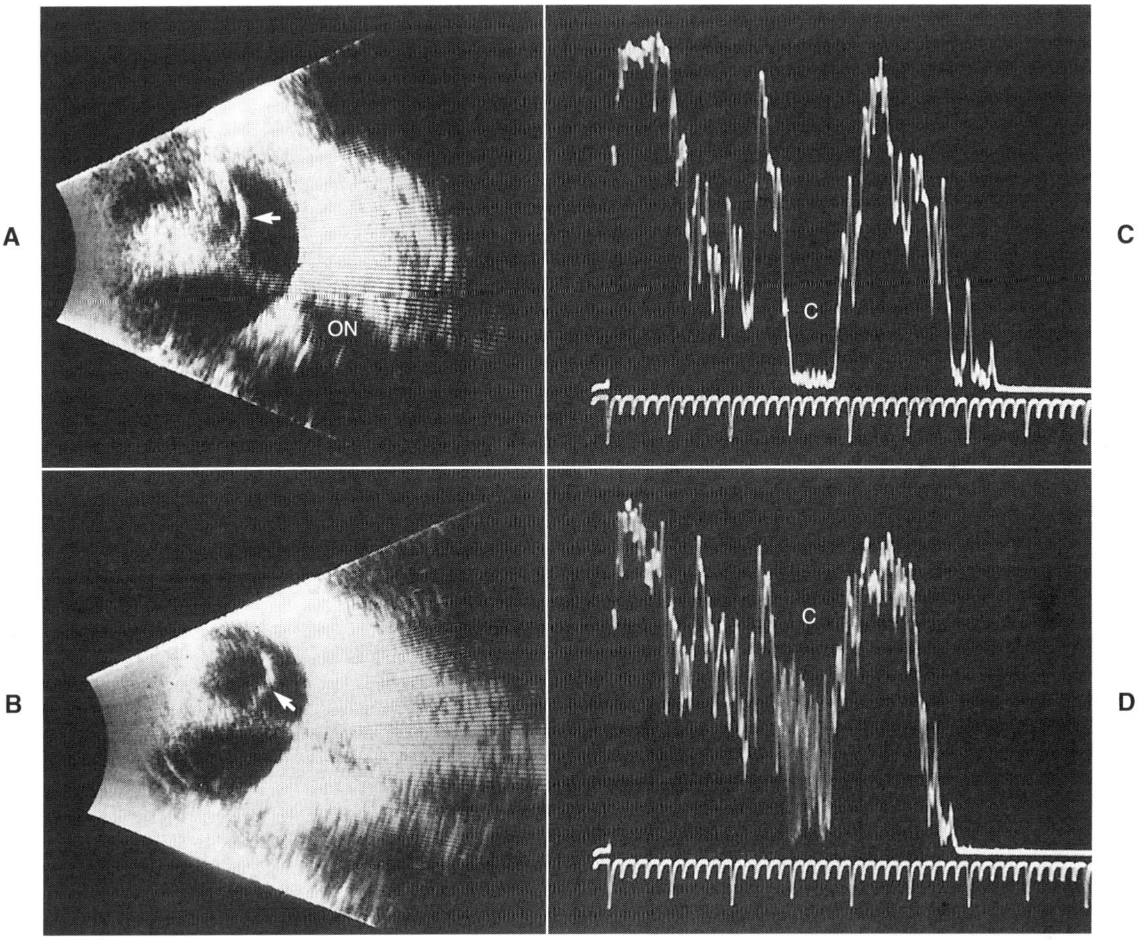

Figure 5-99 Stage V ROP. Longitudinal B-scan echograms (**A** and **B**) show dense, membranous opacities anteriorly and tightly closed funnel-shaped retinal detachment posteriorly inserting into optic nerve *(ON)*. A large retinal loop *(arrow)* is present anteriorly. A-scan echograms (**C** and **D**) show hemorrhage and cholesterol *(C)* in subretinal space. **C,** A-scan at Tissue Sensitivity setting. **D,** A-scan at slightly increased gain. At this higher setting, movement of the subretinal opacities results in blurred spikes. (From Green RL, Byrne SF: Diagnostic ophthalmic ultrasound, in Ryan SJ [ed]: *Retina.* ed 3, St Louis, Mosby, 2001, p 289.)

cally similar to peripheral retinal cysts. Hemorrhage and/or cholesterol debris sometimes may be detected in the subretinal space (Figure 5-99).[13,73] Many eyes with severe stage V ROP are shorter than normal[73] (see Table 5-2).

Persistent Hyperplastic Primary Vitreous

Persistent hyperplastic primary vitreous (PHPV) has a characteristic clinical appearance consisting of a small cornea and prominent ciliary processes. In most cases, PHPV is a unilateral condition.[69] Echography usually shows a shorter than normal globe, although it may be normal in some patients. The lens is often thin, and there may be irregularity of the posterior capsule (Figure 5-100). A retrolental membrane can sometimes be demonstrated on the posterior surface of the lens. In PHPV, a vitreous band (persistent hyaloid vessel) may be seen extending from the posterior lens capsule to the optic disc (see Table 5-2). Very often, this band is extremely thin and difficult to identify along its entire course (Figure 5-101); in other situations, it can be extremely thick and easy to demonstrate (Figure 5-102). In addition, vascularity can sometimes be identified within the patent blood vessels that may be present within this band.

In PHPV, the band can produce a traction retinal detachment in the peripapillary region (Figure 5-103); in more advanced cases, a total retinal detachment may occur. A thick band secondary to persistent hyaloid structures can sometimes be confused with a tightly closed, funnel-shaped retinal detachment. The identification of a small area of traction posteriorly, however, can often help rule out the presence of a total retinal detachment.

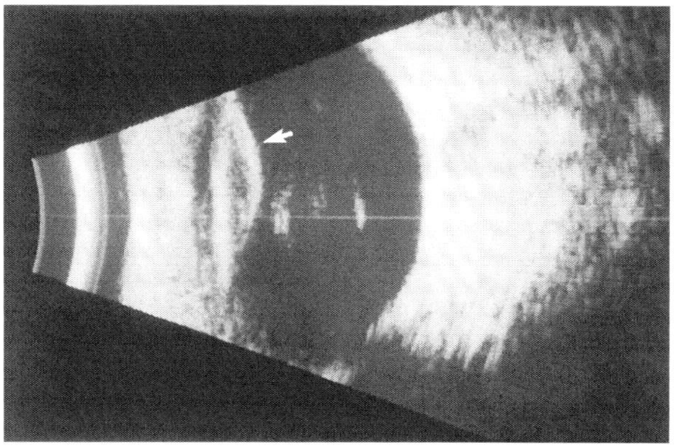

Figure 5-100 PHPV. B-scan echogram shows small globe and thin lens *(arrow)*. There is also a thin membrane adherent to the posterior lens capsule that cannot be distinguished from lens in this echogram. (From Green RL, Byrne SF: Diagnostic ophthalmic ultrasound, in Ryan SJ [ed]: *Retina*. ed 3, St Louis, Mosby, 2001, p 289.)

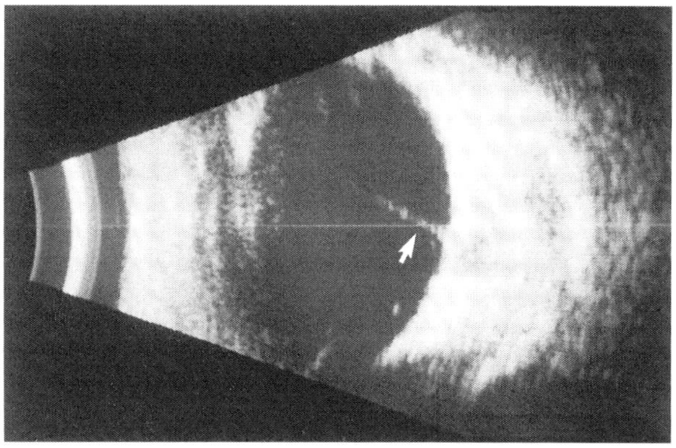

Figure 5-101 PHPV with thin band. Longitudinal B-scan shows thin band *(arrow)* extending from optic disc into vitreous cavity.

A

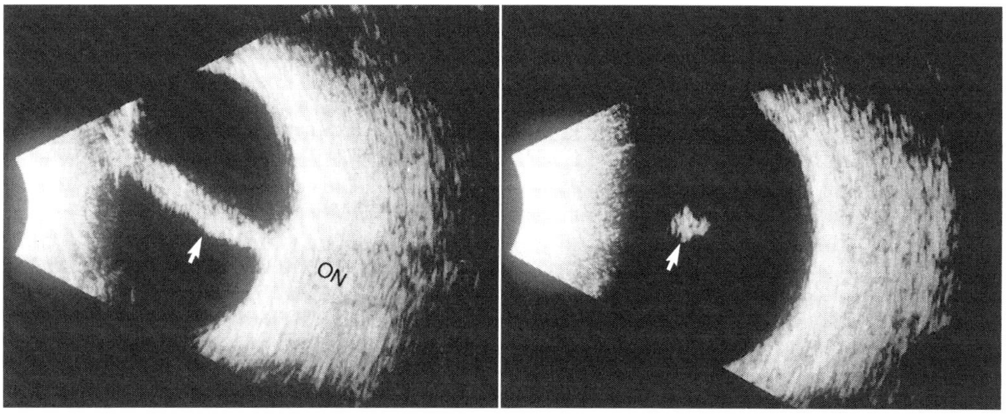

B

Figure 5-102 PHPV with thick band. **A,** Longitudinal B-scan shows thick echo-dense band *(arrow)* extending from anterior aspect of eye to optic nerve *(ON)*. **B,** Transverse B-scan shows cross-section of thick band.

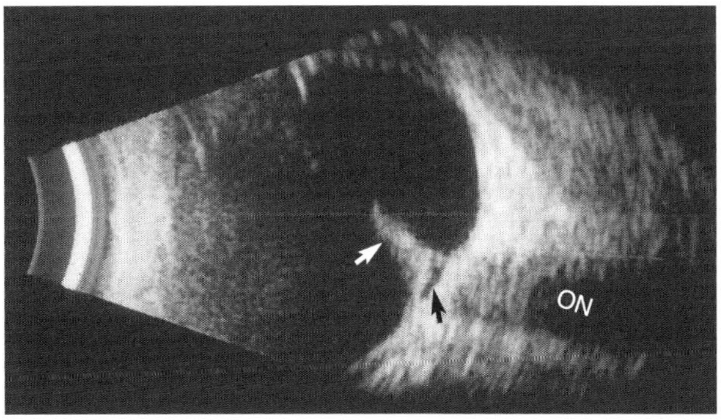

Figure 5-103 PHPV with focal traction retinal detachment. Longitudinal B-scan demonstrates attachment of thick band at optic nerve and shallow peripapillary traction retinal detachment *(black arrow)*. *ON*, Optic nerve. Entire length of band could not be displayed in one section.

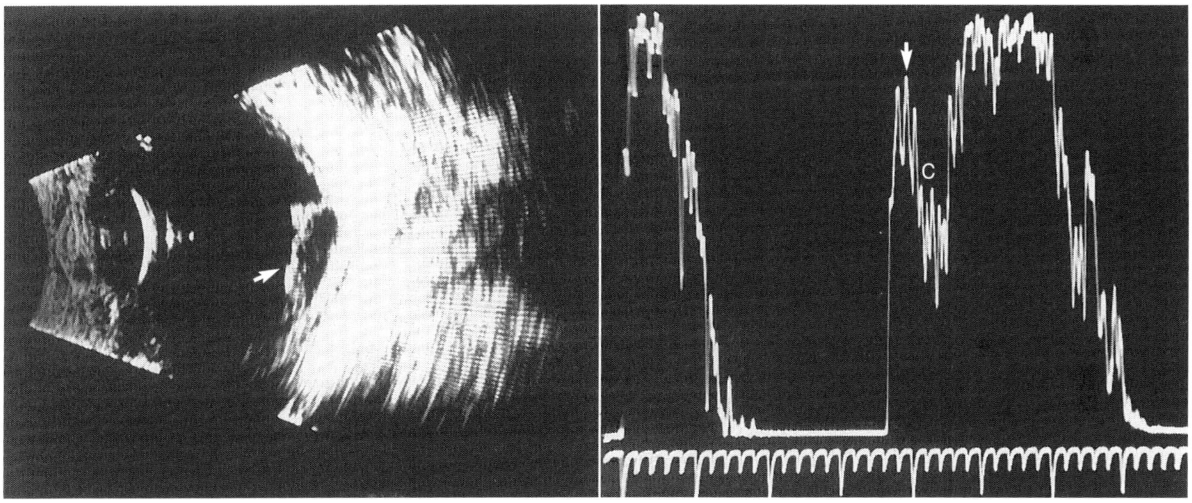

Figure 5-104 Early Coats' disease. **A,** Vertical macula B-scan echogram shows localized dome-shaped exudative retinal detachment at the macula *(arrow)*. **B,** A-scan shows multipeaked spike from thickened retina *(arrow)* and medium reflective spikes from subretinal cholesterol *(C)*. (From Green RL, Byrne SF: Diagnostic ophthalmic ultrasound, in Ryan SJ [ed]: *Retina.* ed 3, St Louis, Mosby, 2001, p 290.)

Coats' Disease

Coats' disease is typically a unilateral condition characterized by an exudative retinal detachment.[39] In the early stages, multiple, localized, shallow retinal detachments may be detected (Figure 5-104). In more severe cases, total detachment of the retina can occur. In these eyes, areas of marked retinal thickening can sometimes be demonstrated. Also characteristic of this condition is the presence of cholesterol in the subretinal space[38,61] (Figure 5-105; see also Table 5-2 and Figure 3-25).

Toxocariasis

See Table 5-2 and p 203 in Chapter 6 for a review of toxocariasis.

Cysticercosis

See Table 5-2 and p 203 in Chapter 6 for a review of cysticercosis.

Medulloepithelioma (Diktyoma)

This rare tumor, which has been described mainly in children,[104] often appears as a whitish mass within the ciliary body.[27] Echographically, these lesions are most often dome-shaped, highly reflective, and moderately vascular. The internal structure is generally somewhat irregular and multiple cystic spaces can often be demonstrated[27] (Figure 5-106; see also Table 5-2). Certain forms of medulloepithelioma also contain cartilage, producing echoes of extremely high reflectivity. It has also been reported that

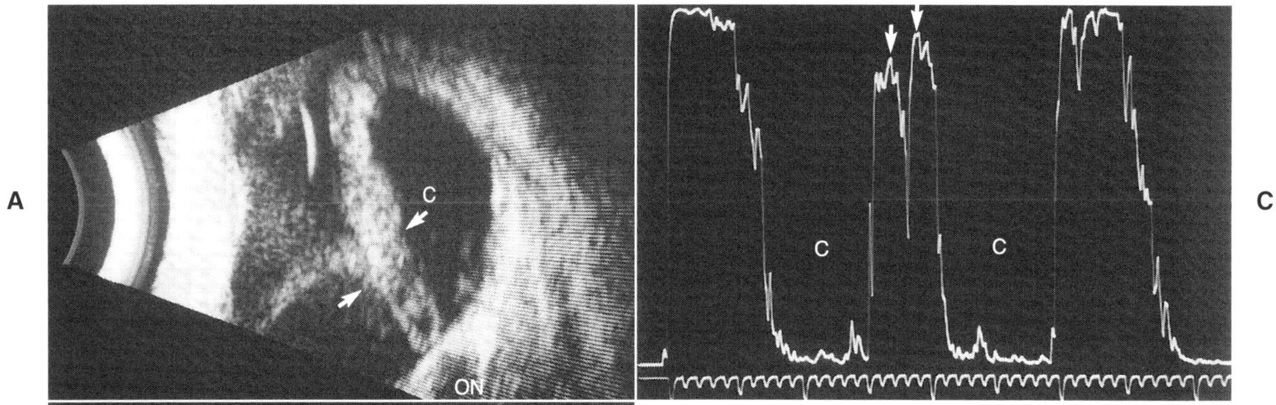

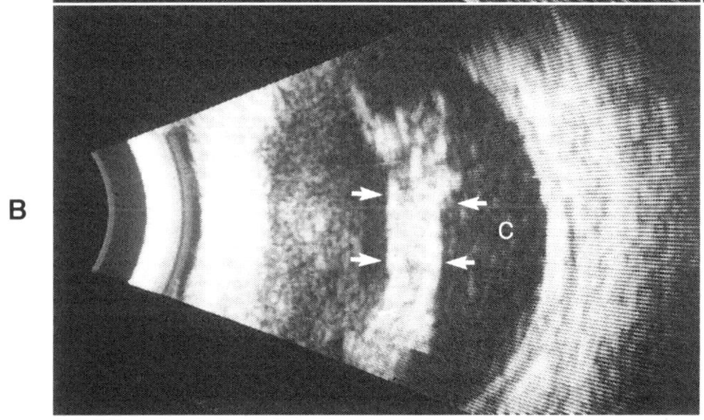

Figure 5-105 Advanced Coats' disease. **A,** Longitudinal B-scan echogram shows funnel-shaped retinal detachment *(arrows)* and opacities from subretinal cholesterol *(C)*. *ON,* Optic nerve. **B,** Transverse B-scan view through temporal globe shows marked thickening of detached retina *(arrows)*. **C,** A-scan shows marked thickening of detached retina *(arrows)* and low reflective echoes from cholesterol in the subretinal space *(C)*. A-scan at increased gain level (echogram not shown) displayed typical medium-reflective spikes from the subretinal cholesterol. (From Green RL, Byrne SF: Diagnostic ophthalmic ultrasound, in Ryan SJ [ed]: *Retina.* ed 3, St Louis, Mosby, 2001, p 291.)

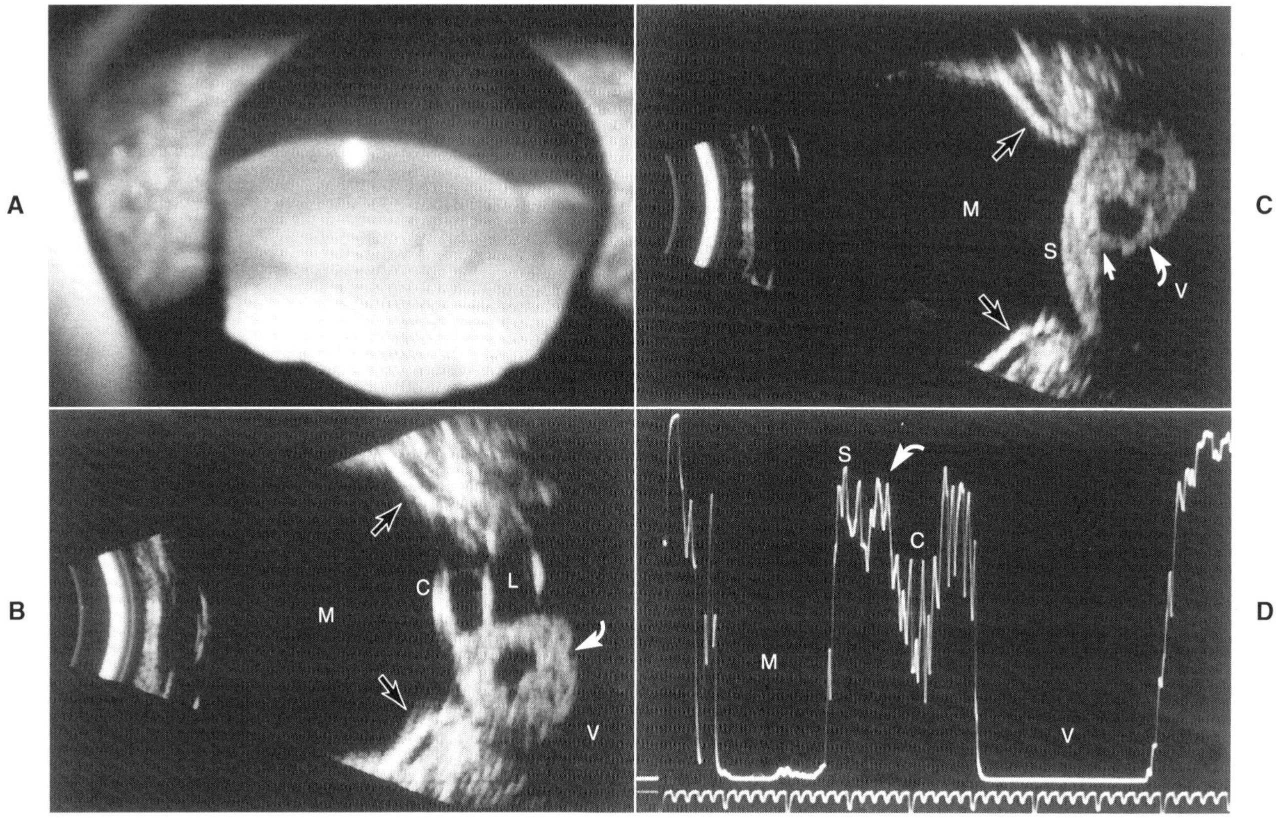

Figure 5-106 Medulloepithelioma of ciliary body (immersion technique). **A,** External photograph shows vascularized mass behind the lens. **B,** Axial B-scan echogram shows rounded ciliary body mass *(curved arrow)* containing large cystic space adjacent to lens *(L)*. *M,* Methylcellulose; *open arrows,* surface of scleral shell; *C,* cornea; *V,* vitreous cavity. **C,** Longitudinal B-scan view with patient's eye rotated so that ciliary body is centered beneath probe shows mass *(curved arrow)*. Posterior margin of mass is noted by *small arrow*. Note cystic cavities within lesion. *S,* Sclera; *open arrows,* surface of scleral shell. **D,** A-scan of ciliary body lesion *(curved arrow)* displays mainly high internal reflectivity with medium spike height from cystic area *(C)*. *S,* Sclera.

these tumors can shed cells into the vitreous, developing into cysts.[106]

REFERENCES

1. Alward WM, Byrne SF, Hughes JR, et al: Dislocated lens nuclei simulating choroidal melanomas. *Arch Ophthalmol* 1989;107:1463.
2. Barr CC, Zimmerman LE, Curtin VT, et al: Bilateral diffuse melanocytic uveal tumors associated with systemic malignant neoplasms. *Arch Ophthalmol* 1982;100:249.
3. Biswas J, Ahuja VK, Shanmugam MP, et al: Malignant melanoma of the choroid presenting as orbital cellulitis: Report of two cases with a review of the literature. *Orbit* 1999;18:123.
4. Brown GC, Shields CL: Choroidal osteoma, in Ryan SJ (ed): *Retina*. vol 1. St Louis, Mosby, 1989, p 749.
5. Buettner H: Varix of the vortex ampulla simulating a choroidal melanoma. *Am J Ophthalmol* 1990;109:607.
6. Byrne SF: Differential diagnosis of disciform lesions using standardized echography, in Hillman JS, LeMay MM (eds): *Ophthalmic Echography*. Dordrecht, Dr W Junk, 1984, p 149.
7. Byrne SF: Standardized echography of the eye and orbit. *Neuroradiology* 1986;28:618.
8. Callanan DG, Lewis ML, Byrne SF, et al: Choroidal neovascularization associated with choroidal nevi. *Arch Ophthalmol* 1993;111:789.
9. Cham MC, Pavlin CJ: Ultrasound detection of posterior scleral bowing in young patients with choroidal melanoma. *Can J Ophthalmol* 2000;35:263.
10. Chan TKJ, Atta HR, Scott GB: Ossification in choroidal melanoma (case report). *Br J Ophthalmol* 1995;79:705.
11. Chang TS, Byrne SF, Gass JDM, et al: Echographic findings in benign reactive lymphoid hyperplasia of the choroid. *Arch Ophthalmol* 1996;114:669.
12. Char DH, Ljung BM, Miller T, et al: Primary intraocular lymphoma (ocular reticulum cell sarcoma) diagnosis and management. *Ophthalmology* 1988;95:625.
13. Clarkson JG, Jacobson SG, Byrne SF, et al: Evaluation of eyes with stage-5 retinopathy of prematurity. *Graefes Arch Clin Exp Ophthalmol* 1989;227:332.
14. Cockerman GC, Hidayat AA, Bijwaard KE, et al: Re-evaluation of "reactive lymphoid hyperplasia of the uvea"—an immunohistochemical and molecular analysis of 10 cases. *Ophthalmology* 2000;107:151.
15. Cogan DG, Kuwabara T: Focal senile translucency of the sclera. *Arch Ophthalmol* 1959;62:604.
16. Coleman DJ: Reliability of ocular tumor diagnosis with ultrasound. *Trans Am Acad Ophthalmol Otolaryngol* 1973;77:677.
17. Coleman DJ, Abramson DH, Jack RL, et al: Ultrasonic diagnosis of tumors of the choroid. *Arch Ophthalmol* 1974;91:344.
18. Coleman DJ, Lizzi FL, Jack RL: *Ultrasonography of the Eye and Orbit*. Philadelphia, Lea & Febiger, 1977.
19. Coleman DJ, Lizzi FL: Computer-processed acoustic spectral analysis. *Trans Am Acad Ophthalmol Otolaryngol* 1977:83;725.
20. Coleman DJ, Lizzi FL: Computerized ultrasonic tissue characterization of ocular tumors. *Am J Ophthalmol* 1983:96:165.
21. Coleman DJ, Lizzi FL, Silverman RH, et al: Regression of uveal malignant melanomas following cobalt-60 plaque: Correlates between acoustic spectrum analysis and tumor regression. *Retina* 1985;5:73.
22. Daubert GL, Puklin JE: Intraoperative ultrasound to document proper plaque placement in treating choroidal melanoma. *Ophthalmology* 1989;96(Sept suppl):107.
23. Farah ME, Byrne SF, Hughes JR: Standardized echography in uveal melanoma with scleral or extraocular extension. *Arch Ophthalmol* 1984;102:1482.
24. Finger PT, Byrne SF, Moshefi DM, et al: Retrobulbar oedema after ophthalmic plaque radiotherapy. *Br J Ophthalmol* 1993;77:604.
25. Font RL, Spaulding AG, Zimmerman LE: Diffuse malignant melanoma of the uveal tract: A clinicopathologic report of 54 cases. *Trans Am Acad Ophthalmol Otolaryngol* 1968;72:877.
26. Forster DJ, Cano MR, Green RL, et al: Echographic features of the Vogt-Koyanagi-Harada syndrome. *Arch Ophthalmol* 1990;108:1421.
27. Foster RE, Murray TG, Byrne SF, et al: Echographic features of medulloepithelioma. *Am J Ophthalmol* 2000;130:364.
28. Fuller DG, Snyder WB, Hutton WL, et al: Ultrasonographic features of choroidal malignant melanomas. *Arch Ophthalmol* 1979;97:1465.
29. Gass JDM: *Stereoscopic Atlas of Macular Diseases—Diagnosis and Treatment*, vol 1, ed 4, St Louis, Mosby, 1997.
30. Gass JDM, Geiser RG, Wilkinson CP, et al: Bilateral diffuse uveal melanocytic proliferation in patients with occult carcinoma. *Arch Ophthalmol* 1990;108:527.
31. Gass JDM, Glatzer RJ: Acquired pigmentation simulating Peutz-Jeghers syndrome—initial manifestation of diffuse uveal melanocytic proliferation. *Br J Ophthalmol* 1991;75:693.
32. Green RL: Echographic diagnosis of large choroidal melanomas, in Hillman JS, LeMay MM (eds): *Ophthalmic Ultrasonography*. Dordrecht, Dr W Junk, 1984, p 15.
33. Green RL: The echographic evaluation of spontaneous vitreous hemorrhage, in Ossoinig KC (ed): *Ophthalmic Echography*. Dordrecht, Dr W Junk, 1987, p 233.
34. Green RL, Byrne SF: Diagnostic ophthalmic ultrasound, in Ryan SJ (ed): *Retina*. ed 2, St Louis, Mosby, 1989, p 191.
35. Green RL: Scleral lesions associated with retroperitoneal fibrosis. Presented at the 18th biennial meeting of the International Society for Diagnostic Ultrasound in Ophthalmoogy (SIDUO), Paris, 2000.
36. Grossniklaus HE, Martin DF, Avery R, et al: Uveal lymphoid infiltration—report of four cases and clinicopathologic review. *Ophthalmology* 1998;105:1265.
37. Haik BG, Siedlecki A, Ellsworth RM, et al: Documented delays in the diagnosis of retinoblastoma. *Ann Ophthalmol* 1985;17:731.
38. Haik BG, Smith ME, Ellsworth RM, et al: Ultrasonography in the diagnosis of advanced Coats' disease, in Ossoinig KC (ed): *Ophthalmic Echography*. Dordrecht, Dr W Junk, 1987, p 428.
39. Haller JA: Coats' disease, in Ryan SJ (ed): *Retina*, vol 2. St Louis, Mosby, 1989, p 491.
40. Hanovar SG, Shields CL, Demirci H, et al: Sclerochoroidal calcification. *Arch Ophthalmol* 2001;119:833.
41. Harbour JW, Murray TG, Byrne SF, et al: Intraoperative echographic localization of Iodine 125 episcleral plaques for posterior uveal melanoma. *Retina* 1996;16:129.
42. Hodes BL: Tissue texture: The histologic basis for standardized A-scan diagnosis in ophthalmology, in White D, Brown RE (eds): *Ultrasound in Medicine*. New York, Plenum Press, 1977, 3B:1895.
43. Hodes BL: Ultrasonographic diagnosis of choroidal malignant melanoma. *Surv Ophthalmol* 1977;22:29.
44. Hodes BL, Choromokos E: Standardized A-scan echographic diagnosis of choroidal malignant melanomas. *Arch Ophthalmol* 1977; 95:593.
45. Jakobiec FA, Sacks E, Kronish JW, et al: Multifocal static creamy choroidal infiltrates: An early sign of lymphoid neoplasia. *Ophthalmology* 1987;94:397.
46. Kline RW, Yeakel PD: Ocular melanoma, I-125 plaques (abstract). *Med Phys* 1987; 14:475.
47. Lizzi FL, Coleman DJ: Ultrasonic spectrum analysis in ophthalmology, in White DN (ed): *Recent Advances in Ultrasound in Biomedicine*, vol 1. Forest Grove, Research Studies Press, 1977, p117.
48. Lizzi FL, Greenebaum M, Feleppa EJ, et al: Theoretical framework for spectrum analysis in ultrasonic tissue characterization. *J Acoust Soc Am* 1983;73:1366.
49. Lim JI, Goldberg MF: Idiopathic sclerochoroidal calcification (case report). *Arch Ophthalmol* 1989;107:1122.
50. Lois N, Shields CL, Shields JA, et al: Cavitary melanoma of the ciliary body—a study of eight cases. *Ophthalmology* 1998;105:1091.
51. Makley TA Jr, Teed RW: Unsuspected intraocular malignant melanomas. *Arch Ophthalmol* 1958;60:475.
52. Martin JA, Robertson DM: Extrascleral extension of choroidal melanoma diagnosed by ultrasound. *Ophthalmology* 1983;90:1554.
53. Minning CA Jr, Davidorf FH: Ossoinig's angle of ultrasonic absorption and its role in the diagnosis of malignant melanoma. *Ann Ophthalmol* 1982;14:564.
54. Morris WR, Haik BG, Osborn D: Intraocular involvement in multifocal fibrosclerosis. *Ophthalmology* 2000;107:962.
55. Moshari A, Cheesman EW, McLean IW: Totally necrotic choroidal and ciliary body melanomas—associations with prognosis, episcleritis, and scleritis. *Am J Ophthalmol* 2001;131:232.
56. Nicholson DH, Byrne SF, Chiu M, et al: Echographic and histologic tumor height measurement in uveal melanoma. *Am J Ophthalmol* 1985;100:454.
57. Osher RH, Abrams GW, Yarian D, et al: Varix of the vortex ampulla. *Am J Ophthalmol* 1981;92:653.

58. Ossoinig KC: Advances in diagnostic ultrasound, in Henkind P (ed): *ACTA:XXIV International Congress of Ophthalmology.* Philadelphia, JB Lippincott, 1983, p 89.
59. Ossoinig KC: How to obtain maximum measuring accuracies with standardized A-scan, in Hillman JS, LeMay MM (eds): *Ophthalmic Ultrasonography.* Dordrecht, Dr W Junk, 1984, p 197.
60. Ossoinig KC: Standardized echography: Basic principles, clinical applications and results. *Int Ophthalmol Clin* 1974;19:128.
61. Ossoinig KC: *Standardized Ophthalmic Echography of the Eye, Orbit and Periorbital Region. A Comprehensive Slide Set and Study Guide.* ed 3, Iowa City, Goodfellow, 1985.
62. Ossoinig KC, Bigar F, Kaefring SL: Malignant melanoma of the choroid and ciliary body: A differential diagnosis in clinical echography. *Bibl Ophthalmol* 1975;83:141.
63. Ossoinig KC: Preoperative differential diagnosis of tumors with echography. I: Physical principles and morphologic background of tissue echograms. *Curr Concepts Ophthalmol* 1974;4:264.
64. Ossoinig KC: Preoperative differential diagnosis of tumors with echography. III: Diagnosis of intraocular tumors. *Curr Concepts Ophthalmol* 1974;4:296.
65. Ossoinig KC, Cennamo G, Green RL, et al: Echographic results in the diagnosis of retinoblastoma, in Thijssen JM, Verbeek AM (eds): *Ultrasonography in Ophthalmology.* Dordrecht, Dr W Junk, 1981, p 103.
66. Ossoinig KC, Lohmeyer M: Choroidal nevi: diagnosis with standardized echography, in Sampaolesi R (ed): *Ultrasonography in Ophthalmology 12.* Dordrecht, Kluwer Academic, 1990, p 173.
67. Ossoinig K, Till P: Methods and results of ultrasonography in diagnosing intraocular tumors, in Gitter KA, Keeney AH, et al (eds): *Ophthalmic Ultrasound.* St Louis, Mosby, 1969, p 294.
68. Packer S, Rotman M, Salanitro P: Radiotherapy of choroidal melanoma with iodine-125. *Ophthalmology* 1980;87:582.
69. Patz A, Palmer EA: Retinopathy of prematurity, in Ryan SJ (ed): *Retina.* ed 2, St Louis, Mosby, 1989, p 509.
70. Pavlin CJ, Japp B, Payne DG, et al: Intraoperative use of ultrasound in the management of choroidal melanomas, in Ossoinig KC (ed): *Ophthalmic Echography.* Dordrecht, Dr W Junk, 1987, p 391.
71. Pavlin CJ, Japp B, Simpson R, et al: Ultrasound determination of the relationship of radioactive plaques to the base of choroidal melanomas. *Ophthalmology* 1989;96:538.
72. Pavlin CJ, Foster FS: *Ultrasound Biomicroscopy of the Eye.* New York, Springer-Verlag, 1995.
73. Pulido J, Byrne SF, Clarkson JG, et al: Evaluation of eyes with stage V retinopathy of prematurity using standardized echography. *Ophthalmology* 1991;98:1100.
74. Ryan SJ, Zimmerman LE, King FM: Reactive lymphoid hyperplasia. An unusual form of intraocular pseudotumor. *Trans Am Acad Ophthalmol Otolaryngol* 1972;76:652.
75. Sanborn GE: Choroidal hemangioma, in Ryan SJ (ed): *Retina.* ed 2, St Louis, Mosby, 1989, p 757.
76. Schachat AP, Robertson DM, Mieler WF, et al: Sclerochoridal calcification. *Arch Ophthalmol* 1992;110:196.
77. Schreiver S, Clememte C, Hintschich C, et al: Standardized echography in multifocal fibrosclerosis (M. Ormond) with orbital and ocular involvement (abstract), in Shammas HJ and Hasenfratz G (eds): *Ultrasound in Ophthalmology.* Regensburg, S. Roderer Verlag, 1998, p 106.
78. Scott IU, Murray TG, Hughes JR: Evaluation of imaging techniques for detection of extraocular extension of choroidal melanoma. *Arch Ophthalmol* 1998;116:897.
79. Shammas HJ: *Atlas of Ophthalmic Ultrasonography and Biometry.* St Louis, Mosby, 1984.
80. Shammas HJ, Boyer DS, Miller JB: Ultrasound characteristics of posterior uveal melanomas treated with cobalt plaque radiotherapy, in Ossoinig KC (ed): *Ophthalmic Echography.* Dordrecht, Dr W Junk, 1987, p 379.
81. Shammas HJ, Dunne S, Fisher YL: *Three-Dimensional Ultrasound Tomography of the Eye.* NovaCoast, Eden Mills, 1998.
82. Shields SR, de Juan E, Machemer R: Ultrasonography of stage IV and V retinopathy of prematurity. *Ophthalmology* 1987; 94(Oct suppl):116.
83. Shields JA, Shields CL, Eagle RC Jr: Mesectodermal leiomyoma of the ciliary body managed by partial lamellar iridocyclectomy. *Ophthalmology* 1989;96:1369.
84. Shields CL, Shields JA, Pankajkumar S: Retinoblastoma in older children. *Ophthalmology* 1991;98:395.
85. Shields JA, Font RL, Eagle RC, et al: Melanotic schwannoma of the choroid. *Ophthalmology* 1994;101:843.
86. Shields JA, Shields CL: *Eyelid and Conjunctival Tumors.* Philadelphia, Lippincott, Williams & Wilkins, 1999.
87. Shields JA: *Diagnosis and Management of Intraocular Tumors.* St Louis, Mosby, 1983.
88. Shields JA, Shields CL: *Intraocular Tumors.* Lippincott Williams & Wilkins, Philadelphia, 1999.
89. Shields CL, Shields JA, Santos MC, et al: Incomplete spontaneous regression of choroidal melanoma associated with inflammation [letter]. *Arch Ophthalmol* 1999;117;1245.
90. Sidoti PA, Valencia M, Chen N, et al: Echographic evaluation of primary cysts of the iris pigment epithelium. *Am J Ophthalmol* 1995; 120:161.
91. Silverman RH, Folberg R, Boldt CH, et al: Correlation of ultrasound parameter imaging with microcirculation patterns in uveal melanomas. *Ultrasound Med Biol* 1997;23:573.
92. Sivalingam A, Shields CL, Shields JA, et al: Idiopathic sclerochoroidal calcification. *Ophthalmology* 1991;98:720.
93. Sneed RS, Byrne SF, Meiler WF, et al: Choroidal effusions associated with malignant choroidal tumors. *Ophthalmology* 1991;98:968.
94. Stallard HB: Radiotherapy for malignant melanoma of the choroid. *Br J Ophthalmol* 1966;50:147.
95. Suan EP, Rubsamen PE, Byrne SF: Bilateral ciliochoroidal detachments after Valsalva maneuver [Case Report]. *Arch Ophthalmol* 1993;111:27.
96. Tabandeh H, Chaudhry NA, Murray TG, et al: Intraoperative echographic localization of Iodine-125 episcleral plaque for brachytherapy of choroidal melanoma. *Am J Ophthalmol* 2000;129:1999.
97. Taylor D, Moore A: Retinoblastoma. *Pediatric Ophthalmology.* Boston, Blackwell Scientific, 1990, p 355.
98. The Collaborative Ocular Melanoma Study Group: Accuracy of diagnosis of choroidal melanomas in the Collaborative Ocular Melanoma Study: Coms Report No 1. *Arch Ophthalmol* 1990;108:1268.
99. Uy HS, Nguyen QD, Arbour J, et al: Sclerosing inflammatory pseudotumor of the eye. *Arch Ophthalmol* 2001;119:603.
100. Valencia M, Green RL, Lopez PF: Echographic findings in hemorrhagic disciform lesions. *Ophthalmology* 1994;101:1379.
101. Verbeek AM: A choroidal oat-cell carcinoma metastasis mimicking a choroidal melanoma, in Thijssen JM, Verbeek AM (eds): *Ultrasonography in Ophthalmology.* Dordrecht, Dr W Junk, 1981, p 131.
102. Ward SD, Byrne BJ, Kincaid MC, et al: Ultrasonographic evidence of mushroom-shaped choroidal metastasis. *Am J Ophthalmol* 2000;130:681.
103. Williams DF, Meiler WF, Lewandowski M, et al: Echographic verification of radioactive plaque position in the treatment of melanomas. *Arch Ophthalmol* 1988;106:1623.
104. Wilson DJ, Green WR: Miscellaneous uveal tumors, in Ryan SJ (ed): *Retina*, vol 1. St Louis, Mosby, 1989, p 767.
105. Witschel H, Font RL: Hemangioma of the choroid: A clinicopathologic study of 71 cases and a review of the literature. *Surv Ophthalmol* 1976;20:415.
106. Yanoff M, Fine BS: *Ocular Pathology*, ed 4, London, Mosby-Wolfe, 1996.
107. Yap EY, Robertson DM, Buettner M: Scleritis as an initial manifestation of choroidal malignant melanoma. *Ophthalmology* 1992; 99:1693.
108. Zimmerman LE: Retinoblastoma and Retinocytoma, in Spencer WH (ed): *Ophthalmic Pathology—An Atlas and Textbook.* Philadelphia, WB Saunders, 1985, p 1292.

William D. Bates

6

Inflammatory Diseases of the Eye

Ultrasound can play an important role in the evaluation of a wide variety of inflammatory conditions affecting the eye (Box 6-1). It may be used to identify specific sites of intraocular inflammation or to help establish the etiology of inflammation. It is especially important when the inflammatory response precludes visualization of the posterior segment. Echography also has been shown to aid in the management and follow-up of patients with inflammatory disease.

Inflammatory disease can have an infectious or noninfectious etiology and may affect the eye in a variety of ways. The inflammation may be diffuse, involving multiple ocular structures, as in endophthalmitis or panophthalmitis. Alternatively, the inflammation may be more localized, as seen in scleritis or in certain inflammatory conditions that involve the choroid. Some of these include Vogt-Koyanagi-Harada syndrome, sympathetic ophthalmia, uveal lymphoid hyperplasia, and Lyme disease.

Unique ultrasound findings may be observed in certain types of ocular infections (e.g., toxocariasis and cysticercosis). In addition, ultrasound has been used to visualize the inflammation that occurs in association with some intraocular tumors (e.g., retinoblastoma or melanoma) and may be useful in the evaluation and treatment of inflammation related to human immunodeficiency virus (HIV) infection (acquired immunodeficiency syndrome [AIDS]).

ENDOPHTHALMITIS

Infectious endophthalmitis is a potentially devastating condition that may occur following intraocular surgery or ocular trauma, or it may develop from an endogenous source elsewhere in the body. Endophthalmitis is clinically suspected when there are signs of inflammation, both externally and within the eye.

Echography is very useful for determining the severity and extent of the infection in eyes with endophthalmitis (Box 6-2). The first step in the evaluation is to assess the vitreous cavity for the presence of inflammatory opacities and membranes. This assessment is facilitated by the use of a high gain setting on both B- and A-scan. On B-scan, these opacities and membranes appear as fine dots and lines of varying density. On A-scan, moderately severe endophthalmitis normally produces a chain of low amplitude spikes from within the vitreous cavity (Figure 6-1). If the opacities are secondary to an anterior locus of infection, they tend to be denser anteriorly than posteriorly. As the infection spreads, however, the opacities usually become more evenly distributed throughout the vitreous cavity. In eyes with posterior vitreous detachment (PVD), the subvitreal space should be carefully inspected using a high gain setting on B-scan since the presence of opacities in the subvitreal space suggests active inflammation (Figure 6-2, *A*). If the posterior hyaloid has not detached prior to the infection, it usually remains attached, presumably because of an inflammatory adhesion between the hyaloid and the retina.

In eyes with endophthalmitis, ultrasound may also detect thickening of the retinochoroid layer as well as exudative and traction retinal detachment (RD). Other findings can include swelling of the optic nerve head and choroidal detachment (Figure 6-2, *B*, *C*, and *D*). One study has shown that the presence of choroidal detachment on the initial evaluation correlates with a poor visual outcome.[6] In some cases of endogenous endophthalmitis, associated choroidal abscesses and/or granulomas have been identified (Figure 6-3). Furthermore, endogenous endophthalmitis in children may present clinically with leukokoria and may be caused not only by bacterial infection but also by other etiologies such as toxocariasis (see p 203) or intraocular cysticercosis (see p 203).

Ultrasound may also be useful in the treatment of endophthalmitis since the echographic findings may help determine the best diagnostic and/or therapeutic approach. For example, the detection of a choroidal detachment may influence the length of the infusion cannula for diagnostic vitrectomy or the depth of needle penetration necessary for diagnostic vitreous aspiration. Furthermore, the discovery of RD may indicate the need for more extensive vitreoretinal surgery than would be necessary for diagnosis and treatment alone.

BOX 6-1

Inflammatory Conditions

Endophthalmitis
Uveitis and vitritis
Scleritis
Vogt-Koyanagi-Harada syndrome
Sympathetic ophthalmia
Uveal lymphoid hyperplasia
Lyme disease
Toxocariasis
Cysticercosis
Acquired immunodeficiency syndrome (AIDS)
Inflammation associated with intraocular tumors

BOX 6-2

Echographic Findings in Endophthalmitis*

Vitreous opacities/membranes
Posterior vitreous detachment
Subvitreal opacities
Macular edema
Retinochoroidal thickening (diffuse)
Retinal traction
Retinal detachment
Subretinal opacities
Choroidal detachment
Suprachoroidal opacities
Choroidal abscess or granuloma
Optic nerve head swelling
Scleral thickening
Episcleral edema
Orbital inflammation

*Some or all of the above findings may be detected in patients with endophthalmitis.

A

B

C

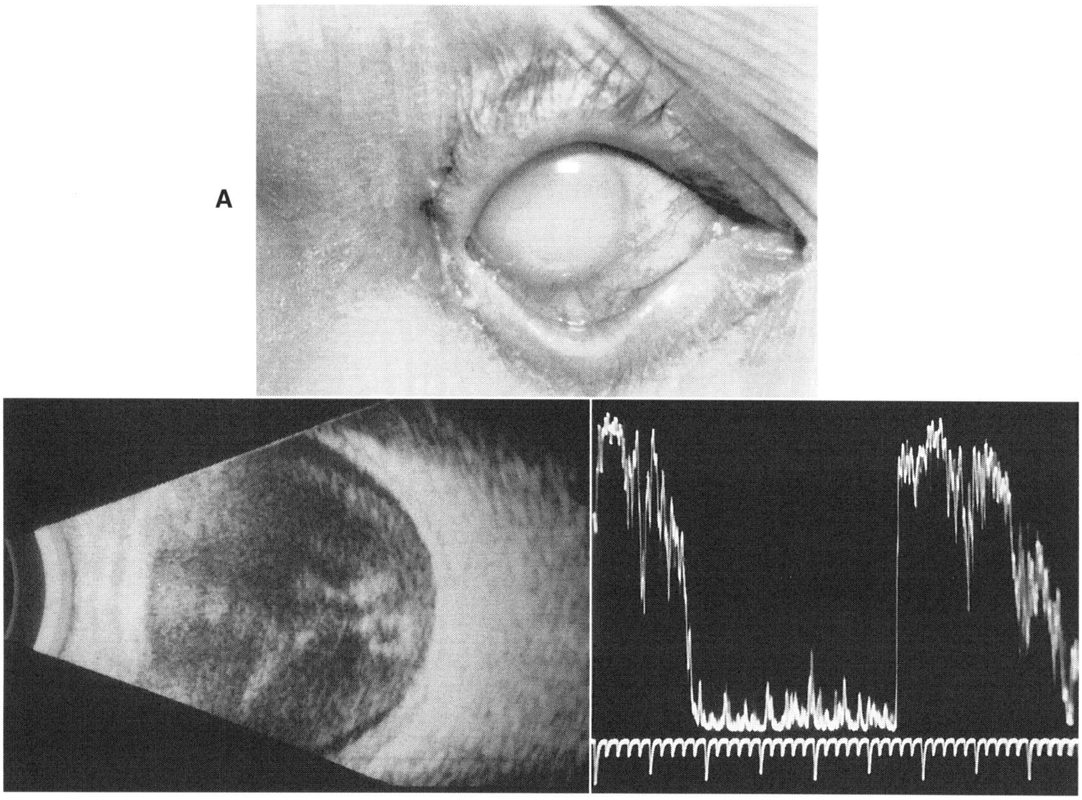

Figure 6-1 Endophthalmitis. **A,** External photograph shows large hypopyon. **B,** Transverse B-scan demonstrates diffuse vitreous opacities with some membrane formation. **C,** A-scan shows low reflective spikes from inflammatory debris in vitreous cavity.

A C B D

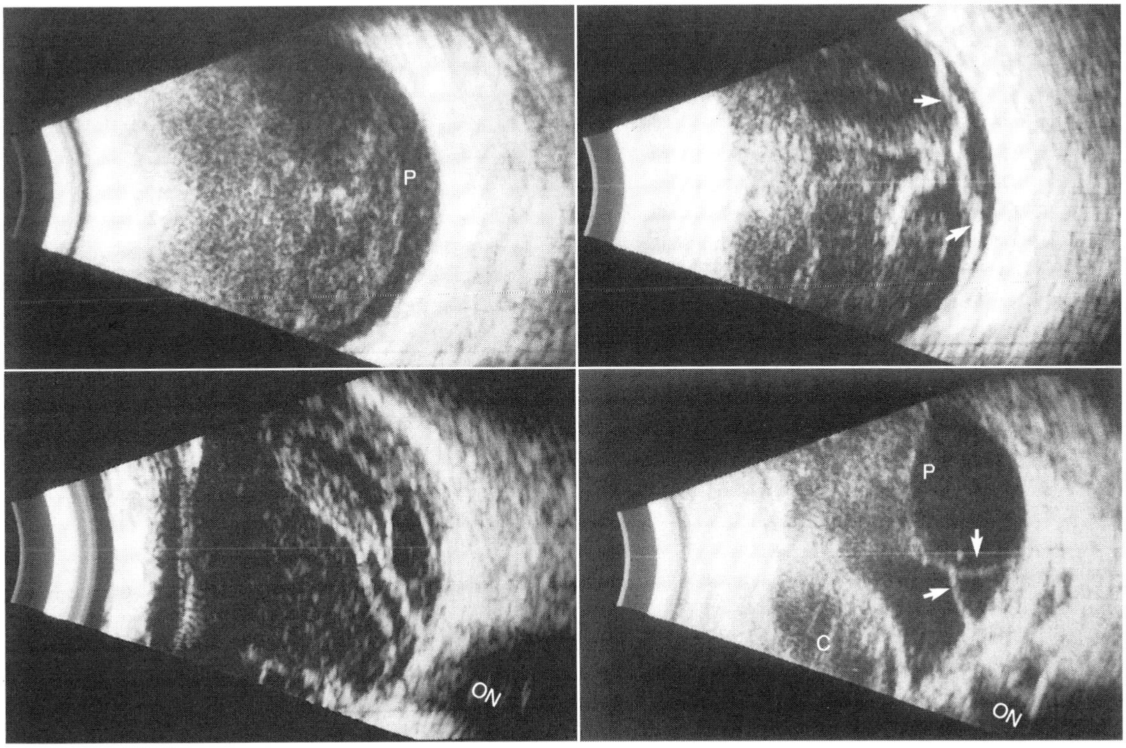

Figure 6-2 Various B-scan findings in endophthalmitis. **A,** Transverse view shows diffuse, mild opacities in subhyaloidal space in association with diffuse vitreous opacities and shallow PVD *(P)*. **B,** Longitudinal scan demonstrates organized vitreous membranes extending to posterior aspect of eye. *ON,* Optic nerve. **C,** Transverse scan demonstrates shallow retinal detachment *(arrows)* with overlying vitreous opacities and membranes. **D,** Longitudinal view along the temporal meridian shows opacities and PVD producing focal, tentlike traction RD at the macula *(arrows)*. Note bullous, nonserous choroidal detachment *(C)*.

A B

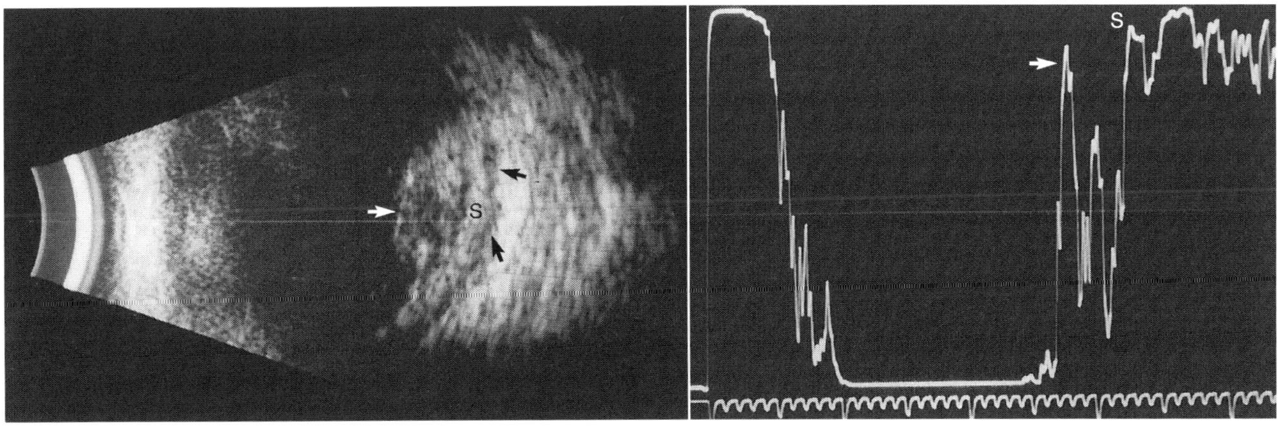

Figure 6-3 Choroidal abscess associated with endogenous endophthalmitis. **A,** Transverse B-scan through peripheral fundus demonstrates dome-shaped lesion *(white arrow)*. Note thickening of adjacent sclera *(S)* and edema of sub-Tenon's space *(black arrows)*. **B,** A-scan shows somewhat irregular internal reflectivity of lesion.

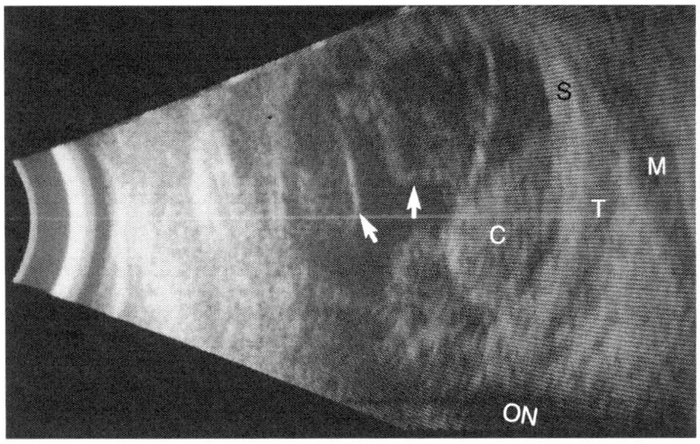

Figure 6-4 Panophthalmitis. Longitudinal B-scan demonstrates dense vitreous opacities and membranes *(arrows)*, nonserous choroidal detachment *(C)*, and diffusely thickened sclera *(S)*. Note also inflammation and thickening of sub-Tenon's space *(T)* and thickening of lateral rectus muscle *(M)*. *ON*, Optic nerve.

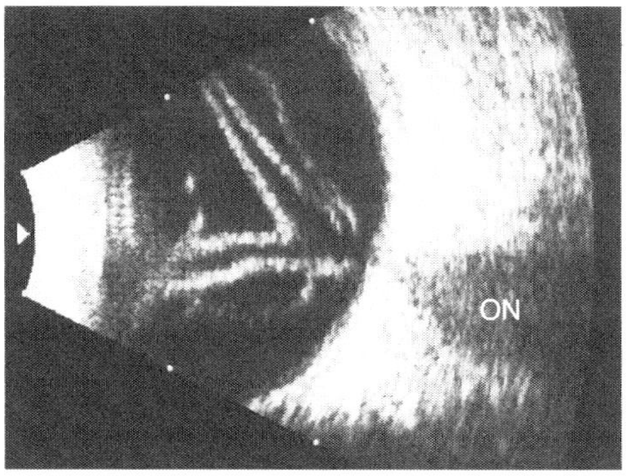

Figure 6-5 Posterior vitreoschisis in eye with uveitis. Longitudinal B-scan shows multiple layers of membranes representing splits in the posterior cortical vitreous. *ON*, Optic nerve.

In some cases, the diagnosis of endophthalmitis may be in question because the clinical presentation is not straightforward. The echographic detection of vitreous opacities in these eyes may be misleading because vitreous hemorrhage may appear echographically similar to inflammatory vitreous debris. However, there are two findings that may be useful in differentiating inflammation from hemorrhage: first, PVDs tend to be more extensive when resulting from hemorrhage than from endophthalmitis; and second, pseudomembrane formation in the inferior portion of the globe (secondary to blood layered by gravity) more commonly occurs with vitreous hemorrhage (see p 45 and Figure 3-4).

The intraocular infection occurring in panophthalmitis, a more advanced form of endophthalmitis, may additionally involve the sclera, episclera, and sometimes the orbital tissues (Figure 6-4).

NONINFECTIOUS UVEITIS AND VITRITIS

Uveitis is an inflammatory condition that may be idiopathic or may be associated with a specific autoimmune disease (e.g., collagen vascular disorders, sarcoidosis, or ankylosing spondylitis). It may affect the anterior and/or the posterior segment of the eye, or both, but ultrasound is generally more useful for the evaluation of posterior uveitis. The echographic findings most commonly seen in posterior uveitis include vitritis, PVD, subvitreal opacities, retinochoroid layer thickening, macular edema, and choroidal detachments. Peripheral vitreous opacities and preretinal membranes can be detected in certain peripheral types of posterior uveitis (i.e., pars planitis).

The noninfectious (sterile) vitritis associated with posterior uveitis produces echographic findings similar to those of infectious endophthalmitis, although there appears to be less vitreous membrane formation in eyes with sterile vitritis. It should be noted, however, that this condition can produce posterior vitreoschisis,[28,29] which can simulate inflammatory vitreous membranes (Figure 6-5).[4]

In some cases, an external infection may produce a sterile vitritis, which can be confused with an infectious endophthalmitis. For example, a sterile vitritis may occur in the presence of an infectious corneal ulcer with sterile hypopyon. This vitritis appears to be due to a spillover of inflammatory cells from the hypopyon into the vitreous cavity, especially in aphakic or pseudophakic eyes. Sterile vitreous opacities also may be associated with either infectious or noninfectious scleritis or with orbital inflammation. In these instances, the echographic findings can mimic an infectious panophthalmitis (see Figure 6-4).

Another cause of intraocular inflammation is lens-induced uveitis. This condition occurs when lens material leaks from a hypermature cataractous lens or is lost in the vitreous cavity during cataract surgery. When the inflammation is secondary to a hypermature cataract, a diffuse vitritis commonly occurs. In some cases, a hypermature lens may leak into the anterior chamber. This may result in opacification of the anterior chamber and a secondary glaucoma. In such cases, immersion ultrasound may demonstrate the hypermature nature of the lens (see Figure 7-3).

Cortical lens material, lens nucleus fragments, or the entire lens nucleus may fall back into the vitreous gel during cataract surgery (see p 106). Inflammatory vitreous opacities and/or membranes are normally associated with retained lens material (see Figures 4-39 and 4-40).

Longstanding uveitis can lead to the formation of cataract and cyclitic membrane (Figure 6-6). In addition, chronic uveitis can cause hypotony, either by shutting down the production of aqueous or by detachment of the ciliary body due to traction from the cyclitic membrane (see p 77). Hypotony produces specific echographic findings such as diffuse thickening of the retinochoroid layer (including the macula), scleral thickening, choroidal detachments, scleral

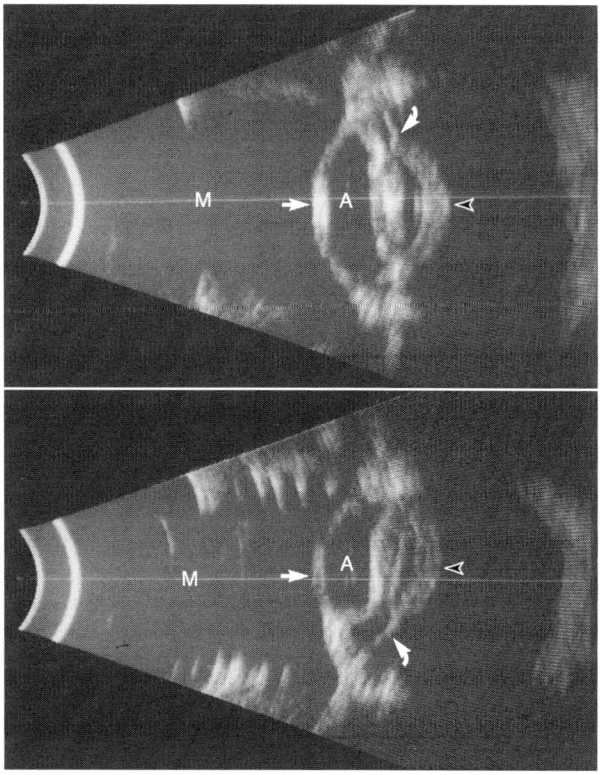

Figure 6-6 Cataract and cyclitic membrane in eye with uveitis (immersion technique). Axial **(A)** and longitudinal **(B)** B-scans show deep anterior chamber *(A)* and dense, swollen cataractous lens *(open arrows)*. Note dense lens nucleus within cataract in **A.** *Curved arrows* indicate cyclitic membrane extending between lens and ciliary body, possibly on surface of zonules. *M*, Methylcellulose within scleral shell.

folds, and shortened axial eye length measurements (see p 216).

Treatment for posterior uveitis often includes the injection of steroids in sub-Tenon's space. Ultrasound can be used in these eyes to localize the injected steroid material, thus ensuring proper needle placement.[13] There have been cases in which steroids were inadvertently injected into the vitreous cavity (see Figure 4-41).

SCLERITIS

Scleritis is an inflammatory condition that can affect either the anterior or posterior aspect of the eye or both. This disorder can be idiopathic; it may be secondary to systemic diseases (e.g., rheumatoid arthritis), or it can have an infectious etiology.[26] Scleritis usually results in thickening of the sclera, although thinning can occur in more chronic stages. Patients with scleritis often present with severe ocular pain, usually with other associated inflammatory signs and symptoms. Clinically, the diagnosis of anterior scleritis is usually straightforward, whereas the assessment of posterior scleral inflammation can be quite challenging. In fact, posterior scleritis has generally been considered a diagnosis of exclusion. However, the ability of ultrasound to image the sclera now provides a more reliable means to evaluate and diagnose scleritis, especially in the posterior segment.

Posterior Scleritis

The clinical presentation of posterior scleritis often includes severe pain, periocular inflammation, and visual loss. Signs of this condition may include choroidal folds, serous retinal detachment, swollen optic disc, and orbital inflammation (e.g., proptosis and lid swelling).[23] Occasionally, a subretinal mass may also be visible. It should be mentioned, however, that a certain number of patients present with minimal clinical findings.

The most important ultrasound finding in this condition is thickening of the sclera. The scleral thickening can vary in degree and can be either diffuse or localized (i.e., nodular).[1,9,17] The thickened sclera is usually highly reflective, with regular internal structure, and in most cases, there is an associated inflammatory reaction in the episcleral region, resulting in distention and swelling of sub-Tenon's space. Frequently, thickening of the retinochoroid layer can also be identified.

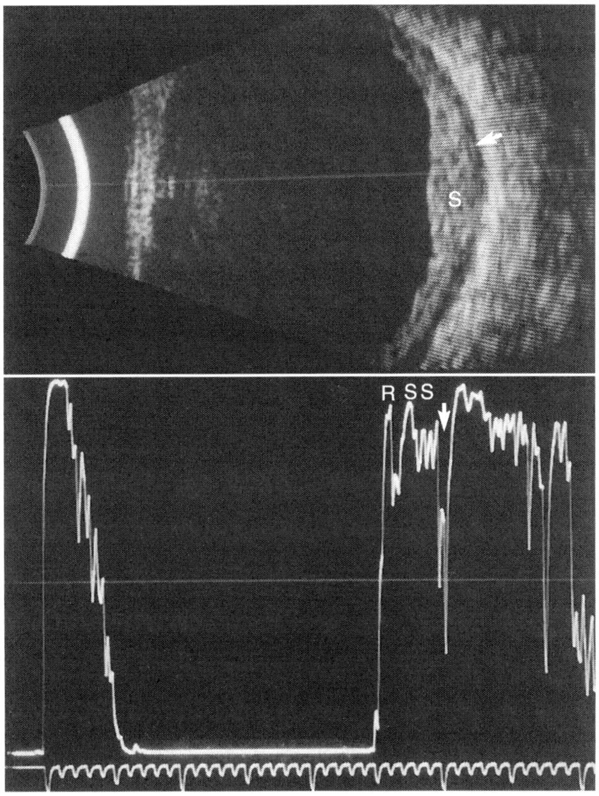

Figure 6-7 Diffuse posterior scleritis. **A,** Transverse B-scan echogram shows diffuse thickening of retinochoroid layer and sclera *(S)*. *Arrow* indicates diffuse infiltration in sub-Tenon's space. **B,** A-scan shows highly reflective thickening of retinochoroid layer *(R)* and sclera *(S)*. Arrow shows medium reflectivity from infiltration in sub-Tenon's space. (From Green RL, Byrne SF: Diagnostic ophthalmic ultrasound, in Ryan SJ [ed]: *Retina.* ed 3, St Louis, Mosby, 2001, p 261.)

Diffuse Posterior Scleritis

Diffuse posterior scleritis presents as a diffuse thickening of the posterior sclera that is usually most prominent in the temporal aspect of the eye. It is typically associated with diffuse retinochoroid layer thickening, as well as episcleral infiltration and/or edema (Figures 6-7 and 6-8). When it occurs in the peripapillary region, the episcleral inflammation causes distention of sub-Tenon's space, producing the "T-sign"[19] on B-scan (Figure 6-9). Choroidal and ciliary body detachments may also occur, which may result in angle closure and secondary glaucoma. Serous retinal detachments have also been identified. Associated orbital findings may include myositis (see Chapter 15), optic neuritis (see Chapter 16), and diffuse soft tissue inflammation (see Chapter 17).

Nodular Posterior Scleritis

Nodular posterior scleritis may present clinically as an elevated choroidal mass, thus mimicking an intraocular tumor.[9] In addition, these patients may present with little or no pain, further obscuring the clinical diagnosis of scleritis.[1] This lesion causes focal expansion of the ocular wall, extending both within and outside of the normal confines of the globe. The thickened sclera in these nodular lesions exhibits predominantly high reflectivity with regular internal structure. As in the diffuse form, there may also be thickening of the retinochoroid layer, as well as edema or inflammatory infiltration in sub-Tenon's space adjacent to the lesion (Figure 6-10). Echographically, nodular scleritis is easily differentiated from melanoma, although sometimes it may be confused with a highly reflective choroidal tumor (e.g., hemangioma or metastatic carcinoma).[17]

Anterior Scleritis

The diagnosis of anterior scleritis can typically be made by the clinical signs of conjunctival injection, intense redness of the sclera, and tenderness to touch. Anterior scleritis is similar to posterior scleritis in that it can present in a diffuse or nodular manner. Ultrasound plays less of a role in this group of patients since the diagnosis can usually be made on a clinical basis. Ultrasound, however, can show diffuse

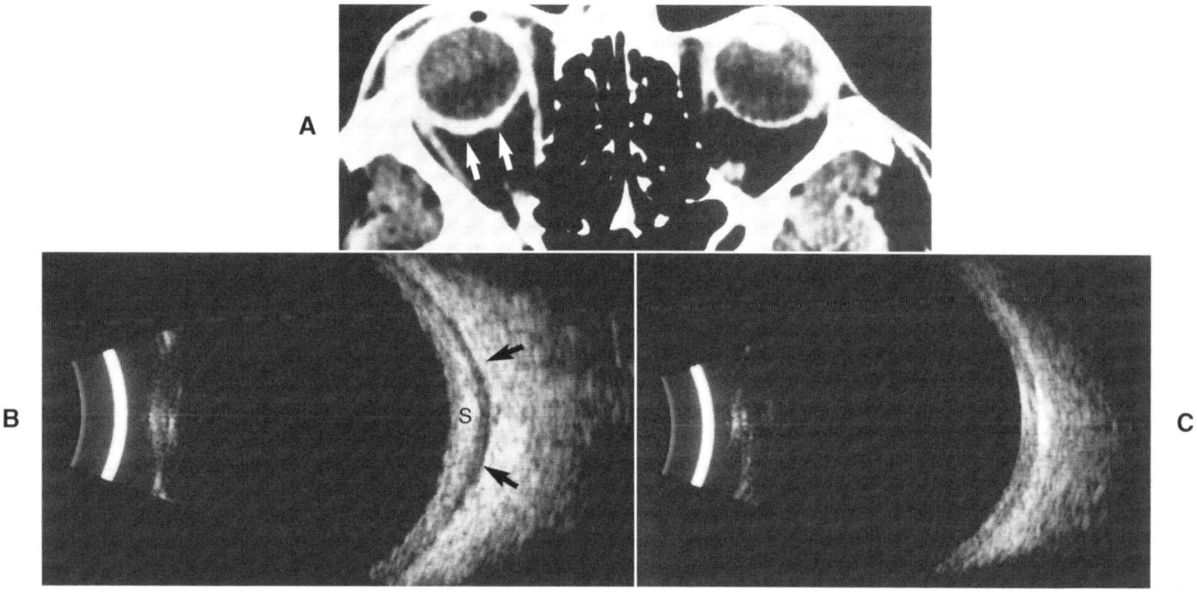

Figure 6-8 Diffuse posterior scleritis. **A,** Axial CT scan demonstrates diffuse thickening of posterior ocular wall in the right eye *(white arrows)*. **B,** Transverse B-scan of right eye shows diffuse thickening of retinochoroid layer and sclera *(S)* and edema of sub-Tenon's space *(black arrows)*. **C,** Transverse B-scan of left eye displays normal thickness of retinochoroid layer and sclera.

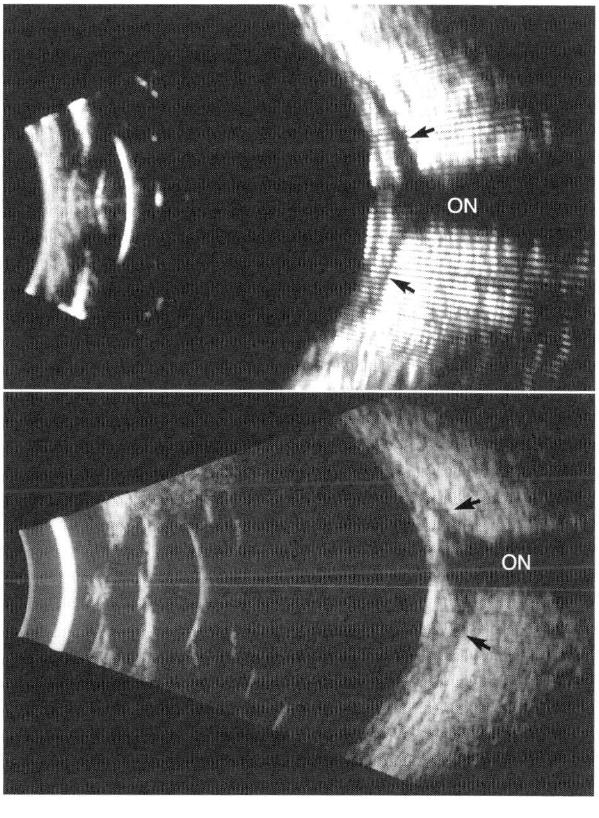

Figure 6-9 Axial B-scans demonstrating "T-sign" in two different patients with diffuse posterior scleritis. The T-sign is formed by distension of sub-Tenon's space *(arrows)* occurring around the optic nerve *(ON)*.

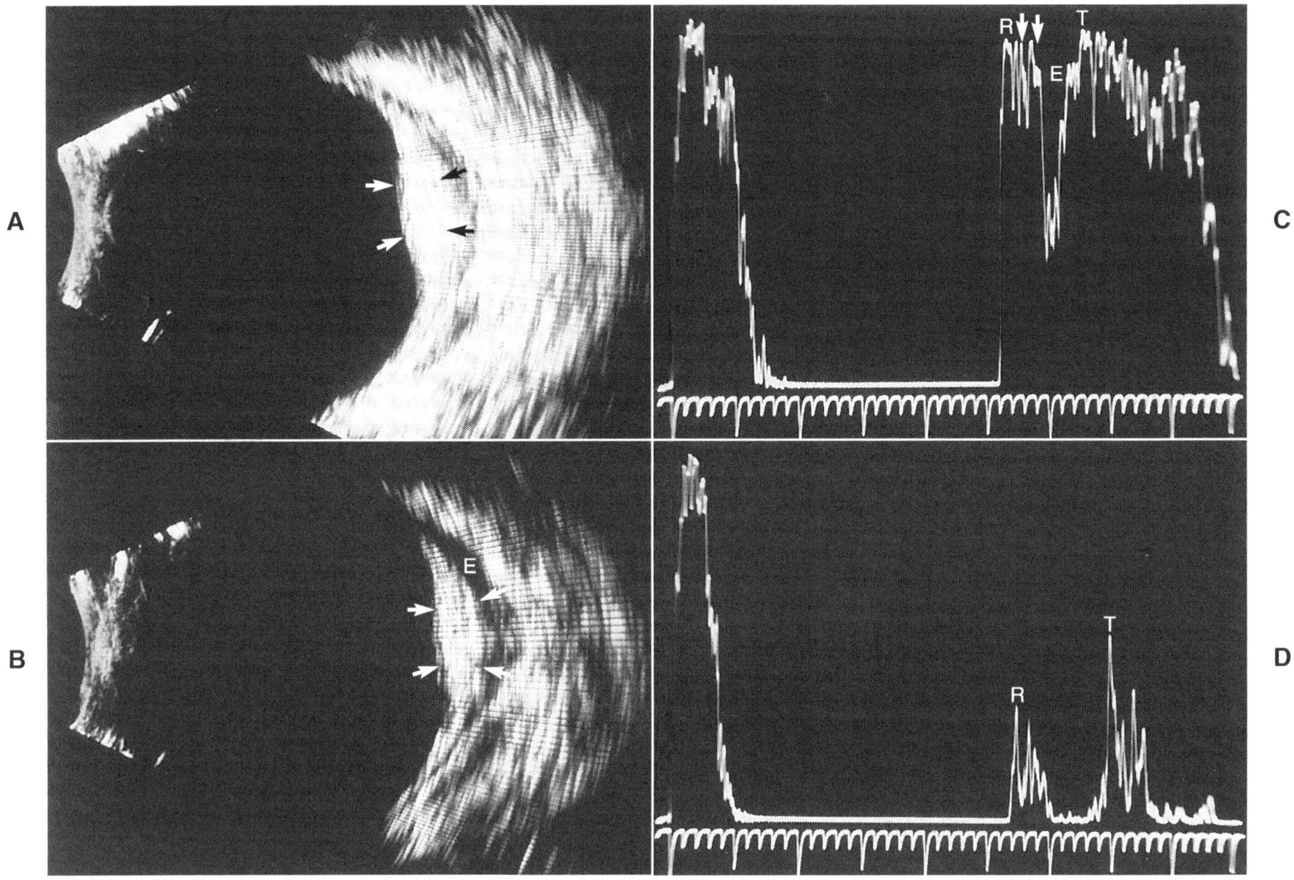

Figure 6-10 Posterior nodular scleritis. B- and A-scan echograms show marked, localized thickening of sclera that clinically presented as an intraocular mass. Transverse B-scans at high gain **(A)** and reduced gain **(B)** show the markedly thickened retinochoroid layer *(white arrows)* and sclera *(black arrows)* expanding both within and outside of the globe. Note moderately echolucent area adjacent to the sclera *(E)* corresponding to inflammation in sub-Tenon's space. A-scan at Tissue Sensitivity **(C)** shows high reflectivity of thickened retinochoroid layer *(R)* and sclera *(arrows)*, as well as medium reflectivity of the infiltrated sub-Tenon's space *(E)*. *T*, Tenon's capsule. **D,** A-scan at reduced gain shows thickness of lesion between retina *(R)* and Tenon's capsule *(T)*. (From Green RL, Byrne SF: Diagnostic ophthalmic ultrasound, in Ryan SJ [ed]: *Retina*. ed 3, St Louis, Mosby, 2001, p 284.)

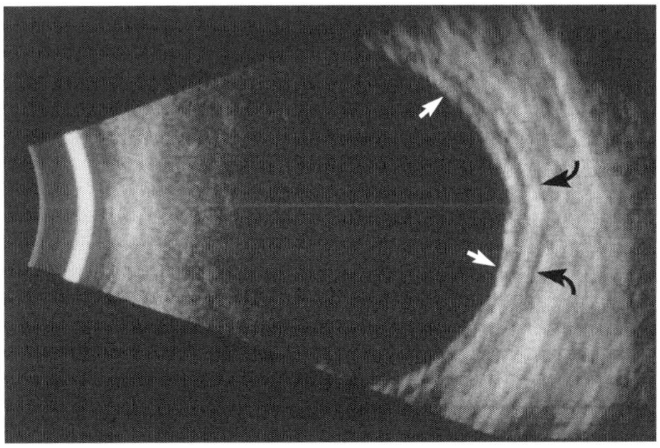

Figure 6-11 Anterior scleritis. Transverse B-scan view through peripheral aspect of eye shows diffuse thickening of sclera and mild edema of sub-Tenon's space *(curved black arrows)*, as well as shallow ciliochoroidal detachment *(straight white arrows)*.

thickening of the anterior sclera, as well as the presence of shallow ciliochoroidal detachments (Figure 6-11). In some cases, these findings can be better documented using high-resolution ultrasound (see p 233).

In the chronic or necrotizing form of this disease, scleral thinning may occur, leading to scleral bulging (i.e., staphyloma). The underlying darkly pigmented uveal tissue can sometimes be seen and may simulate a pigmented tumor such as a melanoma. Therefore, in chronic scleritis, ultrasound can be useful for identifying these staphylomas and ruling out an intraocular tumor (Figure 6-12).

Scleritis Associated with Intraocular Tumors

Scleritis has been known to occur in association with intraocular tumors, including choroidal melanoma (see Figures 5-9 and 5-18) and metastatic carcinoma. Scleral in-

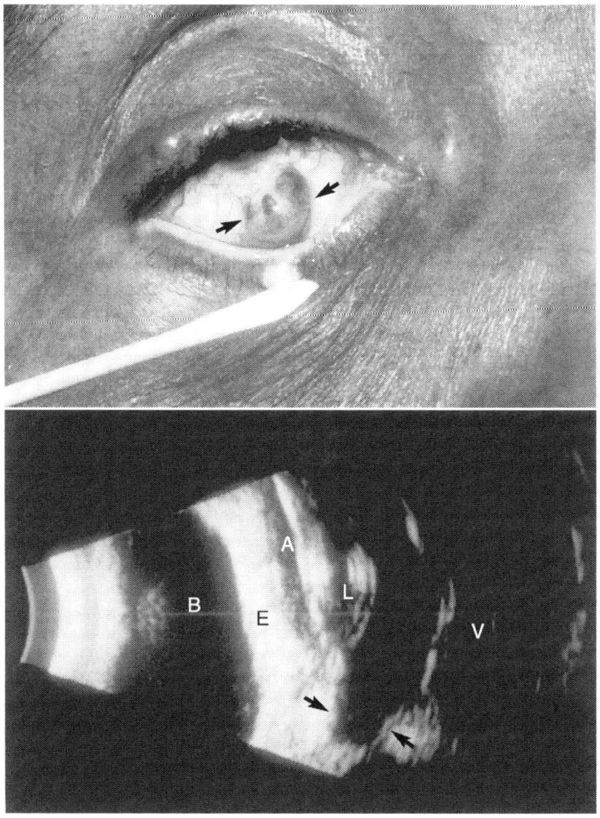

Figure 6-12 Anterior staphyloma in an eye with necrotizing scleritis. **A,** External photograph shows large, dark lesion inferior to limbus *(arrows)*. **B,** Immersion B-scan obtained with balloonlike device *(B)* placed over closed eyelid *(E)*. Echogram shows large staphyloma *(black arrows)* inferior to anterior chamber *(A)* and lens *(L)*. *V,* Vitreous cavity.

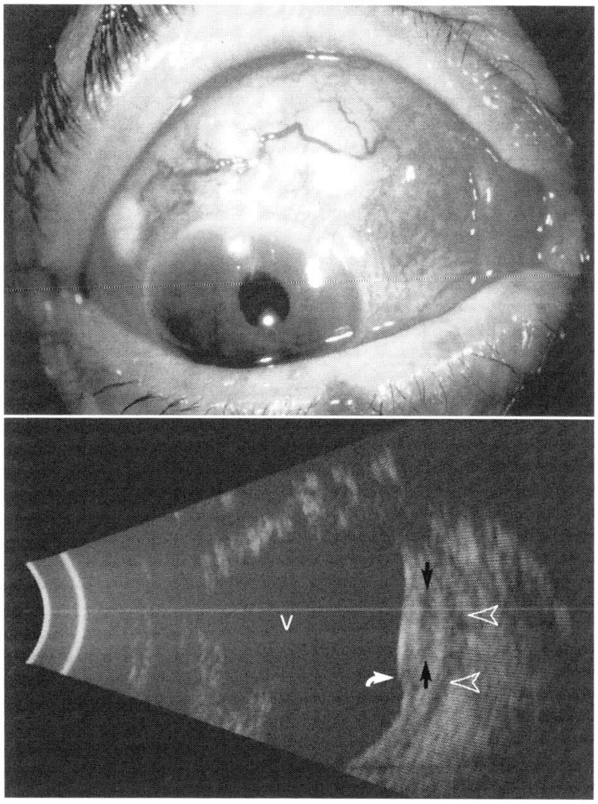

Figure 6-13 Infectious scleritis. **A,** External photograph demonstrates abscess formation superior to limbus. **B,** Transverse B-scan view through the superior anterior aspect of the eye shows intrascleral abscess *(straight black arrows)*. *Curved white arrow* displays diffuse thickening of underlying choroid. *Open arrows* indicate diffuse episcleral inflammation. *V,* Vitreous cavity.

flammation is most likely secondary to tumor necrosis. Episcleral and/or orbital involvement may also be present in these cases.

Infectious Scleritis

Infectious scleritis occurs less frequently than the idiopathic or autoimmune forms of the disorder. Anterior infectious scleritis has been associated with corneal ulcers and the excision of pterygia, as well as with infected scleral buckles and glaucoma-filtering shunts (see p 221). Infectious posterior scleritis can occur as an extension of anterior scleritis, or more rarely, it may develop from an endogenous source.

The echographic findings of infectious scleritis are similar to those of noninfectious forms of scleritis, although the intraocular and orbital inflammation may be more severe. Abscesses can be present within the sclera[31] (Figure 6-13), the choroid (see Figure 6-3), and even the orbit. The ability of ultrasound to aid in the diagnosis, however, can be limited in the presence of implanted foreign material (e.g., scleral buckle or glaucoma-filtering shunt) in that the sound attenuation from these materials may prevent imaging of the affected sclera. Whenever there is the possibility of an infected buckle, the ultrasound examination should focus on areas adjacent to the buckle to look for inflammatory changes that are not masked by the foreign material (Figure 6-14).

INFLAMMATORY CONDITIONS OF THE CHOROID

Diffuse choroidal thickening secondary to inflammatory infiltration may be observed in a number of conditions such as Vogt-Koyanagi-Harada syndrome (VKH), sympathetic ophthalmia, and uveal lymphoid infiltration.* Some of these disorders may also be associated with thickening of the sclera, serous RD, and vitritis, as well as with episcleral and orbital lesions.

*References 3, 5, 7, 11, 12, 18, 21.

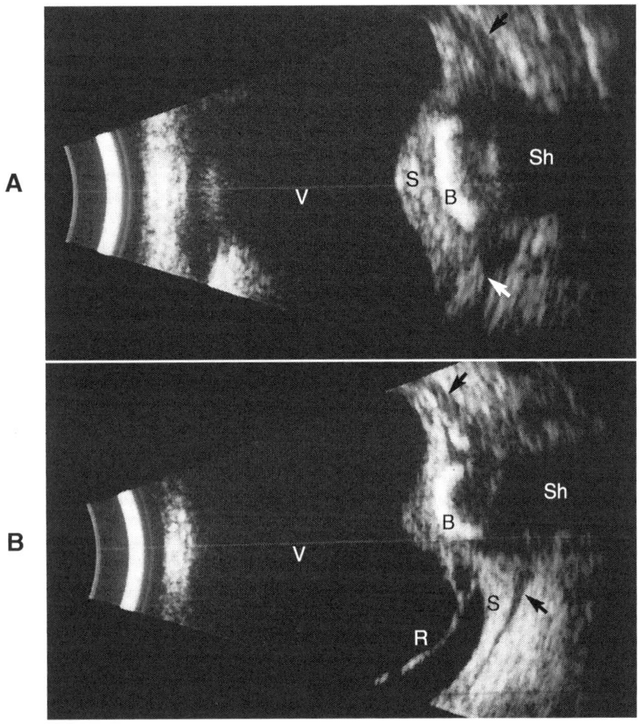

Figure 6-14 Infectious scleritis associated with scleral buckle. Transverse **(A)** and longitudinal **(B)** B-scans show curved echodense scleral buckle *(B)* indenting the globe and producing shadowing *(Sh)*. Inflammation and thickening of episclera are seen adjacent to the buckle *(arrows)*. Note thickening of sclera *(S)* overlying and adjacent to the buckle. Detached retina *(R)* extends posteriorly from the buckle. *V*, Vitreous cavity.

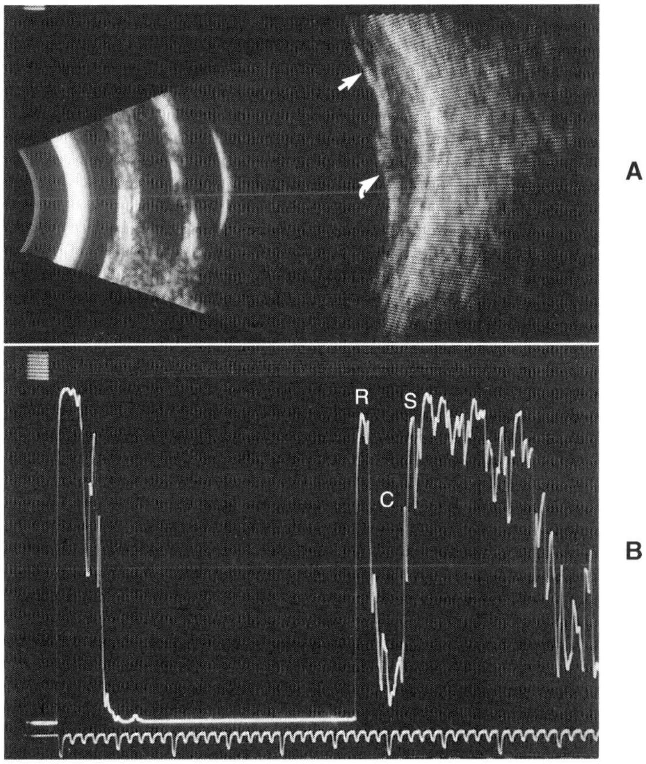

Figure 6-15 Vogt-Koyanagi-Harada syndrome. **A,** Vertical macula B-scan view demonstrates diffuse thickening of posterior choroid *(curved arrow)* and shallow serous RD *(straight arrow)* extending from superior margin of the lesion. **B,** Corresponding A-scan demonstrates low internal reflectivity of thickened choroid *(C)*. *R*, Retina; *S*, sclera.

BOX 6-3

Clinical and Echographic Differential Diagnosis of VKH Syndrome

Posterior scleritis
Sympathetic ophthalmia*
Idiopathic posterior uveitis
Lyme disease*
Relapsing polychondritis*
Uveal lymphoid hyperplasia (see p 153)*
Lymphoma (see p 151)*
Leukemia (see p 154)*
Diffuse malignant melanoma of the choroid (see p 136)*
Metastatic carcinoma (see p 143)
Uveal effusion syndrome (see p 82)

*Inflammatory conditions that exhibit diffuse, low to medium reflective choroidal thickening, similar to VKH.

Vogt-Koyanagi-Harada Syndrome

Vogt-Koyanagi-Harada (VKH) syndrome is a systemic disorder that often includes ocular involvement. This condition is usually bilateral, although the findings may be asymmetric. The primary ophthalmologic features of VKH include anterior and posterior uveitis, serous detachment of the retina, changes in the retinal pigment epithelium, and hyperemia of the optic disc.[27]

Several conditions can mimic VKH clinically (Box 6-3). In addition, VKH may have an atypical presentation, and in some cases, opaque ocular media may preclude adequate visualization of the fundus. In all of these instances, ultrasound can be helpful for either confirming or ruling out the diagnosis of VKH. Moreover, ultrasound may be able to detect abnormalities in an eye with a normal fundus appearance. These findings can be important for confirming bilateral involvement in patients who clinically appear to have only unilateral disease.[12]

The most important echographic finding in VKH is diffuse, low to medium reflective thickening of the choroid. This thickening is generally most pronounced in the peri-

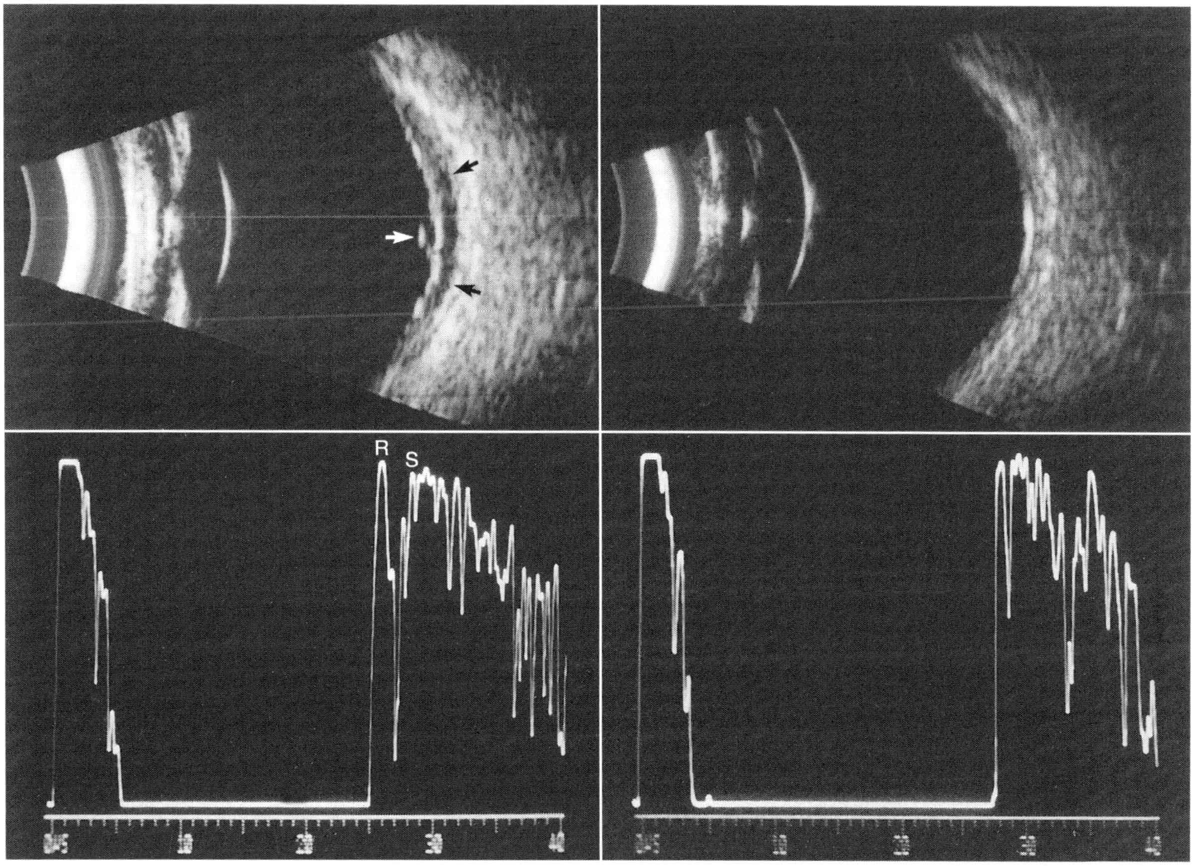

Figure 6-16 Vogt-Koyanagi-Harada syndrome before (**A** and **B**) and after (**C** and **D**) corticosteroid therapy. **A,** Vertical macula B-scan section shows diffuse thickening of posterior choroid *(black arrows)* and focal overlying serous retinal detachment *(white arrow)*. **B,** Corresponding A-scan shows low internal reflectivity of thickened choroid. *R,* Retina; *S,* sclera. Vertical macula B-scan **(C)** and corresponding A-scan **(D)** demonstrate nearly complete resolution of choroidal thickening and retinal detachment following treatment.

papillary region (Figure 6-15). From there, it usually extends to the equator, where the choroid becomes progressively thinner. In some patients, the infiltration may also involve the ciliary body. Other echographic features of this disease may include serous RD, mild vitreous opacities, and thickening of the sclera and/or episclera.

The echographic differential diagnosis of VKH includes a number of conditions (see Box 6-3). Although many of these disorders can demonstrate low to medium internal reflectivity, other clinical and echographic findings will usually allow accurate differentiation.

Ultrasound can also be incorporated into the management of patients with VKH. The usual clinical method for monitoring the response to corticosteroid therapy is the documentation of an improvement in signs and symptoms.[11] However, if a cataract or other media opacity limits visualization of the fundus, then these clinical findings may not be an accurate means of assessing resolution of the inflammation. In these cases, ultrasound can document a decrease in choroidal thickening and/or serous detachment of the retina (Figure 6-16). Also, when the ocular media are clear, the presence of residual choroidal thickening may not be clinically apparent, despite the resolution of other signs and symptoms. Therefore, ultrasound can be used as another clinical marker for determining the response to therapy and as a gauge for tapering the steroid treatment.

Sympathetic Ophthalmia

Sympathetic ophthalmia is a rare condition that can occur after penetrating injury or intraocular surgery. Although sympathetic ophthalmia is a bilateral condition, the symptoms are often most evident in the noninjured (sympathizing) eye. The primary echographic finding is diffuse, low to medium reflective thickening of the choroid (Figure 6-17). Choroidal thickening can also be detected in the traumatized eye if it is not too disorganized. Other associated findings can include vitreous opacities, serous RD, and

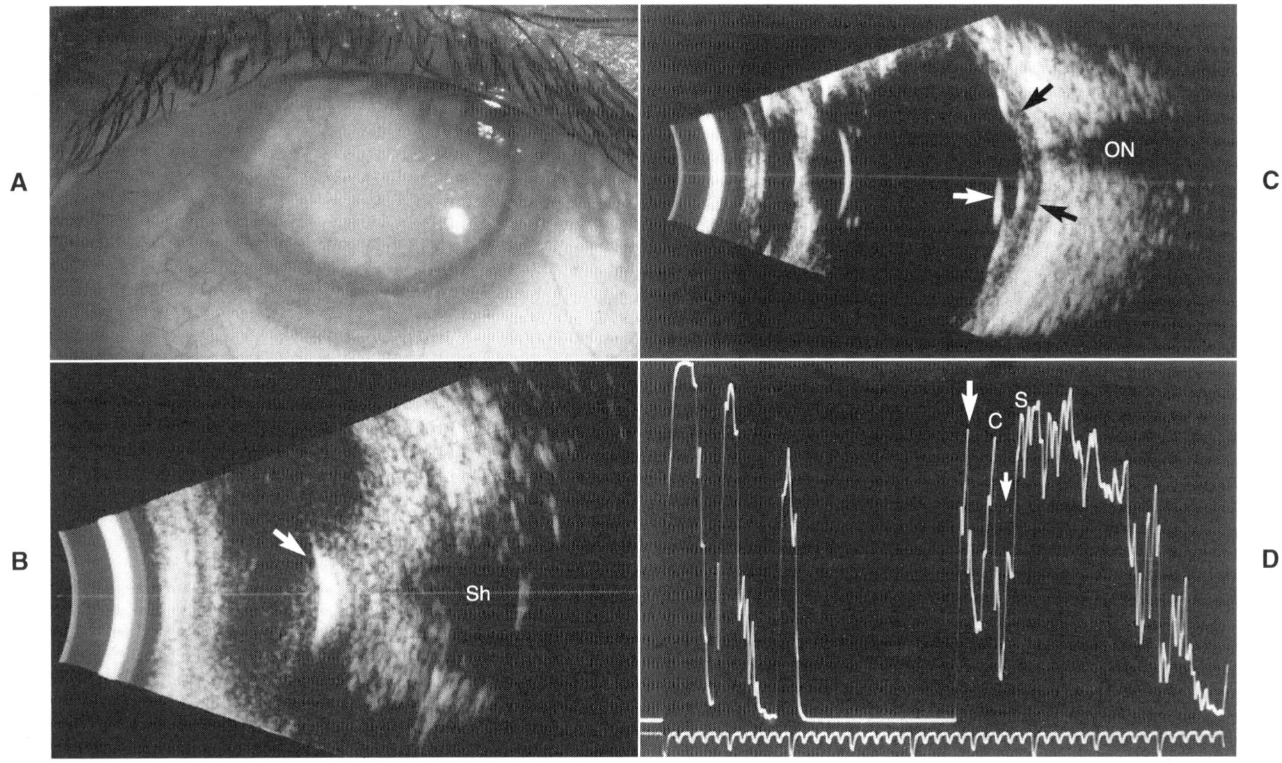

Figure 6-17 Sympathetic ophthalmia following penetrating foreign body injury. **A,** External photograph of injured eye demonstrating dense opacification of anterior vitreous. **B,** Transverse B-scan from eye shown in **A** demonstrates large intraocular foreign body *(arrow)* surrounded by dense vitreous opacities. *Sh,* Shadowing from foreign body. **C,** Horizontal axial B-scan of fellow eye demonstrates diffuse thickening of posterior choroid *(black arrows)* and shallow retinal detachment overlying macula *(white arrow)*. *ON,* optic nerve. **D,** Corresponding A-scan through macula shows retinal detachment *(large white arrow)* and low to medium reflective choroidal thickening *(small white arrow)*. *C,* Surface of choroid; *S,* sclera.

scleral thickening. Ultrasound can also be used to monitor choroidal thickness to determine the response to therapy.

The clinical and echographic findings for sympathetic ophthalmia are similar to those of other disorders, although they most closely resemble the features of VKH. Sympathetic ophthalmia, however, occurs almost exclusively following penetrating ocular trauma or previous ocular surgery.[11]

An unusual form of sympathetic ophthalmia has recently been described. The patient presented with a bilateral, diffuse, granulomatous infiltration involving primarily the retina and retinal pigment epithelium and a history of scleral buckle surgery in one eye.[33] On B-scan, there was pronounced, diffuse thickening of the retina and retinal pigment epithelium, especially in the peripapillary region, giving the false impression of an enlarged optic cup (Figure 6-18). No serous retinal detachment was detected. The internal reflectivity of the thickened tissue was primarily medium-high.

Uveal Lymphoid Hyperplasia

This unilateral lymphoproliferative disorder presents as a diffuse or nodular amelanotic choroidal lesion with low to medium internal reflectivity on echography. The clinical and echographic features of this disorder are described in detail in Chapter 5 (see p 153).

MISCELLANEOUS CONDITIONS ASSOCIATED WITH INFLAMMATION OF THE CHOROID, RETINA, AND RETINAL PIGMENT EPITHELIUM (RPE)

There are some isolated reports of inflammatory conditions associated with significant choroidal thickening. One of these conditions is Lyme disease, one report of which described diffuse, bilateral, low to medium reflective choroidal thickening,[8] similar to that of VKH. Another disorder that has been associated with diffuse choroidal thickening is relapsing polychondritis. In one case, the patient presented with bilateral medium to high reflective choroidal thickening. In the more severely affected eye, there was also an associated scleral thickening (Figure 6-19), as well as a serous retinal detachment.[2]

Mild choroidal thickening can occur secondary to other inflammatory conditions, including endopthalmitis (see p 191), uveitis (see p 194), and scleritis (see p 195).

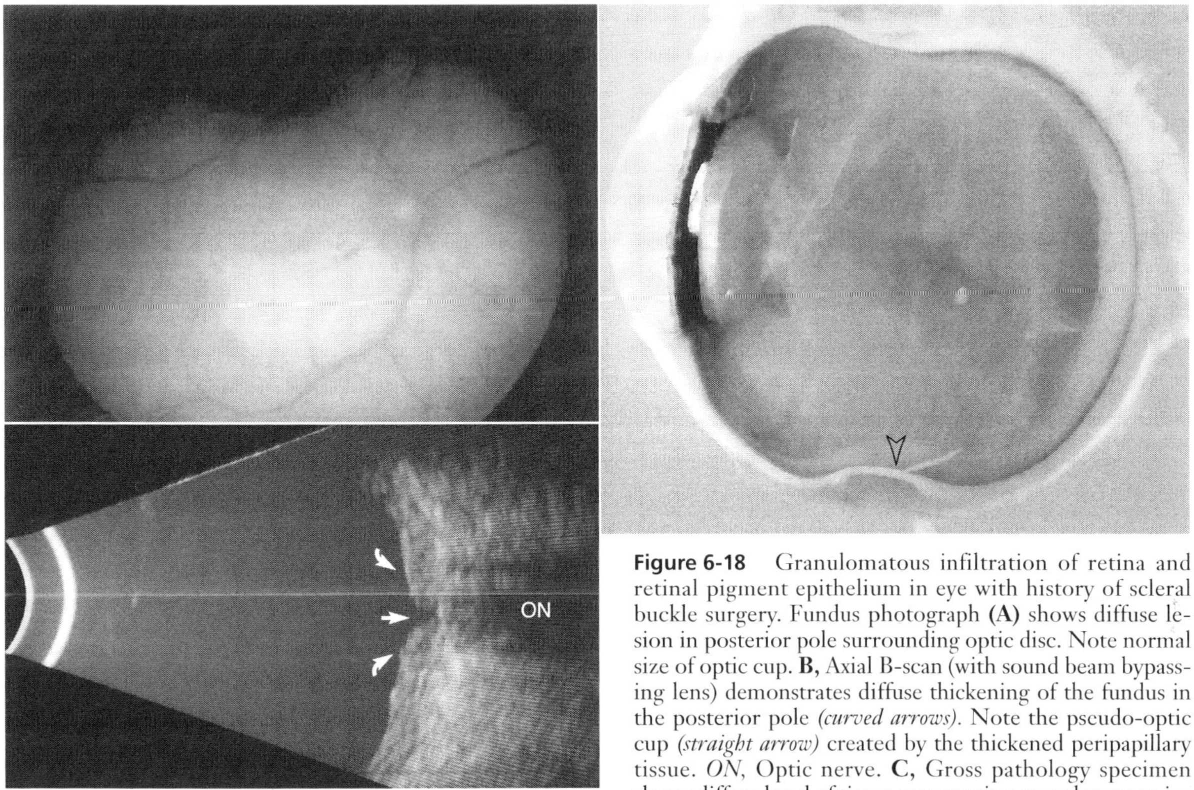

Figure 6-18 Granulomatous infiltration of retina and retinal pigment epithelium in eye with history of scleral buckle surgery. Fundus photograph **(A)** shows diffuse lesion in posterior pole surrounding optic disc. Note normal size of optic cup. **B,** Axial B-scan (with sound beam bypassing lens) demonstrates diffuse thickening of the fundus in the posterior pole *(curved arrows).* Note the pseudo-optic cup *(straight arrow)* created by the thickened peripapillary tissue. *ON,* Optic nerve. **C,** Gross pathology specimen shows diffuse band of tissue representing granulomatous infiltration that primarily involves retina and pigment epithelium. *Open arrow,* Scleral buckle. (**A** and **C** from Wang RC, Zamir E, Dugel PU, et al: Progressive subretinal fibrosis and blindness associated with multifocal granulomatous chorioretinitis—a variant of sympathetic ophthalmia. *Ophthalmology.* In press.)

Toxocariasis

Toxocariasis may present clinically as a whitish lesion in the posterior or peripheral fundus, or as a leukokoria (see Table 5-2) secondary to diffuse inflammation of the vitreous. Although there are no pathognomonic echographic criteria for toxocariasis, three characteristics that are common to these infections have been identified in eyes with clear media, as well as in eyes with endophthalmitis that had opaque media.[32] These echographic findings are (1) mildly to moderately elevated granulomatous lesions that may be calcified, (2) vitreous membranes extending from the granulomatous lesion to the posterior pole, and (3) posterior traction RD or retinal fold (Figures 6-20 and 6-21).

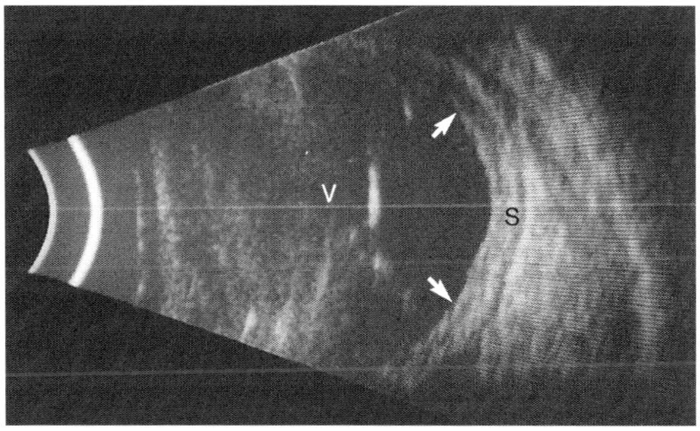

Figure 6-19 Relapsing polychondritis. Longitudinal B-scan demonstrates diffuse thickening of choroid *(arrows)* and sclera *(S)*. *V,* Vitreous cavity.

Cysticercosis

Cysticercosis may present as a whitish mass in the posterior aspect of the eye, with secondary inflammation of the vitreous. When the vitreous inflammation is severe, the patient may present with leukokoria (see Table 5-2). The echographic appearance is quite characteristic, with one or more well-outlined, oval-shaped cysts located within the vitreous cavity and/or the subretinal space.[10,24] The scolex of the parasite appears as a very highly reflective, echodense nodule attached to the inner wall of the cyst (Figure 6-22). Some investigators have reported movement of the cyst during kinetic evaluation.[24]

A

B

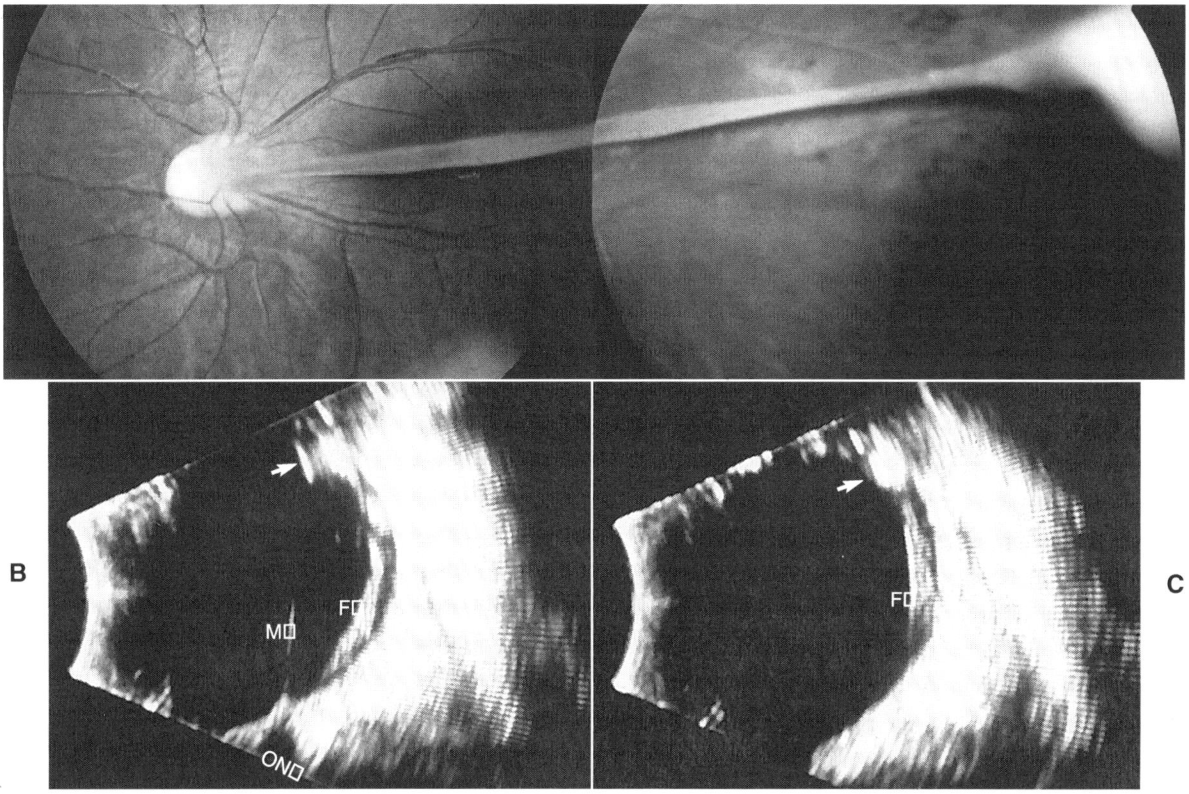

C

Figure 6-20 Toxocariasis. **A,** Fundus photograph montage shows a retinal fold extending from the optic disc to a peripheral granuloma. **B,** Longitudinal B-scan demonstrates the dense nodular peripheral granuloma *(arrow)* shown in **A.** A thin membrane *(M)* and retinal fold *(F)* extend from the granuloma back to the optic nerve *(ON)*. **C,** More anterior longitudinal B-scan better shows the granuloma and adjacent retinal fold. (From Green RL, Byrne SF: Diagnostic ophthalmic ultrasound, in Ryan SJ [ed]: *Retina.* ed 3, St Louis, Mosby, 2001, p 291.)

A

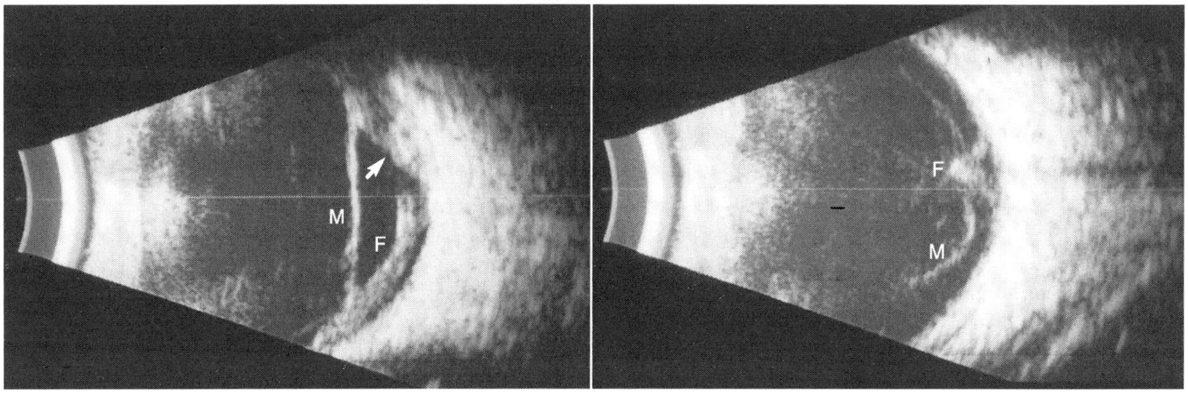

B

Figure 6-21 Toxocariasis. **A,** Longitudinal B-scan shows an elevated peripheral granuloma *(arrow)*. A thick membrane *(M)* extends from the peripheral granuloma to the posterior aspect of a radial traction retinal fold *(F)*. **B,** Transverse B-scan shows cross-section of open traction retinal fold with inflammatory membrane attached to apex.

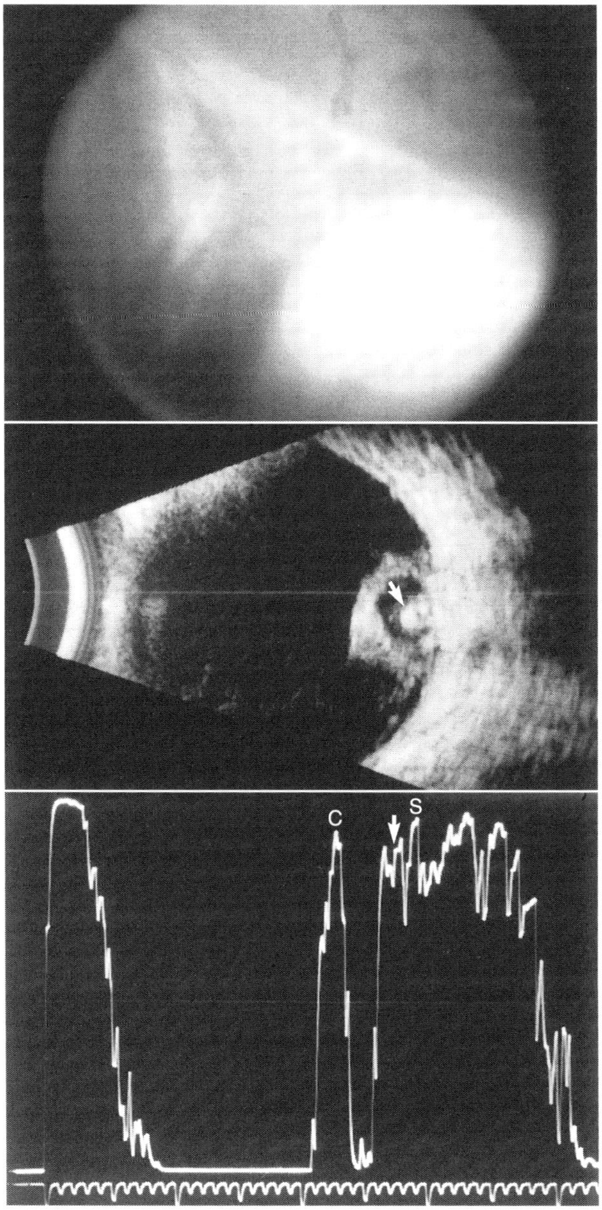

Figure 6-22 Intraocular cysticercosis. **A,** Fundus photograph shows elevated, nonpigmented lesion in inferior aspect of eye. **B,** Transverse B-scan echogram shows subretinal cyst containing dense nodule *(arrow)* corresponding to scolex of the organism that typically attaches to the inner cyst wall. **C,** A-scan echogram shows highly reflective spike from anterior cyst wall *(C)* and thick, high spike from the scolex *(arrow)*. *S,* Sclera.

Acquired Immunodeficiency Syndrome (AIDS)

In recent years, AIDS has created multiple new clinical problems affecting the eye. Many different opportunistic infections can occur that may lead to a devastating visual outcome. The various infections can include cytomegalovirus (CMV), toxoplasmosis, *Pneumocystis carinii,* syphilis,

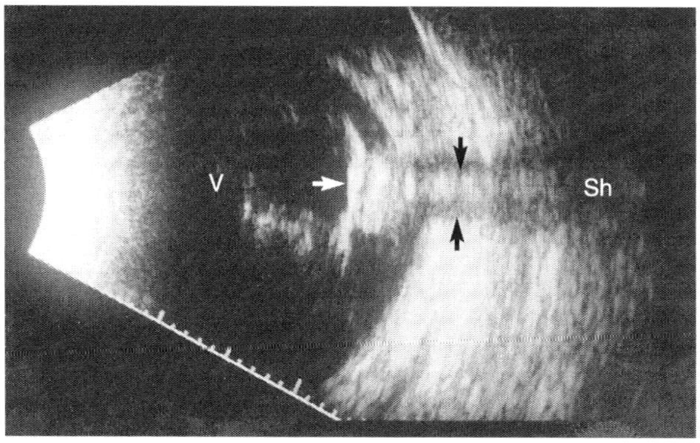

Figure 6-23 Gancyclovir implant in a patient with CMV retinitis. Very anterior transverse B-scan shows echo-dense implant *(white arrow)* followed by chain of multiple signals *(black arrows)* and shadowing *(Sh)*. *V,* Vitreous cavity.

tuberculosis, herpes simplex, and herpes zoster. Fortunately, however, recent improvements in medical therapy have significantly lessened the incidence and severity of these opportunistic infections.

Although there are no specific echographic findings in the patient with AIDS, different infections present in unique forms, and ultrasound can be useful in the diagnosis and management of these patients.

CMV retinitis usually presents with flat, creamy lesions in the posterior pole. In some cases, these lesions are treated with a gancyclovir implant. Although ultrasound is not helpful in diagnosing CMV, the implant does exhibit a rather specific echographic appearance (Figure 6-23).

Herpes infections are associated with certain forms of retinal necrosis. Herpes simplex is most commonly associated with acute retinal necrosis (ARN). Herpes zoster, however, is the primary etiologic agent of progressive outer retinal necrosis (PORN), the form of retinal necrosis usually seen in patients with AIDS. In both of these conditions, mild to moderately dense vitreous opacities may be present, and retinal detachments frequently occur (Figure 6-24). Swelling of the retrobulbar optic nerve can be seen in some patients.

Tuberculosis and syphilis, typically rare ocular disorders, are now being seen more frequently because of AIDS. Clinically, they usually present with an anterior and/or posterior uveitis. There may also be a choroiditis in the case of tuberculosis, or a chorioretinitis in syphilis. These disorders may produce diffuse thickening of the retinochoroid layer and/or focally elevated fundus lesions[20] (Figure 6-25). The echographic findings are similar to the inflammatory changes seen in posterior uveitis (see p 194). In one case of tertiary syphilis, a markedly thickened optic nerve was demonstrated[22] (Figure 6-26).

Ocular toxoplasmosis in the immunocompromised patient may present with a focal retinitis, although it may be

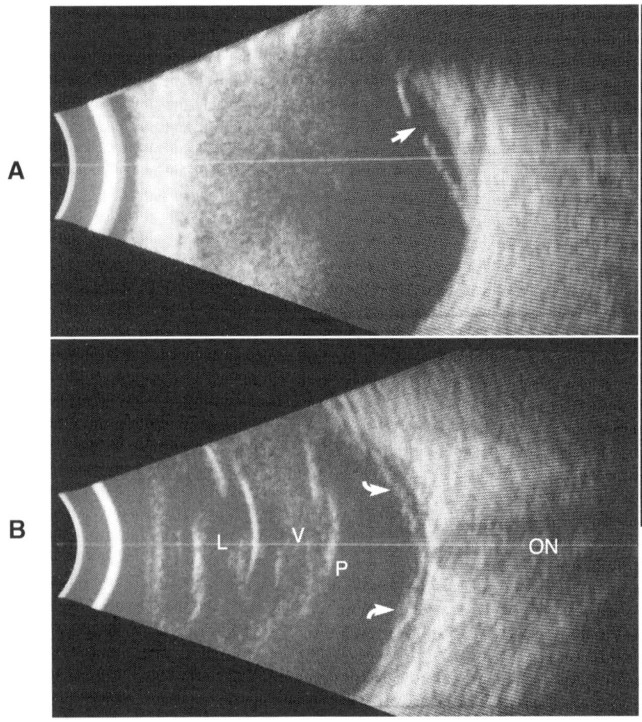

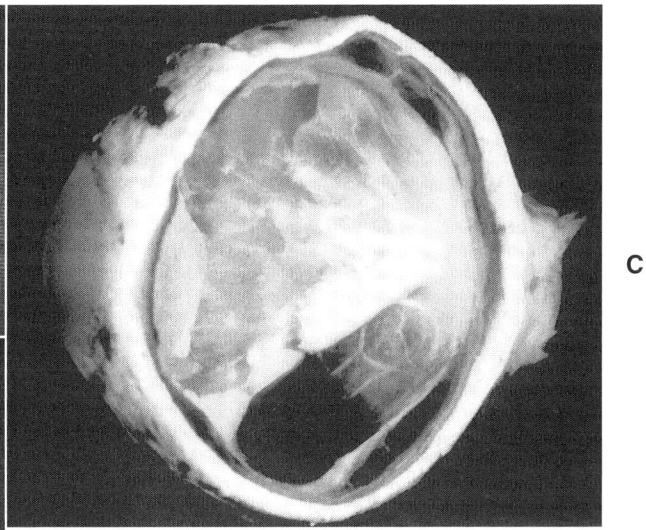

Figure 6-24 Acute retinal necrosis. **A,** Anterior longitudinal B-scan view shows necrotic retinal hole *(arrow)* in shallow retinal detachment. **B,** Axial B-scan displays vitreous opacities *(V)*, PVD *(P)*, and shallow, diffuse posterior retinal detachment *(curved arrows)*. *L*, Lens; *ON*, optic nerve. **C,** Gross pathology specimen demonstrates organized vitreous and shallow, diffuse retinal detachment.

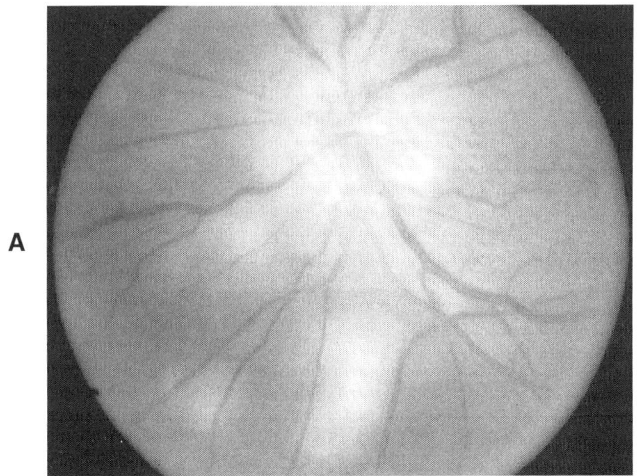

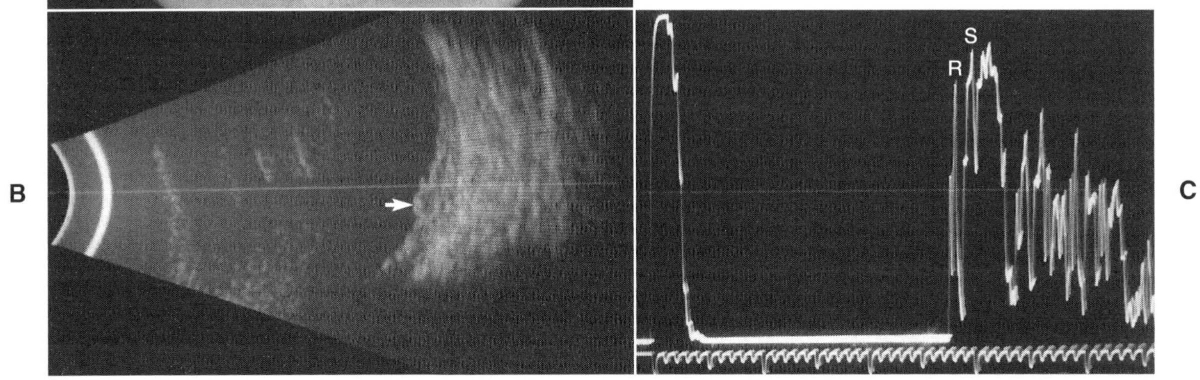

Figure 6-25 Miliary tuberculosis. **A,** Fundus photograph shows multiple cream colored, mildly elevated lesions in the posterior pole. **B,** B-scan echogram demonstrates mildly elevated lesion with slightly irregular surface contour *(arrow)*. **C,** Corresponding A-scan displays mildly elevated lesion with low internal reflectivity. *R*, Retina; *S*, sclera.

A

B

C

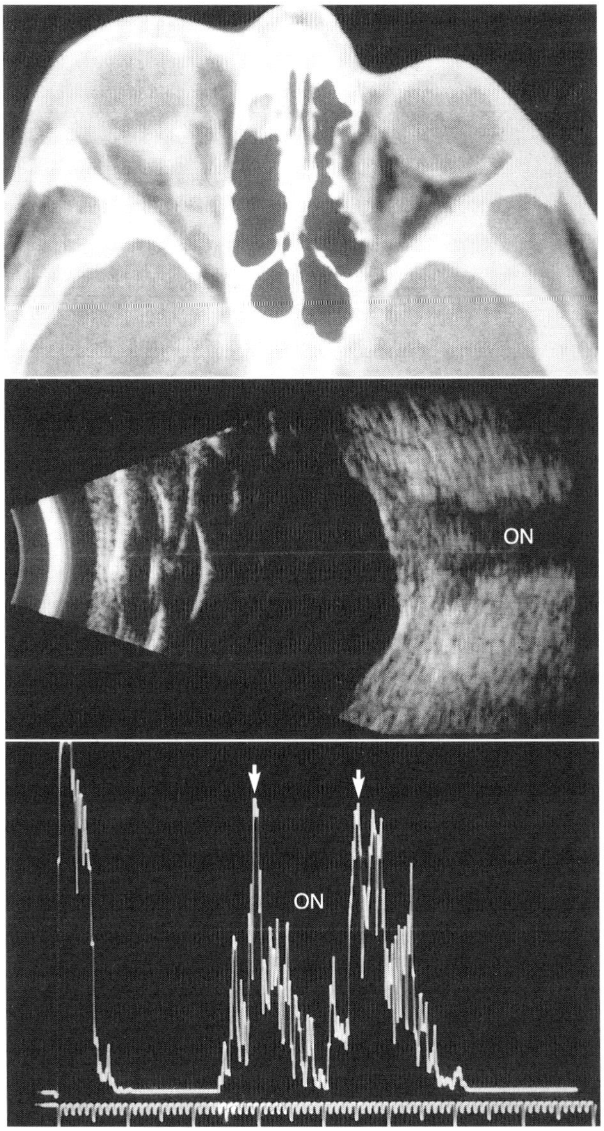

Figure 6-26 Syphilitic optic neuritis in a patient with AIDS. **A,** Axial CT scan demonstrates proptosis of right eye and marked thickening of retrobulbar optic nerve. **B,** Axial B-scan shows marked, irregular thickening of the optic nerve *(ON)*. **C,** A-scan shows marked thickening of optic nerve with low to medium internal reflectivity. *Arrows,* Perineural sheath. (**A** from Kronish JW, Johnson TE, Gilberg SM: Orbital infections in patients with human immunodeficiency virus infection. *Ophthalmology* 1996;103:1485.)

a diffuse process in patients with AIDS.[25] Vitreous opacities and PVD may also be present. Other findings can include papillitis, as well as orbital involvement.

Ultrasound may demonstrate mild to moderately elevated fundus lesions. Echographic findings can also include vitreous opacities and strands, as well as PVD. Elevation of the optic disc has been demonstrated, as well as orbital inflammation, including myositis (see p 396) and enlargement of the retrobulbar optic nerve with increased subarachnoid fluid (see p 419).

Inflammation Associated with Ocular Tumors

Certain intraocular tumors can be associated with inflammation, whereas others may mimic an inflammation by their clinical presentation (pseudoinflammation). In both instances, the confusing clinical and echographic findings may lead to misdiagnosis. Some systemic malignancies can also produce a secondary intraocular inflammatory response that is unrelated to a metastatic intraocular tumor.

Tumors that sometimes develop inflammation include choroidal melanoma, metastatic carcinoma, and retinoblastoma. Melanomas have been associated with ciliochoroidal detachments, scleritis, episcleritis and orbital inflammation (see Figures 5-9 and 5-18). These findings can occur with or without extraocular extension of the tumor (see p 120). In metastatic carcinoma, ciliochoroidal detachments have been described when the tumor involves the peripheral choroid and ciliary body[30] (see Figure 5-43). Scleritis may also occur when the tumor simultaneously involves the choroid and adjacent episclera or the orbital tissues. Furthermore, retinoblastoma may produce an orbital cellulitis that may not be related to extraocular extension (see p 180).

Pseudoinflammation occurring secondary to tumor infiltration of the vitreous or the anterior chamber can be seen in retinoblastoma, as well as in intraocular B-cell lymphoma (reticulum cell sarcoma, see p 151). In retinoblastoma, this usually occurs in older children with a diffuse tumor. The clinical presentation may include hypopyon and/or vitritis. Intraocular B-cell lymphoma may also mimic a vitritis secondary to tumor cells within the vitreous cavity.

Certain systemic malignancies (e.g., ovarian and small cell carcinoma) can produce a bilateral diffuse inflammatory infiltration of the choroid that is unrelated to choroidal metastasis. This rare condition, known as bilateral diffuse uveal melanocytic proliferation (BDUMP),[14,16] is typically associated with a low-grade inflammation and cataract (see p 166). Echographically, this condition appears as mild, diffuse thickening of the retinochoroid layer with slightly irregular surface contour.

REFERENCES

1. Benson WE, Shields JA, Tasman W, et al: Posterior scleritis. A cause of diagnostic confusion. *Arch Ophthalmol* 1979;97:1482.
2. Bhagat N, Green RL, Feldon SE, et al: Exudative retinal detachment in relapsing polychondritis—case report and literature review. *Ophthalmology* 2001;108:1156.
3. Chang TS, Byrne SF, Gass JDM, et al: Echographic findings in benign reactive lymphoid hyperplasia of the choroid. *Arch Ophthalmol* 1996;114:669.
4. Chu TG, Lopez PF, Cano MR, et al: Posterior vitreoschisis. An echographic finding in proliferative diabetic retinopathy. *Ophthalmology* 1996;103:315.
5. Cockerham GC, Hidayat AA, Bijwaard KE, et al: Re-evaluation of "reactive lymphoid hyperplasia of the uvea"—an immunohistochemical and molecular analysis of 10 cases. *Ophthalmology* 2000;107:151.
6. Dacey MP, Valencia M, Lee MR, et al: Echographic findings in infectious endophthalmitis. *Arch Ophthalmol* 1994;112:1325.
7. Desroches G, Abrams GW, Gass JDM: Reactive lymphoid hyperplasia of the uvea: A case with ultrasonographic and computed tomo-

graphic studies. *Arch Ophthalmol* 1983;101:725.
8. DiBernardo C, Schachat A, Fekrat S: *Ophthalmic Ultrasound—A Diagnostic Atlas*. New York, Thieme, 1998, p 68.
9. Finger PT, Perry HD, Packer, et al: Posterior scleritis as an intraocular tumor. *Br J Ophthalmol* 1986;74:121.
10. Fishman M, Kerman B, Foxman S: Intraocular cysticercosis: Migratory, in Ossoinig KC (ed): *Ophthalmic Echography*. Dordrecht, Dr. W Junk, 1987, p 285.
11. Forster DJ, Cano MR, Green RL, et al: Echographic features of the Vogt-Koyanagi-Harada syndrome. *Arch Ophthalmol* 1990;108:1421.
12. Forster DJ, Green RL, Rao NA: Unilateral manifestation of Vogt-Koyanagi-Harada syndrome in a 7-year-old child. *Am J Ophthalmol* 1991;111:380.
13. Freeman WR, Green RL, Smith RE: Echographic localization of corticosteroids after periocular injection. *Am J Ophthalmol* 1987;103:281.
14. Gass JDM: *Stereoscopic Atlas of Macular Diseases*, ed 4, St Louis, Mosby, 1997, p 238.
15. Gass JDM, Geiser RG, Wilkinson CP, et al: Bilateral diffuse uveal melanocytic proliferation in patients with occult carcinoma. *Arch Ophthalmol* 1990;108:527.
16. Gass JDM, Glatzer RJ: Acquired pigmentation simulating Peutz-Jeghers syndrome—initial manifestation of diffuse uveal melanocytic proliferation. *Br J Ophthalmol* 1991;75:693.
17. Green RL: Echographic diagnosis of posterior scleritis, in Ossoinig, KC (ed): *Ophthalmic Echography*. Dordrecht, Dr. W Junk, 1987, p 515.
18. Grossniklaus HE, Martin DF, Avery R, et al: Uveal lymphoid infiltration—report of four cases and clinicopathologic review. *Ophthalmology* 1998;105:1265.
19. Harr DL, Quencer RM, Abrams GW: Computed tomography and ultrasound in the evaluation of orbital infection and pseudotumor. *Radiology* 1982;142:395.
20. Illingsworth RS, Wright T: Tubercles of the choroids. *Br Med J* 1948;2:365.
21. Jakobiec FA, Sacks E, Kronish JW, et al: Multifocal static creamy choroidal infiltrates: An early sign of lymphoid neoplasia. *Ophthalmology* 1987;94:397.
22. Kronish JW, Johnson TE, Gilberg SN, et al: Orbital infections in patients with human immunodeficiency virus infection. *Ophthalmology* 1996;103:1483.
23. McCluskey PJ, Watson PG, Lightman S, et al: Posterior scleritis—clinical features, systemic associations, and outcome in a large series of patients. *Ophthalmology* 1999;106:2380.
24. Moragrega E: Ultrasonic diagnosis of intraocular cysticercus, in Hillman JS, LeMay MM (eds): *Ophthalmic Ultrasonography*. Dordrecht, Dr. W Junk, 1984, p 191.
25. Nussenblatt RB, Whitcup SM, Palestine AG: *Uveitis—Fundamentals and Clinical Practice*, ed 2, St Louis, Mosby, 1996.
26. Riono WP, Hidayat AA, Rao NA: Scleritis—a clinicopathologic study of 55 cases. *Ophthalmology* 1999;106:1328.
27. Rubsamen PR, Gass JDM: Vogt-Koyanagi-Harada syndrome. Clinical course, therapy, and long-term visual outcome. *Arch Ophthalmol* 1991;109:682.
28. Schwartz SD, Alexander R, Hiscott P, et al: Recognition of vitreoschisis in proliferative diabetic retinopathy. A useful landmark in vitrectomy for diabetic traction retinal detachment. *Ophthalmology* 1996;103:323.
29. Seabag J: Diabetic vitreopathy (editorial). *Ophthalmology* 1996;103:205.
30. Sneed RS, Byrne SF, Meiler WF, et al: Choroidal effusions associated with malignant choroidal tumors. *Ophthalmology* 1991;98:968.
31. Taravella MJ, Johnson DW, Petty JG, et al: Infectious posterior scleritis caused by *Pseudallescheria boydii*. *Ophthalmology* 1997;104:1312.
32. Wan WL, Cano MR, Pince KJ, et al: Echographic characteristics of ocular toxocariasis. *Ophthalmology* 1987;94(Oct Suppl):135.
33. Wang RC, Zamir E, Dugel PU, et al: Progressive subretinal fibrosis and blindness associated with multifocal granulomatous chorioretinitis—a variant of sympathetic ophthalmia. *Ophthalmology*. In press.

William D. Bates

7 Glaucoma

As a result of improvements in ultrasound instrumentation, as well as significant advances in the treatment of glaucoma, the role of echography has become increasingly important in the evaluation of glaucoma patients. In addition, the indications for echography in this field are continually expanding.

The assessment of optic nerve cupping in the presence of opaque ocular media was one of the initial indications for the use of ultrasound in glaucoma.[9] Ultrasound subsequently has proved to be helpful in the differentiation and diagnosis of angle closure glaucoma, secondary glaucoma, and congenital (infantile) glaucoma. It is now commonly employed for the management of patients with glaucoma shunt surgery,[23] and it has become indispensable for the evaluation and management of complications following all types of glaucoma surgery.

New ultrasound technologies have emerged in recent years, including ultrasound biomicroscopy (UBM)[27,28] and color Doppler imaging.[21,22] These techniques now provide a better understanding of the pathophysiology of certain types of glaucoma and, in some cases, can aid in the diagnosis and management of these disorders (see Chapter 8 and Chapter 14).

OPTIC DISC

B-scan can provide a useful and reliable estimation of optic cup size in eyes with opaque ocular media. The technique for optic nerve head evaluation, as described on p 431 in Chapter 16, emphasizes the importance of positioning the probe so that the sound beam bypasses the lens, thereby maximizing resolution of the optic rim.

Although the assessment of cup size is somewhat unreliable for small and medium-sized cups, the detection of large cups has been shown to be relatively accurate[9] (Figure 7-1). In certain cases, however, the estimation of cup size may be especially challenging, such as when a large cup has a shallow, saucer-like shape. In these eyes, the resolution of the ultrasound system may be insufficient to resolve the borders of the optic rim, and therefore the enlarged cup may not be recognized. Additionally, membranes inserting into or overlying the optic disc may prevent echographic imaging of the optic cup. Consequently, the detection of a large cup can be considered a reliable finding; but if not detected, the diagnosis cannot be excluded.

When a large cup is detected, the possibility of a deep, congenital physiologic cup should be considered. Comparison with the fellow eye, provided the cup can be visualized with ophthalmoscopy, can usually help determine whether the echographic findings represent glaucomatous changes.

Pseudocupping of the optic disc can occur. This can be seen in eyes with marked, diffuse thickening of the retina and/or choroid surrounding the optic disc. The result is a cavity or depression overlying the optic nerve head that can mimic a large optic cup on B-scan (see Figure 6-18). Differentiation can usually be made, however, by comparing the thickness of the retinochoroid layer in the peripapillary region to other areas of the fundus and/or the fellow eye.

CONGENITAL GLAUCOMA

The clinical diagnosis of congenital glaucoma is generally established by the assessment of intraocular pressure, evaluation of the optic nerve, the measurement of corneal diameter, and gonioscopy (Figure 7-2). Diagnostic challenges arise because early optic disc cupping may be difficult to detect, corneal diameter and gonioscopy may be normal, and visual fields analysis is not possible. Also, the intraocular pressure may be normal at the time of examination under anesthesia, and the intraocular pressure may be influenced by the anesthetic agent.

Ultrasound biometry can be helpful for establishing the diagnosis of glaucoma in borderline cases and for monitoring the condition during treatment. Studies have shown a close correlation between longstanding changes in intraocular pressure and the axial eye length measurement.[3,24,30] Therefore changes in axial length may be the best indicator of the success or failure of glaucoma therapy.

The immersion technique is generally preferable to the contact method for detecting subtle changes in the length of the smaller eyes characteristic of the pediatric population (see p 259 and Table 10–1). In addition, B-scan examination can help evaluate and monitor the contour of the posterior ocular wall to determine if a posterior staphyloma is developing. It should be noted that as eyes with congenital glaucoma enlarge, the anterior chamber depth increases and lens

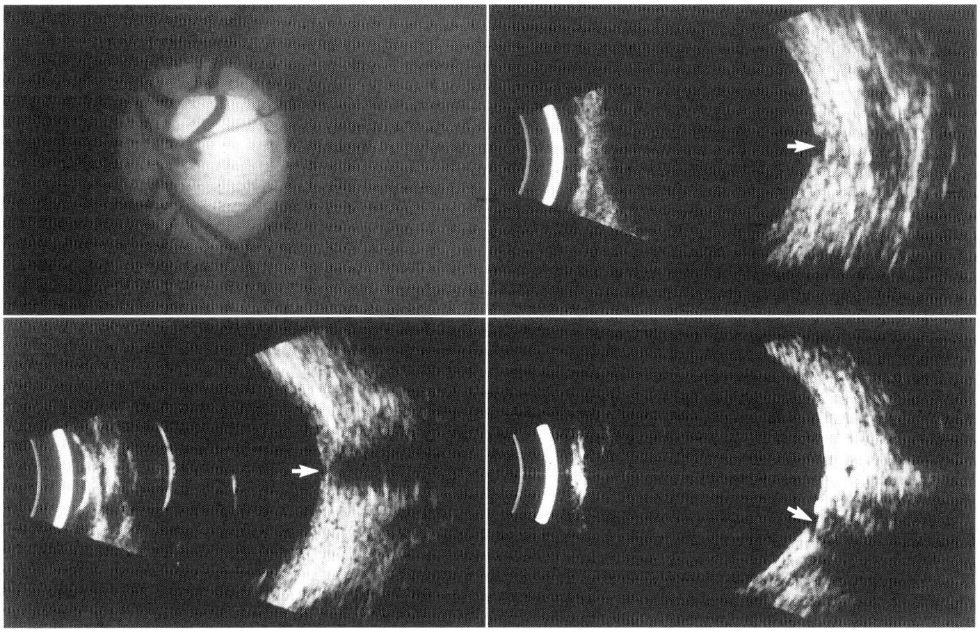

Figure 7-1 Large optic cup displayed in various B-scan views. **A,** Fundus photograph showing large optic cup. **B,** Optic cup is rather indistinct in vertical axial B-scan orientation. Cup is shown better in vertical transverse **(C)** and longitudinal 12-o'clock **(D)** views. *Arrows,* Optic cup.

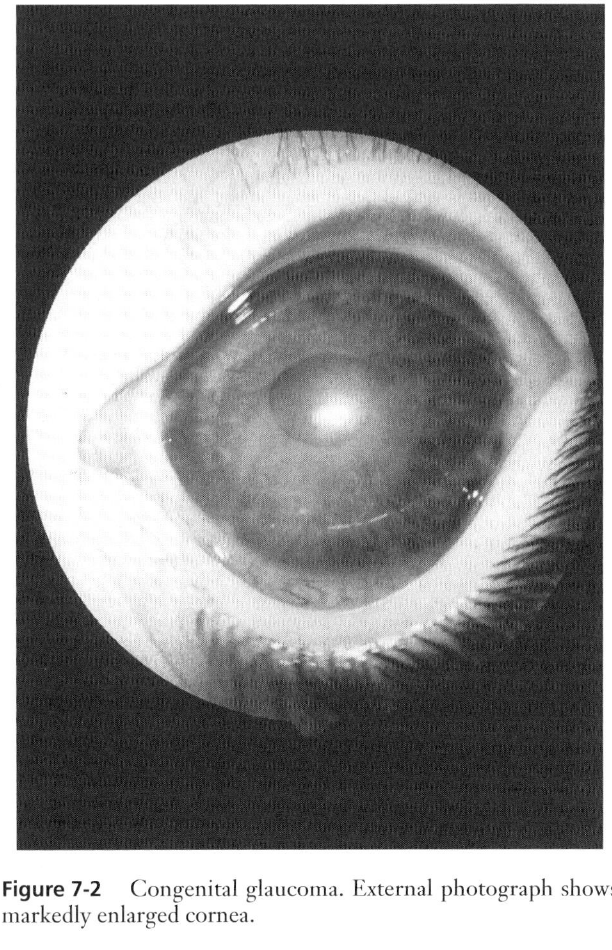

Figure 7-2 Congenital glaucoma. External photograph shows markedly enlarged cornea.

thickness decreases. This observation is helpful in differentiating congenital glaucoma from normal growth of the myopic eye. More recently, UBM has been used to evaluate the anterior segment of eyes with congenital glaucoma (see Chapter 8).[27,28]

Congenital glaucoma may also occur in Sturge-Weber syndrome. In addition to measuring axial eye length, ultrasound can demonstrate the diffuse choroidal hemangiomas that are often present in these eyes (see p 147).

ANGLE CLOSURE GLAUCOMA

Clinical findings of angle closure glaucoma include increased intraocular pressure, pain, redness, corneal edema, blurred vision, and a mid-dilated pupil. In these patients, gonioscopy typically shows a very narrow or closed anterior chamber angle. Corneal edema and, in some cases, cataract formation may prevent adequate visualization of the fundus.

In eyes with primary acute angle closure glaucoma, ultrasound can be used to document certain anatomic characteristics. These include a relatively shallow anterior chamber and short axial eye length, as well as diffuse thickening of the retinochoroid layer and sclera. In addition, these eyes often have somewhat thickened lenses, especially in the presence of cataractous changes. The echographic findings may also be valuable for identifying eyes with potentially occludable anterior chamber angles.

Ultrasound can also be helpful in identifying the many causes of secondary angle closure glaucoma, including intraocular tumors (see p 212), phacomorphic glaucoma (see

> **BOX 7-1**
> **Causes of Secondary Glaucoma**
> Lens abnormalities
> Pigmentary dispersion
> Intraocular tumors
> Intraocular hemorrhage
> Ciliochoroidal effusions
> Elevated episcleral venous pressure
> Inflammatory diseases

below), malignant glaucoma (see p 216), ciliochoroidal effusion (see p 216), intraocular hemorrhage (see p 213), iris bombe (see p 213), retinopathy of prematurity (see p 184), and persistent hyperplastic primary vitreous (see p 185).

Newer ultrasound technology, using higher frequency probes, allows a more detailed examination of anterior segment structures (see Figure 2-33 and Chapter 8). As a result, the mechanisms of angle closure glaucoma are now better understood. These newer techniques can also aid in the diagnosis of certain types of angle closure glaucoma, such as plateau iris (see p 229).

SECONDARY GLAUCOMA

There are many causes of secondary glaucoma in which ultrasound can be useful for both diagnosis and management (Box 7-1).

Lens Abnormalities

Phacolytic Glaucoma

Phacolytic glaucoma is a form of open angle glaucoma associated with a hypermature cataractous lens. Clinically, these patients present with an acute onset of monocular pain and redness. Slit-lamp examination of the anterior chamber shows a heavy flare and the presence of small crystals in the aqueous. In some cases, however, complete opacification of the anterior chamber occurs. It has been suggested that the material in the anterior chamber is a macrophagic response to extruded lens protein.[32] An immersion ultrasound examination usually demonstrates a thinner than normal lens and may also show displacement of the nucleus within the otherwise liquefied cortical material (Figure 7-3).

A less common variation of phacolytic glaucoma occurs when the lens has dislocated posteriorly into the vitreous and has undergone phacolysis. Vitreous reaction may prevent adequate visualization, and ultrasound can demonstrate the hypermature nature of the dislocated lens (see Figure 5-77).

Phacomorphic Glaucoma (Intumescent Lens)

Swelling of a cataractous lens produces phacomorphic glaucoma, a type of angle closure glaucoma with pupillary

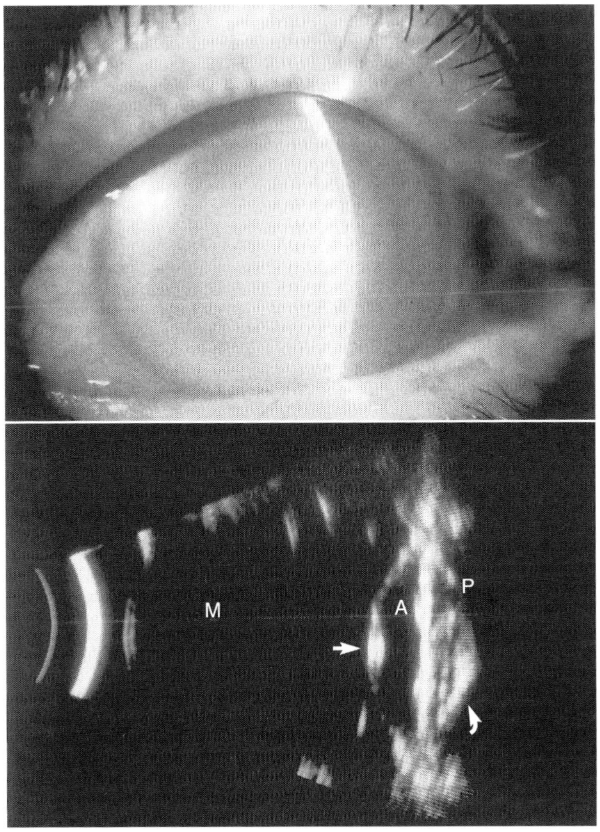

A

B

Figure 7-3 Phacolytic glaucoma in eye with hypermature cataractous lens. **A,** Slit-lamp photograph shows complete opacification of anterior chamber secondary to leakage of proteinaceous lens material. **B,** Immersion vertical axial B-scan of anterior segment demonstrates deep, clear anterior chamber *(A)* and a thin, cataractous lens with inferior displacement of the lens nucleus *(curved arrow)* within the otherwise liquefied cortical material. *M,* Methylcellulose within scleral shell. *P,* Posterior lens capsule.

block. An immersion ultrasound examination can detect shallowing of the anterior chamber and thickening of the cataractous lens (Figures 7-4 and 7-5).

Dislocated Lens

Dislocation of the lens anteriorly into the pupil or anterior chamber may result in acute narrow angle glaucoma secondary to pupillary block. If the cornea becomes opacified as a result of corneal edema, ultrasound can demonstrate the anterior displacement of the lens and rule out any posterior segment abnormalities (see Figure 7-5).

Pigmentary Glaucoma

Pigmentary glaucoma appears to occur secondary to pigmentary dispersion, presumably caused by mechanical rubbing of the lens zonules against the posterior iris pigment epithelium.[32] UBM has greatly contributed to the understanding of the pathophysiology of this disorder and its management (see p 230).

A 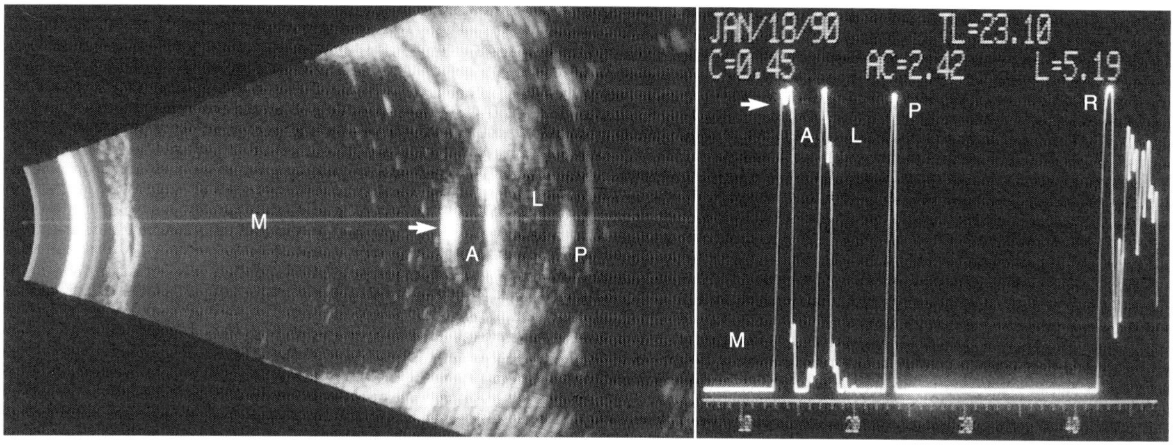 B

Figure 7-4 Phacomorphic glaucoma. Axial immersion B-scan **(A)** and immersion A-scan axial eye length measurement **(B)** demonstrate thickened cataractous lens *(L)* and shallowing of the anterior chamber *(A)*. *M*, Methylcellulose within scleral shell; *arrow*, cornea; *P*, posterior lens capsule; *R*, retina.

A 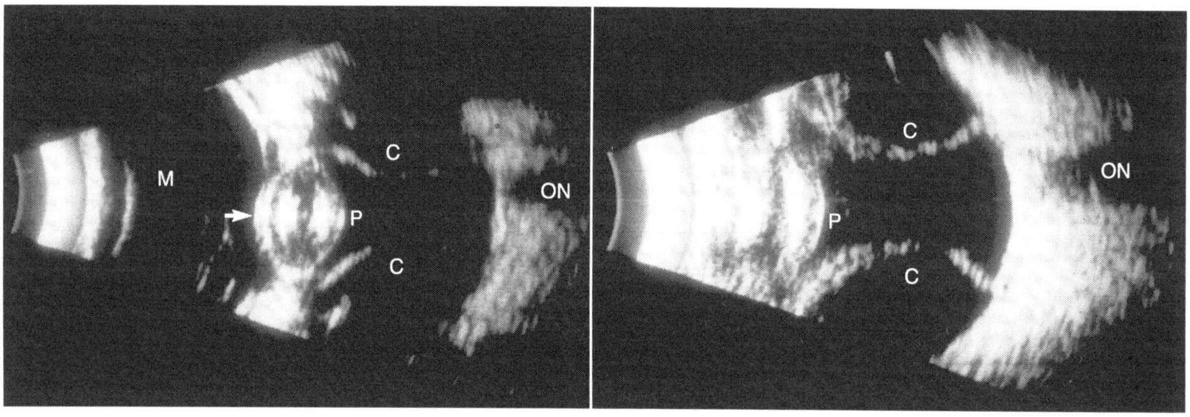 B

Figure 7-5 Anterior dislocation of intumescent lens. **A,** Immersion axial B-scan shows markedly thickened, densely cataractous lens dislocated anteriorly with complete flattening of the anterior chamber. Large, serous ciliochoroidal detachments *(C)* are also shown. *M*, Methylcellulose within scleral shell; *arrow*, cornea; *P*, posterior lens capsule, *ON*, optic nerve. **B,** Contact axial B-scan better demonstrates large ciliochoroidal detachments that caused the anterior dislocation of the intumescent lens.

Intraocular Tumors

Glaucoma is associated with a variety of intraocular tumors, the most common of which is uveal melanoma. The mechanism of glaucoma depends on whether the tumor involves the anterior or posterior segment. Glaucoma caused by anterior segment tumors may be secondary to direct invasion of the tumor into the anterior chamber angle or to angle closure. Posterior segment tumors, on the other hand, usually produce a form of angle closure glaucoma when they become very large and displace the lens/iris diaphragm anteriorly.

Anterior Segment Tumors

Benign and malignant tumors of the anterior segment may cause a secondary glaucoma. Primary cysts of the iris pigment epithelium, although rarely associated with secondary angle closure glaucoma, can be detected and differentiated from solid tumors with ultrasound (see pp 170 and 232). Secondary cysts (epithelial implantation cysts) may occur after surgery or trauma and are more likely than are primary cysts to cause glaucoma (see p 170). Solid benign tumors of the anterior segment that can be associated with glaucoma include iris nevi, melanocytomas, benign adenomas, and uveal lymphoid hyperplasia (with iris and/or ciliary body involvement) (see Chapter 5). Uveal melanoma is the most common malignant tumor of the anterior segment, although metastatic carcinoma and lymphoma can occur as well. A unique form of ciliary body melanoma, in which the tumor invades the ciliary body in a circumferential manner, has been referred to as ring melanoma.

Posterior Segment Tumors

Large choroidal melanoma is the most common type of posterior segment tumor that results in glaucoma. Ultrasound can often show a very large tumor pressing against the lens (see Figure 5-87). In rare cases, metastatic tumors to the choroid are associated with secondary glaucoma (see Figure 5-44).

Intraocular Tumors of Childhood

RETINOBLASTOMA

When a child presents with glaucoma in the presence of opaque ocular media, the diagnosis of retinoblastoma should be considered. The causes of glaucoma in patients with retinoblastoma include neovascularization of the iris, angle closure caused by massive retinal detachment, and obstruction of the anterior chamber angle by inflammatory cells or necrotic tumor tissue.[32] Ultrasound has proved to be very reliable in the diagnosis of retinoblastoma, largely because of the presence of calcium within the tumor (see p 180). In addition, ultrasound can differentiate retinoblastoma from other causes of leukokoria that may be associated with glaucoma, including Coats' disease (see p 187), persistent hyperplastic primary vitreous (PHPV) (see p 185), and retinopathy of prematurity (ROP) (see p 184). The most common cause of glaucoma in these cases is secondary angle closure. In Coats' disease, the angle closure may be secondary to a massive exudative retinal detachment that causes shallowing of the anterior chamber. In both ROP and PHPV, shallowing of the anterior chamber may be caused by contracture of retrolental fibrous membranes.[32]

MEDULLOEPITHELIOMA

Medulloepitheliomas are primary tumors of childhood that arise from the nonpigmented ciliary epithelium. A large number of these cases are associated with glaucoma. Ultrasound usually shows a well-defined ciliary body mass (see p 187).

NEUROFIBROMATOSIS

Glaucoma can be associated with neurofibromatosis, especially the peripheral form that includes not only intraocular tumors but also plexiform lesions of the lid (see p 315). Intraocular lesions can involve the iris, ciliary body, and choroid (see p 155).

Intraocular Hemorrhage

Intraocular hemorrhage can cause glaucoma in a variety of ways. This can occur from hyphema or longstanding vitreous hemorrhage, as well as from massive subvitreal, subretinal,[11] or suprachoroidal hemorrhage.

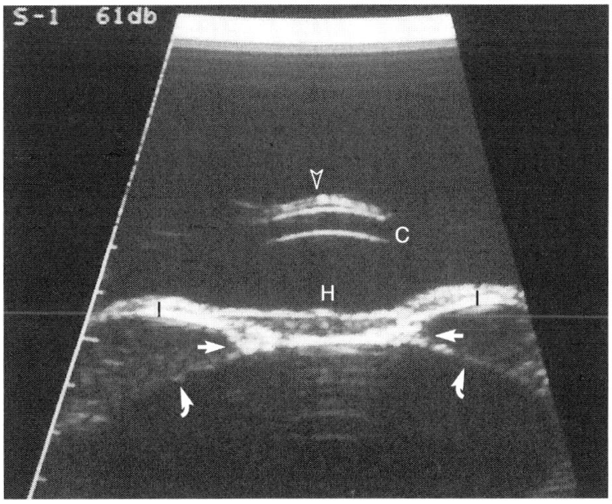

Figure 7-6 Anterior chamber hyphema and iris bombe. High-resolution axial B-scan (20 MHz) shows shallow hyphema *(H)* and forward bowing of iris *(I)*. Note adhesion of iris at pupillary margins *(straight arrows)* to anterior lens capsule *(curved arrows)*. *C*, Cornea; *open arrow*, surface of probe balloon tip on cornea. (Courtesy Rhonda Waldron, MMSc, COMT, Atlanta, Georgia.)

Hyphema

A large blood clot in the anterior chamber can mechanically occlude the trabecular meshwork, producing secondary open angle glaucoma. Ultrasound can be especially helpful when corneal blood staining prevents visualization of the anterior and posterior segments (Figure 7-6; see also Figure 4-1).

Vitreous Hemorrhage

In longstanding vitreous hemorrhage, red blood cells degenerate and become less pliable (ghost cells). In addition, macrophages can ingest the contents of the red blood cells. When the anterior hyaloid is disrupted, these ghost cells and macrophages can enter the anterior chamber and accumulate in the trabecular meshwork, causing elevation of the intraocular pressure (hemolytic/ghost cell glaucoma). Ultrasound can be useful for the diagnosis of this disorder by demonstrating diffuse opacities in the vitreous cavity. It should be noted that in the vitrectomized eye, a very high gain setting may be needed to detect diffuse, mild hemorrhage in the vitreous cavity (see Figure 4-45, *C* and *D*).

Subvitreal Hemorrhage

Occasionally, a massive subvitreal hemorrhage can push the vitreous body forward, causing shallowing of the anterior chamber and secondary angle closure glaucoma. Ultrasound can demonstrate the very dense nature of the subvitreal hemorrhage and forward displacement of the posterior hyaloid (see Figure 3-10).

A

B

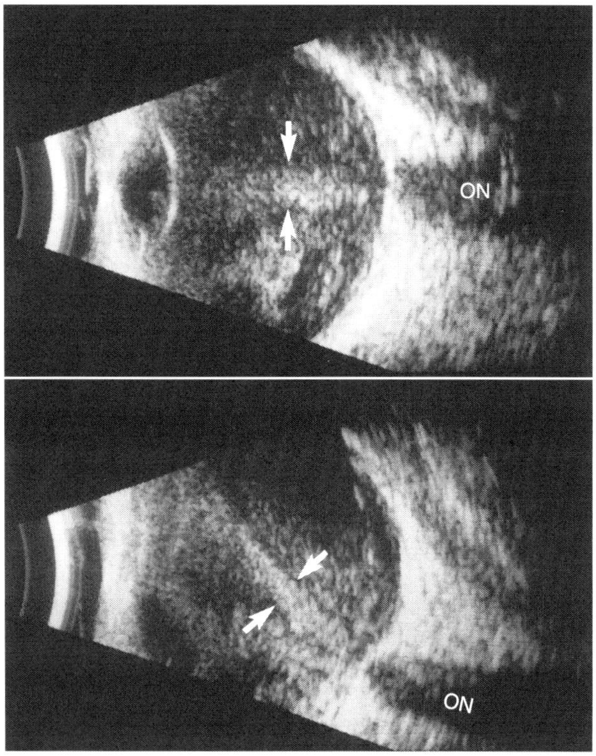

Figure 7-7 Massive subretinal hemorrhage secondary to age-related macular degeneration producing angle closure glaucoma. Axial (**A**) and longitudinal (**B**), B-scans show a total, closed, funnel-shaped retinal detachment *(arrows)* extending between posterior surface of the lens and the optic nerve *(ON)*. Note dense subretinal opacities.

Subretinal and Suprachoroidal Hemorrhage

Massive subretinal and/or suprachoroidal hemorrhage can displace the iris-lens diaphragm anteriorly, producing a secondary angle closure glaucoma. Ultrasound can demonstrate these detachments and the underlying hemorrhage. The most common cause of massive subretinal hemorrhage is age-related macular degeneration (Figure 7-7; see also p 159). Other causes include subretinal hemorrhage associated with intraocular tumors, the most common of which is choroidal melanoma. Although rare, massive subretinal hemorrhage secondary to a metastatic lung carcinoma to the choroid can also occur (see Figure 5-44).

Massive suprachoroidal hemorrhage usually develops either at the time of intraocular surgery (expulsive hemorrhage) or after severe penetrating trauma. Delayed suprachoroidal hemorrhage can also occur following intraocular surgery, most often after glaucoma surgery. The ultrasound characteristics of suprachoroidal hemorrhages are explained later in this chapter, as well as in Chapters 3 and 4.

Ciliochoroidal Effusion

Ciliochoroidal detachment can cause a forward rotation of the lens-iris diaphragm and angle closure glaucoma in a number of conditions.[12] These include uveal effusion syndrome, nanophthalmos, toxic reaction to systemic medications, arteriovenous fistulae (see below), and certain inflammatory disorders (see p 198). Angle closure secondary to ciliochoroidal effusion has also been shown to occur after scleral buckling procedures (see p 109), glaucoma surgery (see p 216), and panretinal photocoagulation.

Uveal Effusion Syndrome

Uveal effusion syndrome is characterized by spontaneous uveal effusions that produce thickening and detachment of the choroid and ciliary body, as well as serous retinal detachment. Glaucoma can occur if angle closure is present. In these cases, ultrasound typically shows a moderately short eye, diffusely thickened sclera, and detachment of the choroid and retina (see Figure 3-69).

Nanophthalmos

Nanophthalmos may present with ciliochoroidal detachments, similar to those seen in uveal effusion syndrome. Nanophthalmos is characterized by a very small eye with a shallow anterior chamber and unusually thick sclera. These eyes have a tendency to develop postoperative or spontaneous uveal effusions, which may cause a pupillary block and subsequent angle closure glaucoma. Ultrasound of a nanophthalmic eye typically demonstrates a short axial length and thickened sclera (see p 82).

Toxic Reaction to Systemic Medications

A number of cases have been reported in which a toxic reaction to systemic medications produced bilateral, shallow ciliochoroidal detachments (Figure 7-8). This resulted in shallowing of the anterior chamber, increased myopia, and in some cases, angle closure glaucoma. Ultrasound was essential for documenting the etiology of the clinical findings in these unusual cases.[34]

Elevated Episcleral Venous Pressure

A rise in episcleral venous pressure can produce an increase in intraocular pressure, resulting in glaucoma.[29] Conditions known to produce this phenomenon include arteriovenous fistulae and malformations (see pp 355 and 365), thyroid ophthalmopathy (see p 396), and Sturge-Weber syndrome (see p 147).

Arteriovenous Fistulae and Malformations

Arteriovenous fistulae and malformations include carotid-cavernous and dural-cavernous sinus fistulae and arteriovenous malformations of the orbit. These conditions produce increased arterial blood flow in the orbit, resulting in orbital soft tissue congestion and venous stasis.[1,29] Clinically, these patients may present with proptosis, characteristic dilatation of episcleral blood vessels, and frequently, increased intraocular pressure. Choroidal effusions with secondary angle

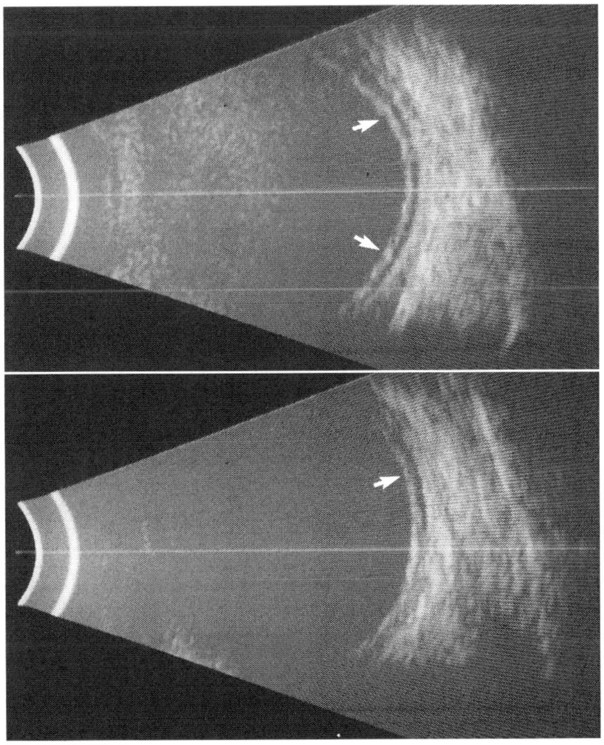

Figure 7-8 Annular ciliochoroidal detachments secondary to toxic reaction from systemic medication. Transverse **(A)** and longitudinal **(B)** B-scans demonstrate shallow, annular, peripheral ciliochoroidal detachments *(arrows)*. The patient also had shallow anterior chambers, increased myopia, and secondary angle closure glaucoma.

closure can also occur in these patients. Ultrasound can be useful both for diagnosing these disorders and for demonstrating the presence of choroidal effusions.

Thyroid Ophthalmopathy

Increased intraocular pressure can develop as a result of elevated episcleral venous pressure in patients with thyroid ophthalmopathy. This increased venous pressure is caused by the obstruction of venous outflow produced by orbital congestion. Inflammation and fibrosis of the extraocular muscles can also contribute to increased intraocular pressure in patients with thyroid ophthalmopathy, leading to a mechanical restriction of ocular motility and a rise in intraocular pressure when eye movement is attempted (especially with upgaze).[29] Ultrasound has proved to be very effective for evaluating this disorder, particularly when the patient does not present with the typical signs of thyroid ophthalmopathy. The findings usually include bilateral extraocular muscle thickening and orbital soft tissue swelling (see p 396).

Inflammatory Diseases

Inflammatory diseases can produce secondary glaucoma in a number of ways. Anterior uveitis can lead to anterior synechiae, resulting in increased intraocular pressure. Posterior synechiae can produce iris bombe and secondary angle closure glaucoma. Angle closure can also be caused by ciliochoroidal detachments associated with posterior scleritis or by inflammatory infiltration of the ciliary body in disorders such as Vogt-Koyanagi-Harada syndrome (VKH) (see p 200) and sympathetic ophthalmia (see p 201).

Anterior Uveitis

Anterior uveitis can produce anterior synechiae that may lead to secondary angle closure. These anterior synechiae are best demonstrated with high resolution B-scan (see p 230). Posterior synechiae can also develop, producing adhesions of the iris to the crystalline or pseudophakic lens. This can result in iris bombe and angle closure glaucoma, secondary to pupillary block. Ultrasound can demonstrate the anterior bowing of the iris and can rule out an underlying cyst or solid mass (see Figure 7-6 and Chapter 8).

Posterior Scleritis

Posterior scleritis can produce choroidal effusions, resulting in angle closure glaucoma. Ultrasound can show the diffusely thickened sclera typically seen in this disorder, as well as the anterior effusions (see p 195 and Figure 6-11).

Vogt-Koyanagi-Harada Syndrome/ Sympathetic Ophthalmia

Both VKH and sympathetic ophthalmia are characterized by diffuse inflammatory infiltration of the choroid. When the uveal inflammation involves the periphery of the eye, thickening of the peripheral choroid and ciliary body can cause anterior rotation of the ciliary body and iris. This can lead to shallowing of the anterior chamber and secondary angle closure glaucoma. Ultrasound is an ideal method of showing the diffuse thickening of the choroid (see Figure 6-15) and ciliary body (see p 77).

NORMAL-TENSION GLAUCOMA

Although the pathogenesis of glaucomatous damage in normal-tension glaucoma is unknown, in recent years, color Doppler ultrasound has provided an increased understanding of this disorder.[17,19] The use of color Doppler imaging to measure blood flow velocities in the ophthalmic artery, central retinal artery, and posterior ciliary arteries has shown that eyes with normal-tension glaucoma have an increased vascular resistance distal to the ophthalmic artery. This implies that the glaucomatous damage in these patients may have a vasogenic etiology resulting in reduced blood flow to the optic nerve. Ongoing studies utilizing color Doppler imaging may further clarify the pathogenesis of normal-tension glaucoma and may assist in the development of new treatments for this disorder (see Chapter 14).

COMPLICATIONS OF GLAUCOMA SURGERY

Certain surgical complications that are unique to or that occur more commonly after glaucoma surgery include malignant glaucoma, hypotony, and choroidal hemorrhage. Endophthalmitis secondary to infected filtering blebs can also occur.[5,20] Ultrasound has become an indispensable tool for the evaluation and management of these complications.

Malignant Glaucoma

Shallowing of the anterior chamber associated with normal or high intraocular pressure sometimes presents as a complication following glaucoma surgery. Traditionally the diagnosis of malignant glaucoma has been made once other possible causes of these findings have been excluded (i.e., suprachoroidal hemorrhage and pupillary block). This complication is generally believed to be a result of misdirection of aqueous into the vitreous cavity. The misdirected aqueous is thought to produce pockets of fluid behind the vitreous body, displacing the vitreous forward and resulting in shallowing of the anterior chamber and increased intraocular pressure. No imaging technique, including ultrasound, has been able to demonstrate this phenomenon. One echographic study, however, of patients with a clinical diagnosis of malignant glaucoma showed that all of the patients demonstrated peripheral annular ciliochoroidal detachments.[10] The investigators concluded that these peripheral detachments may simulate aqueous misdirection.

Annular Ciliochoroidal Detachment

Annular ciliochoroidal detachments have been found as a postoperative complication of glaucoma surgery. They are associated with a shallow anterior chamber and normal to high intraocular pressure, apparently caused by anterior rotation of the ciliary body-iris diaphragm. The clinical presentation of these detachments is similar to that of malignant glaucoma (aqueous misdirection) and can be difficult or impossible to detect with ophthalmoscopy. Ultrasound is the key tool for confirming the diagnosis of annular peripheral ciliochoroidal detachments (although concurrent aqueous misdirection cannot be excluded).[10] These peripheral detachments can usually be imaged using contact techniques by directing the sound beam to the far peripheral aspect of the eye (see Figure 7-8 and Figure 3-61). Immersion techniques, however, using both conventional and UBM instrumentation, may more elegantly demonstrate the ciliary body detachment (see p 230 and Figure 3-62). A recently introduced high resolution B-scan (20 MHz) probe, using a contact stand-off technique, also appears to be an easy, safe, and effective method of demonstrating the ciliary body detachments in these cases (Figure 7-9). The medical or surgical management of these detachments can be readily monitored with ultrasound.

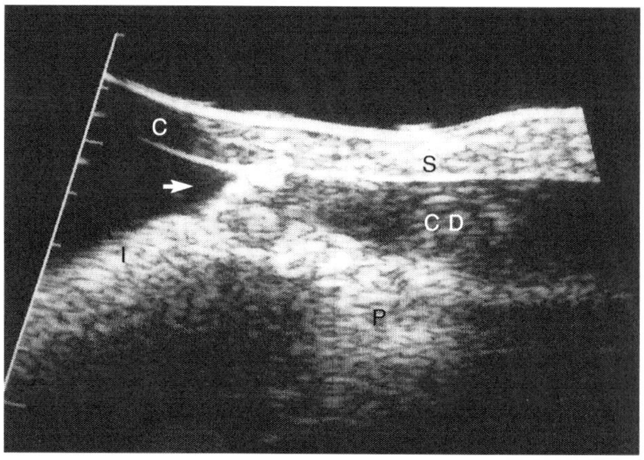

Figure 7-9 Ciliary body detachment. High resolution B-scan (20 MHz) (longitudinal view) through ciliary body and peripheral aspect of anterior chamber shows significant ciliary body detachment *(CD)*. Note the presence of echoes within the supraciliary space indicating hemorrhage and/or inflammation. *C*, Cornea; *arrow*, anterior chamber angle; *I*, iris; *P*, pars plicata; *S*, sclera. (Courtesy Rhonda Waldron, MMSc, COMT, Atlanta, Georgia.)

Hypotony

Although low intraocular pressure commonly occurs after glaucoma surgery, persistent hypotony can lead to serious ocular sequelae. Low pressure is often associated with a shallow anterior chamber that, in most cases, is due to overfiltration of aqueous. This shallowing of the chamber, however, can also be secondary to serous choroidal detachments resulting from the low intraocular pressure. Chronic hypotony can lead to macular abnormalities, including edema, striae and folds ("hypotony maculopathy").[13,18]

In patients with hypotony and opaque ocular media, ultrasound can document the presence of choroidal detachments (see p 74). In addition, chronic hypotony has been shown to cause a decrease in axial eye length measurements (see Chapter 10). Other echographic findings in these eyes include diffuse thickening of the retinochoroid layer and sclera. Ultrasound examination of the macula may, however, show more pronounced thickening of the retinochoroid layer and/or shallow focal detachment of the retina, retinal pigment epithelium or choroid (Figure 7-10). Maculopathy following hypotony may persist even after normal intraocular pressure has been restored. Anecdotal experience with ultrasound, in patients with chronic hypotony, has shown that the scleral thickening remains even after the pressure increases[15] (Figure 7-11). Further studies may help determine the period of time that an eye can tolerate low intraocular pressure before scleral thickening and maculopathy become irreversible.

Chronic hypotony, if not reversed, will ultimately lead to marked shrinkage of the eye. This, in turn, can produce atrophy and degeneration of intraocular structures with calcification of the posterior ocular coats. The ultrasound findings for this process, phthisis bulbi, can be found on p 114.

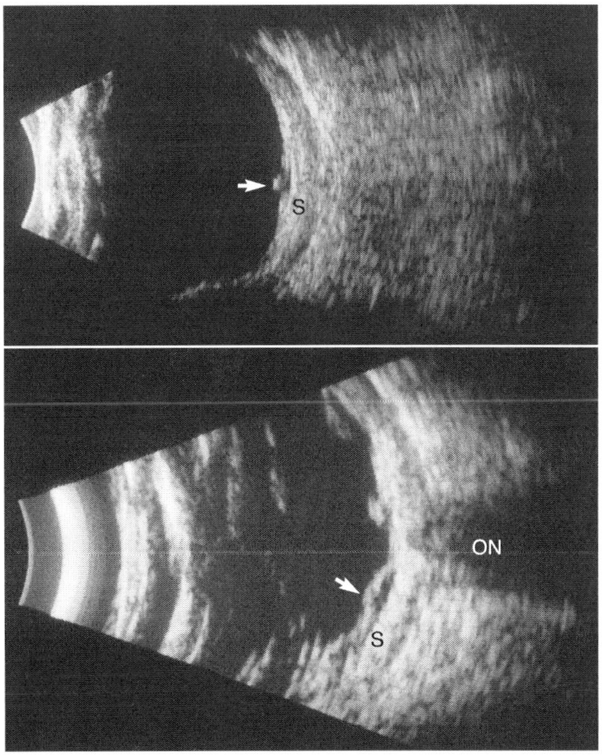

Figure 7-10 Hypotony maculopathy in two different patients. Vertical transverse **(A)** and horizontal axial **(B)** B-scans through macula show diffuse thickening of retinochoroid layer and sclera *(S)* with a focal, dome-shaped membrane *(arrow)*. These membranes may represent focal detachment of the retina, pigment epithelium, or choroid. *ON*, optic nerve.

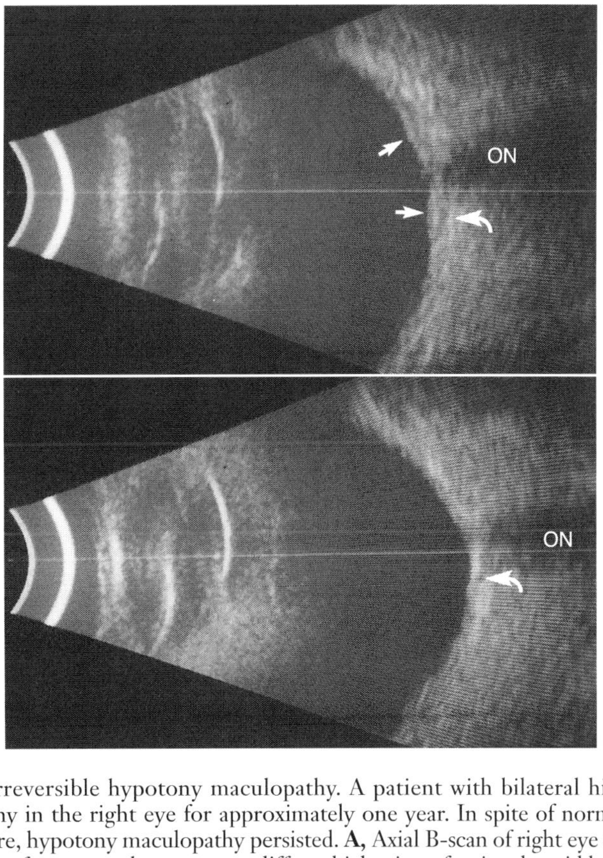

Figure 7-11 Irreversible hypotony maculopathy. A patient with bilateral high myopia had chronic hypotony in the right eye for approximately one year. In spite of normalization of intraocular pressure, hypotony maculopathy persisted. **A,** Axial B-scan of right eye obtained at time of normalization of pressure, demonstrates diffuse thickening of retinochoroid layer and sclera in peripapillary region *(straight arrows)* including the macula *(curved arrow)*. **B,** Axial B-scan of fellow left eye shows significantly longer globe and no appreciable thickening of the retinochoroid layer and sclera. Axial length measurements were 25 mm in the right eye and 28 mm in the left eye.

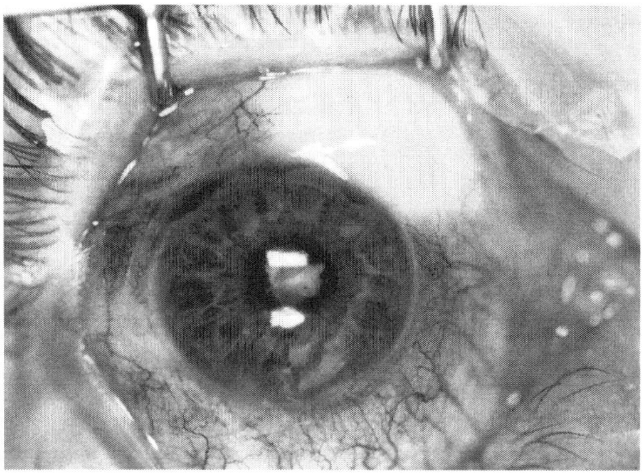

Figure 7-12 External photograph of infected filtering bleb. (Courtesy Dr. Don Minckler, Los Angeles, California.)

Choroidal Hemorrhage

Although massive suprachoroidal hemorrhage (i.e., expulsive hemorrhage) can be an intraoperative complication of any type of intraocular surgery (see Figure 4-34), delayed hemorrhagic choroidal detachments most commonly develop following glaucoma filtering procedures.[16] These delayed lesions usually present within the first few postoperative days but can occur significantly later. The frequency of these hemorrhages appears to increase in eyes that have undergone previous intraocular surgical procedures such as cataract extraction and/or vitrectomy. They are usually accompanied by the onset of severe ocular pain, redness, and in some cases, increased intraocular pressure. The echographic findings for choroidal hemorrhages have been previously described (see p 75). Massive hemorrhagic choroidal detachments may demonstrate apposition (kissing) in the central vitreous cavity (see p 104).

Serial ultrasound examinations can be performed to monitor for regression of the choroidal detachments and status of the retina when the patient is managed conservatively. When surgical intervention is contemplated, however, the ultrasound documentation of suprachoroidal blood clot lysis (see p 106 and Figure 4-38) can be useful for timing the surgical procedure. Studies have shown that the average time required for clot lysis is 14 days.[7]

Endophthalmitis

Endophthalmitis can occur after any type of intraocular surgery. However, patients who have undergone trabeculectomy have a higher incidence of endophthalmitis after the immediate postoperative period because of subsequent infection of the filtering bleb. Inflammation of the filtering bleb (blebitis)[4] (Figure 7-12) and signs of anterior segment inflammation may suggest but do not necessarily indicate the presence of endophthalmitis.[2,5] Conservative management can be undertaken if the inflammation has not extended into the posterior segment.[4,35] In such situations, ultrasound can be used to evaluate the posterior segment for concurrent signs of inflammation (e.g., vitreous opacities and membranes, retinal, and choroidal detachments, see Chapters 3 and 6).

Potential Error in Intraocular Lens Calculations

Successful glaucoma filtering surgery often results in a shortened axial eye length measurement due to the lower intraocular pressure. This can lead to challenges in determining the intraocular lens (IOL) power if subsequent cataract surgery with IOL placement is planned. The problem in these situations is that if the pressure in the eye increases following the cataract procedure, the axial length may also increase, resulting in an unanticipated postoperative myopia. One study compared axial length measurements pre- and post-trabeculectomy as well as following cataract surgery.[6] This small series of patients showed that the axial length decreased after successful trabeculectomy surgery but then increased back toward pre-trabeculectomy values following the cataract surgery. There are no studies to date, however, that address the changes in axial length that occur in eyes with chronic hypotony following cataract surgery.

As previously noted, selection of the IOL power can be quite challenging in patients who have undergone a trabeculectomy or other types of glaucoma filtering surgery. A determination needs to be made in these patients as to the likelihood that the axial length will increase following cataract surgery. In patients with very low intraocular pressure that has persisted for a long period of time, the axial length may not change significantly following cataract surgery. On the other hand, eyes with moderate lowering of pressure following trabeculectomy may revert back to pre-trabeculectomy axial length values following cataract surgery. As a result of these possible scenarios, adjustments in the IOL power to be used may be necessary.

GLAUCOMA-FILTERING IMPLANT DEVICES (SHUNTS)

The surgical implantation of drainage devices has been used increasingly in recent years in the management of complicated glaucomas. Several somewhat similar devices are currently used. Each consists of a tube that extends from the anterior chamber (or in some cases the vitreous cavity) to a plate located on the sclera, beneath the conjunctiva and Tenon's capsule. These devices differ in size and shape, as well as in the materials from which they are constructed. They either have an open, unobstructed drainage tube or a pressure-regulating valve. When a device does not include a pressure valve, an absorbable suture is typically placed around the drainage tube at the time of surgery. Absorption of the suture over time allows a gradual lowering of the intraocular pressure to prevent complications that can occur from a sudden drop in pressure.

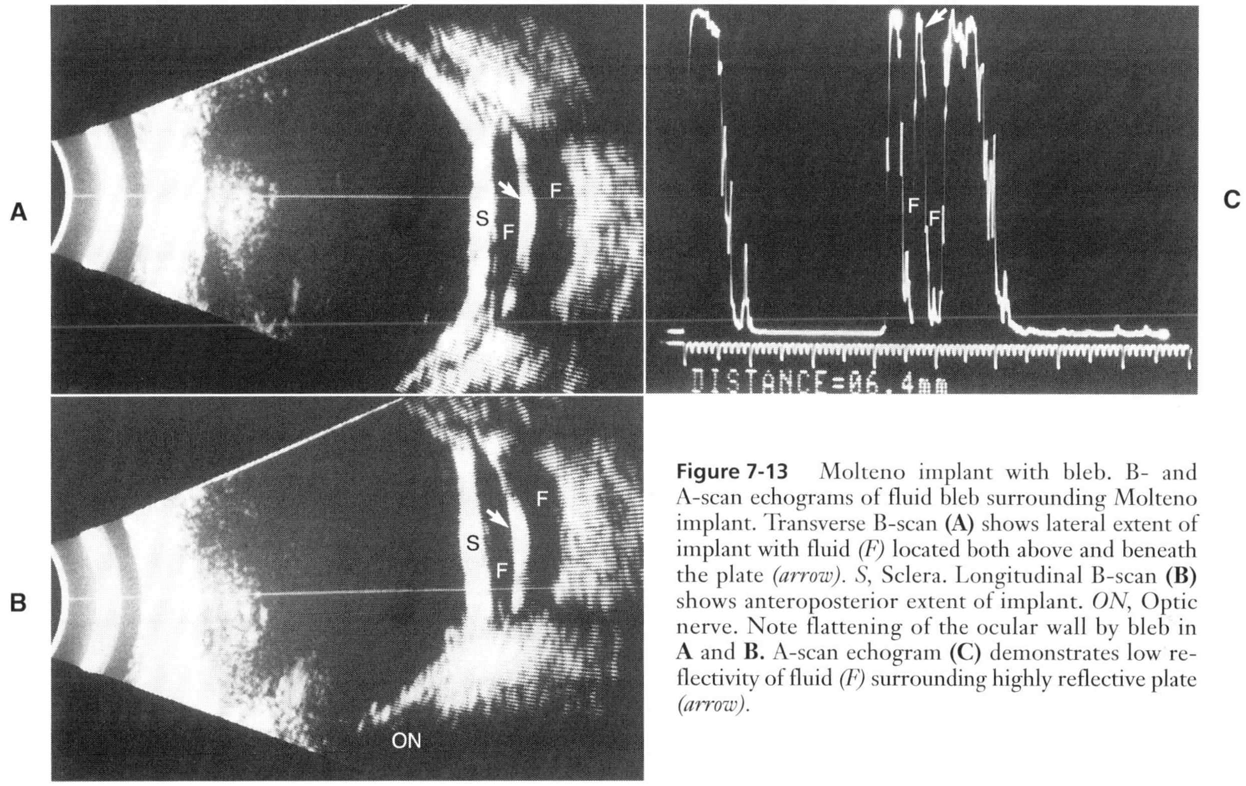

Figure 7-13 Molteno implant with bleb. B- and A-scan echograms of fluid bleb surrounding Molteno implant. Transverse B-scan **(A)** shows lateral extent of implant with fluid *(F)* located both above and beneath the plate *(arrow)*. *S*, Sclera. Longitudinal B-scan **(B)** shows anteroposterior extent of implant. *ON*, Optic nerve. Note flattening of the ocular wall by bleb in **A** and **B.** A-scan echogram **(C)** demonstrates low reflectivity of fluid *(F)* surrounding highly reflective plate *(arrow)*.

After the plate is inserted, a capsule forms around it, thus providing a potential space in which a fluid bleb can be contained. Because the plate is often placed in a relatively posterior position on the globe, the bleb can be difficult to observe clinically. In such situations, ultrasound can be used to image the plate and determine if a bleb has been created.[23]

On B-scan, the bleb appears as an echolucent region adjacent to (underlying and/or overlying) the plate.[14,23] Flattening or indentation of the adjacent sclera is sometimes noted. B-scan localization of the bleb and plate is best achieved with the use of both transverse and longitudinal scans (see Chapter 2). The transverse view shows the lateral extent of the plate (for example, from the 12:30 to 2:30 clock positions), whereas the longitudinal view demonstrates the posterior extent relative to the optic nerve. On A-scan, the plate is represented as a highly reflective spike just posterior to the scleral spike. The fluid bleb exhibits very low (cystlike) internal reflectivity in contrast to the highly reflective spike from the plate (Figure 7-13). Localization of the plate can be challenging if no bleb is present because the highly reflective plate (e.g., Molteno implant) may be difficult to distinguish from the normal highly reflective sclera and orbital soft tissues. For the Molteno implant, plate location is best identified by noting shadowing produced by the thick edges of the plate (Figure 7-14).

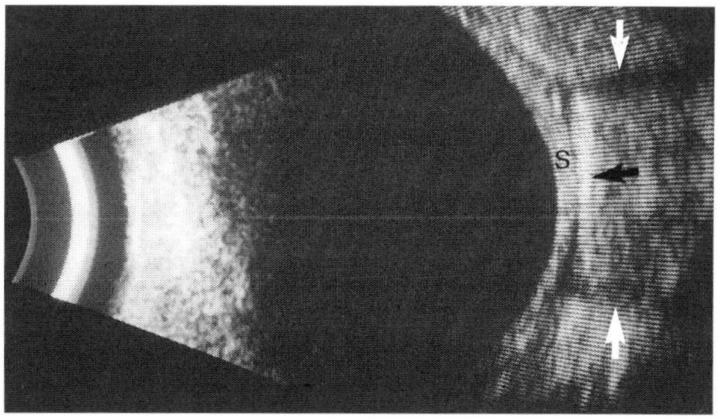

Figure 7-14 Molteno plate without bleb. Transverse B-scan shows highly reflective plate *(black arrow)* adjacent to sclera *(S)*. Note thin areas of shadowing *(white arrows)* produced by edges of plate. (From Lloyd MA, Minckler DS, Heuer DK: Echographic evaluation of glaucoma shunts. *Ophthalmology* 1993;100:921.)

The echographic detection of a bleb correlates well with the patency of a drainage tube, although bleb size has not been shown to correlate with intraocular pressure.[23] In some cases, very large blebs are associated with high intraocular pressure, and conversely, shallow blebs may be present when the pressure is low. Nevertheless, the echographic findings are very important for the postoperative management of these patients. For example, if the intraocular pressure is

A

B

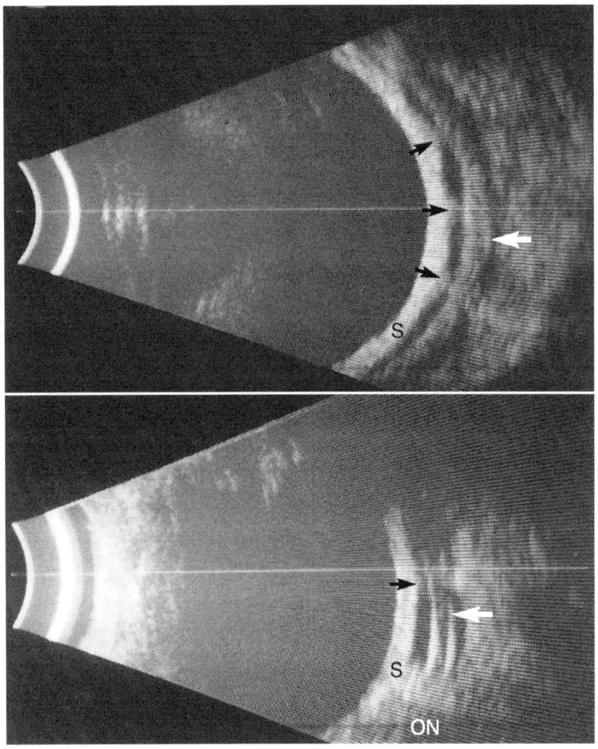

Figure 7-15 Baerveldt implant with bleb. **A,** Transverse B-scan demonstrates thick, circumferential band representing silicone Baerveldt plate *(white arrow)*. Echolucent region on either side of band indicates fluid bleb. Note the scalloped appearance of the bleb due to fibrous tissue growth through fenestration holes in plate *(black arrows)*. *S*, Sclera. **B,** Longitudinal B-scan shows plate *(white arrow)* and bleb extending posteriorly toward optic nerve *(ON)*. On B-scan, the silicone Baerveldt plate normally appears relatively echolucent as in **B.** The more echodense appearance in **A** is due to a slightly oblique section to emphasize the scalloped nature of the bleb.

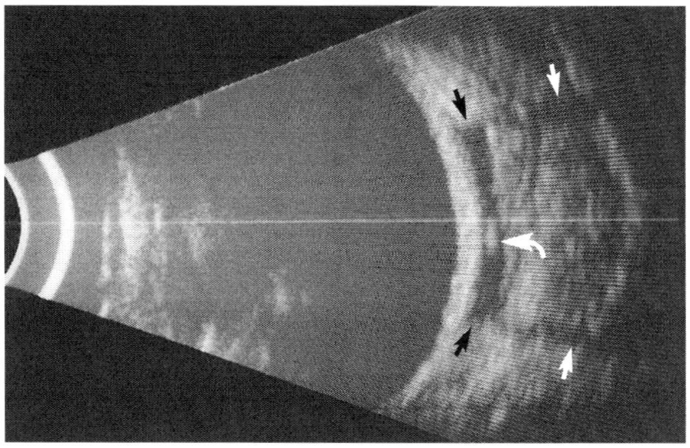

Figure 7-16 Ahmed implant without bleb. Transverse B-scan shows lateral extent of silicone plate *(black arrows)*. Note dense echo in center of plate *(curved arrow)* representing implant valve. *White arrows*, Thin regions of shadowing produced by edges of plate.

high and ultrasound detects no bleb, this may indicate that the ligature has not absorbed or the drainage tube is plugged or kinked. On the other hand, high pressure in the presence of a bleb may indicate that the eye is in a hypertensive, encapsulated bleb phase. This is a period of time, usually 1 to 3 months postoperatively, when high pressure can occur in the presence of a functioning tube. However, this could also mean that further medical or surgical treatment is indicated.

The absence of a bleb in the presence of low intraocular pressure may indicate insufficient aqueous production, excessive flow around the tube, or detachment of the choroid or retina. Alternatively, if the pressure is low and a bleb is present, there is likely to be excessive flow through the bleb walls.

Several different drainage devices are currently being used in the treatment of complicated glaucomas. The single plate Molteno implant was the first glaucoma filtering device developed.[25,26] This device was subsequently redesigned with two plates to increase the surface area of the bleb. With the double-plate Molteno implant, ultrasound can demonstrate a plate and bleb adjacent to the globe both supratemporally and supranasally.

Another drainage device currently in use is the Baerveldt implant.[33] In this implant, the plate is made of silicone (see p 112); therefore it appears significantly thicker and less reflective on ultrasound than the Molteno implant. As a result, the plate is sometimes difficult to distinguish from the surrounding bleb. The initial Baerveldt implants produced very large blebs, often causing marked flattening of the globe. More recent versions of the Baerveldt implant have been designed with multiple perforations of the plate. These perforations allow fibrous bands to grow between the bleb walls, thus limiting the size of the bleb. On B-scan, the bleb created by these perforated plates has a scalloped appearance (Figure 7-15).

The Ahmed implant, also made of silicone, has a pressure-sensitive valve that eliminates the need for a slow releasing ligature around the tube.[8] On B-scan, the Ahmed plate appears similar to the Baerveldt plate, although the contour of its anterior surface is somewhat irregular. The valve within the plate can also be demonstrated (Figure 7-16).

The Schocket tube shunt is a drainage device that uses a tube extending from the anterior chamber to a silicone band that completely encircles the globe.[31] In many cases, the encircling band is already present from previous retinal detachment surgery (i.e., a scleral buckle; see p 109). Ultrasound is generally not very effective in assessing the function of the Schocket device because sound attenuation from the encircling band prevents adequate imaging of the filtering bleb.

Anterior chamber hyphemas and/or hypopyons can produce drainage of blood or inflammatory cells into a filtering

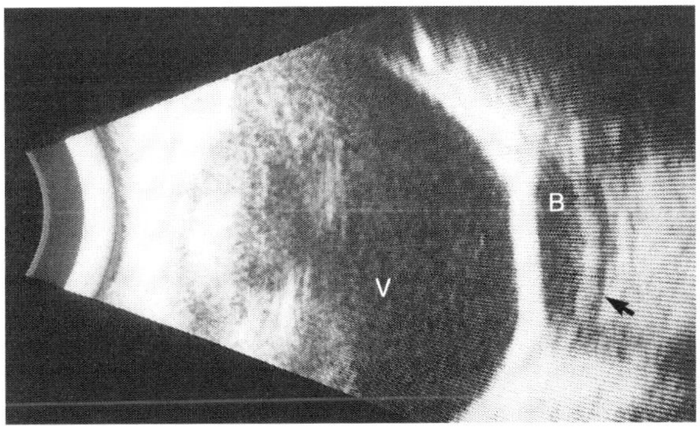

Figure 7-17 Molteno implant with hemorrhagic bleb. Transverse B-scan displays Molteno plate *(black arrow)* and blood within the bleb *(B)*. Note also diffuse hemorrhage within vitreous cavity *(V)*. (From Lloyd MA, Minckler DS, Heuer DK: Echographic evaluation of glaucoma shunts. *Ophthalmology* 1993;100:924.)

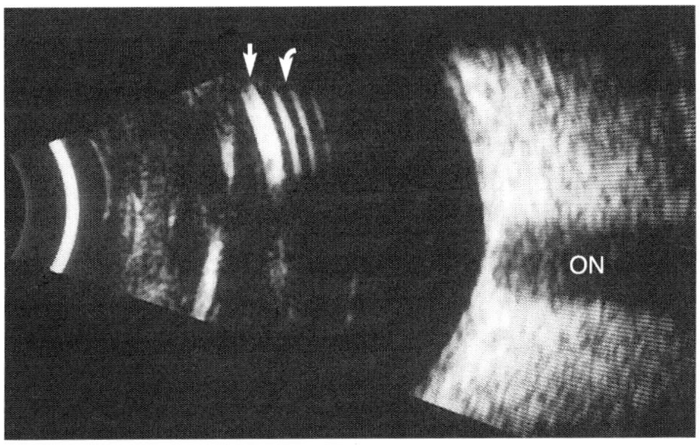

Figure 7-18 Molteno tube through pars plana. Axial B-scan of aphakic eye shows tube *(straight arrow)* extending from pars plana into anterior vitreous cavity. Multiple signals *(curved arrow)* extend posterior to tube. *ON*, Optic nerve. (From Lloyd MA, Minckler DS, Heuer DK: Echographic evaluation of glaucoma shunts. *Ophthalmology* 1993;100:924.)

bleb. When this occurs, B-scan can detect opacities within the bleb (Figure 7-17).

In some situations, clinical signs may suggest infection of the sclera adjacent to the filtering device. The ability of ultrasound to evaluate the sclera in this region is, however, somewhat limited because of sound attenuation from the plate. However, the existence of an occult infection may be suggested by the demonstration of scleral and/or episcleral thickening adjacent to the plate and bleb (see p 199 and Figure 6-14).

The tube placed in the anterior chamber with glaucoma filtering devices usually cannot be imaged with traditional contact B-scan instrumentation. High resolution B-scan instruments, on the other hand, can often localize these tubes and, in some cases, can determine whether they are patent. Tubes are sometimes inserted into the anterior vitreous cavity through the pars plana rather than into the anterior chamber. When this occurs, contact B-scan can often demonstrate the anterior aspect of the tube (Figure 7-18).

REFERENCES

1. Atta HR, Dick AD, Byrne SF, et al: Venous stasis orbitopathy—a clinical and echographic study. *Br J Ophthalmol* 1996;80:129.
2. Ayyala RS, Bellows AR, Thomas JV, et al: Bleb infections. Clinically different courses of "blebitis" and endophthalmitis. *Ophthalmic Surgery and Lasers* 1997;28:452.
3. Bluth K: Ultrasonic biometry in congenital glaucoma, in Hillman JS, LeMay MM (eds): *Ophthalmic Ultrasonography*. Dordrecht, Dr W Junk, 1984, p 191.
4. Brown RH, Yang LH, Walker SD, et al: Treatment of bleb infection after glaucoma surgery. *Arch Ophthalmol* 1994;112:57.
5. Ciulla TA, Beck AD, Topping TM et al: Blebitis, early endophthalmitis, and late endophthalmitis after glaucoma-filtering surgery. *Ophthalmology* 1997;104:986.
6. Cashwell FL, Martin CA: Axial length decrease accompanying successful glaucoma filtration surgery. *Ophthalmology* 1999;106:2308.
7. Chu TG, Cano MR, Green RL: Massive suprachoroidal hemorrhage with retinal apposition. *Arch Ophthalmol* 1991;109:1575.
8. Coleman AL, Hill R, Wilson MR, et al: Initial clinical experience with the Ahmed glaucoma valve implant. *Am J Ophthalmol* 1995;102:894.
9. Darnley-Fisch DA, Byrne SF, Hughes JR, et al: Contact B-scan echography in the assessment of optic nerve cupping. *Am J Ophthalmol* 1990;109:59.
10. Dugel PU, Heuer DK, Thach AB: Annular peripheral choroidal detachment simulating aqueous misdirection after glaucoma surgery. *Ophthalmology* 1997;104:439.
11. El Baba F, Jarrett WH, Harbin TS, et al: Massive hemorrhage complicating age-related macular degeneration. *Ophthalmology* 1986; 93:1581.
12. Fourman S: Angle-closure glaucoma complicating ciliochoroidal detachment. *Ophthalmology* 1989;96:646.
13. Gass JDM: Hypotony maculopathy, in Bellows JC (ed): *Contemporary Ophthalmology honoring Sir Stewart Duke-Elder*. Baltimore, Williams & Wilkins, 1972, p 343.
14. Green RL, Lloyd MA, Minckler DS, et al: Echographic evaluation of Molteno implants. ARVO Abstracts. *Invest Ophthalmol Vis Sci* 1991;2:746.
15. Green RL: Chronic hypotony. Personal communication, 2001.
16. Gressel MG, Parrish RK, Heuer DK: Delayed nonexpulsive suprachoroidal hemorrhage. *Arch Ophthalmol* 1984;102:1757.
17. Harris A, Sergott RC, Spaeth, et al: Color Doppler analysis of ocular vessel blood velocity in normal-tension glaucoma. *Am J Ophthalmol* 1994;118:642.
18. Jampel HD, Pasquale LR, DiBernardo CL: Hypotony maculopathy following trabeculectomy with mitomycin C. *Arch Ophthalmol* 1992;110:1049.
19. Kaiser HJ, Schoetzau A, Stumpfig D, et al: Blood-flow velocities of the extraocular vessels in patients with high-tension and normal-tension primary open-angle glaucoma. *Am J Ophthalmol* 1997; 123:320.
20. Kangas TA, Greenfield DS, Flynn HW, et al: Delayed-onset endophthalmitis associated with conjunctival filtering blebs. *Ophthalmology* 1997;104:746.
21. Lieb WE, Flaharty PM, Sergott RC, et al: Color Doppler imaging provides accurate assessment of orbital blood flow in occlusive carotid artery disease. *Ophthalmology* 1991;98:548.
22. Lieb WE: Color Doppler imaging of the eye and orbit. *Radiol Clin North Am* 1998;36:1059.
23. Lloyd MA, Minckler DS, Heuer DK: Echographic evaluation of glaucoma shunts. *Ophthalmology* 1993;100:919.
24. Massin M, Pellat B: Ultrasonic biometry in congenital glaucoma—a clinical study, in Hillman JS, LeMay MM (eds): *Ophthalmic Ultrasonography*. Dordrecht, Dr W Junk, 1984, p 191.
25. Minckler DS, Heuer DK, Hasty B, et al: Clinical experience with the single-plate Molteno implant in complicated glaucomas. *Ophthalmology* 1988;95:1181.

26. Molteno ACB: New implant for drainaåge in glaucoma: clinical trial. *Br J Ophthalmol* 1969;53:606.
27. Pavlin CJ, Foster FS: *Ultrasound Biomicroscopy of the Eye.* New York, Springer-Verlag, 1995.
28. Pavlin CJ, Foster FS: Ultrasound Biomicroscopy: high-frequency ultrasound imaging of the eye and microscopic resolution. *Radiol Clin North Am* 1998;36:1059.
29. Phelps CD, Thompson HS, Ossoinig KC: The diagnosis and prognosis of atypical carotid-cavernous fistula (red-eyed shunt syndrome). *Am J Ophthalmol* 1982;93:423.
30. Sampaolesi R, Caruso R: Ocular echometry in the diagnosis of congenital glaucoma. *Arch Ophthalmol* 1982;100:574.
31. Schockett SS, Lakjanpal V, Richards RD: Anterior chamber tube shunt to an encircling band in the treatment of neovascular glaucomas. *Ophthalmology* 1982;89:1188.
32. Shields, B: *Textbook of Glaucoma.* ed 4, Baltimore, Williams & Wilkins, 1998.
33. Sidoti PA, Dunphy TR, Baerveldt G, et al: Experience with the Baerveldt glaucoma implant in treating neovascular glaucoma. *Ophthalmology* 1995;102:32.
34. Soylev MF, Green RL, Feldon SE: Choroidal effusion as a mechanism for transient myopia induced by hydrochlorothiazide and triamterene. *Am J Ophthalmol* 1995;120:395.
35. Wolner B, Leibmann JB, Sassan JW, et al: Late bleb-related endophthalmitis after trabeculectomy with adjunctive 5-fluorouracil. *Ophthalmology* 1991;98:1053.

8

Charles J. Pavlin, F. Stuart Foster

Ultrasound Biomicroscopy of the Eye

The use of ultrasound frequencies in the 40 to 100 MHz range is a relatively new development in ultrasound imaging of the eye. This technique has been developed in the authors' laboratories over the past several years,[19,23,29] progressing from the theoretical description of the basic science required, past the first in vitro experiments in eye bank eyes, to the construction of an instrument capable of clinical use. Investigators have established a broad clinical experience with this instrument in normal patients and patients with ocular disease. The term *ultrasound biomicroscopy (UBM)* is applied to this technique because of its similarities to optical biomicroscopy, i.e., the observation of living tissue at microscopic resolution. This chapter will summarize the theoretical basis of the technology and illustrate the application of this tool in clinical ophthalmology and ophthalmic research.

THEORETICAL CONSIDERATIONS AND DEVELOPMENT OF THE ULTRASOUND BIOMICROSCOPE

Mechanical waves and vibrations occur over a wide range of frequencies called the *acoustic spectrum.* This spectrum extends from the familiar audible range (10 to 20,000 Hz) to the range of phonons (>10_{12} Hz), which comprise the vibrational states of matter. This chapter considers the development and application of a new class of ultrasound imaging systems that use very high frequency ultrasound in the range from 40 to 100 MHz. Such systems have provided subsurface detail with resolution that approaches that of optical microscopy and is not available using any other imaging means.

Resolution

The current limits of clinical imaging result from the need to provide maximum resolution versus the need for the ultrasound beam to penetrate the eye and, to a certain extent, the orbit. In an ultrasound imaging system, the lateral resolution can be related via diffraction theory to the full width of the ultrasound beam at half maximum amplitude (FWHM) and is given by the equation:

$$\text{FWHM} = cf/(\upsilon\, d) = \lambda\ (\text{f-number}) \qquad (1)$$

where c is the speed of sound, f is the focal length of the transducer, υ is the frequency of ultrasound, d is the diameter of the focused transducer, λ is the wave length, and f-number is the ratio of the focal length to the diameter of the transducer. Figure 8-1 represents a plot of resolution as defined by equation 1 for transducers with f-numbers of 1.0, 2.0, and 4.0. A typical ophthalmic transducer with a frequency of 10 MHz and an f-number of 4.0 would have lateral resolution of 600 μm at the focus (Figure 8-1, *point a*). Equation 1 allows the examiner almost unlimited freedom in achieving arbitrarily high resolution by simply selecting the appropriate frequency. For example, to achieve a 60 μm resolution, an operating frequency of 60 MHz and an f-number of 2.0 could be chosen, as shown in Figure 8-1, *point b.* This is approximately 10 times the resolution obtained with conventional ophthalmic ultrasound instrumentation.

The trade-off for this increase in resolution is a loss of penetration. All human tissues exhibit ultrasound attenuation coefficients that increase with frequency. Assuming an attenuation coefficient of 0.5 dB/mm MHz, which is consistent with typical soft tissues,[8] the maximum penetration that could be achieved for a 10 MHz system is approximately 50 mm for an 80 dB dynamic range. For the 60 MHz system, penetration is only 5 mm (Figure 8-2). This reinforces the need to optimize transducer sensitivity and performance in UBM systems development.

Scanner Design

In an ultrasound biomicroscope, essential component blocks are identical to those of a conventional B-mode imaging system except that the operating frequency is

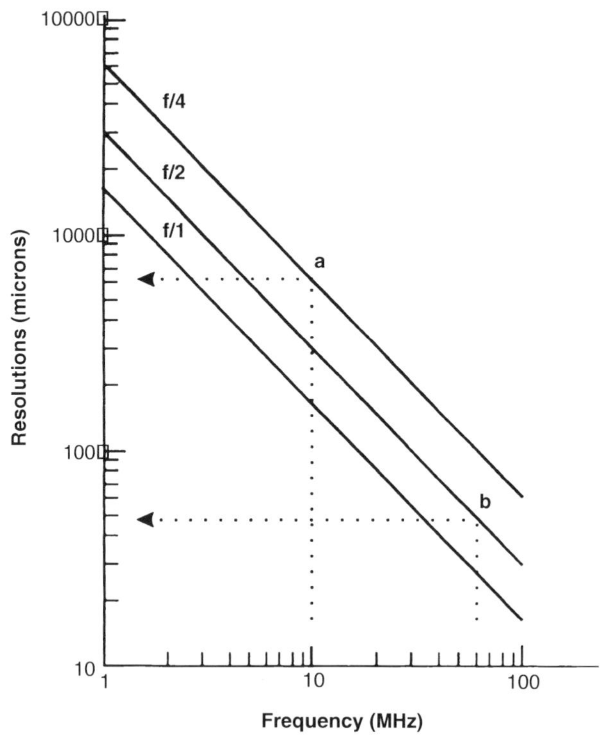

Figure 8-1 Plot of resolution vs. frequency for transducers with various f-numbers. (From Pavlin CJ, Foster FS: *Ultrasound Biomicroscopy of the Eye.* New York, Springer Verlag, 1994, p 14.)

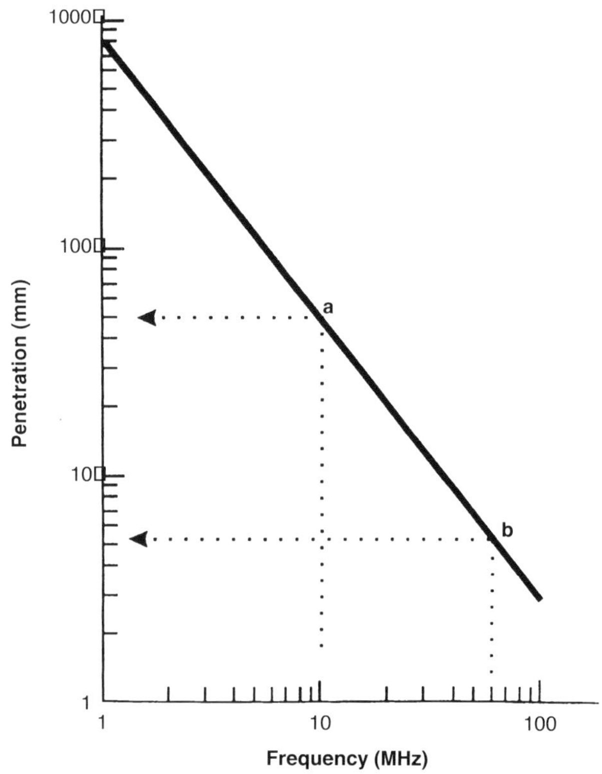

Figure 8-2 Plot of depth of penetration vs. frequency for a system with a dynamic range of 80 dB. (From Pavlin CJ, Foster FS: *Ultrasound Biomicroscopy of the Eye.* New York, Springer Verlag, 1994, p 14.)

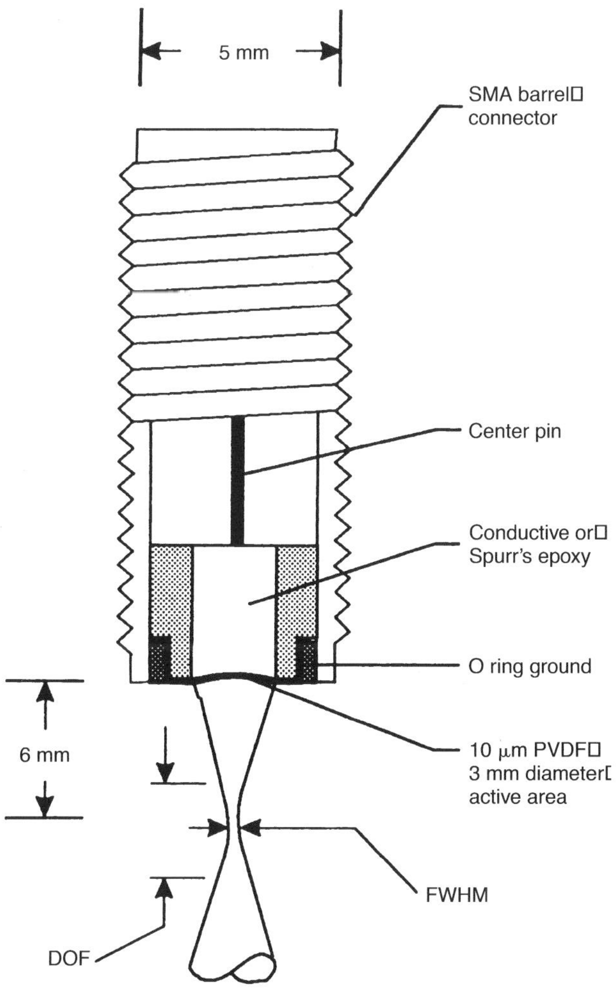

Figure 8-3 A high frequency PVDF transducer. The width of the beam at the focus is given in equation 1.

approximately an order of magnitude higher. A 40 to 100 MHz transducer is moved linearly over the imaging field (typically 4 to 8 mm), collecting radiofrequency (rf) data at each position. A monocycle high voltage 40 to 100 MHz pulse is used to excite the transducer. The rf signal is received and amplified in proportion to the depth from which it originated, using a time-gain circuit. This compensates for the attenuation of the ultrasound beam in the tissue. After the signal is processed to enhance the low-level signals, a section of the detected signal corresponding to the focal zone is digitized by a special high-speed scan converter, stored, and displayed as brightness on a video monitor. The servo motion system and electronics are controlled and synchronized by a computer. More detailed quantitative analysis of rf signals can be performed using a digitizing oscilloscope interfaced to the computer. B-mode imaging is currently performed at 5 to 10 frames/second. Additional details on the scanner design are provided in the literature.[6,29,33]

Transducers

The development of high-frequency transducers has been central to the progress achieved in ultrasound biomicroscopy. The piezoelectric polymer polyvinylidene diflouride (PVDF) and copolymer polyvinylidene diflouride/triflouroethylene materials are used for external imaging applications such as the eye (Figure 8-3). Such transducers produce short, wide bandwidth pulses with good sensitivity. Note that the highest resolution, defined as FWHM in equation 1, is only achieved at the focus. The depth of field (DOF), defined as the range of depth over which the beam remains well focused, must also be considered. In general the DOF increases with the square of the f-number. F-numbers ranging from 2 to 4 represent a good compromise between DOF and resolution. Typical UBM transducers have f-numbers of 2.0 to 3.0. The choice of transducer parameters will clearly have a significant impact on image quality; therefore it is necessary to optimize transducer characteristics for each application to obtain the best compromise for resolution, contrast, and DOF.

CLINICAL USE OF ULTRASOUND BIOMICROSCOPY

High-resolution ultrasound scans used in this chapter have been performed with the original instrument constructed in the authors' laboratories and the commercial instrument based on this design (Paradigm, Salt Lake City, Utah). The laboratory instruments have frequencies between 40 and 100 MHz. The commercial instrument uses a 50 MHz transducer that provides a good compromise between resolution and penetration.

Technique

The technique of eye examination using UBM is similar to conventional B-scan examination of the anterior segment (see p 37). A fluid immersion technique is required to provide an adequate standoff from the structures being examined. This is necessary to avoid distortion of the image close to the transducer and to prevent contact of the transducer and the eye. A series of eye cups (see Appendix D) are used to hold the eyelids open and allow more rapid patient preparation. These eye cups resemble those used in conventional ophthalmic ultrasound (see Figure 2-30), with a lip that slides under the eyelids and holds the cup in place. They differ from biometry eye cups in that they are shallower and have a distinct flair that allows a good view of precisely where the scanning head is being placed. Figure 8-4 shows an examination being performed with one of these eye cups. 1% methylcellulose is an excellent coupling medium with sufficient viscosity to prevent fluid loss during the examination. Air bubbles have to be carefully avoided, both in the fluid and on the concave surface of the transducer. Air bubbles can be removed by immersing the transducer in water and wiping the surface gently with a swab.

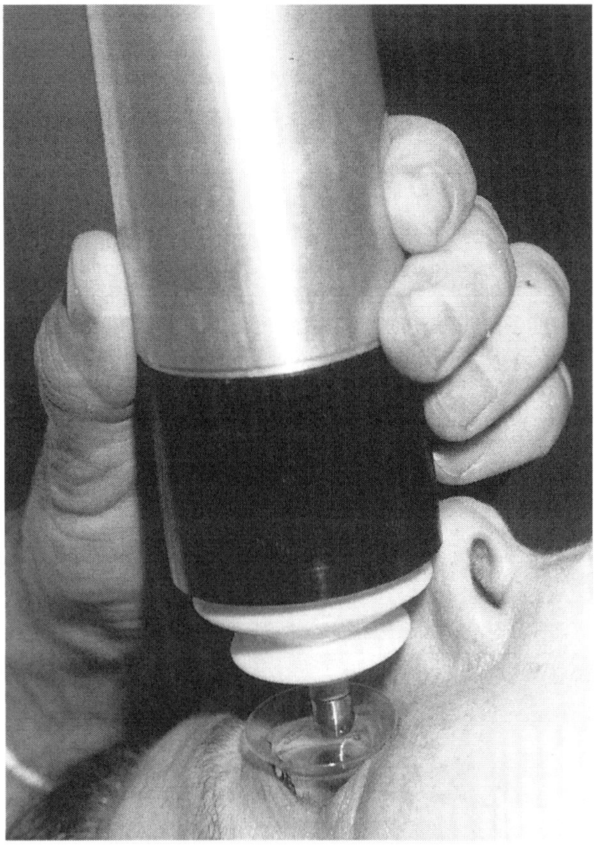

Figure 8-4 An examination with UBM using a flared eye cup.

Unlike conventional 10 MHz B-scan, high frequency transducers are generally not covered by a membrane. A membrane would provide excessive sound attenuation and defeat the purpose of doing examinations at this frequency. Since the transducer is constantly moving, contact with the eye and resulting corneal abrasion must be carefully avoided. The presence of an articulated arm is invaluable in improving control of the scanning head. A technique that involves resting part of the examiner's hand on the patient's forehead is also valuable in this regard. Careful attention must be paid to the screen image to prevent the scanning head from getting too close to the eye. In practice, contact with the eye has been an extremely rare occurrence.

Any part of the eye that can be approached directly over the surface can be examined. The cornea and anterior segment structures are easily examined in any meridian. The conjunctiva, underlying sclera, and peripheral retina can be evaluated by rotating the eye as far as possible away from the region being examined. This allows imaging posterior to the muscle insertions with somewhat greater range temporally because of anatomic considerations. Any adnexal structures with exposed surfaces can be examined. Penetration through the skin is not as good as that through conjunctiva because of the attenuation caused by keratinized epithelium. Examination of structures such as the posterior pole of the eye is not possible at the present time.

Measuring Ocular Structures

Ultrasound biomicroscopy improves the ability to accurately measure ocular structures. Measurement accuracy is improved by UBM, which has an axial resolution 5 to 10 times that of conventional 10 MHz ultrasound. Measurements are performed on the screen during the examination using electronic calipers. Stored images can be transferred to a computer via an image capture board and measured using imaging software. Measuring a structure accurately with ultrasound requires knowledge of the speed of sound in the structure being examined. Little is known of the true speed of sound in these structures, particularly at these frequencies. A speed of sound of 1,540 m/sec has been used to make the majority of measurements. This speed is used in conventional ultrasound scanning to measure distances in most tissue. A speed of 1,640 m/sec is generally used for the cornea, and can be used for the sclera as well since it is similar in structure. Greater precision will require studies to determine the true speed of sound in ocular tissue at high frequencies.

Conventional ultrasound is capable of measuring relatively large distances such as anterior chamber depth (see Chapter 10). However, UBM increases the measurement accuracy of such structures because the shorter wavelength allows a finer positioning of end points and the exact measurement position can be defined more precisely. A number of ocular structures, such as the ciliary body, sclera, and iris, cannot be measured as precisely by other techniques because of inadequate resolution and the inability to differentiate these structures from adjacent tissue. UBM allows clarification of borders and, thus, allows accurate measurement. For example, UBM presents the unique ability to measure iris thickness at various positions in living human eyes. Current imaging techniques are inadequate for this purpose because of lower axial resolution and difficulty in differentiating the posterior iris from the anterior lens surface.

Normal Ocular Structures

Because a large number of structures that can be imaged have not previously been imaged in the living eye, it is useful to define a number of measurement parameters that can be used for future comparison between normal and pathologic eyes.[21] Modifications and additions have been made as this method has been brought to bear on various ocular problems. Some of these measurement sites are shown diagrammatically in Figure 8-5. Measurement sites are defined in terms of fixed anatomic landmarks such as the scleral spur, tip of the ciliary processes, etc., to allow reproducibility in the future.

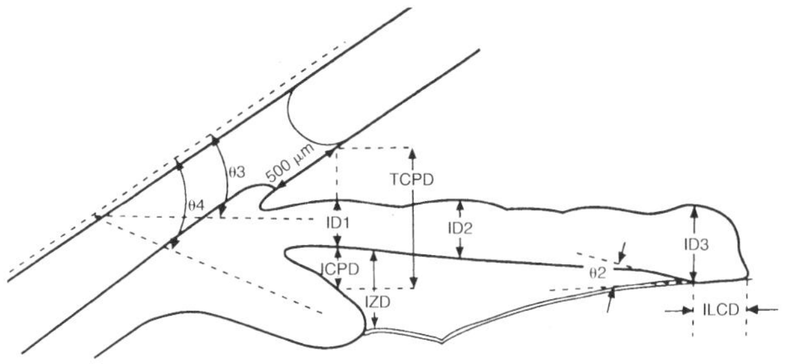

Figure 8-5 UBM measuring positions shown on a diagrammatic cross-section of the eye. The scleral spur is used for a fixed reference point. Trabecular-ciliary process distance (TCPD) is measured on a line extending from a point 500 μm from the scleral spur perpendicularly through the iris to the ciliary process. Iris thickness (ID1-3) can be measured at any position. Iris-zonule distance (IZD) is measured at a point just clearing the ciliary process. Length of iris-lens contact (ILCD) can be measured. Various angles can also be measured as shown in the diagram. *ICPD*, Iris-ciliary process distance. (From Pavlin CJ, Harasiewicz K, Foster FS: Ultrasound biomicroscopy of anterior segment structures in normal and glaucomatous eyes. *Am J Ophthalmol* 1992;113:384.)

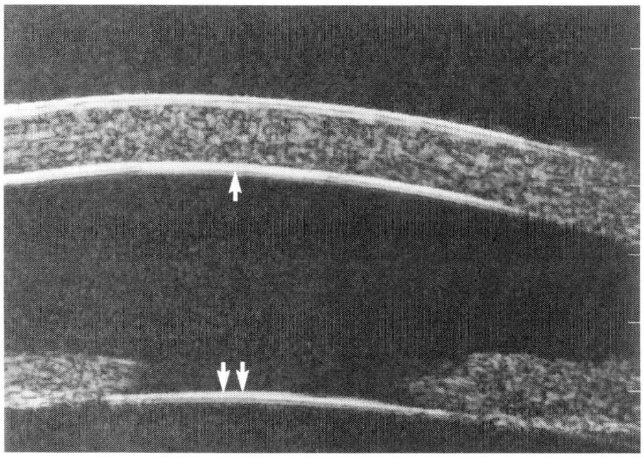

Figure 8-6 UBM image of the central anterior chamber. The cornea displays reflections from the epithelial surface, Bowman's membrane, and Descemet's membrane. The anterior chamber depth can be measured from the inner corneal surface *(arrow)* to the anterior lens capsule *(double arrow)*. (From Pavlin CJ, Harasiewicz K, Foster FS: Ultrasound biomicroscopy of anterior segment structures in normal and glaucomatous eyes. *Am J Ophthalmol* 1992;113:384.)

Cornea

A typical corneal cross-section is shown in Figure 8-6, which shows the central anterior chamber. The corneal layers can be differentiated. The epithelium forms a smooth surface line that is thickened in the presence of edema. The epithelium can be differentiated from Bowman's membrane, which forms a highly reflective line just below that of the epithelium. The corneal stroma reveals an internal reflectivity that is lower than that found in the more irregular collagen distribution of the sclera. This difference allows definition of the corneoscleral junction. The endothelium cannot be differentiated from Descemet's membrane, but together they form a single highly reflective line at the posterior corneal margin. Greater definition of corneal structure can be achieved using higher frequency transducers.

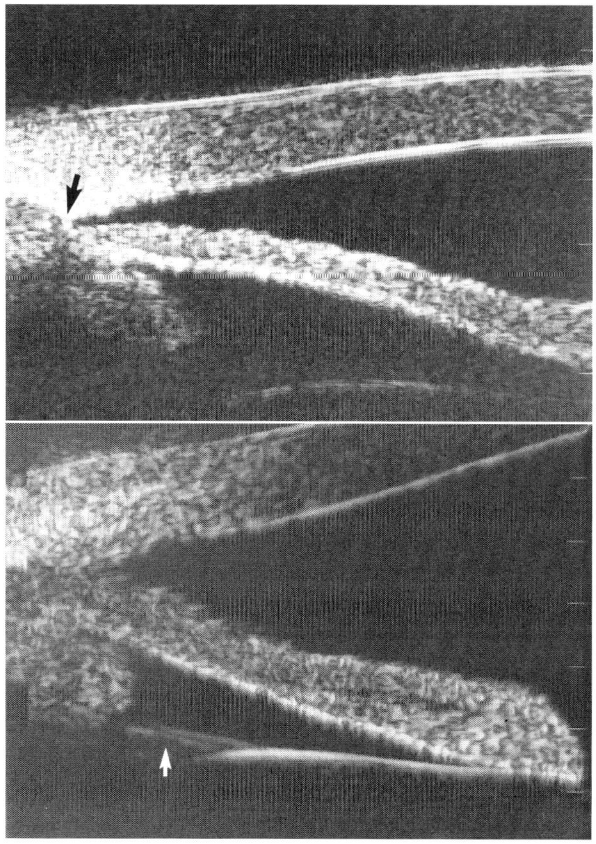

A

B

Figure 8-7 **A,** Typical UBM radial cross-section section through the angle region. The image is taken through a ciliary process. The scleral spur *(arrow)* is an important landmark. **B,** UBM cross-section image through the angle. The anterior zonule is clearly displayed *(arrow)*. (From Pavlin CJ, Foster FS: *Ultrasound Biomicroscopy of the Eye*. New York, Springer Verlag, 1994, p 49.)

Anterior Chamber

Anterior chamber depth (ACD) is easily measured using ultrasound biomicroscopy (see Figure 8-6). Measuring the axial distance from the internal corneal surface to the lens surface is facilitated by the ease of distinguishing the iris from the lens surface. This can be difficult in eyes with very small pupils using conventional ultrasound. Measurement of anterior chamber depth is not confined to the axial position; it can be taken from any point on the endothelial surface to either the iris or lens surface. This provides an improved ability to define the profile of the entire anterior chamber.

Angle Region

Figure 8-7 represents cross-sections through the angle region. These scans were made along the temporal meridian, through a typical ciliary process, and as vertically as possible, as determined by observing the screen image. The corneoscleral junction and scleral spur can be distinguished consistently with UBM. These structures are important in maintaining orientation in the angle region. The scleral spur, in particular, is a very useful landmark, presenting a constant reference point for measurement in the angle region.

Angle Opening

Previous methods of measuring the angle opening have been largely qualitative in nature. One suggested technique for quantifying angle measurements is based on ultrasound biomicroscopy.[21,34] A point 500 μm from the scleral spur would correspond to the anterior aspect of the trabecular meshwork. A line perpendicular to the plane of the trabecular meshwork is extended from this point to the opposing iris. The length of this line is then measured. This measurement is the "angle opening distance" (AOD). Angular measurements in degrees are easily made but difficult to define because of anatomic variations in angle configuration. The angle formed with the apex at the iris recess and the arms passing through the point on the meshwork 500 μm from the scleral spur and the point on the iris perpendicularly opposite is termed the *trabecular-iris angle (Ø1)*. Ultrasound methods have been used in the past to attempt a quantitative measure of the angle of iris opening.[14] Conventional ultrasound, however, lacks the resolution required to define the subtle variations in curvature found in the peripheral angle and these methods provide a gross estimate at best. The ability of ultrasound biomicroscopy to image a cross-section of the angle structures with sufficient resolution to appreciate these variations allows the first truly quantitative method of angle assessment. This method is not restricted by corneal clarity or iris configuration. The ability to observe the angle opening in the context of its surrounding structures aids in clarifying the reason for angle closure.

Iris

The iris normally shows variations in thickness. Histologic studies show that it is generally thinnest at the iris root and thickest near the pupillary margin. In addition, there are variations in thickness depending on the presence of crypts, and the state of dilation or constriction of the pupil. The pupil size is constantly variable within a small range in the absence of pharmacologic agents. The position of iris measurement can be defined with reference to the scleral spur. The iris epithelium forms a constant highly reflective layer on the posterior iris surface. This highly reflective line defines the posterior iris border and can be quite useful when differentiating intra-iris lesions from lesions behind the iris. The zone of iris-lens contact can be measured. Volumetric measurements are possible by tracing the iris profile on a computer and calculating the area of the iris. This can then be projected to a full 360 degrees. Iris curvature can be measured by extending a line from the iris root to the iris tip and measuring the deviation of the iris epithelium from this line.[30]

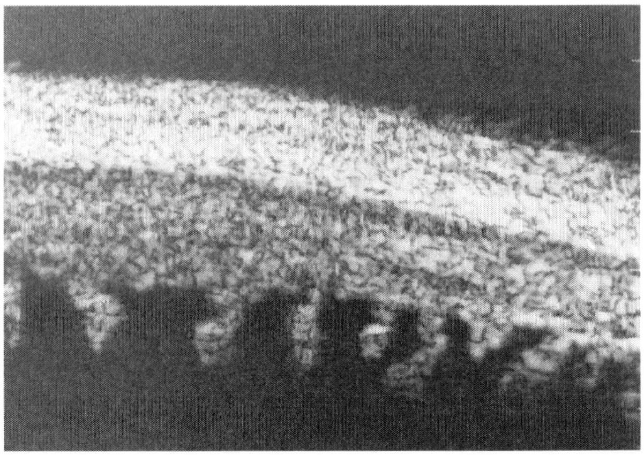

Figure 8-8 UBM image demonstrating the ciliary processes (perpendicular to image shown in Figure 8-7). The variability of the ciliary processes is displayed.

Ciliary Body

The ciliary body is well defined by UBM. The ciliary processes can be quite variable in configuration and length. The appearance of the ciliary body will vary depending on whether the sound beam is passing through a process or a valley between processes. During the examination, either of these views can be produced, as desired. Figure 8-8 shows an image at right angles to the view shown in Figure 8-7 and displays the variable configuration of the ciliary processes and the valleys between them.

The distance between the anterior trabecular meshwork and the ciliary process is an important measurement. This distance is defined as the length of a line starting 500 μm from the scleral spur on the trabecular meshwork and extending perpendicularly through the iris to the ciliary process. This distance defines the port through which the iris must traverse and has implications as to the potential maximum angle opening. The ciliary sulcus is defined as the space between the anterior surface of the ciliary processes and the posterior iris surface.

Zonule

The entire posterior chamber cannot always be defined with UBM. The posterior zonule and vitreous face can be resolved in some shallow chambered eyes but not consistently in eyes with chambers of average or greater depth. The anterior zonule and lens surface, however, can be consistently visualized in all eyes (see Figure 8-7, *B*). The zonule inserts smoothly into the surface of the lens but is occasionally more irregular, which may indicate the degree of zonular tension.

ULTRASOUND BIOMICROSCOPY IN OCULAR DISEASE

Since UBM is a new nonspecific imaging tool, it is suitable for examination of a large range of diseases that fall within the penetration limits of this technique. It is particularly useful in those conditions in which structural abnormalities are present, i.e., those conditions that produce rearrangement of normal anatomy. Glaucoma and intraocular tumors are two areas in which UBM provides particularly useful information. The use of conventional ultrasound for glaucoma is described in Chapter 7 and for intraocular tumors in Chapter 5.

Glaucoma

Several types of glaucoma are caused by structural abnormalities of the anterior segment of the globe. This is particularly true of angle closure glaucoma and infantile glaucoma. The ability of UBM to image structural abnormalities on a much finer scale than has previously been possible provides us with a quantitative new tool for research and clinical assessment of glaucomatous disease. Examples of use in glaucoma are provided.

Pupillary Block

In pupillary block the iris assumes a convex profile due to the pressure differential between the posterior and anterior chambers. The convex contour of the iris in a case of pupillary block is noted in Figure 8-9. Following iridotomy, the profile changes to a much straighter configuration. Previous studies have been done to define the iris profile. Tiedeman provided a theoretical analysis to predict the iris profile.[35] An optical technique (Scheimpflug technique) has been described to define the iris profile.[1] UBM presents a relatively easy method of accomplishing this task and allows definition of the entire iris profile to the iris root. Interestingly, the degree of iris-lens contact is relatively small in pupillary block, as the iris is lifted off the lens. Thus, the block is not related to the area of contact. The area of iris-lens contact becomes even smaller when the pupil dilates. Anatomic angle closure in the dark, resulting in pupillary block, occurs rapidly and relates to increased iris thickness and increased anterior bowing as the iris tip moves towards the iris root.[37] A dark room provocative test can be done utilizing UBM to detect whether anatomic angle closure occurs in the dark.[10,22]

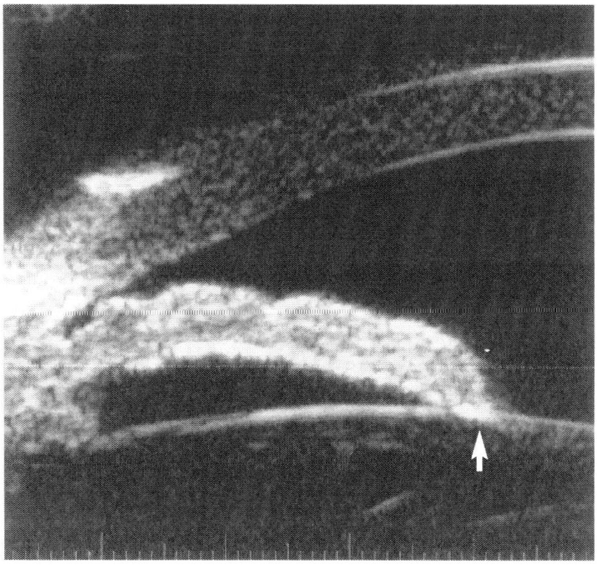

Figure 8-9 UBM image in a case of pupillary block. The iris is bowed forward. The angle is narrow but open. The iris-lens contact is minimal *(arrow)*.

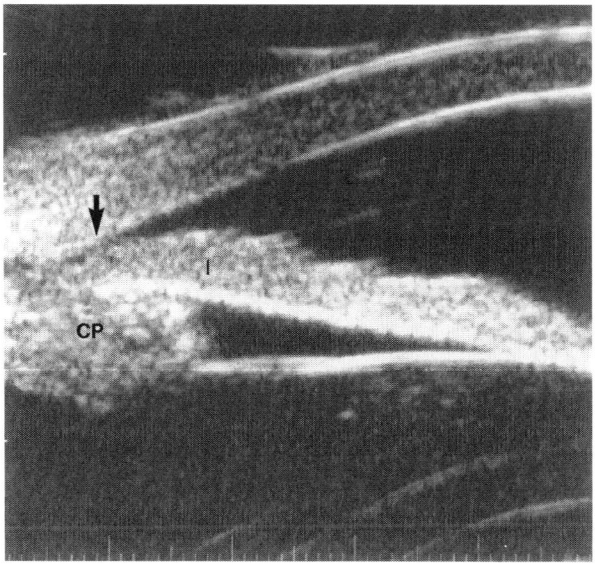

Figure 8-10 UBM image in a case of plateau iris syndrome. The ciliary processes *(CP)* are forward, closing the ciliary sulcus and supporting the peripheral iris *(I)*. The iris profile is straight, but the peripheral angle is narrow *(arrow)*.

Plateau Iris Syndrome

UBM has been used to elucidate the etiology of plateau iris syndrome.[26] In plateau iris syndrome, the ciliary processes are anatomically anterior, closing the ciliary sulcus and providing structural support behind the peripheral iris (Figure 8-10). This prevents this portion of the iris from falling away from the trabecular meshwork following iridectomy. A good way of looking at this phenomenon is that the ciliary processes and the trabecular meshwork form a port through which the iris thickness must pass. The smaller this port and/or the thicker the iris in this region, the greater the degree of angle closure. In studies of this disease, anterior chamber depth, trabecular-ciliary process distance, and

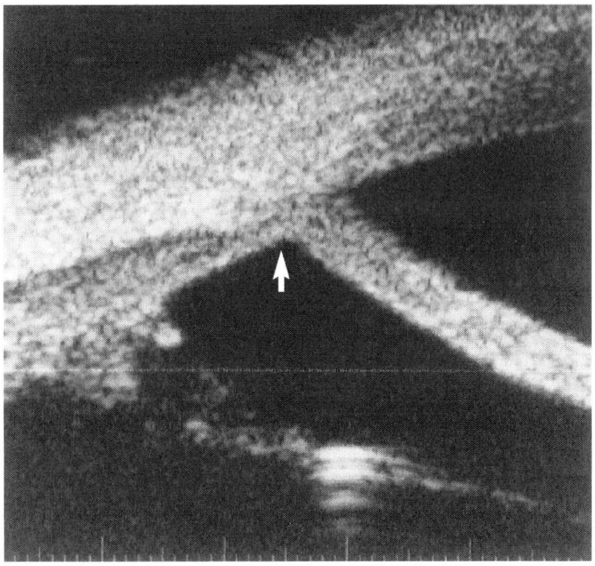

Figure 8-11 UBM image showing a closed angle due to anterior synechiae. The iris has an angled appearance *(arrow).*

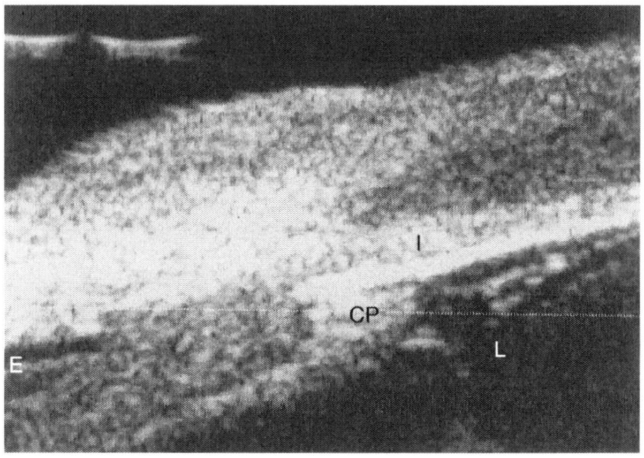

Figure 8-12 UBM image in a case of malignant glaucoma. A supraciliary effusion *(E)* is present. The ciliary processes *(CP)* and iris *(I)* are rotated forward closing the angle. The lens margin *(L)* is just medial to the ciliary process.

iris-zonule distance were all significantly smaller than that found in normals. In studies of plateau iris in the dark and after pilocarpine administration, it was demonstrated that the distance between the ciliary processes and trabecular meshwork remained constant with iris thickness being the only variable contributing to angle narrowing.[20]

Anterior Synechiae

Total angle closure by synechiae is illustrated in Figure 8-11. The iris takes an angular form as opposed to the smooth curve of pupillary block. The state of the angle behind synechia can be defined by UBM. This may improve the ability to assess the prognosis in these cases. It is difficult to differentiate complete appositional closure from synechial closure, but UBM is capable of defining an extremely small split between the iris and the trabecular meshwork.

Iris Rotation

In patients with extremely shallow anterior chambers such as those seen in spherophakia, the iris can be rotated forward, directly narrowing the angle in the absence of pupillary block.

Supraciliary Effusions and Malignant Glaucoma

Supraciliary effusions that cannot be detected by conventional ultrasound can be imaged by UBM.[17] These effusions occur in a variety of conditions including inflammatory disease and vein occlusions, and following retinal detachment surgery.[28,39] Supraciliary effusions produce rotation of the ciliary processes and iris around the scleral spur. This can result in angle closure, particularly if the angle is narrow to begin with. Most cases of malignant glaucoma have supraciliary effusions and anteriorly rotated ciliary processes[12,36] (Figure 8-12). It is likely that effusions play a major role in the clinical manifestation of this condition (see p 216).

Pigmentary Dispersion

Pigmentary dispersion syndrome is characterized by loss of pigment from the pigment epithelial layer of the iris and subsequent pigment deposition in the trabecular meshwork, leading to glaucoma. The concept of reverse pupillary block[30] implies temporary reversal of the pressure differential in the anterior and posterior chambers, producing posterior bowing of the iris and leading to iris-zonule contact with mechanical pigment loss. UBM has shown that accommodation produces posterior iris bowing, which is reversed by iridotomy.[24] Other factors, including blinking and exercise, have also been considered possible causes.[11] Examination of patients with this condition should include observation of the effects of accommodation on iris profile. This can be accomplished by having the patient change fixation from a target on the ceiling to a near target, using the eye not being examined (Figure 8-13).

Filtering Surgery

Figure 8-14 illustrates the ability of UBM to analyze the state of filtering procedures. This figure shows a patent opening continuous with a distinct scleral split and a functioning bleb. The internal surgical opening can be consistently visualized and the state of the filtering bleb assessed.[38] Filtering blebs show variable internal reflectivity, most likely dependent on the distribution of fluid in the episcleral tissue.

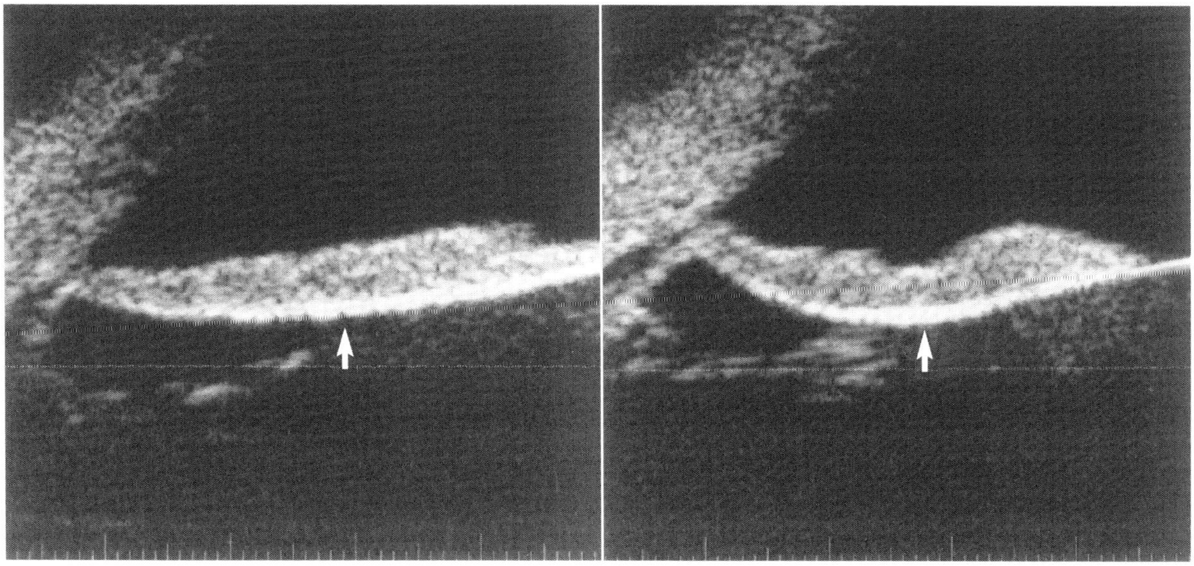

A B

Figure 8-13 UBM images of pigmentary glaucoma. With distance fixation **(A)** the iris is slightly bowed posteriorly *(arrow)*. With accommodation **(B)**, bowing of the posterior iris increases markedly *(arrow)*. (From Pavlin CJ, Foster FS: *Ultrasound Biomicroscopy of the Eye*. New York, Springer Verlag, 1994, p 19.)

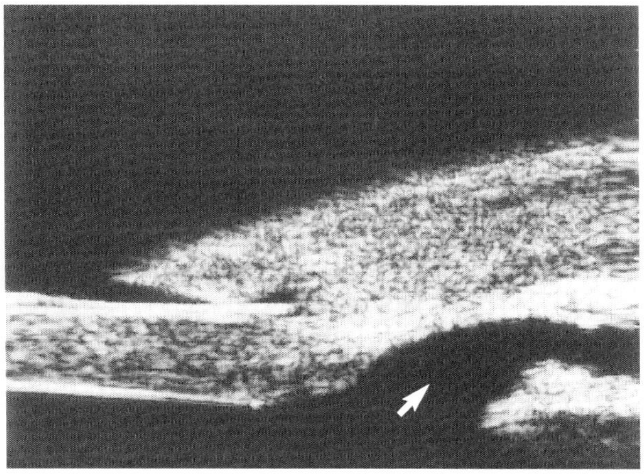

Figure 8-14 UBM image following filtering surgery. The internal ostium and trans-scleral pathway are imaged *(arrow)*. The bleb shows diffuse reflectivity from edematous episcleral tissue. (From Pavlin CJ, Harasiewicz K, Foster FS: Ultrasound biomicroscopy of anterior segment structures in normal and glaucomatous eyes. *Am J Ophthalmol* 1992;113:387.)

Anterior Segment Tumors

UBM is a very useful adjunct in the management of anterior segment tumors.[25] UBM provides a clear image of even the smallest anterior segment lesions. The ability to measure these lesions accurately adds the dimension of depth to the criteria for demonstrating growth. The ability to determine the underlying structure of the tumor allows improved classification and the ability to determine ciliary body involvement. When observation is elected, lesions may be followed with greater precision. Where surgical intervention is indicated, information gained is helpful in planning the approach.

Iris Tumors

The presence of a typical morphologic appearance on UBM may be helpful as a diagnostic sign. Several small, minimally elevated lesions involving the peripheral iris and clinically considered nevi have a similar appearance on

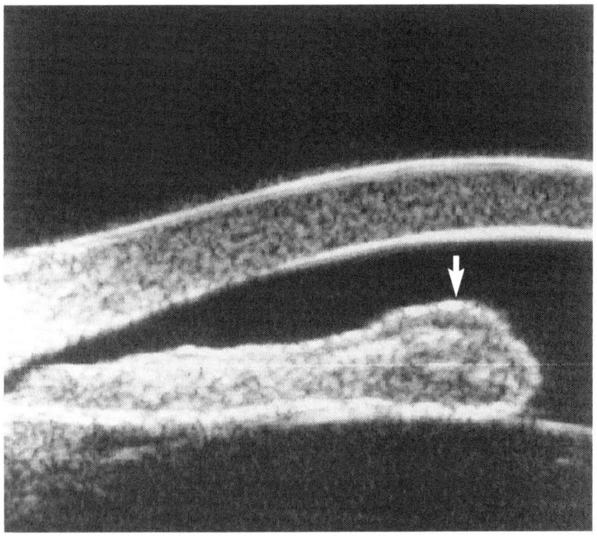

Figure 8-15 UBM image demonstrating iris nevus at the pupillary margin. A low reflective surface plaque is present *(arrow)*.

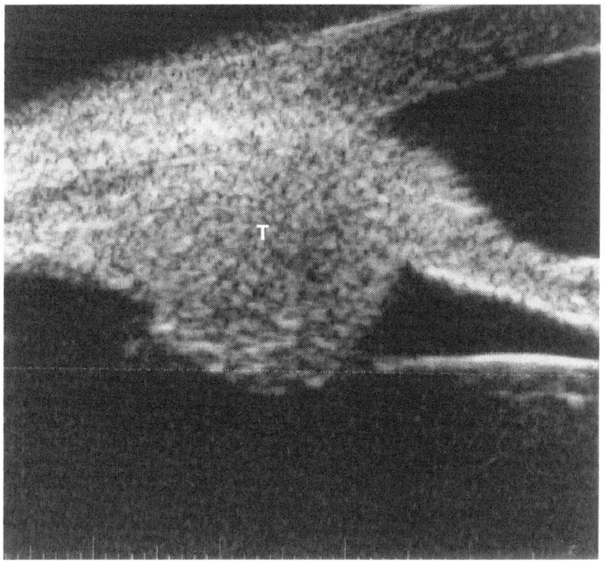

Figure 8-16 UBM image showing ciliary body tumor *(T)* with regular, medium reflectivity. The peripheral iris is involved.

UBM. They share the ultrasound biomicroscopic appearance of a small moderately thickened iris lesion, not extending past the iris root. There is frequently a hypoechoic layer on the surface of these lesions, possibly indicating that the superficial layer is involved with the closely spaced cells of a surface plaque (Figure 8-15).

It is difficult to be too specific as to histologic diagnosis with ultrasound, even with the added detail presented by UBM. Resolution is not at the level that can differentiate individual cells. Malignant melanomas of the iris can be quite variable in their clinical and ultrasonic presentation. UBM can be helpful in a number of ways. Internal reflectivity varies considerably, depending on the degree of vascularity and the patterns of internal cellular structure. Some melanomas show a linear internal pattern, others show a uniform reflectivity, still others show a large degree of internal vascularity. Margins can be defined, which is especially important for assessing ciliary body involvement. Histology has shown good correlation between the ultrasound margin and the histologic margin. The posterior pigment epithelial layer can be assessed for evidence of breakthrough. Serial measurements are invaluable for assessing growth. A change in shape of the lesion can also be imaged. Evidence of internal seeding can be defined. Some iris melanomas have a component that is under the iris and can be hidden from view. UBM can image these regions. If iridocyclectomy is performed, UBM provides an additional method of assessing the iridocyclectomy bed for evidence of recurrence.

Ciliary Body Tumors

Ciliary body tumors can be assessed easily, although large tumors (<4 mm in depth) cannot be completely imaged because of sound attenuation. Small lesions that cannot be detected by conventional ultrasound can be defined by UBM. Larger ciliary body lesions are detectable by conventional ultrasound (see Chapter 5), but UBM shows improved internal detail of the superficial part of the tumor and frequently allows a more precise localization of the posterior and lateral boundaries (Figure 8-16). This information is important if iridocyclectomy is considered as a possible treatment. Extrascleral extension can be localized in relation to the tumor and frequently a transscleral connection imaged.

Cysts

Cysts are clearly imaged by UBM.[2,25] The usual clinical presentation of an iridociliary cyst is an elevation of the peripheral iris without iris involvement. The typical ultrasound biomicroscopic appearance of a thin-walled cyst with no internal reflectivity (Figure 8-17) is diagnostic and essentially eliminates any question of whether a lesion is a cyst or a solid tumor. Small cysts are also found occasionally, either as an isolated finding on examination for some other clinical indication, or in association with solid lesions of the iris or ciliary body.[5]

Peripheral Choroidal Tumors

The anterior aspect of anteriorly located choroidal tumors can be imaged by UBM.[13] Although it is often impossible to measure these tumors through their greatest thickness, valuable information can be gained regarding the anterior extent of the lesion and the involvement of anterior segment structures. This is particularly important if radioactive plaque treatment is contemplated, as it provides a guide for placement of the anterior margin of the plaque.

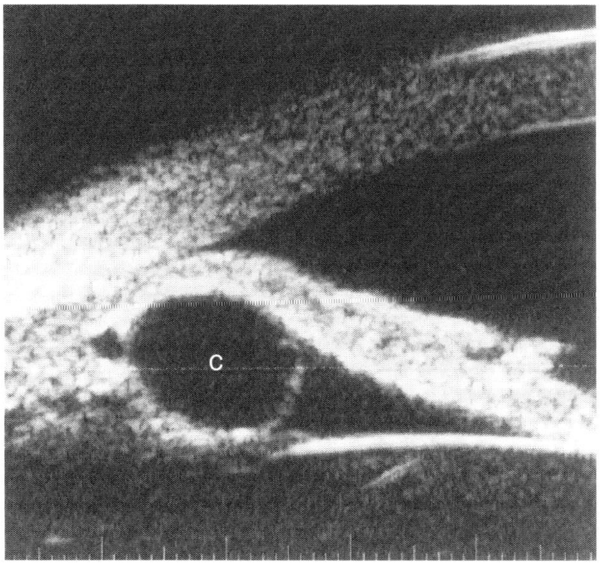

Figure 8-17 UBM image showing iridociliary cyst *(C)*. Note the cyst wall and lack of internal echoes indicating fluid. Local angle closure is present.

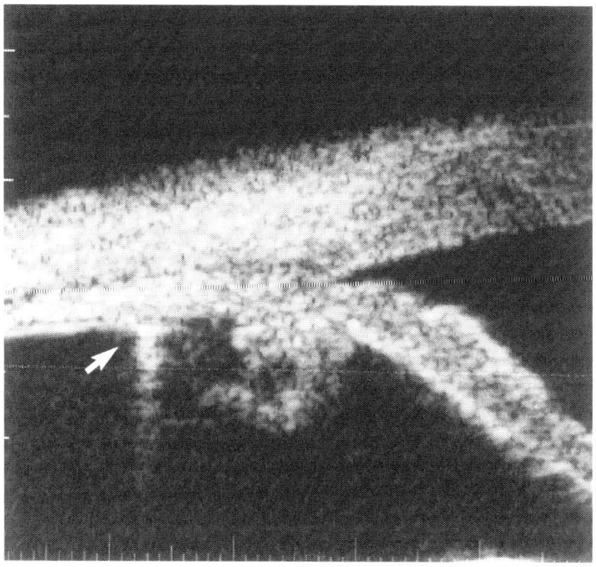

Figure 8-18 UBM image showing IOL haptic *(arrow)*. Note that the haptic is displaced over the pars plana.

Imaging the internal structure of the anterior aspect of the tumor can also provide helpful differential diagnostic information. In cases of extrascleral extension, the relationship of the tumor to the extrascleral component can be defined, and frequently the trans-scleral connection is imaged.

Corneal and Scleral Disease

UBM can be helpful in patients with opaque corneas prior to transplantation.[15] Anterior segment details, such as the depth of the anterior chamber, state of the angle, presence of anterior synechiae, and intraocular lens positioning, can be determined preoperatively. Intracorneal abnormalities can also be imaged. Corneal edema can be assessed and measured. An arc scanner recently developed uses a transducer path that follows the corneal curvature, allowing imaging of the entire cornea in one sweep. This instrumentation has allowed construction of three-dimensional depth maps of corneal thickness, epithelial thickness, and depth of intracorneal incisions.[31] It is likely to be helpful in assessing results and complications of refractive surgery. UBM is also useful in scleritis, allowing differentiation between extrascleral and intrascleral disease and allowing assessment of the degree of scleral thinning.[18]

Intraocular Lens Complications

UBM can easily evaluate the position of intraocular lens haptics. This is very useful in assessing malpositioned lenses[27] (Figure 8-18) and the source of intraocular bleeding and in determining haptic freedom if removal or repositioning is required.[32]

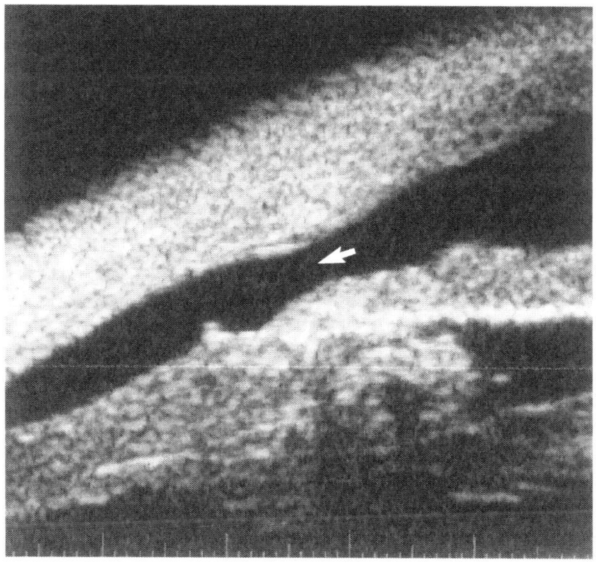

Figure 8-19 UBM image demonstrating cyclodialysis cleft *(arrow)*. The cleft is open in this image.

Hypotony and Trauma

UBM can image cyclodialysis clefts even when the anterior chamber is shallow and the cyclodialysis cleft is not obvious with gonioscopy.[7] There is always 360 degrees of supraciliary fluid present in these cases. The region of the cleft is usually obvious from the displacement of the iris root from the scleral spur (Figure 8-19). Other causes of hypotony in which UBM can provide useful information include occult wound leaks and ciliary body membranes. In other trauma problems, UBM can image the state of the anterior chamber under traumatic opacities[3] and detect small foreign bodies that are

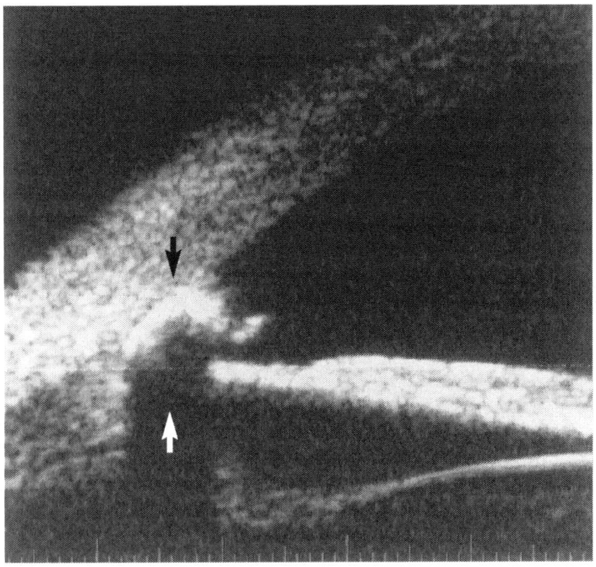

Figure 8-20 UBM image showing foreign body in the angle *(black arrow)*. Note high reflectivity and shadowing of posterior structures *(white arrow)*.

difficult to image using conventional techniques[4] (Figure 8-20). For the use of conventional ultrasound in hypotony, see p 216 and for anterior segment trauma, see pp 87 and 93.

Conjunctival and Adnexal Disease

UBM can provide valuable information in the differential diagnoses of tumors, judging the depth of conjunctival and limbal lesions and imaging canalicular conditions.[9]

SUMMARY AND FUTURE DIRECTIONS

UBM presents a new method of imaging the anterior segment of the eye at high resolution. Its strengths lie in its ability to produce cross-sections of the living eye at microscopic resolution without violating the integrity of the globe. Although histologic assessment of various disease types is sometimes available from pathology specimens, this usually occurs at a late stage in the disease and is susceptible to the inevitable distortions of the preparation process. UBM, although lacking the resolution of optical microscopy, provides images in living eyes without affecting the internal relationships of the structures imaged. This method has proven valuable in both clinical practice and ophthalmic research. New methods of using high frequency ultrasound are in development including three-dimensional imaging, Doppler,[16] and the use of contrast agents. These developments should extend the use of this technique to new areas.

ACKNOWLEDGMENTS

The authors would like to acknowledge the contribution of Michael Sherar, Brian Starkoski, and Kasia Harasiewicz to the development of this imaging system.

REFERENCES

1. Anderson R, Jin G, Wright MM: The physiological characteristics of relative pupillary block. *Am J Ophthalmol* 1991;111:344.
2. Augsburger JJ, Affel LL, Benarosh DA: Ultrasound biomicroscopy of cystic lesions of the iris and ciliary body. *Trans Am Ophthalmol Soc* 1996;94:259.
3. Berinstein DM, Gentile RC, Sidoti PA, et al: Ultrasound biomicroscopy in anterior ocular trauma. *Ophthalmic Surg Lasers* 1997;28:201.
4. Deramo VA, Shah GK, Baumal CR, et al: Ultrasound biomicroscopy as a tool for detecting and localizing occult foreign bodies after ocular trauma. *Ophthalmology* 1999;106:301.
5. Fine N, Pavlin CJ: Primary cysts in the iridociliary sulcus: ultrasound biomicroscopic features of 210 cases. *Can J Ophthalmol* 1999;34:325.
6. Foster FS, Pavlin CJ, Harasiewicz KA, et al: Advances in ultrasound biomicroscopy. *Ultrasound Med Biol* 2000;26:1.
7. Gentile RC, Pavlin CJ, Liebmann JM, et al: Diagnosis of traumatic cyclodialysis by ultrasound biomicroscopy. *Ophthalmic Surg Lasers* 1996;27:97.
8. Hill C: *Physical Principles of Medical Ultrasonics.* London, Ellis Howood Limited, 1986.
9. Hurwitz JJ, Pavlin CJ, Hassan A: Proximal canalicular imaging utilizing ultrasound biomicroscopy A: normal canaliculi. *Orbit* 1998;17:27.
10. Ishikawa H, Esaki K, Liebmann JM, et al: Ultrasound biomicroscopy dark room provocative testing: a quantitative method for estimating anterior chamber angle width. *Jpn J Ophthalmol* 1999;43:526.
11. Liebmann JM, Tello C, Chew SJ, et al: Prevention of blinking alters iris configuration in pigment dispersion syndrome and in normal eyes [see comments]. *Ophthalmology* 1995;102:446.
12. Liebmann JM, Weinreb RN, Ritch R: Angle-closure glaucoma associated with occult annular ciliary body detachment. *Arch Ophthalmol* 1998;116:731.
13. Maberly DA, Pavlin CJ, McGowan HD, et al: Ultrasound biomicroscopic imaging of the anterior aspect of peripheral choroidal melanomas. *Am J Ophthalmol* 1997;123:506.
14. Makabe R: Comparative studies of the width of the anterior chamber angle using echography and gonioscopy. *Klin Montasbl Augenheilkd* 1989;194:6.
15. Milner MS, Liebmann JM, Tello C, et al: High-resolution ultrasound biomicroscopy of the anterior segment in patients with dense corneal scars. *Ophthalmic Surg* 1994;25:284.
16. Pavlin CJ, Christopher DA, Burns PN, et al: High-frequency Doppler ultrasound examination of blood flow in the anterior segment of the eye. *Am J Ophthalmol* 1998;126:597.
17. Pavlin CJ, Easterbrook M, Harasiewicz K, et al: An ultrasound biomicroscopic analysis of angle-closure glaucoma secondary to ciliochoroidal effusion in IgA nephropathy. *Am J Ophthalmol* 1993;116:341.
18. Pavlin CJ, Easterbrook M, Hurwitz JJ, et al: Ultrasound biomicroscopy in the assessment of anterior scleral disease. *Am J Ophthalmol* 1993;116:628.
19. Pavlin CJ, Foster FS: Ultrasound biomicroscopy. High-frequency ultrasound imaging of the eye at microscopic resolution. *Radiol Clin North Am* 1998;36:1047.
20. Pavlin CJ, Foster FS: Plateau iris syndrome: changes in angle opening associated with dark, light, and pilocarpine administration. *Am J Ophthalmol* 1999;128:288.
21. Pavlin CJ, Harasiewicz K, Foster FS: Ultrasound biomicroscopy of anterior segment structures in normal and glaucomatous eyes [see comments]. *Am J Ophthalmol* 1992;113:381.
22. Pavlin CJ, Harasiewicz K, Foster FS: An ultrasound biomicroscopic dark-room provocative test. *Ophthalmic Surg* 1995;26:253.
23. Pavlin CJ, Harasiewicz K, Sherar MD, et al: Clinical use of ultrasound biomicroscopy. *Ophthalmology* 1991;98:287.
24. Pavlin CJ, Macken P, Trope GE, et al: Accommodation and iridotomy in the pigment dispersion syndrome. *Ophthalmic Surg Lasers* 1996;27:113.
25. Pavlin CJ, McWhae JA, McGowan HD, et al: Ultrasound biomicroscopy of anterior segment tumors. *Ophthalmology* 1992;99:1220.
26. Pavlin CJ, Ritch R, Foster FS: Ultrasound biomicroscopy in plateau iris syndrome. *Am J Ophthalmol* 1992;113:390.
27. Pavlin CJ, Rootman D, Arshinoff S, et al: Determination of haptic position of transsclerally fixated posterior chamber intraocular lenses by ultrasound biomicroscopy [see comments]. *J Cataract Refract Surg* 1993;19:573.

28. Pavlin CJ, Rutnin SS, Devenyi R, et al: Supraciliary effusions and ciliary body thickening after scleral buckling procedures. *Ophthalmology* 1997;104:433.
29. Pavlin CJ, Sherar MD, Foster FS: Subsurface ultrasound microscopic imaging of the intact eye. *Ophthalmology* 1990;97:244.
30. Potash SD, Tello C, Liebmann J, et al: Ultrasound biomicroscopy in pigment dispersion syndrome [see comments]. *Ophthalmology* 1994;101:332.
31. Reinstein DZ, Silverman RH, Raevsky T, et al: Arc-scanning very high-frequency digital ultrasound for 3D pachymetric mapping of the corneal epithelium and stroma in laser in situ keratomileusis. *J Refract Surg* 2000;16:414.
32. Rutnin SS, Pavlin CJ, Slomovic AR, et al: Preoperative ultrasound biomicroscopy to assess ease of haptic removal before penetrating keratoplasty combined with lens exchange. *J Cataract Refract Surg* 1997;23:239.
33. Sherar M, Starkoski B, Taylor WB, et al: A 100 MHz B-scan ultrasound backscatter microscope. *Ultrason Imaging* 1989;11:95.
34. Tello C, Liebmann J, Potash SD, et al: Measurement of ultrasound biomicroscopy images: intraobserver and interobserver reliability. *Invest Ophthalmol Vis Sci* 1994;35:3549.
35. Tiedeman S: A physical analysis of factors that determine the contour of the iris. *Am J Ophthalmol* 1991;111:338.
36. Trope GE, Pavlin CJ, Bau A, et al: Malignant glaucoma. Clinical and ultrasound biomicroscopic features. *Ophthalmology* 1994;101:1030.
37. Woo EK, Pavlin CJ, Slomovic A, et al: Ultrasound biomicroscopic quantitative analysis of light-dark changes associated with pupillary block. *Am J Ophthalmol* 1999;127:43.
38. Yamamoto T, Sakuma T, Kitazawa Y: An ultrasound biomicroscopic study of filtering blebs after mitomycin C trabeculectomy. *Ophthalmology* 1995;102.1770.
39. Yuki T, Kimura Y, Nanbu S, et al: Ciliary body and choroidal detachment after laser photocoagulation for diabetic retinopathy. A high-frequency ultrasound study. *Ophthalmology* 1997;104:1259.

9

Paul T. Finger

Three-Dimensional Ultrasound of the Eye

Three-dimensional ultrasonography (3DUS) combines sequential two-dimensional (2D) digital image acquisition (tomograms) with computerized reconstruction software. Computer-assisted image processing allows ocular pathology to be viewed in 3D. Three-dimensional reconstruction can allow the entire surface of an intraocular tumor to be visualized, its topographic anatomy rendered, and its volume calculated. Interactive analysis (sectioning) of the scanned 3D volume image block allows for examination of unique oblique and coronal views (Table 9-1).[2,6,12] These capabilities have already been found helpful for evaluating episcleral plaque placement and extrascleral extension of choroidal melanoma.[11,19]

Future prospects for ophthalmic 3D imaging include the potential for new and unique findings in ocular and orbital oncology, as well as in vitreoretinal diseases. In addition, 3D imaging should play an important role in telemedicine.

INSTRUMENTATION

The one commercially available ophthalmic 3D ultrasound system (3D i-scan, [OTI] Ophthalmic Technologies Inc, Toronto, Ontario) utilizes a conventional 10 MHz B-scan transducer combined with a motorized, rotating holder and computerized image processing (Figure 9-1). The data from 60, 90, or 180 serial B-scan images are acquired while the transducer rotates (in angular increments of 3, 2, or 1 degrees, respectively). These images are imported into a computer for processing to form a 3D volume image (Figure 9-2).

Three-dimensional volume image blocks are displayed on the computer screen. The polyhedral display format used by OTI has been used for other 3DUS applications in radiology.[15] The initial 3D volume image block is 41 mm deep by 37.5 mm high by 37.5 mm wide. The polyhedron consists of six fixed planes, which define the boundaries of the scanned volume image block, plus movable planes created by the operator. By moving two or more planes, the observer slices into the 3D volume image block, much like a pathologist slices into a paraffin block. But, unlike the pathologist, the observer can reform the block or slice it from two or more directions at the same time. For example, Romero et al retrospectively obtained an oblique ultrasound image of extrascleral extension (of a uveal melanoma) in an effort to match its corresponding histopathologic section (Figure 9-3).[19]

It is important to note that 3DUS probes operate at 10 MHz and offer an axial resolution of 0.1 mm, as in conventional B-scan ultrasound.[1] The acquisition time for obtaining serial B-scan images is currently 5 to 7.5 seconds per scan sequence. Sound velocities used to perform measurements with the OTI machine are 1,550 m/s, ± 3%.

INTRAOCULAR TUMORS

3DUS can be particularly helpful in the diagnosis and management of intraocular tumors. This technique has been used for the diagnosis of extrascleral extension,[19] for imaging radioactive plaques during implantation,[11] and for clinicopathologic correlation in retinoblastoma.[21] The accuracy and reproducibility of 3DUS for measurements (especially volume) of choroidal melanomas have been studied.[18]

Topography and Volumetric Analysis

Ocular oncologists have traditionally used conventional A- and B-scan ultrasound to assess a tumor's apical height, considered the most reliable indicator of growth or post-treatment shrinkage. In addition, 2D B-scan has been used indirectly to assess a tumor's topography and volume.[13] The development of 3DUS now allows for an easier and more accurate method of evaluating both tumor topography and volume, and can enhance the measurement of apical height.

The procedures used to measure tumor volume and to perform topographic mapping are essentially the same, but the information is processed differently by the computer software. The procedure involves outlining multiple, successive, parallel cross-sectional slices of the tumor volume

TABLE 9-1

2D vs. 3D Ultrasound*

Characteristics	2D Ultrasound	3D Ultrasound
Axial resolution	0.1	0.1
Lateral resolution	0.3	0.3
Linear analysis	Yes	Yes
Spatial analysis	No	Yes
Initial image	2D real-time	2D real-time
Dynamic examination	Yes	No
Acquisition time	5 to 15 minutes	5 to 7.5 seconds
Images acquired	5 to 10	60 to 180
Static record	2D files/2D slices	3D files/2D slices
Replay possible	No	Yes
3D reconstruction	No	Yes
Image rotation	No	Yes
Coronal/oblique sections	No	Yes
Volumetric analysis	No	Yes
Topographic mapping	No	Yes

*Both 2D and 3D ultrasound instruments use a 1D MHz probe.

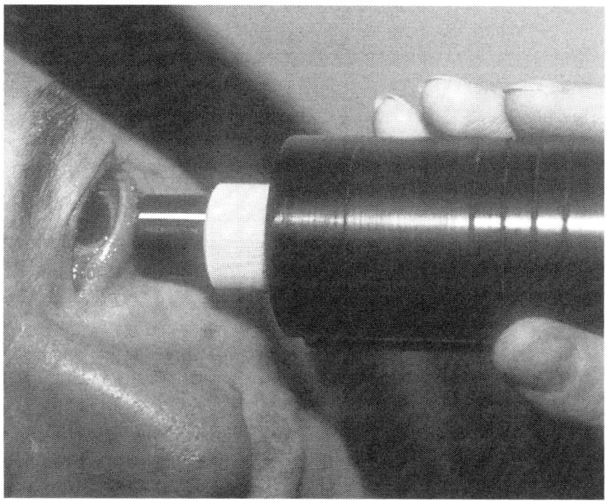

Figure 9-1 Photograph of the OTI B-scan probe. The probe is contained within a motorized, rotating holder and is rotated to acquire multiple sequential 2D images.

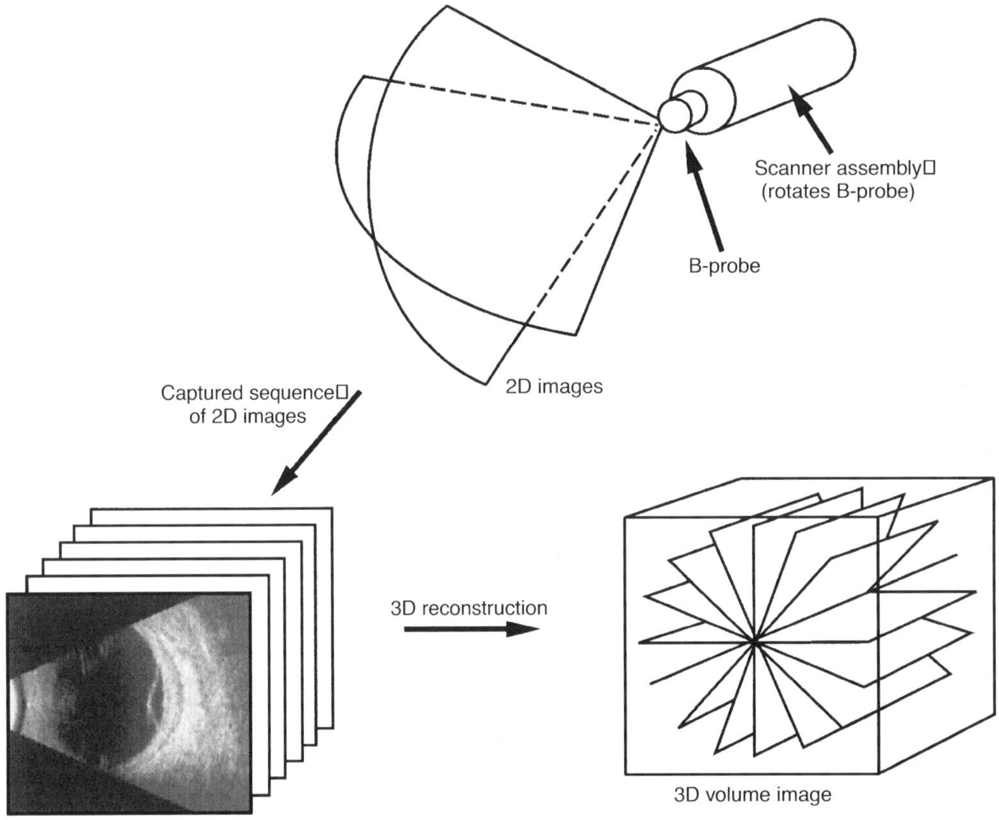

Figure 9-2 Schematic drawing shows rotation of the B-scan probe to acquire multiple, sequential 2D images for computer storage. Software is used to construct a polyhedral volume image (volume image block) that appears on the computer screen for interactive analysis. (Courtesy Ophthalmic Technologies, Inc, Toronto, Canada.)

A 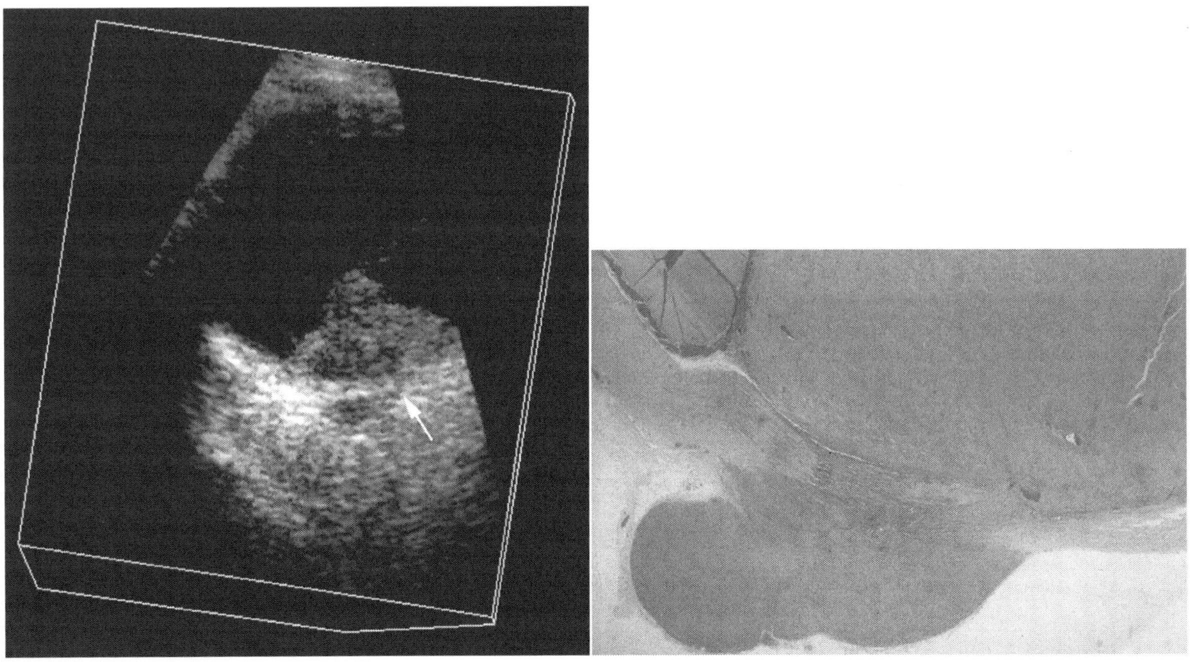 B

Figure 9-3 3DUS echogram and histopathology of choroidal melanoma with extrascleral extension. **A,** 3DUS echogram shows an "oblique" slice through the volume image block that corresponds to the histopathologic section **(B).** Note the path of the tumor through the sclera *(arrow).* **B,** Histopathologic section of tumor showing extrascleral extension and tumor extension through sclera.

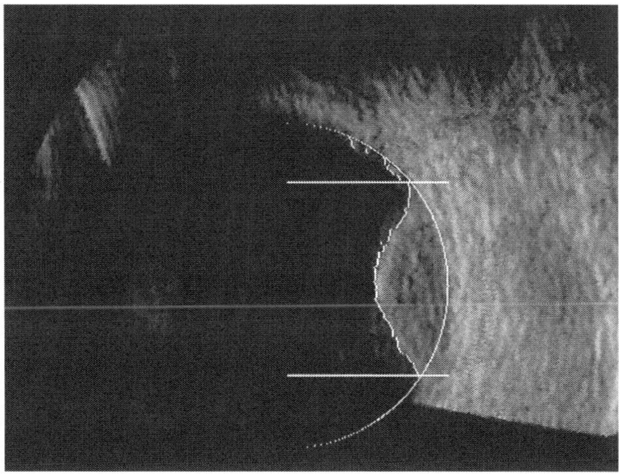

Figure 9-4 3DUS topographic mapping of a choroidal melanoma. The retinal and scleral surfaces of a tumor slice obtained from the volume image block are manually outlined. This procedure is performed on multiple serial slices to calculate tumor volume. This process will be automated in the future.

image block. The number of slices to be analyzed ranges from 60 to 180. Currently, each slice presented on the screen must be outlined manually (Figure 9-4). For tissue volume, a single numeric value is provided; for topography, the results are presented in a graphic three-dimensional form.

Topographic renderings of intraocular tumors, using 3DUS, provide the ability to view the entire surface of the tumor, thereby enhancing the detection of subtle changes along the tumor's surface.[20] This is because each 3D rendering provides thousands of measurements of lesion thickness and cross-sectional extent (Figure 9-5). This can be especially helpful for measuring the apical height of intraocular tumors. Traditionally, the apical height measurement has been obtained with A-scan or an interpolated 2DUS B-scan image.[4,5] These approaches, however, require the examiner to identify the apex of the tumor by dynamically scanning across the tumor surface. With 3DUS, on the other hand, 60 to 180 2DUS image slices are individually outlined and a multitude of points near the tumor surface are obtained. Because the tumor apex is accurately localized on the topographic map (see Figure 9-5), the apical height measurement becomes more objective and less dependent on examiner skill. This technique for localizing the tumor apex is also helpful when the location of the apex changes because of growth or regression. With 3DUS, future software refinements will allow a computer algorithm to search the topographic thickness map to identify the original tumor apex location in relation to the margins of the lesion, thus minimizing errors.

Despite clinical reliance on apical height measurements, most tumors grow volumetrically.[11,15] As previously described, a volumetric measurement can simply be a single number in cubic measure. With further study, tumor volumes may be found to be better predictors of a change in tumor size, as well as of metastatic potential. There are currently no comparative or prospective clinical studies that have examined these potentials.

An experienced observer performing topographic and volumetric analysis typically takes from 1 to 2 hours to outline 60 to 180 2D slices. This procedure of outlining the retinal/tumor surfaces and defining the sclera is subjective (see Figure 9-4); but this process will become less subjective with the use of a computer software process called autosegmentation. By this method, a computer will be programmed to identify the retinal and scleral surfaces, thus increasing the speed and accuracy of outlining the two-dimensional slices.

Choroidal Melanoma

In addition to topographic and volumetric analysis, there are a number of other ways in which 3DUS may prove useful in the evaluation of choroidal melanomas. Coronal and oblique sections through the tissue block are uniquely helpful in the diagnosis and management of these tumors. An example is when a subretinal hemorrhage obscures an underlying melanoma both clinically and with conventional ultrasound. In such cases, repeated analysis of oblique and coronal views obtained with 3DUS can help differentiate blood from tumor. The examiner can also use 3DUS to detect an eccentric or occult collar button by scrolling back and forth through serial sections of the tumor.

The diagnosis of extrascleral extension is another area in which 3DUS is particularly beneficial.[19] In these cases, coronal and oblique reconstructions allow evaluation of the presence, degree, and relative location of extraocular extension. The reliability of 3DUS in this regard has

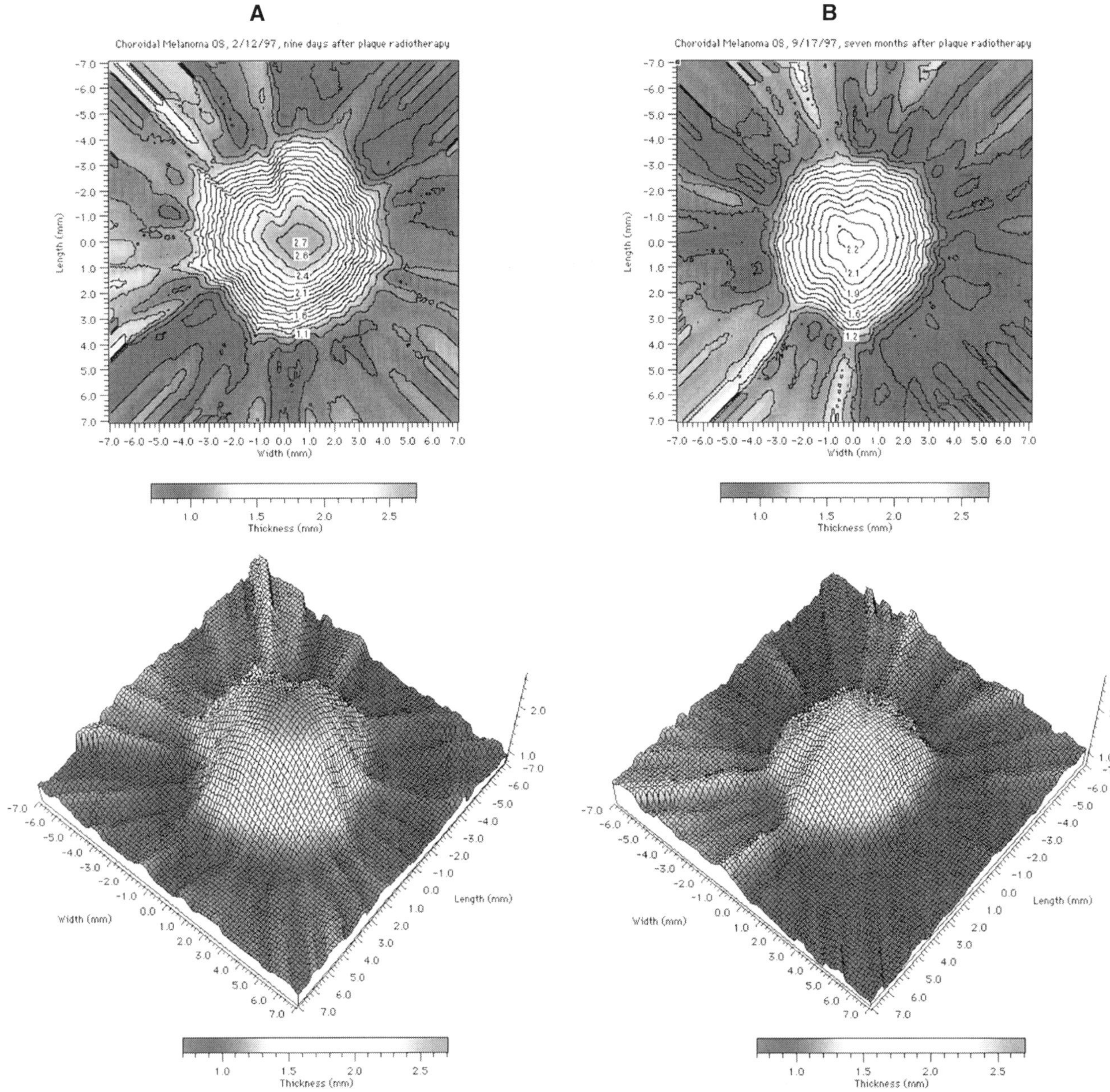

Figure 9-5 Topographic surface rendering of a choroidal melanoma from 3DUS images. The tumor is imaged before **(A)** and 7 months after **(B)** palladium-103 ophthalmic plaque radiation therapy. (Courtesy Dr. Ray Iezzi, Detroit, Michigan.)

been confirmed by sonopathologic correlation. This was achieved by interactively analyzing the stored volume image block to recreate the same plane of section used by the pathologist (see Figure 9-3). As a result, 3DUS can increase confidence in the diagnosis of extraocular tumor extension and may affect the management.[8]

3DUS may also aid in the assessment of choroidal melanomas by quantifying areas of cystic or necrotic tumor and by evaluating internal reflectivity. These capabilities may become even more useful as morphology is linked to tumor behavior.[3,17]

Retinoblastoma

3DUS may play a particularly important role in the evaluation of retinoblastoma. Because children are typically examined under sedation or general anesthesia, the ability to acquire and subsequently analyze the stored volume image block is invaluable. In addition, 3DUS vividly reveals intratumoral calcification and the associated 3D orbital shadows produced by the calcium. The demonstration of calcification is a major diagnostic finding in retinoblastoma (Figure 9-6).

Known risk factors for metastasis of retinoblastoma include optic nerve invasion, choroidal infiltration, and or-

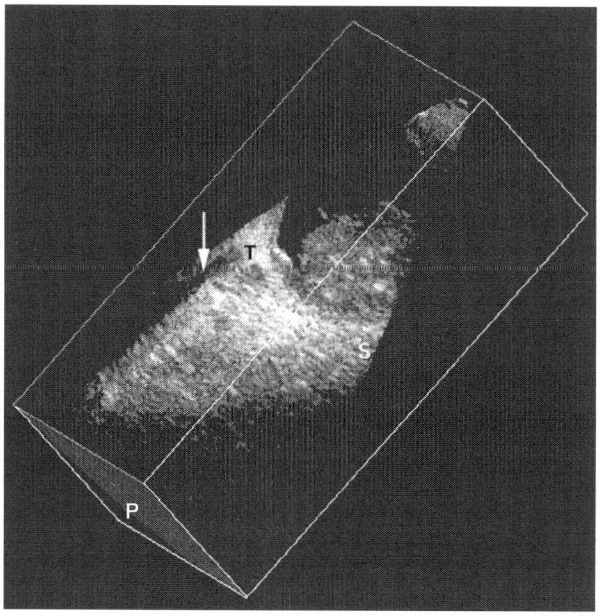

Figure 9-6 3DUS volume image block of retinoblastoma with calcification. Simultaneous sections in the plane of the optic nerve *(arrow)* and tumor show their relative location. *T*, Temporal; *S*, superior; *P*, posterior.

bital extension.[16] Coronal sectioning of the optic nerve with 3DUS offers a new perspective for evaluation of this structure. Topographic mapping offers the potential to quantify choroidal invasion. Furthermore, the ability to examine suspicious areas of sclera with repetitive interactive analysis using coronal and oblique sectioning, should enhance the detection of extrascleral extension.

3DUS for Ophthalmic Plaque Radiation Therapy

Ultrasound is helpful for ophthalmic plaque localization in the treatment of intraocular tumors.[14] While a standard B-scan probe can be rotated by hand to evaluate all of the plaque walls and their proximity to the sclera, 3DUS automates that process and allows the surgeon to replay the entire rotation. Interactive analysis of the stored volume image block has allowed "quartering" of the plaque. This quartering technique provides for the simultaneous assessment of two perpendicular tumor-plaque margins (Figure 9-7, *A*). In addition, coronal sections can be useful for judging proximity of the plaque to the optic nerve (Figure 9-7, *B*).[10,11]

3DUS has also been used to image radioactive seeds within eye plaques.[11] In current practice, determining seed-to-tumor apex distance requires calculations with a number of assumptions (plaque position on the sclera, thickness of the sclera, and constancy of tumor thickness during treatment).[8] In vivo measurements, both prior to and after ophthalmic plaque radiation therapy, will help define the dose delivered to the tumor. In addition, calculation of the actual dose to the tumor and normal ocular structures using 3DUS may help define the actual dose thresholds for radiation complications.[9] Finally, the time needed to obtain a 3D volume image block is much less than that required by conventional B-scan using dynamic scanning. With 3DUS, interactive analysis of the volume image block can be performed at a safe distance from the radioactive plaque.

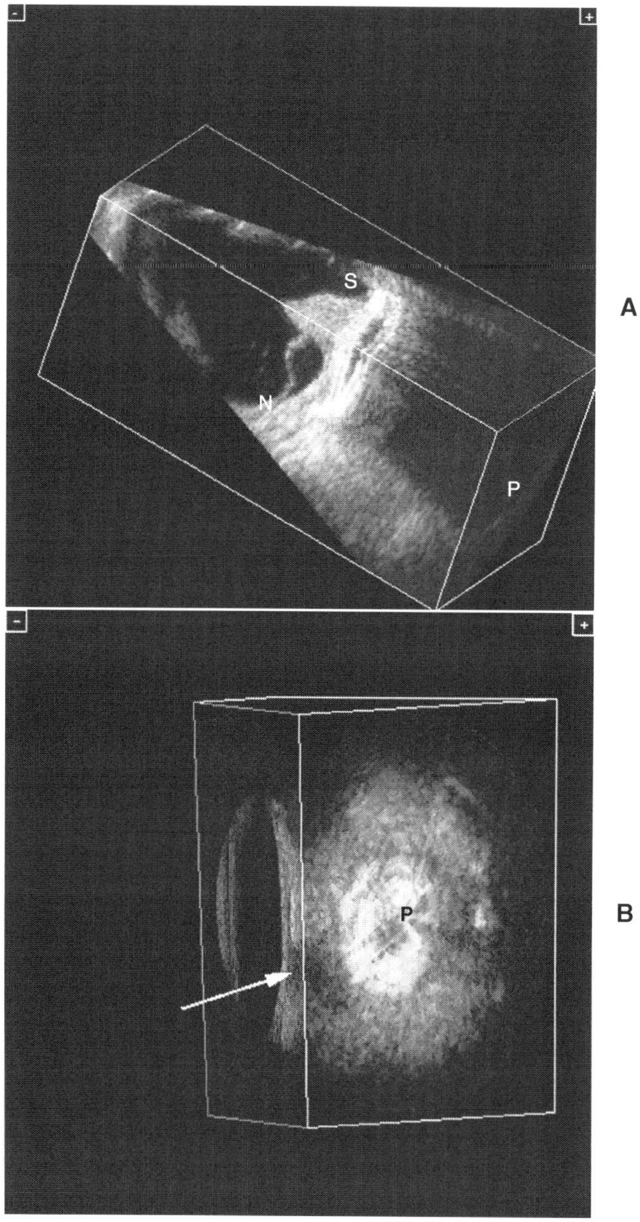

Figure 9-7 3DUS evaluation of choroidal melanoma with radioactive plaque. **A,** Interactive analysis of plaque position beneath tumor simultaneously reveals the temporal and inferior margins. The plaque is "quartered" with simultaneous nasal-temporal and inferior-superior cuts. *S*, Superior; *N*, nasal; *P*, posterior. **B,** Unique coronal section demonstrates the back of the plaque *(P)* adjacent to the optic nerve *(arrow)*.

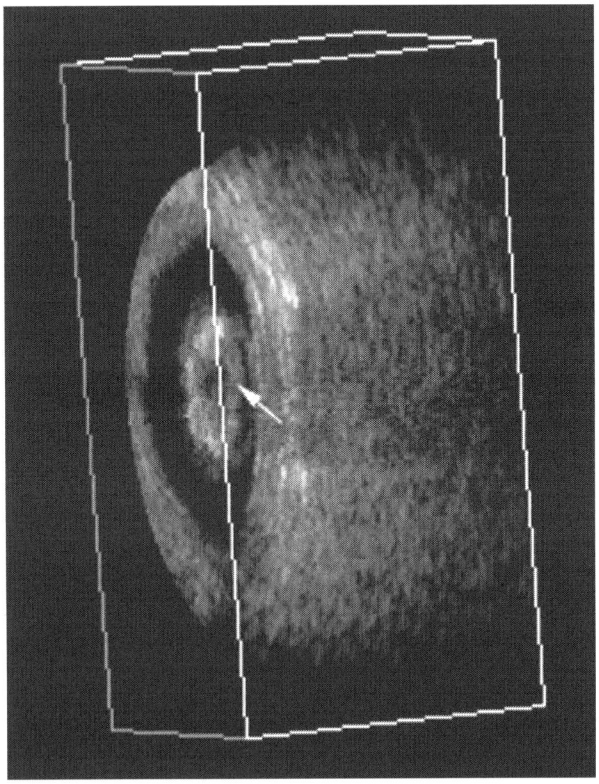

Figure 9-8 Dislocated crystalline lens imaged by 3DUS. Interactive analysis allowed a cut at the lens equator and a perpendicular slice creating a lens quarter. This quartering technique allows the nucleus and cortex to be shown in two separate planes *(arrow)*.

VITREORETINAL DISEASE

Vitreous opacities (hemorrhage, asteroid hyalosis, floaters, and inflammatory debris) are best evaluated during the dynamic, conventional B-scan examination. With this method, the mobility of the opacities can be readily assessed. 3DUS, on the other hand, can create a unique volumetric recording of the quantity and position of the opacities. This capability can be particularly helpful for the follow up of these eyes.

Similarly, the mobility of a dislocated crystalline lens is best demonstrated using conventional B-scan. However, interactive sectioning of the 3D volume image block of the lens allows quartering to create a unique and diagnostic perspective (Figure 9-8).

Retinal Detachment

3DUS is particularly helpful for evaluating retinal detachment. In one case, a 3D volume image block was sliced to demonstrate a coronal view of an open funnel retinal detachment (Figure 9-9). Retinal surgeons can use 3DUS to evaluate the shape of the funnel and document any subretinal elements of traction prior to surgery. The ultrasonographer need not mentally construct a 3D image, because the retinal detachment is both visible on the screen and available for analysis. These capabilities become more important when there is no ophthalmoscopic view of the fundus.[7]

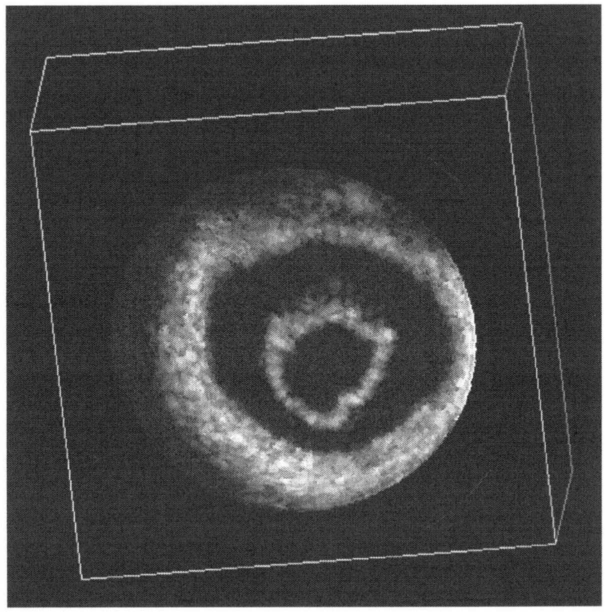

Figure 9-9 3DUS analysis of funnel-shaped retinal detachment. Coronal section shows cross-section of the open funnel. Scrolling anterior or posterior along the retina allows the funnel to be visualized.

Choroidal Detachment

Evaluation of choroidal detachments can be aided by 3DUS reconstructions. Combinations of standard, coronal and oblique sections can be used to reveal the multifaceted shapes of choroidal detachment that are seen beneath a retinal detachment (Figure 9-10).

ADVANTAGES AND LIMITATIONS OF OPHTHALMIC 3DUS

With conventional 2D ultrasound, the ultrasonographer typically takes from 5 to 15 minutes to evaluate the eye dynamically while performing a mental 3D reconstruction (see Table 9-1).[4,5] In contrast, after dynamic examination, 3DUS involves acquiring 60 to 180 sequential 2D images that are stored with each transducer rotation. Computer software then uses this information to reconstruct a 3D volume image block (see Figure 9-2). Without further contact with the patient, the entire examination can either be played back repeatedly (with the same perspective) or rotated and viewed from any orientation. This is quite different from conventional 2D ultrasound that typically involves the acquisition and storage of five or more representative 2D images.[1,4,5]

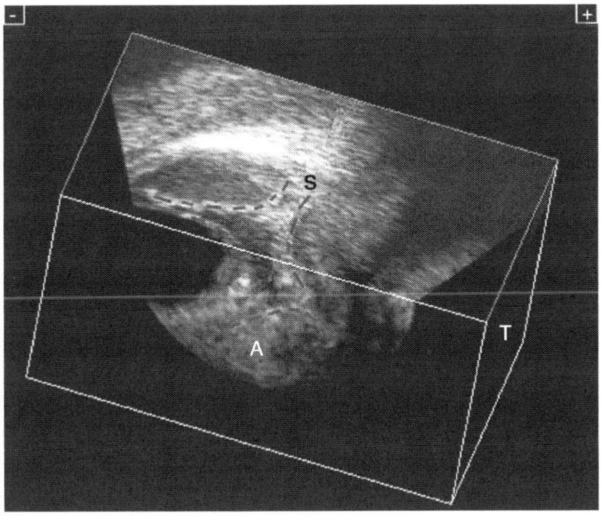

Figure 9-10 Hemorrhagic choroidal detachment imaged with 3DUS. Coronal and oblique sections reveal scalloped shape of choroidal detachments. *Dotted lines*, Surface of choroidal detachments; *A*, anterior; *T*, temporal; *S*, superior. (Courtesy Dr. Julian Garcia, New York, New York.)

The interactive ability to rotate and slice a 3D volume image block allows for the analysis of unique coronal and oblique perspectives. These views were not previously obtainable with 2D ultrasound because of limitations in probe placement due to the orbital bone and other anatomic structures (see Table 9-1). As with evaluation of the static 2D images, retrospective evaluation of the 3D volume image block does not reproduce the dynamic nature of the original ultrasound examination. In fact, the quality of the reconstructed 3D volume image block is exquisitely sensitive to movement of either the patient's eye or the ultrasonographer's hand during the 5- to 7.5-second image acquisition cycle. In practice, multiple 3D data sets are usually acquired and reviewed until the reconstructed volume is free of motion artifacts.

FUTURE DIRECTIONS AND THE INTERNET

The Internet has revolutionized everyday life, and telemedicine is rapidly becoming a reality. Teleradiology has led the way because radiographic images lend themselves to being transmitted from a remote facility to the radiologist. In these cases, the ability to replay the 3DUS, as well as the ability of the observer to evaluate the scanned tissues interactively, are likely to make this format invaluable. Clearly, telemedicine will make the unique talents of ultrasound specialists available to more patients around the world.

At this time, 3DUS should be viewed as an emerging technology that offers unique capabilities for improving ophthalmic practice and patient care.

REFERENCES

1. Byrne SF, Green RL: *Ultrasound of the Eye and Orbit.* St. Louis, Mosby, 1992.
2. Coleman DJ, Katz L, Lizzi FL: Isometric, three-dimensional viewing of ultrasonograms. *Arch Ophthalmol* 1975;93:1362.
3. Coleman DJ, Rondeau MJ, Silverman RH, et al: Correlation of microcirculation architecture with ultrasound backscatter parameters of uveal melanoma. *Eur J Ophthalmol* 1995;5:96.
4. COMS Study Group: Echography (Ultrasound) Procedures for the Collaborative Ocular Melanoma Study (COMS), Report No. 12, Part I. *J Ophthalmic Nurs Technol* 1999;18:143.
5. COMS Study Group: Echography (Ultrasound) Procedures for the Collaborative Ocular Melanoma Study (COMS), Report No. 12, Part II. *J Ophthalmic Nurs Technol* 1999;18:219.
6. Downey DB, Nicolle DA, Levin MF, et al: Three-dimensional ultrasound imaging of the eye. *Eye* 1996;10:75.
7. Endo K, Kato S, Fukushima H, et al: Usefulness of three-dimensional ultrasonography for invisible fundus [letter]. *Br J Ophthalmol* 2000;84:1080.
8. Finger PT: Radiation therapy for choroidal melanoma. *Surv Ophthalmol,* 1997;42(3):215.
9. Finger PT: Tumour location affects the incidence of cataract and retinopathy after ophthalmic plaque radiation therapy. *Br J Ophthalmol* 2000;84:1068.
10. Finger PT, Iezzi R, Esteveo ML, et al: Diode-light transillumination for ophthalmic plaque localization around juxtapapillary choroidal melanomas. *Int J Radiat Oncol Biol Phys* 1999; 44:887.
11. Finger PT, Romero JM, Rosen RB, et al: Three-dimensional ultrasonography of choroidal melanoma: localization of radioactive eye plaques. *Arch Ophthalmol* 1998;116:305.
12. Fisher Y, Hanutsaha P, Tong S, et al: Three-dimensional ophthalmic contact B-scan ultrasonography of the posterior segment. *Retina* 1998;18:251.
13. Gosbell AD, Barry WR, Favilla I: Computer-aided volume measurement of choroidal melanomas. *Aust N Z J Ophthalmol* 1987;15:349.
14. Harbour JW, Murray TG, Byrne SF, et al: Intraoperative echographic localization of iodine 125 episcleral radioactive plaques for posterior uveal melanoma. *Retina* 1996;16:129.
15. Iezzi R, Rosen RB, Tello C, et al: Personal computer–based 3-dimensional ultrasound biomicroscopy of the anterior segment. *Arch Ophthalmol* 1996;114:520.
16. Kopelman JE, McLean IW, Rosenberg SH: Multivariate analysis of risk factors for metastasis in retinoblastoma treated by enucleation. *Ophthalmology* 1987;94:371.
17. Pe'er J, Rummelt V, Mawn L, et al: Mean of the ten largest nucleoli, microcirculation architecture, and prognosis of ciliochoroidal melanomas. *Ophthalmology* 1994;101:1227.
18. Romero JM, Finger PT, Rosen RB, et al: Three-dimensional ultrasound for measurement of choroidal melanomas. *Arch Ophthalmol* 2001;119:1275.
19. Romero JM, Finger PT, Iezzi R, et al: Three-dimensional ultrasonography of choroidal melanoma: Extrascleral extension. *Am J Ophthalmol* 1998;126:842.
20. Rosen RB, Iezzi R, Romero J, Finger P: Topography Mapping. In Shammas JH, Dunne S, Fisher Y: *Three-Dimensional Ultrasound Topography of the Eye.* Eden Mills, Ontario, NovaCoast, 1998, p 197.
21. Shammas JH, Dunne S, Fisher Y: *Three-Dimensional Ultrasound Tomography of the Eye.* Eden Mills, Ontario, NovaCoast, 1998.

10

Paul T. Finger

Axial Eye Length Measurements (A-Scan Biometry)

The measurement of axial eye length (AEL) is the most common ultrasound procedure performed in ophthalmology and is the primary component of intraocular lens (IOL) power calculations.[8,18,31,43] This chapter will describe the contact and immersion examination techniques for measuring eye length[2,12,37] (Figure 10-1). It will also cover different types of instrumentation and the use of appropriate instrument settings. Solutions to various problems and the avoidance of pitfalls will also be addressed. This chapter will also discuss the use of A-scan biometry in the diagnosis and management of certain ocular conditions (e.g., congenital glaucoma and nanophthalmos).

STANDARD AXIAL EYE LENGTH DIMENSIONS

The accuracy of AEL measurements, using A-scan ultrasound, is generally accepted to be within 0.1 mm.[1,3] Standard values for the AEL and the various ocular components (i.e., cornea, anterior chamber, and lens) have been established. A review of several studies using different measurement techniques shows that the axial length of the normal eye is approximately 23.6 mm.* It has also been shown that the majority of axial lengths range from 22.0 mm to 24.5 mm[22] and that in most individuals, the difference in AEL measurement between right and left eyes is within 0.3 mm.[8,24,40]

Average values have also been determined for corneal thickness, anterior chamber depth, and thickness of the crystalline lens.[19,21] The established value for average corneal thickness is 0.55 mm. The anterior chamber depth in phakic eyes has been found to measure 3.24 mm (±0.44 mm),[21] and the thickness of the cataractous lens is 4.63 mm.[19] It has also been shown that the thickness of the cataractous lens increases and the anterior chamber depth decreases with age.[19]

*References 1, 3, 19, 21, 22, 36, 41, 42.

In children, A-scan biometry has become increasingly important, both for IOL calculations and for management of congenital glaucoma. Various studies have been performed to establish standard axial length values in the pediatric population (Table 10-1).[11,13,16,46]

INSTRUMENTATION

A variety of A-scan equipment is available for AEL measurements. Some instruments are specifically dedicated to AEL measurements (i.e., biometers), whereas others have capabilities for both diagnostic and biometric examinations (Figure 10-2). Most available biometers provide accurate measurements as long as proper technique is used.

Certain features are recommended when choosing among the instrumentation that is currently available (Box 10-1). Most importantly, an instrument should have a screen display that can be continually monitored. In addition to the echogram, the display should ideally include a numerical reading of the AEL measurement, as well as values for the anterior chamber depth, lens thickness, and vitreous length. Certain instruments additionally provide values for the average and/or standard deviation of multiple measurements obtained from a given eye. Contact and immersion capabilities are beneficial, as are manual and automatic measurement modes.

In addition, some instruments provide the ability to change the sound velocity setting from preset values, which can be helpful in certain situations (see pp 246 and 266). Also, most newer machines allow the storage of multiple echograms for subsequent review and critiquing, so that scans of poor quality can be deleted and repeated, if necessary.

The majority of biometric A-scan instruments are digitized, which allows individual echograms to be frozen and, in some instruments, one or more echograms to be stored. Most of these machines have a foot pedal that is depressed to

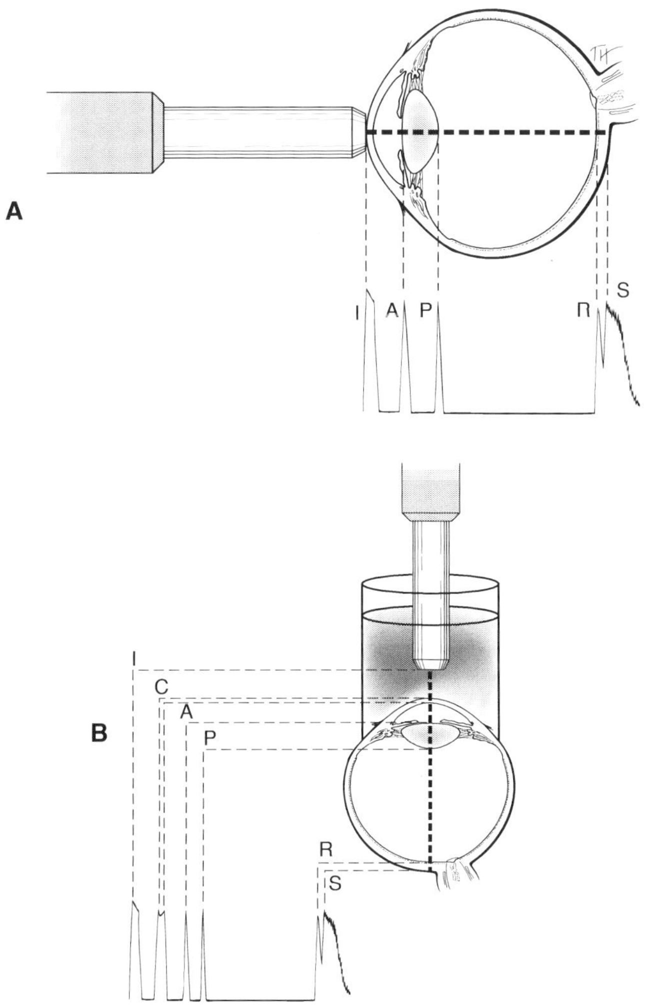

Figure 10-1 Techniques for contact **(A)** and immersion **(B)** A-scan AEL measurements. In both methods, the sound beam is directed along the visual axis, through the center of the lens, perpendicular to the macula. **A,** Probe is placed directly on cornea. *I,* Initial spike corresponding to probe tip on cornea; *A,* anterior lens capsule; *P,* posterior lens capsule; *R,* retina; *S,* sclera. **B,** Probe is placed in fluid within immersion shell (not touching cornea). *I,* Initial spike corresponding to tip of probe in fluid; *C,* cornea; *A,* anterior lens capsule; *P,* posterior lens capsule; *R,* retina; *S,* sclera.

freeze a given scan. The foot pedal is beneficial because it frees the examiner's hands to perform other functions.

Documentation of measurements is important and can be accomplished with a photograph of the echogram. Many of the newer biometers also offer the option of a printer, which can provide less expensive documentation of findings. Also, many of these biometers are programmed with a variety of formulas to facilitate calculation of the IOL power.

Probes

The first generation of contact biometers used water-filled probes with a soft membranous tip. The purpose of the soft tip was to minimize corneal indentation. Water-filled probes, however, must be filled with distilled water, and in the process, small air bubbles can become trapped in the

TABLE 10-1

Normal Axial Length Values

Age	Axial Length (in mm)
Newborn	17.02
10-45 days	17.22
46-75 days	18.77
76-120 days	19.43
5-9 months	20.09
10-18 months	20.14
19-36 months	22.01
4-5 years	22.78
6-7 years	22.56
8-10 years	23.12

Modifed from Grignolo A, Rivara A: Biometry of the human eye from the sixth month of pregnancy to the tenth year of life, in J Vanysek (ed): *Diagnostica Ultrasonica in Ophthalmologia,* Brno, Czechoslovakia, Universita J.E. Purkynje, 1968, p 251.

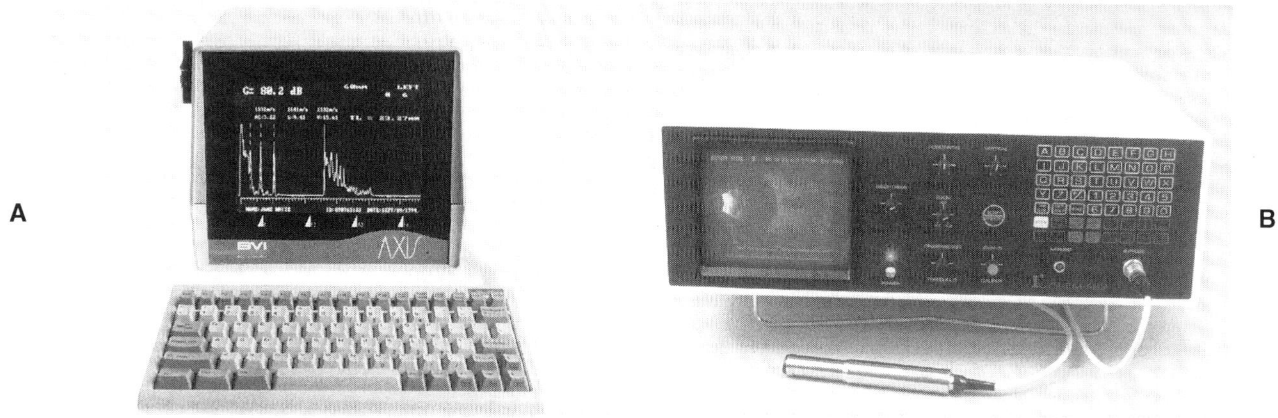

Figure 10-2 Instruments used for A-scan biometry. **A,** BVI Axis (BV International, Clermont-Ferrand, France) is primarily used for AEL measurements. **B,** I^3 ABD-X (Innovative Imaging, Inc, Sacramento, California) can be used for both AEL measurements and diagnostic echography.

BOX 10-1

Recommended Features of Biometry Instrumentation

- Screen display
- Contact and immersion capabilities
- Choice of average or individual sound velocity settings
- Adjustable sound velocity settings
- Four or more measuring gates (which are moveable on frozen echogram)
- Numeric values displayed for anterior chamber depth, lens thickness, vitreous length, average and standard deviation of the AEL measurements

From Byrne SF: *A-scan Axial Length Measurements—A Handbook for IOL Calculations.* Mars Hill, NC, Grove Park Publishers, 1995, p 10.

water chamber. These bubbles can result in erroneous AEL readings.

Newer biometers use a solid probe that requires less maintenance and avoids many of the problems inherent in water-filled probes (Figure 10-3). The solid tip probe, however, can more easily indent the cornea, resulting in a shortened AEL reading. Nevertheless, in most cases, the probe can be applied with minimal pressure, thereby minimizing corneal compression.

Most biometry probes function at an operating frequency of 10 to 12 MHz, providing adequate resolution for obtaining accurate measurements. Some of these probes emit a focused sound beam, whereas others emit a nonfocused beam (see p 6).

INSTRUMENT SETTINGS

The settings on most instruments include (1) measurement mode, (2) eye type, (3) position of electronic gates or cursors, and (4) gain. Familiarity with the settings on a particular instrument is important so the proper adjustments can be made.[5,8]

Measurement Mode (Automatic vs. Manual)

Most of the newer biometry instruments provide a choice of automatic or manual measuring modes. In the automatic mode, the instrument (rather than the examiner) selects the scan to be measured. The automatic acquisition of an echogram is often accompanied by an audible tone. These automated features can allow the examiner to concentrate on the mechanics of technique while relying on the instrument to indicate when proper sound beam alignment has been achieved. Furthermore, the automatic mode can be beneficial for performing more rapid measurements in an otherwise normal cataractous eye. Although these automatic features require minimal technical skill, it is important that the examiner be able to interpret the echograms selected by the instrument.

Some biometers also provide a semiautomatic or dense cataract mode that can be used when the examiner is having difficulty in displaying a distinct, high spike from the posterior lens capsule or retina. In this mode, the instrument parameters for spike height and smoothness are somewhat relaxed compared to those used for the fully automatic mode.

A manual scanning mode can also be used. For this mode, the examiner determines when a scan is to be measured, depresses a foot pedal to freeze the image, and positions the gates at the desired spikes. It should be noted, though, that in some instruments, it is necessary to preposition the gates prior to freezing the echogram. The manual mode may be helpful for examining aphakic and pseudophakic eyes, as well as phakic eyes in which measurements are difficult to obtain using the automatic mode. With the manual mode, more time can be taken to align the sound beam along the visual axis to select the best scan for measurement.

A

B

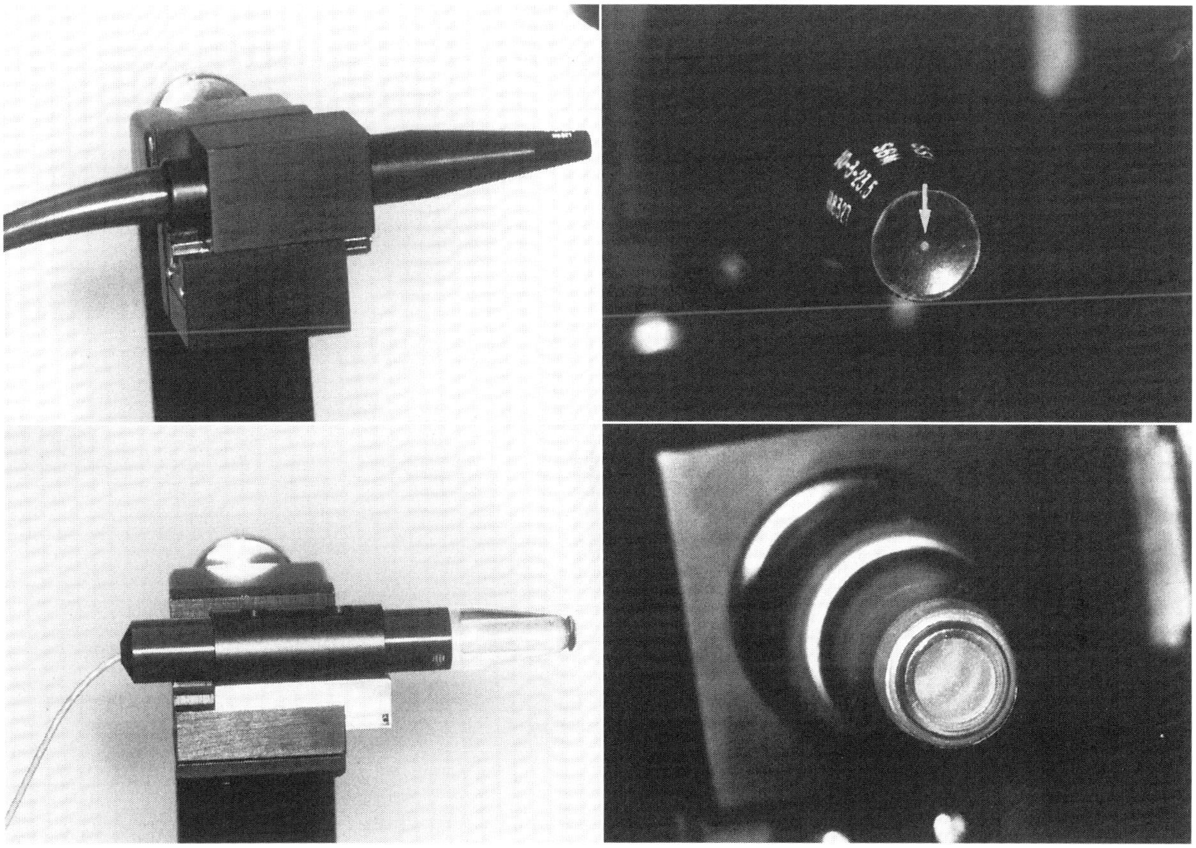

Figure 10-3 Solid and water-filled probes mounted in spring-loaded sleeve for applanation technique. **A,** Solid-tip probe has fixation light in center of probe *(arrow)*. **B,** Water-filled probe with rubber membrane on surface.

TABLE 10-2

Sound Velocities for Eye Length Measurements

INDIVIDUAL OCULAR MEDIA	
Medium	**Velocity (m/sec)**
Cornea	1,641
Aqueous/vitreous	1,532
Crystalline lens	1,641*
Solid tissue	1,550
IOL Implants	See Table 10-3
Silicone oil	980-1,040
EYE TYPES	
Eye Type	**Velocity (m/sec)**
Aphakia	1,532
Phakia (average)	1,550
Pseudophakia	1,532 (see p 255)

*This value may decrease with age (see p 253).

Eye Type (Sound Velocity)

As discussed in Chapter 1, ultrasound measurements are calculated according to the speed at which the sound wave travels through a given medium. The use of appropriate sound velocity settings is essential for obtaining accurate AEL measurements (Table 10-2). The velocity setting on the instrument should always be checked prior to beginning the examination.

When measuring a phakic eye, some instruments use an average sound velocity setting of 1,550 m/sec, which takes into account the faster sound speed in lens (1,641 m/sec), as compared to aqueous and vitreous (1,532 m/sec). This average sound velocity assumes a constant relationship between the lens thickness and the depth of the anterior chamber. Although this method is sufficient for measuring the normal phakic eye (see p 252), slight errors may occur when the lens is inordinately thin or thick or when the eye is very short or very long.[3,20] In these cases, more accurate measurements can be obtained with instruments that measure the components separately at their appropriate sound velocities and then add these individual values together for the final reading.

If an incorrect eye type (sound velocity setting) is used, an erroneous measurement will occur. The correct value can be determined, however, without remeasuring the eye by using the velocity conversion equation[8,20] (see p 262).

Gates

Gates are electronic markers or cursors on the screen display that provide measurements of the distance between

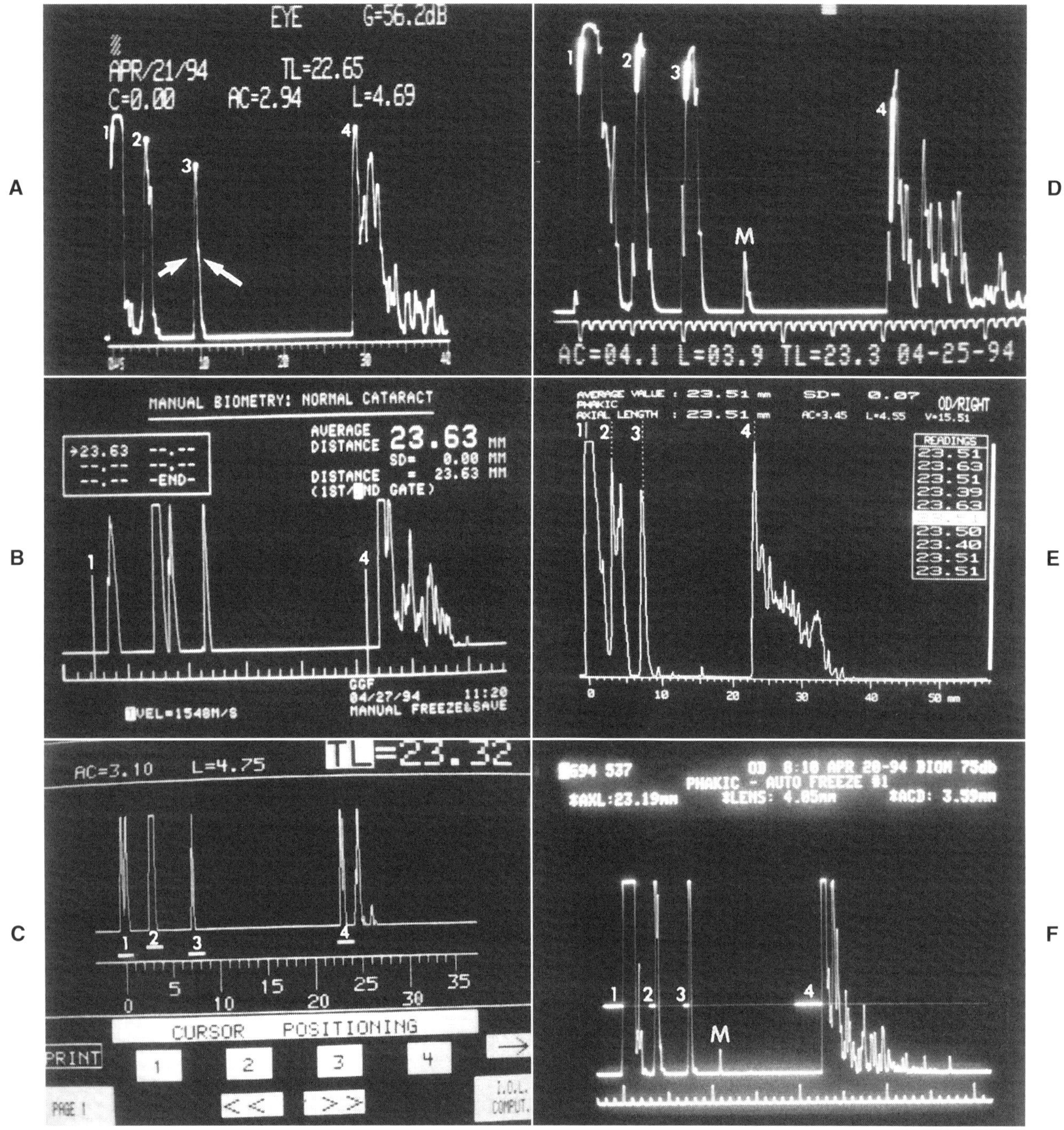

Figure 10-4 Normal contact axial A-scans shows proper positioning of gates. Echograms were obtained from six different phakic eyes using instruments with varying types and number of gates. **A,** Mini A-scan (4 gates). *Small arrow,* Ascending limb or leading edge of spike; *large arrow,* descending limb of spike; *1,* corneal gate (initial spike); *2,* anterior lens capsule gate; *3,* posterior lens capsule gate; *4,* retinal gate. **B,** Sonomed A-2500 biometer (2 gates). **C,** Paxial biometer (4 gates). **D,** Ophthascan S, B/A-scan (4 gates). *M,* Multiple signal. **E,** Ocuscan biometer (4 gates). **F,** I[3] ABD-X, B/A-scan (4 gates). Note that gates are positioned on either the ascending limb or peak of each spike but are never placed on the descending limb of a spike. (From Byrne SF: *A-scan Axial Length Measurements—A Handbook for IOL Calculations.* Mars Hill, NC, Grove Park Publishers, 1995, p 20.)

A 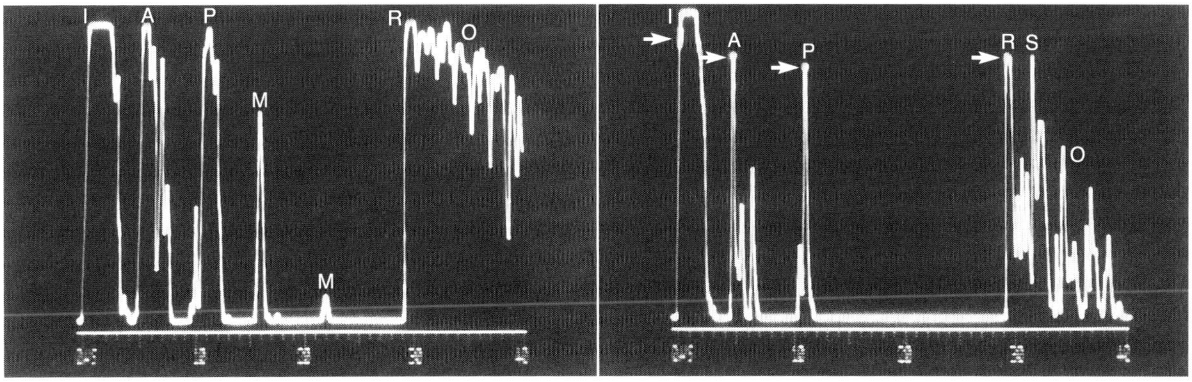 B

Figure 10-5 Contact axial A-scans from phakic eye at high gain **(A)** and reduced gain **(B)**. *I*, Initial spike; *A*, anterior lens capsule; *P*, posterior lens capsule; *M*, multiple signals; *R*, retina; *S*, sclera; *O*, orbital fat; *arrows*, gates. (From Byrne SF: *A-scan Axial Length Measurements—A Handbook for IOL Calculations*. Mars Hill, NC, Grove Park Publishers, 1995, p 22.)

two or more anatomic interfaces. In the automatic mode (see p 246), gate position is usually determined by the instrument, whereas in the manual mode, it is selected by the examiner.

An ultrasound instrument can have two to four gates. Aphakic and pseudophakic eyes are measured with either two or three gates, depending on the instrument (see p 255), and the phakic eye can be measured with as few as two or as many as four gates (Figure 10-4; see also p 252).

Significant measurement errors can result from incorrect gate placement. Incorrect placement can occur when either automatic or manual measurement modes are employed and when using either the contact or the immersion technique (see pp 253 and 260). Constant monitoring of the echogram for proper gate placement is essential.

Instruments that employ only two gates and do not allow changes in the preset sound velocity settings cannot provide a separate value for the lens thickness. However, there are circumstances in which this measurement is necessary. For instance, some formulas require a lens thickness measurement for accurate calculation of the IOL power.[28] In such situations, the two gates can be placed on the anterior and posterior lens capsule spikes and the velocity conversion equation can be used to derive the lens thickness (see p 262).

Gain Setting

The gain is defined as the degree of echo amplification in an ultrasound system. The adjustable gain setting controls the effective sound beam width, sensitivity, resolution, and depth of penetration (see p 8).

At the beginning of an examination, the gain should be placed at a relatively high level. A high gain setting should be used initially to align grossly the sound beam with structures along the visual axis and to assess the overall appearance of the echogram. Ideally, the gain should then be reduced to a medium level to improve resolution of the spikes (Figure 10-5).

Errors can occur when the gain is set too high or too low. With a very high gain setting, instruments that measure between the peaks of the spikes may yield a slightly short reading. Conversely, at a very low gain setting, the amplitude of the retinal spike may decrease to the point that the adjacent scleral spike may be mistaken for the retinal spike, resulting in a long reading. Occasionally, however, the use of a higher or lower gain setting may be necessary (see pp 256 and 265).

EXAMINATION PROCEDURES FOR A-SCAN BIOMETRY

Accurate AEL measurements can be facilitated by using a systematic approach for each examination. Many errors can be attributed to a breakdown of procedures or shortcuts taken during the examination. All examinations should begin with the examiner taking a history and explaining the examination to the patient. The patient should be positioned for the particular type of examination (i.e., contact or immersion) and instrument settings should be adjusted appropriately. The examination is then performed. Whenever possible, both eyes should be measured for comparison. At the conclusion of the examination, the eye is cleansed and the results are double-checked for accuracy.

Because there are advantages and disadvantages to both the contact and the immersion methods, one may be more appropriate than the other in certain situations. Although both methods can yield accurate results, it is generally believed that the immersion technique produces the most precise measurements. This is due to the potential error of corneal compression inherent in the contact technique. Four investigations comparing AEL using both contact and immersion techniques in the same patients have reported mean values ranging from 0.14 to 0.36 mm longer with the immersion technique than with the contact method.[1,36,41,42] These two methods will be discussed in detail later in this chapter.

Keratometry

The keratometer is used to measure the radius of curvature of the anterior corneal surface. These measurements (k-readings) are usually performed in conjunction with A-scan biometry to calculate the IOL power for cataract surgery. Keratometry readings should always be obtained prior to the AEL measurement. This is because A-scan biometry may cause mild distortion of the corneal mires, resulting in inaccurate k-readings. It is important that the keratometry instrument be calibrated frequently to help assure accurate readings.

History-Taking

A history should be taken prior to any biometry examination. Information to be obtained includes any previous ocular surgery, as well as known intraocular abnormalities. For example, it is important to know if the eye is pseudophakic or contains silicone oil since these conditions require the use of specific sound velocities and examination techniques (see pp 255 and 265). A history of diabetes or age-related macular degeneration raises the possibility of detachment or thickening of the macula that may result in a short AEL measurement. Furthermore, a history that includes a scleral buckling procedure indicates that the eye may measure significantly longer than the fellow eye.

Patient Preparation

After the biometry procedure is explained to the patient and the patient is questioned about any allergies to eye drops, anesthetic drops are instilled. The patient is positioned according to the measurement method to be used (see pp 259 and 260). The main instrument settings (measurement mode, eye type, gate position, and gain) should be checked just before the examination (see p 246).

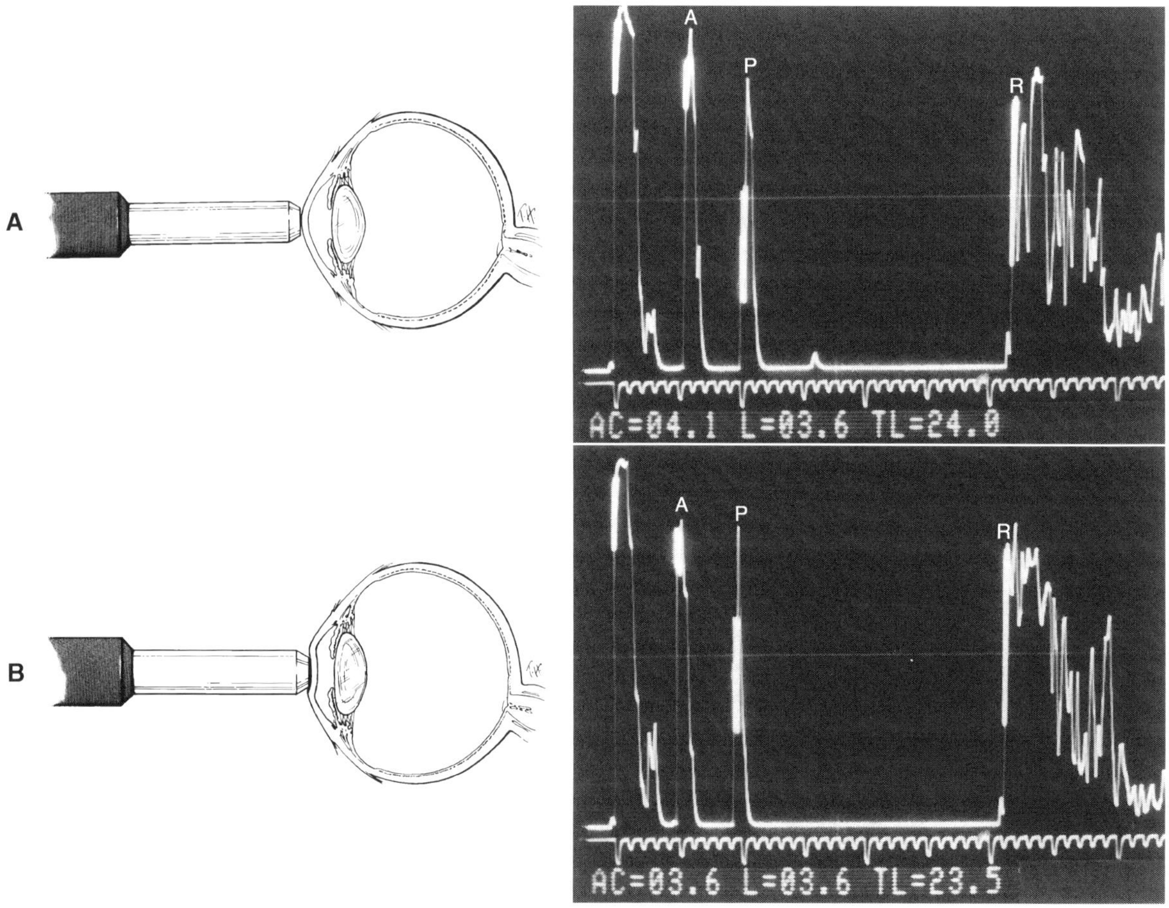

Figure 10-6 Correct (no compression) and incorrect (compression) placement of probe on cornea. **A,** Schematic drawing and echogram show correct measurement when probe just touches but does not indent cornea. The anterior chamber depth = 4.1 mm and the AEL = 24.0 mm. *A*, Anterior lens capsule; *P*, posterior lens capsule; *R*, retina. **B,** schematic drawing and echogram of same eye with corneal indentation. The anterior chamber depth and the axial length are both decreased by 0.5 mm.

Prior to each use, the probe should be cleaned appropriately and the probe tip inspected to ensure that it is dry with no fluid adherent to the surface. After the probe and instrument settings have been assessed, the patient is instructed to fixate in primary gaze, preferably at the light within the probe. Whenever possible, both eyes should be measured to help avoid errors.

Contact Technique

Using the contact technique, the AEL is measured with the probe placed gently on the center of the cornea and the sound beam directed toward the macula. This technique can be performed either by placing the probe in a chin rest device (applanation method) or by holding the probe by hand (hand-held method).

Steps should always be taken to minimize both corneal compression and corneal abrasion. This can be achieved by obtaining a measurement as soon as the probe touches the center of the cornea. The probe is then removed from the eye, and the patient is asked to blink to keep the cornea moist. This on-and-off procedure is repeated several times until at least three high-quality readings have been obtained. During each reading, the anterior chamber depth should be evaluated since the chamber shallows when the cornea is indented (Figure 10-6; see also p 269). The use of intermittent probe contact also lessens the likelihood of a corneal abrasion. Damage to the corneal epithelium can result from excessive pressure or manipulation of the probe on the corneal surface.

Prior to each measurement, it is important to make certain that no ointment or excess fluid (e.g., anesthetic drops or tears) is present on the cornea. This is because even small amounts of fluid on the cornea may lead to an erroneously long AEL reading (Figure 10-7; see also p 256).

Applanation Method

For the applanation method, a chin rest apparatus is used, with the probe secured within a holder or sleeve. If available, a pressure-sensitive probe holder can be used to help minimize corneal compression. The patient is seated upright, with the chin positioned firmly in the chin rest and the forehead pressed against the headrest (Figure 10-8). The patient is instructed to fixate in primary gaze at the tiny fixation light located within the center of the probe tip (see Figure 10-3). Initially, the joystick is retracted as far away

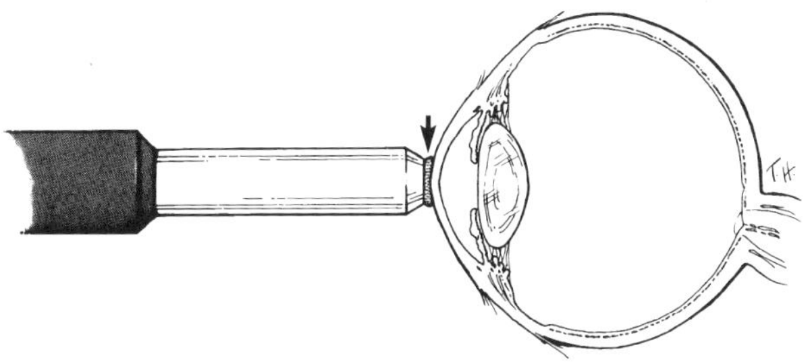

Figure 10-7 Fluid meniscus between probe tip and cornea *(arrow)*. The presence of such fluid will result in an abnormally long AEL measurement.

A

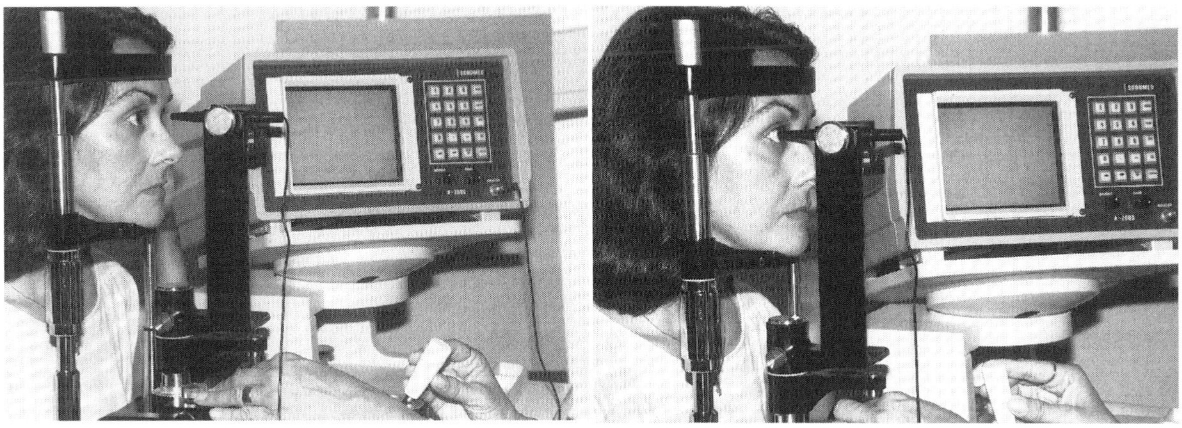

B

Figure 10-8 Applanation technique. **A,** Joystick is fully retracted, with probe away from eye prior to measurement. **B,** Joystick is advanced, just until probe touches corneal surface.

A

B

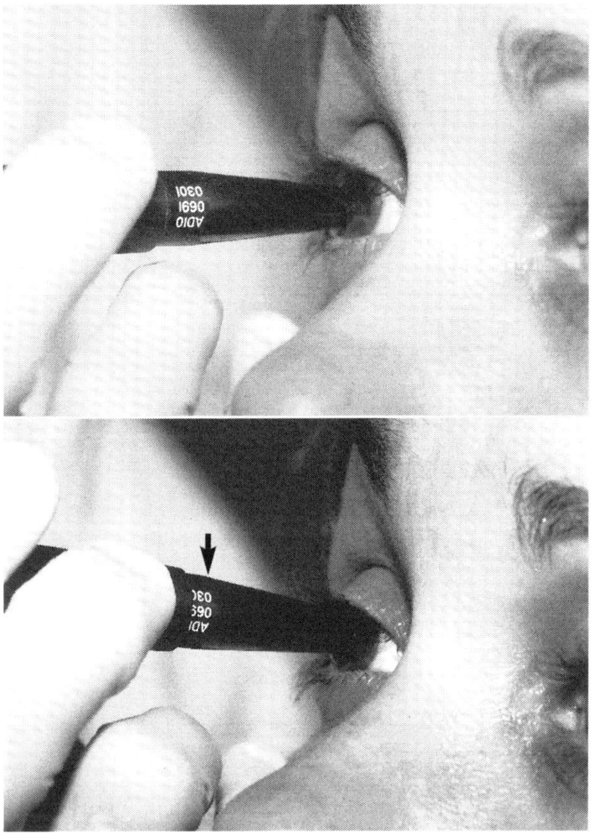

Figure 10-9 Contact, hand-held method using solid probe in pressure-sensitive sleeve. **A,** Probe in gentle contact with cornea. **B,** Corneal compression. Note partial obscuration of numbers *(arrow)* as probe retracts into sleeve. (From Byrne SF: *A-scan Axial Eye Length Measurements—A Handbook for IOL Calculations.* Mars Hill, NC, Grove Park Publishers, 1995, p 29.)

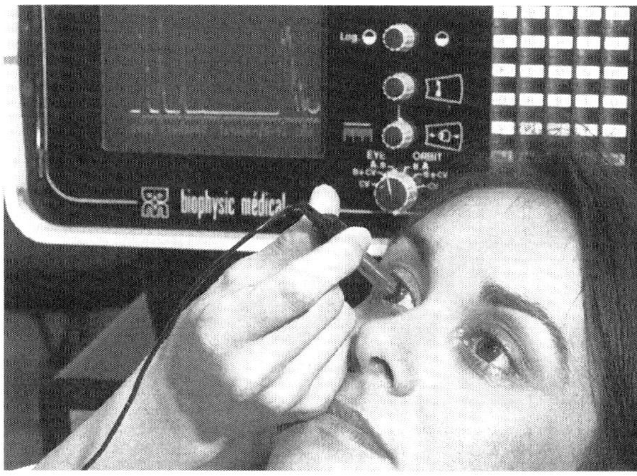

Figure 10-10 Patient positioned for contact, hand-held technique. Patient is reclined and eye being measured is positioned near the screen.

from the eye as possible. The joystick is then advanced until the probe gently touches the center of the cornea.

Hand-Held Method

Extra caution must be exercised when a hand-held technique is employed because the cornea is more easily compressed with this technique than with the applanation method. For hand-held measurements, the patient is either seated upright or reclined. Some examiners prefer to use a probe mounted in a pressure-sensitive sleeve (similar to that used for the applanation method) to help lessen corneal compression (Figure 10-9). For the pressure-sensitive sleeve to function as intended, the patient must be examined in an upright or semireclined position. When a pressure sensitive sleeve is not employed, the patient should be reclined. This facilitates placement of the examined eye near the screen for optimum hand/eye coordination (Figure 10-10) and provides better support for the probe.

Measurement of the Phakic Eye (Contact Technique)

Accurate AEL measurements can usually be obtained from a normal cataractous eye within a few minutes. However, if the cataract is extremely dense, sound attenuation (see p 265) may cause weakening of the retinal and scleral spikes, resulting in a more difficult, prolonged examination. In this situation, the use of a manual mode or a semiautomatic (dense cataract) mode (see p 246) is preferable to the use of a fully automatic mode.

The first spike in the echogram, the initial spike, represents the probe tip on the cornea and is always present in the echogram. In addition to the initial spike, four additional primary spikes are displayed from the phakic eye: anterior lens capsule, posterior lens capsule, retina, and sclera. The scleral spike is then followed by a chain of spikes that originate from the orbital fat behind the eye (see Figures 10-1 and 10-5). All four primary spikes should be as smooth, steeply rising, and as high as possible. If one or more spikes are indistinct or of much lower amplitude than the others, the sound beam may not be properly aligned along the visual axis.

Either a manual or an automatic measurement mode can be used to measure the normal, phakic eye (see p 246). However, it is always best to use a manual mode for difficult examinations or whenever an abnormality is suspected or is known to be present. The phakic eye type setting is employed for the examination.

A-scan biometers generally measure the phakic eye in one of two ways. Some use a preset, average sound velocity setting (1,550 m/sec)[1,26,27] and two gates; others use individual sound velocity settings and four gates to measure each component of the eye separately.[30,31] When two gates are employed, the anterior gate is placed at the initial spike and the posterior gate is positioned at the retinal spike. For the four-gate method, gates are placed at the initial spike, the anterior lens capsule spike, the posterior lens capsule spike, and the retinal spike (see Figure 10-4, *A*). With the four-gate method, the anterior chamber depth is measured using 1,532 m/sec, the lens is measured using 1,641 m/sec, and the vitreous is measured using 1,532 m/sec. The biometer then automatically combines these individual measurements to determine the AEL measurement. The use of

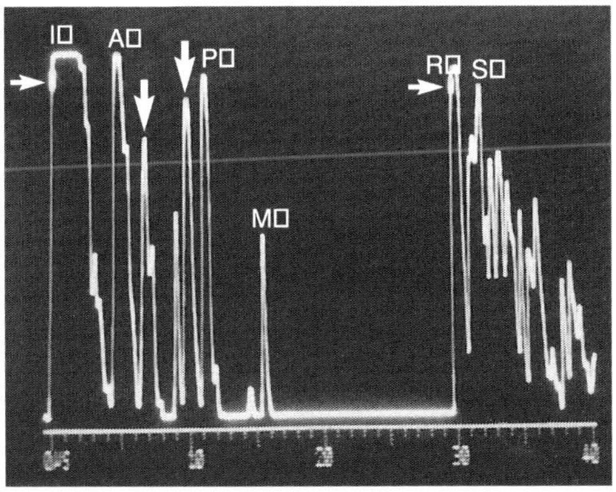

Figure 10-11 Contact axial A-scan showing dense cataract. Note the presence of abnormal spikes *(vertical arrows)* between anterior *(A)* and posterior *(P)* lens capsule spikes. *Arrows*, Gates; *I*, initial spike; *M*, multiple signal; *R*, retina; *S*, sclera.

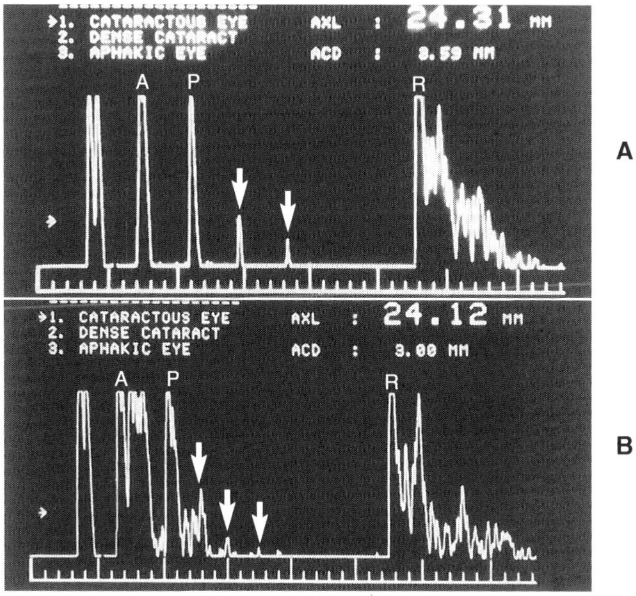

Figure 10-12 Contact axial A-scans from two different patients showing multiple signals produced by the lens. **A,** Low reflective multiple signals *(arrows)*. *A*, Anterior lens capsule; *P*, posterior lens capsule; *R*, retina. **B,** Multiple signals *(arrows)* are more irregularly spaced and numerous due to the very dense nature of the cataract.

individual sound velocity settings and four gates may provide more consistent and accurate AEL readings than use of a two-gate method with an average sound velocity.

Another method has been developed for measuring the phakic eye.[26-28] This method uses two gates, as just described, and the aphakic sound velocity setting (1,532 m/sec) in lieu of the average phakic sound velocity setting (1,550 m/sec). Once the AEL measurement is obtained, a corrected axial length factor (CALF)[23,28] is then added to account for the crystalline lens. This factor is based on changes in lens thickness and sound velocity that occur with age. The average CALF value for most cataract patients is 0.32 mm.[28]

When a phakic eye is measured, spikes may be displayed in the echogram in addition to those used for the measurement. These additional spikes, which may occur between the anterior and posterior lens capsule spikes, are due to interfaces within a cataractous lens (Figure 10-11). Spikes may also appear along the vitreous baseline, caused either by artifacts (multiple signals [see p 466]) or by actual abnormalities in the vitreous cavity.

In biometry of the phakic eye, the majority of multiple signals encountered are due to reverberations between the probe and the crystalline lens. Multiple signals are usually highly reflective and evenly spaced along the vitreous baseline, declining in height from left to right. These signals disappear at reduced gain levels (see Figure 10-5) and typically produce more motion than spikes originating from true intraocular interfaces. Multiple signals are usually few in number when the lens is clear or there is a cataract of only moderate density. However, they may be more numerous when a cataract is extremely dense. In some cases, multiple signals produce low reflective spikes similar in appearance to those of vitreous opacities (Figure 10-12). In the phakic eye, these weakly reflective echoes usually occur just to the right of the posterior lens capsule spike. To distinguish such artifactual spikes from those produced by actual vitreous opacities, the probe can be placed on the conjunctiva, with the sound beam directed anteriorly across the vitreous cavity, avoiding the lens. With the sound beam bypassing the lens in this way, the multiple signals will no longer be present (see Figure 1-11). When, however, the spikes originate from vitreous opacities, they will continue to be displayed. Should repositioning the probe fail to determine the nature of these low reflective echoes, a B-scan examination can be employed to evaluate the posterior segment of the eye more thoroughly.

Abnormal vitreous spikes can occur from a number of conditions. The two most common conditions encountered during biometry are asteroid hyalosis (Figure 10-13) and vitreous hemorrhage (see p 45).

When abnormal spikes are present, either within the lens or along the vitreous baseline, caution should be exercised in using the automatic mode since the instrument may place one or more gates on the wrong spikes, resulting in an erroneous measurement (Figure 10-14; see also p 247).

Measurement of the Aphakic Eye (Contact Technique)

The aphakic eye is generally easy to measure because of the absence of the lens. For this same reason, however, the sound beam can more easily be misdirected in the aphakic

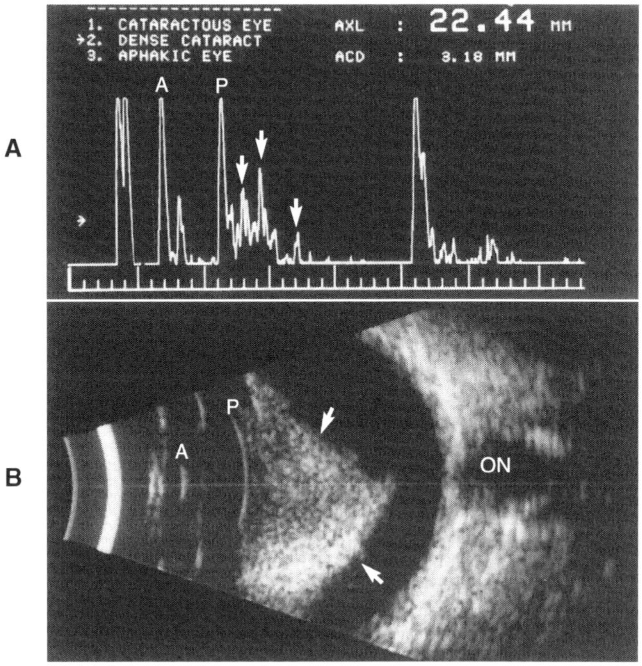

Figure 10-13 Asteroid hyalosis. **A,** Contact axial A-scan showing medium-low reflective spikes *(arrows)* from asteroid bodies. *A,* Anterior lens capsule; *P,* posterior lens capsule. **B,** Axial B-scan of same eye showing dense opacities within vitreous cavity *(arrows)*. *ON,* Optic nerve.

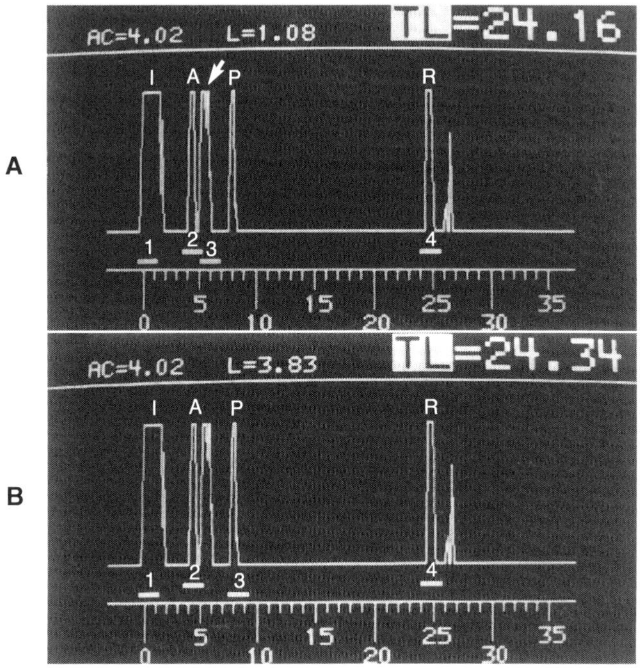

Figure 10-14 Erroneous AEL measurement using automatic measurement mode (contact technique). The gates appear as bars beneath the spikes (*1,* initial spike; *2,* anterior lens capsule; *3,* posterior lens capsule; *4,* retina). **A,** Erroneous automatic measurement. Gate 2 is properly positioned beneath the anterior lens capsule spike *(A)*, but gate 3 is incorrectly placed beneath a high spike from within the cataractous lens *(arrow)*. Note that the lens thickness measures only 1.08 mm and the AEL measurement = 24.16 mm. *I,* Initial spike; *P,* posterior lens capsule; *R,* retina. **B,** Correct measurement using manual mode. Gate 3 has been repositioned beneath the true posterior lens capsule spike. The correct lens thickness = 3.83 mm, and the AEL measurement = 24.34 mm.

eye than in the phakic eye, in which the lens spikes help to guide the sound beam along the visual axis.

In the aphakic echogram, the two lens spikes are replaced by a single spike representing the iris, the posterior lens capsule, or the anterior vitreous face. The aphakic echogram thus consists of the initial spike, a spike from the iris/posterior lens capsule/anterior vitreous face spike, and spikes from the retina and sclera (Figure 10-15). In these eyes, it is suggested that the manual measurement mode be used to help ensure alignment of the sound beam along the visual axis. The aphakic eye type (1,532 m/sec) is used for the measurement. Using two gates, the anterior gate is placed at the initial spike and the posterior gate at the retinal spike. Some instruments provide three gates, with the second gate placed at the iris/posterior lens capsule/anterior vitreous face spike to measure anterior chamber depth.

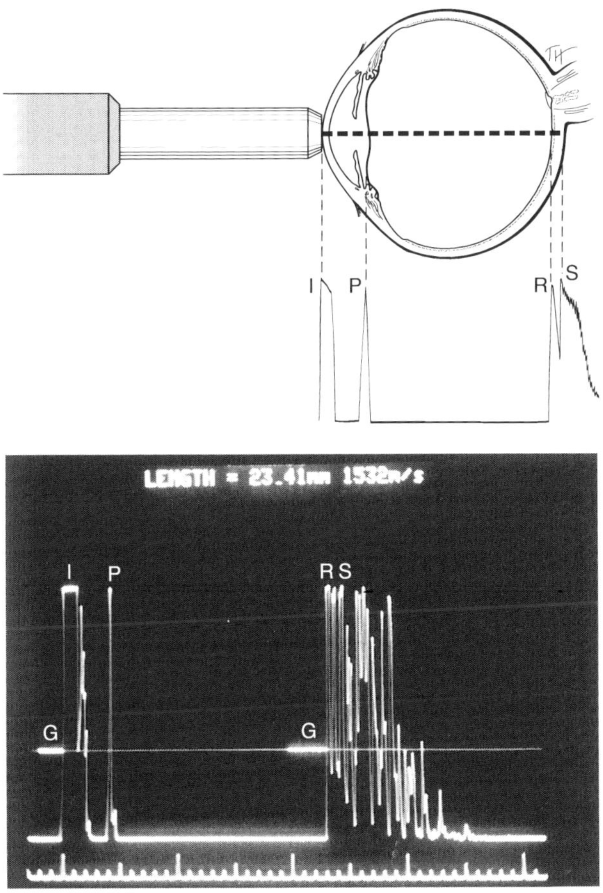

Figure 10-15 Contact axial A-scan of aphakic eye. A single spike is produced from the posterior lens capsule *(P)* in this example. *I*, Initial spike; *R*, retina; *S*, sclera; *G*, gates. (From Byrne SF: *A-scan Axial Length Measurements—A Handbook for IOL Calculations.* Mars Hill, NC, Grove Park Publishers, 1995, p 33.)

Measurement of the Pseudophakic Eye (Contact Technique)

Measurement of the pseudophakic eye requires knowledge of the IOL composition and awareness of the artifactual signals in the echogram produced by the IOL. Although most IOLs were initially made of polymethylmethacrylate (PMMA), silicone or acrylic lenses are primarily used today. Because the sound velocity of these materials varies significantly, it is important to identify the composition of the IOL to facilitate the use of an appropriate correction factor for the AEL measurement.

Holladay has described two methods for determining the correction factors to be used for the measurement of pseudophakic eyes.[26,27] One method employs simple correction factors and can be used for eyes of average length (Table 10-3). The other method, for longer and shorter eyes, requires knowing the thickness of the IOL.

Measurement of the pseudophakic eye is performed with the manual mode using the aphakic eye type setting (1,532 m/sec). The pseudophakic echogram consists of the initial spike and a very high reflective spike from the IOL, as well as spikes from the retina and sclera. In addition, the implant spike is followed by a chain of highly reflective artifactual spikes (multiple signals) along the vitreous baseline. These signals are caused by reverberations occurring between the probe tip and the surface of the implanted lens. Using a two-gate system, the anterior gate is placed at the initial spike and the posterior gate is placed at the retinal spike (Figure 10-16). Some instruments provide three gates, with the second gate positioned at the lens implant spike to measure anterior chamber depth. The true AEL is determined by adding the appropriate correction factor for the IOL composition (e.g., PMMA, silicone, or acrylic) to the measured value (Figure 10-17; see also Table 10-3).[8,26-28]

The presence of multiple signals in the pseudophakic echogram is a potential source of error because one of these signals may be mistaken for the retinal spike, resulting in a falsely short measurement. If the automatic mode is used for these measurements, the instrument may be unable to identify the true retinal spike; therefore, the manual mode is recommended. The position of the retinal gate should be observed closely to ensure proper placement. Mistakes are

TABLE 10-3

Average Correction Factors for Pseudophakic Eyes

Implant Composition	Sound Velocity (m/sec)	Correction Factor (mm)
PMMA	2,720	+0.4 mm
Silicone	980	−0.8 mm
	1,090	−0.6 mm
Acrylic	1,900	+0.3 mm
	2,120	+0.2 mm

Modified from Byrne SF: *A-scan Axial Length Measurements—A Handbook for IOL Calculations.* Mars Hill, NC, Grove Park Publishers, 1995, p 68.

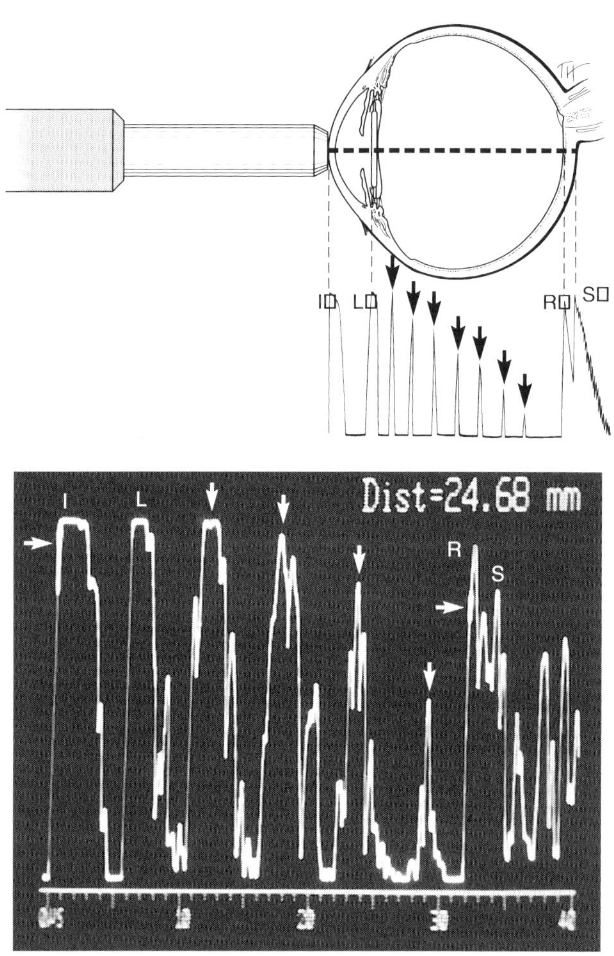

Figure 10-16 Contact axial A-scan of pseudophakic eye. The IOL *(L)* produces a very highly reflective spike. Note highly reflective multiple signals *(vertical arrows)* from reverberations occurring between IOL and probe tip. *I*, Initial spike; *horizontal arrows*, gates; *R*, retina; *S*, sclera. (Echogram from Byrne SF: *A-scan Axial Length Measurements—A Handbook for IOL Calculations*. Mars Hill, NC, Grove Park Publishers, 1995, p 34.)

most easily made in short eyes, in which the multiple signals may be superimposed on the retinal spike. In such cases, the retina can be localized by observing the screen as the gain is decreased. This results in disappearance of the multiple signals and persistence of the higher reflective retinal spike (Figure 10-18).

The average correction factors listed in Table 10-3 can be used to determine the true axial length of a pseudophakic eye when composition of the IOL is known.[26,27] The AEL is measured using the aphakic sound velocity setting (1,532 m/sec), and the appropriate factor is then added or subtracted. These values are intended for use in eyes of average length. Very short or very long eyes necessitate the use of a formula requiring knowledge of the IOL thickness.[28]

Potential Sources of Error with the Contact Method

It is important to understand the potential sources of error with the contact technique. These include corneal compression, a fluid meniscus between probe and cornea, and misalignment of the sound beam.

The most common potential error with the contact technique is corneal compression that results in a shortened AEL measurement. To minimize this error, a gentle on-and-off technique is recommended. Experience has shown that it is more difficult to control compression of the cornea when using the hand-held technique than when using the applanation method. Some examiners, however, prefer the hand-held method. To minimize compression with this technique, it may be helpful to view the cornea from the side. Significant compression can usually be detected by monitoring the anterior chamber depth. When the cornea is indented, anterior chamber depth decreases, indicating that compression is occurring (see Figure 10-6).

A fluid meniscus trapped between the tip of the probe and the cornea may result in a falsely long reading.[8,37] This can occur if a small drop of fluid is retained on the probe

A C

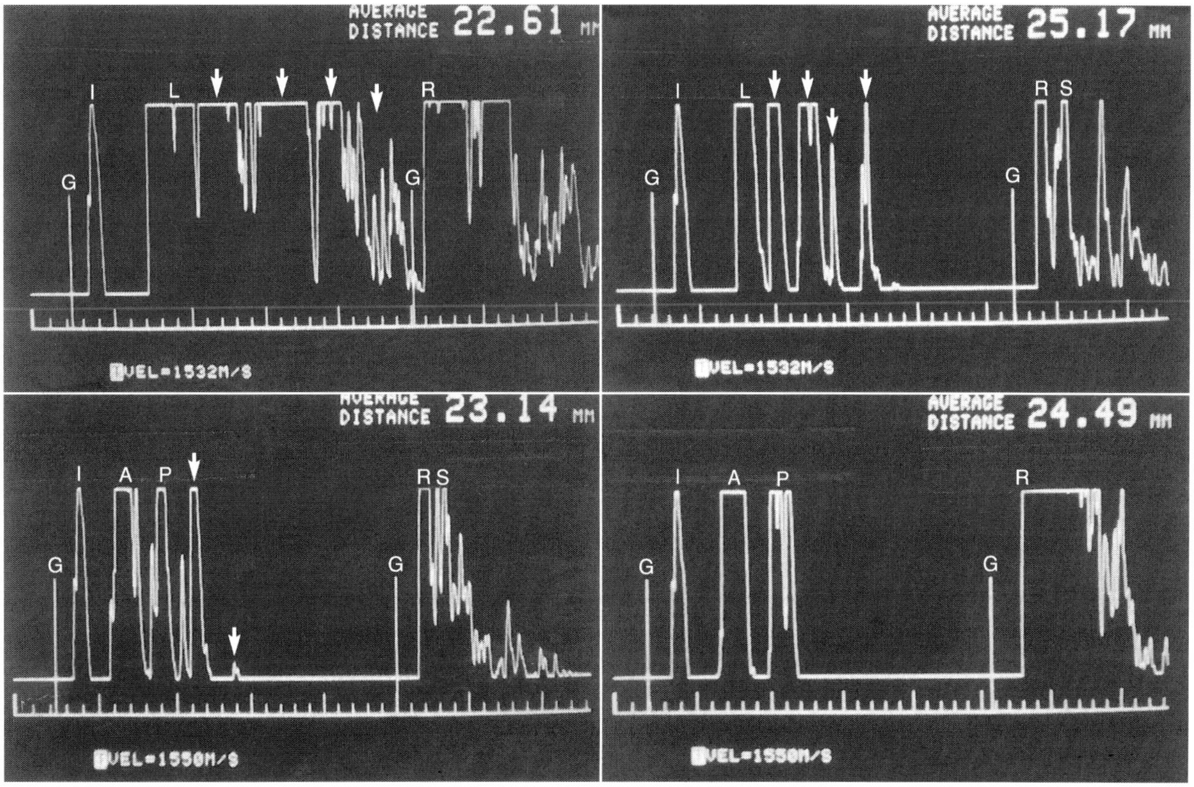

B D

Figure 10-17 Contact axial A-scans from two pseudophakic patients with different types of IOLs. Both patients are pseudophakic in only one eye and phakic in the fellow eye. Patient 1: PMMA implant **(A)** and normal, phakic fellow eye **(B).** Patient 2: Silicone implant **(C)** and normal, phakic fellow eye **(D).** Both pseudophakic eyes were measured using a sound velocity of 1,532 m/sec with the addition of an appropriate correction factor. The phakic eyes were measured using an average sound velocity of 1,550 m/sec. **A,** Patient 1. Measurement of eye with PMMA IOL = 22.61 mm. The correction factor for PMMA (+0.4 mm) is added: 22.61 + 0.4 = 23.01 mm. *I,* Initial spike; *L,* lens implant; *arrows,* multiple signals; *R,* retina; *G,* gates. **B,** Patient 1. Measurement of phakic fellow eye = 23.14 mm. Note that the actual difference in AEL between the two eyes is only 0.13 mm. *I,* Initial spike; *A,* anterior lens capsule; *P,* posterior lens capsule; *arrows,* multiple signals; *R,* retina; *S,* sclera; *G,* gates. **C,** Patient 2. Measurement of eye with silicone IOL = 25.17 mm. The correction factor for silicone IOL at 980 m/sec (0.8 mm) is subtracted: 25.17 mm − 0.8 mm = 24.37 mm. **D,** Patient 2. Measurement of phakic fellow eye = 24.49 mm. Note that the actual difference in the AEL of the two eyes in **C** and **D** is only 0.12 mm. (From Byrne SF: *A-scan Axial Length Measurements–A Handbook for IOL Calculations.* Mars Hill, NC, Grove Park Publishers, 1995, p 36.)

tip, if there is an unusually thick tear film, or if ointment is present in the eye (see Figure 10-7). Therefore, just prior to the measurement, the examiner should check to make certain that the probe tip is dry, that excess tears have been wiped from the eye, and that no ointment has been previously applied.

In some cases, misalignment of the sound beam can occur with the use of the contact method, resulting in a significant error. Proper alignment of the sound beam can be facilitated, however, by first localizing the optic disc and then shifting the sound beam temporally toward the macula (Figure 10-19).

As previously mentioned, other important sources of error include improper gate position (most often associated with the use of the automatic measurement mode, see pp 253 and 260) and incorrect eye type settings (see p 247).

Immersion Technique

The immersion technique is becoming increasingly popular as demands for greater accuracy in postoperative visual acuity increase and as its advantages become better known. This method employs a small water bath to avoid placing

A

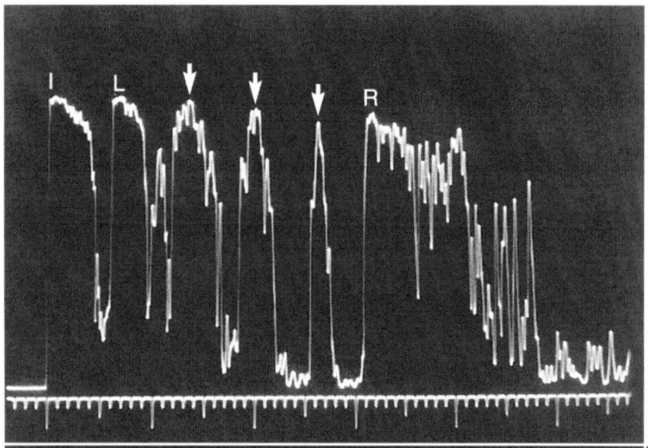

Figure 10-18 Contact axial A-scans of pseudophakic eye (PMMA implant) at high **(A)**, medium **(B)**, and very low **(C)** gain settings. **A,** Multiple signals *(arrows)* nearly reach the retinal spike *(R)*. *I,* Initial spike; *L,* lens implant. **B,** At lower gain, multiple signals decrease in height. Spikes from the retina and sclera *(S)* are clearly displayed. **C,** At very low gain, multiple signals begin to disappear whereas retinal and scleral spikes persist. (From Byrne SF: *A-scan Axial Length Measurements—A Handbook for IOL Calculations.* Mars Hill, NC, Grove Park Publishers, 1995, p 38.)

B

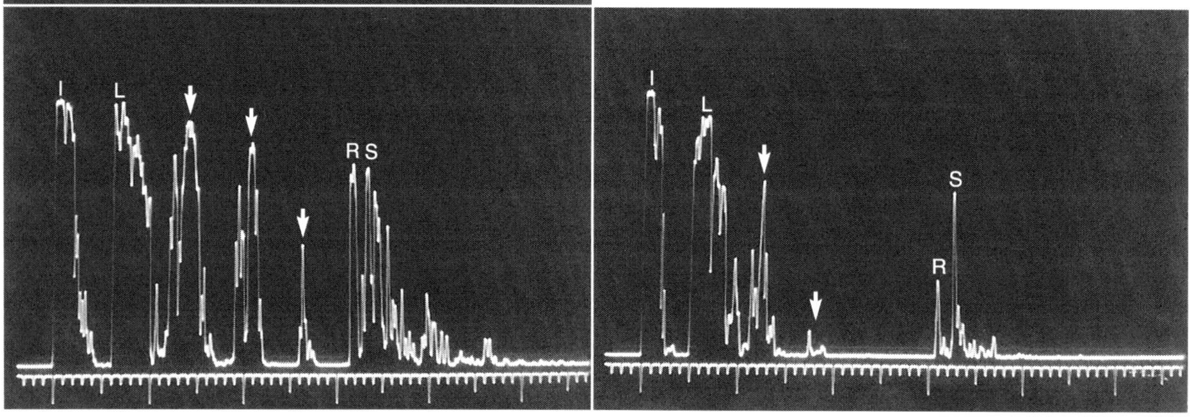

C

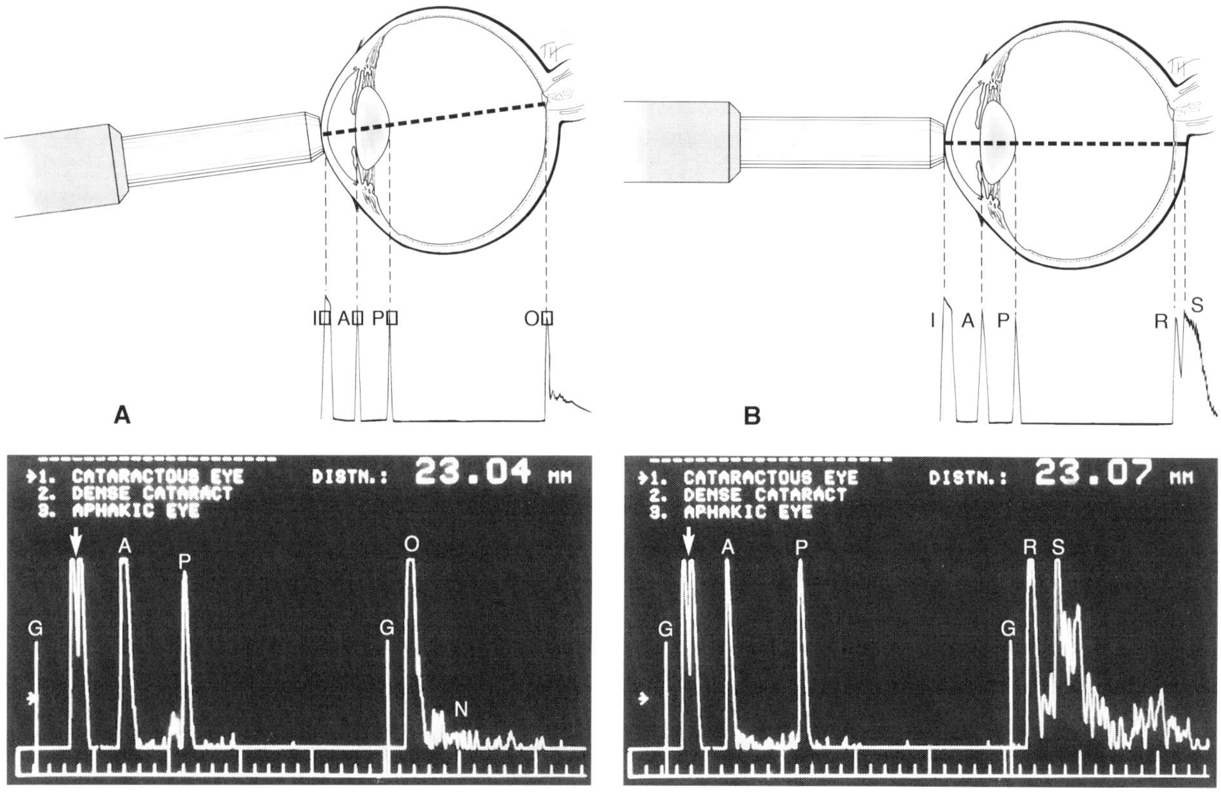

Figure 10-19 Localization of macula technique. Contact AEL measurement to optic nerve **(A)** and to macula **(B)** in same eye. **A,** Sound beam directed perpendicular to optic disc. Note that low reflective spikes appear behind the globe as the sound beam passes along the optic nerve *(N)*. *Arrow,* Initial spike; *A,* anterior lens capsule; *P,* posterior lens capsule; *O,* optic disc; *G,* gates. **B,** Sound beam is now properly directed perpendicular to retina *(R)* at the macula. Note that spikes from the orbital tissues are higher reflective as compared with the lower reflectivity obtained from the optic nerve in **A.** Also note that the scleral spike *(S)* is now displayed.

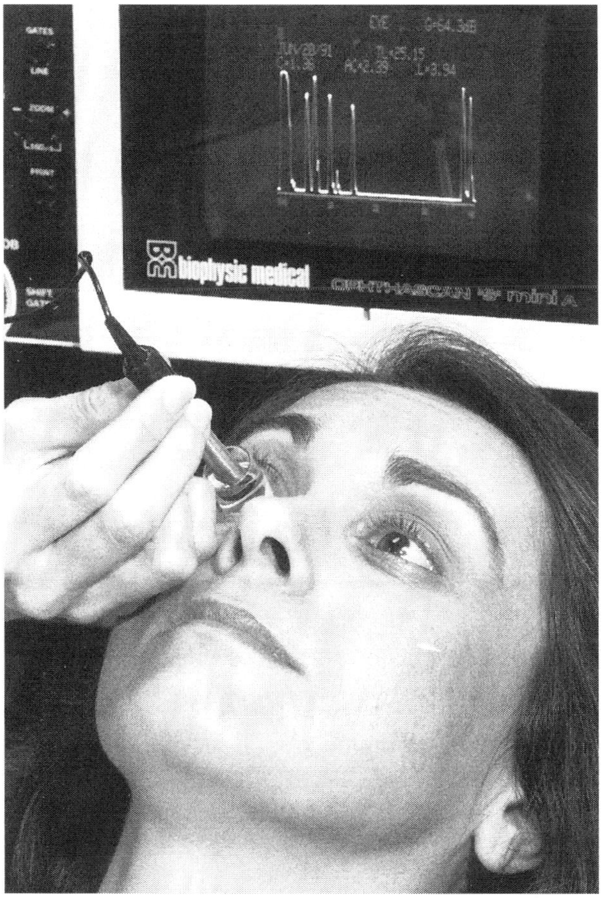

Figure 10-20 Immersion examination technique. Patient is reclined with head positioned near the screen. The A-scan probe is immersed within the fluid overlying the cornea.

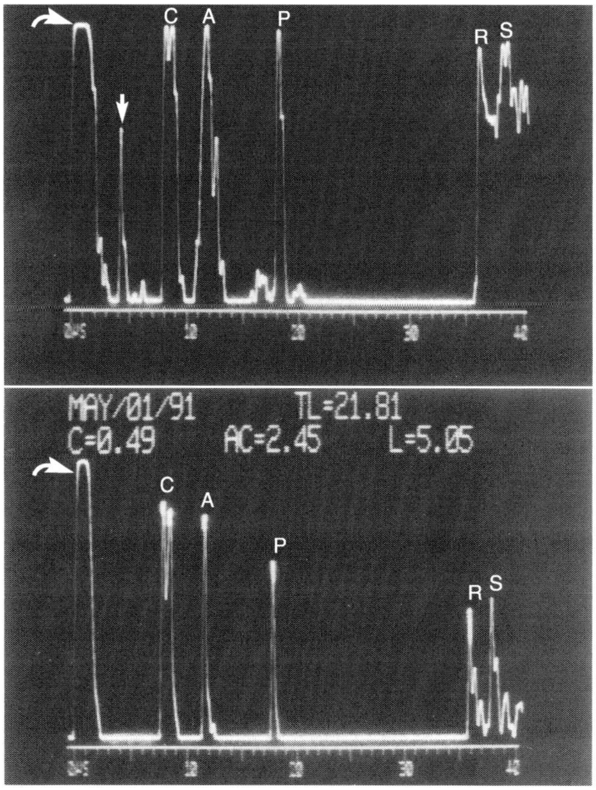

Figure 10-21 Immersion axial A-scans from same eye. **A,** High gain (Tissue Sensitivity) setting. *Curved arrow,* Initial spike corresponding to probe tip within fluid; *straight arrow,* small air bubble within fluid; *C,* cornea; *A,* anterior lens capsule; *P,* posterior lens capsule; *R,* retina; *S,* sclera. **B,** Reduced gain setting with gates properly positioned on spikes. Corneal thickness = 0.49 mm; anterior chamber depth = 2.45 mm; lens thickness = 5.05 mm; AEL measurement = 21.81 mm. Note that this instrument provides five gates: two for cornea, two for lens, and one for retina.

the probe directly on the cornea.[8,37] The obvious advantage of this technique is that the cornea cannot be compressed. In addition, the display of a separate corneal spike (not present in the contact method) may facilitate alignment of the sound beam along the visual axis. The availability of both contact and immersion methods allows the examiner to choose the most suitable technique for a given situation.

The immersion technique is generally performed with the patient reclined and the eye to be measured positioned close to the screen. After topical anesthetic drops are instilled, a small plastic cylinder (i.e., scleral shell; see Appendix D) is inserted between the lids and filled about two-thirds full of methylcellulose (Figure 10-20; see also Figure 10-1). Air bubbles within the methylcellulose should be avoided as this can lead to erroneous measurements (see Potential Sources of Error on p 260).

For measurement of the phakic eye, the phakic eye type setting and either the automatic or manual measurement mode can be used. Using a high gain setting initially, the examiner immerses the probe into the fluid just until an echogram is displayed. With the patient fixating on a target in primary gaze, the sound beam is directed perpendicular to the center of the cornea along the visual axis. This results in the display of a double-peaked corneal spike and single-peaked spikes from the anterior and posterior lens surfaces, retina, and sclera. Once steeply rising, highly reflective spikes are displayed from these interfaces at high gain, the decibel level is reduced slightly for improved resolution (Figure 10-21). As the gain is turned down, the displayed spikes decrease in height, necessitating close observation of the screen to ensure that all spikes remain as high and distinct as possible. It may be necessary to adjust the position of the probe during this procedure to maintain perpendicular sound beam incidence.

A measurement is taken when peaks of the displayed spikes are at their maximum height, although in some cases, the height of the spikes may decrease slightly from left to right. At least three high-quality echograms should be obtained from the examined eye. Measurements are usually made electronically, using gates (see p 247). As for the contact method, measurements can be obtained using two gates and an average sound velocity setting or by using four gates and discrete sound velocities for the aqueous, lens, and vitreous (see Table 10-2). With any immersion technique, the first gate is positioned at the corneal spike rather than the initial spike (which represents the tip of the probe).

As previously described for the contact method, another way to measure the phakic eye is to use the aphakic eye type setting and add a CALF to the measured axial length value[23,28] (see p 253).

Measurement of the aphakic or pseudophakic eye with the immersion technique employs many of the same principles as the contact method (see p 255). It should be re-emphasized that the manual measurement mode and aphakic eye type setting should be used for measurement of both the aphakic and pseudophakic eye.

Another type of scleral shell (Prager shell; see Appendix D) that has become available in recent years may simplify the performance of the immersion technique for some examiners.[8] This shell is designed so that the probe can be secured by a set screw, allowing the probe and shell to function as one unit. The probe is inserted into the shell and secured with its tip located approximately ⅛ inch from the bottom of the shell. The shell (with probe attached) is placed over the cornea, and balanced salt solution is injected through a port on the side of the shell (Figure 10-22). As the patient gazes at the light within the fixed probe, the sound beam is easily aligned along the visual axis. An advantage of this shell is that it allows the immersion examination to be performed with the patient sitting upright rather than reclined. Such positioning can be desirable when a patient is confined to a wheelchair, is otherwise unable to tolerate a reclined position, or their eye contains silicone oil (see p 265).

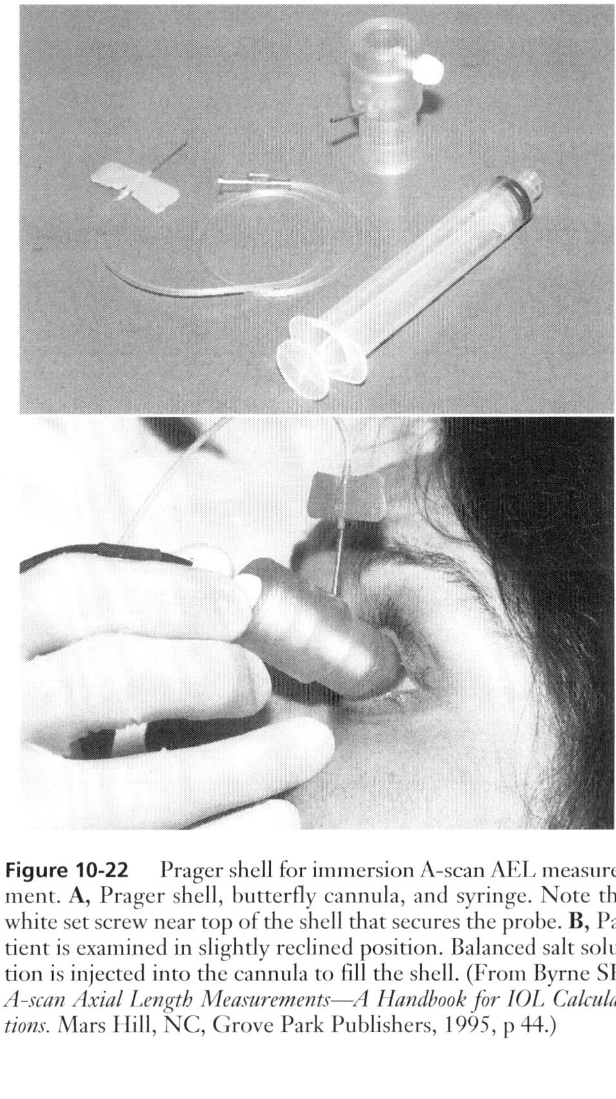

A

B

Figure 10-22 Prager shell for immersion A-scan AEL measurement. **A,** Prager shell, butterfly cannula, and syringe. Note the white set screw near top of the shell that secures the probe. **B,** Patient is examined in slightly reclined position. Balanced salt solution is injected into the cannula to fill the shell. (From Byrne SF: *A-scan Axial Length Measurements—A Handbook for IOL Calculations.* Mars Hill, NC, Grove Park Publishers, 1995, p 44.)

Potential Sources of Error with the Immersion Technique

The primary source of error with the immersion technique is the presence of small air bubbles within the fluid between the probe and cornea. These bubbles can result in the display of additional spikes in the echogram to the left of the corneal spike (Figure 10-23). Misinterpretation of one of these spikes as the corneal spike can result in a falsely long measurement. This potential error can be avoided, however, by identifying the double-peaked corneal spike to ensure proper gate placement. If too many bubbles are present or if a bubble persistently adheres to the surface of the cornea, it may be necessary to remove and reapply the scleral shell and then to add fresh methylcellulose.

As previously mentioned, the other primary potential source of error includes improper gate position, most often associated with use of the automatic measurement mode (Figure 10-24; see also Figure 10-14). Errors can also occur due to the selection of an inappropriate eye type (sound velocity) setting (see p 246).

Concluding the Examination

The examination may be concluded once multiple, consistent readings have been obtained. Generally, an average of three or more high-quality echograms are used to determine the final AEL reading. Ideally, the AEL readings from multiple echograms should be within 0.2 mm. Additional echograms should be obtained if greater variability is noted.

Both the echograms and the accompanying numerical data should be evaluated for accuracy. If errors are detected (e.g., incorrect gate position or sound velocity settings, see p 247), the examination may have to be repeated. In addition, if discrepancies in measurements larger than 0.3 mm are found between the two eyes, further testing (e.g., B-scan examination, see p 263) should be considered. Repeat examination by a second examiner may also be helpful when measurements are inconsistent.

After the examination, the eye should be cleansed of excess fluid or irrigated to remove methylcellulose used for the immersion technique.

A B

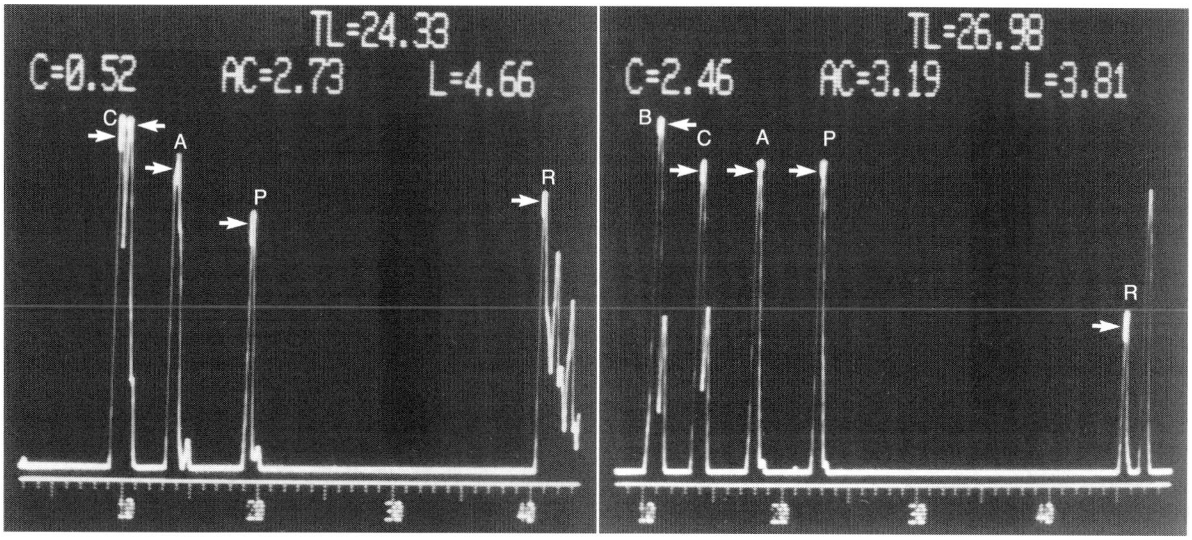

Figure 10-23 Immersion axial A-scans from same eye showing proper **(A)** and improper **(B)** gate placement. **A,** Correct gate placement yields an AEL measurement of 24.33 mm. *C,* Cornea; *A,* anterior lens capsule; *P,* posterior lens capsule; *R,* retina. *Arrows,* Gates. **B,** First corneal gate is placed on peak of small air bubble *(B)* within fluid, causing incorrect AEL reading of 26.98 mm. Note that this instrument provides five gates: two for cornea, two for lens, and one for retina. The initial spike was shifted to the left and is not visible.

A B

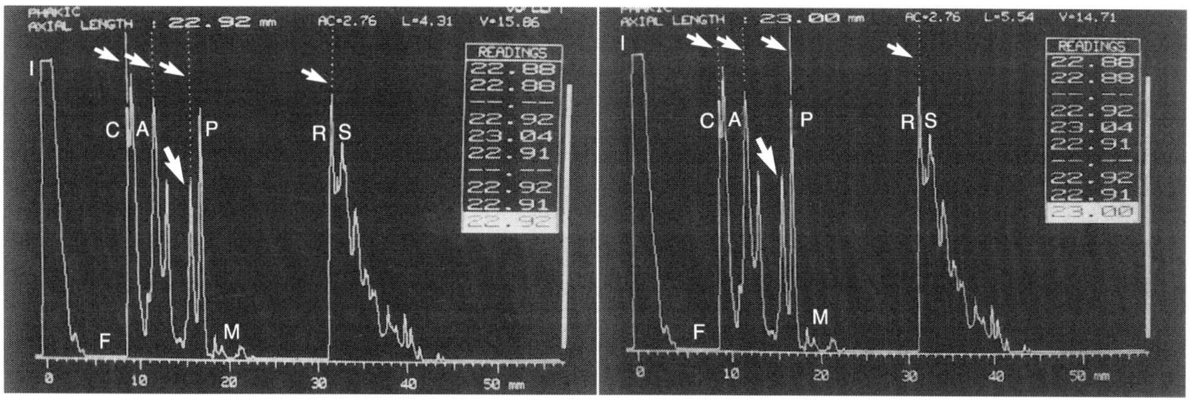

Figure 10-24 Immersion axial A-scans from the same eye demonstrating incorrect gate placement with use of automatic mode. **A,** Incorrect gate placement with automatic mode. **B,** Correct gate placement with manual mode. Measurements were performed using four gates. **A,** The instrument misinterpreted a spike originating from the lens nucleus *(large arrow)* for the posterior lens capsule *(P)*. The AEL = 22.92 mm. *I,* Initial spike representing probe tip in fluid *(F); C,* cornea; *A,* anterior lens capsule; *M,* multiple signals; *R,* retina; *S,* sclera; *small arrows,* gates. **B,** With manual mode, gate for posterior lens capsule is properly positioned and correct AEL measurement = 23.00 mm. (From Byrne SF: *A-scan Axial Length Measurements—A Handbook for IOL Calculations.* Mars Hill, NC, Grove Park Publishers, 1995, p 44.)

TROUBLESHOOTING

Inadequate Patient Fixation

One challenge that may occur during the biometry examination is a patient's inability to maintain steady fixation. In such situations, the first step is to ask the patient if he or she can be made more comfortable. In many cases, merely modifying the head or body position is all that is needed to solve the problem.

Inadequate patient fixation can be related to poor visual acuity in one or both eyes. If the cataract in the examined eye is extremely dense, the patient may be unable to clearly visualize the fixation light within the probe. In this event, it may be helpful to patch the fellow eye to eliminate distractions. A patient who is still unable to visualize the light can be asked to gaze at another target with the fellow eye. If necessary, an assistant can hold a fixation target, such as a penlight, at close range to be viewed by the fellow eye. If the patient has poor visual acuity bilaterally and adequate fixation cannot be attained, proper sound beam alignment will be difficult to achieve.

Other techniques may be required if the patient has strabismus, nystagmus or marked blepharospasm. When the examined eye is strabismic, the gaze of the fellow eye should be adjusted to bring the examined eye as close as possible to primary gaze. In the unlikely event that fixation near primary gaze cannot be achieved, it may be necessary to examine the eye from an unconventional position (e.g., from the side). When a patient has nystagmus or blepharospasm, additional contact readings may be required to ensure accuracy, although an immersion technique (see p 259) is generally recommended in these cases to help prevent corneal abrasion. In fact, the immersion technique should always be considered whenever a patient has difficulty maintaining fixation, since this procedure often proves easiest and most accurate in such circumstances.

Incorrect Sound Velocity Settings

As previously mentioned (see p 247), accurate measurements can only be obtained if the correct sound velocity setting is used. This may apply to the entire AEL measurement or to the measurement of individual ocular components.

Errors in AEL measurements can occur if the wrong eye type (sound velocity setting) is chosen for the examination. For example, if the phakic eye type setting is mistakenly used to measure an aphakic eye, an erroneously long AEL measurement will result. Problems in measurement can also occur if an instrument does not allow changes in the sound velocity from preset values. This can be especially problematic when measuring eyes containing silicone oil since the sound velocity of the oil is much slower than that of the vitreous (see Table 10-2). Furthermore, instruments that employ only two gates and do not allow changes in the preset sound velocity settings cannot provide a separate value for lens thickness. In all of these circumstances, the velocity conversion equation can be used to derive the correct values.

Velocity Conversion Equation

The velocity conversion equation[8,20] (VCE) is useful for obtaining a correct measurement when an inappropriate sound velocity is used during the examination. The correct measurement is obtained by dividing the correct sound velocity (Vc) by the incorrect sound velocity used for the measurement (Vm), multiplied by the measurement obtained:

$$\text{correct value} = \text{Vc/Vm} \times \text{measurement}$$

To determine the true axial length measurement (TAL) using the VCE, divide the correct sound velocity (Vc) by the incorrect sound velocity setting that had been used for the measurement (Vm) and then multiply by the incorrect (apparent) axial length reading (AAL)[20]:

$$\text{TAL} = \text{Vc/Vm} \times \text{AAL}$$

For example, an aphakic eye was measured using an incorrect sound velocity of 1,550 m/sec rather than the correct aphakic velocity of 1,532 m/sec. The erroneous (apparent) axial length reading obtained was 25.0 mm. To determine the correct (true) axial length measurement:

$$1{,}532/1{,}550 \text{ m/sec} \times 25.0 \text{ mm} = 24.71 \text{ mm}$$

To determine the true lens thickness (TLT) using a two-gate system with unadjustable sound velocity settings, divide the correct sound velocity (Vc) by the incorrect sound velocity that had been used for the measurement (Vm) and then multiply by the incorrect (apparent) measurement (AM):

$$\text{TLT} = \text{Vc/Vm} \times \text{AM}$$

For example, lens thickness was measured with a two-gate instrument with nonadjustable sound velocity settings using the aphakic eye type (1,532 m/sec) rather than the correct lens velocity (1,641 m/sec). The erroneous (apparent) lens reading was 4.5 mm. To determine the correct (true) lens thickness measurement:

$$1{,}641/1{,}532 \text{ m/sec} \times 4.5 \text{ mm} = 4.8 \text{ mm}$$

Intraocular Lesions

Intraocular lesions (e.g., dense cataracts, asteroid hyalosis, retinal detachment, macular lesions, and posterior staphylomas) can interfere with the ability to obtain accurate AEL measurements.[33] Certain findings in the patient's history may suggest particular intraocular pathology that may be encountered during the examination. These include a history of high myopia, previous cataract or vitreoretinal surgery, diabetic retinopathy, and macular degeneration. There are also certain clues that may be noted during the biometry examination that may suggest the presence of an intraocular lesion (Box 10-2).

BOX 10-2

A-Scan Findings Suggestive of an Intraocular Lesion

Unexplained spikes along the vitreous baseline
Inability to display distinct, high retinal spike
Abnormal separation of retinal spike from scleral spike
Inconsistent AEL measurements in examined eye (>0.2 mm)
Variation in AEL measurement compared to fellow eye (>0.3 mm)

From Byrne SF: *A-scan Axial Length Measurements—A Handbook for IOL Calculations.* Mars Hill, NC, Grove Park Publishers, 1995, p 68.)

Whenever intraocular pathology is suspected, a B-scan examination should be performed to detect any abnormalities that may affect the AEL measurement. In many cases, B-scan may assist in obtaining the measurements. A good rule of thumb is whenever the posterior segment cannot be visualized with ophthalmoscopy, the eye should be screened with B-scan prior to biometry.

Posterior Staphyloma

The presence of a posterior staphyloma may complicate the biometry examination, and it should be considered whenever there is a history of high myopia. Posterior staphylomas often cause an irregular shape of the ocular wall, resulting in an inability to display a distinct, high retinal spike, and thus potentially leading to a significant error in the A-scan measurement. These staphylomas are often located in the peripapillary region, adjacent to but not centered on the macula.

Because the deepest portion of the staphyloma may be located eccentric to the macula, the measurement may be longer than the true axial length along the visual axis. In addition, the macula may be located on the slope of the staphyloma, thereby resulting in oblique sound beam incidence to the macula (Figure 10-25). Localization of the macula and the display of a distinct, high retinal spike can be very difficult in these eyes.[6,8]

A posterior staphyloma is suggested whenever a distinct, high retinal spike is difficult to display and AEL readings are long and inconsistent in the eye being measured (i.e., differing by more than 0.2 mm). In addition, if a distinct retinal spike and consistent measurements are obtained but the probe appears to be directed eccentric to the macula (e.g., nasally), the possibility of a posterior staphyloma should be considered. Since staphylomas are typically bilateral and asymmetric in depth, the fellow eye will usually also measure longer than normal with readings between the two eyes generally varying by more than 0.3 mm (see p 268).

In an eye with a suspected posterior staphyloma, immersion A-scan may allow for a more accurate measurement. The presence of a separate corneal spike in the echogram may assist in better aligning the sound beam along the visual axis (see p 259). However, even with the immersion technique, a distinct, high retinal spike may not be obtainable. When this occurs, it may be necessary to be satisfied with a retinal spike that is less distinct and of lower amplitude for the measurement than is generally acceptable.

B-scan can be of great assistance in the measurement of eyes with posterior staphylomas. It can be used to demonstrate the shape of the posterior ocular wall and the relationship of the macula to the staphyloma. The AEL measurement can also be obtained from the B-scan echogram (using an immersion technique).[7] Measurements are made with either electronic gates (cursors) or by superimposing a vector A-scan on the B-scan echogram[6-8] (Figure 10-26; see also p 122).

In some severely staphylomatous eyes, it can be helpful to use a combination of A- and B-scan techniques for the AEL measurement. The anterior chamber depth and lens thickness are first measured with either contact or immersion A-scan techniques. Although these measurements are most easily obtained using an instrument with four gates, a two-gate system can still be used by incorporating the use of the velocity conversion equation (see p 262). Once these values are obtained, B-scan is then used to measure the length of the vitreous cavity. A horizontal axial B-scan echogram (see p 21) is obtained. One electronic cursor is placed at the posterior lens capsule echo and a second cursor is positioned at the surface of the macula. The A-scan measurements for lens and anterior chamber and the B-scan measurement for the vitreous cavity are then added together to determine the final axial length reading (Figure 10-27).

A

B

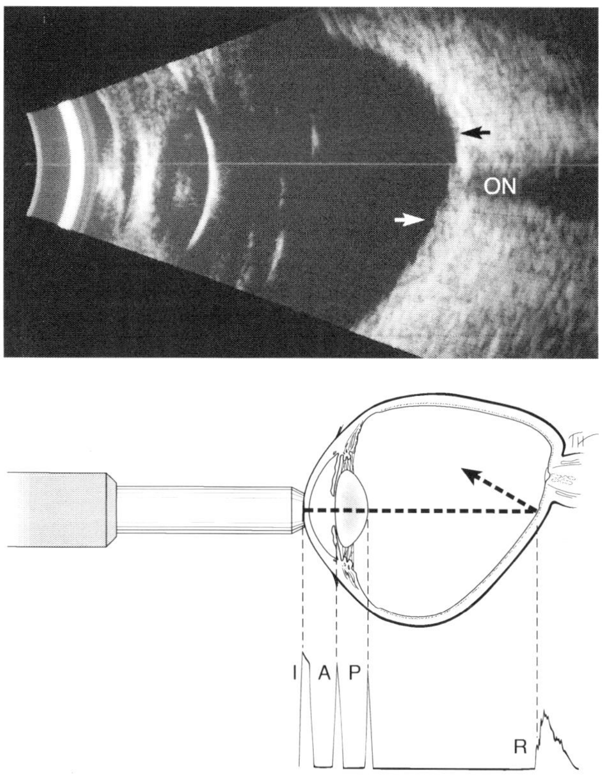

Figure 10-25 Posterior staphyloma located eccentric to the macula. **A,** Horizontal axial B-scan demonstrates posterior staphyloma with deepest portion *(black arrow)* nasal to optic nerve *(ON)*. Note that the globe is angulated in region of macula *(white arrow)*. **B,** Schematic drawing shows posterior staphyloma located eccentric to macula and contact A-scan echogram. Because of angulation of the globe wall temporal to the nerve, a portion of the sound beam is refracted away from the probe. This results in a poorly defined retinal spike *(R)*. *I*, Initial spike; *A*, anterior lens capsule; *P*, posterior lens capsule.

Macular Lesions

The presence of an elevated macular lesion can complicate the biometry examination. These lesions may prevent the display of a distinct retinal spike and often cause a shortened AEL measurement. Lesions of the macula that may

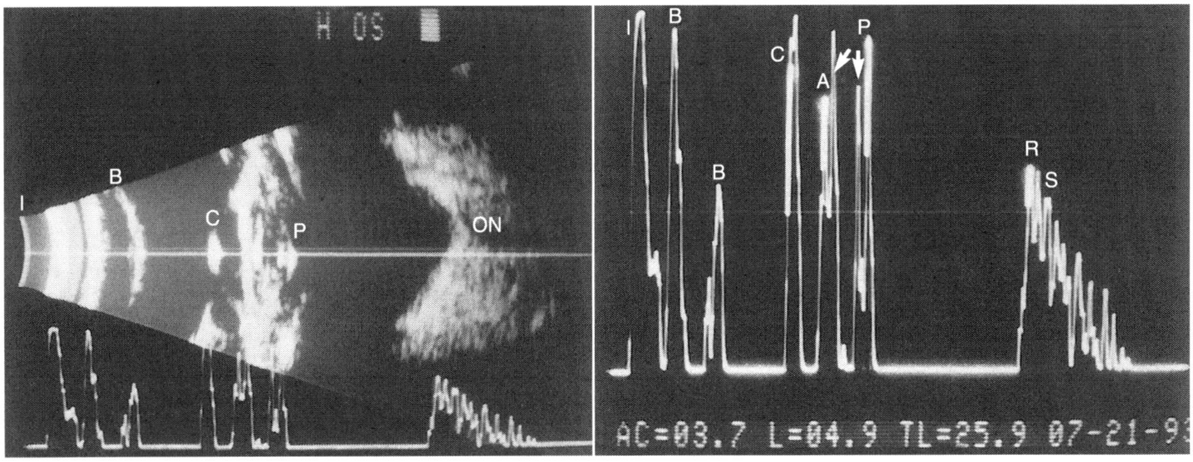

Figure 10-26 AEL measurement of an eye with a posterior staphyloma using immersion B-scan and corresponding vector A-scan. Macula is located on slope of staphyloma. **A,** Horizontal axial B-scan shows deep staphyloma with its base at optic nerve *(ON)*. Line from vector A-scan is positioned along visual axis to macula. *I*, Initial line representing probe tip in fluid; *B*, bubbles in fluid; *C*, cornea; *P*, posterior lens capsule. **B,** Vector A-scan (from **A**) indicates AEL measurement of 25.9 mm. *I*, Initial spike; *B*, bubbles in fluid; *C*, cornea; *A*, anterior lens capsule; *arrows*, spikes within lens corresponding to dense nuclear sclerosis; *P*, posterior lens capsule; *R*, retina; *S*, sclera. (From Byrne SF: *A-scan Axial Length Measurements—A Handbook for IOL Calculations*. Mars Hill, NC, Grove Park Publishers, 1995, p 66.)

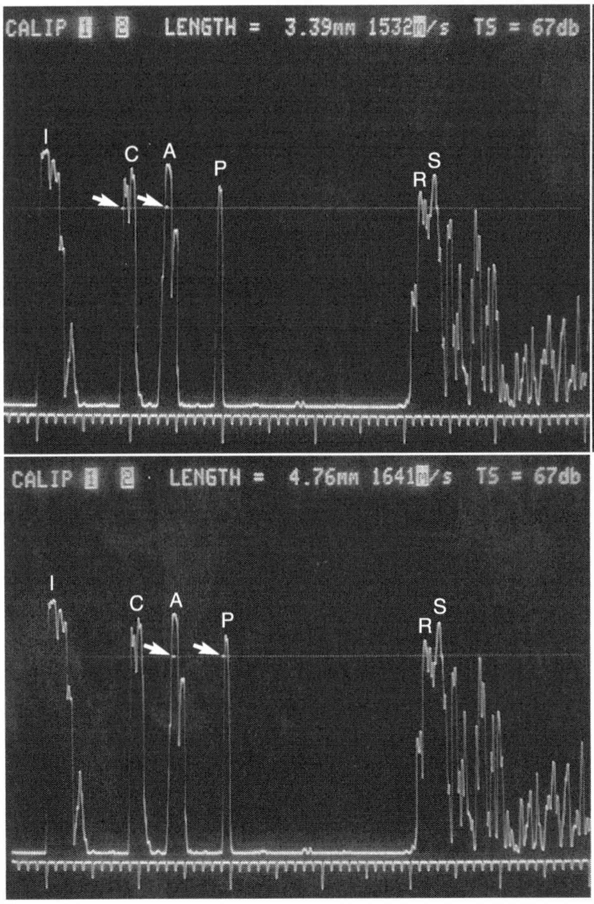

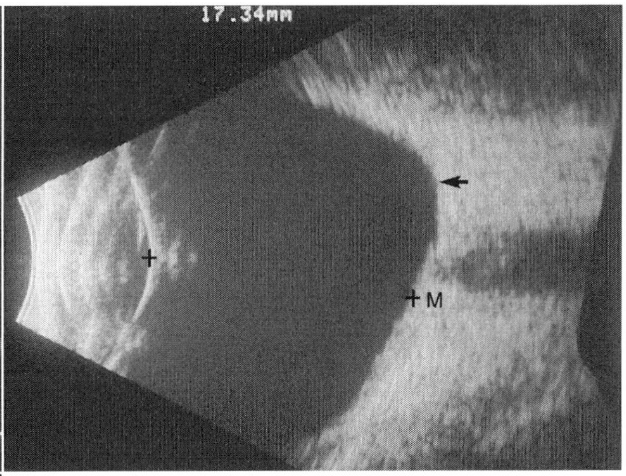

Figure 10-27 AEL measurement of an eye with posterior staphyloma eccentric to the macula using a combination of immersion A-scan (**A** and **B**) and contact B-scan **(C)**. **A,** Immersion A-scan measurement of anterior chamber depth = 3.39 mm. I, Initial spike; *white arrows*, gates; *C*, cornea; *A*, anterior lens capsule; *P*, posterior lens capsule; *R*, retina; *S*, sclera. **B,** Immersion A-scan measurement of anterior chamber depth = 4.76 mm. **C,** Horizontal axial B-scan shows posterior staphyloma with deepest portion *(black arrow)* nasal to optic nerve *(ON)*. Note angulation of globe in region of macula *(M)* and placement of electronic cursors *(black crosses)* at posterior lens capsule and macula for measurement of vitreous length. The AEL measurement = 25.49 mm (3.39 + 4.76 + 17.34 mm).

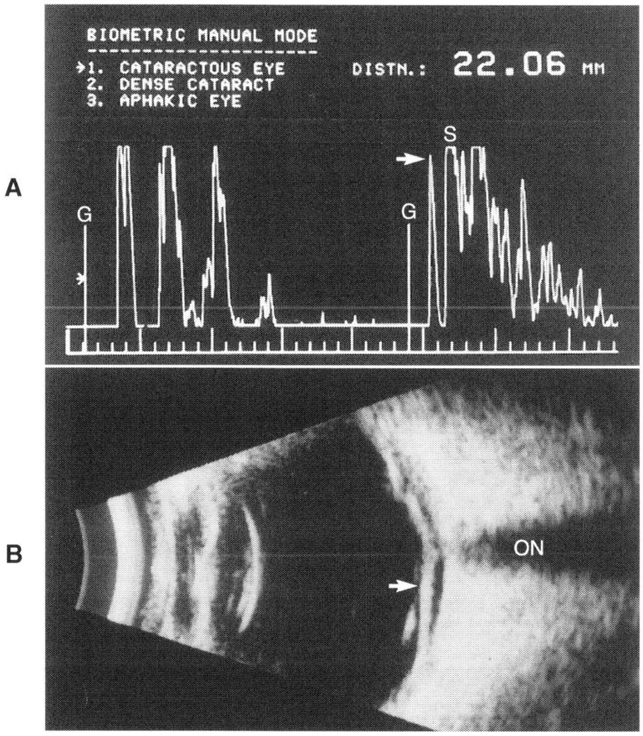

Figure 10-28 Shortened AEL measurement due to retinal detachment involving the macula. **A,** A-scan shows retinal spike *(arrow)* separated from sclera *(S)*. *G,* Gates. AEL = 22.06 mm (1.0 mm shorter than normal fellow eye). **B,** Horizontal axial B-scan shows retinal detachment in macular region *(arrow)*. *ON,* Optic nerve.

affect AEL measurements include macular edema (see p 67), disciform lesions secondary to AMD, and tumors (see Chapter 5). A macular lesion should be suspected if there is difficulty in displaying a steeply rising, high retinal spike or if the AEL in the measured eye is shorter than the fellow eye by 0.3 mm or more. In addition, the distance between the retinal and scleral spikes may appear greater than normal.

The B-scan examination can be helpful for demonstrating the presence of a macular lesion (see p 28) and, in some cases, can establish its etiology. If it is determined that the macular lesion is only temporary (e.g., macular edema), it may be necessary to add a correction factor to the measurement to account for eventual flattening of the lesion. Measurement of the fellow eye can be useful in choosing the correction value for these eyes.[6]

Retinal Detachment

Retinal detachment involving the macula produces shortening of the AEL compared with the fellow eye. Retinal detachment should be suspected when a wider than normal distance between the retinal and scleral spikes is encountered. If a retinal detachment is suspected, a B-scan examination is indicated (Figure 10-28).

Vitreous Lesions

Dense opacities and membranes in the vitreous cavity, especially when located near the retina, can potentially be mistaken for the retinal spike, resulting in erroneous measurements. The two most common vitreous conditions that may be encountered during the biometry examination are asteroid hyalosis[18] (see Figure 10-13) and vitreous hemorrhage (see p 45). Asteroid hyalosis can be especially problematic because of the medium to high spikes that are produced by the calcium particles in this condition. These spikes can easily be mistaken for the retinal spike, particularly when the automatic measurement mode is used. Asteroid hyalosis should always be suspected when one or more abnormal spikes appear along the vitreous baseline and artifactual spikes (i.e., multiple signals) have been excluded.

Intraocular air or gas bubbles from previous ocular surgery can lead to a measurement error, in some cases preventing the AEL measurement altogether. A small to medium-sized bubble situated along the path of the visual axis can produce a spike of extremely high reflectivity and may cause shadowing (see pp 109 and 466). In some cases, it may be possible to dislodge the bubble from the visual axis by having the patient change his or her head or body position.

Dense Cataract

Strong sound attenuation, produced by very dense cataracts, can significantly impair the ability to display spikes from the various interfaces along the visual axis. In this circumstance, a maximum gain setting may be required to obtain spikes of sufficient height from the posterior lens capsule and retina.

Extremely strong sound attenuation may occur when there is dense calcification of the crystalline lens. This may result in shadowing of the posterior ocular structures (see p 466), thus preventing measurement of the AEL (Figure 10-29). In such circumstances, it may be necessary to use readings obtained from the fellow eye for the IOL power calculations. It is important to remember, however, that the AEL measurement used should always be considered in the context of the patient's refractive history.

Silicone Oil

In recent years, silicone oil has become increasingly useful as a tamponade in the vitreous cavity for complicated retinal detachment surgery.[10,34,44] The lower sound velocity of silicone oil must be taken into account if AEL measurements are performed for subsequent cataract surgery.[34,35] This low sound velocity can result in pronounced sound attenuation and difficulty in identifying the retinal spike. In addition, if proper sound velocities are not used, erroneously long AEL measurements will be obtained. The sound velocity of silicone oil that is most commonly used in the United States today is 1,040 m/sec (5,000 centistokes). The velocity may vary, however, depending on the particular silicone oil used (e.g., 980 m/sec [1,000 centistokes]).

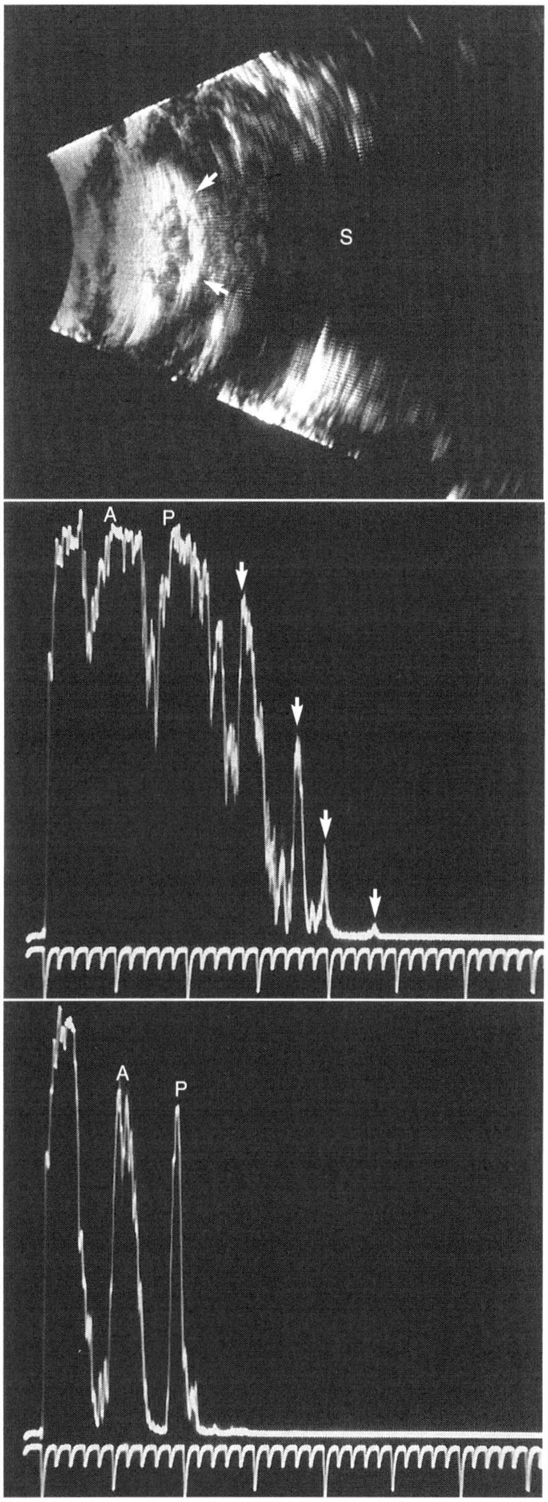

Figure 10-29 Totally calcified, cataractous lens (contact technique). **A,** Axial B-scan shows echo-dense, oval lens *(arrows)*. Note wide shadow posterior to lens *(S)* and absence of echoes from posterior ocular wall. **B,** Axial A-scan at high gain shows very highly reflective spikes from anterior *(A)* and posterior *(P)* lens capsules. Note multiple signals of decreasing height *(arrows)* following lens spikes, as well as lack of echoes from posterior ocular wall. **C,** A-scan at lower gain setting. Only spikes from anterior and posterior lens surfaces can be displayed.

In order to facilitate measurement of a silicone-filled eye, it is recommended that the patient be seated upright. This is because the silicone oil placed at the time of surgery may not completely fill the vitreous cavity. If the AEL measurement is carried out with the patient recumbent, the silicone oil, which is usually lighter than vitreous, may move toward the front of the eye, thus creating a fluid-filled space between the bubble of silicone oil and the retina in the posterior pole. When this occurs, it becomes difficult to differentiate a spike produced by the posterior surface of the silicone bubble from that produced by the retina. This may then result in a falsely short AEL reading. With the patient in an upright position, however, the silicone oil bubble typically remains in contact with the posterior retina, which facilitates correct localization of the retinal spike.

For accurate AEL measurements in eyes containing silicone oil, it is recommended that the various ocular components (e.g., anterior chamber, lens and vitreous cavity) be measured separately using four gates and appropriate sound velocities (Figure 10-30; see also Table 10-2). This method of measurement requires that the instrument used allow the sound velocity settings to be changed from preset values.

If the biometer provides only preset sound velocities, an AEL measurement can still be obtained using the velocity conversion equation (VCE)[8,20] (see p 262). If the instrument has four gates, the VCE is used to correct the vitreous length measurement. If, on the other hand, the instrument has only two gates, the VCE is used to correct measurements for both the lens and vitreous length. In the example of a two-gate machine, the anterior chamber depth, lens thickness, and vitreous length are first measured individually using the aphakic eye type setting (1,532 m/sec). The VCE is then applied to obtain correct measurements for the lens and vitreous cavity. Finally, the individual values are combined to determine the AEL measurement. Because of these limitations, it is important to obtain the refractive history and the AEL of the fellow eye whenever possible.

To use the VCE as just described, measure the AEL with a sound velocity of 1,532 m/sec as follows:

1. Measure the anterior chamber depth. Place the first gate at the initial spike (contact method) or the separate corneal spike (immersion method) and the second gate at the anterior lens capsule spike. Record the anterior chamber depth.
2. Measure the apparent lens thickness. Place the first gate at the anterior lens capsule spike and the second gate at the posterior lens capsule spike. Record the apparent lens thickness.
3. Measure the apparent vitreous length. Place the first gate at the posterior lens capsule spike and the second gate at the retinal spike. Record the apparent vitreous length.
4. Apply the velocity conversion equation:
   a. True lens thickness = 1,641/1,532 m/sec × measured lens thickness
   b. True vitreous length = 1,040/1,532 m/sec × measured vitreous length

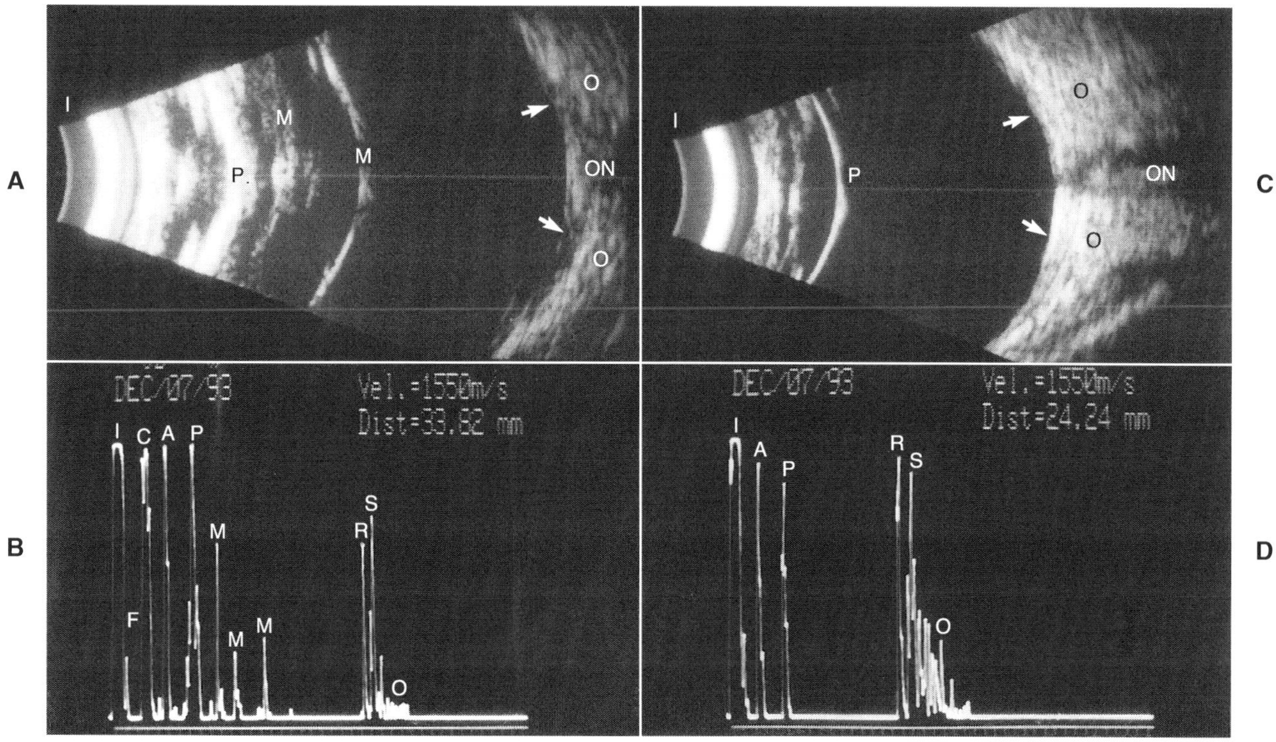

Figure 10-30 Erroneous AEL measurement of eye containing silicone oil. Contact and immersion axial B-scan and A-scan echograms from patient with phakic, silicone oil-filled eye (**A** and **B**) and phakic fellow eye (**C** and **D**). Both eyes were measured using two gates and sound velocity of 1,550 m/sec. Note differing appearance and length of echograms from the two eyes. **A,** Horizontal axial B-scan echogram at high gain. Silicone oil produces long, attenuated echogram due to slow sound velocity of oil. Attenuation is apparent by decreased number and brightness of echoes from posterior ocular wall *(arrows)* and orbital fat *(O)*. *I,* Initial line; *P,* posterior lens capsule; *M,* multiple signals; *ON,* optic nerve. **B,** Immersion A-scan axial length measurement (with compressed screen expansion) = 33.82 mm. *I,* Initial spike representing probe tip in fluid; *F,* fluid; *C,* cornea; *A,* anterior lens capsule; *P,* posterior lens capsule; *M,* multiple signals; *R,* retina; *S,* sclera; *O,* orbital fat. **C,** Horizontal axial B-scan echogram at medium gain. *I,* Initial spike; *P,* posterior lens capsule; *arrows,* posterior ocular wall; *O,* orbital fat; *ON,* optic nerve. **D,** Contact A-scan axial length measurement (with compressed screen expansion) = 24.24 mm. *I,* Initial spike; *A,* anterior lens capsule; *P,* posterior lens capsule; *R,* retina; *S,* sclera; *O,* orbital fat. The eye containing silicone oil erroneously measures 9.58 mm longer than normal fellow eye due to use of an incorrect sound velocity setting. (From Byrne SF: *A-scan Axial Length Measurements—A Handbook for IOL Calculations.* Mars Hill, NC, Grove Park Publishers, 1995, p 48.)

c. Add the true values for lens thickness and vitreous length to that of the measured anterior chamber depth

The following example utilizes the VCE in calculating the AEL measurement in an eye with silicone oil (four gate system with preset sound velocities). The anterior chamber depth = 3.5 mm (using 1,532 m/sec), the lens thickness = 4.7 mm (using 1,641 m/sec) and the *apparent* vitreous length = 24.3 mm (using 1,532 m/sec). Therefore, the *true* axial length = 3.5 mm + 4.7 mm + (1,040/1,532 × 24.3 mm) = 24.7 mm.

The least preferred method of measuring an eye filled with silicone oil is to use only two gates and an average sound velocity setting. Hoffer has published a range of average sound velocities (based on silicone oil with a sound velocity of 980 m/sec) to be used for eyes of varying lengths.[20] His investigation has shown that the average sound velocity for an eye of average length (23.5 mm) is 1,139 m/sec in a phakic eye and 1,052 m/sec in an aphakic eye.

To determine the IOL power to be implanted in an eye with silicone oil, one must also consider the refractive index of the oil compared to that of normal vitreous. The refractive index of silicone oil varies according to the manufacturer and is different from that of the normal vitreous. This difference necessitates a correction to determine the power of posterior chamber implant to be used when silicone oil replaces normal vitreous. A formula has been devised to correct for this change in refractive index that indicates how much power needs to be added to the IOL power calculation.[39] It has been shown that approximately 3.5 diopters should be added to the calculated IOL power when a posterior chamber convexplano PMMA lens is used in an eye of average length. This assumes, however, that the refractive index of the silicone oil in the eye is 1.4034. Additional correction factors may be necessary if IOL implants with a configuration other than convexplano are used. However, if removal of the silicone oil is planned, it is not necessary to use these correction factors.

An AEL measurement often cannot be obtained from an eye containing emulsified silicone oil. Emulsification results in the production of small droplets of silicone that can completely fill the vitreous cavity.[8] These small droplets can produce such highly reflective echoes and strong sound attenuation that it may be impossible to display a spike from the retina. In these situations, or whenever there is difficulty in obtaining a measurement from an eye containing silicone oil, measurements from the fellow eye, if possible, can be used. However, the patient's refractive history should be taken into account.

Due to the obvious difficulty of obtaining accurate AEL measurements of an eye containing silicone oil, it is recommended that biometry be obtained prior to insertion of the oil whenever possible.

MINIMIZING ERRORS

There are many potential sources of error in performing A-scan biometry that can lead to a short or long measurement (Box 10-3). To minimize such errors, one must be constantly vigilant, and the examination must be performed in a systematic fashion (i.e., taking a thorough history, positioning the patient properly, verifying the instrument settings, and using appropriate examination techniques). Certain findings observed during the biometry examination may also suggest a potential error in measurement (see Box 10-2).

A useful method for minimizing errors is to routinely compare the AEL measurement with the patient's refraction. In myopic eyes, a relatively long AEL is usually observed whereas in hyperopic eyes, the AEL is relatively short (see p 244). It is noteworthy, however, that increased cataract formation can cause lenticular, as opposed to axial myopia.

In addition to the refraction, the AEL should be correlated with the corneal curvature (k-readings). For example, long eyes generally have relatively flat k-readings, whereas shorter eyes are typically associated with relatively steep k-readings.

Consistent measurements of the examined eye are one indication that accurate measurements are most likely being achieved. A rule of thumb is that the measurements obtained from a given eye should not vary by more than 0.2 mm. Variability greater than 0.2 mm may indicate a problem with alignment of the sound beam or the presence of a lesion located along the visual axis. One way of monitoring for variability is to store multiple scans and evaluate their quality while comparing the anterior chamber depth and lens thickness, and observing the standard deviation. With this procedure, undesirable scans and measurements can be eliminated and replaced as needed (Figures 10-31 and 10-32). If the quality of the scans does not explain the cause of the variability, then further investigation including diagnostic B-scan may be necessary.

BOX 10-3

Causes of Erroneously Short and Long AEL Measurements

Short Measurement

Corneal compression (contact method)
Sound velocity too slow
Corneal gate to right of corneal spike
Retinal gate incorrectly positioned at spike in vitreous cavity
Gain set too high
Lens measured too thin
Macular thickening/detachment
Misalignment of the sound beam

Long Measurement

Air bubble in fluid bath (immersion method)
Fluid bridge (contact method)
Sound velocity too fast
Retinal gate to right of retinal spike
Gain set too low
Lens measured too thick
Posterior staphyloma eccentric to macula
Misalignment of the sound beam

Modified after Byrne SF: *A-scan Axial Length Measurements—A Handbook for IOL Calculations.* Mars Hill, NC, Grove Park Publishers, 1995, p 24.

As previously mentioned, in most patients, the difference in AEL between fellow eyes is generally within 0.3 mm. Since greater differences may indicate an error in measurement, it is suggested that both eyes be measured whenever possible. If a difference between the two eyes is found, the history should be reviewed. In some cases, a difference in eye length can be explained by a variation in refraction that existed prior to development of the cataract (anisometropia). A longer AEL may also be related to previous ocular surgery, such as a scleral buckling procedure.[4,17] A shorter axial length reading, on the other hand, may occur because of a macular lesion such as cystoid macular edema or age-related macular degeneration (see p 68).

Another situation that may produce a shorter AEL reading in one eye than in the other is when the eye being measured has a lower intraocular pressure. This can be due to trabeculectomy surgery or to inflammation resulting in hypotony. In these eyes, a decrease in globe size may occur secondary to lowered intraocular pressure[9] (see p 216).

When measurements between the two eyes are disparate and yet scans are easily obtained and of high quality, a physiologic difference in eye length is more likely present than is an intraocular abnormality. Nevertheless, if the differ-

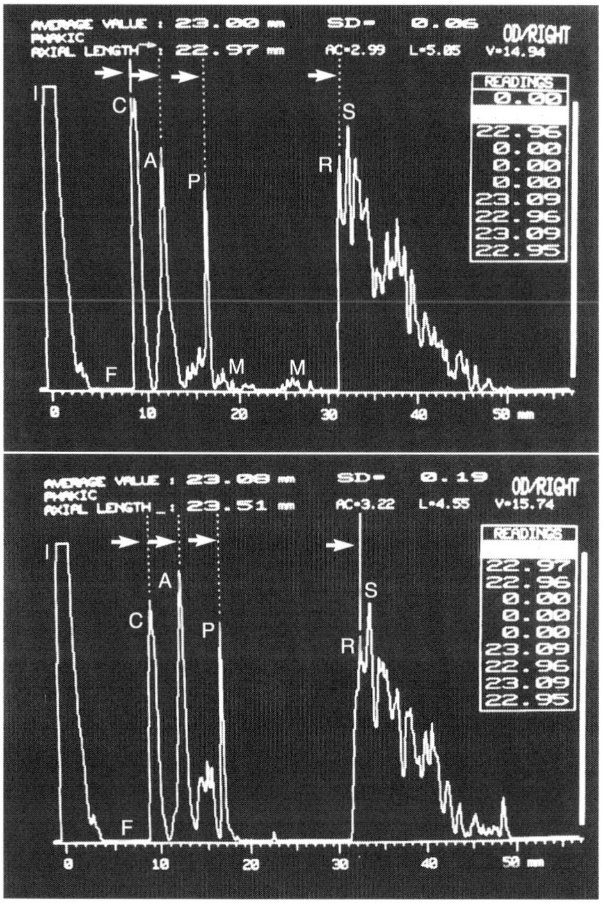

Figure 10-31 Immersion axial A-scans (from same patient) shows correct **(A)** and incorrect **(B)** sound beam alignment. **A,** Correct sound beam alignment is indicated by double-peaked corneal spike *(C)*, and regular decrease in height of spikes from lens and retina. *I*, Initial spike representing probe tip in fluid; *F*, fluid; *A*, anterior lens capsule; *P*, posterior lens capsule; *M*, multiple signals; *R*, retina; *S*, sclera; *arrows*, gates. **B,** Incorrect sound beam alignment. Nonperpendicular sound beam incidence is indicated by single-peaked rather than double-peaked corneal spike, disproportionately high anterior lens capsule spike, and indistinct retinal spike. Note that the properly aligned A-scan **(A)** is 0.54 mm shorter than the improperly aligned A-scan **(B).** (From Byrne SF: *A-scan Axial Length Measurements—Handbook for IOL Calculations.* Mars Hill, NC, Grove Park Publishers, 1995, p 45.)

ence is not clearly explained by the ocular history, it is suggested that the readings be checked by another examiner or an immersion technique be used. In some situations, a diagnostic B-scan examination may be necessary to explain the disparity in measurements. Furthermore, in the case of a shorter AEL occurring due to low intraocular pressure following trabeculectomy or uveitis, it may be necessary to adjust the axial length value used for IOL calculations. This adjustment is based on whether the intraocular pressure and, therefore, the axial length are expected to increase following cataract surgery (see p 216).

It is important to re-emphasize that AEL readings can be

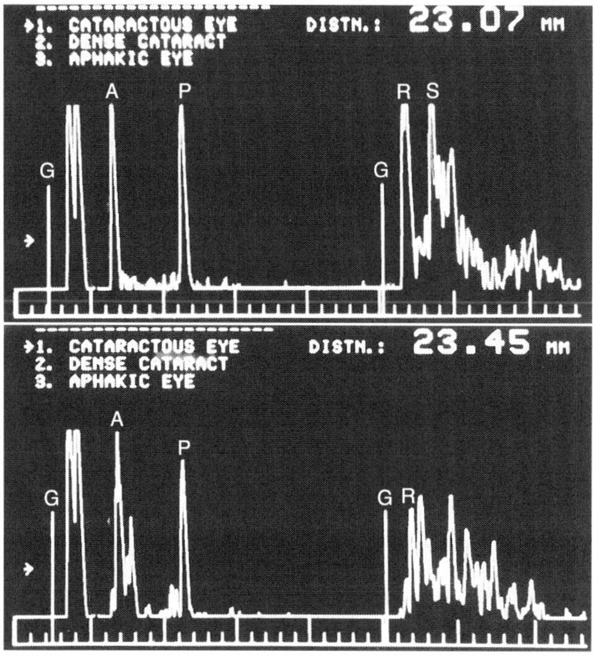

Figure 10-32 Contact axial A-scans (from same patient) shows correct **(A)** and incorrect **(B)** sound beam alignment. **A,** High-quality scan with sound beam perpendicular to both anterior *(A)* and posterior *(P)* lens capsules as well as retina *(R)*. *S*, Sclera; *G*, gates. Note that the lens and retinal spikes are steeply rising and maximally high. The AEL = 23.07 mm. **B,** Sound beam is directed obliquely to posterior lens capsule and retina. Note that the AEL erroneously = 23.45 mm (0.38 mm longer than the correct measurement in **A**).

very reproducible yet inaccurate. For example, if corneal compression occurs during each scan, a consistently short AEL measurement may be obtained in spite of normal-appearing echograms. This potential problem can be avoided by removing the probe from the cornea between scans and carefully monitoring anterior chamber depth (see p 251). Another situation where consistent yet inaccurate readings may be obtained is when an eye with a posterior staphyloma located eccentric to the macula is measured (see p 263).

IOL CALCULATIONS

IOL power calculation formulas require the measurement of AEL and corneal power, as well as an IOL constant.[22,25,27] Some formulas also require measurement of the anterior chamber depth, lens thickness, and corneal diameter.[25,27] Errors in any of these measurements can lead to an unanticipated postoperative refractive error (Box 10-4). In addition to meticulous measurements, optimum postoperative results require personalization of the IOL constant.[27]

One of the most common, yet preventable, sources of error is a problem in recording and transferring data (i.e., transposition errors). Such errors can be avoided by routinely rechecking the values that are obtained, recorded, and used for the IOL power calculation. In addition, documentation

> **BOX 10-4**
> ## Unanticipated Postoperative Refractive Errors
> **Potential Sources of Error**
> AEL measurement incorrect
> Anterior chamber depth not as anticipated
> Keratometry measurement incorrect
> IOL power calculation incorrect
> Mislabeled IOL
> Transposition of data

of all measurements should be retained in the patients record.

UNANTICIPATED POSTOPERATIVE REFRACTIVE ERRORS

When the desired refractive goal is not attained, a complete investigation should be implemented (see Box 10-4). This assessment should generally include re-evaluation of the biometry and keratometry readings, postoperative position of the IOL (e.g., in-the-bag or ciliary sulcus), and the formula used for the original IOL power calculations.

Calibration of both the biometer and the keratometer can be checked. The AEL can be remeasured and the anterior chamber depth measured to determine if the postoperative depth corresponds with the estimated lens position (ELP).[8,28,45] The postoperative k-readings can also be compared to preoperative values. Finally, the IOL power calculations can be recomputed to ensure that the correct lens constant was used and that the planned postoperative refraction was included in the computations.

One of the first steps when investigating an unexpected postoperative refractive error is to remeasure the AEL. An error of only 0.1 mm in the measurement of an eye of average length results in approximately 0.25 diopters of postoperative refractive error. This same degree of error has an even greater impact on the postoperative refraction in a very short eye and is of less significance in a very long eye. When possible, remeasurement should be performed by the same examiner using the same equipment and examination techniques employed for the preoperative examination. Also, it must be remembered that the sound velocity of the implant in the pseudophakic eye must be considered when remeasuring the AEL after surgery (see p 255).

DIAGNOSTIC USES OF AXIAL EYE LENGTH MEASUREMENTS

In addition to its use for IOL calculations, AEL measurements can be helpful in the diagnosis and monitoring of certain conditions. These include congenital disorders such as nanophthalmos (see p 82) and microphthalmos. Some eyes with small corneas may be clinically suspected of being microphthalmic when the axial length actually may be normal or long. The use of biometry for congenital glaucoma has also become increasingly important (see p 209). Other conditions for which AEL measurements may be necessary include phthisis bulbi (see p 114), pseudoexophthalmos (see p 284), or pseudoenophthalmos. In patients with leukokoria, AEL measurements can help identify or rule out specific disorders (see Chapter 5). In addition, biometry can help differentiate axial from lenticular myopia.[29] In all of the above situations, ultrasound can be used to monitor for further increase in axial eye length.[14,15]

B-scan examination can help detect the presence and location of posterior staphylomas (see p 263) and can be used to measure the vertical and horizontal dimensions of an eye. In some situations, the axial length may be normal, but other dimensions of the globe may be large or small, indicating an abnormal shape. The detection of a globe with irregular contour can be particularly important prior to cataract or strabismus surgery.

CLEANING AND CALIBRATION OF BIOMETRY INSTRUMENTS

Probes should be cleaned with a disinfecting solution between each patient examination. It is important, however, that the probe tip be thoroughly rinsed with water or saline prior to the next examination to avoid corneal injury. Additionally, ultrasound probes should never be subjected to heat, which can damage the sensitive piezoelectric crystal located near the probe tip. Calibration of the instrument should be checked periodically according to the manufacturer's specifications.

REFERENCES

1. Artaria LG: Messung der bulbeslange mit verschiednen ultraschallgeraten. *Klin Monatsbl Augenheilkd* 1986;188:492.
2. Binkhorst RD: The accuracy of ultrasonic measurement of the axial length of the eye. *Ophthalmic Surg* 1981;12:363.
3. Binkhorst RD: *Intraocular Lens Power Calculation Manual for IBM and Compatible Personal Computers*, ed. 4, New York, RD Binkhorst, 1987.
4. Burton TC, Herron BE, Ossoinig KC: Axial length changes after retinal detachment surgery. *Am J Ophthalmol* 1977;83:83.
5. Byrne SF: *A-scan Biometry* (video tape). COVE series. San Francisco, American Academy of Ophthalmology, 1988.
6. Byrne SF, Green RL: *Ultrasound of the Eye and Orbit*. St Louis, Mosby, 1992, p 215.
7. Byrne SF: Improving A-scans. *Ocular Surgery News* 1994;12:86.
8. Byrne SF: *A-scan Axial Eye Length Measurements—A Handbook for IOL Calculations*. Mars Hill, NC, Grove Park Publishers, 1995.
9. Cashwell FL, Martin CA: Axial length decrease accompanying successful glaucoma filtration surgery. *Ophthalmology* 1999; 106:2307.
10. Clemens S, Kroll P, Rochels R: Ultrasonic findings after treatment of retinal detachment by intravitreal silicone instillation. *Am J Ophthalmol* 1984;98:369.
11. Coleman DJ, Lizzi FL, Franzen LA, et al: A determination of the velocity of ultrasound in cataractous lenses, in Gitter KA, Keeney AH, Sarin LK, Meyer D (eds): *Ophthalmic Ultrasound*. St Louis, Mosby, 1969, p 246.
12. Coleman DJ, Lizzi FL, Jack RL: *Ultrasonography of the Eye and Orbit*. Philadelphia, Lea & Febiger, 1977, p 91.

13. Fledelius HC: The growth of the eye from the age of 10 to 18 years. A longitudinal study including ultrasound oculometry, in Thijssen JM, Verbeek AM (eds): *Ultrasonography in Ophthalmology*. Dordrecht, Dr W Junk, 1981, p 211.
14. Francois J, Goes F: Comparative study of ultrasonic biometry of emmetropes and myopes with special regard to the heredity of myopia, in Gitter KA, Keeney AH, Sarin LK, et al (eds): *Ophthalmic Ultrasound*. St Louis, Mosby, 1969, p 165.
15. Francois J, Goes F: Oculometry of progressive myopia. *Bibl Ophthalmol* 1975;83:277.
16. Grignolo A, Rivara A: Biometry of the human eye from the sixth month of pregnancy to the tenth year of life, in Vanysek J (ed): *Diagnostica Ultrasonica in Ophthalmologia*. Brno, Universita J.E. Purkyne, 1968, p 251.
17. Harris MJ, Blumenkranz MS, Wittpenn J, et al: Geometric alterations produced by encircling scleral buckles: Biometric and clinical considerations. *Retina* 1987;7:14.
18. Hoffer KJ: Preoperative cataract evaluation, in Caldwell DR (ed): *Transactions of the New Orleans Academy of Ophthalmology*. New York, Raven Press, 1988, p 24.
19. Hoffer KJ: Axial dimension of the human cataractous lens. *Arch Ophthalmol* 1993;111:914.
20. Hoffer KJ: Ultrasound velocities for axial length measurement. *J Cataract Refract Surg* 1994;20:554.
21. Hoffer KJ: Biometry of 7500 cataractous eyes. *Am J Ophthalmol* 1981;99:360.
22. Hoffer KJ: The Hoffer Q formula: A comparison of theoretic and regression formulas. *J Cataract Refract Surg* 1993;18:118.
23. Hoffer KJ: Modern IOL power calculations: Avoiding errors and planning for special circumstances. *AAO Focal Points* 1999;17:3.
24. Holladay JT, Prager TC, Chandler TY, et al: A three-part system for refining intraocular lens power calculations. *J Cataract Refract Surg* 1988;14:17.
25. Holladay JT, Prager TC, Chandler TY, et al: Improving the predictability of IOL power calculations. *Arch Ophthalmol* 1998;104:539
26. Holladay JT, Prager TC: Accurate ultrasonic biometry in pseudophakia [letter]. *Am J Ophthalmol* 1989;107:189.
27. Holladay JT, Prager TC: Accurate ultrasonic biometry in pseudophakia [letter]. *Am J Ophthalmol* 1993;115:536.
28. Holladay JT: Standardizing constants for ultrasonic biometry, keratometry and intraocular lens power calculations. *J Cataract Refract Surg* 1997;23:1356.
29. Jampolsky A, Flom B: Transient myopia associated with anterior displacement of the crystalline lens [case report]. *Am J Ophthalmol* 1955;36:81.
30. Jansson F, Kock E: Determination of the velocity of ultrasound in the human lens and vitreous. *Acta Ophthalmol* 1962;40:420.
31. Jansson F, Sundmark E: Determination of the velocity of ultrasound in ocular tissues at different temperatures. *Acta Ophthalmol* 1961;39:899.
32. Kendall CJ: *Ophthalmic Echography*. Thorofare, NJ, Slack, 1990, p 102.
33. Martin RG, Safir A: Asteroid hyalosis affecting the choice of intraocular lens implant. *J Cataract Refract Surg* 1987;13:62.
34. Meldrum ML, Aaberg TM, Patel A, Davis J: Cataract extraction after silicone oil repair of retinal detachments due to necrotizing retinitis. *Arch Ophthalmol* 1996;114:885.
35. Milauskas AT, Marney S: Pseudo axial length increase after silicone lens implantation as determined by ultrasonic scans. *J Cataract Refract Surg* 1988;14:400.
36. Olsen T, Nielsen PJ: Immersion versus contact in the measurement of axial length by ultrasound. *Acta Ophthalmologica* 1989;67:101.
37. Ossoinig KC: Standardized echography: Basic principles, clinical applications and results. *Int Ophthalmol Clin* 1979;19:127.
38. Ossoinig KC: *Standardized Ophthalmic Echography of the Eye, Orbit and Periorbital Region. A Comprehensive Slide Set and Study Guide*. ed 3, Iowa City, Goodfellow, 1985, p 12.
39. Patel AS: IOL power selection for eyes with silicone oil used as vitreous replacement (abstract #163, p 41). *Symposium on Cataract and Refractive Surgery*, April 1-5, 1995, San Diego.
40. Retzlaff JA, Sanders DR, Kraff MC: *Lens Power Calculations—a Manual of Ophthalmologists and Biometrists*, ed 3, Thorofare, NJ, Slack, 1990.
41. Schlenz J, Kammann J: Comparison of contact and immersion techniques for axial length measurement and implant power calculation. *J Cataract Refract Surg* 1989;15:425.
42. Shammas HJF: A comparison of immersion and contact techniques for axial length measurements. *Am Intraocular Implant Soc J* 1984;10:444.
43. Shammas HJ: *IOL Power Calculations—Avoiding the Errors*. Glendale, News Circle Publishing, 1996.
44. Shugar JK, de Juan E Jr, McCuen BW II, et al: Ultrasonic examination of the silicone-filled eye: Theoretical and practical considerations. *Graefes Arch Clin Exp Ophthalmol* 1986; 224:361.
45. Sorenson AL, Holladay JT, Kim T, et al: Ultrasonographic measurement of induced myopia associated with capsular bag distention syndrome. *Ophthalmology* 2000;107:902.
46. Tane S, Kohno J: Ultrasonic biometry of the sagittal growth of eyes in children, in Hillman JS, LeMay MM (eds): *Ophthalmic Ultrasonography*. Dordrecht, Dr W Junk, 1984, p 277.

THE ORBIT

INTRODUCTION

Standardized Echography of the orbit is a highly sophisticated and accurate method for detecting and differentiating orbital lesions. This method, developed and described by Dr. Karl Ossoinig, uses the standardized A-scan and contact B-scan to evaluate mass lesions of the orbit, as well as disorders of the extraocular muscles and optic nerve. Additionally, Doppler ultrasound is used to assess blood flow within certain orbital lesions. Although computed tomography (CT) and magnetic resonance imaging (MRI) have greatly advanced imaging of the orbit and periorbital regions, ultrasound continues to provide important information to aid in the diagnosis and management of orbital disorders.

Ultrasound is noninvasive, can be performed readily in the office setting, and is ideal for screening the orbits to determine when other procedures are indicated. The unique features of ultrasound that make it so useful for intraocular examinations play an equally important role in the orbit. The high resolution of echography provides reliable and accurate assessment of orbital structures. The small, easily maneuverable ultrasound probes allow the evaluation of orbital lesions with unusual configurations and locations. Additionally, echography continues to be the best method for determining the histologic architecture of lesions in vivo.

One of the important advances of echography is its ability to assess the kinetic properties of orbital lesions. Ultrasound is also an important adjunct in the examination of small children, since it can often be performed without sedation and does not expose the patient to radiation. Similarly, echography is ideal for the follow-up of lesions where serial examinations may be necessary. Another advantage is that ultrasound is typically performed or supervised by an ophthalmologist; this can be beneficial in settings where the radiologist does not have a great deal of experience in evaluating orbital disorders.

Although ultrasound has many advantages, it does have limitations and should be viewed as only one of several tests that may contribute to the diagnosis and management of orbital disorders. One disadvantage is that lesions located near the orbital apex may not be reliably evaluated. This is because the high frequency sound waves necessary for adequate resolution of ocular and orbital structures have limited penetration into the posterior orbit. CT and MRI may provide a better overall view of the orbit and periorbital cavities and can show these areas simultaneously. Furthermore, it is easier for most ophthalmologists to interpret CT or MRI scans. For these reasons, it is suggested that orbital ultrasound be used in conjunction with other imaging techniques, bearing in mind the advantages and disadvantages of each, so that the best results can be achieved.

INDICATIONS

The indications for orbital echography have continually grown as the accuracy and capabilities of the instrumentation and examination techniques have improved. Ultrasound is indicated whenever signs or symptoms of orbital disease are present (Table II-1).

TABLE II-1

Indications for Orbital Examination

Signs and Symptoms

Unilateral or bilateral exophthalmos
Enophthalmos
Globe displacement
Lid abnormalities
Ptosis
Retraction
Swelling
Ecchymosis
Palpable or visible masses
Chemosis
Motility disturbances; diplopia
Pain
Optic disc edema
Optic atrophy
Chorioretinal folds

Additional Indications

Tissue differentiation of mass lesions
Clarification of CT or MRI findings
Assessment of blood flow within lesions
Follow-up studies

William D. Bates

11 Examination Techniques for the Orbit

The orbital examination is divided into three major portions: (1) orbital soft tissue assessment; (2) extraocular muscle evaluation; and (3) retrobulbar optic nerve examination. In this chapter, the techniques that are used to detect, differentiate, and measure mass lesions of the orbital soft tissue and periorbital regions are addressed.[1-7] Techniques for evaluating the extraocular muscles and optic nerves are described in Chapters 15 and 16.

The marked heterogeneity of the orbital soft tissue, comprised of fat, connective tissue septa, nerves, and blood vessels, results in echograms that are very high reflective (A-scan) and echo-dense (B-scan) (Figure 11-1). Two approaches are used to evaluate the orbit: (1) transocular (i.e., examination through the globe), and (2) paraocular (i.e., examination next to the globe). The transocular route is used to detect lesions located within the posterior and mid-aspects of the orbital cavity, whereas the paraocular technique is most helpful for lesions located within the lids or anterior orbit (Figure 11-2, *A* and *B*). Since most orbital lesions have a more homogeneous composition than the normal soft tissue, they usually produce an easily recognizable defect in the echogram (Figure 11-3, *A* and *B*).

A systematic approach using both standardized A-scan and contact B-scan should be employed to detect an orbital mass lesion quickly and reliably. Lesions that are large enough to produce signs or symptoms of orbital disease are normally easily detected with echography. The exception to this is when a lesion is confined to the posterior orbit, where detection is always more difficult.

The importance of being familiar with echographic findings in the normal orbit cannot be overemphasized. The heterogeneous nature of the normal orbit can cause slight variations in a given echogram. Also, minor differences in normal findings can occur from one patient to another. Therefore, it is recommended that the echographer gain as much experience as possible in examining the normal orbit before attempting to evaluate patients with suspected orbital disease. Initially the orbital examination may be quite lengthy, but as experience is gained, the examination can be performed within a few minutes.

POSITIONING THE PATIENT

To begin the examination, the patient is reclined, with his or her head positioned close to the screen of the instrument (see Figure 2-1). Topical anesthetic drops are instilled bilaterally, as it is best to routinely examine both orbits. This is important because confirmation of whether an echogram is normal or abnormal can sometimes be made only by comparing with the uninvolved (normal) orbit. Furthermore, orbital disease sometimes may clinically appear to be unilateral when, in fact, it is bilateral.

B-SCAN TECHNIQUES

Specific techniques using both transocular and paraocular approaches have been developed to facilitate three-dimensional thinking. These techniques include the use of transverse, longitudinal, and axial views.

Transocular Approach

Transocular B-scan techniques are most useful to demonstrate mid- and posterior orbital lesions. A combination of transverse, longitudinal, and axial views are used for transocular scanning.

Transverse Scans (Transocular Approach)

The probe is placed on the globe with the longest diameter of the oval-shaped probe face positioned parallel (i.e., tangential) to the limbus. In this way, the back-and-forth movement of the transducer is parallel to the limbus. The sound beam then oscillates across the opposite fundus and orbit, producing a circumferential slice (i.e., cross-section). This orientation is appropriate for showing the lateral extent of a lesion (e.g., extending from 1- to 3-o'clock meridians, from 8- to 10:30-o'clock meridians, and so forth) (Figure 11-4).

As in the globe, the designation of the transverse scan is determined by the meridian that lies in the center of the scanned section. For example, if the probe is held vertically with its face centered on the 9-o'clock

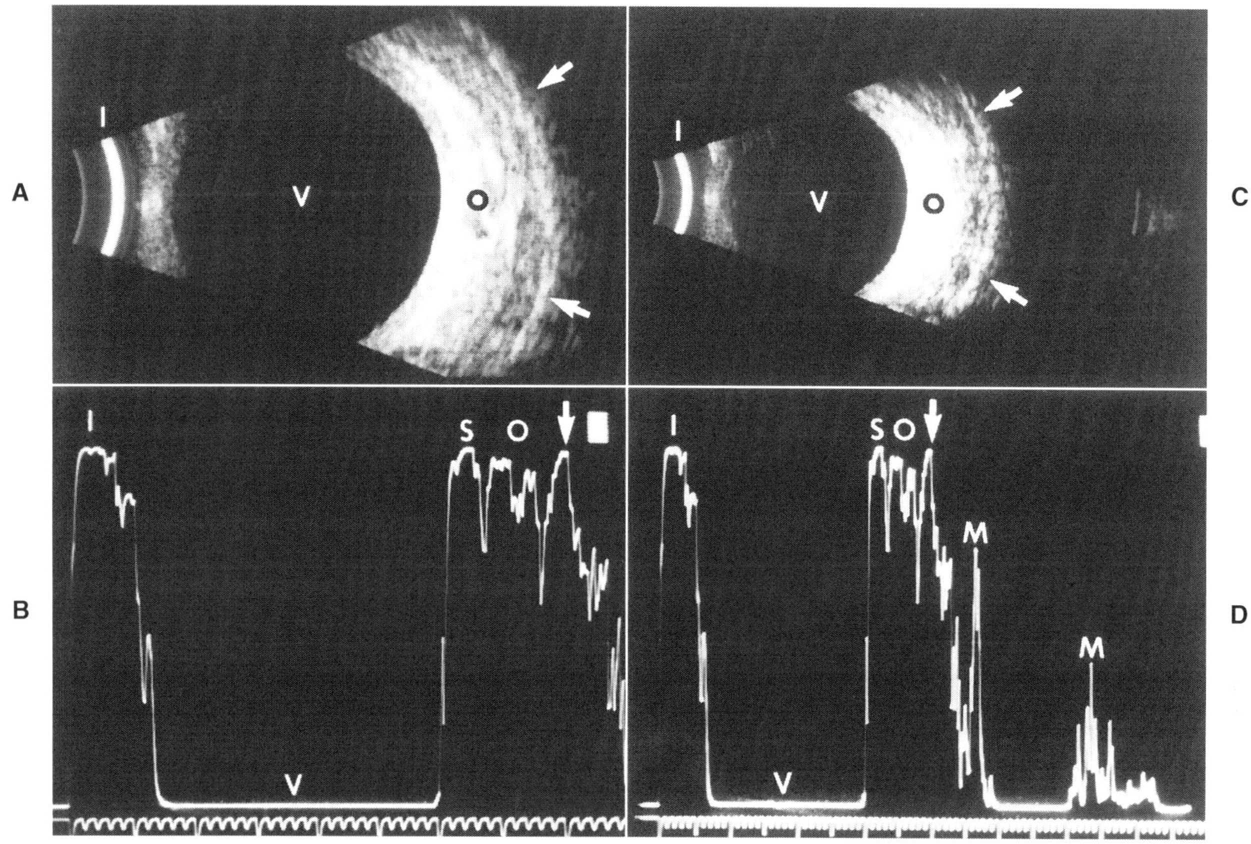

Figure 11-1 B- and A-scan echograms of normal eye and orbit. Horizontal screen expansion for globe (**A** and **B**) and orbit (**C** and **D**). *I*, Initial line (B-scan) and initial spike (A-scan); *V*, vitreous cavity; *S*, sclera; *O*, orbital soft tissue; *arrows*, orbital bone. The normal orbital tissue is extremely high reflective on A-scan and echo-dense on B-scan. In orbital examinations, the screen expansion for orbit is always used for A-scan, but either the globe or orbital screen expansion may be used for B-scan. Note that there are two multiple signals *(M)* shown in echogram **D.** The first signal is due to reverberations between the sclera and the orbital bone. The second multiple signal is caused by reverberations occurring between the probe and the sclera. Such artifacts are commonly seen when the orbital screen expansion on the A-scan is used.

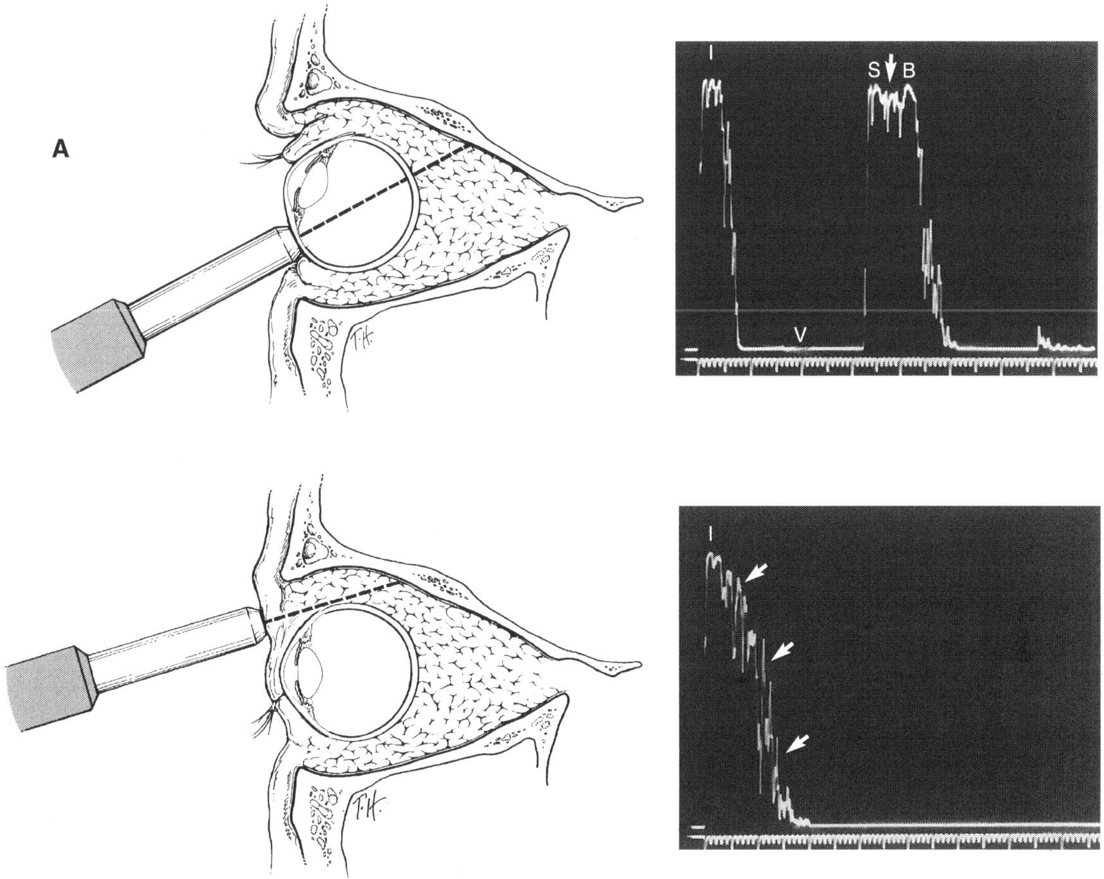

Figure 11-2 Transocular and paraocular A-scan **(A)** and B-scan (**B,** p 278) examination of a normal orbit. **A,** A-scan echograms taken at Tissue Sensitivity. *Top,* Transocular approach. *I,* Initial spike; *V,* vitreous cavity; *S,* sclera, *arrow,* normal soft tissue; *B,* orbital bone. *Bottom,* paraocular approach with probe placed on closed lid and sound beam directed into anterior orbit. *I,* Initial spike followed by chain of highly reflective spikes *(arrows)* from normal orbit. Spike chain decreases in height at steep angle due to strong sound attenuation caused by normal tissue.

Continued

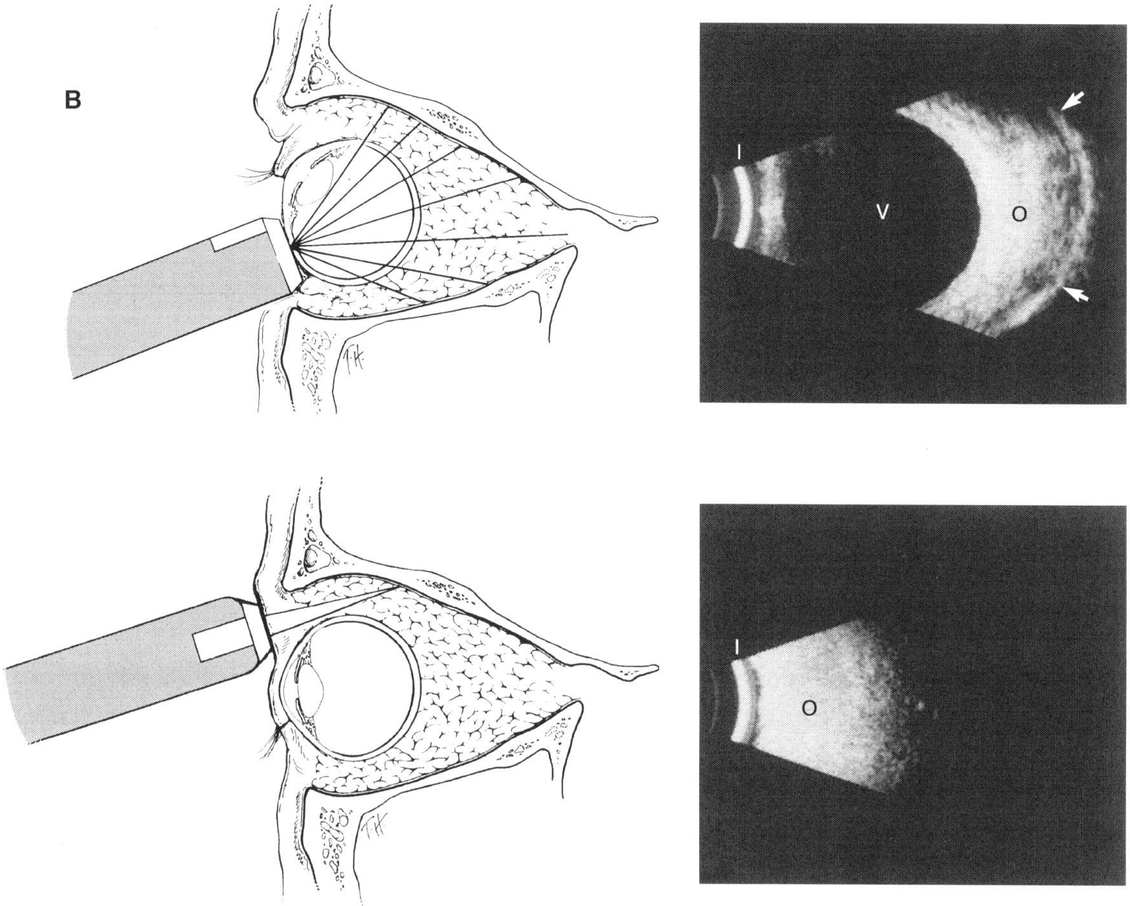

Figure 11-2, cont'd **B,** B-scan echograms obtained with medium-high gain setting. *Top*, Transocular approach. *I*, initial line; *V*, vitreous cavity; *O*, orbital soft tissue; *arrows*, orbital bone. *Bottom*, Paraocular approach. *I*, Initial line; *O*, orbital soft tissue.

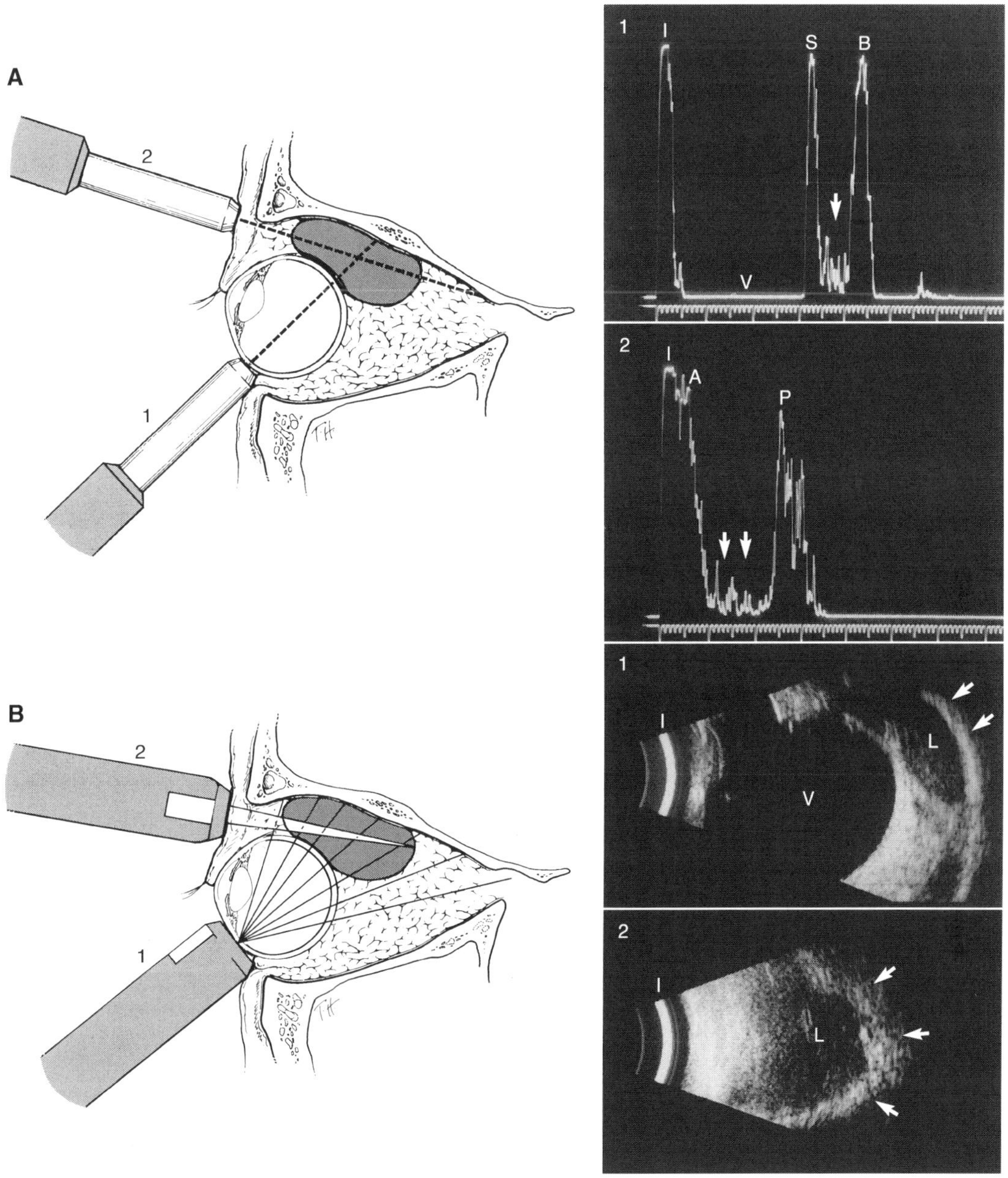

Figure 11-3 Transocular and paraocular A-scan **(A)** and B-scan **(B)** examination of orbital mass. **A,** A-scan echograms taken at Tissue Sensitivity. *1,* Transocular approach. *I,* Initial spike; *V,* vitreous cavity; *S,* sclera; *arrow,* internal lesion spikes; *B,* orbital bone. *2,* Paraocular approach. *I,* Initial spike corresponding to probe tip on lid; *A,* anterior surface spike of lesion; *arrows,* internal lesion spikes; *P,* posterior surface spike of lesion. The transocular approach is used to measure a lesion's maximal thickness, and the paraocular approach is used to measure its maximal depth into the orbit. **B,** B-scan echograms obtained using medium gain setting. *1,* Transocular approach. *I,* Initial line; *V,* vitreous cavity; *L,* lesion; *arrows,* bone. *2,* Paraocular approach. *I,* Initial line corresponding to probe face on lid; *arrows,* posterior surface of lesion.

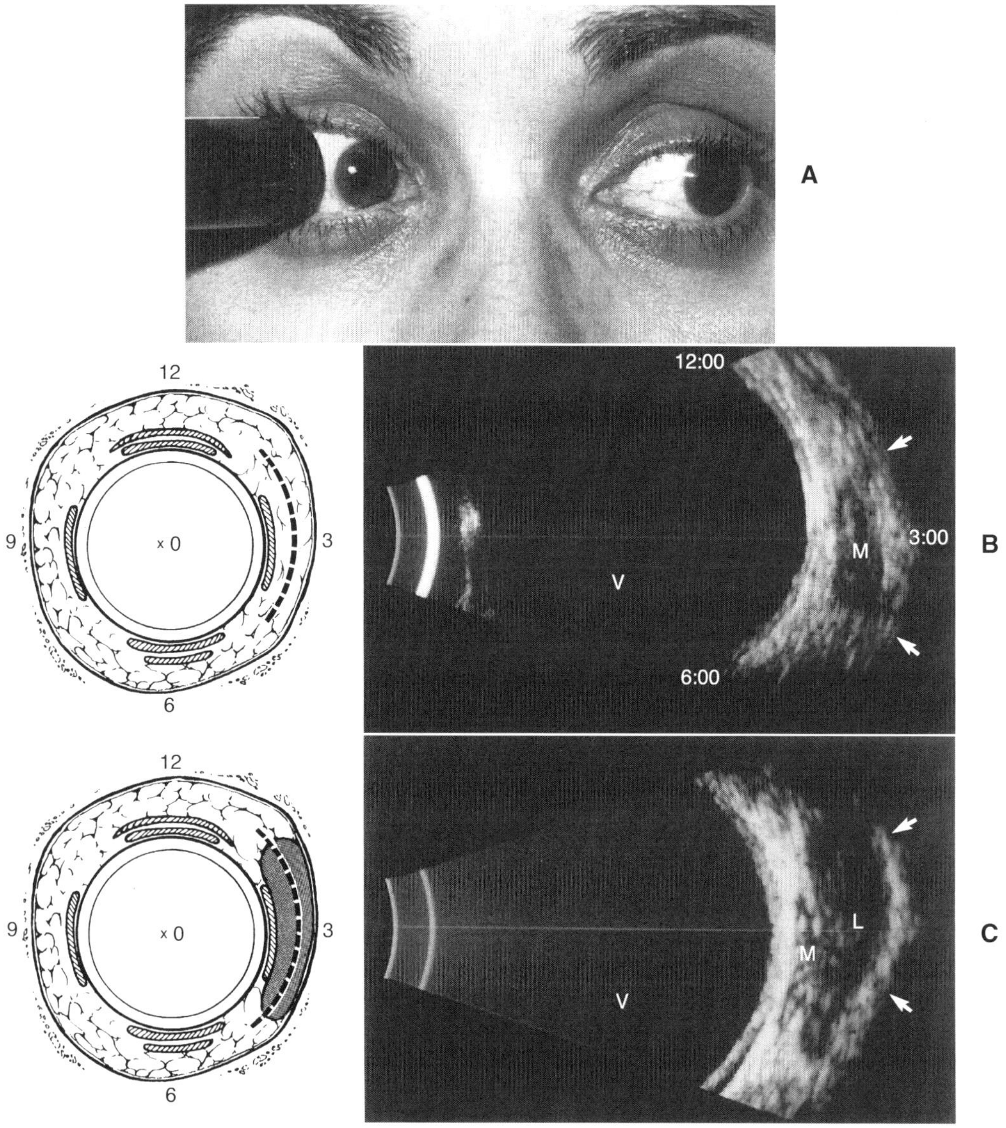

Figure 11-4 Vertical transverse B-scan examination (transocular approach) of 3-o'clock meridian. **A,** The patient fixates toward the examined meridian. The probe marker is directed superiorly. **B,** Normal orbit. **C,** Extraconal tumor. *V,* Vitreous cavity; *M,* medial rectus muscle; *L,* lesion; *arrows,* orbital bone. Note that the medial rectus muscle is compressed by the mass in the bottom echogram.

meridian, the 3-o'clock meridian is displayed in the center of the echogram; this probe position is called a transverse scan of the 3-o'clock meridian. If the probe is placed in a horizontal manner at the 6-o'clock limbus, the sound beam sweeps perpendicularly across the 12-o'clock meridian; this is called a transverse scan of the 12-o'clock meridian.

By convention, horizontal transverse scans (i.e., transverse scans of the 12- or 6-o'clock meridians) are performed with the probe marker oriented toward the patient's nose, so the upper part of the echogram represents the nasal portion of the orbit. Vertical transverse scans (i.e., transverse scans of the 3- or 9-o'clock meridians) are performed with the marker directed superiorly, so the top of the echogram represents the upper portion of the orbit.

Oblique transverse scans (e.g., transverse scans of the 1:30-, 4:30-, 7:30-, or 10:30-o'clock meridians) are performed with the marker directed toward the upper portion of the orbit (see Figure 2-6 and Table 2-1). An oblique scan is the designation for a transverse view of any meridian other than 12:00, 3:00, 6:00, and 9 o'clock.

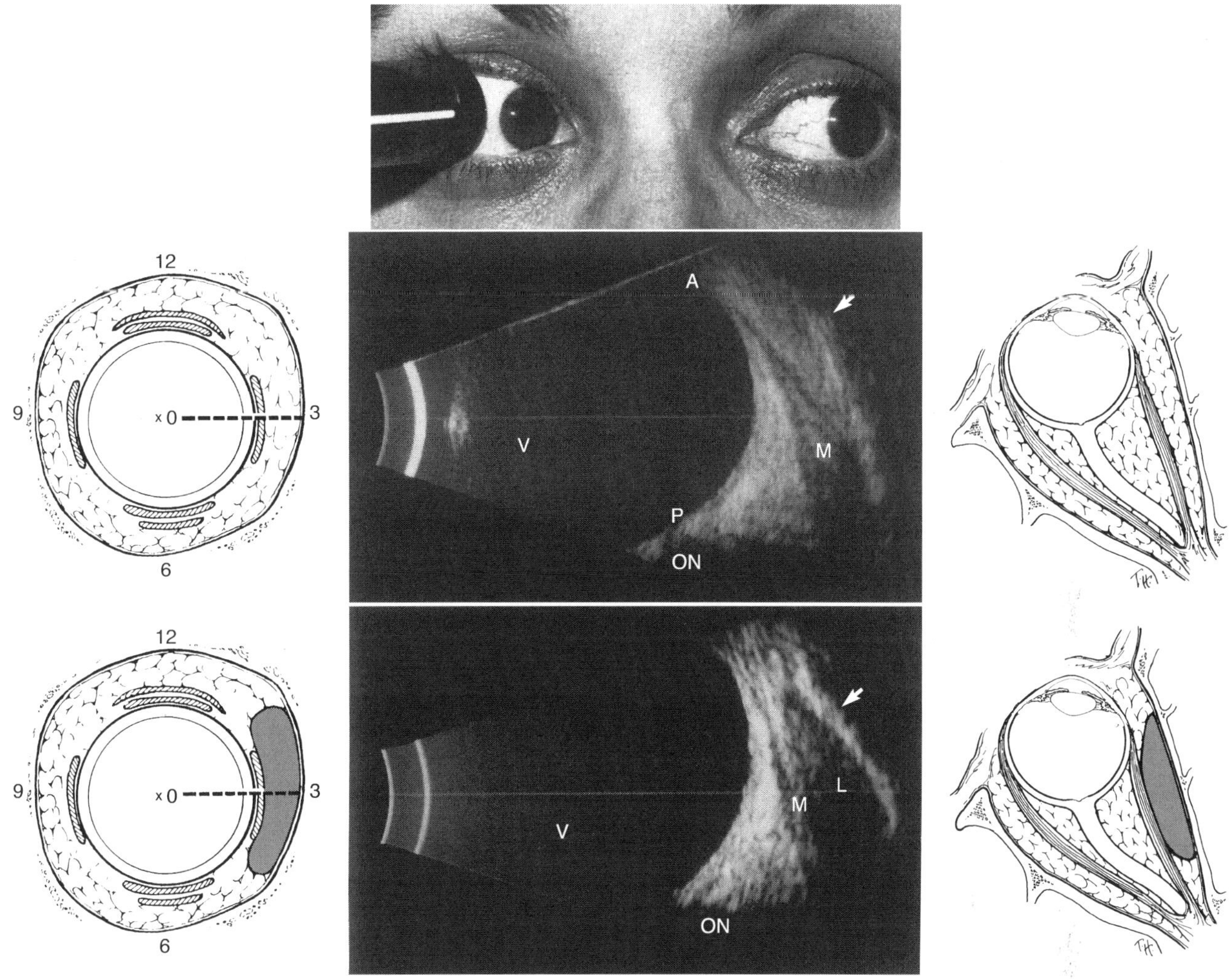

Figure 11-5 Longitudinal B-scan examination (transocular approach) of 3-o'clock meridian. *Top*, The patient fixates toward the examined meridian. The probe marker is directed toward the center of the cornea and the 3-o'clock meridian. *Center*, Normal orbit. *Bottom*, Extraconal tumor (same lesion as in Figure 11-4). *V*, Vitreous cavity; *A*, anterior aspect of globe; *P*, posterior aspect of globe; *ON*, optic nerve; *M*, medial rectus muscle; *L*, lesion; *arrow*, orbital bone.

Longitudinal Scans (Transocular Approach)

A three-dimensional conception of the orbit is greatly enhanced with the use of longitudinal B-scan echograms. Longitudinal scans are performed with the probe rotated 90 degrees from the position used for the transverse scan. This means that the longest diameter of the oval-shaped probe face is placed perpendicular (rather than parallel) to the limbus. The sound beam then sweeps along the meridian that is located opposite to the probe, rather than across the meridian, as in the transverse scan. Consequently, the longitudinal scan provides an anteroposterior view of the orbit and of a lesion (Figure 11-5).

In a longitudinal scan, the marker is always directed toward the center of the cornea and the meridian that is being examined (see Figure 2-8 and Table 2-1). This results in the posterior orbit being displayed on the lower portion of the screen and the anterior orbit being displayed on the upper portion of the screen. The designation of the longitudinal scan is simply by the meridian that is being examined. For example, if the probe is placed on the 4-o'clock meridian of the globe, the sound beam sweeps along the 10-o'clock meridian; this is called a longitudinal scan of the 10-o'clock meridian.

Axial Scans (Transocular Approach)

The axial orientation is the third type of probe position. An axial scan is performed with the patient fixating in primary gaze and with the probe face centered on the cornea. The sound beam is then directed through the center of the lens and the optic nerve. As mentioned previously, this scan is often the easiest to interpret because it displays a lesion in relationship to the globe and optic nerve.

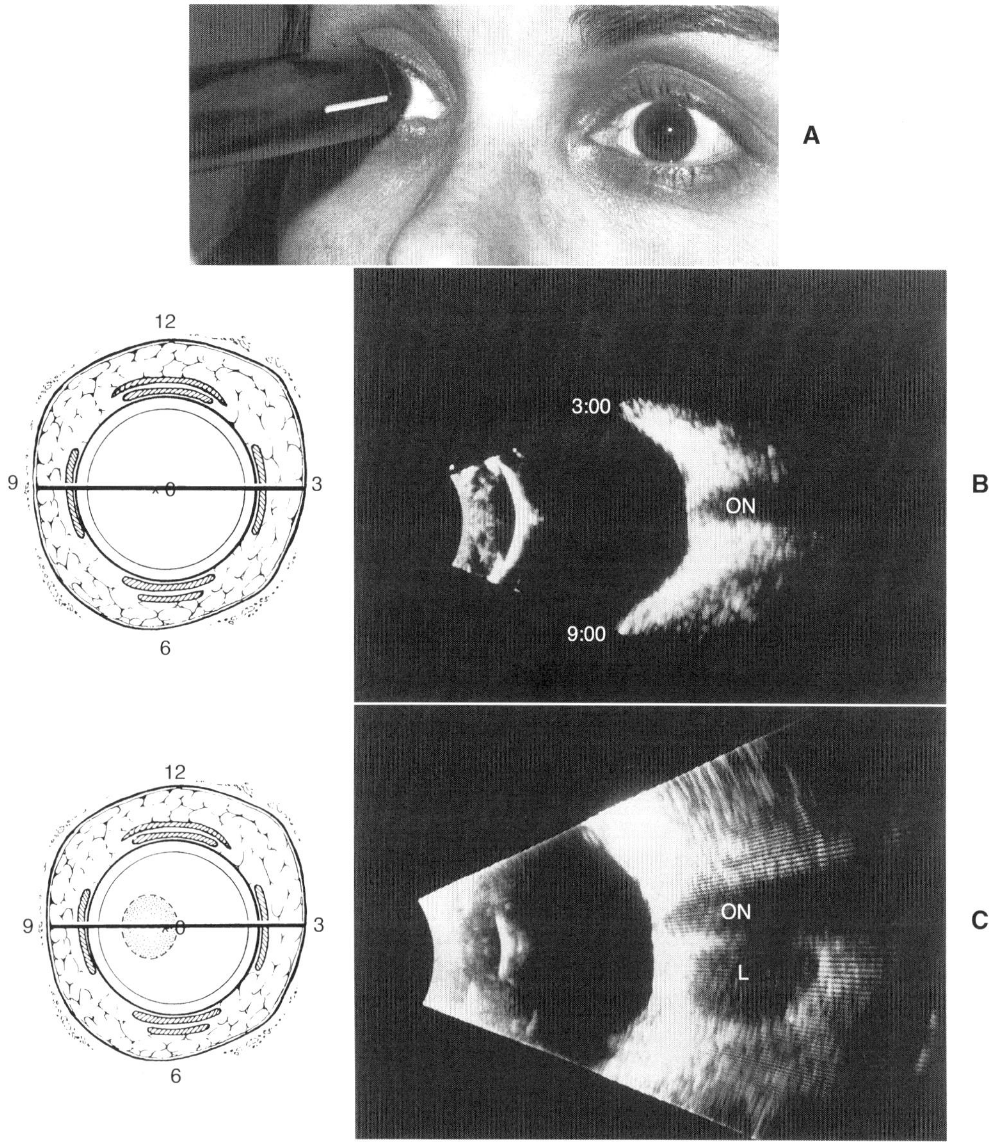

Figure 11-6 Horizontal axial B-scan examination. **A,** The patient fixates in primary gaze. The probe marker is directed nasally. **B,** Normal orbit. **C,** Intraconal orbital mass. Note that the lesion *(L)* is located temporal to the optic nerve *(ON)*.

When a horizontal axial scan is performed, the sound beam sweeps through the 3- and 9-o'clock meridians, and the marker is oriented toward the patient's nose (Figure 11-6). In a vertical axial scan, the sound beam sweeps through the 12- and 6-o'clock meridians, and the marker is oriented superiorly. With an oblique axial scan (e.g., the sound beam sweeps through the 1:30- to 7:30- or the 10:30 to 4:30-meridians), the marker is always oriented toward the upper of the two meridians being examined (see Table 2-1).

Paraocular Approach

Paraocular B-scan techniques may be helpful to demonstrate anterior lesions in relationship to the globe and orbital wall. The paraocular approach can be employed with both transverse and longitudinal probe orientations. Methylcellulose should be applied to the lids as a coupling medium whenever the paraocular approach is used.

Transverse Scans (Paraocular Approach)

The probe is placed on the patient's closed eyelid, between the globe and orbital rim, with the longest diameter of the oval-shaped probe face oriented parallel to the orbital wall. The sound beam then sweeps back and forth across the lid and anterior orbit (i.e., tangential to the globe and parallel to the orbital rim). The echographer shifts the probe back and forth between globe and bone to evaluate fully the region beneath the probe. With the transverse scan, the lateral extent and posterior border of an anterior lesion can be demonstrated (Figure 11-7).

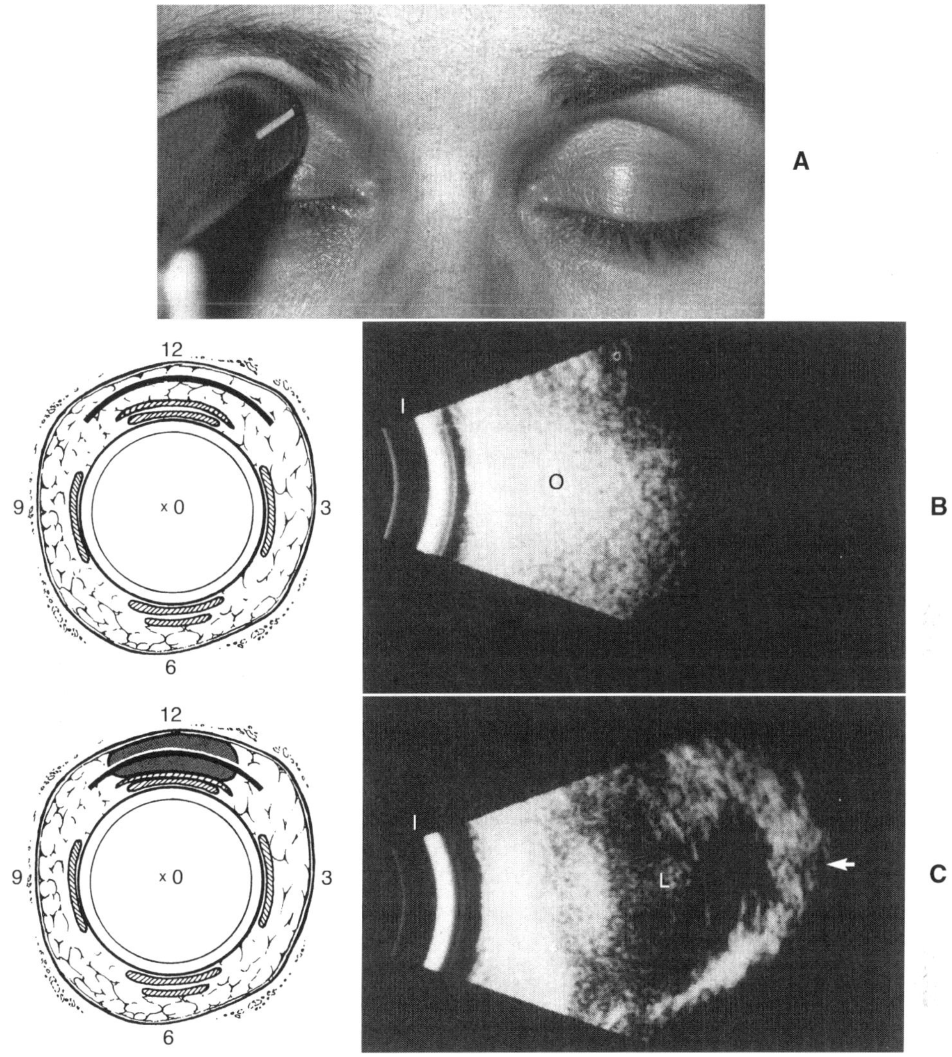

Figure 11-7 Horizontal transverse B-scan examination (paraocular approach) of orbit at 12-o'clock. **A,** The probe is positioned on the upper lid. The probe marker is directed nasally. **B,** Normal orbit *(O)*. **C,** Superior orbital mass lesion *(L)*. *Arrow,* Posterior surface of lesion.

The designation of the transverse scan is determined by the meridian that lies in the center of the echogram (just beneath the probe). For example, if the probe is held horizontally with its face centered on the lid at the 12-o'clock position, the echogram is called a paraocular transverse scan of the 12-o'clock meridian. Vertical and oblique transverse scans are also designated by where the probe is positioned. The marker is oriented as previously described. With horizontal scans (i.e., probe at the 12- or 6-o'clock positions), the marker is directed nasally; with vertical (i.e., probe at 3- or 9-o'clock positions) and oblique scans, the marker is directed superiorly (Figure 11-8, *A*).

Longitudinal Scans (Paraocular Approach)

As in the transverse paraocular approach, the probe face is placed on the patient's closed eyelid between the globe and orbital rim. The probe face, however, is rotated 90 degrees from the transverse position, so that the longest diameter of the oval-shaped probe face is now orientated perpendicular to the orbital rim. The sound beam thus sweeps back and forth (i.e., perpendicularly) between the globe and orbital wall. This scanning view may allow simultaneous display of the peripheral globe and an anterior lesion, depending on probe position (Figure 11-9).

Designation of the longitudinal scan is according to the meridian being examined. For example, if the probe is placed at the 1:30 position, the echogram is called a paraocular longitudinal scan of the 1:30-o'clock meridian.

When performed along any meridian between the 3- and 9-o'clock meridians (i.e., superiorly), the probe marker should be directed to the bony wall (away from the globe) in the meridian scanned. However, when this technique is performed on any inferior meridian, the probe marker should be oriented toward the center of the globe (Figure 11-8, *B*).

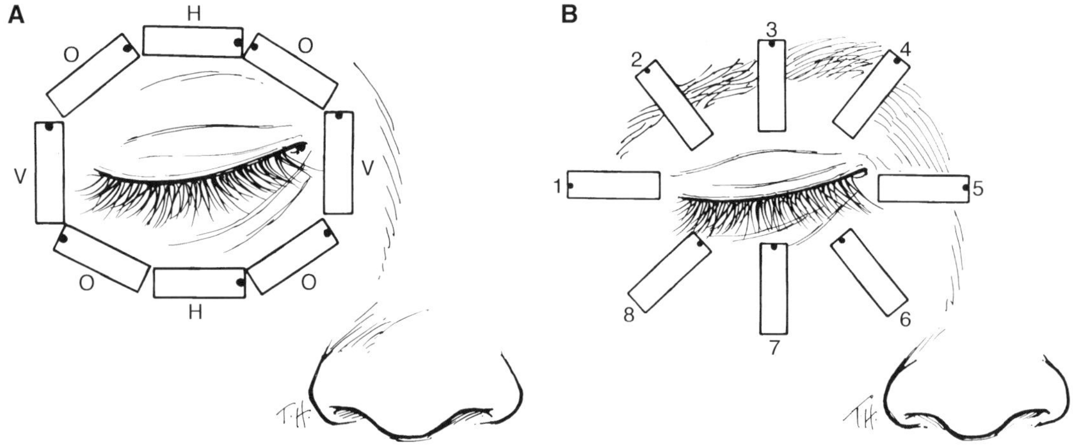

Figure 11-8 Various paraocular B-scan probe positions showing marker orientation. **A,** Transverse positions. Horizontal *(H)*, marker nasal; vertical *(V)*, marker superior; oblique *(O)*, marker superior (e.g., marker directed toward 10:30- or 1:30-o'clock meridians). **B,** Longitudinal positions. The marker is directed toward the orbital rim in positions *1-5* and toward the globe in positions *6-8*. This system ensures that all lesions are displayed in proper anatomic position in the echogram (e.g., above globe if located superiorly, and below globe if located inferiorly).

BASIC EXAMINATION FOR LESION DETECTION

B-Scan Screening

The orbital screening examination can be performed with B- as well as with A-scan. The transocular and, in some cases, the paraocular approach is used for B-scan screening.

Systematic examination techniques are used for B-scan screening of the orbit. The examination is performed initially with transverse scans (transocular approach) of the four major meridians, with the examiner using a medium-high gain setting. Methylcellulose is applied to the probe or eye surface, and the probe is placed directly on the globe.

The superior portion of the orbit is scanned first, with the patient's gaze directed toward the 12-o'clock meridian. The probe is oriented horizontally, with its face placed next to the inferior limbus and centered on the 6-o'clock meridian (i.e., horizontal transverse scan of the 12-o'clock meridian), with the marker directed nasally. With the probe positioned near the limbus, the posterior aspect of the superior orbit is examined initially. The probe is then shifted toward the lower fornix, thereby screening progressively more anterior aspects of the superior orbit (Figure 11-10). As the probe is being shifted, the echographer continuously monitors the echogram to detect any abnormalities.

After the superior orbit has been examined with this procedure, the nasal orbit is examined by having the patient look medially. The probe is placed in a vertical orientation, with its face centered near the temporal limbus (i.e., transverse scan of the 3-o'clock meridian of the right orbit or the 9-o'clock meridian of the left orbit). Again, the probe is shifted from limbus to fornix, thereby scanning the entire nasal half of the orbit. Similar maneuvers are then performed for the inferior and temporal aspects of the orbit.

Longitudinal scans (transocular approach) also can be performed to evaluate the soft tissue and are useful for assessing the lacrimal gland region. The axial approach should also be used to evaluate the retrobulbar space. This position is especially helpful for the detection of lesions that are located near the posterior ocular wall, the optic nerve, or elsewhere in the muscle cone. Vertical and horizontal axial scans (with the lens and the nerve centered) are performed first.

When the axial approach is employed, the retrobulbar space can be more completely evaluated by tilting the probe slightly so that the sound beam just bypasses the optic nerve (i.e., para-axial). With a horizontal axial scan the probe is tilted slightly up and then down, and with a vertical axial scan the probe is tilted nasally and temporally (Figure 11-11). Careful comparison should always be made between the two orbits.

If the examination is normal, the echographer may wish to measure the axial lengths to determine if a large or small eye is producing pseudoexophthalmos or pseudoenophthalmos. Additionally, a Valsalva maneuver may be performed to look for an orbital varix that may be visible only when filled (see p 359, Figure 13-18, and Color Plate 10).

Compressibility of the soft tissues should also be assessed during the screening procedure. This is accomplished by

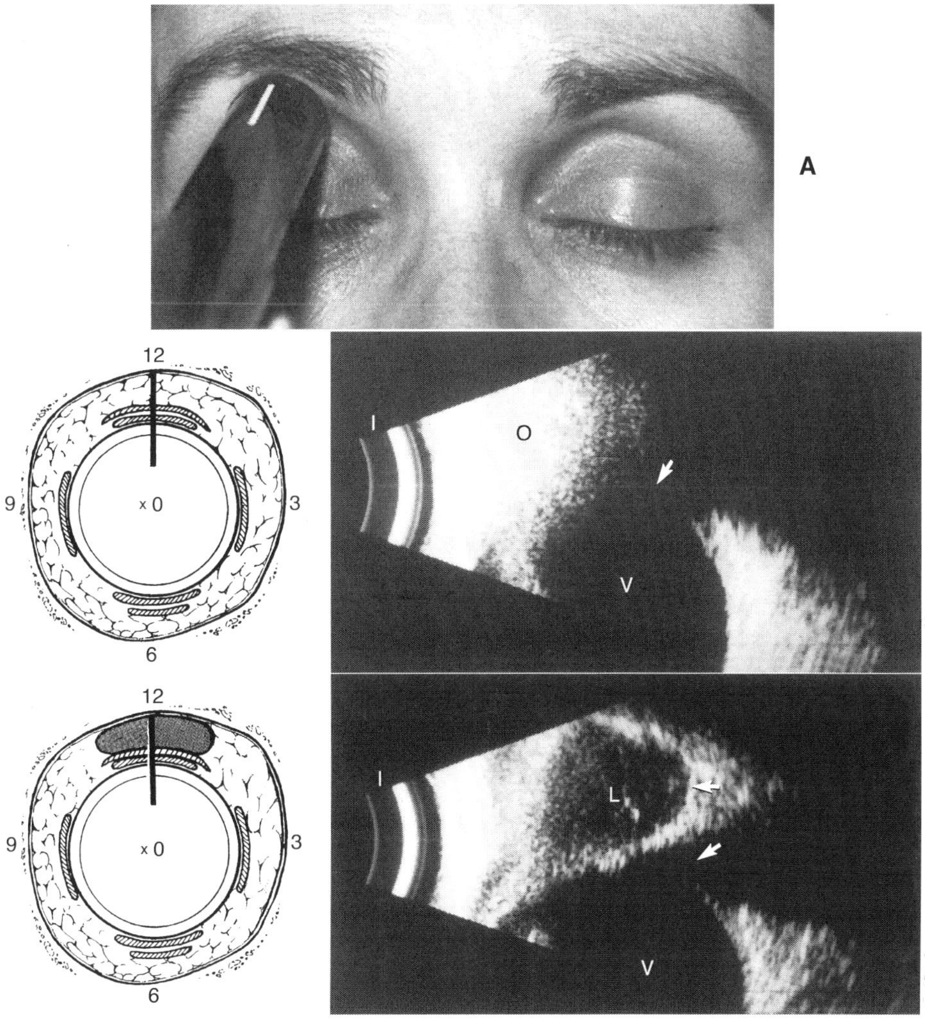

Figure 11-9 Longitudinal B-scan examination (paraocular approach) of superior orbit at 12-o'clock. **A,** The probe is positioned on the upper lid. The probe marker is directed toward 12-o'clock. **B,** Normal orbit *(O)*. **C,** Superior orbital mass lesion *(L)* (same lesion as in Figure 7-7). Note that paraocular longitudinal scans are obtained with the sound beam directed simultaneously through peripheral globe and paraocular tissue. *V,* Vitreous cavity; *black arrow,* posterior surface of lesion; *white arrows,* area of globe surface not imaged due to oblique sound beam incidence.

pressing the probe lightly on the globe. Normal orbital soft tissue is easily compressible, which results in appreciable narrowing of the orbital echogram.

Because of the large size of most B-scan probes, paraocular screening with B-scan is not as reliable as with the smaller A-scan probe. Therefore, paraocular B-scan screening is performed routinely only if A-scan is unavailable.

A-Scan Screening

The standardized Tissue Sensitivity gain setting is used throughout the orbital examination (see Figure 1-12); the screen expansion for orbit is selected (see Figure 11-1). Both transocular and paraocular approaches are used for A-scan screening.

Transocular Approach

The transocular approach is used first. Probe placement and movement for this technique are very similar to that utilized for the globe. As in the globe examination, the 12-o'clock meridian is examined initially. The patient fixates toward 12-o'clock, and the probe is placed at the 6-o'clock limbus, with the sound beam directed toward the posterior orbit. The probe is then shifted along this

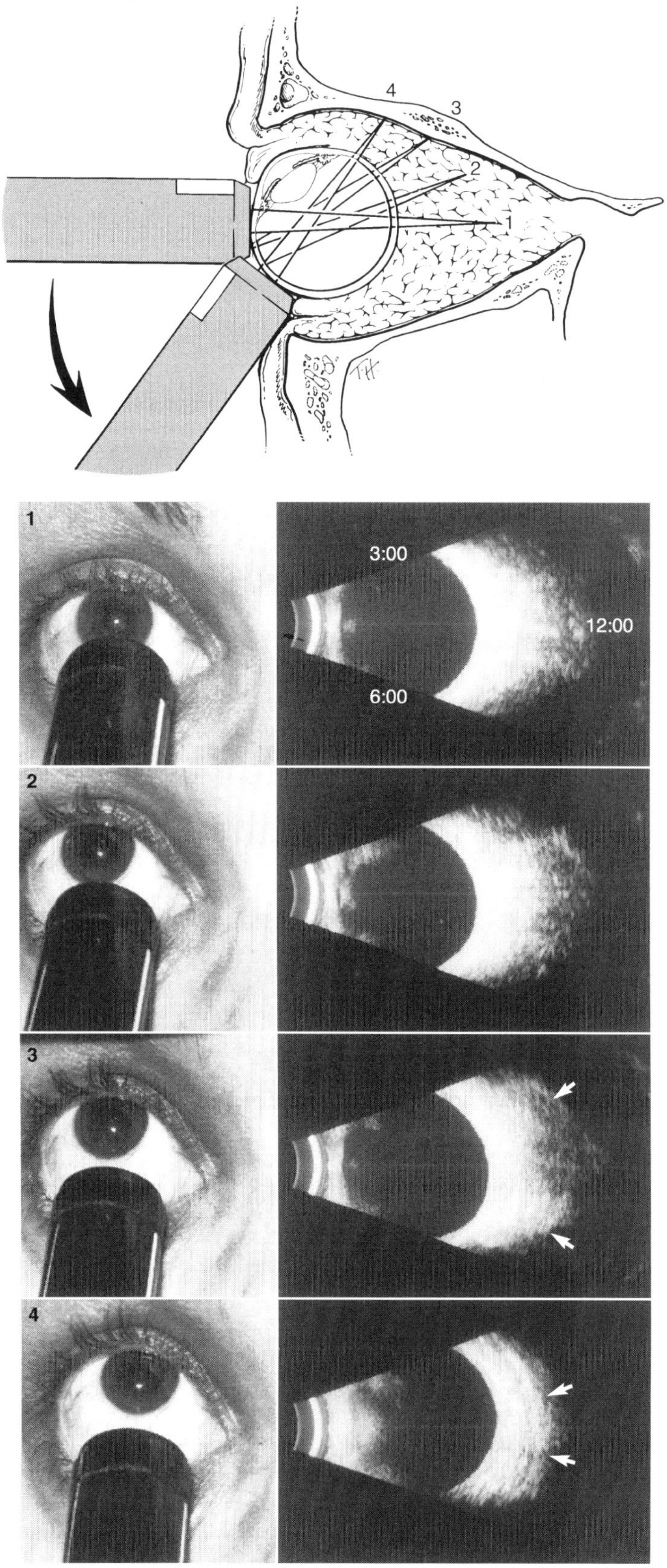

Figure 11-10 Transocular B-scan screening of superior orbit from posterior *(1)* to anterior *(4)* using horizontal transverse probe orientation. Note that the probe marker is oriented nasally. *Arrows,* Orbital bone.

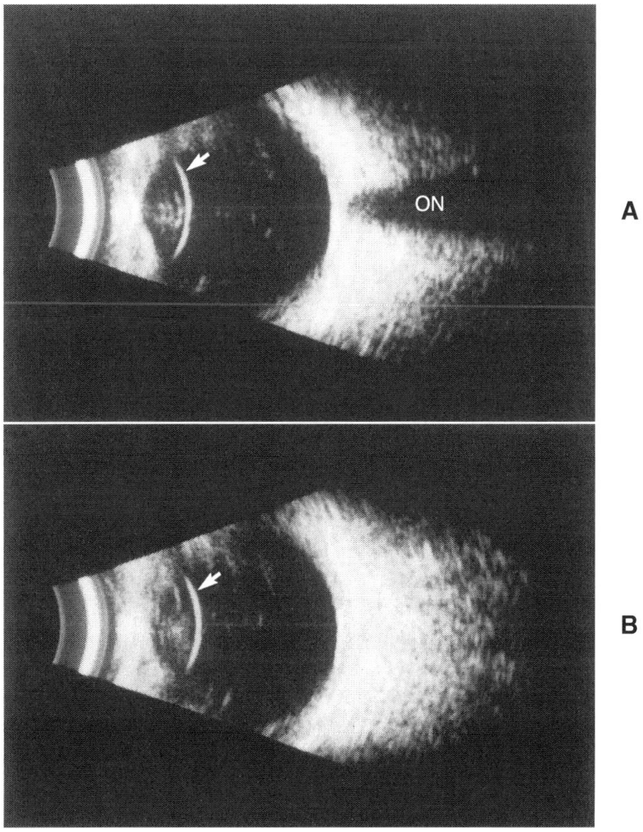

Figure 11-11 Axial and para-axial B-scan echograms of retrobulbar orbit with probe on cornea (fixation in primary gaze). **A,** Axial view shows optic nerve *(ON)* and surrounding orbital soft tissue. *Arrow,* Posterior lens capsule. **B,** Para-axial scan with sound beam shifted slightly to examine orbit just adjacent to optic nerve.

meridian into the fornix as the display is continuously monitored for the appearance of any abnormalities (Figure 11-12). During this procedure, small "defects" originating from the normal orbital fissures, extraocular muscles, optic nerve, and so forth, may be detected. To ensure that these normal findings are not mistaken for an actual lesion, it is helpful to anticipate where they may occur and to compare them immediately with the same area of the fellow orbit. The same limbus-to-fornix shifting procedure is repeated in seven additional meridians, moving temporally around the globe (as in the intraocular examination), until the entire orbital cavity has been examined (see Figure 2-14).

Unless markedly enlarged, the extraocular muscles and optic nerves are not well displayed during the basic A-scan screening examination. This is because of oblique sound beam incidence to the sheaths as the patient fixates away from the probe. Instead, these structures are examined separately with the patient fixating in primary gaze, as described in Chapters 15 and 16.

The normal lacrimal sac may produce a small defect in the echogram when the probe is placed near the fornix temporally and with the sound beam directed toward the nasal aspect of the anterior orbit (see Figure 12-26). The normal lacrimal sac may be more easily detected when the globe is proptotic than when it is in normal position or is enophthalmic.

Careful attention should be given to the posterior orbit, because the detection of lesions in this area can be more difficult. It may be helpful to shift the probe additionally in an arc-like manner along the limbus and to compare carefully with the fellow orbit. The superior orbital fissure is best displayed with the probe placed near the inferonasal limbus, whereas the inferior orbital fissure is shown with the probe positioned supranasally (Figure 11-13).

Paraocular Approach

A-scan screening with the paraocular approach is used to evaluate the lids and the anterior orbit. It is also useful for evaluating the lacrimal system and the periorbital sinuses.

Methylcellulose is applied to the closed lids as a coupling medium to ensure sufficient sound penetration. Using slight but firm pressure, the probe is placed first on the upper lid at the 12-o'clock position, with the sound beam

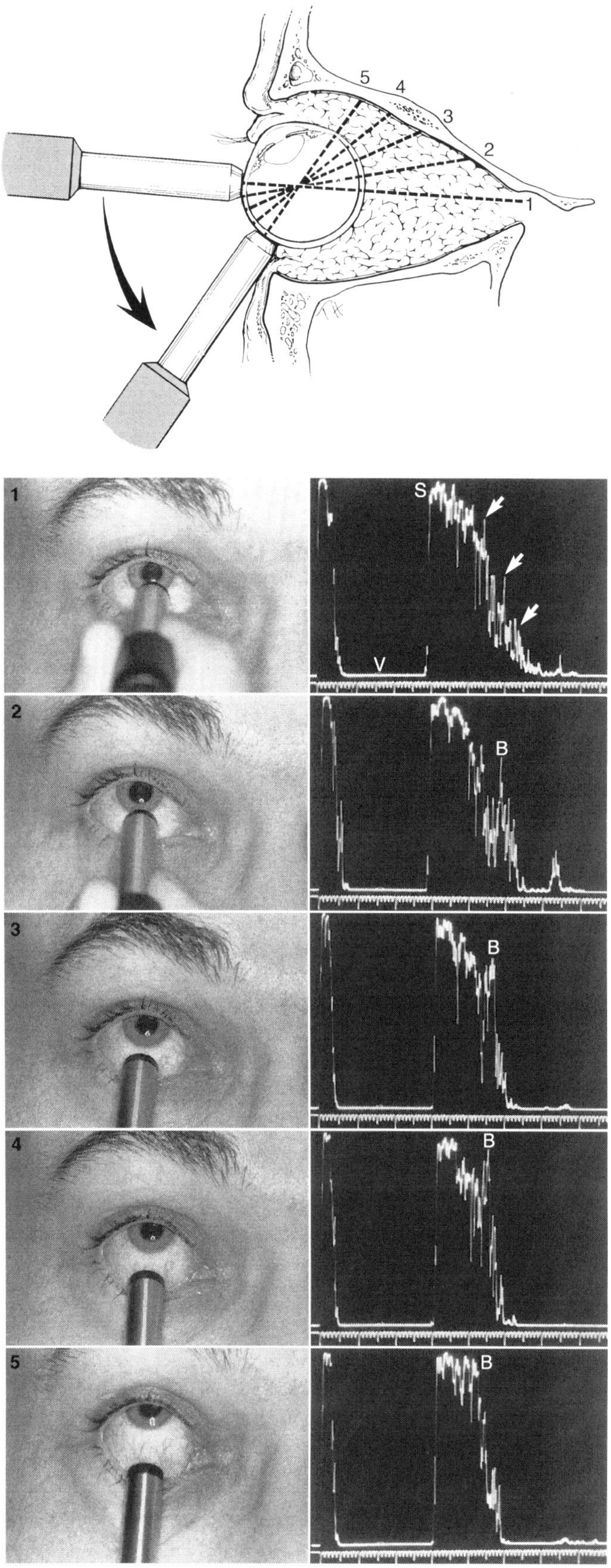

Figure 11-12 Transocular A-scan screening of superior orbit. As patient fixates superiorly, the probe is shifted along the 6-o'clock meridian (thereby examining the 12-o'clock meridian). With probe at limbus *(1)*, the sound beam is aimed toward the orbital apex. As probe is shifted toward lower fornix *(5)*, orbital echogram narrows and bone spike becomes higher. *V*, Vitreous cavity; *S*, sclera; *arrows*, orbital soft tissue spikes decrease in amplitude due to sound attenuation; *B*, orbital bone. This limbus to fornix shifting is performed in eight meridians to screen the entire orbital cavity.

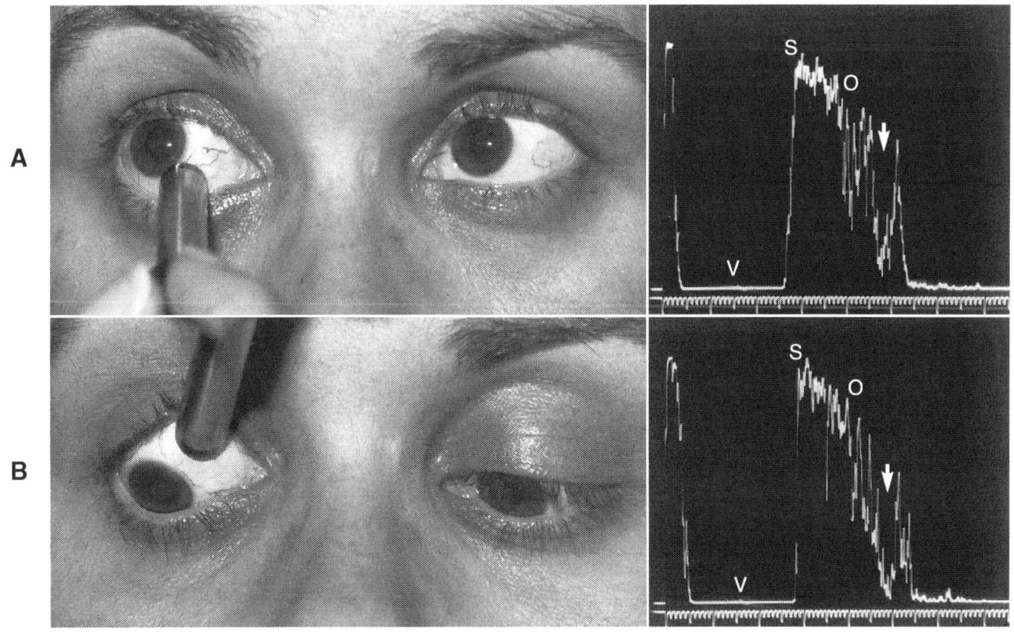

Figure 11-13 A-scan examination of superior and inferior orbital fissures. **A,** Superior orbital fissure displayed with probe placed inferonasally. **B,** Inferior orbital fissure displayed with probe placed supranasally. *V,* Vitreous cavity; *S,* sclera; *O,* orbital soft tissue; *arrow,* fissure.

directed through the globe (toward the 6-o'clock meridian). The probe is then slowly redirected away from the globe and toward the adjacent orbit and proximal bony orbital wall. Finally, the sound beam is aimed posteriorly toward the orbital apex (Figure 11-14). This same globe-to-bone maneuvering is repeated in seven more meridians, moving temporally around the orbit.

The sinuses (maxillary, ethmoid, and frontal sinuses) are specifically evaluated during the paraocular screening examination. The probe is directed perpendicular to the bony wall that overlies the sinus cavity. No echoes are produced from the normal air-filled sinus, as air totally reflects the sound waves. However, when there is mucosal swelling, the sinus is filled with fluid, or solid tissue is present, abnormal echoes appear to the right of the paraocular pattern (Figure 11-15).

The lacrimal system can also be examined with the paraocular approach. The lacrimal sac is evaluated with the probe placed in the medial canthal region (3-o'clock position for the right eye, 9-o'clock position for the left eye), as described in Figure 12-26. The lacrimal gland can be evaluated using the paraocular approach, with the probe placed supratemporally (see Figure 12-17).

SPECIAL EXAMINATION TECHNIQUES FOR LESION DIFFERENTIATION

As in the globe, topographic, quantitative, and kinetic techniques have been developed to localize, differentiate, and measure orbital mass lesions.[1-3] All techniques should be performed systematically for best results (Box 11-1).

Topographic echography determines location, shape, size, and border character of a lesion. It is also used to monitor contour of the globe and bony orbital walls. Quantitative echography reveals data relating to histologic composition and is used to evaluate internal structure, reflectivity, and sound attenuation. Kinetic echography evaluates properties of motion such as consistency, internal blood flow, and mobility.

Topographic Echography: Location, Shape, Size, and Borders

The evaluation of topographic properties is the first step in the differentiation of an orbital mass. Topography is assessed with a combination of B- and A-scan techniques and the use of transocular and/or paraocular approaches, depending on lesion location. Masses that are confined to the lids or the extreme anterior orbit may be assessable only by a paraocular route, whereas those confined to the muscle cone usually must be evaluated with a transocular approach. Conversely, large lesions that extend both anteriorly and posteriorly can normally be evaluated with a combination of the two approaches. B-scan assessment is essential for evaluating and documenting lesion topography, and A-scan examination can be an important adjunct.

Location, Size, and Shape

The accurate localization of a mass is essential because its position (e.g., lacrimal fossa, muscle cone, subperiosteal

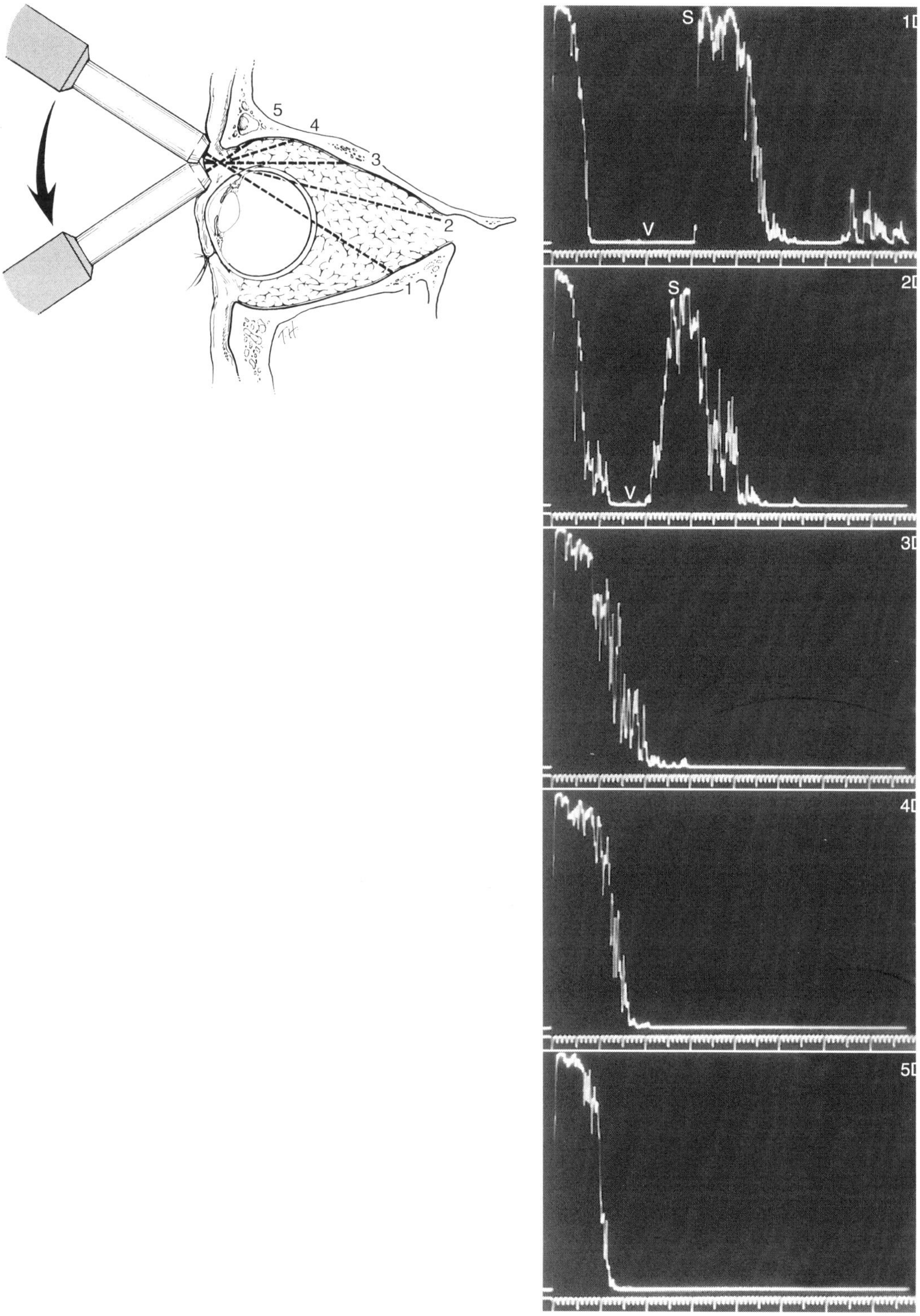

Figure 11-14 Paraocular A-scan screening of superior orbit. Probe is shifted between globe *(1)* and orbital wall *(5)* along the 12-o'clock meridian. *1*, Sound beam directed through globe, perpendicular to sclera *(S)*. *V*, Vitreous cavity. *2*, Sound beam angled through peripheral globe (oblique incidence to sclera, *S*). *3-5*, Normal paraocular echograms.

A

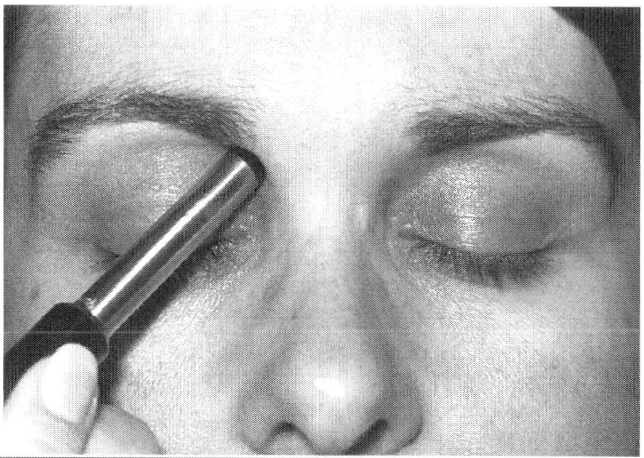

B

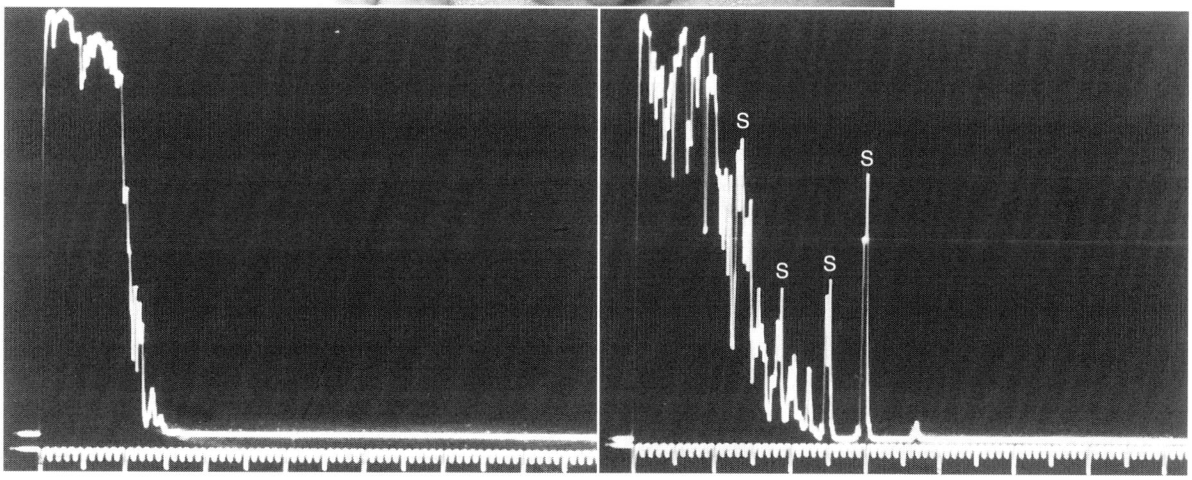

C

Figure 11-15 Examination of the frontal sinus with paraocular A-scan approach. **A,** The A-scan probe is directed toward the frontal sinus. **B,** Normal sinus. No echoes are received from the normally air filled sinus. **C,** Abnormal sinus echoes *(S)*, indicating the presence of fluid, mucosal swelling, or other abnormal tissue.

BOX 11-1

Differentiation of Orbital Mass Lesions*

Topographic

Location: Position, meridians
Shape
Borders
Contour abnormalities
  Bone: Excavation, defects, or hyperostosis
  Globe: Indentation or flattening

Quantitative

Internal reflectivity: Spike height
Internal structure: Histologic architecture
Sound attenuation: Absorption or shadowing

Kinetic

Consistency: Soft vs. hard
Vascularity: Blood flow
Mobility: Of lesion or its contents

*When an orbital mass is detected, these properties are assessed for lesion differentiation.

space) may be an important factor in differentiation. Additionally, the position of the lesion may influence the clinical management (e.g., surgical approach). Location, size, and shape are first evaluated with the two-dimensional B-scan.

A transocular, transverse probe orientation is used initially to assess a lesion's lateral extent, shape, and thickness. The patient fixates toward the lesion, and the probe is placed on the globe at the limbus opposite the lesion. The probe is shifted between limbus and fornix until the center of the lesion is displayed (see Figure 11-4).

The longitudinal approach is then applied to add more information by displaying the lesion in long section. This position also displays the shape of the lesion as well as its posterior extension into the orbit. As in the transverse scan, the patient fixates toward the lesion, and the probe is placed on the globe opposite the lesion. The probe is initially positioned close to the limbus and is then shifted toward the fornix as needed to best display the lesion in maximal extent (see Figure 11-5).

The final step in the topographic B-scan assessment is the use of an axial scan. This orientation is helpful to document the relationship of a lesion to the globe wall, optic nerve, extraocular muscles, and orbital bone. The information derived from the transverse, longitudinal, and axial approaches is then combined for a complete topographic overview (Figure 11-16).

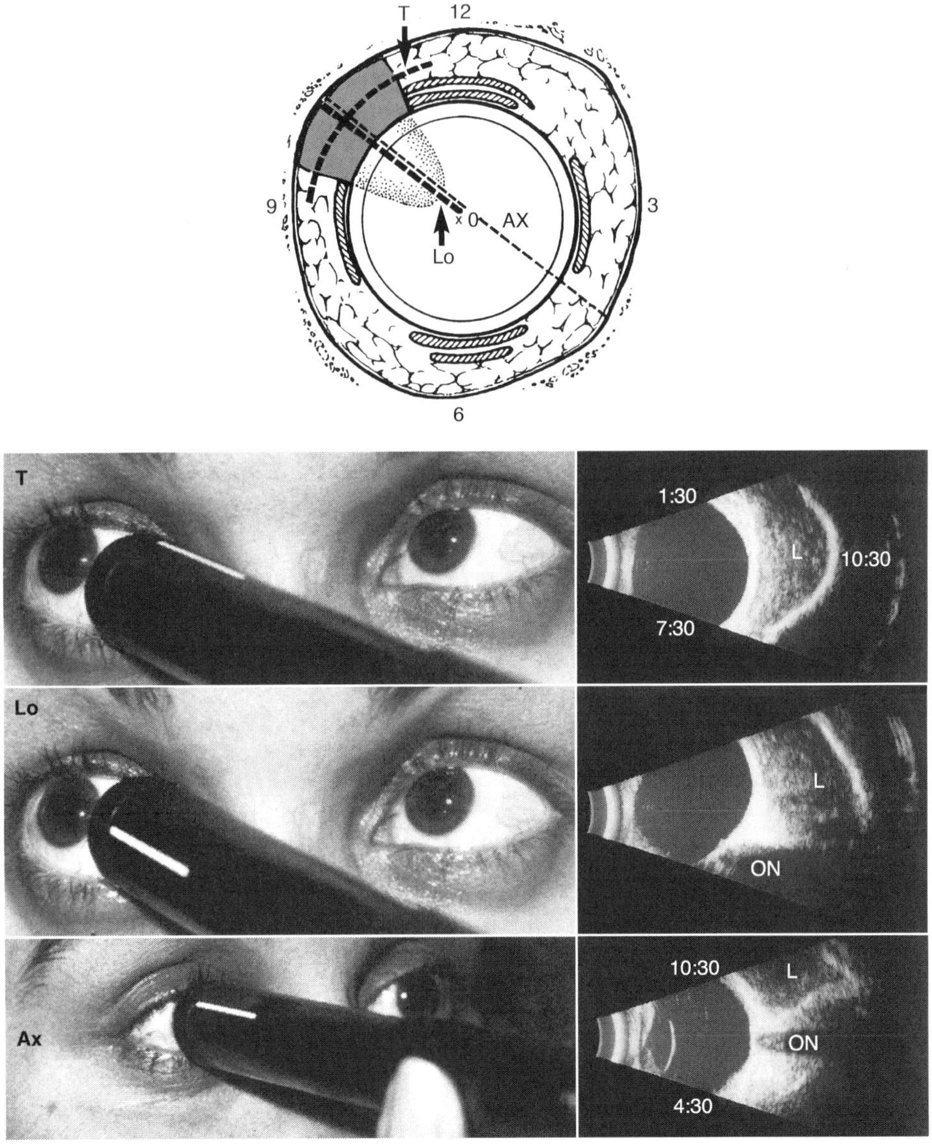

Figure 11-16 Topographic evaluation of large supratemporal mass lesion using transocular approach. *T*, Transverse scan shows lateral extent of lesion *(L)*. *Lo*, Longitudinal scan shows radial extent of lesion. *ON*, Optic nerve. *Ax*, Axial scan shows relationship of lesion to globe and optic nerve. Drawing shows sound beam orientation through lesion.

When a lesion is very large, it may not be possible to display its entire extent in one transverse or longitudinal view. In such cases, it may be helpful to move the probe so as to image both central and peripheral aspects of the lesion (Figure 11-17).

For very anterior lesions, it may be advantageous to use the paraocular B-scan approach, rather than transocular, for the evaluation of topography. Again, a combined approach, utilizing both transverse and longitudinal views, provides the most information (Figure 11-18).

A-scan complements B-scan in the assessment of a lesion's location, size, and shape. In addition, A-scan can provide measurements of a lesion's maximal thickness and posterior extent into the orbit (Figure 11-19; see also Figure 11-3, *A*). By using these various A- and B-scan techniques, the echographer can mentally construct a three-dimensional image of a lesion and can usually classify its shape as round, oval, spindle, or irregular.

Borders

Echographically, a lesion's borders are characterized as well outlined (i.e., well circumscribed) or poorly outlined (i.e., indistinct or diffuse). Lesions that are very well outlined (e.g., with a capsule or pseudocapsule) usually demonstrate a smooth, regular contour and rounded shape on B-scan and a distinct, high posterior surface spike on A-scan. This posterior surface spike can be either single- or double-peaked (Figure 11-20).

In contrast, poorly outlined lesions usually have an indistinct, irregular contour on B-scan and produce a less

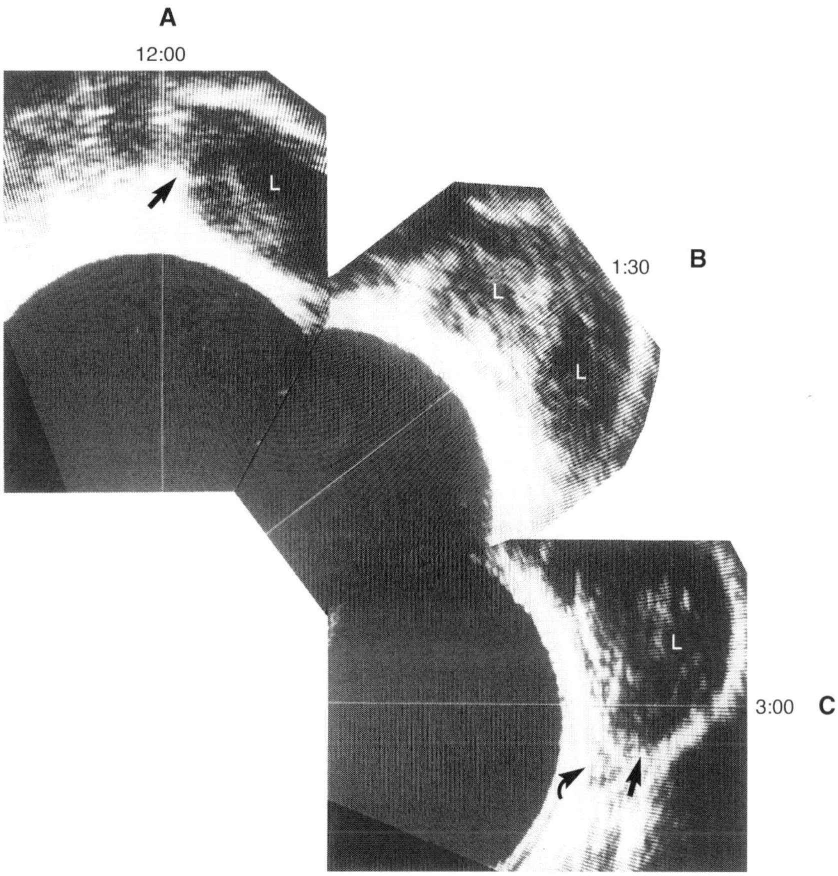

Figure 11-17 Transverse B-scan montage (transocular approach) of large supratemporal mass (left orbit) to document entire lateral extent. **A,** Horizontal scan of 12-o'clock meridian shows upper edge *(arrow)* of lesion *(L)*. **B,** Oblique scan of 1:30-o'clock meridian shows central portion of lesion. **C,** Vertical scan of 3-o'clock meridian shows inferior edge of lesion *(straight arrow)*. *Curved arrow,* Cross-section of lateral rectus muscle. Note that the smooth, rounded borders of the lesion are shown as the tumor margins are centered in echograms **A** and **C.**

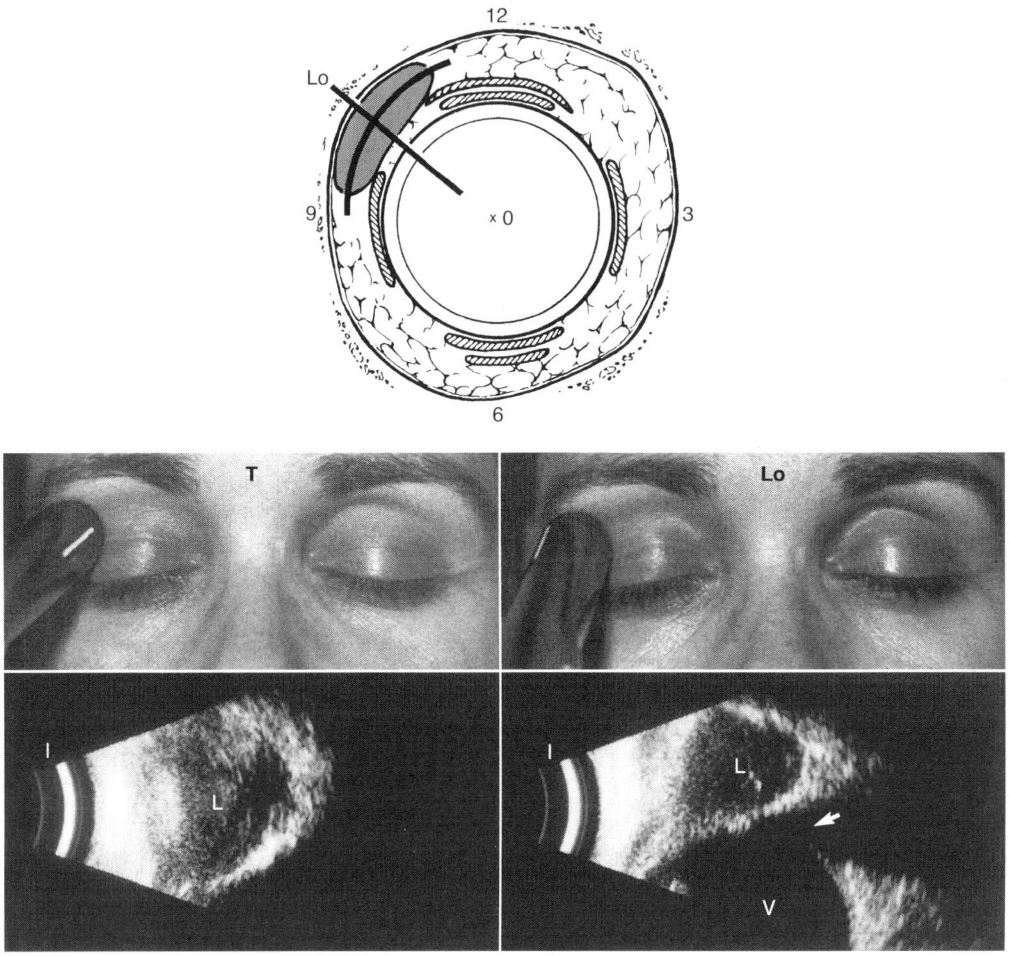

Figure 11-18 Topographic evaluation of supratemporal mass lesion using paraocular B-scan approach. Transverse approach *(T)* shows cross-section of lesion *(L)*. *I*, Initial line. Longitudinal approach *(Lo)* shows long section of lesion *(L)*. *V*, Vitreous cavity; *arrow*, area of globe surface not imaged due to oblique sound beam incidence. Drawing shows sound beam orientation through lesion.

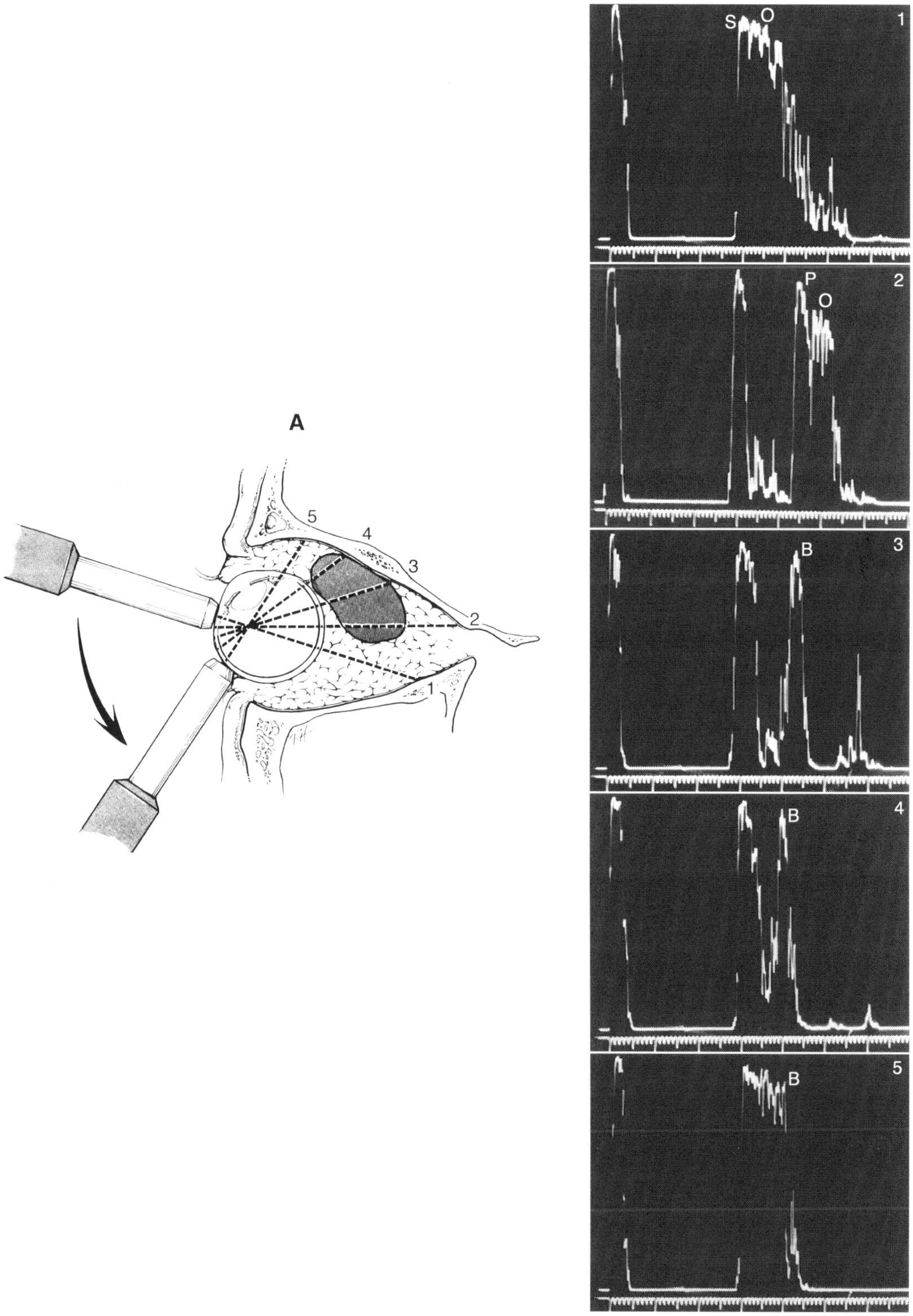

Figure 11-19 Topographic A-scan evaluation of retrobulbar **(A)** and anterior **(B)** mass lesions. **A,** Transocular evaluation of retrobulbar mass. Probe is shifted to localize lesion, assess posterior border character, and determine maximal thickness. *1,* With probe at limbus, sound beam is aimed posteriorly, bypassing lesion; *S,* sclera; *O,* orbital soft tissue. *2,* Sound beam encounters lesion and is directed perpendicular to posterior border *(P)* in area not adjacent to bone. *3,* Sound beam is shifted more anteriorly, relatively perpendicular to orbital bone *(B)*. *4,* Sound beam is angled through anterior aspect of lesion, perpendicular to bone. *5,* Sound beam is directed anterior to mass, perpendicular to bone.

Continued

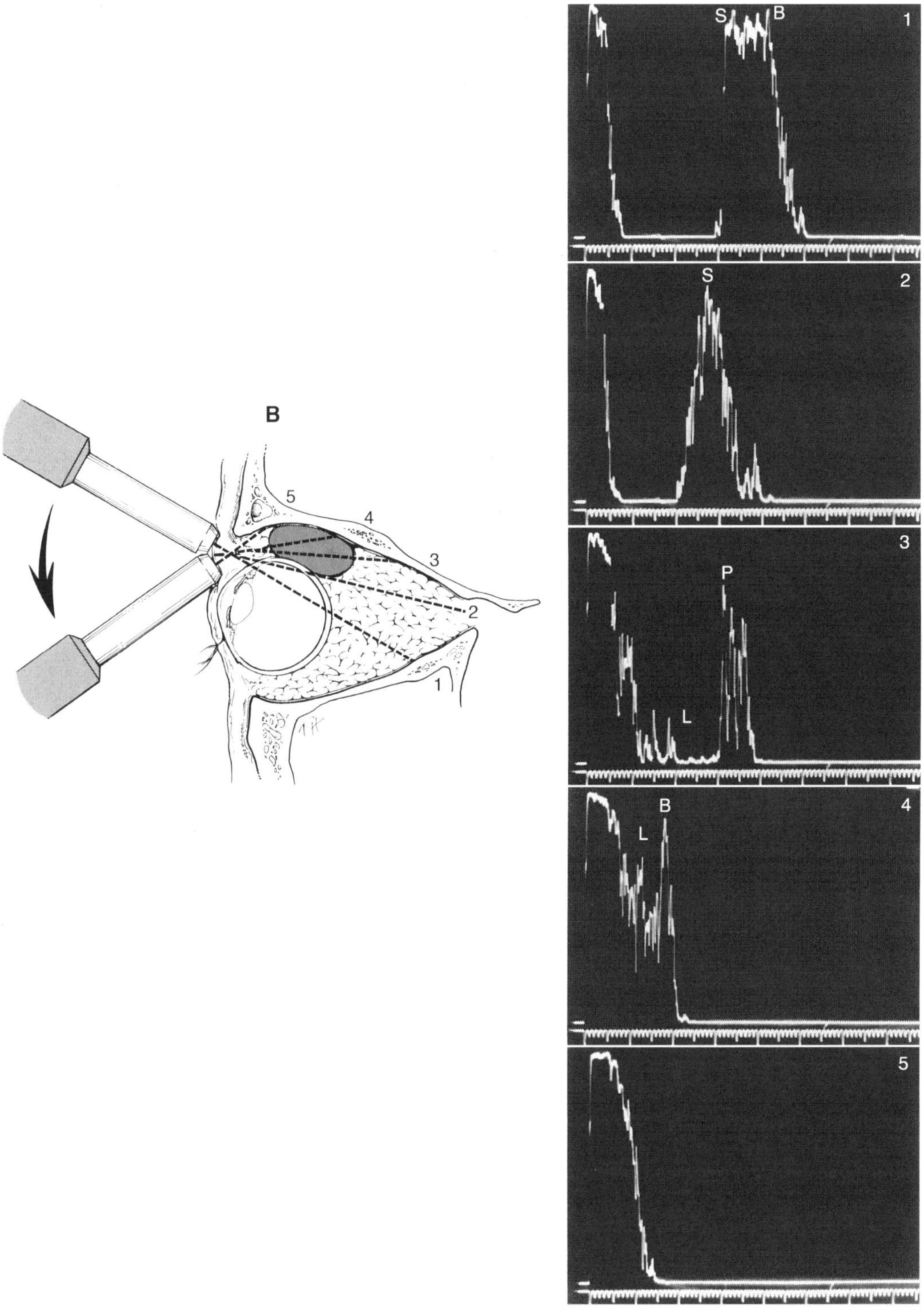

Figure 11-19, cont'd **B,** Paraocular evaluation of anterior mass. Probe is angled between globe and bone to localize lesion, assess posterior border spike, and determine maximal depth into orbit. *1,* Sound beam is first directed through globe; *S,* sclera; *B,* orbital bone. *2,* Sound beam is shifted toward lesion but is now oblique to sclera *(S)*. *3,* Sound beam is now perpendicular to posterior border *(P)* of lesion *(L)* in area of maximal depth in orbit. *4,* Probe is angled through lesion anteriorly, more perpendicular to bone *(B)*. *5,* Beam is directed anterior to lesion, toward bone.

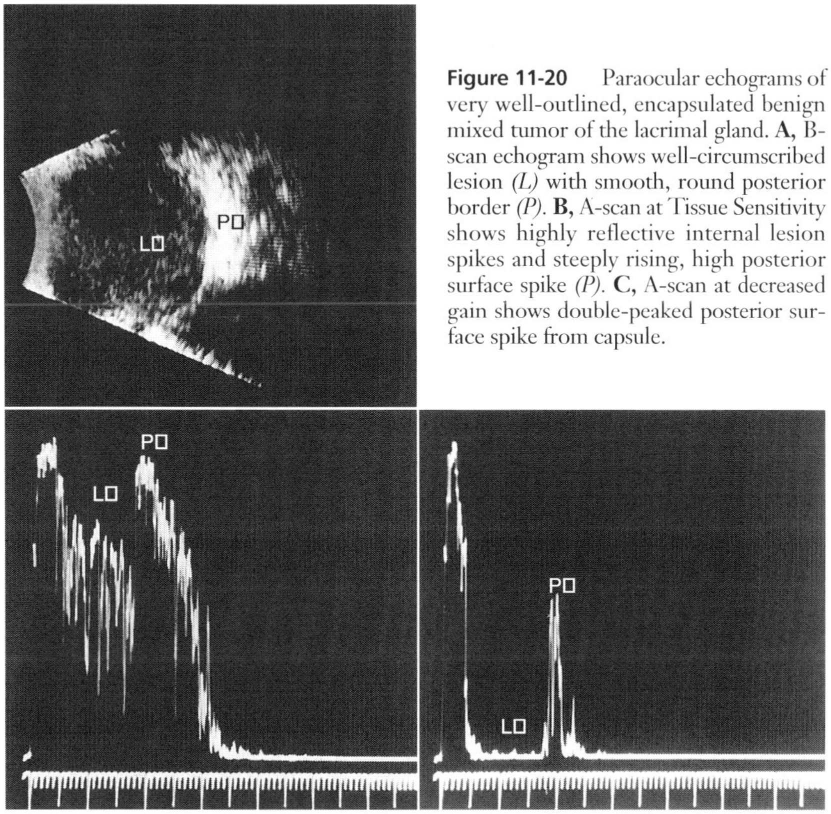

Figure 11-20 Paraocular echograms of very well-outlined, encapsulated benign mixed tumor of the lacrimal gland. **A,** B-scan echogram shows well-circumscribed lesion *(L)* with smooth, round posterior border *(P)*. **B,** A-scan at Tissue Sensitivity shows highly reflective internal lesion spikes and steeply rising, high posterior surface spike *(P)*. **C,** A-scan at decreased gain shows double-peaked posterior surface spike from capsule.

distinct, lower reflective posterior surface spike on A-scan (Figure 11-21). Occasionally, sound attenuation can limit the assessment of a lesion's border characteristics. If a mass produces strong sound attenuation, the amplitude of its posterior border echoes are likely to be significantly reduced and thus more difficult to evaluate.

When assessing the borders of a lesion on A-scan, the surface being evaluated should not be situated adjacent to the bony orbital wall. Therefore, anterior lesions or those located more posteriorly, close to the orbital bone, must be evaluated with a paraocular approach. This directs the sound beam through the mass perpendicular to its posterior surface and parallel to the orbital wall. If, however, a lesion is confined to the muscle cone, it is usually necessary to use the transocular approach to evaluate its borders (see Figures 11-3, *A*, and 11-19, *A*).

Contour Changes in Globe and Bone

When pressure is exerted on the globe by a large mass, B-scan may show flattening or indentation of the ocular wall. Chorioretinal folds in the same area also may be visible by ophthalmoscopy. Globe indentation can be associated with a variety of orbital conditions such as tumors, cysts, enlarged muscles, or optic nerve, as well as hemorrhage or abscess. Changes in contour of the bony orbital walls also may be detected (Figure 11-22).

Immersion Technique

Small lesions that are located superficially on the conjunctiva, within the lid, or within the anterior orbit can be examined by means of an immersion technique. In such anterior lesions, the immersion method may provide the only reliable means of evaluating acoustic properties as well as thickness. A scleral shell, placed directly over the lesion, is filled with methylcellulose (see Appendix D). Both A- and B-scan examinations can be performed, with techniques that are similar to those used for immersion examination of the globe (Figure 11-23; see also p 37 and Figure 2-30).

Quantitative Echography: Reflectivity, Internal Structure, and Sound Attenuation

Once the topographic characteristics of a lesion have been assessed, quantitative echography is performed to determine reflectivity, i.e., the strength of a lesion's internal echoes. This information correlates with the lesion's histologic architecture such as the character of cellular substance; the number, size, and distribution of cell aggregates; and the presence of large interfaces such as blood vessels, connective tissue septa, calcification, and so forth.

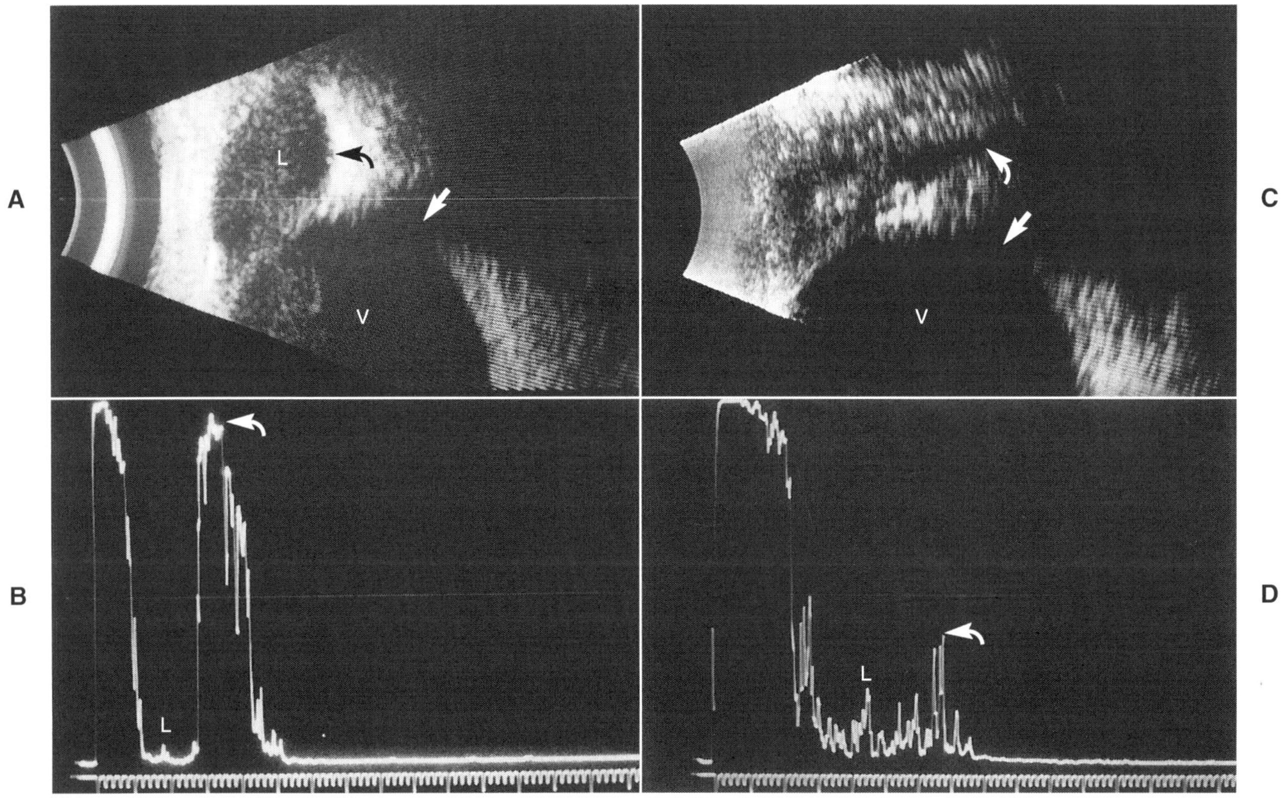

Figure 11-21 Paraocular longitudinal B-scans and paraocular A-scans from very well-outlined inclusion cyst (**A** and **B**) and poorly outlined pseudotumor (**C** and **D**) located in anterior orbit. *L*, Lesion; *curved arrows*, posterior surface of mass; *straight arrows*, area of globe wall not shown well due to oblique sound beam incidence; *V*, vitreous cavity.

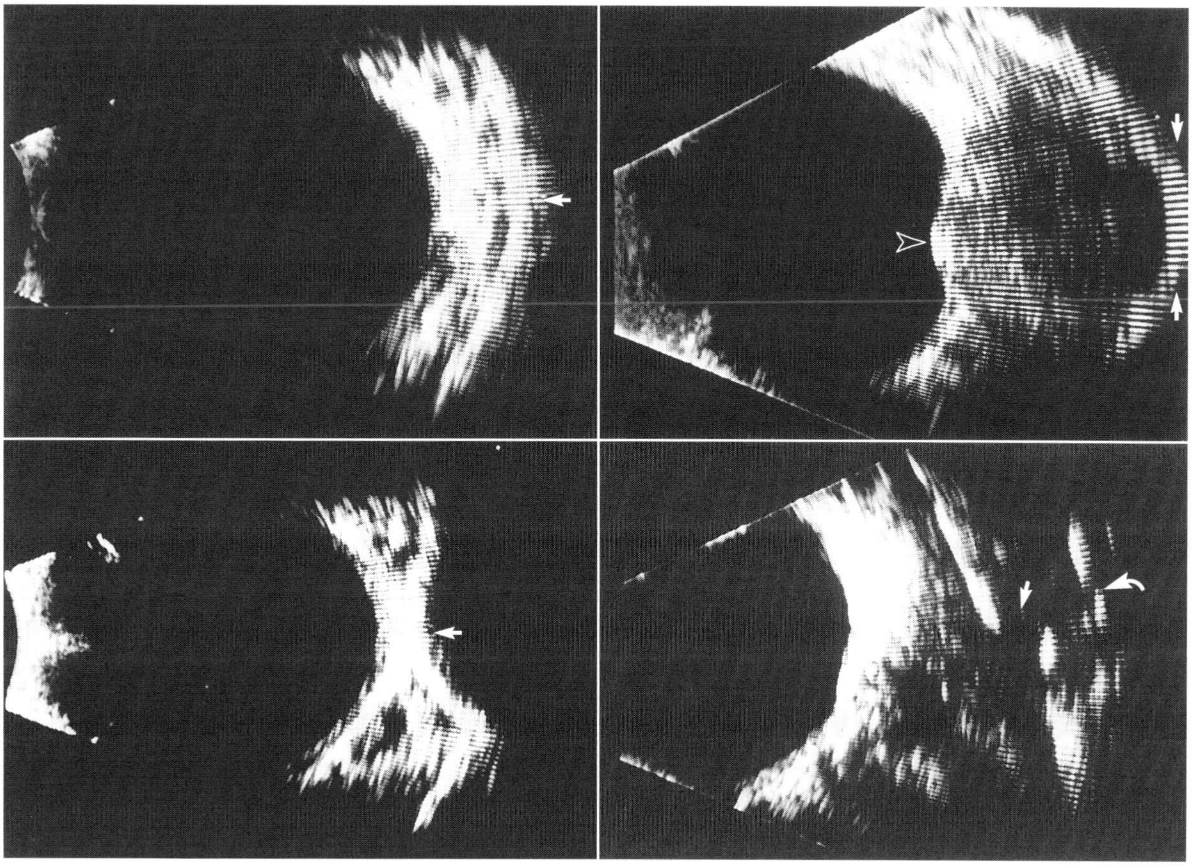

A C B D

Figure 11-22 B-scan montage showing alteration in contour of globe and orbital bone. **A,** Concave shape of normal globe and orbital bone *(arrow)*. **B,** Hyperostotic bone due to fibrous dysplasia is convex *(arrow)*. **C,** Large benign mixed tumor of lacrimal gland is indenting globe *(open arrow)* and excavating bony orbital bone *(closed arrows)*. **D,** Carcinoma has broken through medial wall of orbit causing bone defect *(straight arrow)*. *Curved arrow,* Echoes from tumor in sinus.

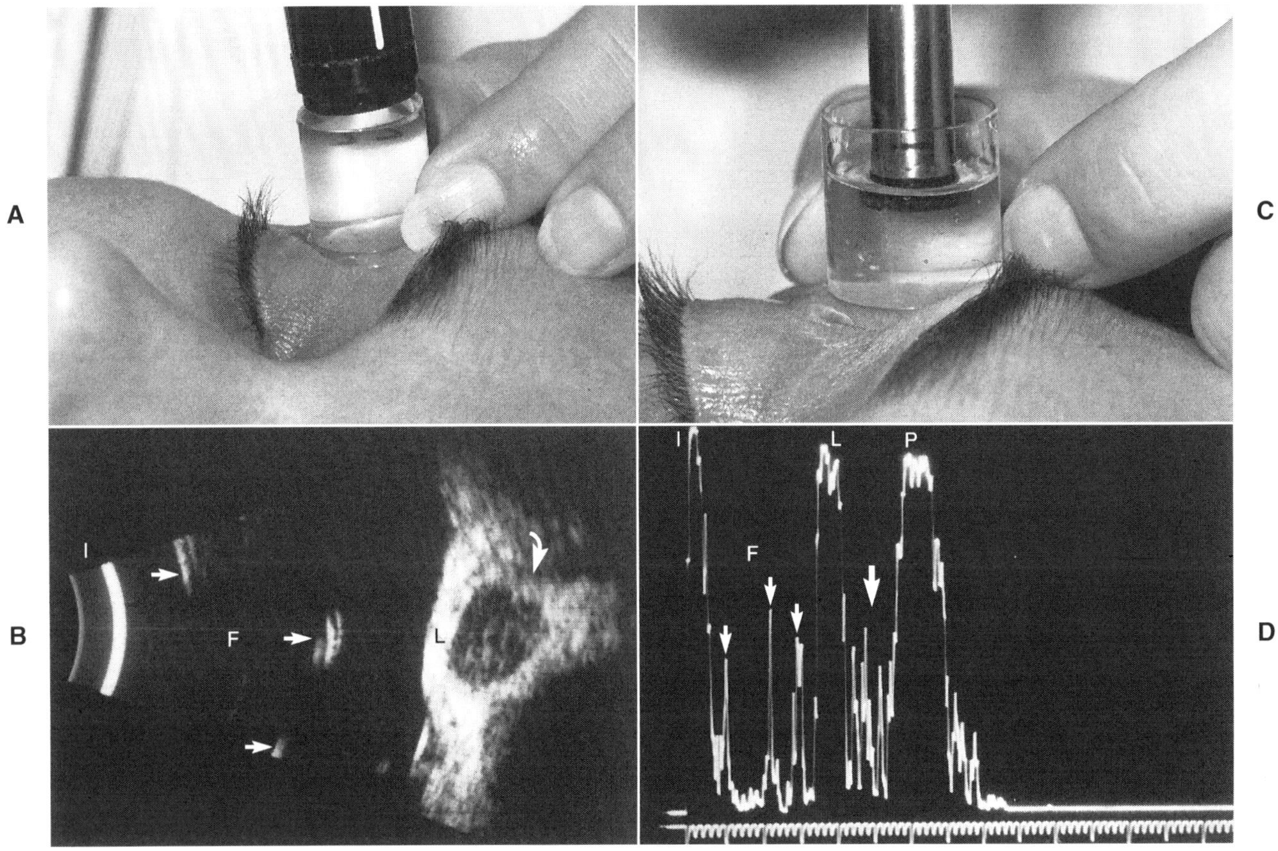

Figure 11-23 Immersion technique through closed lid with B-scan (**A** and **B**) and A-scan (**C** and **D**) for evaluation of an anterior lesion. A small plastic cylinder (i.e., scleral shell) is firmly placed on the lid and is filled with methylcellulose. **B,** B-scan echogram shows well-outlined, anterior lesion *(curved arrow)* adjacent to lid surface *(L)*. *I,* Initial line corresponding to probe face; *F,* fluid (methylcellulose) in scleral shell; *small arrows,* air bubbles. **D,** Corresponding immersion A-scan of lesion. *I,* Initial spike corresponding to probe tip; *F,* fluid within scleral shell; *small arrows,* air bubbles; *L,* lid; *large arrow,* lesion; *P,* posterior surface spike.

Reflectivity

Reflectivity is evaluated by observing the spike height on A-scan and the signal brightness on B-scan. On A-scan, using the Tissue Sensitivity gain setting, reflectivity is judged by estimating the height or amplitude of the internal lesion spikes in relation to the vitreous baseline (0%) and the top of the initial spike (100%). Lesions may be classified into one of several reflectivity groups (Figure 11-24; see also Table 2-3). If a lesion is very large, reflectivity should be assessed more anteriorly, usually within the first 10 to 15 microseconds of the internal lesion spikes. This is necessary to judge accurately a lesion's reflectivity because sound attenuation causes a progressive reduction in the amplitude of more posterior spikes.

Reflectivity may be more precisely determined by measuring spike height on A-scan than by estimating signal brightness on B-scan. The echographer should be cautious in judging reflectivity from B-scan because it does not provide a standardized gain setting as does the standardized A-scan with Tissue Sensitivity. Furthermore, the signal display characteristics, such as gray scale, dynamic range, lines of resolution, etc., may vary from one B-scan instrument to another. In order to assess the significance of a lesion's signal brightness on B-scan, it is necessary to compare it with the normal highly reflective (echo-dense) orbital soft tissue and the very low reflective (echolucent) vitreous cavity. A lesion's internal reflectivity, in comparison to these known tissues, is assessed in terms of different degrees of echo density. The most useful quantitative information obtained with B-scan is in those lesions that are extremely echo-dense (Figure 11-25) and those that are echolucent (see Figure 12-34).

Internal Structure

Internal structure refers to degrees of variation in histologic architecture within a lesion. This is evaluated by noting differences in the height and length of the A-scan spikes and, to a limited extent, differences in echo density on B-scan. Such variations can occur within a single echogram or within different echograms from the same lesion. Regular

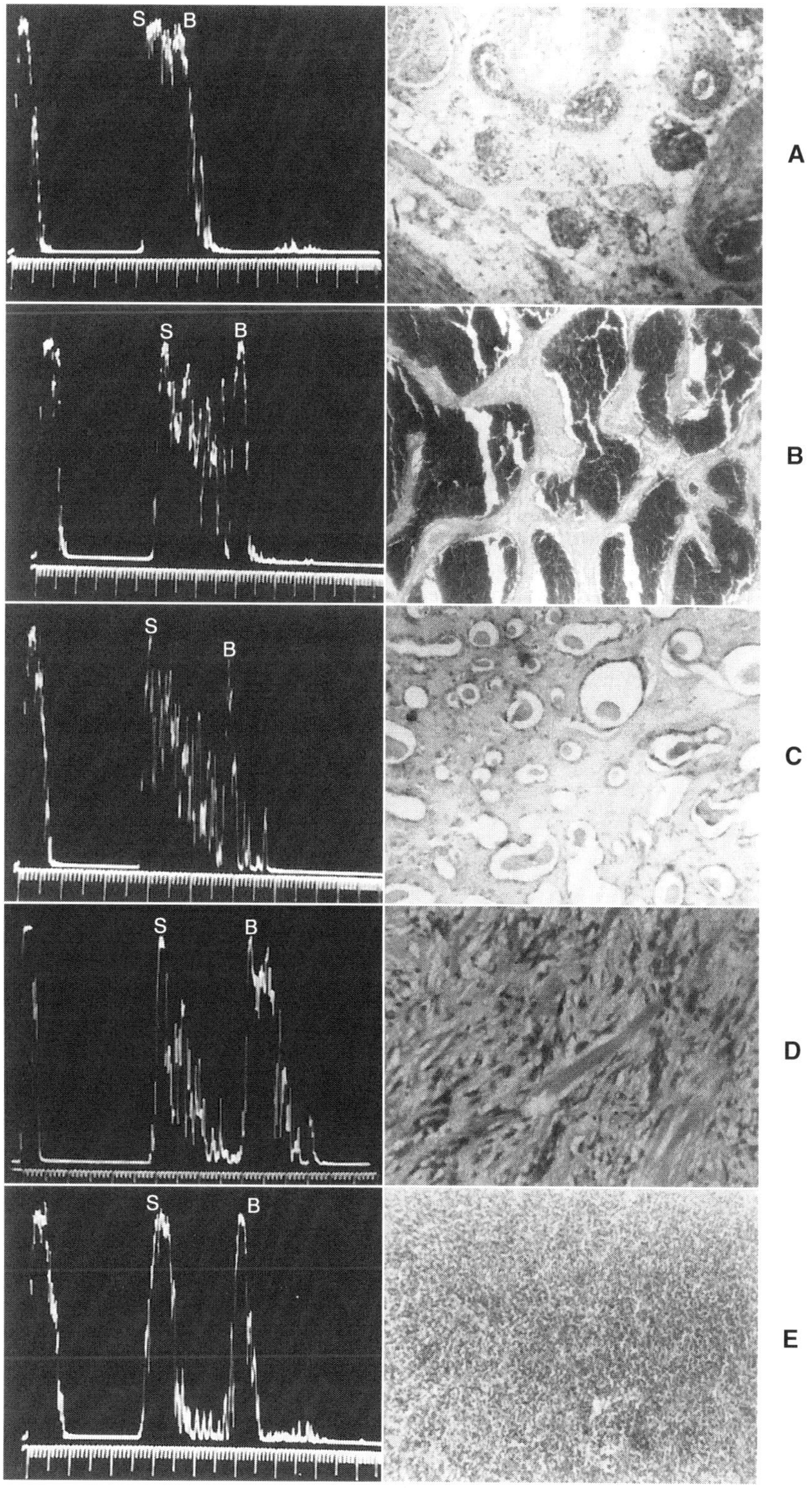

Figure 11-24 Standardized A-scan echograms and histopathology of normal orbit and four different orbital tumors (all at ×100 magnification). Echograms were obtained with a transocular approach and perpendicular sound beam incidence to sclera *(S)* and orbital bone *(B)*. **A,** Normal orbital soft tissue. Heterogeneous tissue (comprised of fat, connective tissue septa, and so forth) produces extremely high reflectivity. **B,** Cavernous hemangioma. Multiple, large, blood-filled spaces produce high reflectivity. **C,** Benign mixed tumor. Multiple, small cystic cavities filled with mucinous material produce medium-high reflectivity. **D,** Hemangiopericytoma. Moderately heterogeneous histologic architecture produces medium reflectivity. **E,** Lymphoma. Homogeneous, densely cellular lesion produces low reflectivity.

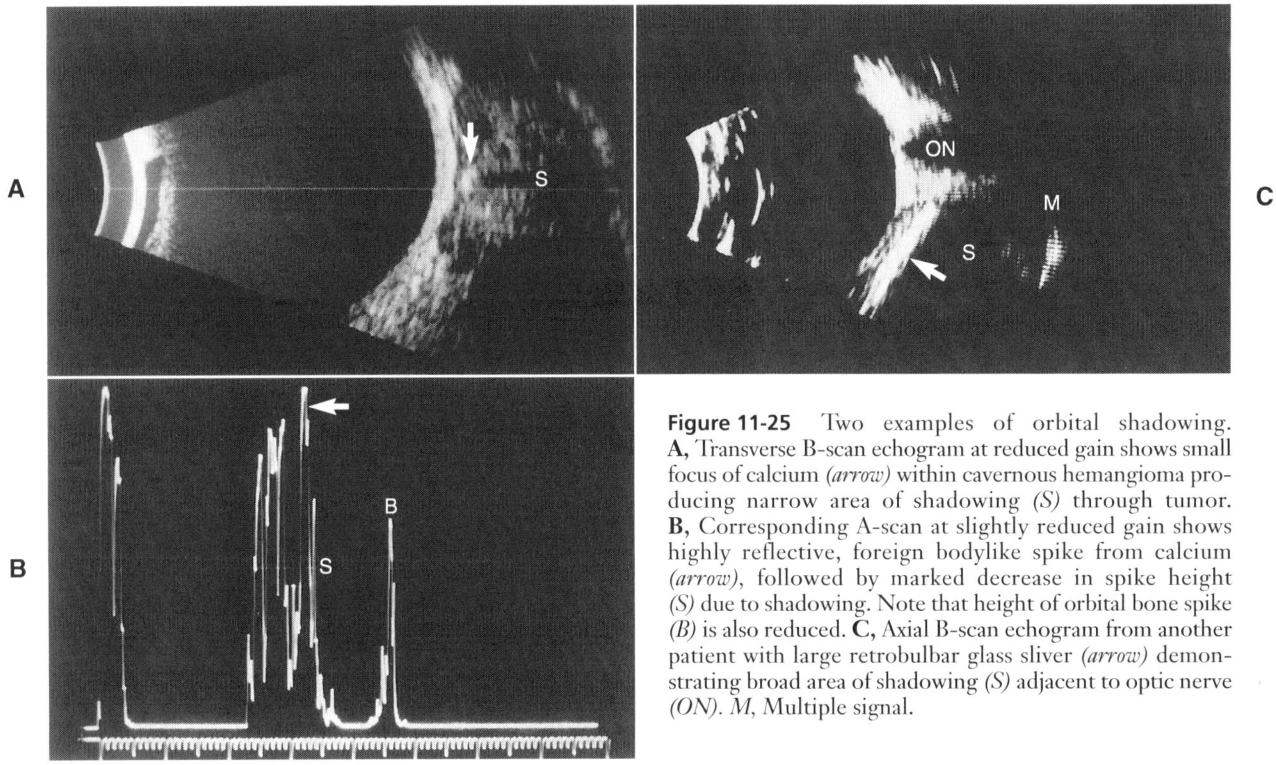

Figure 11-25 Two examples of orbital shadowing. **A,** Transverse B-scan echogram at reduced gain shows small focus of calcium *(arrow)* within cavernous hemangioma producing narrow area of shadowing *(S)* through tumor. **B,** Corresponding A-scan at slightly reduced gain shows highly reflective, foreign bodylike spike from calcium *(arrow)*, followed by marked decrease in spike height *(S)* due to shadowing. Note that height of orbital bone spike *(B)* is also reduced. **C,** Axial B-scan echogram from another patient with large retrobulbar glass sliver *(arrow)* demonstrating broad area of shadowing *(S)* adjacent to optic nerve *(ON)*. *M,* Multiple signal.

internal structure, indicating homogeneous architecture, is represented by little or no variation in the height and length of spikes on A-scan and a uniform appearance of echoes on B-scan. Conversely, irregular internal structure, indicating heterogeneous architecture, is represented by marked differences in echo appearance (Figure 11-26). In some cases, slight variations can be present and the lesion will be classified as moderately irregular.

Sound Attenuation

Sound attenuation occurs when the sound energy is scattered, reflected, and/or absorbed by a given medium. It may be more pronounced when examining through swollen lids, dense opacities and membranes, or extremely high reflective media such as bone, calcium, or foreign material (e.g., scleral buckle, see p 109).

Sound attenuation is indicated by a decrease in spike height on A-scan and echo density on B-scan. This may occur either within or posterior to a lesion (from left to right in the echogram). On the A-scan, an angle is formed by an imaginary line drawn through the peaks of the internal lesion spikes and the horizontal baseline of the echogram. This is referred to as "angle kappa" by Ossoinig.[5-7] The steeper the angle, the greater the sound attenuation. On B-scan, sound attenuation is indicated by decreasing brightness of the echoes, either within or posterior to a lesion (Figure 11-27).

When evaluating a lesion's angle kappa on A-scan, its reflectivity at Tissue Sensitivity must be considered. Since the ideal spike height for assessing a lesion's angle kappa is a medium level, the gain may need to be changed accordingly. Consequently, if a lesion has high internal reflectivity, the gain may need to be decreased, whereas if a lesion is low reflective, it may need to be increased (Figure 11-28).

Various substances, such as bone, calcium, and most foreign bodies, typically produce very strong sound attenuation (i.e., shadowing). On B-scan, this can result in a marked decrease in signal strength or an actual void posterior to the lesion. On A-scan, shadowing is indicated by a steep angle of sound attenuation (see Figure 11-25). However, when a dense echo source is extremely small, sound attenuation may be subtle or altogether absent.

Kinetic Echography: Consistency, Vascularity, and Mobility

Kinetic echography is used for the dynamic assessment of the motion of or within a lesion. Kinetic characteristics may be evaluated with A-scan, B-scan, and Doppler techniques, depending on the given situation.

Consistency

The firmness (i.e., consistency) of a lesion is assessed by compressibility testing, performed with either A- or B-scan.

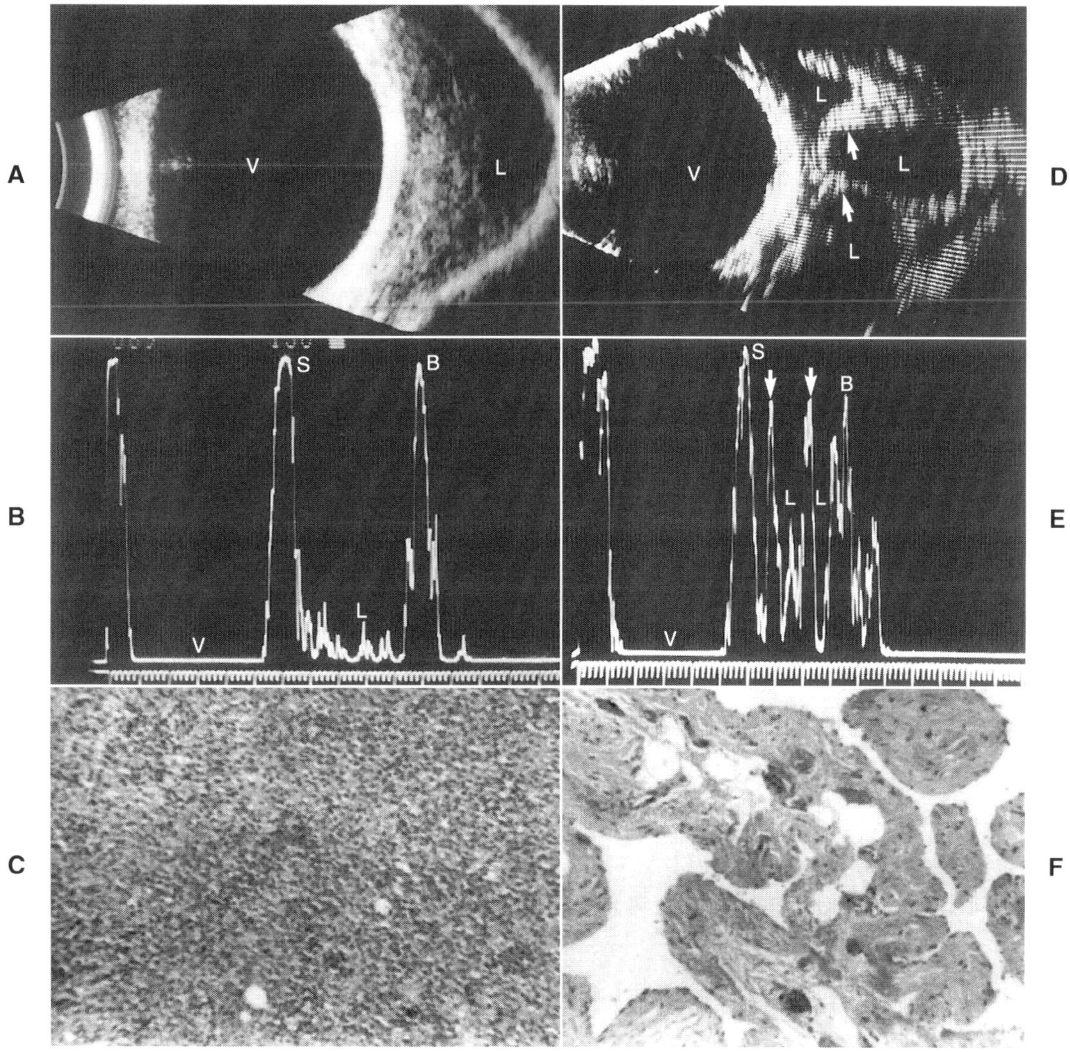

Figure 11-26 Transocular echograms and histopathology from two tumors with regular vs. irregular internal structure. Lymphoma (regular internal structure) demonstrates uniform appearance of internal echoes on both B-scan **(A)** and A-scan **(B)**. *V*, Vitreous cavity; *S*, sclera; *L*, lesion; *B*, bone. Corresponding histopathology of lymphoma **(C)** shows dense cellular composition of tumor (× 100 magnification). Lymphangioma (irregular internal structure) shows marked variation in appearance of internal echoes on both B-scan **(D)** and A-scan **(E)**. *Arrows*, Surfaces of lymphatic spaces. Corresponding histopathology of lymphangioma **(F)** shows irregular nature of tumor architecture (×100 magnification).

A C

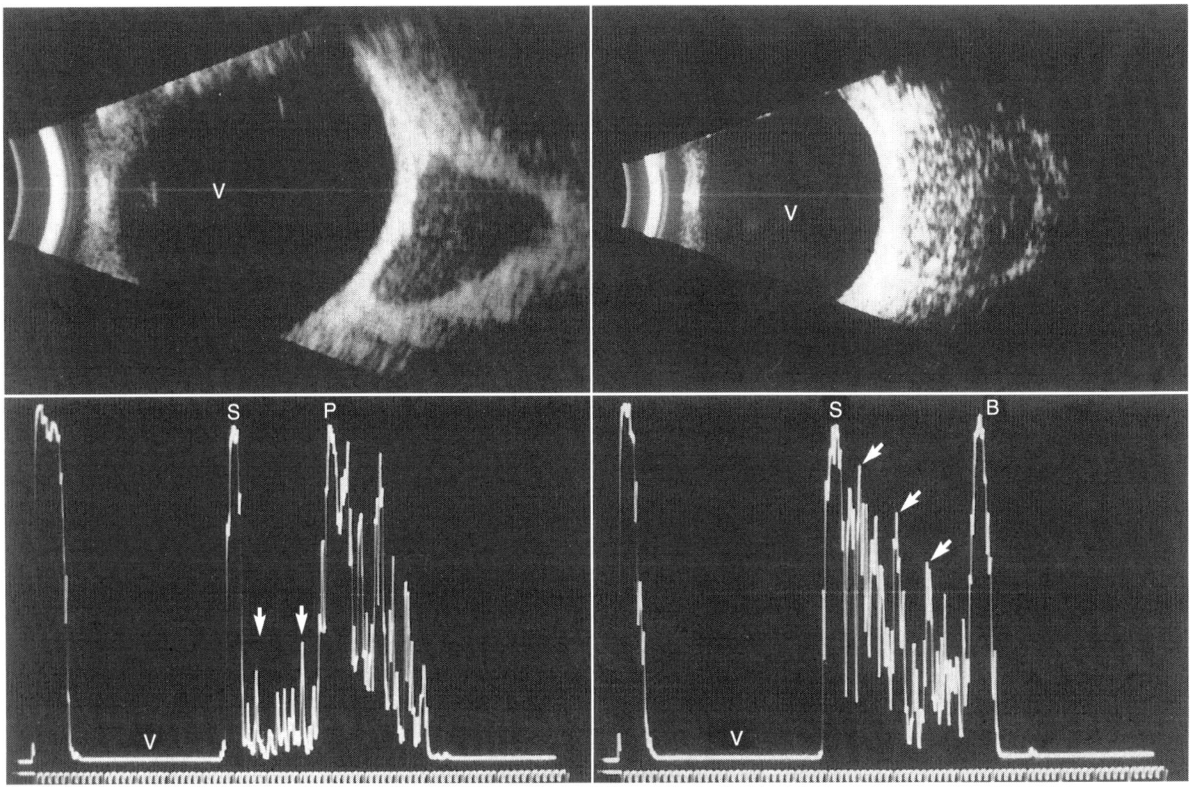

B D

Figure 11-27 Transocular echograms from lymphoma (**A** and **B**) and cavernous hemangioma (**C** and **D**) demonstrate different degrees of sound attenuation. Lymphoma (weak sound attenuation) shows minimal decrease in echo brightness on B-scan **(A)** and consistent spike height on A-scan **(B)**. *V,* Vitreous cavity; *S,* sclera; *arrows,* internal tumor echoes; *P,* posterior tumor surface. Cavernous hemangioma (moderate sound attenuation) shows decreasing brightness of echoes on B-scan **(C)** and decreasing height of internal tumor spikes *(arrows)* on A-scan **(D)**. *B,* Bone.

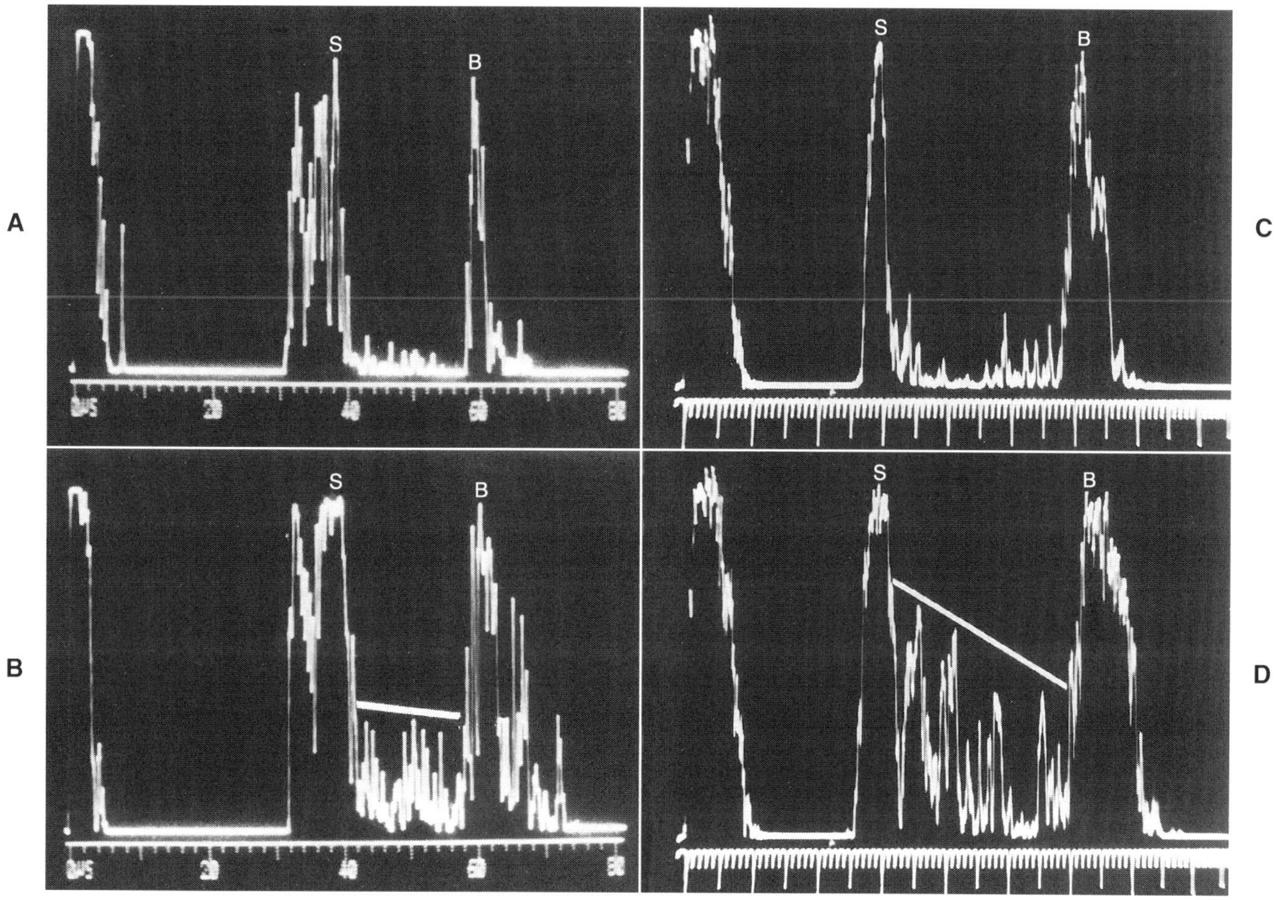

Figure 11-28 Transocular A-scan echograms of two low reflective tumors demonstrate angle kappa by using gain setting that is a few decibels higher than Tissue Sensitivity. Lymphoma at Tissue Sensitivity **(A)** and higher gain **(B)** shows no significant angle kappa with increased gain (note *horizontal line*). Sarcoma at Tissue Sensitivity **(C)** and higher gain **(D)** shows medium angle kappa with increased gain (note *declining line*). *S*, Sclera; *B*, orbital bones.

When possible, the transocular approach should be used for this procedure. First, with the examiner using minimal pressure on the globe, the sound beam is directed perpendicular to the borders of the lesion through its thickest portion. Mild pressure is then exerted against the eye with the probe in an attempt to compress the lesion. As pressure is applied, the screen is monitored to determine whether the lesion decreases in size or shows a change in shape or internal architecture (Figure 11-29). During this maneuver, sound beam orientation may need to be adjusted somewhat to ensure that the probe has not shifted away from the thickest portion of the lesion (which could give a false impression of compressibility). For an anterior lesion, it may be helpful to place a finger firmly on the lid over the lesion to prevent forward displacement during compression testing.

If a lesion is confined to the lid or very anterior orbit, the paraocular approach may be necessary to evaluate consistency (Figure 11-30). When this approach is used, a lesion may be displaced posteriorly and not compressed, thus giving a false impression of firm consistency. In these cases, B-scan examination can be more helpful because it may show changes in the lesion's shape and/or internal character rather than changes in size.

Vascularity

A-scan and B-scan techniques may be useful to determine the presence of blood flow within a lesion. The patient fixates on a target and the lesion is displayed in its maximal thickness. As the probe and eye are held stationary, the internal lesion echoes are observed for the presence of a fast,

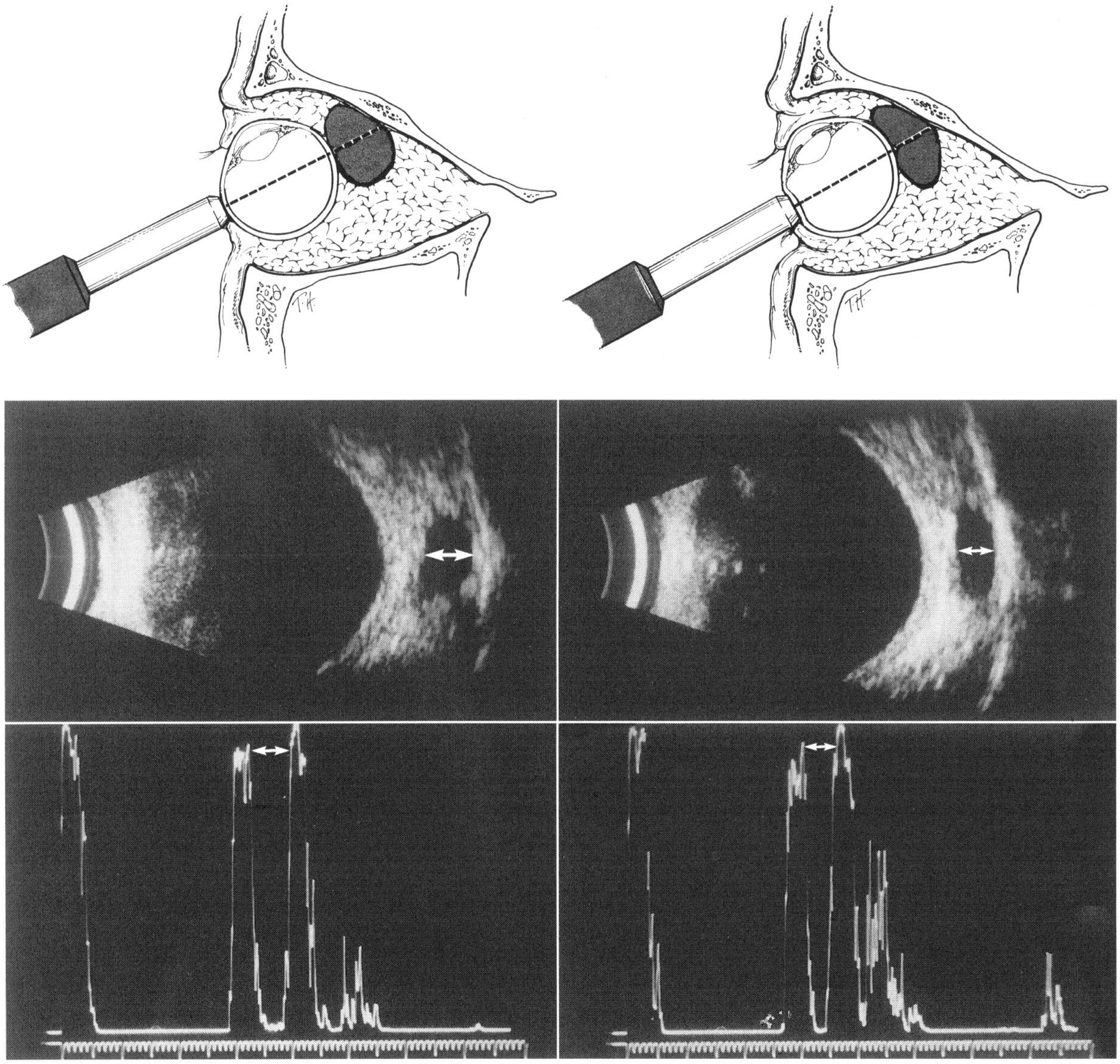

Figure 11-29 Transocular compression test of soft orbital inclusion cyst. Schematic drawings and echograms show cyst prior to *(left)* and during *(right)* compression. Note decrease in size and change in shape of lesion *(arrows)* indicating soft consistency.

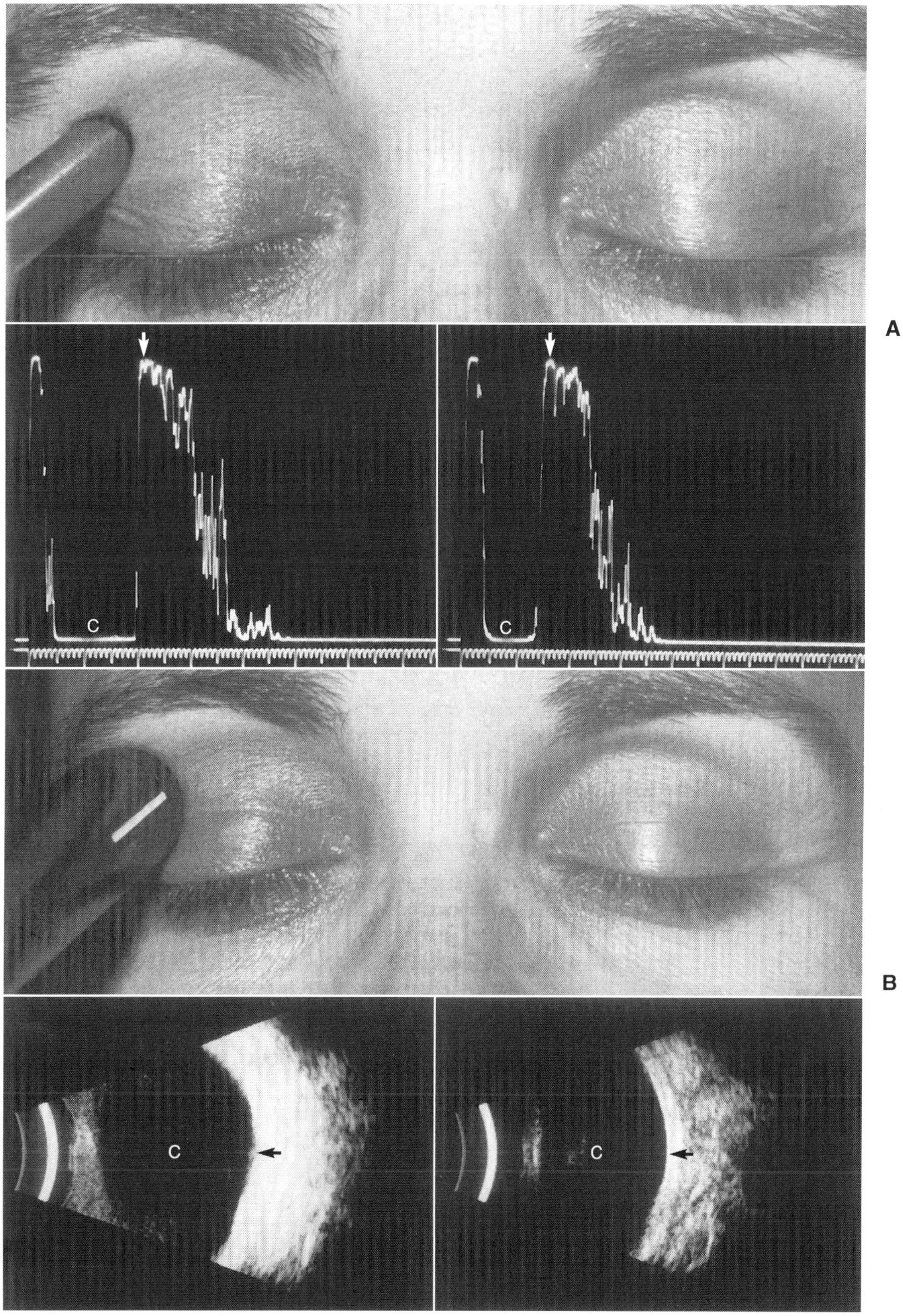

Figure 11-30 Paraocular compression test of large anterior serous orbital cyst with A-scan **(A)** and B-scan **(B)**. Echograms (beneath photographs) were taken prior to *(left)* and during *(right)* compression. Note decrease in size of lesion on A-scan and change in contour on B-scan during compression, indicating soft consistency. *C*, Cyst; *arrows*, posterior surface of lesion.

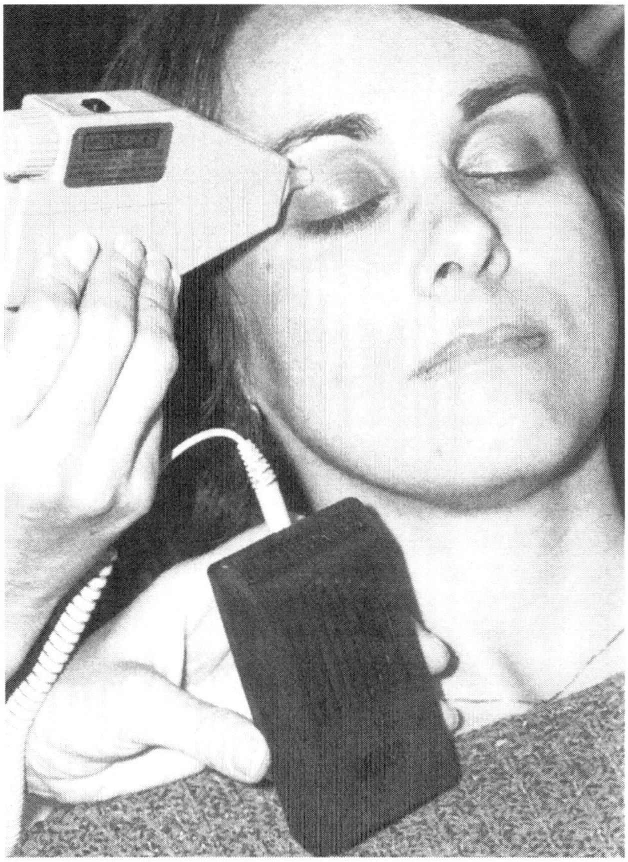

Figure 11-31 Patient being examined with small, nondirectional Doppler instrument.

spontaneous flickering motion. This flickering motion is the result of rapid blood flow through vessels. Such vascularity is commonly present in many orbital lesions and may be a key factor in their correct differentiation (see p 37 and Figures 13-14 and 13-20).

DOPPLER ULTRASOUND EVALUATION

Audio Doppler instrumentation generates a continuous beam of ultrasound, is also used to assess blood flow.[6] Doppler ultrasound detects a shift in the frequency of blood, which is flowing either toward or away from the sound beam. The audio Doppler instrument is best suited for evaluating blood flow within those tumors that are located anteriorly next to the globe by using a paraocular approach. The Doppler response is more difficult to interpret when the transocular approach is used because of competing blood flow from vessels within the retina, choroid, and optic nerve.

A Doppler response can be either directional or diffuse. A directional response, as produced by a normal orbital vessel, disappears as soon as the sound beam is shifted away from the vessel. Conversely, a diffuse response, as produced by a vascularized lesion, persists as the probe is moved over the lesion. In some cases, nonvascular lesions may push normal orbital vessels forward, resulting in a directional response that may be somewhat louder than that detected from the same area of the contralateral normal orbit.

The lesion is first localized with a paraocular A-scan approach to determine its proximity to the globe and bone as well as the meridians that it involves. The Doppler probe is then placed on the closed lid overlying the lesion (Figure 11-31). The examiner listens for a response that indicates blood flow. The probe is then shifted back and forth so as to direct the sound beam throughout the lesion. This maneuver is necessary to determine if the response is diffuse or directional. A pulsatile sound indicates arterial flow, whereas a continuous sound indicates venous flow. If both types of flow are present, a mixed response is obtained. Careful comparison should be made with the same area of the contralateral orbit, using a similar volume level on the Doppler instrument.

Color flow Doppler has also been shown to be useful in evaluating and documenting blood flow within orbital lesions. The instrumentation and examination techniques are explained in detail in Chapter 14.

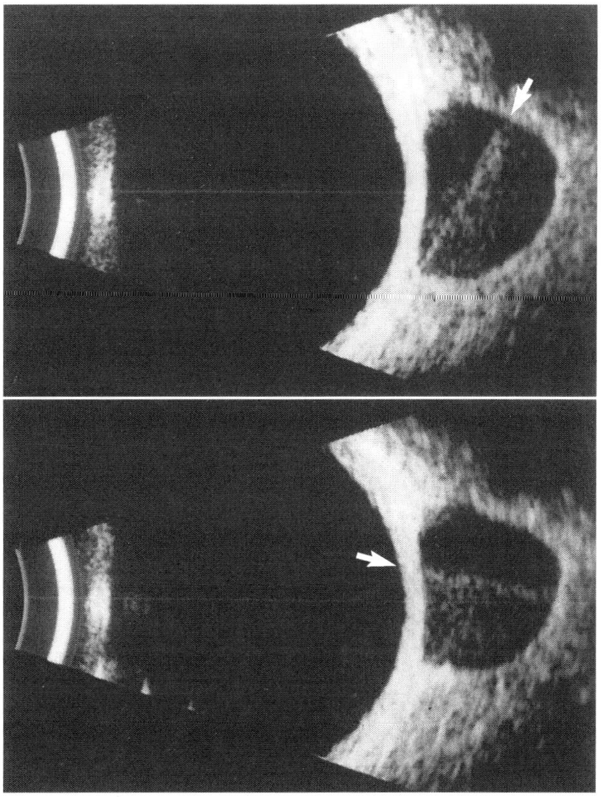

Figure 11-32 Transocular B-scan echograms of well-outlined orbital hematoma demonstrating shifting fluid. **A,** Layered blood *(arrow)* is oriented obliquely with patient in reclined position. **B,** Obvious shift of layered blood *(arrow)* with patient re-examined in sitting position (same probe position as top).

Mobility

The mobility of an orbital lesion or movement of its contents can be evaluated. Lesion mobility is usually best assessed with B-scan by observing the echogram as the patient blinks or performs a saccade. When a lesion is mobile, it moves independently of surrounding normal structures. In contrast, a nonmobile lesion that is attached to the globe, optic nerve, muscle, or bone either does not move or moves in conjunction with normal structures.

Three types of nonvascular movement may occur within a lesion. One is the shifting of fluid levels caused by changes in body position. This may be seen in lesions such as lymphangiomas with hemorrhage, hematomas, and cysts (Figure 11-32). Another type of movement is the continuous, convection-like motion that is sometimes observed in cholesterol within a hematic cyst. This movement is similar to that of cholesterol beneath a longstanding retinal detachment (see p 37 and Figure 3-25). A third type of movement is the aftermovement of nonsolid structures (e.g., septa within a lymphangioma or cystic contents). This is similar to the aftermovement observed with membranes in the globe (see p 36 and Figure 2-27).

REFERENCES

1. Byrne SF: Standardized echography in the differentiation of orbital lesions. *Surv Ophthalmol* 1984;29:226.
2. Byrne SF: Standardized echography of the eye and orbit. *Neuroradiology* 1986;28:618.
3. Byrne SF, Glaser JS: Orbital tissue differentiation with standardized echography. *Ophthalmology* 1983;90:1071.
4. Ossoinig KC: Echography of the eye, orbit, and periorbital region, in Arger PH (ed): *Orbit Roentgenology.* New York, J Wiley & Sons, 1977, p 224.
5. Ossoinig K: The role of clinical echography in modern diagnosis of periorbital and orbital lesions, in Bleeker G (ed): *Proceedings of the 3rd International Symposium on Orbital Disorders.* Amsterdam, Dr W Junk, 1977, p 496.
6. Ossoinig KC: Standardized echography: Basic principles, clinical applications and results. *Int Ophthalmol Clin* 1979;19:127.
7. Ossoinig KC: *Standardized Ophthalmic Echography of the Eye, Orbit and Periorbital Region. A Comprehensive Slide Set and Study Guide,* ed 3, Iowa City, Goodfellow, 1985.

Paul T. Finger

12 Orbital Tumors

Many of the different types of tumors (e.g., vascular, neurogenic, lymphoproliferative, metastatic, etc.) that affect soft tissues in the body also can occur in the orbit. As a result, the clinical diagnosis of an orbital mass may be difficult and the differential diagnosis may be quite extensive. In many cases, however, echography can provide important information augmenting that obtained with other imaging modalities.*

Many of the nonvascular orbital tumors that one can expect to encounter are described in this chapter (Table 12-1), including those that involve the lacrimal system. The vascular tumors and malformations that commonly occur in the orbit are numerous and are described separately in Chapter 13.

The more common orbital lesions can usually be diagnosed reliably with echography. Those that occur less frequently, however, may present a problem in differentiation. Consequently, echography may be able to provide a specific diagnosis in many cases but only a list of likely possibilities in others. Furthermore, some lesions can only be generally categorized as vascular or nonvascular, solid or cystic, and so forth.

PSEUDOTUMOR AND LYMPHOMA (LYMPHOPROLIFERATIVE DISEASES)

Inflammatory mass lesions (i.e., pseudotumors) and lymphoid lesions have a similar appearance echographically and are therefore classified as one entity.[34] Lesions of the pseudotumor/lymphoma group include idiopathic orbital inflammatory masses, granulomatous disorders (e.g., sarcoidosis, Wegener's granulomatosis), reactive and lymphoid hyperplasias, and lymphomas.[45]

The term "pseudotumor" is frequently used to describe a wide spectrum of inflammatory disorders.[28] In this chapter, however, the term is reserved for an inflammatory mass. Other manifestations of inflammatory orbital disease, occurring alone or in conjunction with a pseudotumor, are termed according to the particular structure involved.[28] These include scleritis (see p 195), tenonitis/episcleritis (periscleritis), myositis (see p 396), and perineuritis (see optic neuritis, p 423).[21,24,25,33]

Pseudotumor/lymphomas may be focal or multifocal and can be located anywhere in the orbit. These lesions can be well circumscribed with relatively smooth contour or, more commonly, are diffuse and irregularly shaped (Figures 12-1 and 12-2). In many cases they are attached to orbital structures such as the extraocular muscles, optic nerve, periosteum, or globe (Figure 12-3; see also Figures 12-1 and 12-2).

Lesions of the pseudotumor/lymphoma group are composed of small, densely packed cells, resulting in a homogeneous histologic architecture[34,55] (see Figure 11-24). Consequently, they are usually low to medium reflective with regular internal structure. Typically, they do not produce significant sound attenuation. In some cases, connective tissue septa are present, giving them a slightly irregular appearance (Figure 12-4). Pseudotumor/lymphomas may be nonvascular or can show mild to moderate internal blood flow.

Although the echographic differentiation of pseudotumor from lymphoma cannot be made in most cases, occasionally there are findings that may suggest one diagnosis more than the other. For example, thickening of an adjacent extraocular muscle, edema in sub-Tenon's space, and/or scleritis are more commonly seen with pseudotumor than with lymphoma. On the other hand, lymphomas often seem to be bilateral and mildly compressible, whereas pseudotumors are more frequently unilateral and more firm.

Other highly cellular, homogeneous lesions (e.g., sarcomas) can have a low internal reflectivity similar to that of pseudotumor/lymphoma. However, differentiation sometimes can be made based on history and the clinical examination in combination with other echographic features.

PRIMARY ORBITAL TUMORS

Rhabdomyosarcoma

Rhabdomyosarcoma is the most common primary orbital malignancy of childhood and frequently presents with a rapidly developing exophthalmos.[48] In general, rhabdomyosarcomas are highly cellular, vascularized lesions that echographically may appear very similar to pseudotumor/

*References 4, 6, 13, 14, 19, 26, 35-40.

TABLE 12-1

Differential Diagnosis of Orbital Tumors*

Tumor Type	Shape	Borders	Internal Reflectivity	Internal Structure	Sound Attenuation	Vascularity	Consistency	Bone
Pseudotumor/ lymphoma	Variable	Variable	Low-med	Regular	Weak	+/−	Firm	WNL
Rhabdomyosarcoma	Variable	Variable	Low-med	Irregular	Mod	+	Firm	WNL/defects
Schwannoma (neurilemmoma)	Oval	Well outlined	Low-med	Regular, cystic cavities	Mod	+	Firm	WNL/ excavated
Neurofibroma								
Solitary	Round/oval	Well outlined	Low	Regular	Weak/mod	+/−	Hard	WNL
Plexiform	Irregular	Poorly outlined	High	Irregular	Weak	+	Soft	WNL
Fibrous histiocytoma	Oval	Well outlined	Low-med	Regular	Mod	+/−	Firm	WNL
Metastatic carcinoma								
Infiltrative	Irregular	Poorly outlined	Med-high	Irregular	Weak	−	Hard	WNL/defects
Confined	Variable	Well outlined	Low-med	Regular	Weak/mod	−	Hard	WNL/defects

Med, Medium; *Mod,* moderate; *WNL,* within normal limits.
*This table lists the main echographic findings for the most common orbital tumors.

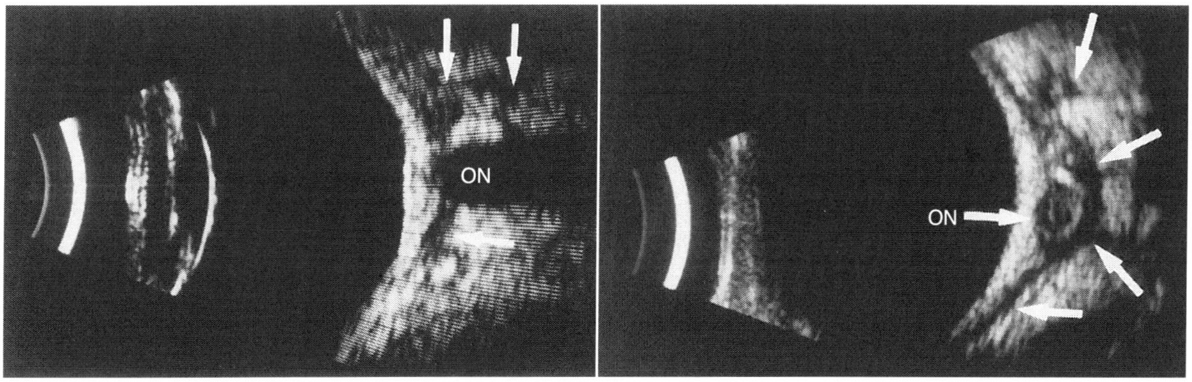

Figure 12-1 Orbital pseudotumor (multifocal). **A,** Vertical axial B-scan echogram displays multiple areas of infiltration in retrobulbar orbit *(arrows). ON,* Optic nerve. **B,** Vertical transverse B-scan through anterior aspect of optic nerve shows lesion infiltrating orbital fat and surrounding nerve.

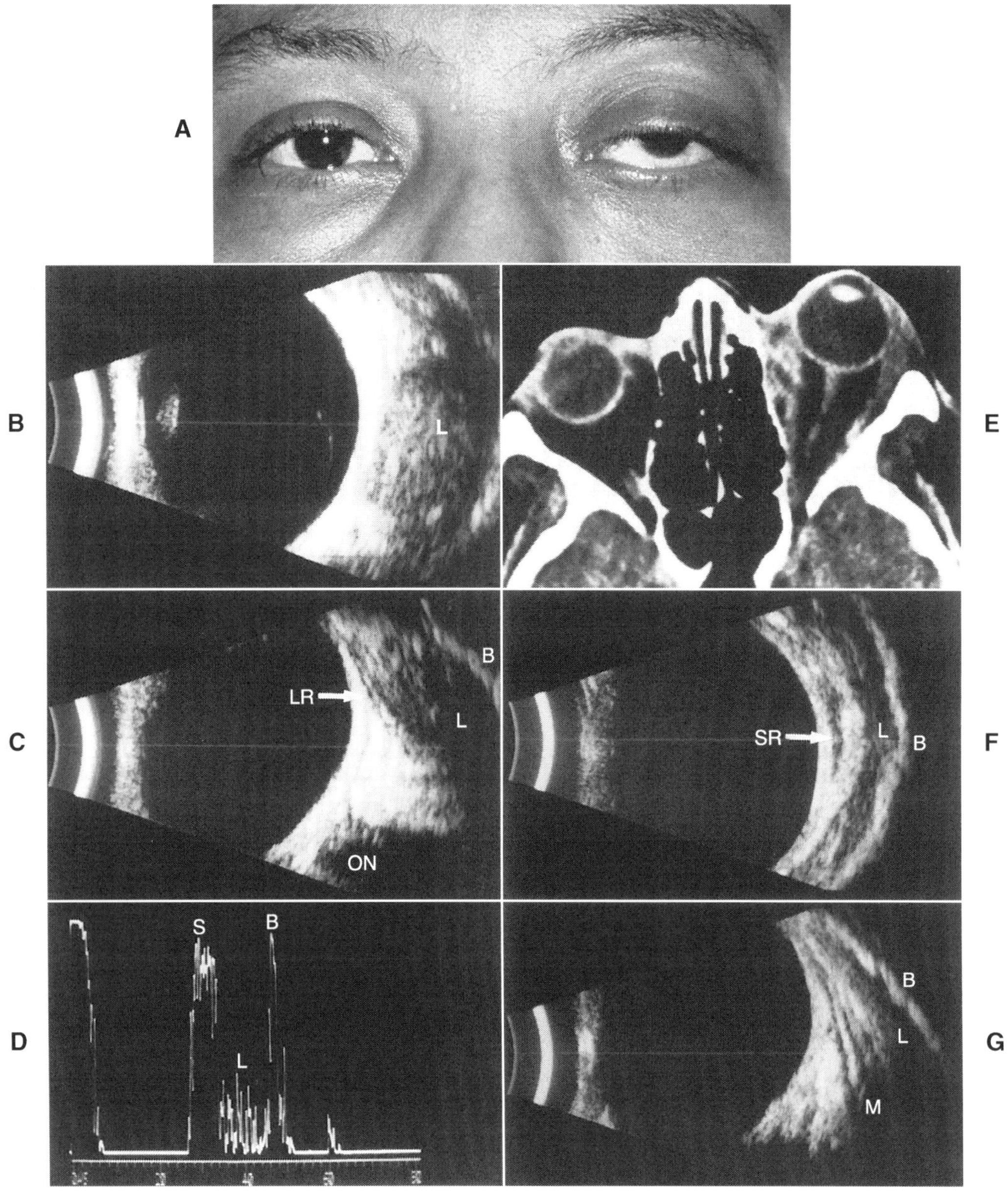

Figure 12-2 Orbital pseudotumor (diffuse). **A,** External photograph showing proptosis of left eye and ptosis of left upper lid. Transocular echograms (**B, C, D, F,** and **G**) show large, diffuse orbital lesion *(L)*. **B,** Transverse B-scan echogram through supratemporal orbit shows large, relatively well-circumscribed mass. **C,** Longitudinal B-scan through temporal orbit shows mass extending posteriorly outside of the muscle cone between lateral rectus muscle *(LR)* and orbital bone *(B)*. *ON,* Optic nerve. **D,** A-scan echogram shows low reflective, regularly structured lesion. *S,* Sclera; *B,* bone. **E,** Axial CT scan demonstrates proptotic left eye and diffuse mass in temporal and medial aspect of left orbit, outside of the muscle cone. **F,** Horizontal transverse B-scan through anterior aspect of orbit superiorly shows diffuse extraconal lesion extending along roof of orbit. *SR,* Superior rectus muscle. **G,** Longitudinal B-scan along 12-o'clock meridian shows lesion extending back into orbit above superior rectus/levator muscle complex *(M)*.

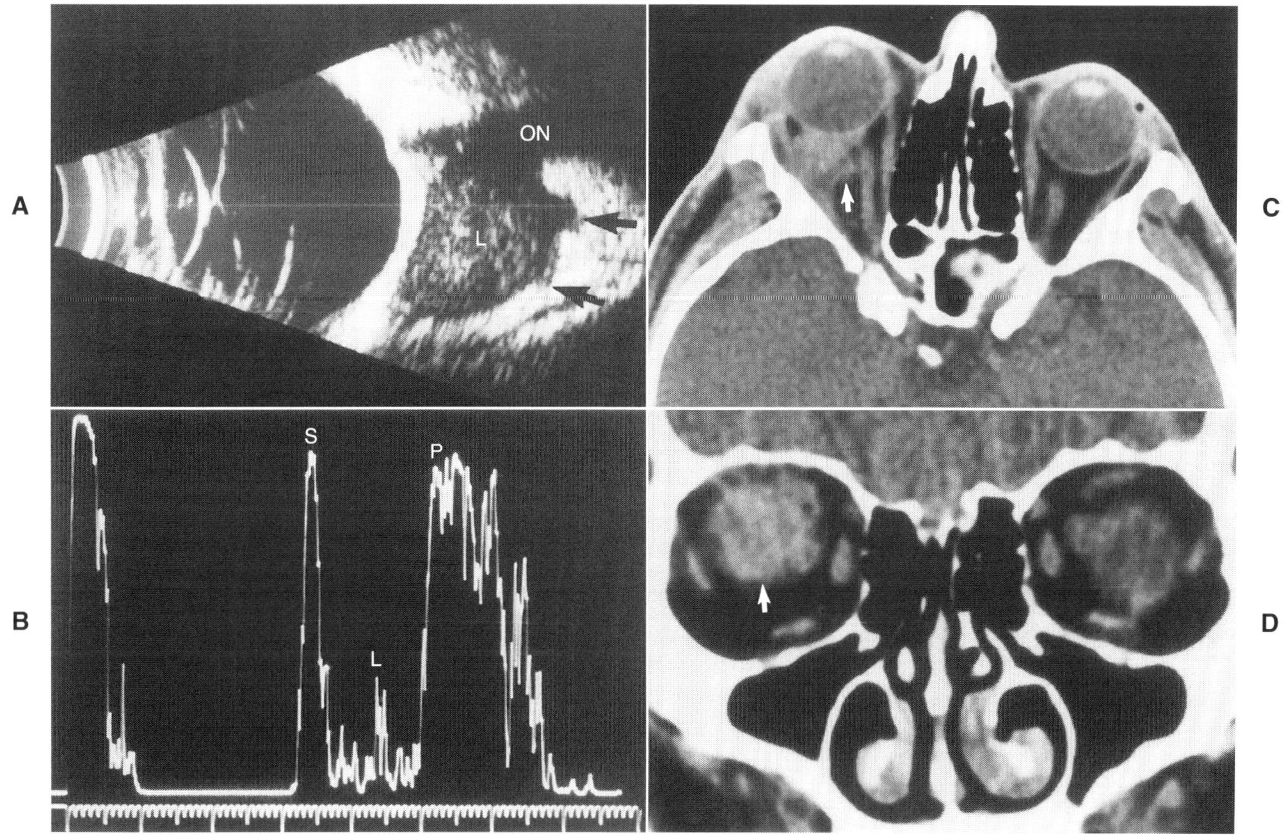

Figure 12-3 Large orbital lymphoma. **A,** Axial B-scan shows lesion *(L)* adjacent to optic nerve *(ON)*. Note irregular posterior contour of mass *(arrows)*. **B**, Transocular A-scan shows low reflective lesion with regular internal structure. *S*, Sclera; *P*, posterior surface spike. Axial **(C)** and coronal **(D)** CT scans show large mass *(arrows)* in supratemporal aspect of orbit.

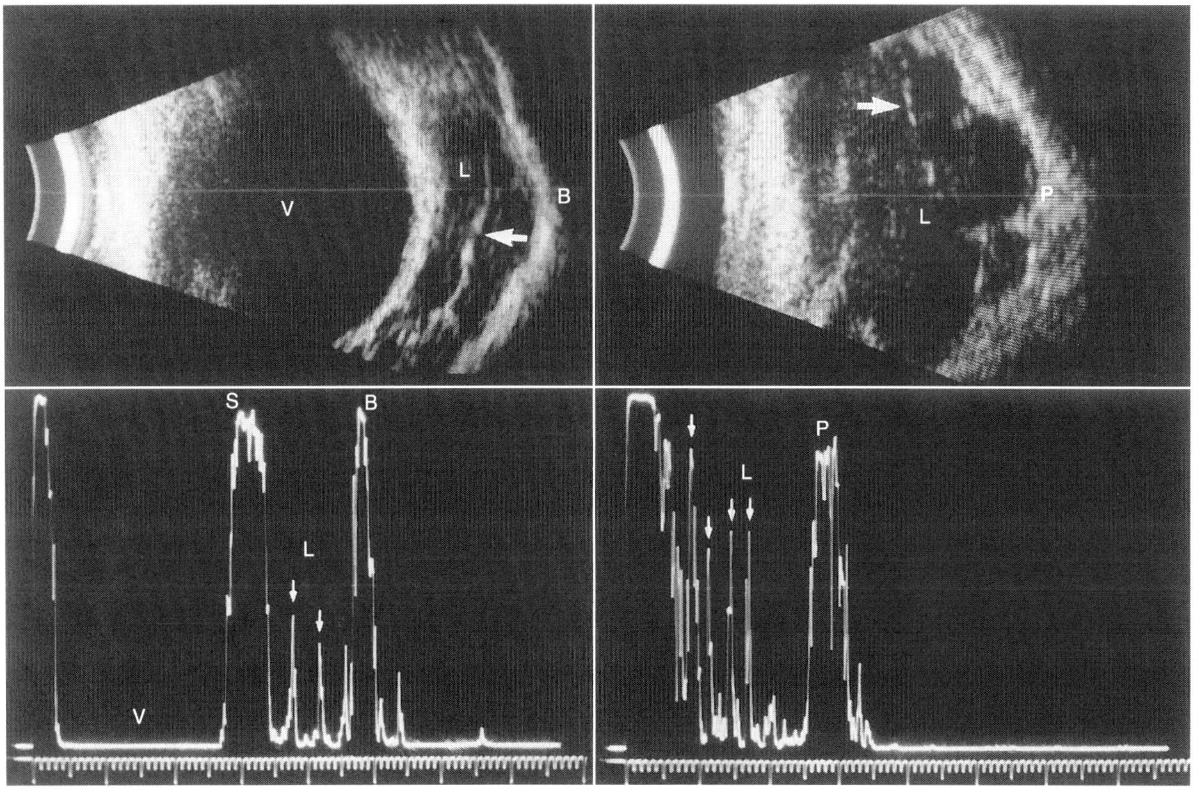

Figure 12-4 Large orbital lymphoma with septa. Transocular (**A** and **B**) and paraocular (**C** and **D**) echograms display large lesion *(L)* with septa. **A,** Transverse B-scan echogram shows diffuse lesion with septum *(arrow)*. *V,* Vitreous cavity; *B,* bone. **B,** A-scan echogram displays very low reflective lesion with distinct spikes from septa *(arrows)*. *S,* Sclera. **C,** Transverse paraocular B-scan shows large mass with septum and irregular posterior border *(P)*. **D,** Paraocular A-scan displays low reflective lesion with multiple spikes from septa. *P,* Posterior surface spike.

lymphomas. However, the echographic features of this tumor usually allow it to be differentiated from the other more common tumors in children, such as capillary hemangioma, lymphangioma with hemorrhage, and dermoid cyst.

Rhabdomyosarcomas can be located anywhere in the orbit. They have previously been reported to most commonly occur superiorly[27] but may be located inferiorly as well. Rhabdomyosarcomas are generally well circumscribed but vary in shape and are often quite large. The bone may be intact or, in more advanced cases, bone defects may be detected. The internal reflectivity is predominantly low to medium, with moderate sound attenuation. Connective tissue septa sometimes can be identified (Figure 12-5). In some cases, the internal structure can be somewhat irregular, with areas of both low and medium reflectivity. Internal blood flow usually can be detected, but the degree may vary significantly from one tumor to another. Similarly, the consistency is generally firm, although these lesions can be moderately compressible. As a rule, the differential diagnosis of any low reflective lesion in a child should include rhabdomyosarcoma.

Schwannoma (Neurilemmoma)

Schwannomas are rare orbital tumors arising from a proliferation of Schwann cells; these tumors can occur as isolated lesions or may be associated with neurofibromatosis.[52] Schwannomas can be located either within the muscle cone or in the extraconal space. These oval, encapsulated lesions appear smooth and well outlined echographically. Schwannomas are generally low to medium reflective and usually have regular internal structure, although cystic cavities are frequently present[9,11] (Figure 12-6). They typically produce moderate sound attenuation and are usually firm with some degree of vascularity.[5] These lesions are not usually associated with bone defects, but bony excavation may occur. A schwannoma can have a similar echographic appearance to a hemangiopericytoma.

Neurofibroma (Solitary Type)

Three cases of the solitary type of neurofibroma[56] have been examined by the authors. All three tumors were located in the supratemporal quadrant of the orbit. The lesions were

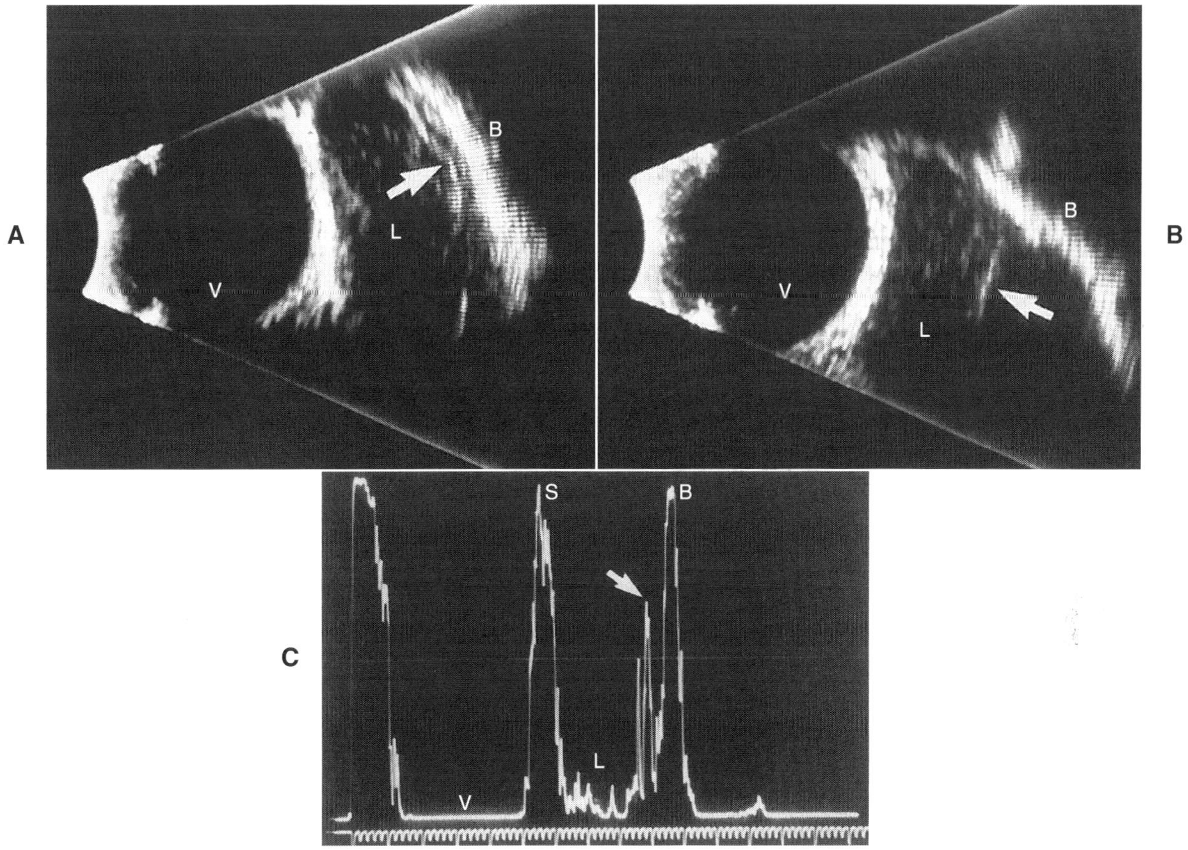

Figure 12-5 Orbital rhabdomyosarcoma. Transocular echograms show large lesion *(L)* with septa *(arrows)* in nasal orbit. **A,** Transverse B-scan displays lesion causing mild flattening of globe. *V,* Vitreous cavity; *B,* bone. **B,** Longitudinal B-scan view demonstrates very large lesion extending from sclera into apex of orbit. **C,** Transocular A-scan echogram shows very low reflectivity with medium-high spike from septum *(arrow)*. *S,* Sclera.

round to oval, hard, and well outlined. Two exhibited low internal reflectivity and mild to moderate sound attenuation, whereas the third tumor was medium to high reflective with strong sound attenuation (Figure 12-7). The internal structure was regular or slightly irregular, and vascularity was mild or absent.

Neurofibroma (Plexiform Type)

Plexiform neurofibromas have a much different appearance than the solitary type, both echographically and histologically.[27] The plexiform neurofibroma is an infiltrative, nonencapsulated lesion and is, therefore, irregularly shaped and poorly outlined on echography. The few plexiform lesions assessed by the authors have shown irregular internal structure with predominantly high internal reflectivity and minimal sound attenuation (Figure 12-8). These lesions are compressible and quite vascularized. In some cases, the extraocular muscles are thickened. The differential diagnosis of this tumor includes capillary (infantile) hemangioma.

Fibrous Histiocytomas

Fibrous histiocytomas are the most common type of mesenchymal tumor occurring in the orbit of adults.[27] This tumor has, in the past, been histologically confused with hemangiopericytoma.[56] Fibrous histiocytomas can occur extraconally or, rarely, may completely fill the orbital cavity. They are generally oval and well outlined and exhibit regular internal structure, low to medium internal reflectivity, and moderate sound attenuation (Figure 12-9). Fibrous histiocytomas are usually noncompressible, vascularized, and not associated with bony abnormalities.

METASTATIC AND SECONDARY TUMORS

Malignant tumors can occur in any area of the orbit, metastasizing from elsewhere in the body, or secondarily invading the orbit from the globe (e.g., retinoblastoma or melanoma [see p 131]). They also can extend into the orbit from adjacent cavities, the skin, or conjunctiva.[46] Metastatic infiltration of the extraocular muscles and

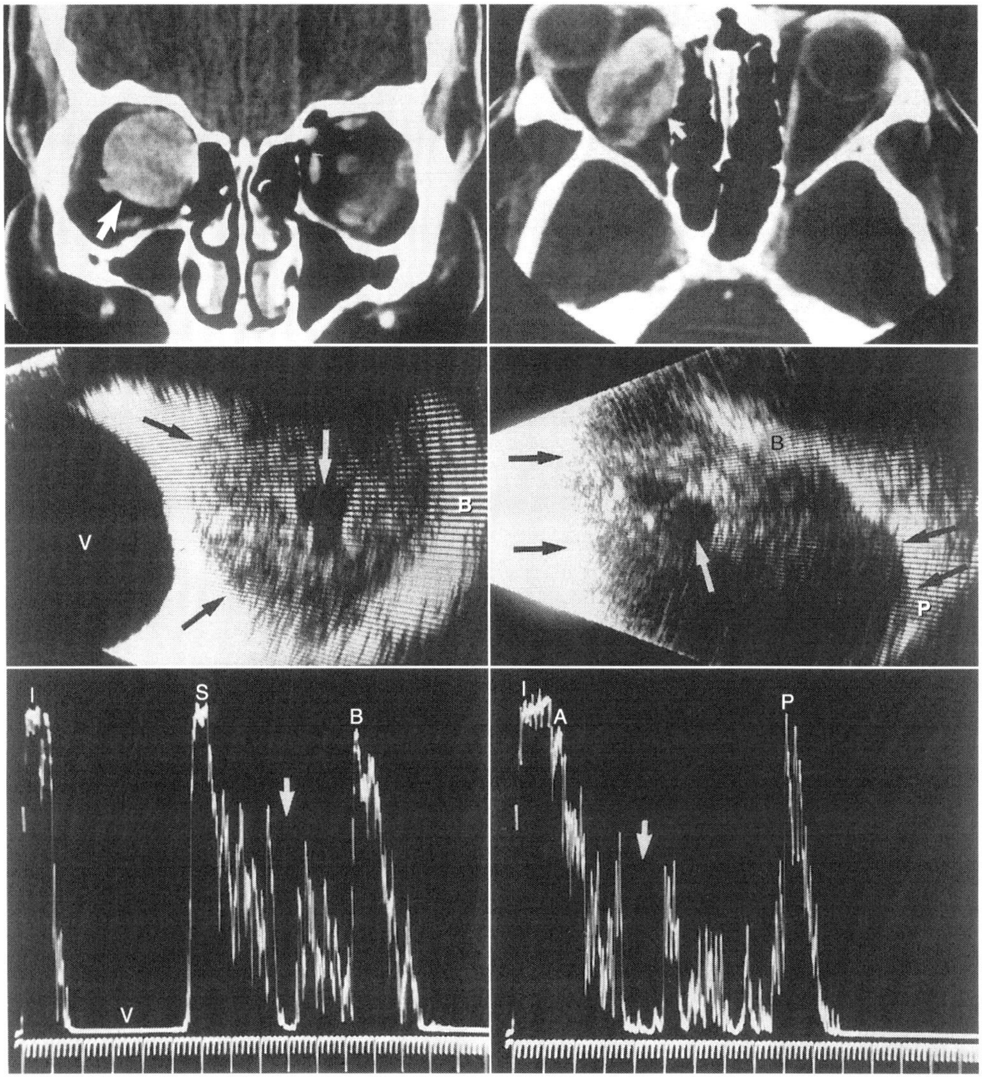

Figure 12-6 Orbital schwannoma. Coronal **(A)** and axial **(D)** CT scans show large mass *(arrows)*, with low-density area centrally. Transocular (**B** and **C**) and paraocular (**E** and **F**) echograms show large tumor with central cystic cavity *(white arrows)*. **B,** Transverse B-scan shows well-circumscribed mass *(black arrows)* and large cystic cavity centrally. *V,* Vitreous cavity; *B,* bone. **C,** A-scan echogram displays medium reflective mass, moderate sound attenuation, and very low reflective cystic cavity. *S,* Sclera. **E,** Transverse paraocular B-scan shows well-circumscribed tumor *(black arrows)* extending posteriorly along orbital bone *(B)*. Note cystic cavities anteriorly. *P,* Posterior border of lesion. **F,** Paraocular A-scan echogram displays medium internal reflectivity, moderate sound attenuation, and large cystic cavity. *A,* Anterior; *P,* posterior surface spikes. (From Byrne SF, Byrne BM: Differential diagnosis of orbital neurilemmoma [schwannoma] with standardized echography, in Ossoinig KC [ed]: *Ophthalmic Echography*. Dordrecht, Dr W Junk, 1987, p 487.)

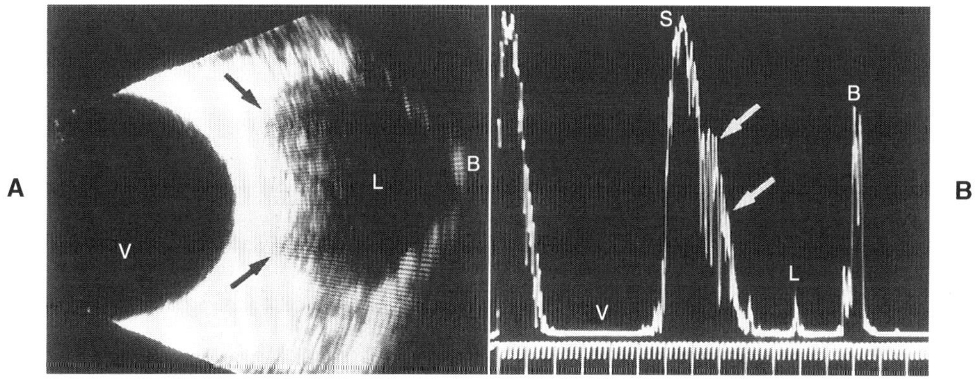

Figure 12-7 Solitary neurofibroma. **A,** Transverse B-scan (at high gain setting) shows oval-shaped lesion *(L)* with smooth borders *(arrows)*. Note marked decrease in brightness of internal echoes and weak appearance of bone *(B)* due to strong sound attenuation. *V,* Vitreous cavity. **B,** Transocular A-scan shows medium reflective lesion producing strong sound attenuation *(arrows)*. Also note decreased height of bone spike due to strong sound attenuation. *S,* Sclera.

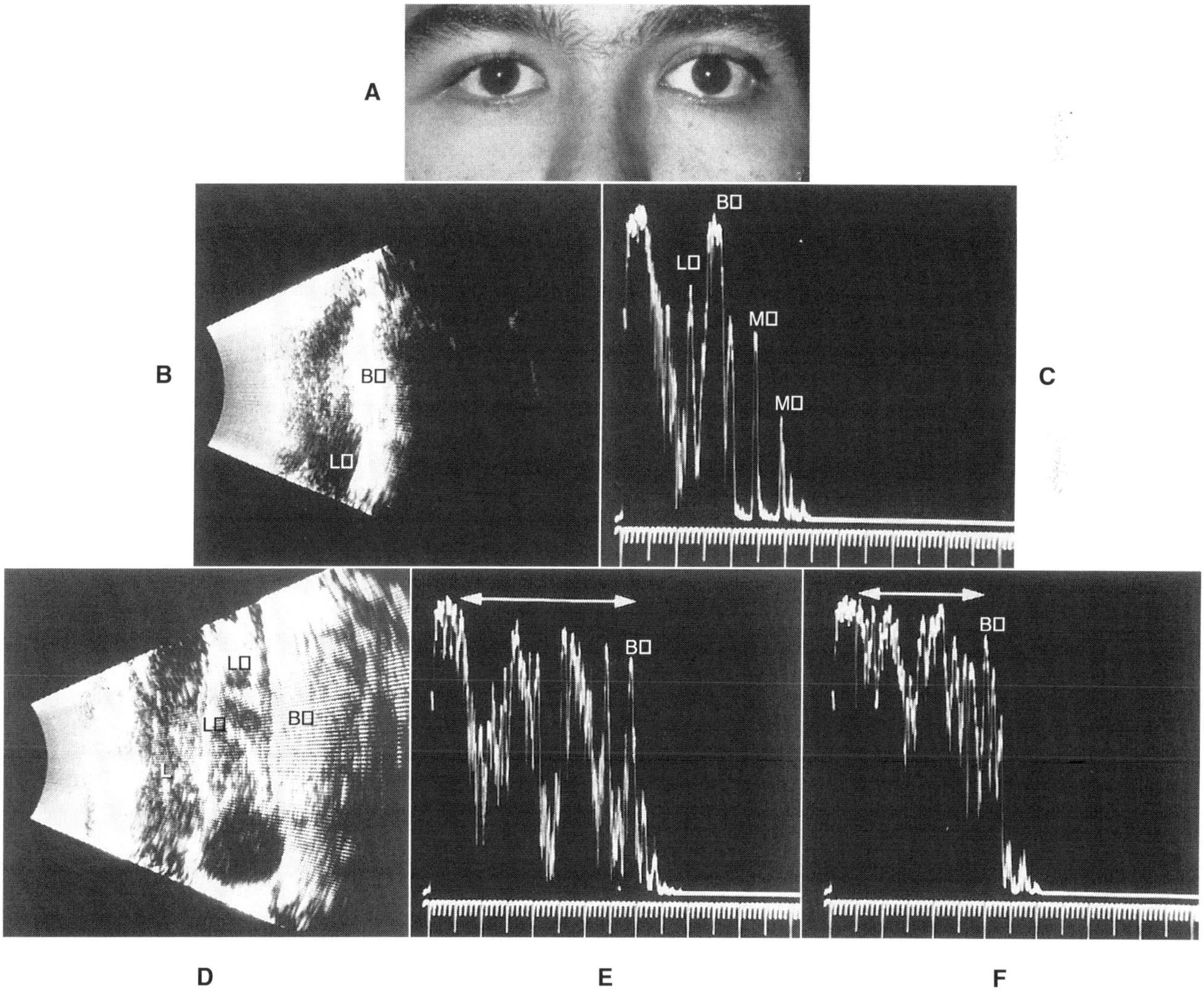

Figure 12-8 Plexiform neurofibroma of right anterior lid and orbit with involvement of temporal fossa. **A,** External photograph showing right upper lid swelling in 28-year-old man. Paraocular echograms display lesion in orbit (**B** and **C**) and temporal fossa (**D** to **F**). **B,** Transverse B-scan echogram shows lesion *(L)* within lid and very anterior aspect of orbit. *B,* Orbital bone. **C,** A-scan shows irregular internal structure of lesion. *B,* Orbital bone; *M,* multiple signals. **D,** B-scan probe is shifted temporal to orbit, overlying temporal fossa. Echogram shows irregular appearance of lesion that fills temporal fossa. *B,* Temporal bone. **E,** A-scan of temporal fossa also demonstrates irregular internal structure of mass. *Double-headed arrow* indicates depth of lesion in fossa between skin and temporal bone. **F,** A-scan during compression testing shows decreased size of mass in temporal fossa *(double-headed arrow)*, indicating very soft consistency.

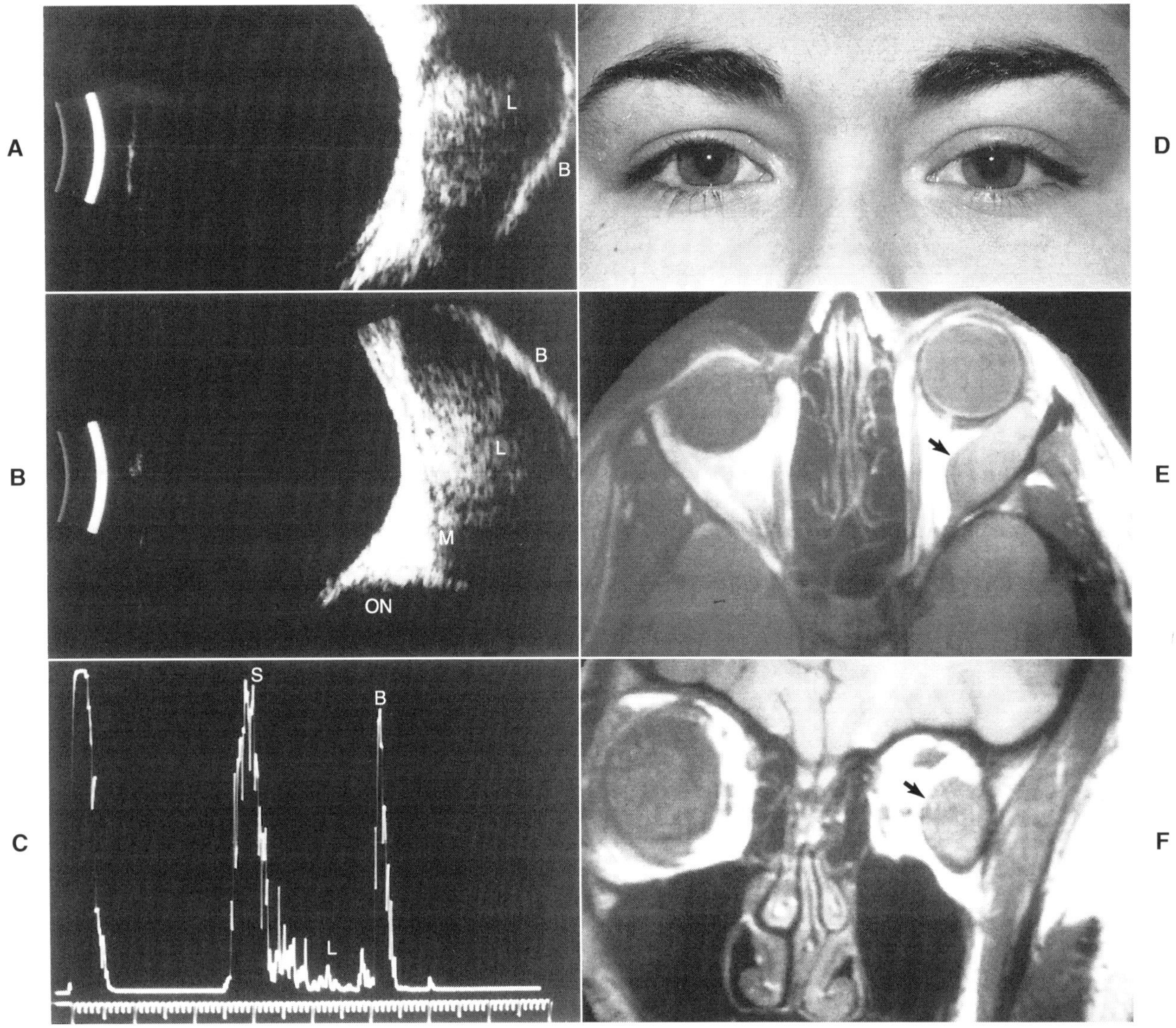

Figure 12-9 Fibrous histiocytoma. Transocular echograms (**A** to **C**) show large orbital lesion *(L)* in temporal orbit. **A,** Vertical transverse B-scan shows well-circumscribed extraconal tumor between globe and orbital bone *(B)*. **B,** Longitudinal B-scan view shows extraconal mass extending posteriorly between lateral rectus muscle *(M)* and orbital bone. **C,** A-scan echogram shows low internal reflectivity and regular structure. *S,* Sclera. **D,** External photograph shows fullness and ptosis of left upper lid. Axial **(E)** and coronal **(F)** MRI scans demonstrate well-circumscribed mass *(arrows)*.

the optic nerve is discussed in Chapters 15 and 16, respectively.

Metastatic tumors are usually infiltrative, although they can appear very well circumscribed, especially when growing within a confined space (e.g., beneath Tenon's capsule or the periosteum). These lesions can invade the orbital walls and produce extensive bony destruction. They are typically hard and nonvascular, and they generally produce weak sound attenuation. The infiltrative metastatic tumors tend to be irregularly shaped and poorly outlined. These neoplasms are most often medium to high reflective with a moderately irregular internal structure (Figure 12-10). Ossoinig has described a V-shaped A-scan pattern for tumors of an infiltrative nature such as metastatic tumors to the orbit[39] (Figure 12-11).

Carcinomas that grow within a confined space are usually more regularly shaped and better outlined than infiltrative tumors. Their shape can vary according to the space in which they are confined. Also, these tumors tend to be more low to medium reflective and regularly structured than the

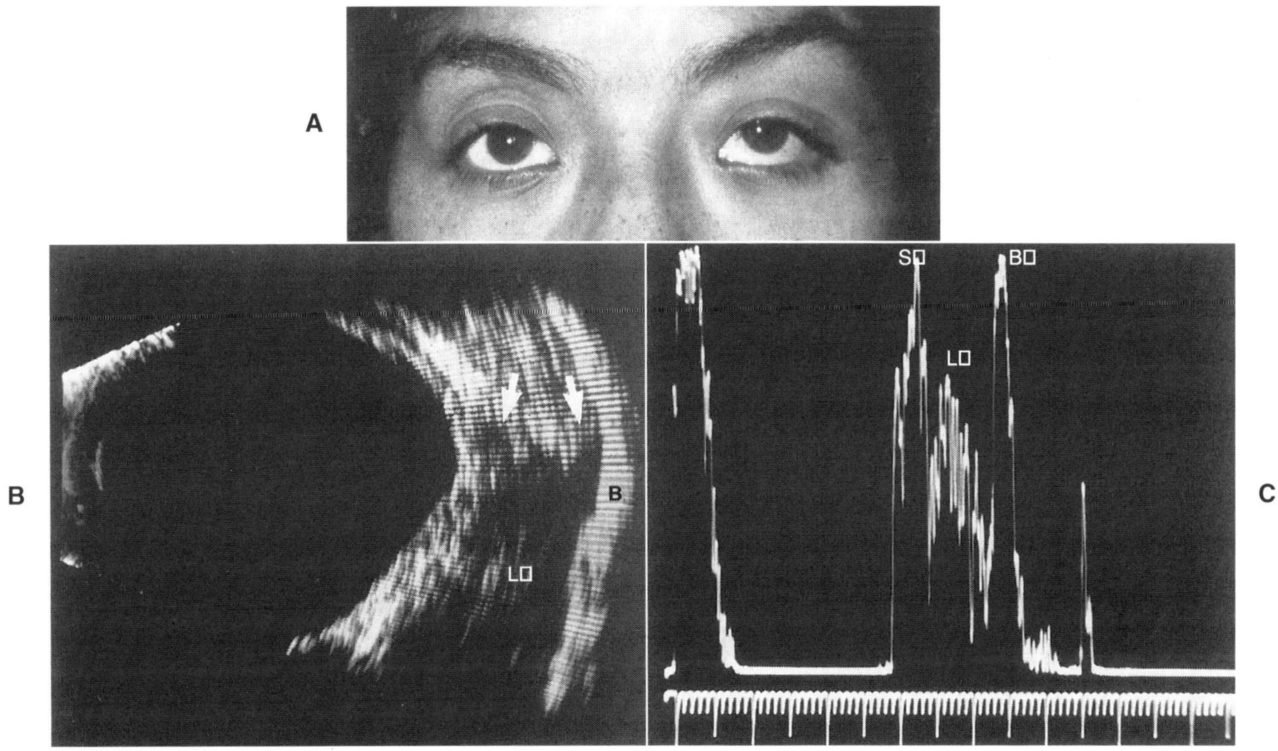

Figure 12-10 Metastatic carcinoma from breast. **A,** External photograph shows slight upward displacement of left eye. **B,** Vertical transverse B-scan echogram through lesion *(L)* located inferotemporally shows irregular contour *(arrows)*. *B,* Bone. **C,** Transocular A-scan shows medium-high reflectivity and irregular structure of lesion. *S,* Sclera.

higher reflective, infiltrative tumors described previously. These lower reflective metastatic tumors sometimes can be difficult to differentiate from pseudotumor/lymphomas.

One case of metastatic renal cell carcinoma[47] and two adenocarcinomas, one from lung and one from colon, have been examined by the authors. The renal cell tumor was oval shaped, well outlined, and highly vascular. The lesion showed medium internal reflectivity with essentially regular internal structure, moderate sound attenuation, and small cystic spaces (Figure 12-12). The two adenocarcinomas were very well outlined and exhibited medium to high internal reflectivity and vascularity. Although these two lesions resembled cavernous hemangiomas in shape and reflectivity, both were hard and significantly indented the globe. In addition, one of these tumors showed bony erosion.

The authors have examined one case of metastatic carcinoid that occurred in the inferior orbit. This tumor indented the globe and had a lobulated configuration. The mass demonstrated low to medium internal reflectivity and regular internal structure. In addition, it produced moderate sound attenuation, was firm in consistency, and showed moderate vascularity (Figure 12-13).

As previously mentioned, secondary tumors can extend into the orbit from the globe (see Chapter 5), lids, and periorbital cavities. These tumors can grow infiltratively or expansively within the orbital cavity. Their internal reflectivity is usually similar to that of the primary tumor[16,21,29,43] (Figures 12-14 through 12-16). Tumors extending into the orbit from adjacent sinus cavities are discussed in Chapter 17.

LACRIMAL SYSTEM DISORDERS

Lacrimal Gland

Echography can make an important contribution in evaluating lesions situated in the lacrimal fossa region.[2,3,41] It is an ideal screening tool for detecting abnormalities and in many instances can augment the information obtained with computed tomography (CT) or magnetic resonance imaging (MRI).

Because a large variety of lesions can occur in the lacrimal fossa region, differentiation can be challenging. The lesions most commonly found in this area include those of inflammatory or lymphoid origin, primary lacrimal gland epithelial tumors, and cysts.[1] Ultrasound can be of great value in helping to differentiate lesions of the pseudotumor/lymphoma group from the epithelial tumors (Table 12-2).

The normal lacrimal gland and surrounding orbital soft tissue are extremely high reflective. As a result of their similar reflectivities, the gland per se usually cannot be delin-

Text continued on p 324.

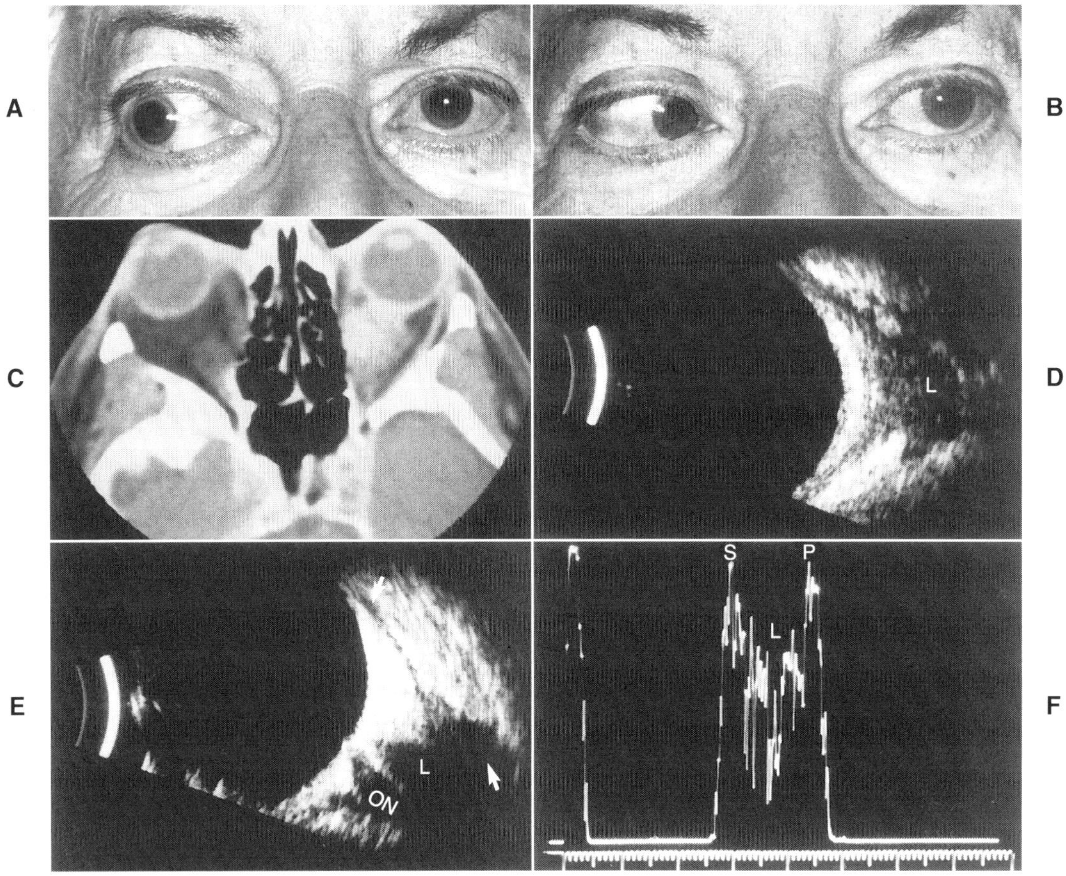

Figure 12-11 Metastatic carcinoma from breast. External photographs (**A** and **B**) show almost total ophthalmoplegia of left eye. **C,** Axial CT scan shows large, poorly defined mass within left orbit. Transocular echograms (**D** to **F**) show large orbital lesion *(L)*. **D,** Transverse B-scan shows irregularly shaped mass conforming to globe and infiltrating orbital soft tissue. **E,** Longitudinal B-scan echogram shows irregularly shaped tumor within muscle cone and around optic nerve *(ON)*. *Arrows,* Medial rectus muscle. **F,** A-scan shows medium-high internal reflectivity of tumor and V shape. *S,* Sclera; *P,* posterior surface spike.

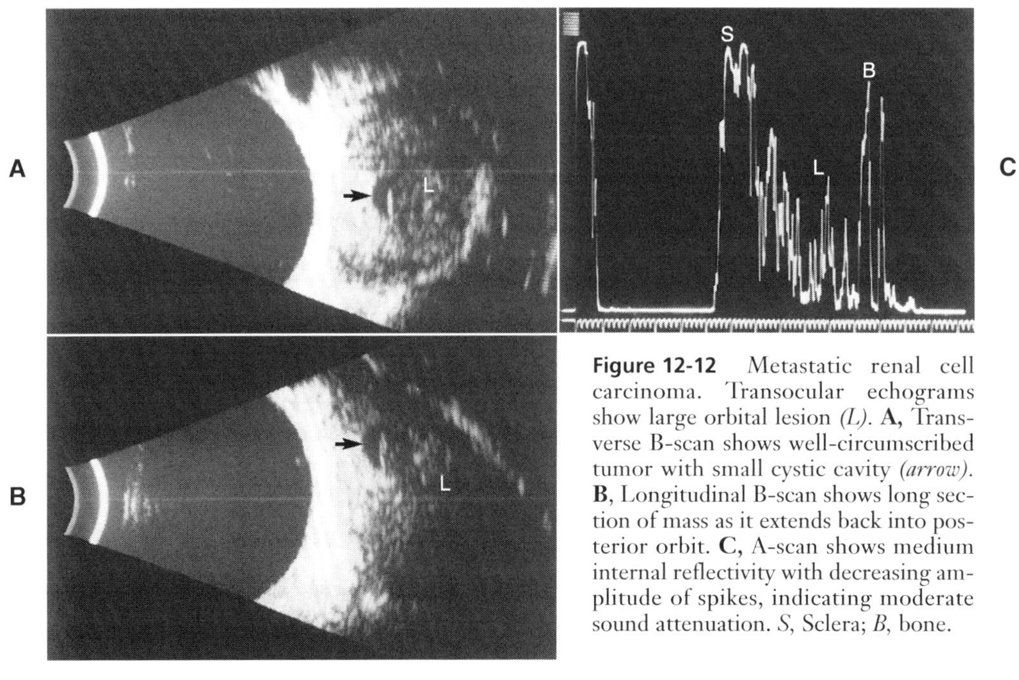

Figure 12-12 Metastatic renal cell carcinoma. Transocular echograms show large orbital lesion *(L)*. **A,** Transverse B-scan shows well-circumscribed tumor with small cystic cavity *(arrow)*. **B,** Longitudinal B-scan shows long section of mass as it extends back into posterior orbit. **C,** A-scan shows medium internal reflectivity with decreasing amplitude of spikes, indicating moderate sound attenuation. *S,* Sclera; *B,* bone.

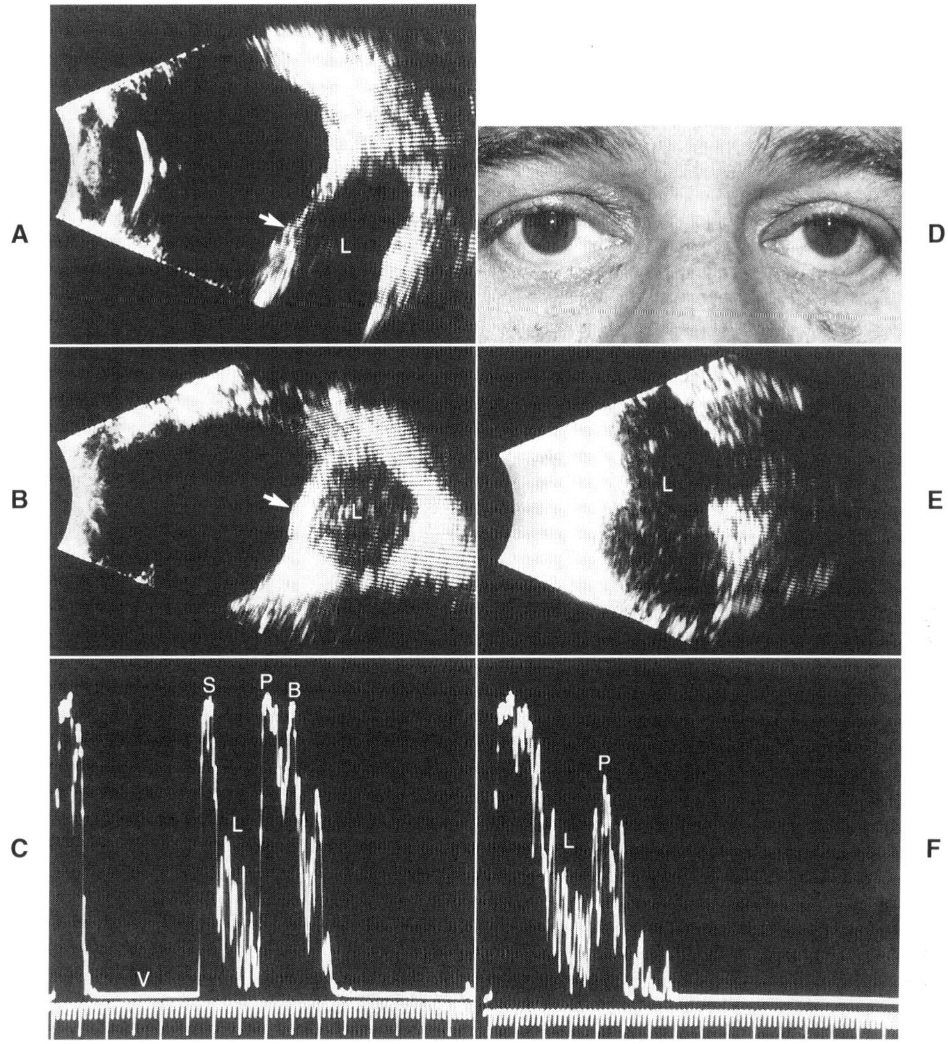

Figure 12-13 Metastatic carcinoid from stomach involving left orbit. Transocular (**A** to **C**) and paraocular (**E** and **F**) echograms show large lesion *(L)* in inferotemporal aspect of left orbit. **A,** Vertical axial B-scan echogram shows well-circumscribed, irregularly shaped retrobulbar mass indenting globe *(arrow)*. **B,** Transverse B-scan through inferior orbit shows cross-section of mass and globe indentation. **C,** A-scan shows medium to low internal reflectivity. *V,* Vitreous cavity; *S,* sclera; *P,* posterior surface spike; *B,* bone. **D,** External photograph shows very mild proptosis of left eye. **E,** Transverse paraocular B-scan shows more lobulated appearance of tumor in this view. **F,** Paraocular A-scan shows medium internal reflectivity. *P,* Posterior surface spike.

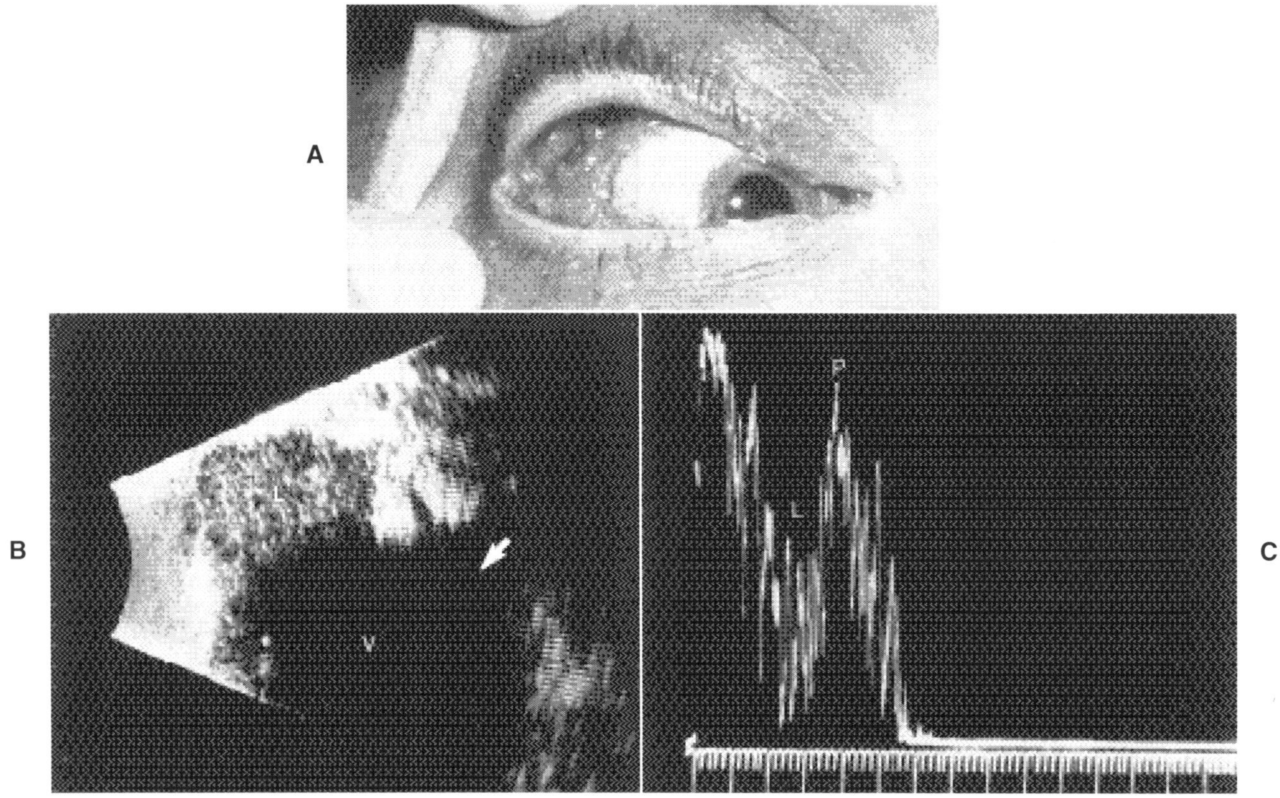

Figure 12-14 Squamous cell carcinoma of conjunctiva with extension into anterior orbit. **A,** External photograph shows large conjunctival mass in fornix. **B,** Longitudinal paraocular B-scan echogram shows lesion *(L)* extending into anterior orbit next to globe. *V,* Vitreous cavity; *arrow,* area of globe wall, not well shown because of edge artifact. **C,** Paraocular A-scan shows medium reflectivity of lesion. *P,* Posterior surface spike.

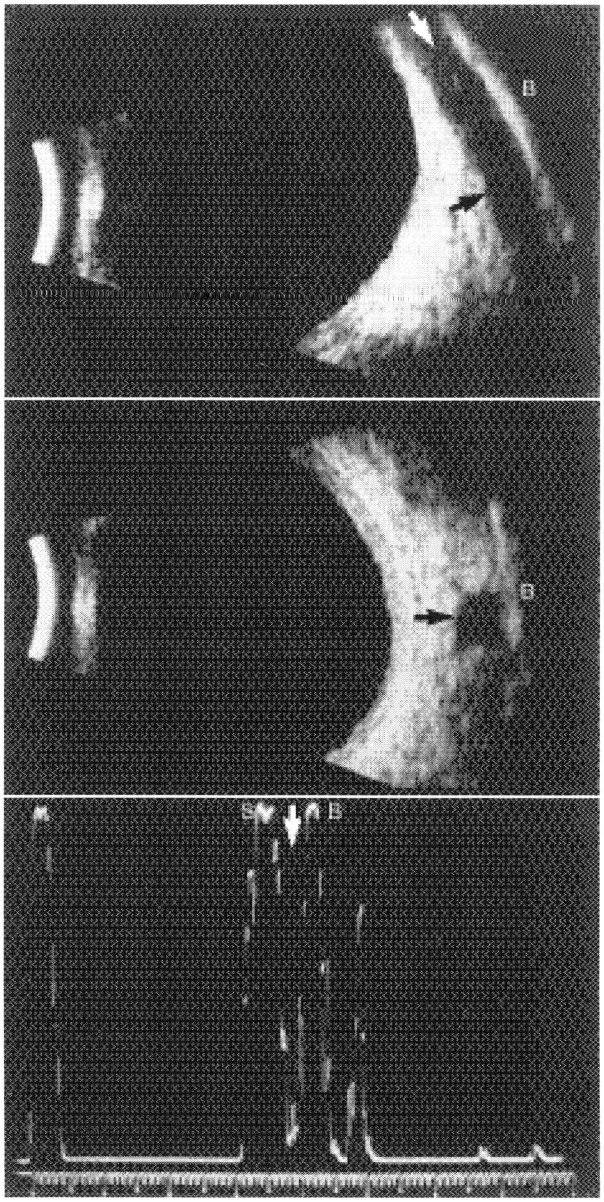

A
B
C

Figure 12-15 Orbital extension of melanoma from skin. Transocular echograms show tubular-shaped lesion *(arrows)* extending back into orbit, presumably along an orbital nerve. **A,** Longitudinal B-scan shows long section of lesion as it extends posteriorly, adjacent to orbital bone *(B)*. **B,** Transverse B-scan shows cross-section of tubular-shaped lesion. **C,** A-scan displays low internal reflectivity and regular structure of mass. The tumor was hard and moderately vascularized. *S,* Sclera; *B,* bone.

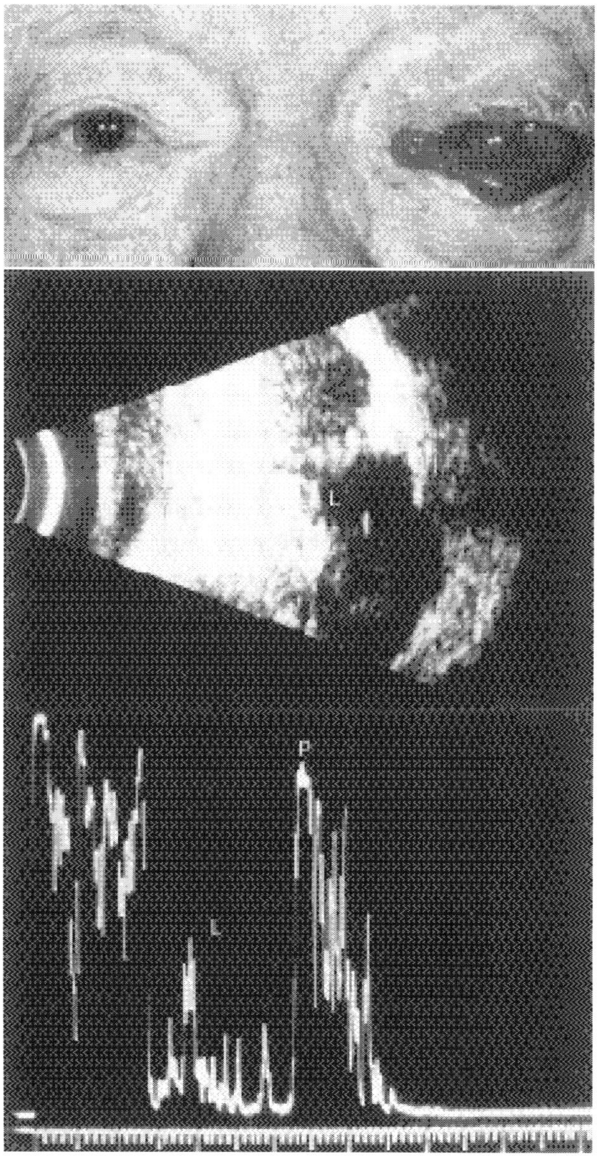

A
B
C

Figure 12-16 Recurrent melanoma following enucleation. **A,** External photograph shows marked hemorrhagic chemosis. **B,** B-scan echogram shows extensive lesion *(L)* with irregular appearance in orbital cavity. **C,** A-scan echogram demonstrates low internal reflectivity of lesion. *P,* Posterior surface spike. The lesion was hard and highly vascularized.

TABLE 12-2

Lacrimal Gland: Pseudotumor/Lymphoma (PL) vs. Benign Mixed Tumors (BMT) and Adenoid Cystic Carcinoma (ACC)*

Tumor Type	Shape	Internal Reflectivity	Internal Structure	Sound Attenuation	Vascularity	Consistency	Unilateral/ Bilateral
PL	Spindle	Low-med	Regular	Weak	+/−	Normal	Either
BMT	Round-oval	Med-high	Regular	Mod	−	Normal/excavated	Unilateral
ACC	Irregular	Med-high	Irregular	Mod/strong	−	Excavated/defects	Unilateral

Med, Medium; *Mod,* moderate; *WNL,* within normal limits.
*The main echographic findings for pseudotumor/lymphomas and the most common epithelial tumors are listed.

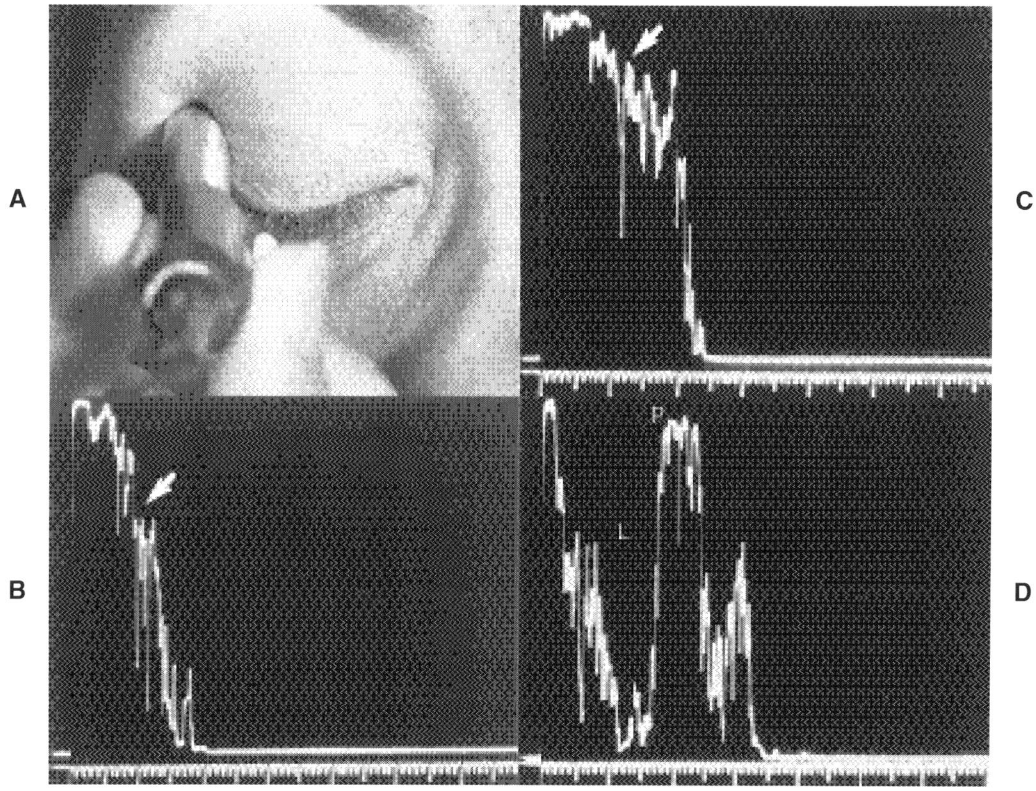

Figure 12-17 Paraocular A-scan technique for evaluating lacrimal gland. **A,** A-scan probe is positioned on the lid overlying lacrimal gland. **B,** Normal appearance of tissue in lacrimal gland region *(arrow)*. **C,** Edema of tissue in lacrimal gland region. **D,** Infiltrated lacrimal gland *(L)*. *P,* Posterior surface spike.

eated from adjacent orbital soft tissue (Figure 12-17).

Benign Mixed Tumor (Pleomorphic Adenoma)

Benign mixed tumors are the most common benign epithelial tumors of the lacrimal gland.[56] These tumors most often involve the orbital lobe of the gland but in rare cases may affect the palpebral lobe.[1] When benign mixed tumors develop within the orbital lobe, they tend to extend farther back into the orbit and can become quite large.[1] In some cases, these lesions cause indentation of the ocular wall, choroidal folds, and bony excavation.[27] However, when involving only the palpebral lobe, the lesion usually remains anterior and does not cause bony abnormalities.[42]

Typically, benign mixed tumors are medium to high reflective with regular internal structure, and they produce moderate sound attenuation[10] (see Figure 11-24). These tu-

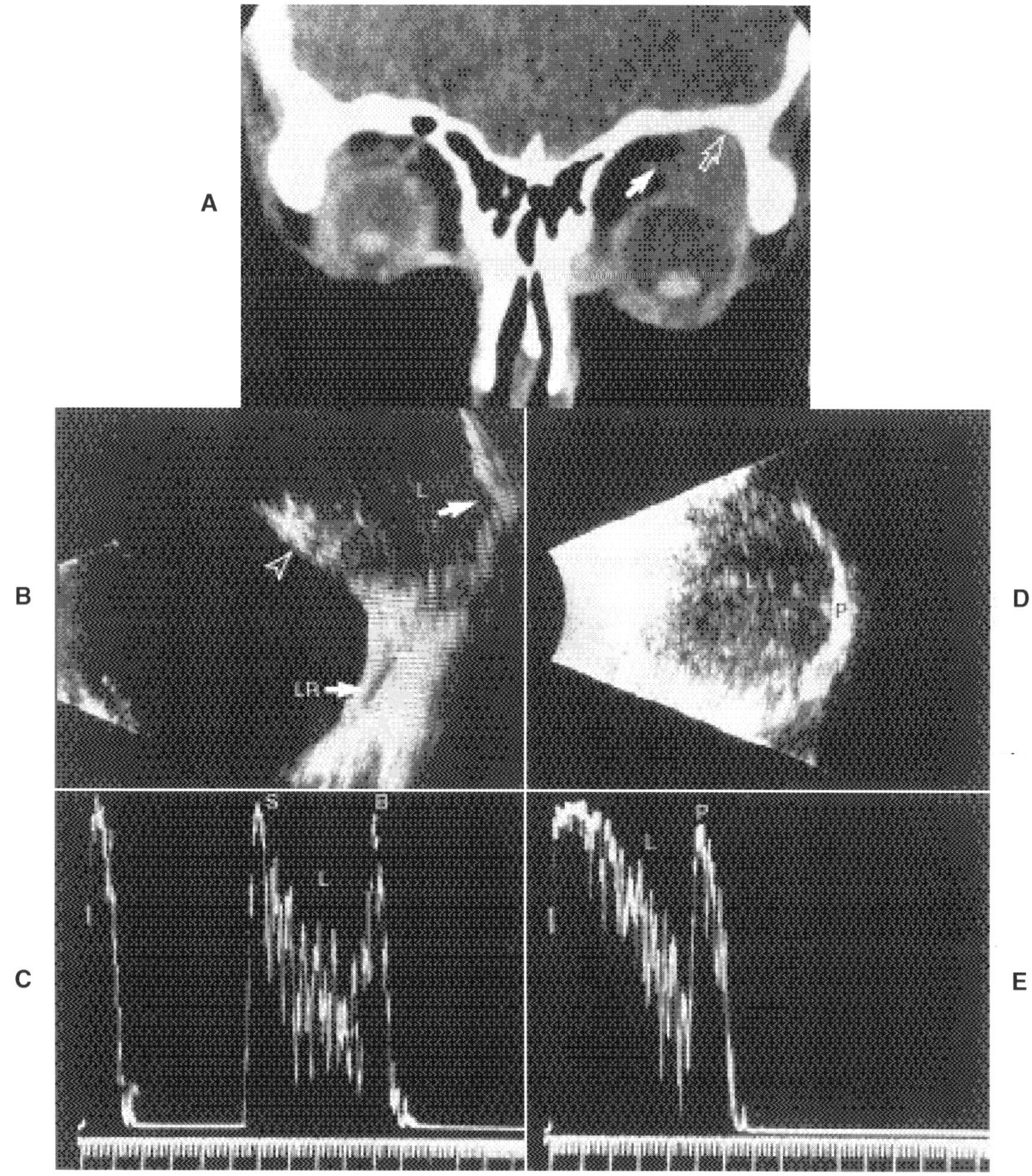

Figure 12-18 Benign mixed tumor. **A,** Coronal CT scan shows mass in left lacrimal gland fossa *(closed arrow)* with bony excavation *(open arrow)*. Transocular (**B** and **C**) and paraocular (**D** and **E**) echograms show large orbital lesion *(L)*. **B,** Vertical transverse B-scan shows well-circumscribed mass in supratemporal orbit. Note indentation of globe *(open arrow)* and excavation of orbital bone *(closed arrow)*. *LR,* Lateral rectus muscle. **C,** A-scan shows medium-high internal reflectivity, regular structure, and moderate sound attenuation. *S,* Sclera; *B,* bone. **D,** Transverse paraocular B-scan demonstrates rounded, smooth posterior surface of tumor *(P)*. **E,** In this view, paraocular A-scan shows higher internal reflectivity; moderate sound attenuation; and distinct, double-peaked posterior surface spike *(P)* from encapsulated lesion.

mors are round to oval and are very well outlined because of the capsule surrounding the tumor (Figure 12-18). They have a very firm consistency, are nonvascular, and may contain one or more small cystic cavities. Very large cystic cavities have been identified in one tumor (Figure 12-19).

Benign mixed tumors can have a shape and reflectivity similar to that of cavernous hemangiomas. Hemangiomas, however, generally have a softer consistency and are rarely found in the lacrimal gland region. Two other lesions that should be considered in the differential diagnosis include

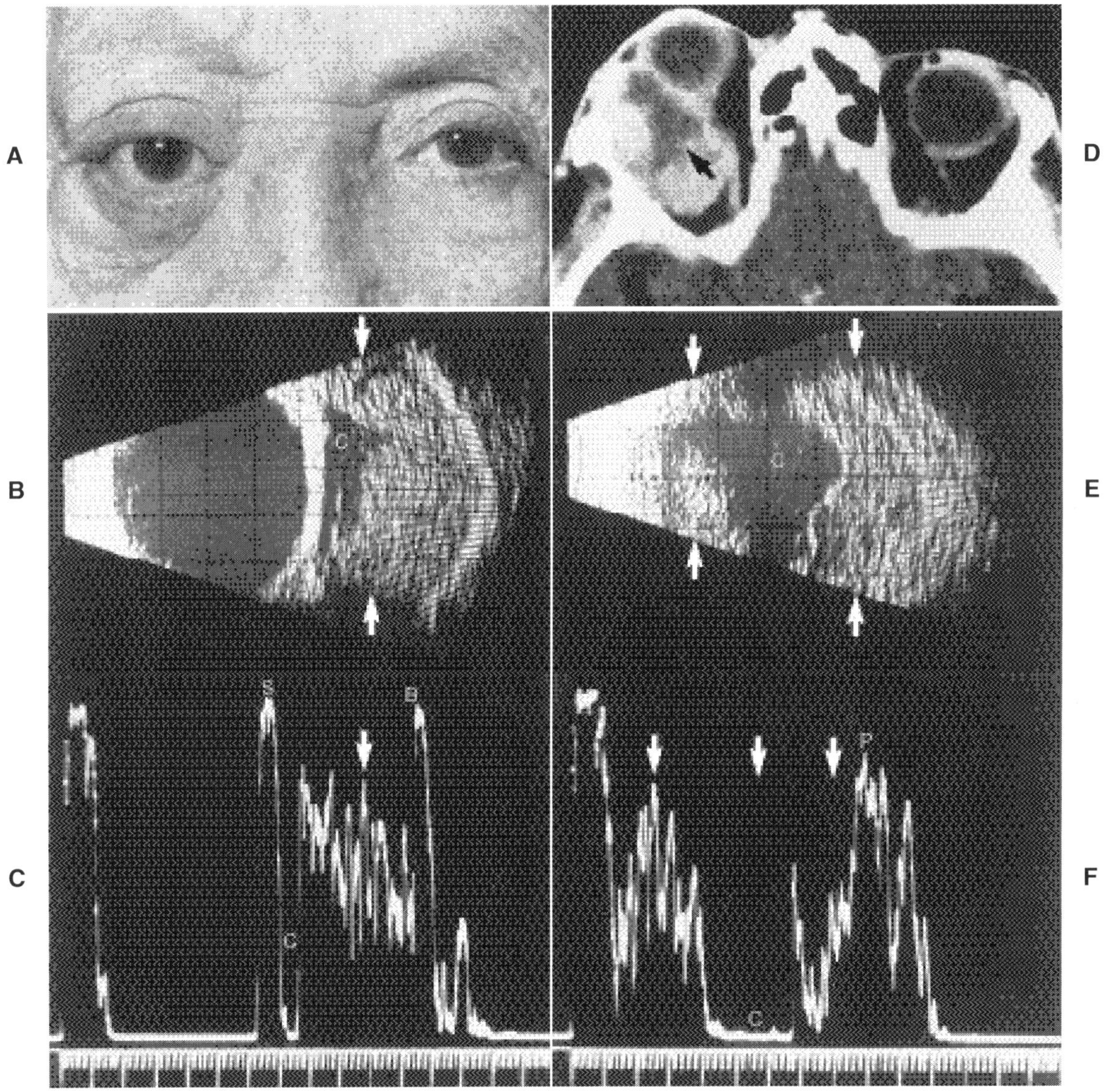

Figure 12-19 Benign mixed tumor with cystic cavities. **A,** External photograph shows proptosis of right eye. Transocular (**B** and **C**) and paraocular (**E** and **F**) echograms show large tumor *(arrows)* containing large cystic cavities *(C)*. **B,** Transverse B-scan shows well-circumscribed mass with cystic cavity next to sclera. **C,** Corresponding A-scan shows medium-high internal reflectivity of tumor with very low reflective cystic cavity. *S,* Sclera; *B,* bone. **D,** Axial CT scan shows large, relatively well-circumscribed tumor with large cystic cavity *(arrow)*. **E,** Transverse paraocular B-scan shows mass with very large cystic cavity. **F,** Paraocular A-scan shows predominantly medium internal reflectivity with very low reflective cystic space in center. *P,* Posterior surface spike.

dermoid cyst and the well-circumscribed form of adenoid cystic carcinoma.

A benign mixed tumor can undergo malignant transformation; echographically, however, this can only be suspected if the tumor breaks out of its capsule.

Adenoid Cystic Carcinoma

Adenoid cystic carcinoma is the second most common epithelial tumor and the most common primary malignant tumor of the lacrimal gland.[56] These tumors are usually infiltrative, although in some cases they can appear well circumscribed. Their internal reflectivity is generally medium to high with an irregular internal structure, although the better-circumscribed lesions may appear more regular. Adenoid cystic carcinomas typically have a hard consistency and are nonvascular. In addition, these lesions usually produce moderate to strong sound attenuation, and cystic cavities can often be identified (Figures 12-20 and 12-21). These tumors frequently affect the bone, causing either excavation or, in some cases, extensive bony destruction. A well-circumscribed adenoid cystic carcinoma may, at times, be difficult to differentiate from a benign mixed tumor or even a dermoid cyst due to their similar acoustic features.

Mucoepidermoid Carcinoma

Mucoepidermoid carcinoma is a rare epithelial tumor of the lacrimal gland[49] that has varied histologic features.[56] Two children and one adult with this tumor have been evaluated by the authors. All three lesions had firm consistency, were relatively well circumscribed, and had predominantly medium to high internal reflectivity. Also, all three lesions had moderately irregular internal structure. Cystic spaces were noted in one case (Figure 12-22). One lesion produced very strong sound attenuation, and significant internal vascularity was not appreciated in any of the tumors. Excavation of the lateral orbital wall and globe indentation were noted in one case. These tumors are difficult to differentiate from other epithelial tumors of the lacrimal gland.[57]

Pseudotumor and Lymphoma (Lymphoproliferative Diseases)

A C E

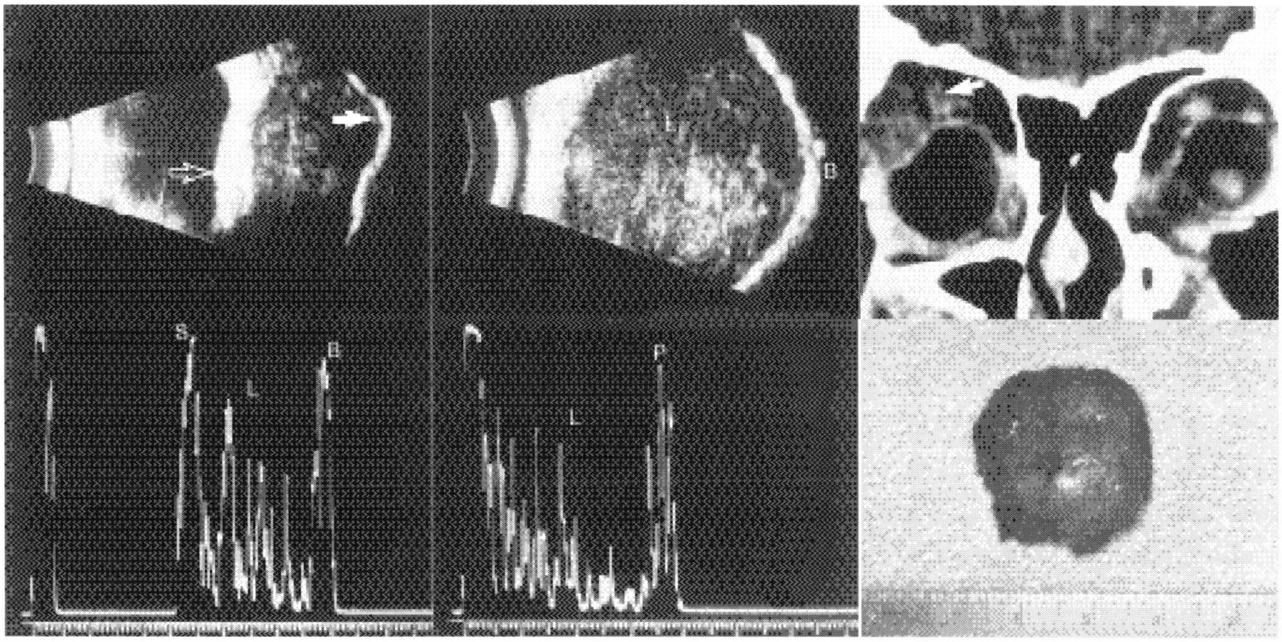

B D F

Figure 12-20 Adenoid cystic carcinoma (circumscribed). Transocular (**A** and **B**) and paraocular (**C** and **D**) echograms shows large orbital lesion *(L)*. **A,** Transverse B-scan shows well-circumscribed mass is indenting the globe *(open arrow)* and excavating the bone *(closed arrow)*. **B,** A-scan shows medium internal reflectivity and moderate sound attenuation. *S*, Sclera; *B*, bone. **C,** Transverse paraocular B-scan with sound beam directed toward bone shows excavation (note concave shape of bone line). **D,** Paraocular A-scan displays medium internal reflectivity of tumor with moderate sound attenuation. *P,* Posterior surface spike. **E,** Coronal CT scan shows large orbital mass *(arrow)* indenting the globe and excavating the adjacent orbital bone. **F,** Gross pathological specimen shows very well-circumscribed tumor.

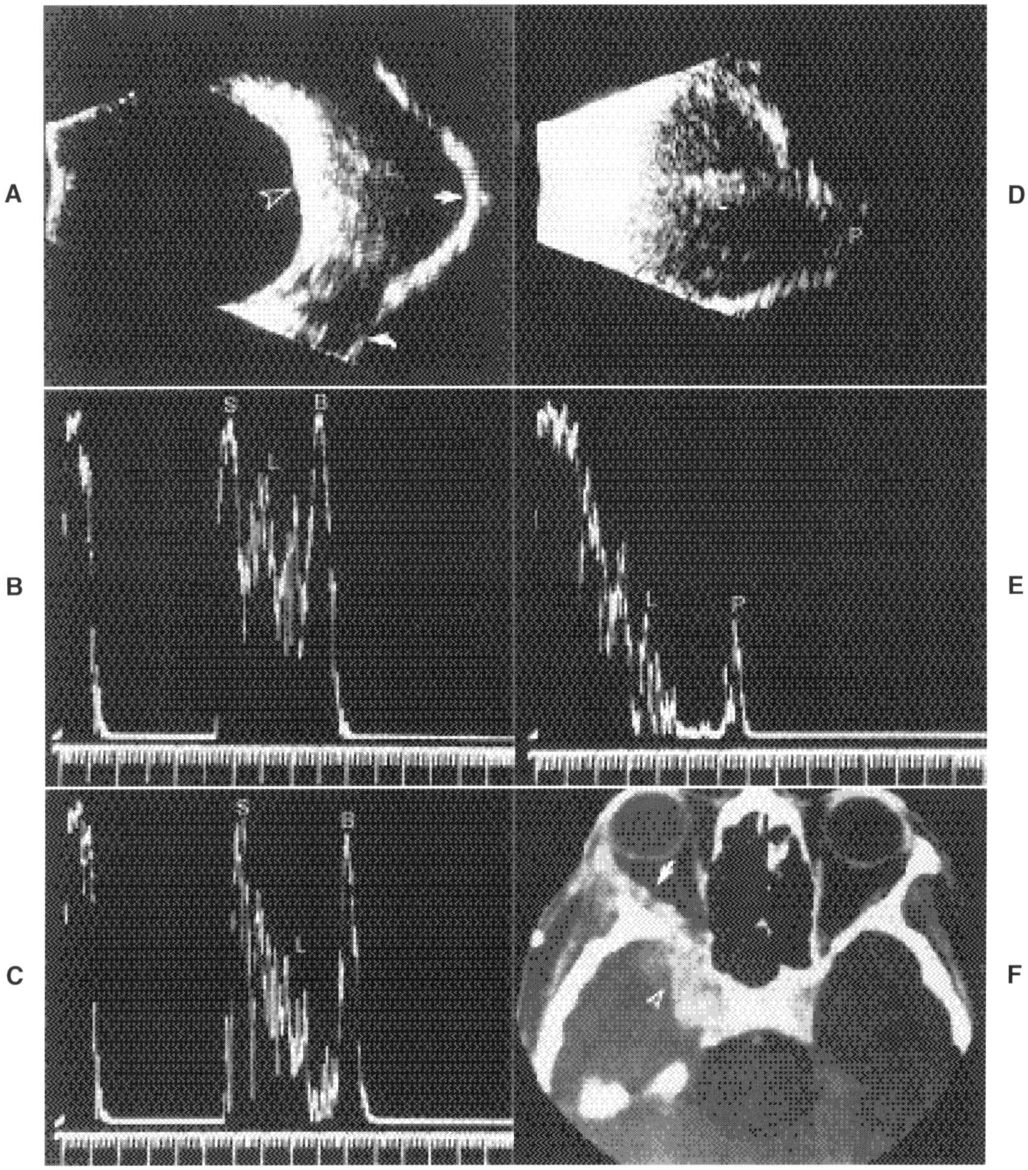

Figure 12-21 Adenoid cystic carcinoma (infiltrative). Transocular (**A** to **C**) and paraocular (**D** and **E**) echograms show large orbital lesion *(L)*. **A,** Transverse B-scan through supratemporal orbit shows extensive tumor with irregular shape inferiorly *(curved arrow)*. Also, note indentation of globe *(open arrow)* and excavation of bone *(closed arrow)*. **B** and **C,** A-scans from two areas of the tumor show predominantly medium reflectivity but moderately irregular internal structure. *S*, Sclera; *B*, bone. **D,** Transverse paraocular B-scan shows poorly defined posterior border *(P)*, indicating infiltrative nature of tumor. **E,** Paraocular A-scan shows medium internal reflectivity with strong sound attenuation in this view. Also note low to medium reflectivity of posterior surface spike *(P)*, indicating lack of encapsulation. **F,** Axial CT scan obtained after biopsy and radiation therapy shows tumor extending posteriorly along lateral orbital wall *(closed arrow)* and into cavernous sinus *(open arrow)*.

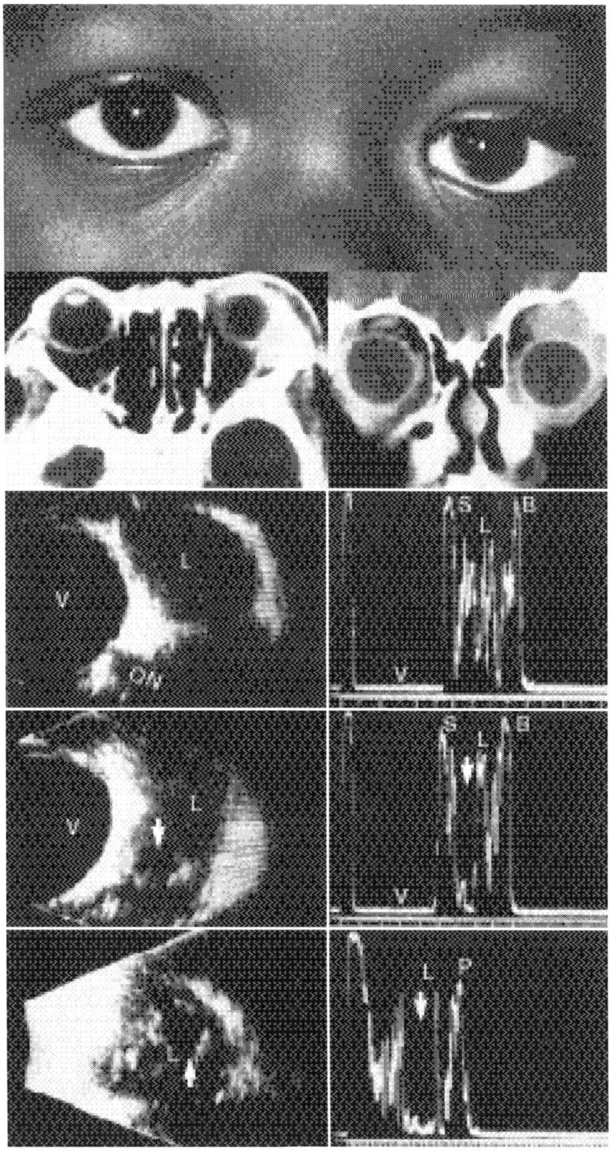

Figure 12-22 Mucoepidermoid carcinoma. **A,** External photograph shows downward displacement of left eye. Axial **(B)** and coronal **(C)** CT scans show extensive orbital mass in left orbit. Transocular (**D** to **G**) and paraocular (**H** and **I**) echograms show large orbital lesion *(L)* containing cystic cavity *(white arrow)* in some views. **D,** Longitudinal B-scan shows well-circumscribed tumor in this view. *V,* Vitreous cavity; *ON,* optic nerve. **E,** Corresponding A-scan shows medium-high reflectivity of lesion. *S,* Sclera; *B,* bone. **F,** Transverse B-scan shows more diffuse, irregularly shaped appearance of tumor and cystic cavity. **G,** Corresponding A-scan shows medium-high internal reflectivity with very low reflectivity of cystic space. **H,** Transverse paraocular B-scan shows irregularly shaped tumor with large cystic cavity centrally. **I,** Corresponding paraocular A-scan shows medium reflectivity of tumor with very low reflective cystic cavity. *P,* Posterior surface spike.

Inflammatory lesions (i.e., pseudotumors) and lymphoid tumors occur quite commonly in the lacrimal fossa region.[51] They can be either unilateral or bilateral. As described earlier, pseudotumor/lymphomas are classified as one entity (pseudotumor/lymphoma) because they have a very similar histologic, and therefore echographic, appearance (see p 310).[34] Lesions in this group include a wide spectrum of conditions, such as idiopathic (nongranulomatous) inflammatory pseudotumor, benign reactive lymphoid hyperplasia, malignant lymphoma, and various types of granulomatous inflammatory processes such as those associated with sarcoidosis.[53]

Most pseudotumor/lymphomas occurring in the lacrimal gland region are irregularly shaped or have a spindlelike configuration on B-scan. On A-scan the posterior border spike can vary from indistinct to well defined. Lesions of this group typically have regular or slightly irregular internal structure and low to medium reflectivity. They produce weak sound attenuation, and septa sometimes can be identified (Figure 12-23). Pseudotumor/lymphomas often show internal vascularity, and their consistency can be either hard or slightly compressible (see p 302). Bony defects and/or excavation are usually not associated with these lesions.[53] Echographically, these lesions can often be shown to be bilateral even though clinically they may appear to be unilateral.

In some cases, pseudotumors exhibit high internal reflectivity. Although these inflammatory lesions are easily distinguished from the low reflective lymphomas, they can be more difficult to differentiate from other lesions that occur in the lacrimal fossa. They may be either well circum-

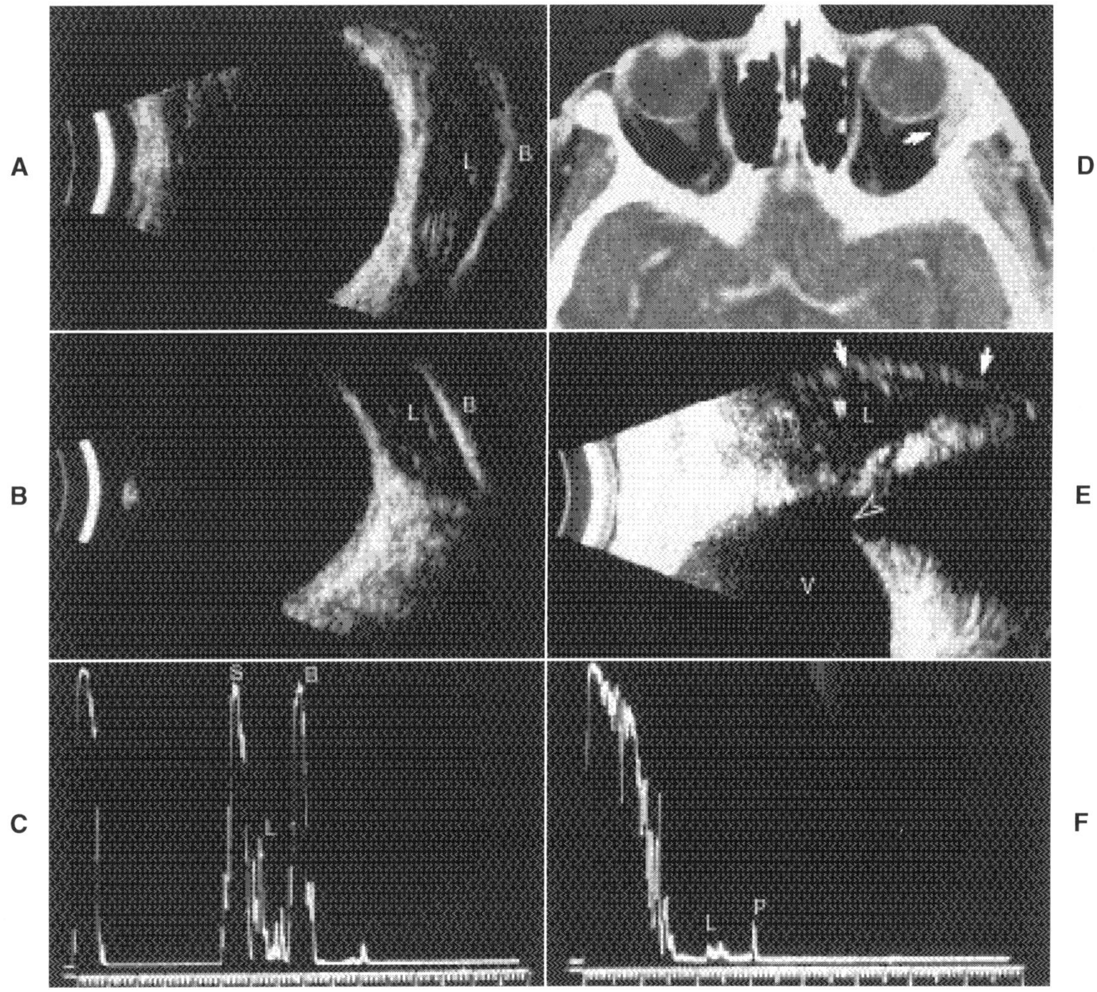

Figure 12-23 Lymphoma involving lacrimal gland. Transocular (**A** to **C**) and paraocular (**E** and **F**) echograms show lesion *(L)* in lacrimal gland region. **A,** Transverse B-scan shows extensive, well-circumscribed tumor next to bone *(B)*. **B,** Longitudinal B-scan displays typical fusiform shape of mass as it extends posteriorly along bone. **C,** A-scan shows low-medium internal reflectivity. *S,* Sclera. **D,** Axial CT scan shows mass in lacrimal gland region *(arrow)*. **E,** Longitudinal paraocular B-scan displays fusiform-shaped tumor extending back into orbit along orbital bone *(closed arrows)*. *V,* Vitreous cavity; *open arrow,* area of globe wall not shown well because of edge artifact. **F,** Paraocular A-scan shows low internal reflectivity and weakly reflective posterior surface spike *(P)*, caused by fusiform shape of mass.

scribed or can have a more diffuse, irregular shape. Characteristics that may help to distinguish these tumors from other lesions in this region include thickening of adjacent extraocular muscles and the presence of vascularity. In addition, they may show an area of inflammatory infiltration surrounding the lacrimal gland (Figure 12-24).

Dacryoadenitis

Acute infection of the lacrimal gland can be difficult to distinguish echographically from inflammatory pseudotumor. Ultrasound may show diffuse, highly reflective, nonvascular enlargement of the lacrimal gland per se, as well as the surrounding orbital soft tissue. In addition, areas of low

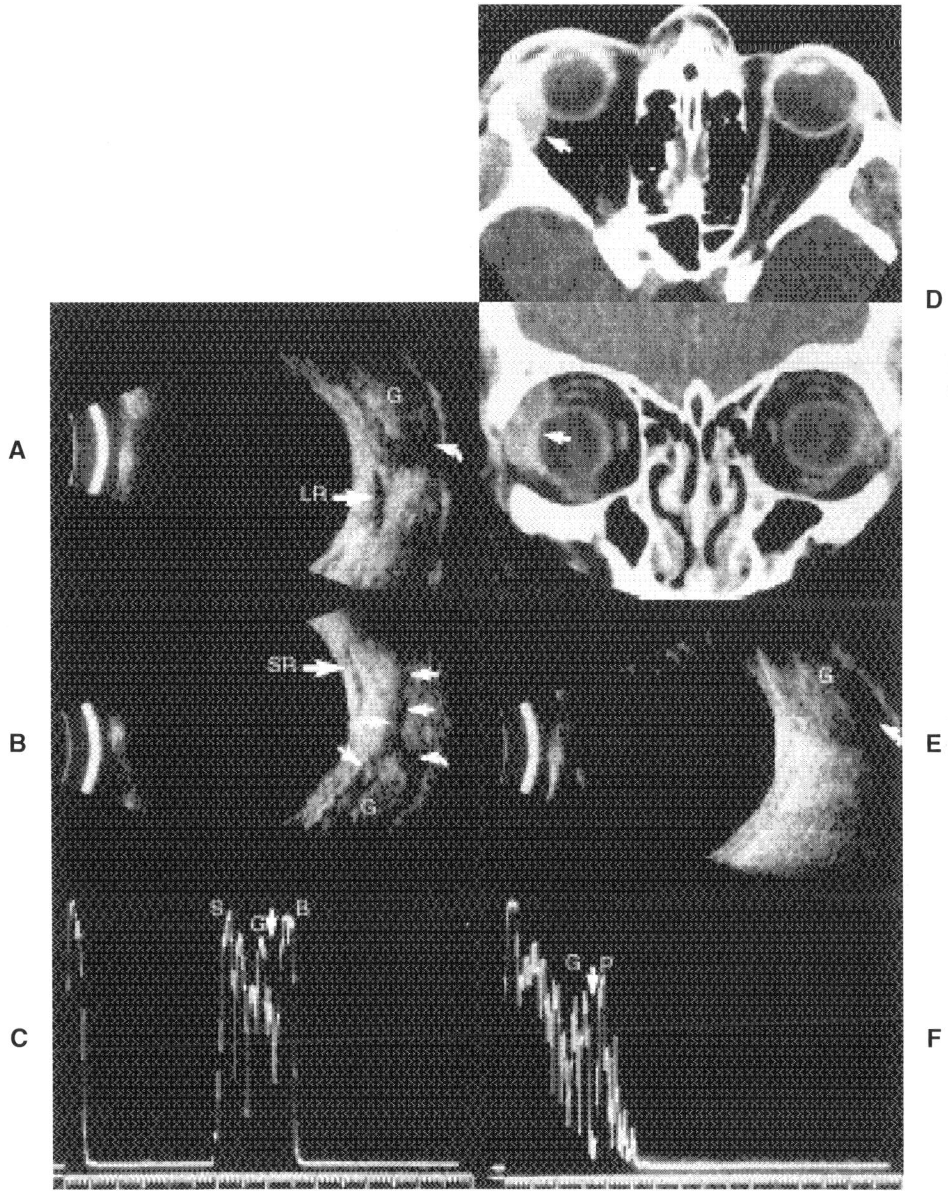

Figure 12-24 Pseudotumor involving lacrimal gland. Transocular (**A, B, C,** and **E**) and paraocular (**F**) echograms show enlarged, inflamed lacrimal gland *(G)*. **A,** Vertical transverse B-scan through temporal orbit shows inferior aspect of enlarged lacrimal gland just above lateral rectus muscle *(LR)*. Note homogeneous appearance of infiltration surrounding lacrimal gland *(curved arrow)*. **B,** Transverse B-scan through supratemporal orbit shows upper aspect of enlarged lacrimal gland and surrounding infiltration next to thickened levator muscle *(small arrows)*. *SR,* Superior rectus muscle. **C,** Transocular A-scan shows high internal reflectivity of gland and lower reflectivity from surrounding infiltration *(arrow)*. *S,* Sclera; *B,* bone. **D,** Axial **(top)** and coronal **(bottom)** CT scans show lesion in lacrimal gland region *(arrows)*. **E,** Longitudinal B-scan shows fusiform shape of enlarged gland and surrounding infiltration *(curved arrow)*. **F,** Paraocular A-scan shows medium-high reflectivity of inflamed gland and low reflectivity of surrounding infiltration. *P,* Posterior surface spike.

reflective infiltration may be present. With follow-up examination, progressive enlargement of a circumscribed, low reflective lesion suggests the development of an abscess (see p 439 and Figure 17-3).

Lacrimal Ductal Cyst (Dacryops)

This is a rare cystic lesion that results from obstruction and ectasia of the lacrimal gland ducts.[27] Dacryops may be unilateral or bilateral and can involve either the palpebral or orbital lobe of the gland.[8] These lesions may be round, oval, or lobulated and are very well outlined. They usually have smooth contour and are very low reflective. Dacryops are nonvascular and soft in consistency. Because these lesions are often small and located anteriorly, their evaluation may be facilitated by using the immersion technique (Figure 12-25; see also Figure 11-23).

Lacrimal Sac

Echography can be useful for evaluating lesions located in the region of the lacrimal sac. In normal situations, the sac can be identified as a small, low reflective structure (Figure 12-26). A dilated sac is much easier to image (Figure 12-27). In addition, this can allow for display of the nasolacrimal duct. The immersion technique also can be helpful for evaluating lesions in this region (see Figure 11-23).

Dacryocystitis

Dacryocystitis is an inflammation of the lacrimal sac.[23] In these cases, ultrasound can demonstrate dilatation of the sac and its opening into the nasolacrimal duct.[18,53] The dilated sac is typically very low reflective, although higher reflectivity may be detected if mucus is present. The demonstration of a mucous plug or layered mucus

A

C

B

D

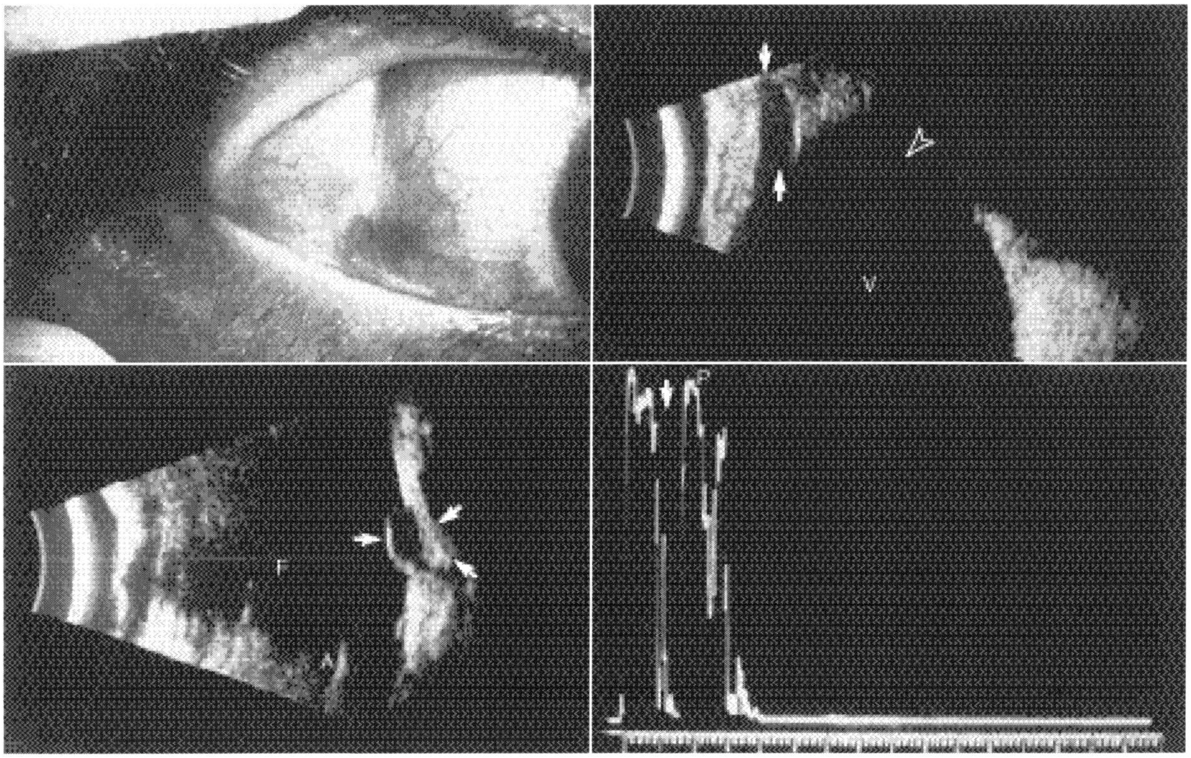

Figure 12-25 Lacrimal ductal cyst (dacryops). **A,** External photograph shows lesion with cystic appearance involving palpebral lobe of lacrimal gland. **B,** Immersion B-scan echogram shows well-outlined, echolucent lesion on surface of globe *(arrows)*. *F,* Fluid within scleral shell; *A,* small air bubble. **C,** Longitudinal paraocular B-scan shows well-outlined, echolucent lesion with cystic appearance *(closed arrows)*. *Open arrow,* area of globe wall not well shown because of edge artifact. *V,* Vitreous cavity. **D,** Paraocular A-scan shows very low reflectivity of lesion *(arrow)*. *P,* Posterior surface spike.

A
C
B
D

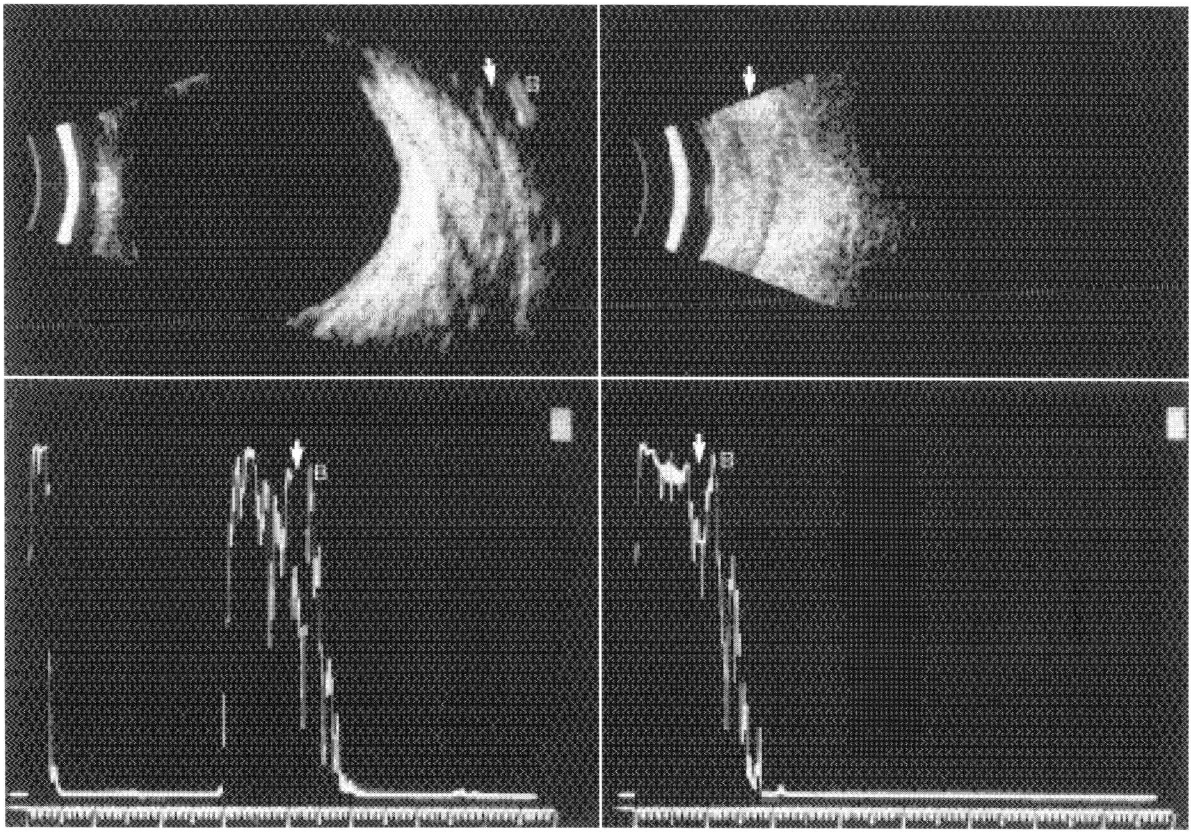

Figure 12-26 Normal lacrimal sac. Transocular (**A** and **B**) and paraocular (**C** and **D**) echograms of sac *(arrows)*. **A,** Longitudinal B-scan through anterior aspect of nasal globe and orbit shows small echolucent area from normal sac. *B,* Lacrimal bone. **B,** Corresponding A-scan shows thin defect from sac. Transverse B-scan **(C)** and A-scan **(D)** were obtained with probes placed in medial canthal region. *Arrow,* Lacrimal sac.

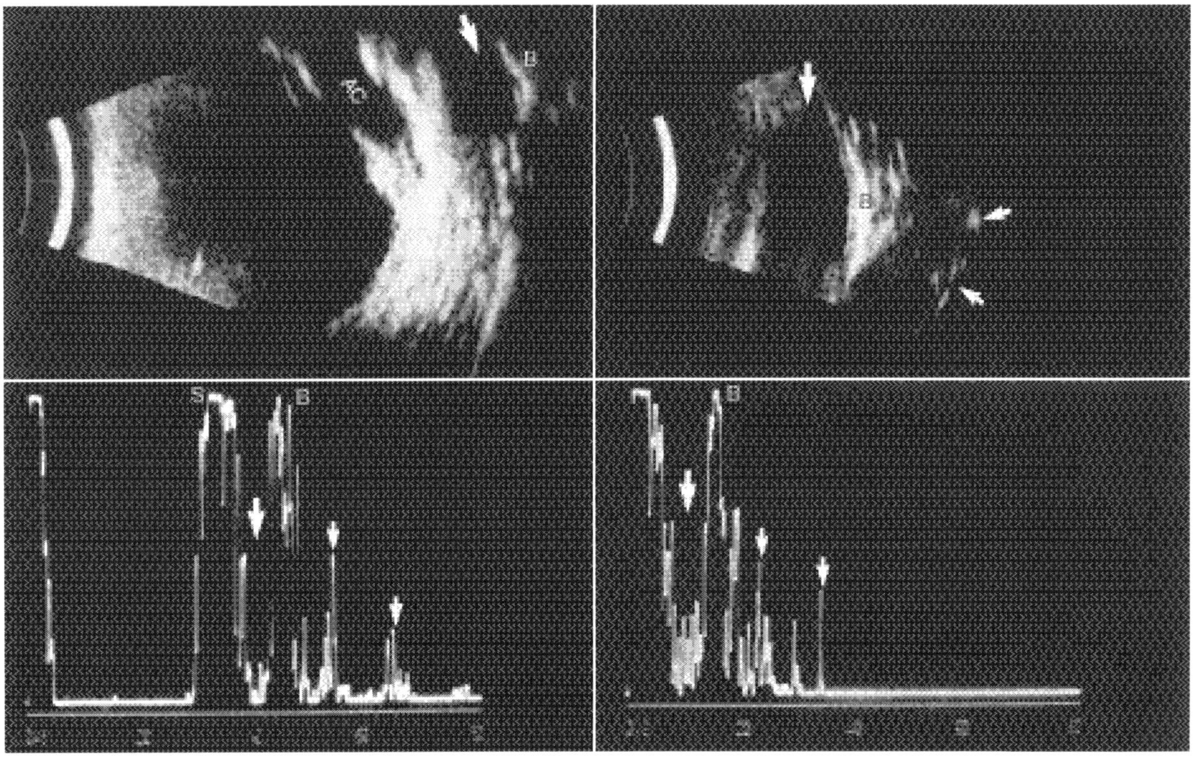

Figure 12-27 Dilated lacrimal sac due to dacryocystitis. Transocular (**A** and **B**) and paraocular (**C** and **D**) echograms show dilated sac *(large arrows)*. **A,** Longitudinal B-scan through anterior aspect of nasal globe and orbit shows enlarged sac. *AC,* Anterior chamber; *B,* lacrimal bone. **B,** Corresponding A-scan shows very low reflectivity of dilated sac. *S,* Sclera; *B,* bone; *small arrows,* multiple signals. **C,** Transverse paraocular B-scan shows enlarged sac next to lacrimal bone. *Small arrows,* Multiple signals. **D,** Corresponding paraocular A-scan shows low internal reflectivity of enlarged sac.

can help to distinguish this condition from a neoplasm (Figures 12-28 and 12-29). These dilated sacs are nonvascular and slightly compressible. A dacryolith may appear as a highly reflective, echo-dense nodule within the dilated sac.[7]

Tumors of the Lacrimal Sac

Tumors of the lacrimal drainage system are rare.[17] Although experience with such lesions is limited, they would be expected to exhibit characteristics similar to those of other orbital tumors, depending on their origin.[44]

CYSTIC LESIONS

Various types of cystic lesions may occur in the orbit (Box 12-1). Most cystic lesions share the common features of smooth contour, round to oval shape, sharp outline, and absence of internal vascularity. As a result, these lesions usually can be easily differentiated from solid tumors.

Dermoid Cyst

The most common orbital cyst is the dermoid, which usually occurs supratemporally or supranasally.[27] These lesions may be located superficially within the lid, at the orbital rim, on the conjunctiva, or within the orbit.

Superficial dermoids most often occur in infants or young children.[50] When a superficial lesion is present, echography may be useful to determine whether it extends posteriorly into the orbit (Figure 12-30).

When dermoids are situated deeper in the orbit, they may not become apparent until later in childhood or early in adulthood.[50] These more posterior cysts may become very large and can erode the adjacent bony wall[27] (Figure 12-31). In other cases, they may actually extend through a small solitary bone defect into adjacent cavities, most often into the temporalis fossa.

Dermoid cysts can be filled with various substances, such as keratin, sebaceous materials, hair follicles, and inflammatory cells.[56] Since their contents are so variable, these lesions can produce many different quantitative characteristics.[12] In general, however, dermoid cysts are predominantly high

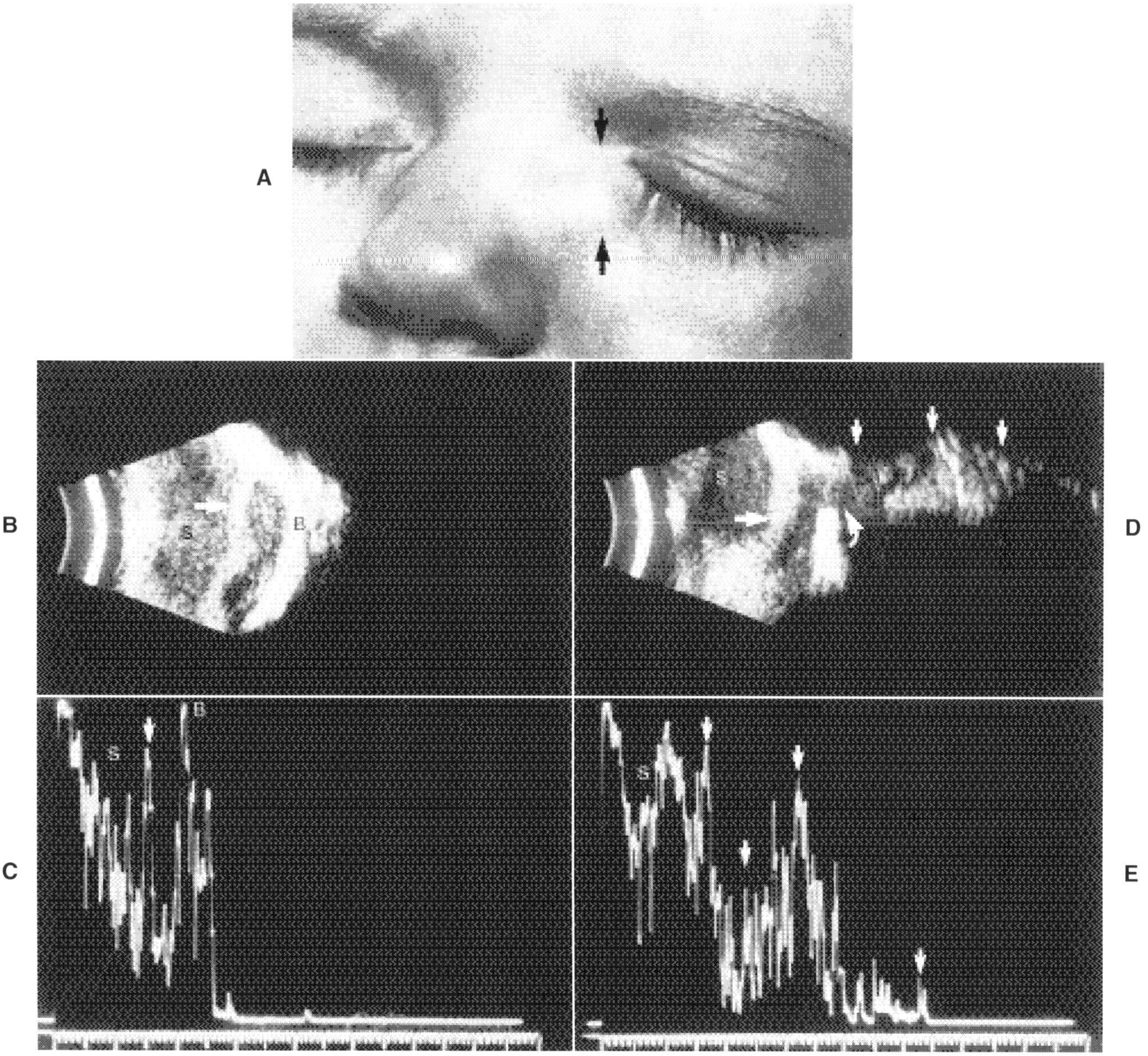

Figure 12-28 Dacryocystitis in newborn. **A,** External photograph shows swelling in region of left lacrimal sac *(arrows)*. Paraocular echograms show dilated sac *(S)*. **B,** Transverse B-scan shows mucous fluid layer *(arrow)* within sac. *B,* Lacrimal bone. **C,** Corresponding A-scan shows medium-high reflectivity of mucus within sac and high reflective spike from surface of layered mucus. **D,** B-scan with probe angled slightly inferiorly shows opening of nasolacrimal duct *(curved arrow)*. Note the layered mucus overlying opening of duct. Chain of echoes *(small arrows)* originates from nasolacrimal duct. **E,** Corresponding A-scan shows medium-high internal reflectivity of sac and chain of spikes from within nasolacrimal duct.

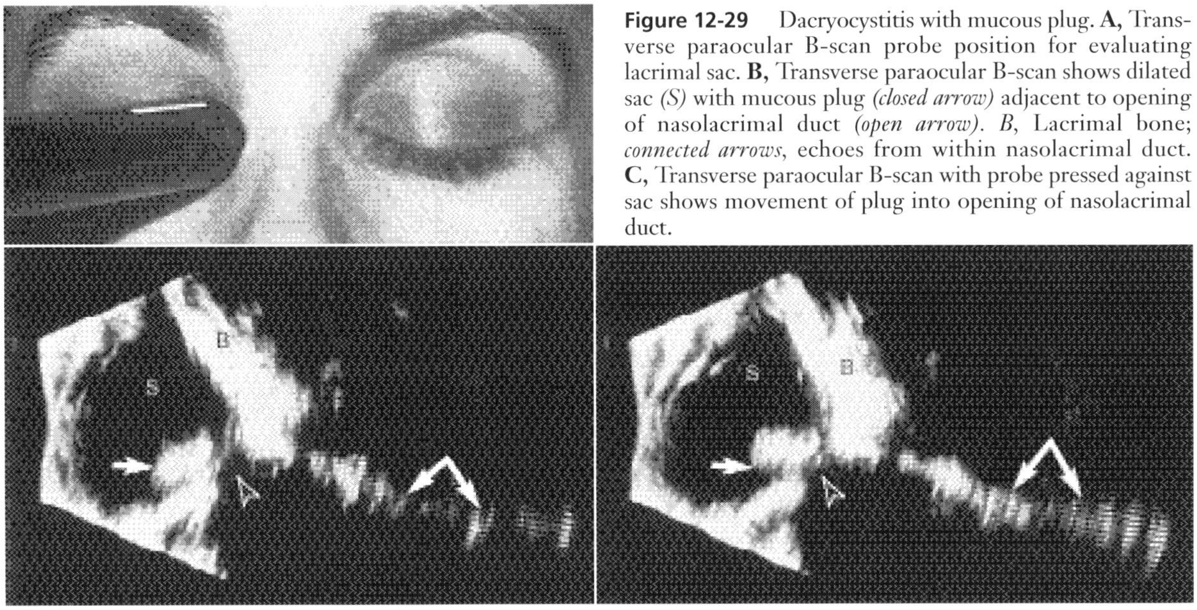

Figure 12-29 Dacryocystitis with mucous plug. **A,** Transverse paraocular B-scan probe position for evaluating lacrimal sac. **B,** Transverse paraocular B-scan shows dilated sac *(S)* with mucous plug *(closed arrow)* adjacent to opening of nasolacrimal duct *(open arrow)*. *B,* Lacrimal bone; *connected arrows,* echoes from within nasolacrimal duct. **C,** Transverse paraocular B-scan with probe pressed against sac shows movement of plug into opening of nasolacrimal duct.

BOX 12-1

Orbital Cystic Lesions

Dermoid cyst
Epidermoid cyst
Dermolipoma
Epithelial inclusion cyst
Hematic cyst
Microphthalmos with cyst
Congenital cystic eye (anophthalmos with cyst)
Teratoma
Lacrimal ductal cyst (see lacrimal gland)
Mucocele (see p 452)

reflective with slightly irregular internal structure. Some dermoids produce marked sound attenuation, whereas others attenuate minimally. These lesions are usually firm to hard in consistency, but recurrent dermoids are typically compressible. Settling of liquid contents may be appreciable in some cases. When located in the lacrimal gland region, a dermoid cyst sometimes can be difficult to distinguish from a benign mixed tumor of the lacrimal gland.

Epidermoid Cyst

Histopathologically, epidermoid cysts differ only slightly from dermoids in that their walls do not contain adnexal structures.[27] Therefore, these two lesions usually cannot be distinguished from one another echographically. One patient with bilateral biopsy-proven epidermoid cysts has been evaluated by the authors.[31] Both lesions were oval and located within the upper lid. They exhibited moderately irregular internal structure with variable reflectivity and sound attenuation (Figure 12-32). These cysts were soft and nonvascular, and aftermovement of the mobile internal lesion echoes was observed.

Dermolipoma

Dermolipomas are fat-filled lesions and thus may be very difficult to distinguish from normal orbital soft tissue. These lesions demonstrate extremely high reflectivity, are often compressible, and are nonvascular (Figure 12-33). If large enough, the cyst wall may be shown as a highly reflective posterior border spike.

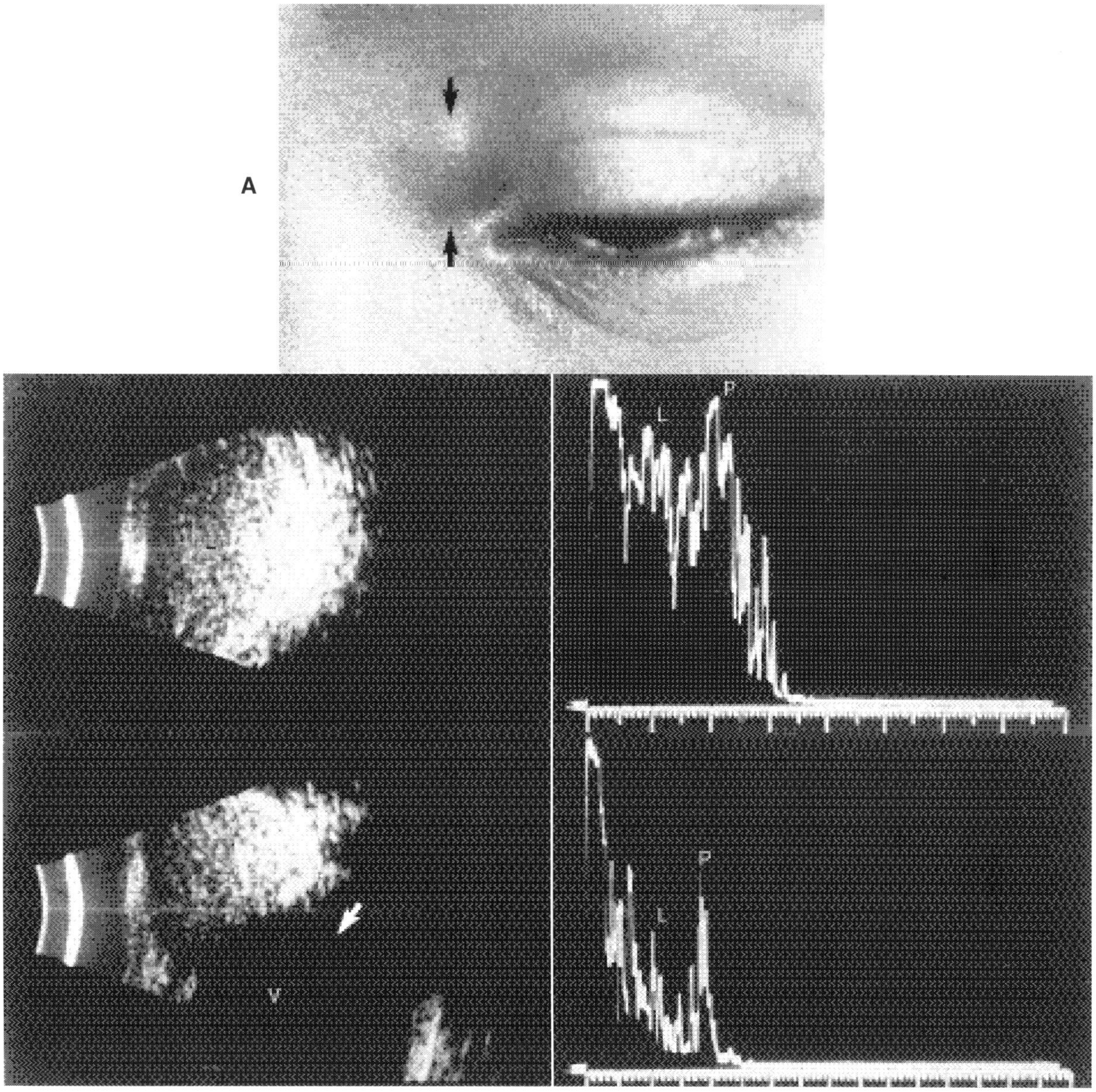

Figure 12-30 Superficial dermoid cyst. **A,** External photograph shows swelling of nasal aspect of left upper lid. Paraocular echograms show lesion *(L)* in anterior orbit. **B,** Transverse B-scan shows very echo-dense lesion. **C,** Longitudinal B-scan shows echo-dense lesion anteriorly adjacent to globe. *V,* Vitreous cavity; *arrow,* area of globe wall not shown well because of edge artifact. **D,** A-scan at Tissue Sensitivity shows high internal reflectivity and highly reflective posterior surface spike *(P)* from cyst wall. **E,** A-scan at reduced sensitivity setting shows distinct nature of posterior surface spike.

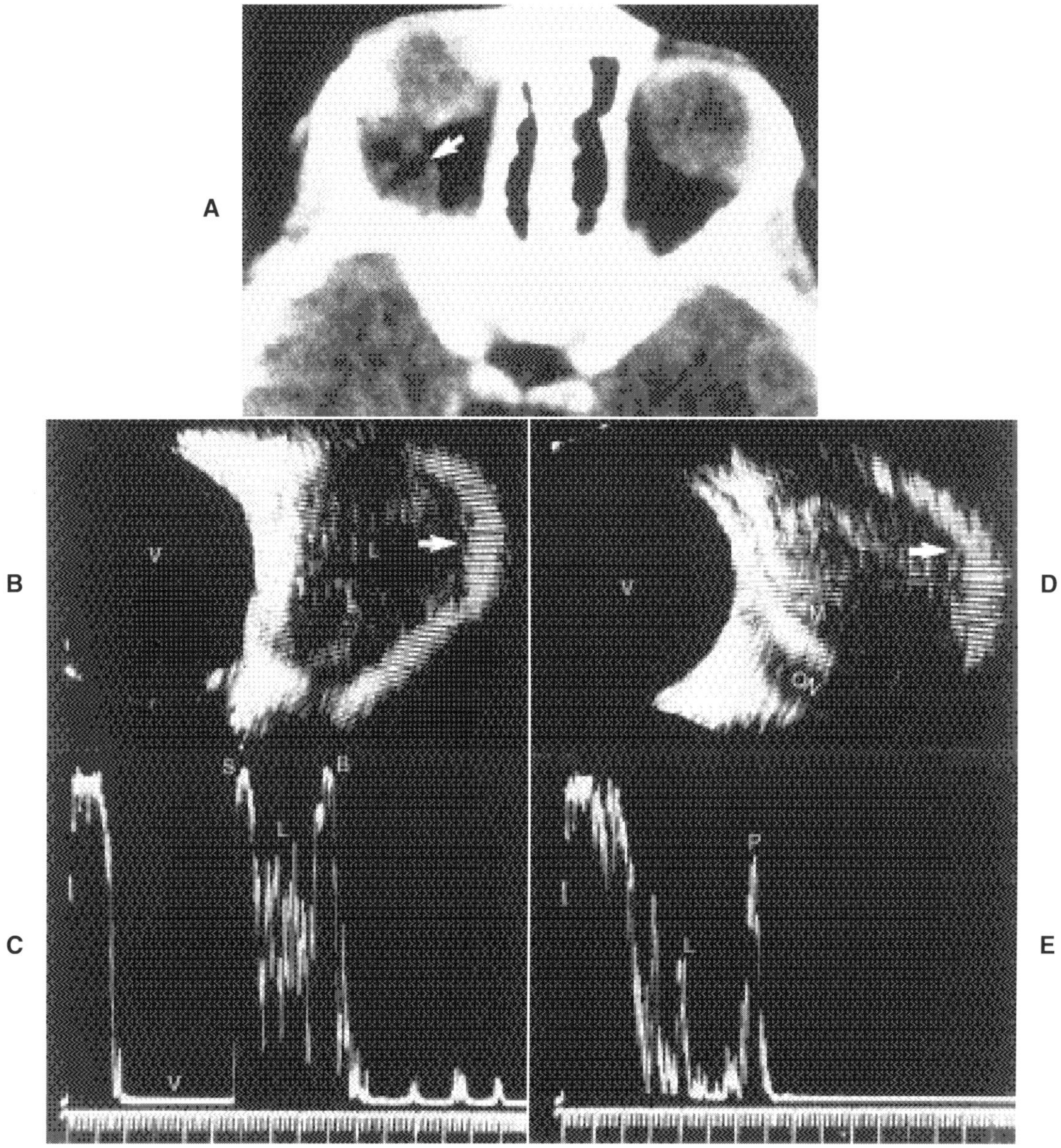

Figure 12-31 Deep dermoid cyst. **A,** Axial CT scan shows large retrobulbar mass *(arrow)* along lateral orbital wall (note mild bony excavation). Transocular (**B** to **D**) and paraocular (**E**) echograms show large orbital lesion *(L)*. **B,** Transverse B-scan displays well-circumscribed mass with excavation of bone *(arrow)*. *V,* Vitreous cavity. **C,** A-scan shows medium-high internal reflectivity. *S,* Sclera; *B,* bone. **D,** Longitudinal B-scan shows well-circumscribed lesion extending into posterior orbit between lateral rectus muscle *(M)* and slightly excavated bone *(arrow)*. Note displacement of optic nerve *(ON)*. **E,** Paraocular A-scan shows more irregular internal structure and strong sound attenuation in this view. Note that posterior surface spike *(P)* from cyst wall is reduced in height as a result of sound attenuation.

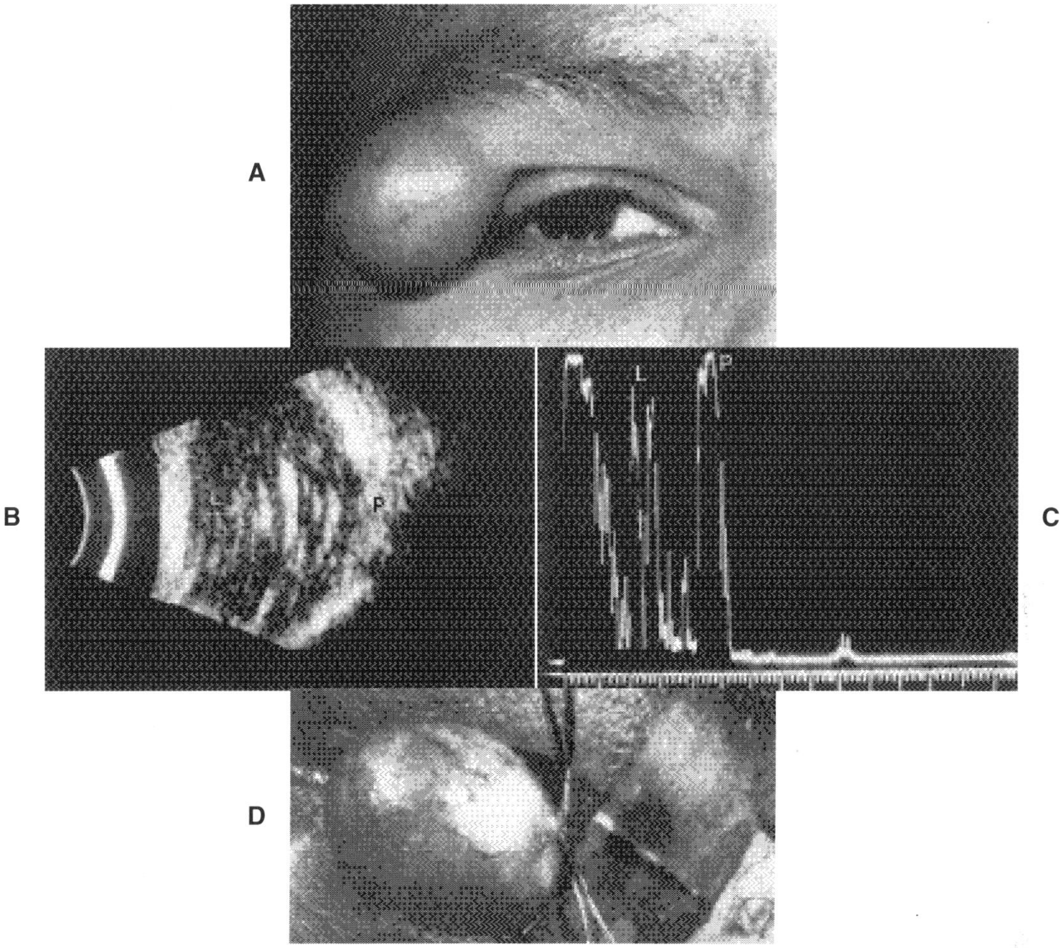

Figure 12-32 Epidermoid cyst. **A,** External photograph shows patient with upper lid swelling supratemporally. **B,** Paraocular transverse B-scan echogram shows well-circumscribed lesion *(L)* with heterogeneous contents. *P,* Posterior border of encapsulated lesion. **C,** Paraocular A-scan echogram of lesion shows irregular internal structure with high spikes from keratin debris within the cyst. Note steeply rising, high double-peaked posterior surface spike from encapsulated lesion. **D,** Photograph shows encapsulated cyst as it was excised from the right upper lid. Histopathologically, this lesion was filled with keratinous material. (Clinical photographs courtesy Dr. Jan Kronish, Delray Beach, Florida.)

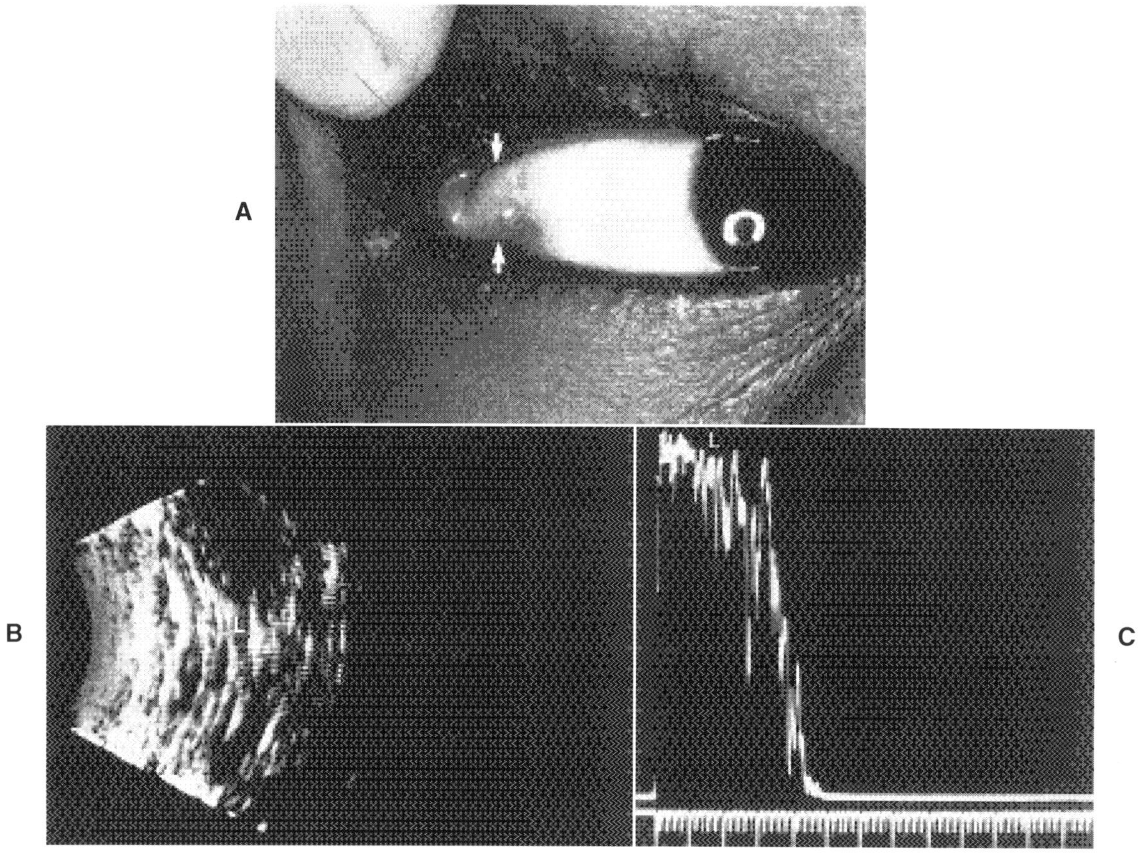

Figure 12-33 Dermolipoma of conjunctiva and orbit. **A,** External photograph showing subconjunctival lesion on temporal aspect of right globe *(arrows)*. **B,** Transverse B-scan echogram displays echo-dense lesion *(L)*. **C,** Paraocular A-scan with probe placed directly on mass shows high internal reflectivity of lesion similar to normal orbital soft tissue.

Epithelial Cyst

Epithelial cysts can arise from conjunctiva and may occur within the orbit. They are usually secondary to previous trauma or surgery where conjunctival or cutaneous epithelium has been inadvertently implanted in the orbit.[32] Less commonly, these lesions are of congenital origin.[56]

These lesions are round with smooth contour and are very well outlined. They are filled with serous fluid or other homogeneous liquid contents and so are very low reflective (Figure 12-34). Epithelial cysts are nonvascular and are typically quite soft. These lesions have been detected anterior to an orbital implant following enucleation (Figure 12-35, *A* and *B*).

Hematic Cyst (Cholesterol Granuloma)

Hematic cyst appears to occur following longstanding subperiosteal hemorrhage.[30] These cysts are located beneath the periosteum in the superior, more temporal aspect of the orbit and are associated with a well-demarcated, solitary bone defect. They are well circumscribed and have a round or oval configuration. The internal reflectivity is generally low, but higher reflective clumps of mobile cholesterol debris sometimes can be identified (Figure 12-36; see also p 37).

Microphthalmos with Cyst

Microphthalmos with cyst results from failure of the fetal fissure to close and is therefore present at birth.[50] The globe is usually deformed and microphthalmic. When these cysts are large and extend anteriorly, they tend to be bluish-gray and to transilluminate well.[56] Large cysts are most often located inferiorly and thus displace the globe upward.

Echographically, the cyst usually appears to be attached to the globe wall. It may communicate directly with the globe or it may be separated from the globe by a thin membrane. These cysts are typically very low reflective; have smooth, round contour; and are very well outlined[22] (Figure 12-37). Additionally, they have a soft consistency and are nonvascular.

Anophthalmos/Congenital Cystic Eye (Anophthalmos With Cyst)

Anophthalmos is a developmental anomaly in which the eye is absent at birth.[15] In these cases, echography shows the or-

Text continued on p 345.

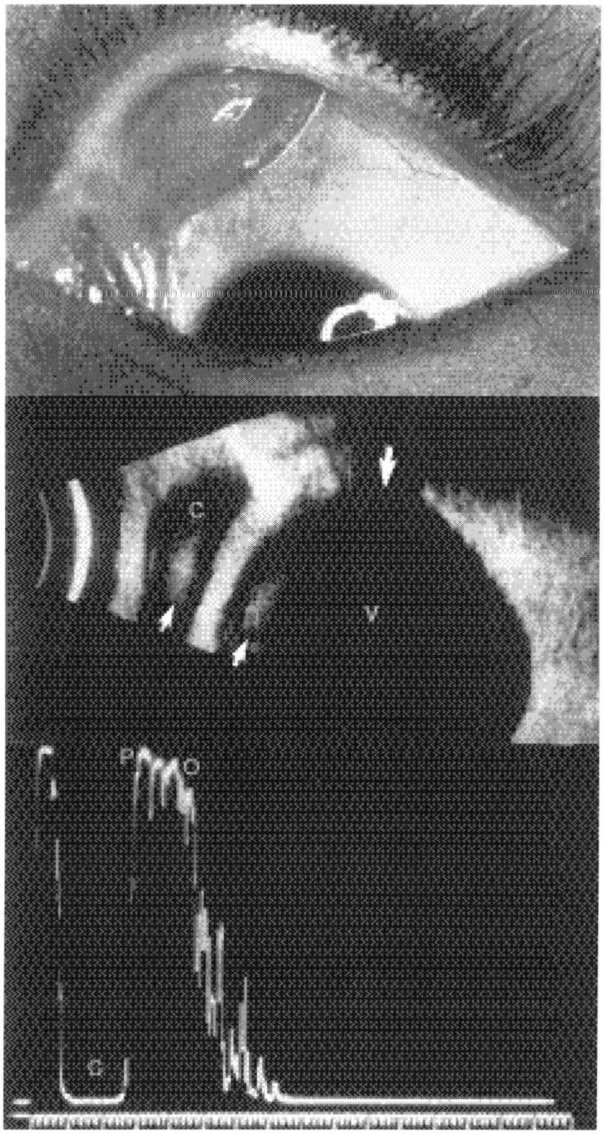

Figure 12-34 Conjunctival epithelial cyst. **A,** External photograph shows cystic lesion in fornix supranasally. **B,** Longitudinal paraocular B-scan echogram shows very well-outlined, echolucent cyst *(C)* along anterior aspect of globe. *V,* Vitreous cavity; *small arrows,* multiple signals within cyst and vitreous cavity; *large arrow,* area of globe wall not shown well because of edge artifact. **C,** Paraocular A-scan shows very low reflective, well-outlined cyst. Note steeply rising, smooth posterior surface spike *(P)* of this encapsulated cyst. *O,* Normal orbital soft tissue behind lesion.

A

B

C

D

E

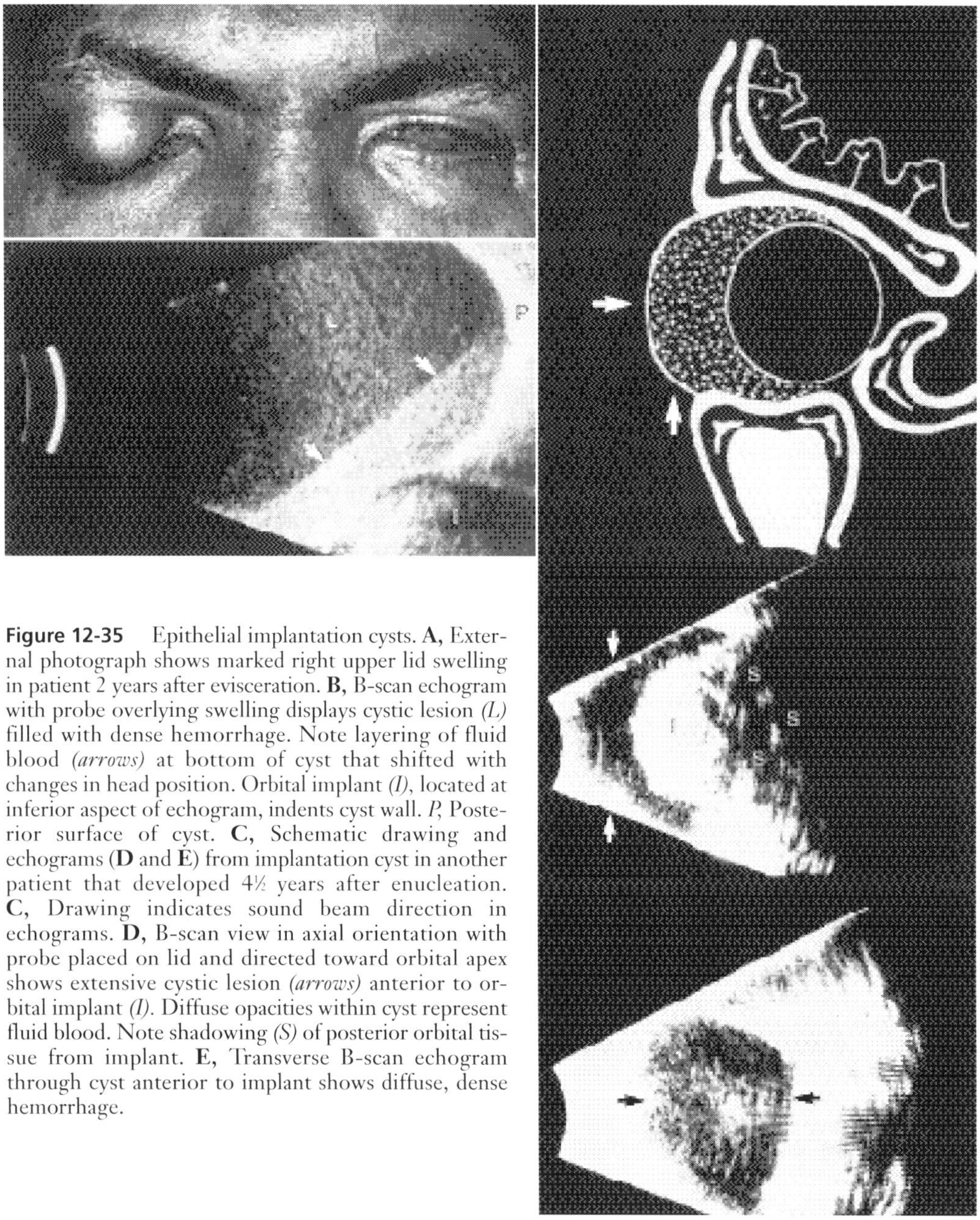

Figure 12-35 Epithelial implantation cysts. **A,** External photograph shows marked right upper lid swelling in patient 2 years after evisceration. **B,** B-scan echogram with probe overlying swelling displays cystic lesion *(L)* filled with dense hemorrhage. Note layering of fluid blood *(arrows)* at bottom of cyst that shifted with changes in head position. Orbital implant *(I)*, located at inferior aspect of echogram, indents cyst wall. *P,* Posterior surface of cyst. **C,** Schematic drawing and echograms (**D** and **E**) from implantation cyst in another patient that developed 4½ years after enucleation. **C,** Drawing indicates sound beam direction in echograms. **D,** B-scan view in axial orientation with probe placed on lid and directed toward orbital apex shows extensive cystic lesion *(arrows)* anterior to orbital implant *(I)*. Diffuse opacities within cyst represent fluid blood. Note shadowing *(S)* of posterior orbital tissue from implant. **E,** Transverse B-scan echogram through cyst anterior to implant shows diffuse, dense hemorrhage.

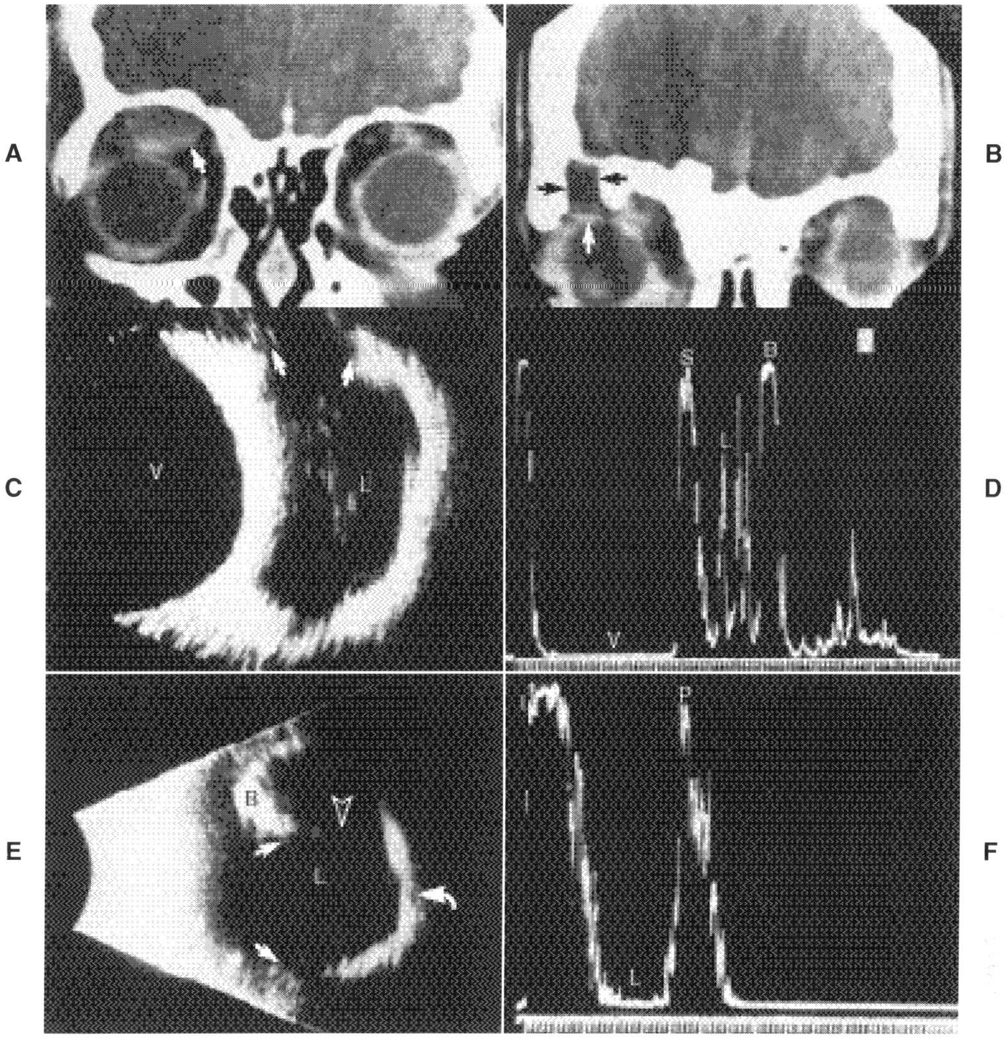

Figure 12-36 Hematic cyst. **A,** Coronal CT scan posterior to bone defect shows smooth mass along roof of orbit *(arrow)*. **B,** Very anterior coronal CT scan shows large bone defect in roof of orbit *(arrows)*. Transocular (**C** and **D**) and paraocular (**E** and **F**) echograms show orbital lesion *(L)* associated with large bone defect supratemporally. **C,** Oblique transverse B-scan view through anterior aspect of supratemporal orbit displays extensive subperiosteal mass with bone defect. *V,* Vitreous cavity; *arrows,* edges of bone defect. **D,** A-scan shows low reflectivity of the lesion with a few higher spikes from large clumps of cholesterol debris (i.e., slightly irregular internal structure). *V,* Vitreous cavity; *S,* sclera; *B,* bone. **E,** Transverse paraocular B-scan shows lesion extending from orbit through large defect in orbital roof *(closed straight arrows)*. *B,* Orbital bone; *open arrow,* bone not shown in this area due to edge artifact; *curved arrow,* layer of bone at base of defect. **F,** Paraocular A-scan shows very low reflectivity of lesion in this view and smooth, high, double-peaked posterior surface spike *(P)* from the cyst wall. *I,* Initial spike.

A

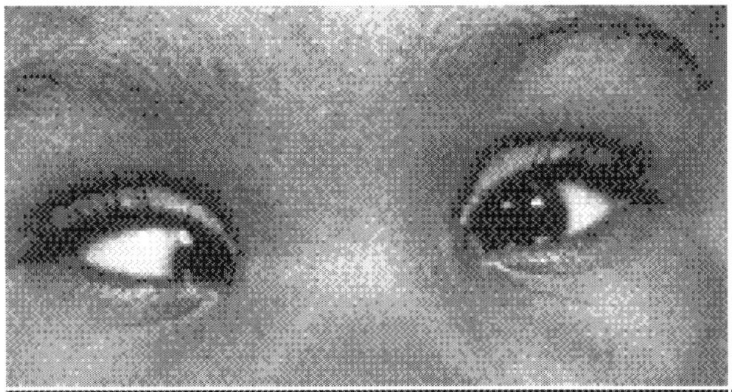

Figure 12-37 Microphthalmos with cyst. **A,** External photograph shows small, esotropic right eye with leukokoria. **B,** Axial B-scan echogram displays small, microphthalmic globe with large echolucent orbital cyst *(C)*. *P*, Posterior lens capsule; *V*, vitreous cavity. **C,** Transverse A-scan shows large, very low reflective cyst posterior to globe. *S*, Sclera; *B*, orbital bone.

B

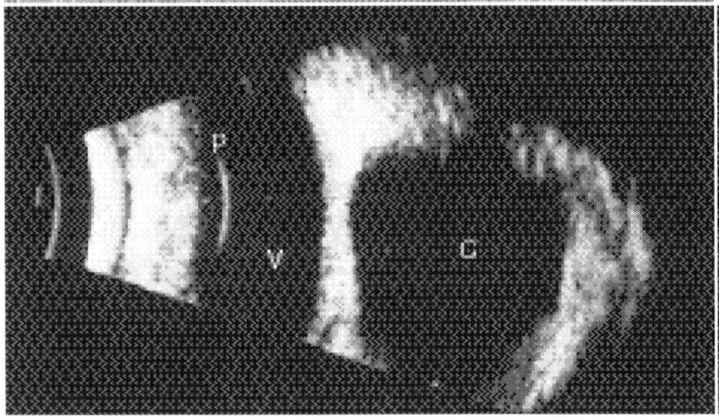

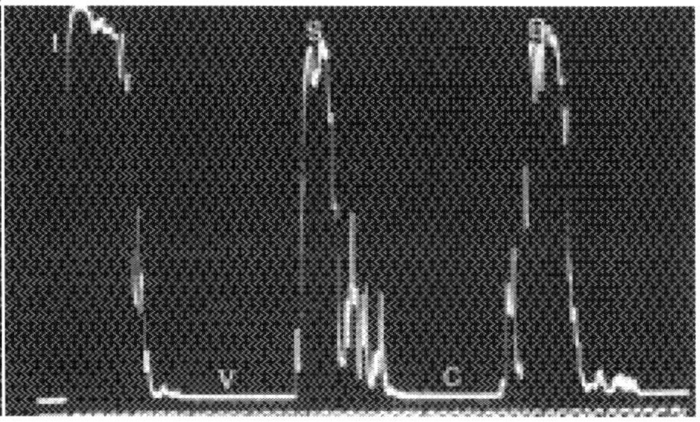

C

A

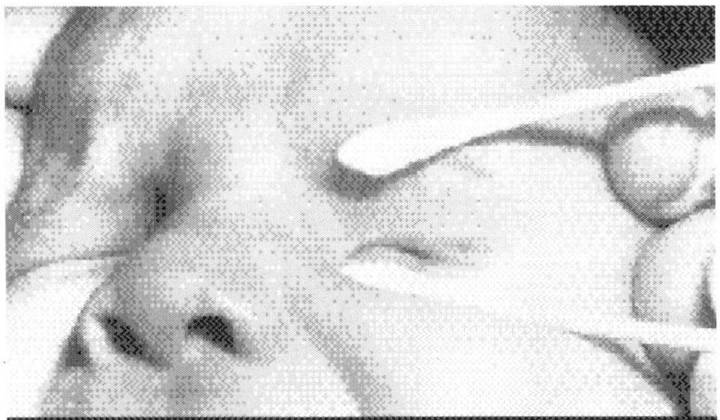

Figure 12-38 Anophthalmos. **A,** External photograph shows newborn whose globes are not detectable clinically. Echograms were obtained with probes placed on lid and sound beam directed toward apex of orbit. B-scan **(B)** and A-scan **(C)** show normal orbital soft tissue *(O)* and no evidence of formed globe. *I*, Initial line (B-scan) and spike (A-scan).

B

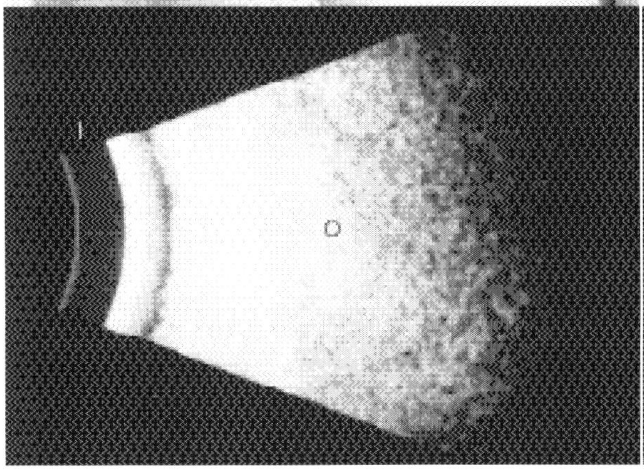

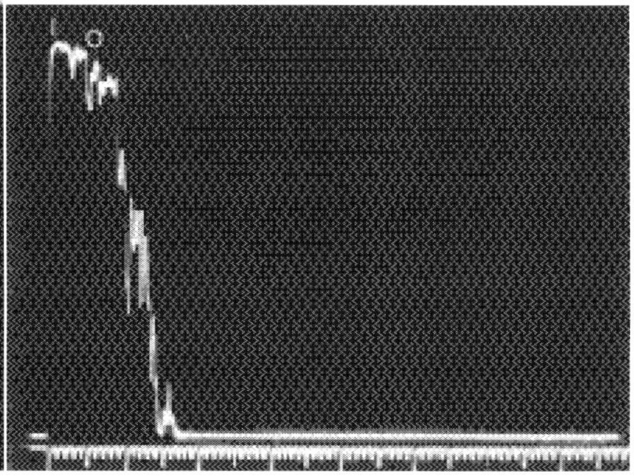

C

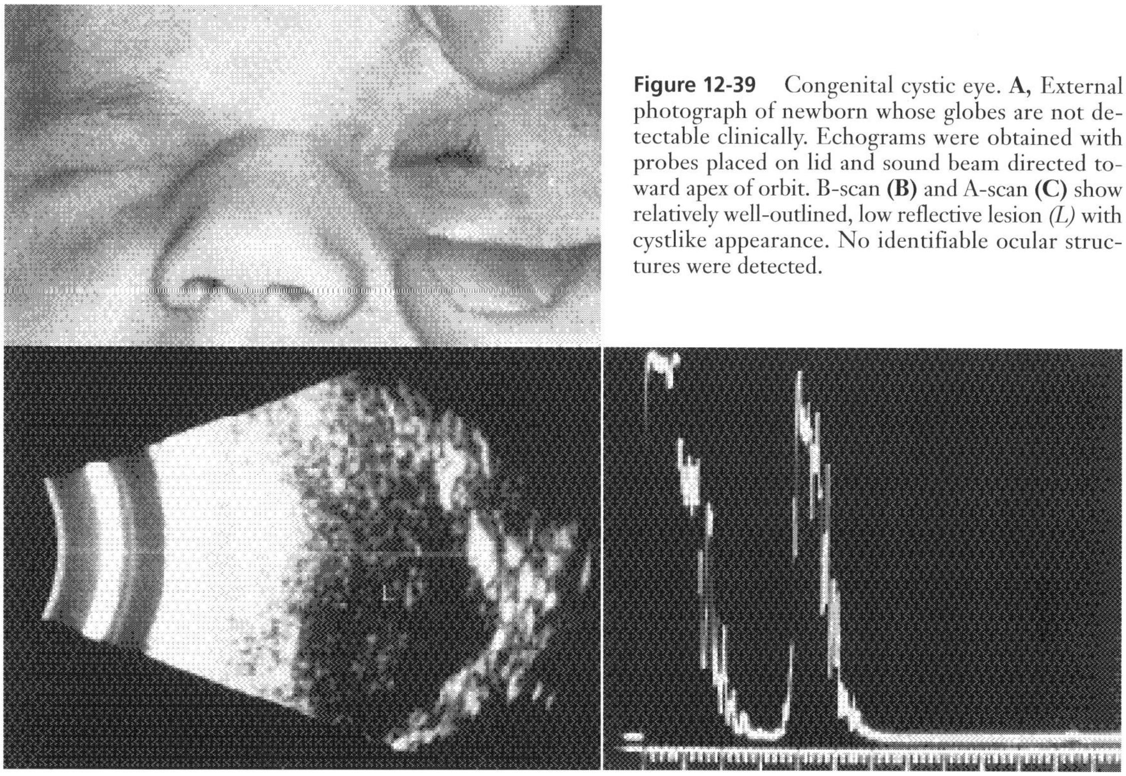

Figure 12-39 Congenital cystic eye. **A,** External photograph of newborn whose globes are not detectable clinically. Echograms were obtained with probes placed on lid and sound beam directed toward apex of orbit. B-scan **(B)** and A-scan **(C)** show relatively well-outlined, low reflective lesion *(L)* with cystlike appearance. No identifiable ocular structures were detected.

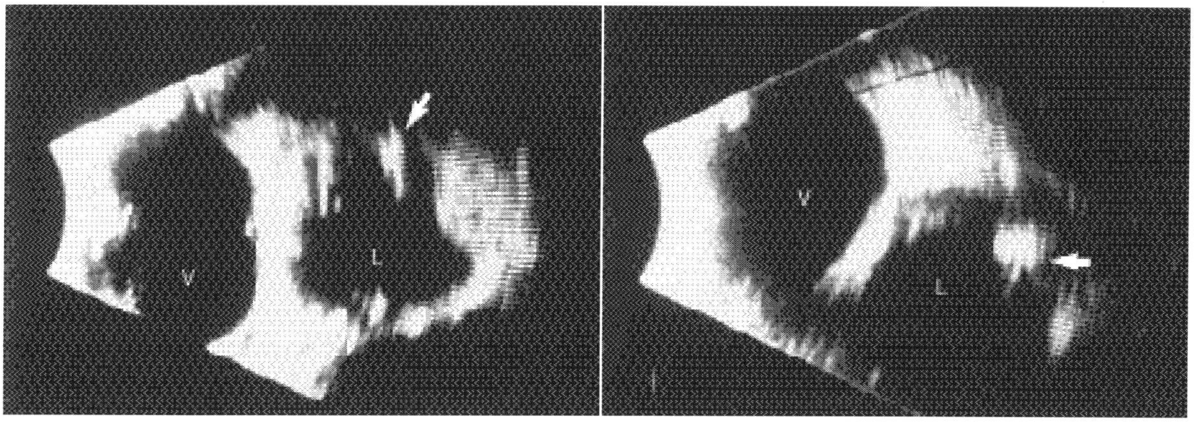

Figure 12-40 Teratoma in newborn. B-scan echograms (**A** and **B**) show well-circumscribed, echolucent cystic lesion *(L)* in posterior orbit. *Arrow,* Calcified nodule within cyst; *V,* vitreous cavity.

bital cavity to be filled with normal-appearing highly reflective soft tissue, but a globe is not detected (Figure 12-38).

Congenital cystic eye is a term that denotes a vestige rather than total absence of an eye.[56] These cystic structures can vary in size and can be located superficially or situated deep within the orbit. When the cyst is visible clinically, it appears as a bluish-colored, soft mass. Echographically, a cystlike lesion is displayed that lacks identifiable ocular structures such as lens and optic nerve (Figure 12-39). In such cases, the extraocular muscles may or may not be detectable.

Teratoma

Teratoma is a congenital lesion that is present at birth.[56] The one case examined by the authors was very large, predominantly low reflective, and well outlined. The lesion also contained a highly reflective calcified nodule (Figure 12-40).

REFERENCES

1. Auran J, Jakobiec FA, Krebs W: Benign mixed tumor of the palpebral lobe of the lacrimal gland—clinical diagnosis and appropriate surgical management. *Ophthalmology* 1988;95:90.
2. Balchunas WR, Quencer RM, Byrne SF: Lacrimal gland and fossa

masses: Evaluation by computed tomography and A-mode echography. *Radiology* 1983;149:751.
3. Bellone G, Gallenga PE: Echography of mixed tumours of the lacrimal gland. *Ophthalmologica* 1973;166:156.
4. Berges O, Vignaud J, Aubin ML: Comparison of sonography and computed tomography in the study of orbital space-occupying lesions. *AJNR* 1984;5:247.
5. Bergin DJ, Parmley V: Orbital neurilemoma. *Arch Ophthalmol* 1988;106:414.
6. Blodi F, Ossoinig KC: Modern diagnosis of orbital tumors, in *Symposium on Diseases and Surgery of the Lids, Lacrimal Apparatus and Orbit.* St Louis, Mosby, 1982, p 129.
7. Bradbury JA, Rennie IG, Parsons MA: Adrenaline dacryolith: Detection by ultrasound examination of the nasolacrimal duct. *Br J Ophthalmol* 1988;72:935.
8. Bullock JD, Fleishman JA, Rosset JS: Lacrimal ductal cysts. *Ophthalmology* 1986;93:1355.
9. Byrne BM, van Heuven WA, Lawton AW: Echographic characteristics of benign orbital schwannomas (neurilemmomas). *Am J Ophthalmol* 1988;106:195.
10. Byrne SF: Standardized echography in the differentiation of orbital lesions. *Surv Ophthalmol* 1984;29:226.
11. Byrne SF, Byrne BM: Differential diagnosis of orbital neurilemmoma (schwannoma) with standardized echography, in Ossoinig KC (ed): *Ophthalmic Echography.* Dordrecht, Dr W Junk, 1987, p 491.
12. Byrne SF, Hughes JR: Orbital dermoid cysts, in Ossoinig KC (ed): *Ophthalmic Echography.* Dordrecht, Dr W Junk, 1987, p 465.
13. Coleman DJ: Modern examination methods of orbital disease. Orbital ultrasonic tomography (B-scan). *Trans Am Acad Ophthalmol Otolaryngol* 1974;78:577.
14. Dallow RL: Ultrasonography of the orbit. *Int Ophthalmol Clin* 1986;26(3):51.
15. Day S: Disorders of the eye as a whole, in Taylor D (ed): *Pediatric Ophthalmology.* Boston, Blackwell Scientific Publications, 1990, p 135.
16. Divine RD, Anderson RL, Ossoinig KC: Metastatic carcinoid unresponsive to radiation therapy presenting as a lacrimal fossa mass. *Ophthalmology* 1982;89:516.
17. Duke-Elder SS, Macfaul PA: In Duke-Elder SS (ed): *System of Ophthalmology: The Ocular Adnexa.* St Louis, Mosby, 1974, p 738.
18. Dutton JJ: Standardized echography in the diagnosis of lacrimal drainage dysfunction. *Arch Ophthalmol* 1989;107:1010.
19. Dutton JJ, Byrne SF, Proia AD: *Diagnostic Atlas of Orbital Diseases.* Philadelphia, WB Saunders Co, 2000.
20. Farah ME, Byrne SF, Hughes JR: Standardized echography in uveal melanomas with scleral or extraocular extension. *Arch Ophthalmol* 1984;102:1482.
21. Feldon SE, Sigelman J, Albert DM, et al: Clinical manifestations of brawny scleritis. *Am J Ophthalmol* 1978;85:781.
22. Fisher YL: Microphthalmus with ocular communicating orbital cyst—ultrasonic diagnosis. *Ophthalmology* 1978;85:1208.
23. Font RL: Eyelids and lacrimal drainage system, in Spencer WH: *Ophthalmic Pathology: An Atlas and Textbook*, ed 3, Philadelphia, WB Saunders Co, 1986, p 2314.
24. Goes F: Ultrasonographic and clinical characteristics of orbital pseudotumors, in Ossoinig KC (ed): *Ophthalmic Echography.* Dordrecht, Dr W Junk, 1987, p 499.
25. Green RL: Echographic diagnosis of posterior scleritis, in Ossoinig KC (ed): *Ophthalmic Echography.* Dordrecht, Dr W Junk, 1987, p 515.
26. Harrie RP: Standardized echography of the orbit (review), in Ossoinig KC (ed): *Ophthalmic Echography.* Dordrecht, Dr W Junk, 1987, p 445.
27. Jakobiec FA, Font RL: Orbit, in Spencer W: *Ophthalmic Pathology: An Atlas and Textbook*, ed 3, Philadelphia, WB Saunders Co, 1986, p 2459.
28. Kennerdell JS, Dresner SC: The nonspecific orbital inflammatory syndromes. *Surv Ophthalmol* 1984;29:93.
29. Kerman BM, Fishman ML: Orbital malignant melanoma with ipsilateral intraocular pathology, in Ossoinig KC (ed): *Ophthalmic Echography.* Dordrecht, Dr W Junk, 1987, p 477.
30. Kersten RC, Kersten JL, Bloom HR, et al: Chronic hematic cyst of the orbit: Role of magnetic resonance imaging in diagnosis. *Ophthalmology* 1988;95:1551.
31. Kronish JW, Sneed SR, Tse DT: Epidermal cysts of the eyelid. *Arch Ophthalmol* 1988;106:270.
32. McCarthy RW, Beyer CK, Dallow RL, et al: Conjunctival cysts of the orbit following enucleation. *Ophthalmology* 1981;88:30.
33. Mottow-Lippa L, Jakobiec FA, Smith M: Idiopathic inflammatory orbital pseudotumor in childhood. Results of diagnostic tests and biopsies. *Ophthalmology* 1981;88:565.
34. Ossoinig KC: Quantitative echography—the basis of tissue differentiation. *J Clin Ultrasound* 1974;2:41.
35. Ossoinig KC: A-scan echography and orbital disease. *Mod Probl Ophthalmol* 1975;14:203.
36. Ossoinig K: Echography of the eye, orbit, and periorbital region, in Arger PH (ed): *Orbit Roentgenology.* New York, John Wiley & Sons, 1977, p 224.
37. Ossoinig K: The role of clinical echography in modern diagnosis of periorbital and orbital lesions, in Bleeker G (ed): *Proceedings of the 3rd International Symposium on Orbital Disorders.* Amsterdam, Dr W Junk, 1977, p 496.
38. Ossoinig KC: Standardized echography: Basic principles, clinical applications and results. *Int Ophthalmol Clin* 1979;19(4):127.
39. *Ossoinig KC: Standardized Ophthalmic Echography of the Eye, Orbit and Periorbital Region. A Comprehensive Slide Set and Study Guide*, ed 3. Iowa City, Goodfellow, 1985, p 47.
40. Ossoinig KC: Preoperative differential diagnosis of tumors with echography. IV: Diagnosis of orbital tumors, in Blodi FC (ed): *Current Concepts in Ophthalmology*, vol 14. St Louis, Mosby, 1974, p 313.
41. Ossoinig KC, Tamayo G: Ultrasonic differential diagnosis of lacrimal-gland tumors. *J Ultrasound Med* 1985;4(suppl):52.
42. Parks SL, Glover AT: Benign mixed tumors arising in the palpebral lobe of the lacrimal gland. *Ophthalmology* 1990;97:526.
43. Rochels R, Nover A: Small choroidal melanoma with diffuse orbital involvement detected and differentiated with standardized echography—with special reference to the reliability of sonography in predicting scleral tumoral infiltration. *Ophthalmologica* 1986;192:39.
44. Rochels R, Scherer U, Nover A, et al: Echographical diagnosis of lacrimal sac tumors, in Ossoinig KC (ed): *Ophthalmic Echography.* Dordrecht, Dr W Junk, 1987, p 551.
45. Rootman J: Inflammatory diseases, in Rootman J: *Diseases of the Orbit.* Philadelphia, JB Lippincott Co, 1988, p 159.
46. Rootman J: Secondary tumors of the orbit, in Rootman J: *Diseases of the Orbit.* Philadelphia, JB Lippincott Co, 1988, p 427.
47. Rootman J, Chan KW: Metastatic and secondary tumors of the orbit, in Rootman J: *Diseases of the Orbit.* Philadelphia, JB Lippincott Co, 1988, p 426.
48. Rootman J, Chan KW: Striated muscle tumors, in Rootman J: *Diseases of the Orbit.* Philadelphia, JB Lippincott Co, 1988, p 335.
49. Rootman J, Dolman P: Carcinoma and pleomorphic adenoma, in Rootman J: *Diseases of the Orbit.* Philadelphia, JB Lippincott Co, 1988, p 403.
50. Rootman J, Lapointe JS: Structural lesions, in Rootman J: *Diseases of the Orbit.* Philadelphia, JB Lippincott Co, 1988, p 481.
51. Rootman J, Lapointe JS: Tumors of the lacrimal gland, in Rootman J: *Diseases of the Orbit.* Philadelphia, JB Lippincott Co, 1988, p 386.
52. Rootman J, Robertson WD: Neurogenic tumors, in Rootman J: *Diseases of the Orbit.* Philadelphia, JB Lippincott Co, 1988, p 319.
53. Rootman J, Robertson W, Lapointe JS: Inflammatory diseases, in Rootman J: *Diseases of the Orbit.* Philadelphia, JB Lippincott Co, 1988, p 172.
54. Scott WE, Fabre JA, Ossoinig KC: Congenital mucocele of the lacrimal sac. *Arch Ophthalmol* 1979;97:1658.
55. Shammas HJ: *Atlas of Ophthalmic Ultrasonography and Biometry.* St Louis, Mosby, 1980.
56. Shields JA: *Diagnosis and Management of Orbital Tumors.* Philadelphia, WB Saunders Co, 1989.
57. Sofinski SJ, Brown BZ, Rao N, et al: Mucoepidermoid carcinoma of the lacrimal gland: Case report and review of the literature. *Ophthalmic Plast Reconstr Surg* 1990;2:148.

William D. Bates

13 Vascular Lesions

Lesions of vascular origin are among the most common orbital abnormalities encountered in echography. In most cases, because of their distinct anatomy and histologic architecture, they can be easily detected and differentiated with Standardized Echography.[2-4,7,13-16]

Color Doppler imaging[10] can also be used to further evaluate these types of lesions (see Chapter 14). Vascular lesions of the orbit are divided into two main groups: neoplasms and malformations[8] (Box 13-1).

VASCULAR NEOPLASMS

Vascular neoplasms commonly occur in both children and adults. Specific echographic criteria are used to differentiate many of these lesions (Table 13-1).

Cavernous Hemangioma

Cavernous hemangiomas are one of the most common tumors in adults.[23] The histologic architecture is heterogeneous because of the multiple blood-filled vascular channels that comprise the tumor. The vascular channels are filled with relatively stagnant blood, and the walls that form the vascular spaces are relatively large interfaces, resulting in high reflectivity.[4,14,18] These highly reflective lesions have regular internal structure and exhibit moderate sound attenuation (see Figure 11-24).

Cavernous hemangiomas are typically situated within the muscle cone, without attachment to the globe or other orbital structures (Figure 13-1). These tumors can become very large (Figure 13-2) and may cause mild flattening of the globe with choroidal folds,[8] but marked indentation of the ocular wall rarely occurs. The lack of significant indentation sometimes can be helpful in distinguishing hemangiomas from other more solid tumors, which often indent the globe to a greater extent. Also, hemangiomas can markedly displace the optic nerve (Figure 13-3).

Cavernous hemangiomas are round to oval and are very well outlined.[6] The capsule that surrounds the tumor produces a well-demarcated border on B-scan and a steeply rising, high posterior surface spike on A-scan (see Figure 13-1). Occasionally, a cavernous hemangioma may be found outside of the muscle cone or even within the lid (Figure 13-4).

Cavernous hemangiomas have a relatively firm consistency, although mild compressibility often can be demonstrated. Ossoinig describes the finding of "delayed compressibility" in these lesions.[15] Because the blood within the cavernous spaces is for the most part stagnant, they exhibit medium-high reflectivity and no internal vascularity[18] (see Color Plate 11). Occasionally, however, a hemangioma may contain mild blood flow within lower reflective cavernous spaces.

Capillary (Infantile) Hemangioma

These lesions can be apparent at birth or may become noticeable at a few months of age.[23] Like cavernous hemangiomas, capillary hemangiomas have very characteristic findings that, in most cases, make the echographic diagnosis straightforward.

The histologic architecture of these lesions is quite mixed. They are composed of capillary-sized blood vessels and endothelial cells, as well as large endothelium-lined ectatic spaces.[22] As a result, pathologists sometimes describe them as mixed capillary/cavernous hemangiomas.[8]

This varied histologic architecture can result in irregular internal structure, although reflectivity is usually high because of the predominance of dense capillaries. In some

BOX 13-1
Vascular Lesions

Neoplasms
- Cavernous hemangioma
- Capillary (infantile) hemangioma
- Lymphangioma
- Hemangiopericytoma

Vascular Malformations
- Carotid-cavernous sinus fistula
- Dural-cavernous sinus fistula
- Superior ophthalmic vein thrombosis
- Orbital varix
- Arteriovenous malformation
- Orbital aneurysm

TABLE 13-1

Differential Diagnosis of Vascular Neoplasms*

Tumor Type	Shape	Borders	Internal Reflectivity	Internal Structure	Sound Attenuation	Vascularity	Consistency
Cavernous hemangioma	Round/oval	Well outlined	High	Regular	Moderate	—	Firm/soft
Capillary hemangioma	Irregular	Poorly outlined	High	Irregular	Variable	+	Soft
Lymphangioma	Irregular	Poorly outlined	Low†	Irregular	Variable	—	Soft; firm (heme)
Hemangio-pericytoma	Round/oval	Well outlined	Medium	Regular	Moderate	+	Hard

*This table lists the main echographic findings for the most common vascular neoplasms of the orbit.
†This lesion is low reflective with highly reflective septi.

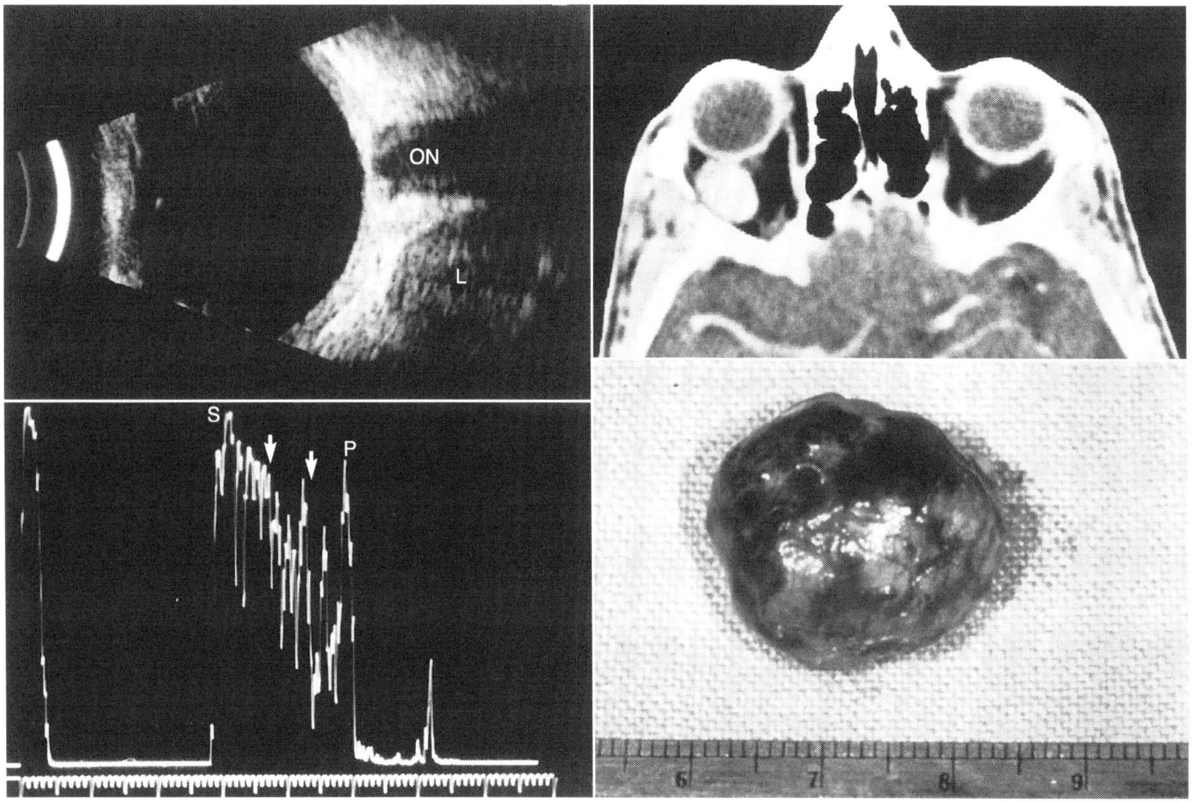

Figure 13-1 Small intraconal cavernous hemangioma. **A,** Horizontal axial B-scan echogram from aphakic eye shows oval-shaped lesion *(L)* situated temporal to optic nerve *(ON)*. **B,** Transocular A-scan echogram shows high reflectivity and moderate sound attenuation *(arrows)*. *P,* Posterior surface spike; *S,* sclera. **C,** Axial CT scan shows well-circumscribed intraconal mass. **D,** Gross pathologic specimen of encapsulated tumor.

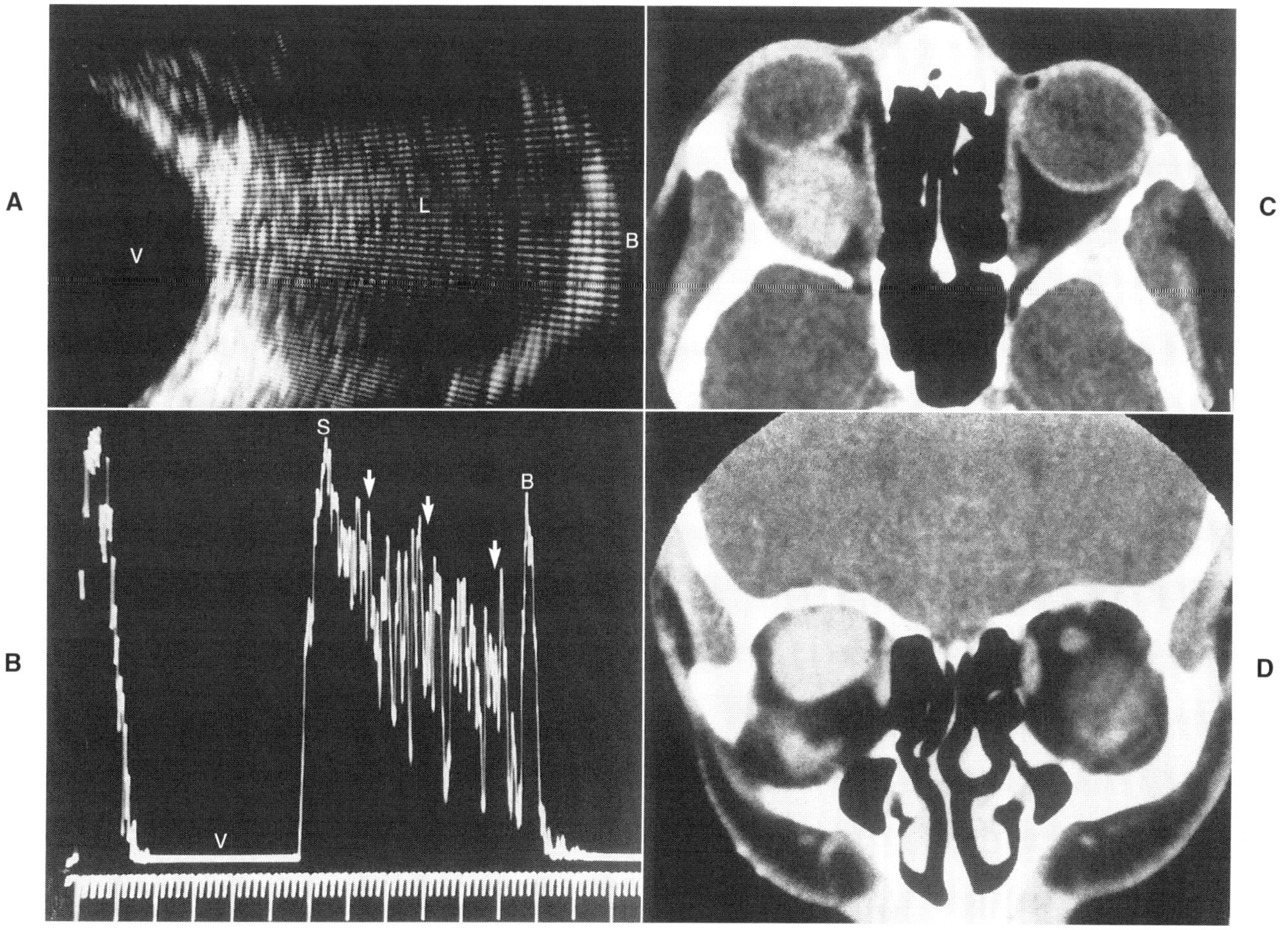

Figure 13-2 Large intraconal cavernous hemangioma. **A,** Transverse B-scan echogram shows oval lesion *(L)* situated between globe and orbital bone *(B)*. *V,* Vitreous cavity. **B,** Transocular A-scan shows high reflectivity and moderate sound attenuation *(arrows)*. *S,* Sclera. Axial **(C)** and coronal **(D)** CT scans demonstrate large orbital tumor in the right orbit.

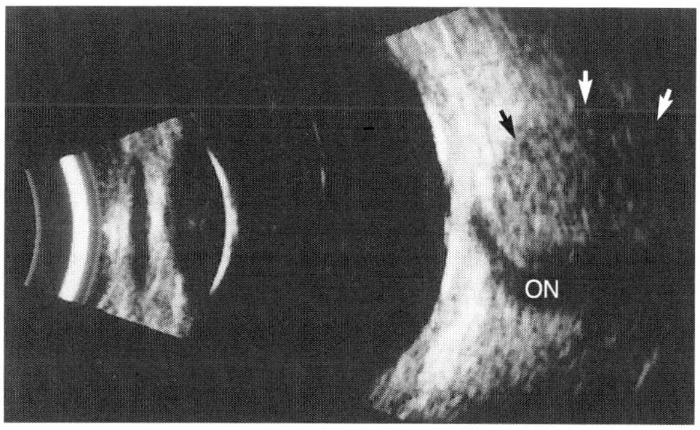

Figure 13-3 Vertical axial B-scan echogram shows cavernous hemangioma *(arrows)* displacing the optic nerve *(ON)* inferiorly.

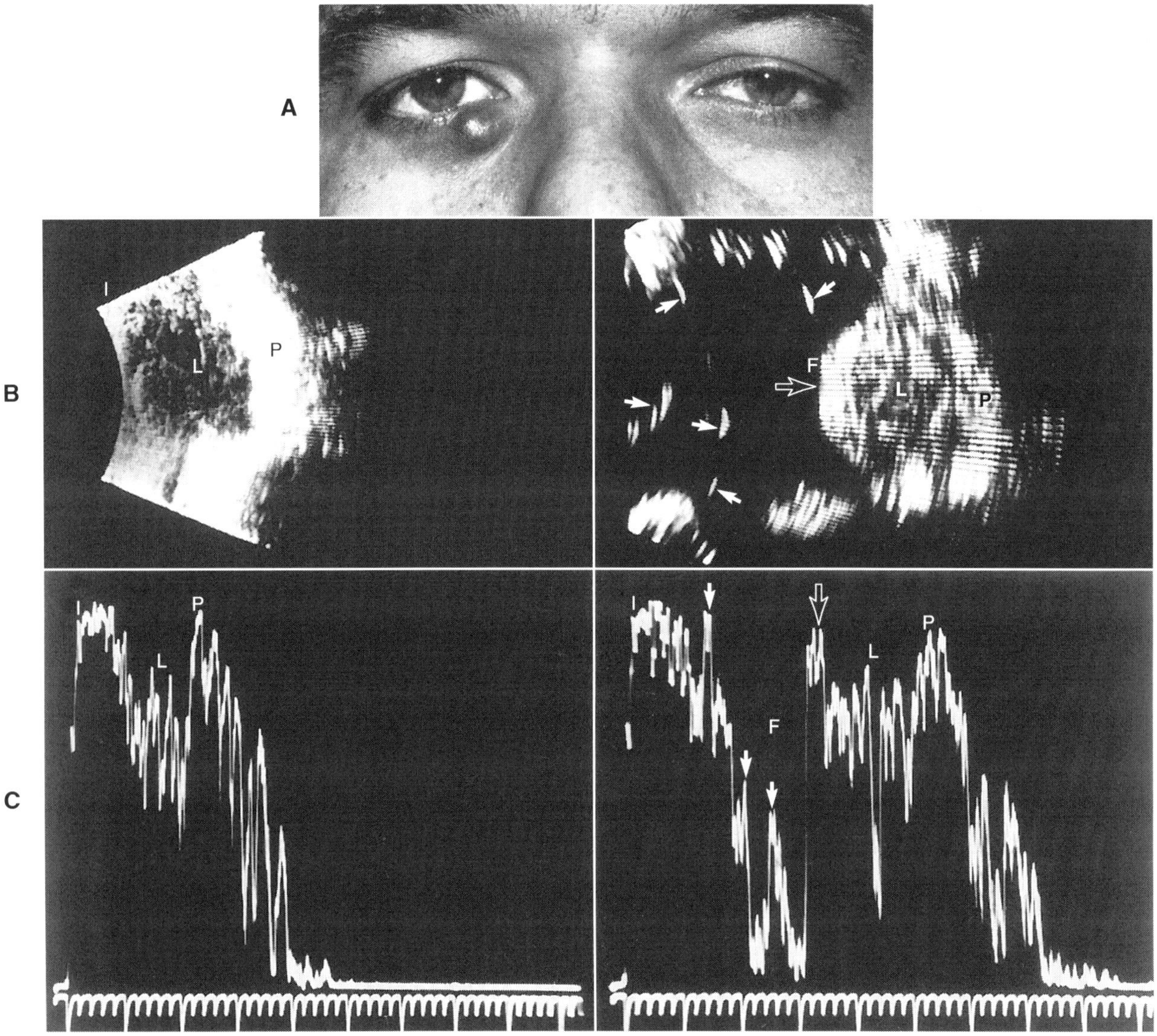

Figure 13-4 Cavernous hemangioma of right lower lid. **A,** External photo shows right lower lid lesion. **B,** Paraocular B-scan echogram shows lesion *(L)* and thick posterior surface *(P)*. *I*, Initial line corresponding to probe face. **C,** Paraocular A-scan echogram shows high reflectivity of lesion and distinct, highly reflective posterior surface spike *(P)*. *I*, Initial spike. **D,** Immersion B-scan view shows well-circumscribed, round lesion near lid surface *(open arrow)*. The initial line is shifted to the left and is not seen. *F*, Fluid (methylcellulose) within scleral shell; *small arrows*, small air bubbles; *P*, posterior surface of lesion. **E,** Immersion A-scan shows highly reflective lesion adjacent to lid *(open arrow)*. *I*, Initial spike; *F*, fluid; *small arrows*, air bubbles; *P*, posterior surface spike.

tumors, areas of lower reflectivity are produced by more cellular portions of the lesion, as well as by large cavernous spaces (Figure 13-5). The cavernous spaces occur most often in more longstanding lesions.[8]

Capillary hemangiomas can be located superficially or deep within the orbit.[21] These tumors are not well circumscribed and therefore typically have indistinct borders (Figure 13-6). Lesions presenting at birth often fill the entire orbital cavity. At this stage the tumors tend to be more highly reflective and therefore may be mistaken for normal orbital soft tissue. However, a widened orbital soft tissue pattern compared with that of the normal fellow orbit should alert the echographer that abnormal vascular tissue may be present. In some cases, there can be thickening of the extraocular muscles and/or mild dilatation of the superior ophthalmic vein.

The key point in diagnosing a capillary hemangioma is the marked internal blood flow, which can be detected with both A-scan and Doppler instruments (see Color Plate 14). Additionally, these lesions are soft and thus are easily compressible.[15,25] As the patient becomes older, capillary hemangiomas normally involute,[9] and vascularity gradually diminishes.

Lymphangioma

Lymphangiomas are detected most often in children and young adults.[16] They may be confined to the orbit or may also involve the conjunctiva and/or lid. These lesions can grow slowly, producing lid swelling or displacement of the globe, or they may present with sudden, acute proptosis secondary to spontaneous hemorrhage.[9]

Histopathologically, lymphangiomas consist of multiple lymph-filled spaces (that are low reflective) with thin, endothelium-lined walls (that are highly reflective). This mixture of low and high reflectivity makes their internal

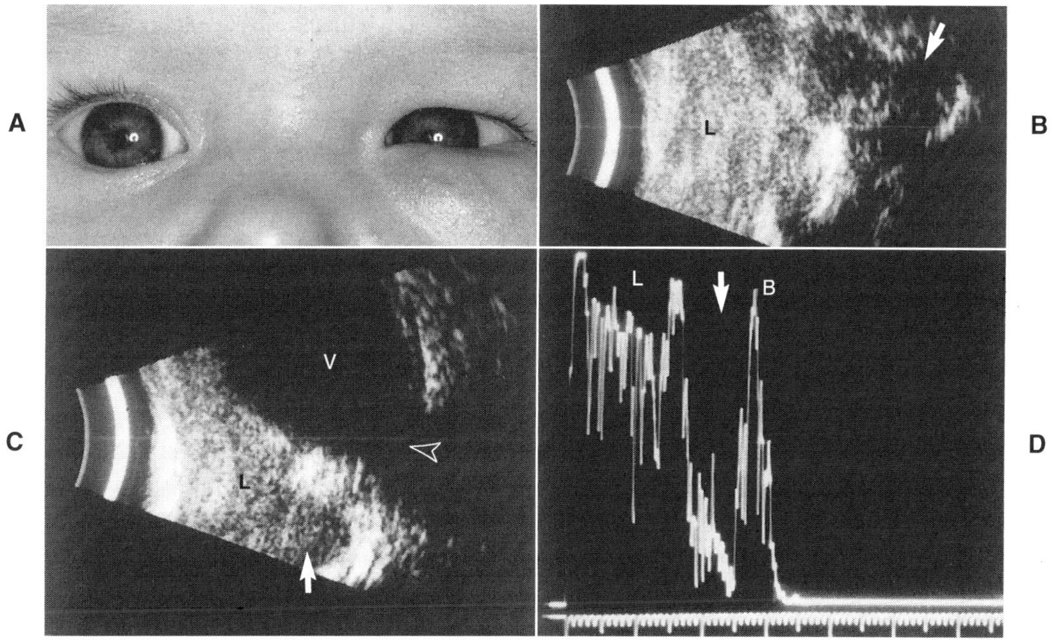

Figure 13-5 Capillary hemangioma. **A,** External photograph shows child with swelling of left lower lid. **B,** Transverse paraocular B-scan echogram shows large, irregularly structured lesion *(L)*. *Arrow,* Large posterior cavernous space. **C,** Longitudinal paraocular B-scan view shows lesion *(L)* beneath globe. Note large posterior cavernous space *(closed arrow)*. *V,* Vitreous cavity; *open arrow,* area of globe wall not shown well because of edge artifact. **D,** Paraocular A-scan echogram shows high reflectivity of lesion *(L)* anteriorly with low reflective cavity posteriorly *(arrow)*. Sound beam is partially directed toward orbital bone *(B)*.

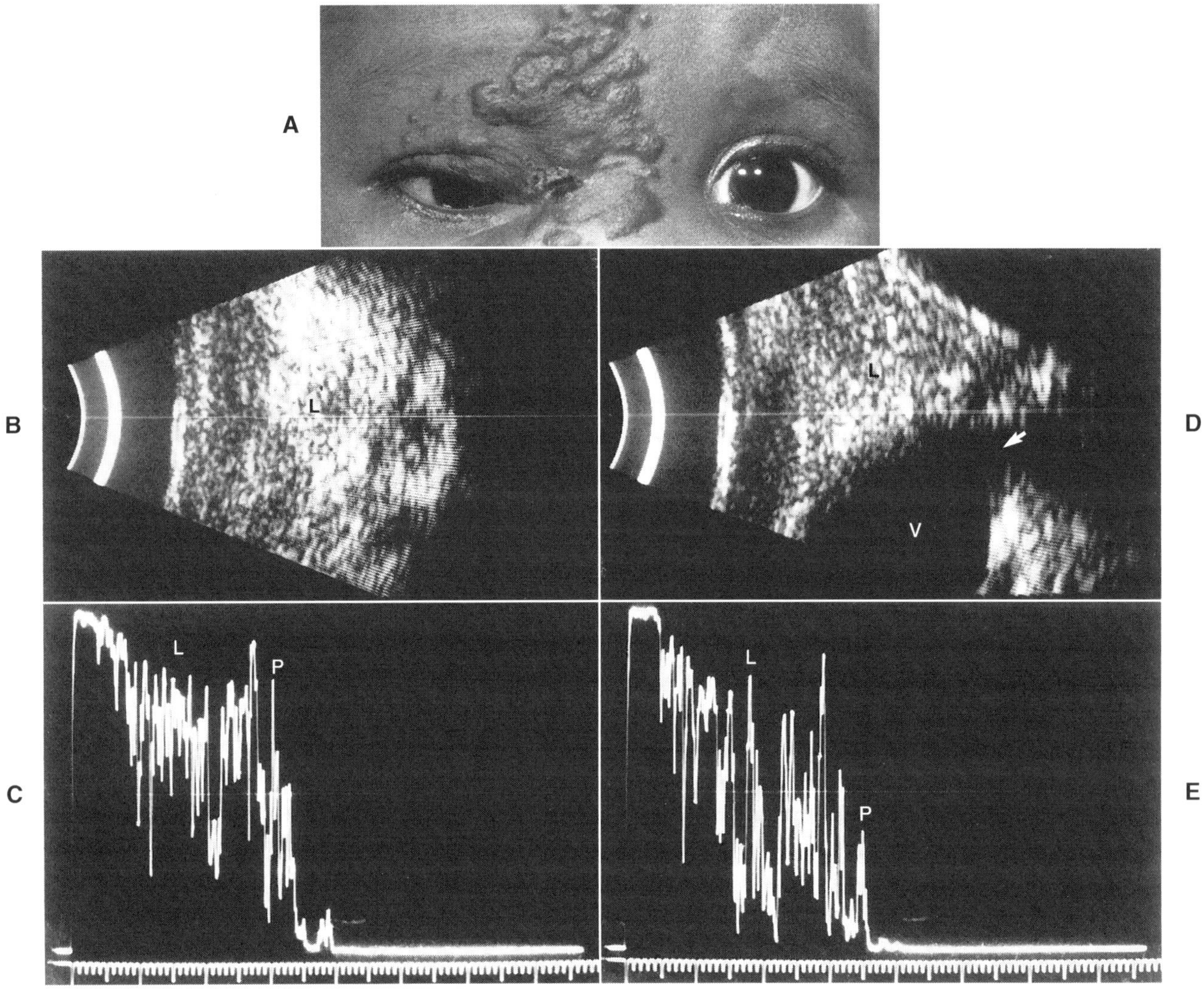

Figure 13-6 Capillary hemangioma. **A,** External photograph shows child with extensive capillary hemangioma of forehead and right upper lid. Paraocular B- and A-scan echograms show large lesion *(L)* within lid and orbit. **B,** Transverse B-scan shows large, diffuse mass. **C,** A-scan shows high reflectivity and indistinct posterior surface spike *(P)*. **D,** Longitudinal B-scan through superior orbit shows lesion *(L)* above globe extending posteriorly. *V,* Vitreous cavity; *arrow,* area of globe wall not shown well because of edge artifact. **E,** Different A-scan position shows more irregular internal structure and weaker reflective posterior surface spike *(P)* in this view.

structure somewhat irregular (see Figure 11-26). In addition, lymphangiomas are usually infiltrative and consequently produce indistinct borders. These tumors can be small and localized but frequently are large and diffuse. Occasionally, a lymphangioma can even fill the entire orbital cavity (Figure 13-7). Similar to capillary hemangiomas, lymphangiomas can have a very soft consistency but do not exhibit internal vascularity as is typically seen in capillary hemangiomas.

When a sudden hemorrhage occurs within a lymphangioma, the cavernous spaces become markedly dilated (Figure 13-8). This blood does not clot and is usually low reflective, although reflectivity is slightly higher than clear lymph (Figure 13-9). In some cases, the blood layers so that a fluid level can be demonstrated within some of the large cavernous spaces (Figure 13-10; see Figure 11-32). Although the lesion can have a very firm consistency immediately after hemorrhage has occurred, it usually becomes more compressible with time.

A lymphangioma with hemorrhage that presents with sudden proptosis must be differentiated from rhabdomyosarcoma. Echographically, the large dilated lymphatic spaces usually allow a lymphangioma to be easily differentiated from the solid, more homogeneous patterns

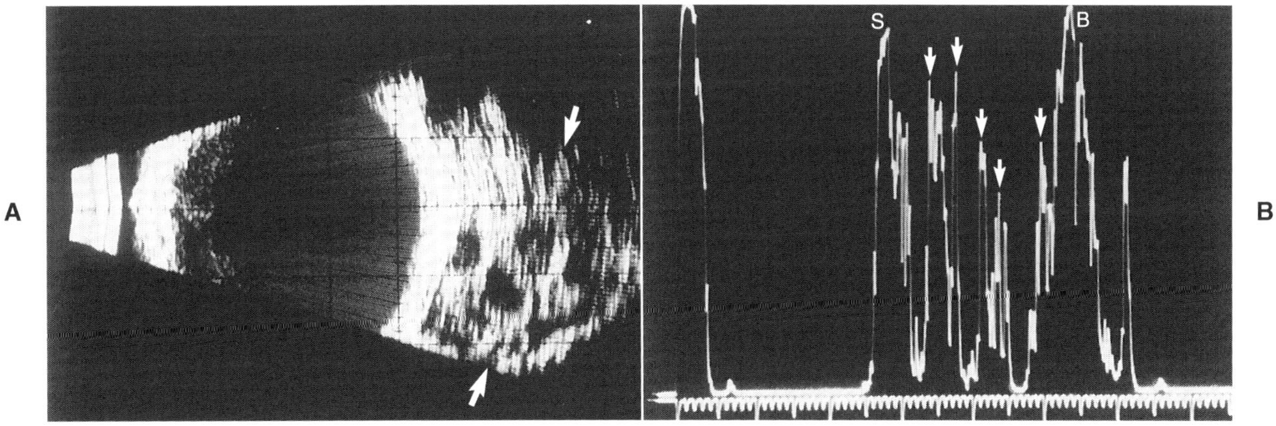

Figure 13-7 Transocular echograms of large orbital lymphangioma. **A,** B-scan view shows large mass *(arrows)* with multiple, dilated lymph-filled spaces. **B,** A-scan view shows lesion between sclera *(S)* and orbital bone *(B)*. Internal structure is irregular due to the multiple, low reflective lymph-filled spaces. *Arrows,* Surfaces of lymphatic spaces.

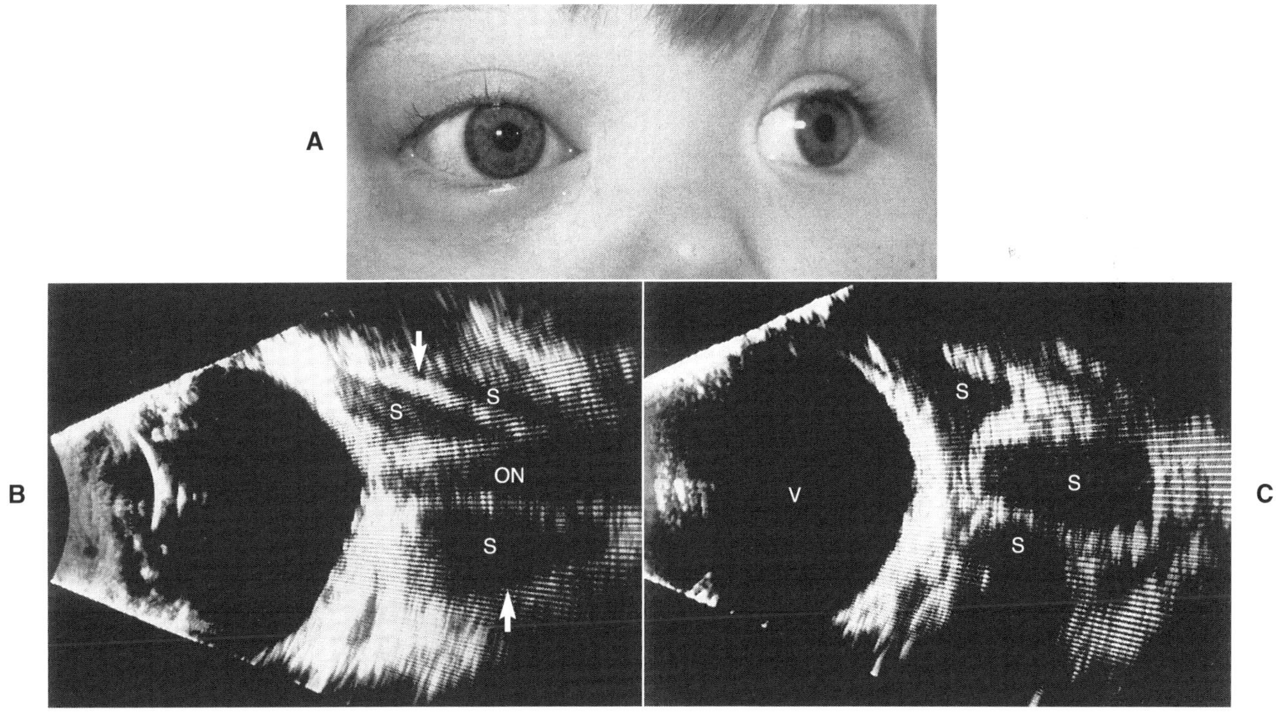

Figure 13-8 Lymphangioma with hemorrhage filling the orbital cavity. **A,** External photograph of child with proptosis of the right eye. **B,** Axial B-scan echogram displays large lesion *(arrows)* with dilated lymph spaces *(S)* surrounding the optic nerve *(ON)*. **C,** Transverse B-scan view through superior orbit shows several large dilated spaces. *V,* Vitreous cavity.

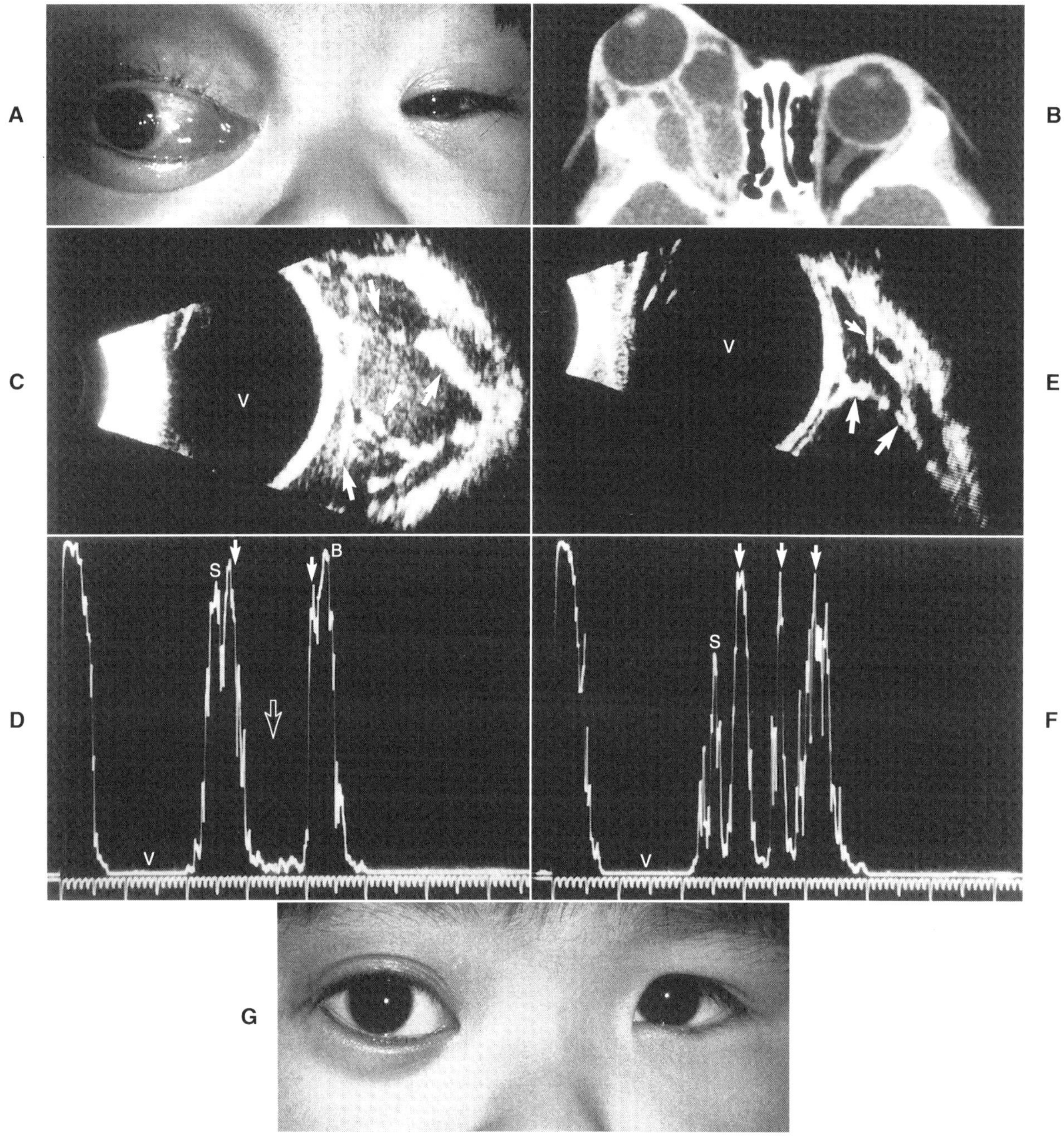

Figure 13-9 Lymphangioma with hemorrhage. **A,** External photograph shows child with marked proptosis of right eye at presentation. **B,** Axial CT scan at presentation shows massive lesion filling right orbit and causing marked proptosis. Transocular echograms (**C** to **F**) demonstrate large mass. *Closed arrows* indicate walls of dilated spaces. **C,** Transverse B-scan echogram displays extensive orbital mass with multiple blood-filled spaces. *V,* Vitreous cavity. **D,** Corresponding A-scan shows low reflective spikes from hemorrhage *(open arrow)* within large space. *S,* Sclera; *B,* bone. **E,** Longitudinal B-scan (at reduced gain setting) through anterior portion of lesion shows smaller spaces. **F,** Corresponding A-scan shows multiple, small, dilated spaces. Note that oblique sound beam incidence results in lower than normal reflectivity of sclera *(S)*. **G,** External photograph of child 4 weeks after drainage of orbital hemorrhage shows decrease in proptosis.

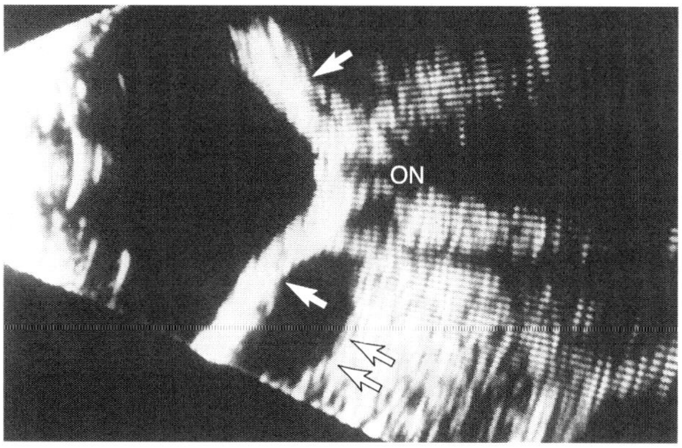

Figure 13-10 Lymphangioma with layered hemorrhage. Axial B-scan echogram at decreased gain shows very extensive retrobulbar lymphangioma with hemorrhage. Note layering of fluid blood *(open arrows)* within markedly dilated lymphatic spaces. Massive dilatation of spaces is causing marked indentation of posterior ocular wall *(closed arrows)*. *ON*, Optic nerve.

seen in a rhabdomyosarcoma (see p 310). Decompression of a lymphangioma is sometimes necessary when the hemorrhage causes marked proptosis. In these cases, ultrasound may help determine the best areas for needle aspiration, and B-scan echography may be used to guide positioning of the needle[24,26] (see Figure 17-4).

Hemangiopericytoma

Hemangiopericytomas are relatively uncommon orbital tumors.[21] They usually occur within the superior portion of the orbit, are round to oval, and are well outlined. The internal reflectivity is predominantly medium, and the internal structure can be regular or slightly irregular[3] (Figure 13-11). In addition, cystic spaces of variable size may be present. These tumors have hard consistency, usually show prominent internal blood flow, and produce moderate sound attenuation (Figure 13-12; see also Color Plate 12). Other tumors that can produce similar echographic findings include schwannomas, fibrous histiocytomas, and the rare metastatic renal cell carcinomas.

Other tumors (e.g., pseudotumor/lymphomas, rhabdomyosarcomas, and fibrous histiocytomas) that are not classified pathologically as vascular lesions can exhibit various degrees of internal blood flow. Consequently, these lesions occasionally can be confused with true vascular neoplasms.

VASCULAR MALFORMATIONS

Cavernous Sinus Fistula

Fistulas within the cavernous sinus can result in dilation and arterialization of the orbital veins, as well as congestion of the orbital soft tissue. Although these fistulas (i.e., shunts) are usually unilateral, bilateral orbital involvement can occur. These fistulas have been classified as either fast flow or slow flow.[19] Generally, a fast flow shunt is due to an internal carotid-cavernous sinus fistula, whereas slow flow shunts are more often associated with dural-cavernous sinus communication.

Carotid-Cavernous Sinus Fistula (Fast Flow)

This type of fistula is usually the result of severe head trauma. It presents with characteristic clinical signs and symptoms and is easily detected with echography. Clinical signs include dilated episcleral blood vessels, pulsatile exophthalmos, chemosis, audible bruit, and, in some cases, increased intraocular pressure.[19,21]

The classic finding is a dilated superior ophthalmic vein that is often undetectable in normal orbits. This vessel typically courses between the superior rectus muscle and the optic nerve as it extends from the supranasal orbit to the superior orbital fissure[11,12] (Figure 13-13). Other orbital findings that can be associated with cavernous sinus fistulas include (1) orbital soft tissue swelling causing widening of the normal orbital soft tissue pattern; (2) mild enlargement of the extraocular muscles, with medium to high reflectivity; and (3) widening of the optic nerve pattern as a result of increased subarachnoid fluid.[19] In addition, ciliochoroidal detachments can be observed in association with this condition.

The vein, depending on the speed of flow within the fistula, can be either mildly or markedly dilated. On A-scan, the dilated vein is typically very low reflective and demonstrates marked blood flow (Figure 13-14; see also Color Plate 9). Pulsation of the vein sometimes can be seen on A- and/or B-scan. Additionally, the audio Doppler response, with the probe placed on the nasal aspect of the upper lid, is markedly positive.[11] The marked blood flow

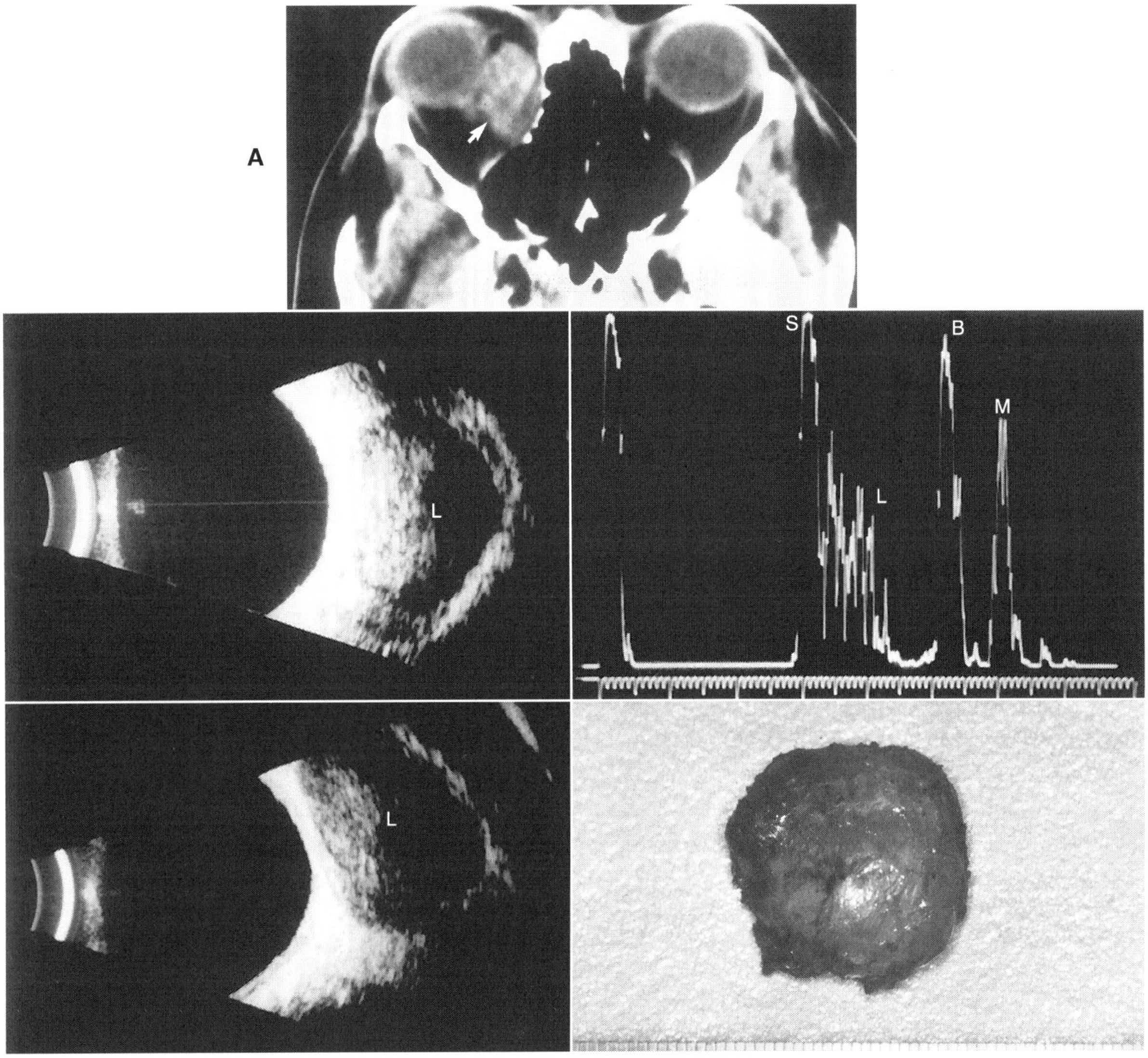

Figure 13-11 Echograms and CT scan of hemangiopericytoma. **A,** Axial CT scan shows large, well-circumscribed orbital mass supranasally *(arrow)*. Transocular echograms show large orbital lesion *(L)* located supranasally. **B,** Transverse B-scan shows well-circumscribed, oval lesion. Note decreasing brightness of internal echoes due to sound attenuation. **C,** Longitudinal B-scan displays well-circumscribed, oval lesion extending back into orbit. **D,** A-scan displays medium internal reflectivity of lesion with relatively strong sound attenuation. *S,* Sclera; *B,* bone; *M,* multiple signal. **E,** Gross pathologic specimen shows well-circumscribed mass.

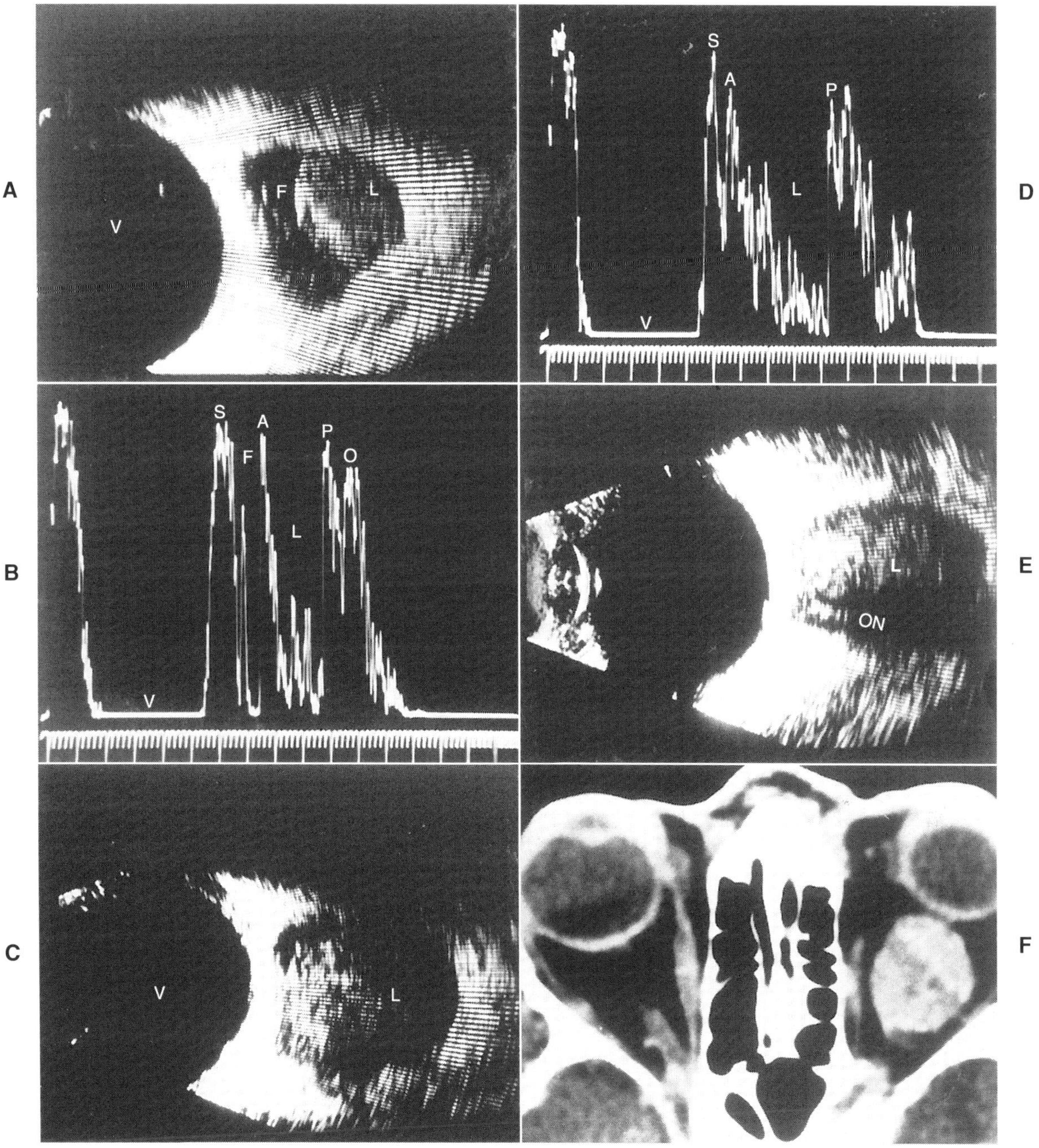

Figure 13-12 Large hemangiopericytoma with cyst examined over 6-month period. All echograms of lesion *(L)* were obtained with a transocular approach. **A,** Initial examination. Transverse B-scan shows intraconal mass with fluid-filled cystic cavity *(F)* anteriorly. *V,* Vitreous cavity. **B,** A-scan corresponding to **A** shows fluid-filled cavity and medium to low reflective, solid lesion. *V,* Vitreous cavity; *S,* sclera; *A,* anterior and *P,* posterior surface spikes of solid portion of lesion; *O,* orbital soft tissue. **C,** Follow-up examination 6 months later shows increased size of lesion and cystic area is no longer present. **D,** A-scan corresponding to **C** shows medium reflectivity and moderately strong sound attenuation. **E,** Vertical axial B-scan from second examination shows lesion above optic nerve *(ON).* **F,** Axial CT scan from time of second examination shows the large, well-circumscribed intraconal mass in the left orbit.

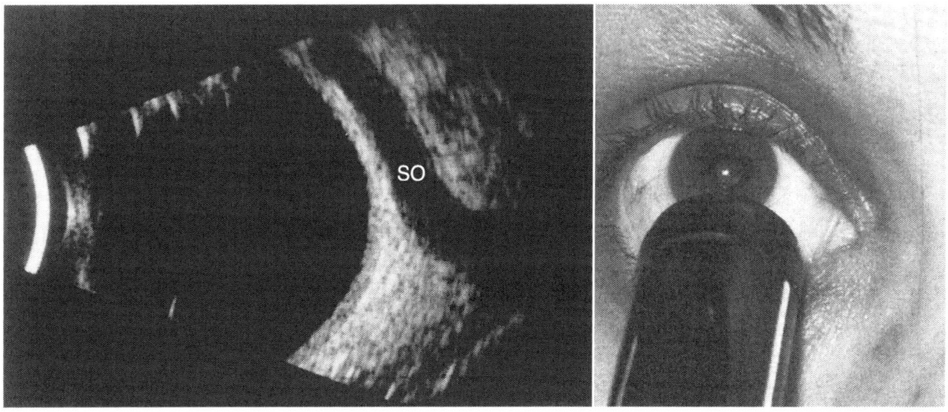

Figure 13-13 Dilated superior ophthalmic vein secondary to carotid-cavernous sinus fistula. **A,** Transverse B-scan view through superior orbit (just above optic nerve) shows superior ophthalmic vein *(SO).* Note that the vein courses from the supranasal aspect of the orbit back toward the orbital apex. **B,** Photograph shows horizontal transverse B-scan probe position for displaying superior ophthalmic vein.

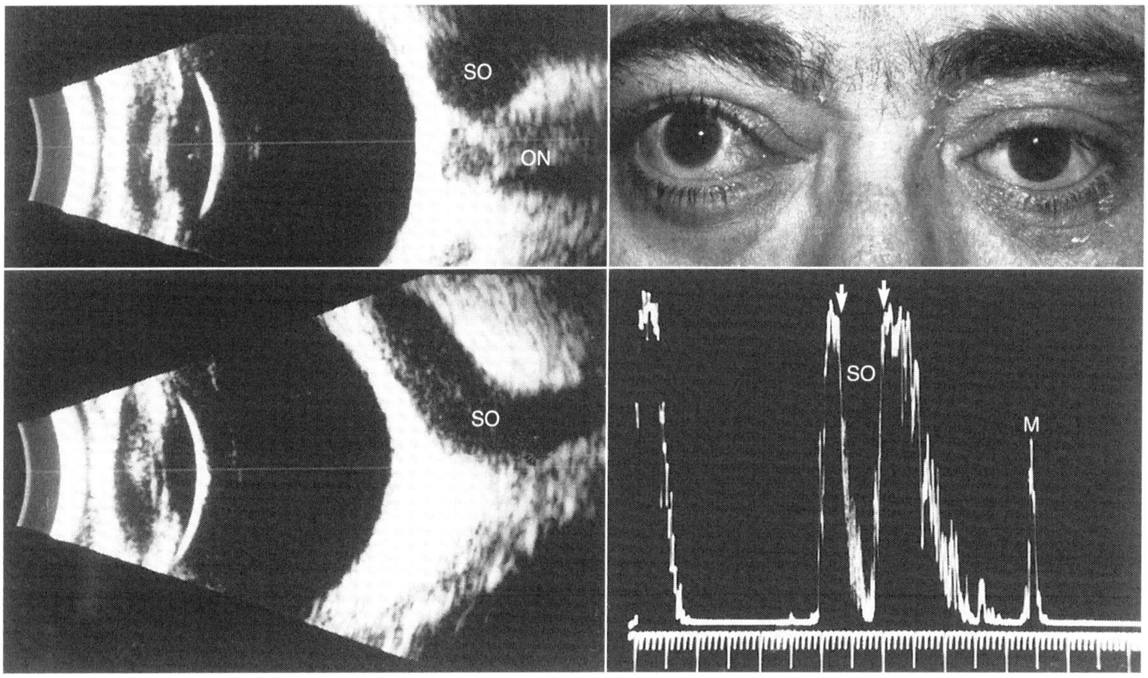

Figure 13-14 Carotid-cavernous sinus fistula involving right orbit following severe head trauma. **A,** Vertical axial B-scan echogram shows cross-section of dilated superior ophthalmic vein *(SO)* above optic nerve *(ON).* **B,** Horizontal para-axial B-scan view (through superior orbit) shows long section of dilated vein. **C,** External photograph shows proptotic globe with dilated episcleral vessels. **D,** A-scan view shows cross-section of dilated vein *(arrows)* with blurred, low reflective spikes from fast-flowing blood. *M,* Multiple signal.

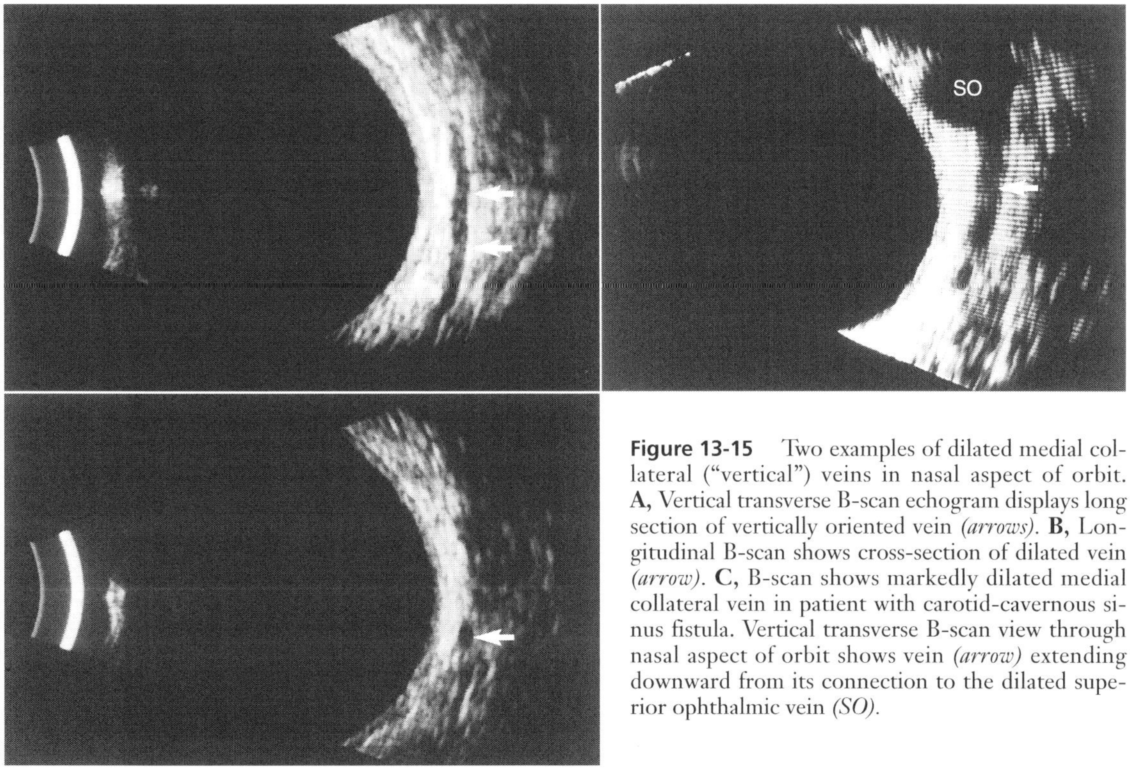

Figure 13-15 Two examples of dilated medial collateral ("vertical") veins in nasal aspect of orbit. **A,** Vertical transverse B-scan echogram displays long section of vertically oriented vein *(arrows)*. **B,** Longitudinal B-scan shows cross-section of dilated vein *(arrow)*. **C,** B-scan shows markedly dilated medial collateral vein in patient with carotid-cavernous sinus fistula. Vertical transverse B-scan view through nasal aspect of orbit shows vein *(arrow)* extending downward from its connection to the dilated superior ophthalmic vein *(SO)*.

through these veins results in a firm consistency during compression testing. Other tributary veins, such as the medial collateral or "vertical" vein described by Ossoinig et al,[17] can also be dilated in this condition (Figure 13-15).

Dural-Cavernous Sinus Fistula (Slow Flow)

This type of fistula, also known as "red eyed shunt syndrome," usually occurs spontaneously in middle-aged to elderly women and causes orbital congestion.[19] These patients typically show dilated episcleral blood vessels, minimal proptosis, and increased intraocular pressure. Furthermore, no bruit or pulsation of the eye is usually detected.

The primary echographic findings in dural-cavernous sinus fistulas include mild to moderate widening of the orbital soft tissue pattern and thickening of the extraocular muscles in the affected orbit[1] (see p 406). The superior ophthalmic vein can be of normal size (and thus undetectable), or it can be moderately dilated (Figure 13-16). In these cases, the internal reflectivity of the dilated vein is usually low to medium, higher than that seen in fast flow carotid-cavernous sinus fistulas. This higher internal reflectivity may be due to partial thrombosis of the low flow fistula, resulting in larger interfaces and thus a more heterogeneous echographic pattern. Audio Doppler ultrasound may show findings similar to the normal fellow orbit, or there may be a low-grade positive response. In cases where the vein is not dilated but the extraocular muscles are enlarged, this condition may appear echographically similar to thyroid ophthalmopathy.

Superior Ophthalmic Vein Thrombosis

Thrombosis of the superior ophthalmic vein can occur in carotid-cavernous sinus fistulas and, as discussed previously, may also be seen in dural-cavernous sinus fistulas. Acute thrombosis of the superior ophthalmic vein can present with proptosis, chemosis, and lid edema.[21] In some instances, thrombosis can cause increased dilatation of the superior ophthalmic vein. Blood flow is usually markedly diminished or totally absent.[17] The clotted blood within the vein produces large interfaces and thus medium-high internal reflectivity (Figure 13-17).

Orbital Varix

Orbital varices are venous malformations that may cause a characteristic intermittent proptosis, which is often exacerbated with bending of the head or performance of a Valsalva maneuver.[23] This increase in venous pressure, caused either by bending over or by the Valsalva maneuver, allows blood to collect passively in the abnormal venous spaces. These patients may eventually become enophthalmic,[20] presumably from fat necrosis due to fluctuation in size of the lesion over time.

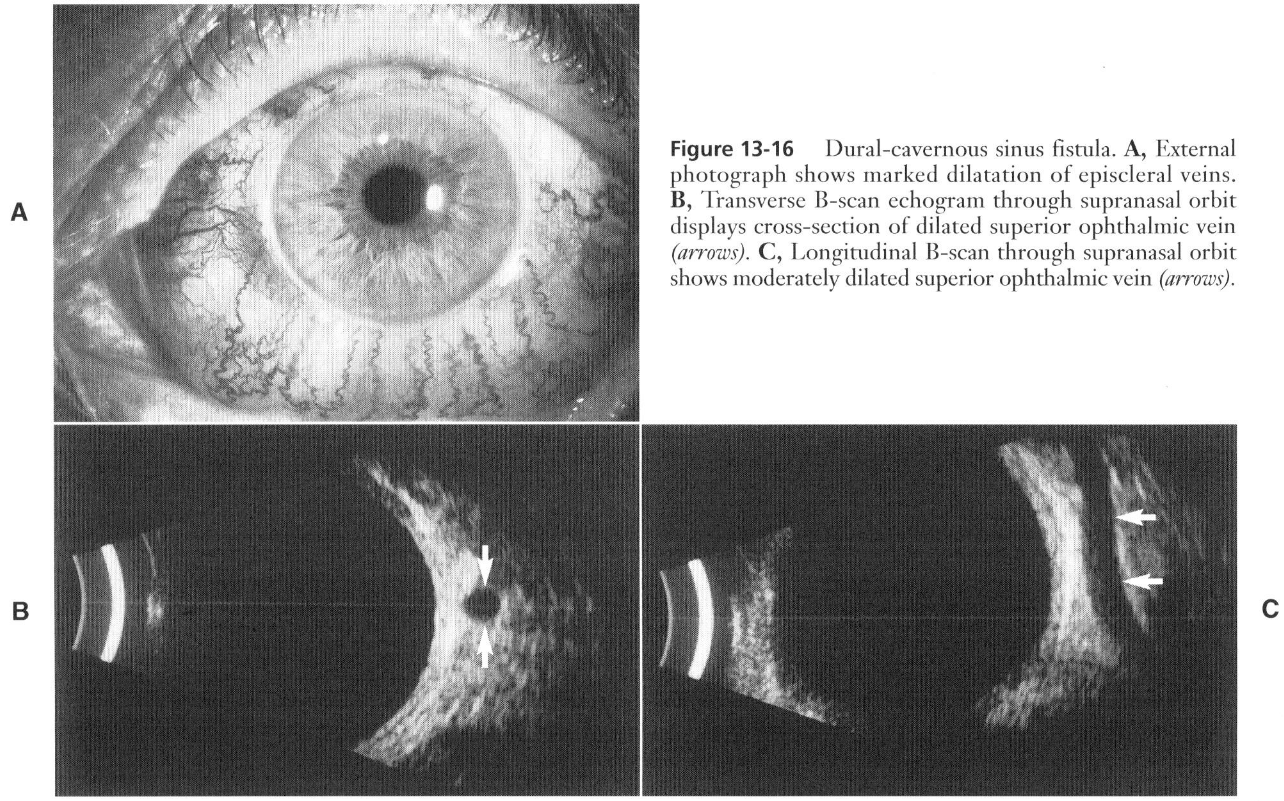

Figure 13-16 Dural-cavernous sinus fistula. **A,** External photograph shows marked dilatation of episcleral veins. **B,** Transverse B-scan echogram through supranasal orbit displays cross-section of dilated superior ophthalmic vein *(arrows)*. **C,** Longitudinal B-scan through supranasal orbit shows moderately dilated superior ophthalmic vein *(arrows)*.

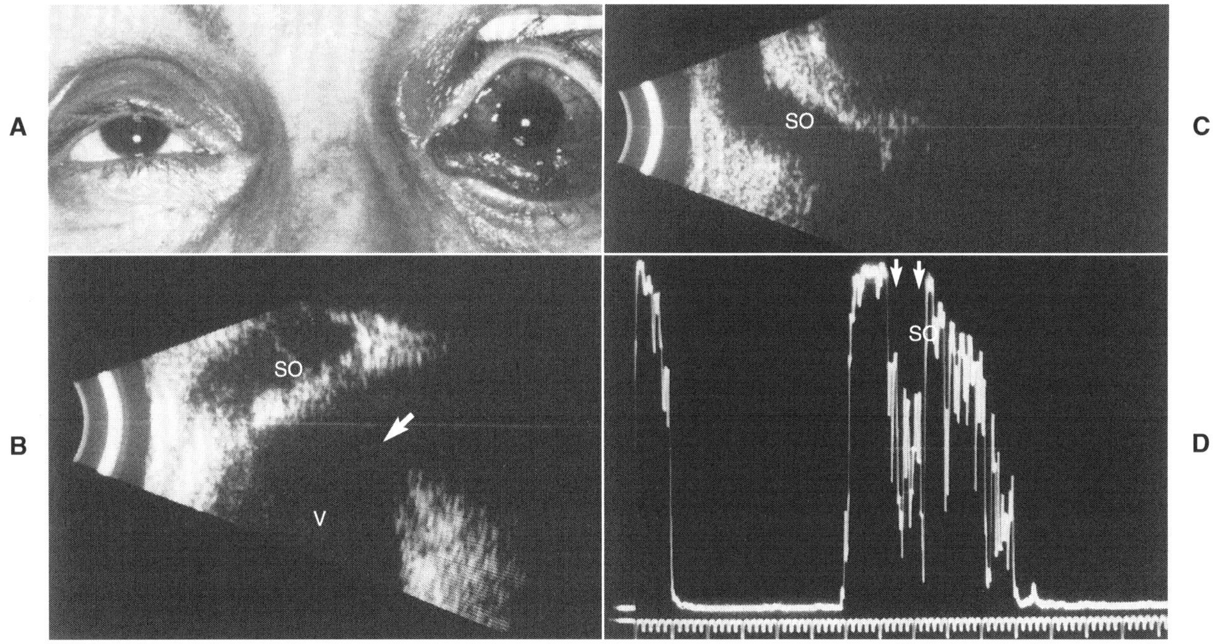

Figure 13-17 Thrombosis of dural-cavernous sinus fistula. **A,** External photograph showing marked conjunctival chemosis and hyperemia of the left eye. Patient also complained of pain and was found to have high intraocular pressure as well as bullous, serous choroidal detachments (not shown). **B,** Longitudinal paraocular B-scan echogram supranasally shows dilated superior ophthalmic vein *(SO)* anterior to globe. *V,* Vitreous cavity; *arrow,* area of globe wall not shown well because of edge artifact. **C,** Transverse paraocular B-scan shows dilated vein. **D,** Transocular A-scan shows medium reflectivity of vein filled with clotted blood. *Arrows,* Wall of vein.

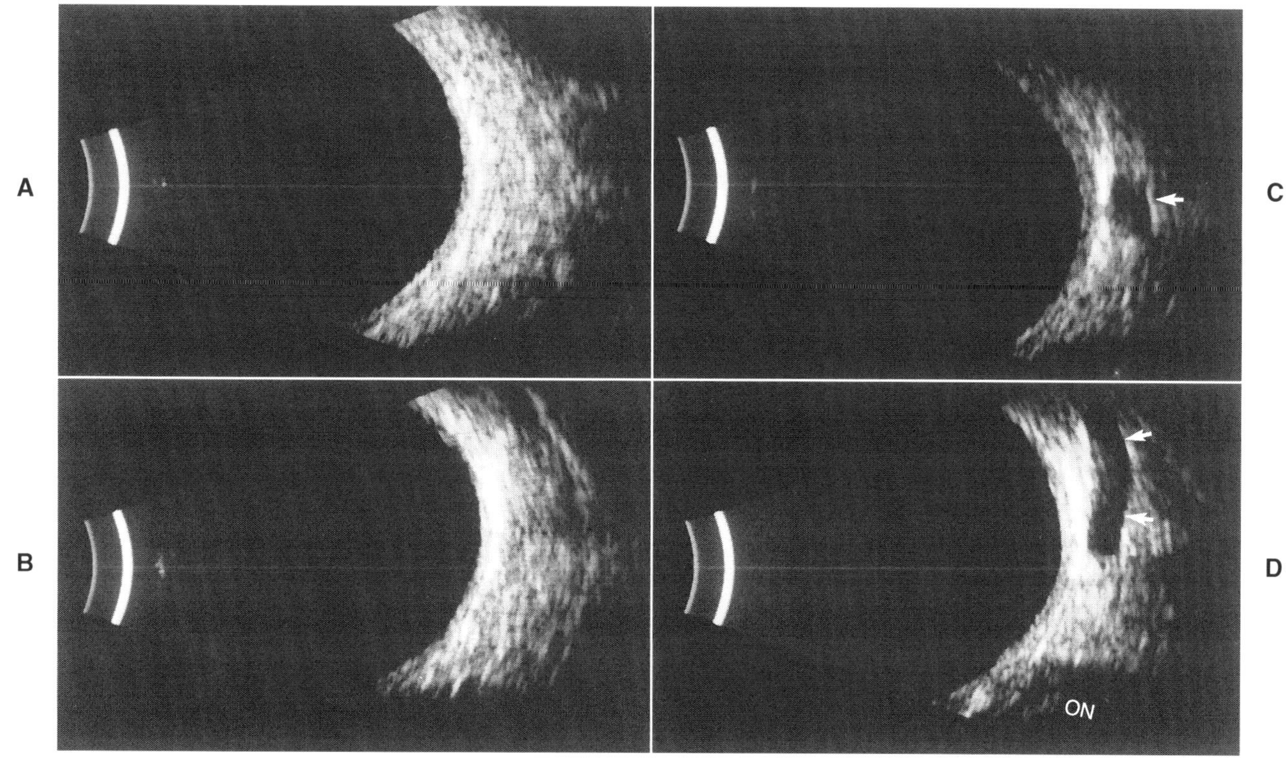

Figure 13-18 Tubular-shaped orbital varix before and during Valsalva maneuver. Transocular B-scan echograms before (**A** and **B**) and during (**C** and **D**) Valsalva maneuver. Transverse **(A)** and longitudinal **(B)** views show normal orbital pattern before Valsalva maneuver with no evidence of varix. **C,** Transverse section shows cross-section of varix *(arrow)* during Valsalva maneuver. **D,** Longitudinal view shows long section of varix *(arrows)* during Valsalva maneuver. *ON,* Optic nerve.

If a varix is collapsed, the lesion may not be detectable during the basic screening examination. However, if the patient then performs a Valsalva maneuver or leans forward, the venous space(s) can fill, resulting in the appearance of a well-outlined, low-to-medium reflective orbital lesion.[15] A varix can have the tubular shape of a blood vessel (Figure 13-18; see also Color Plate 10), or it can appear as a large mass. Varices are usually compressible, but internal vascularity is not appreciable because of their venous supply. In order to detect a varix, in some cases the examiner may need to bend over or actually sit on the floor for proper probe placement. The examiner should be aware that even in normal situations, mild dilation of the superior ophthalmic veins can occur in both orbits when the patient bends forward. Thrombosis of an orbital varix also can occur[5] (Figure 13-19, *A* and *B*).

A

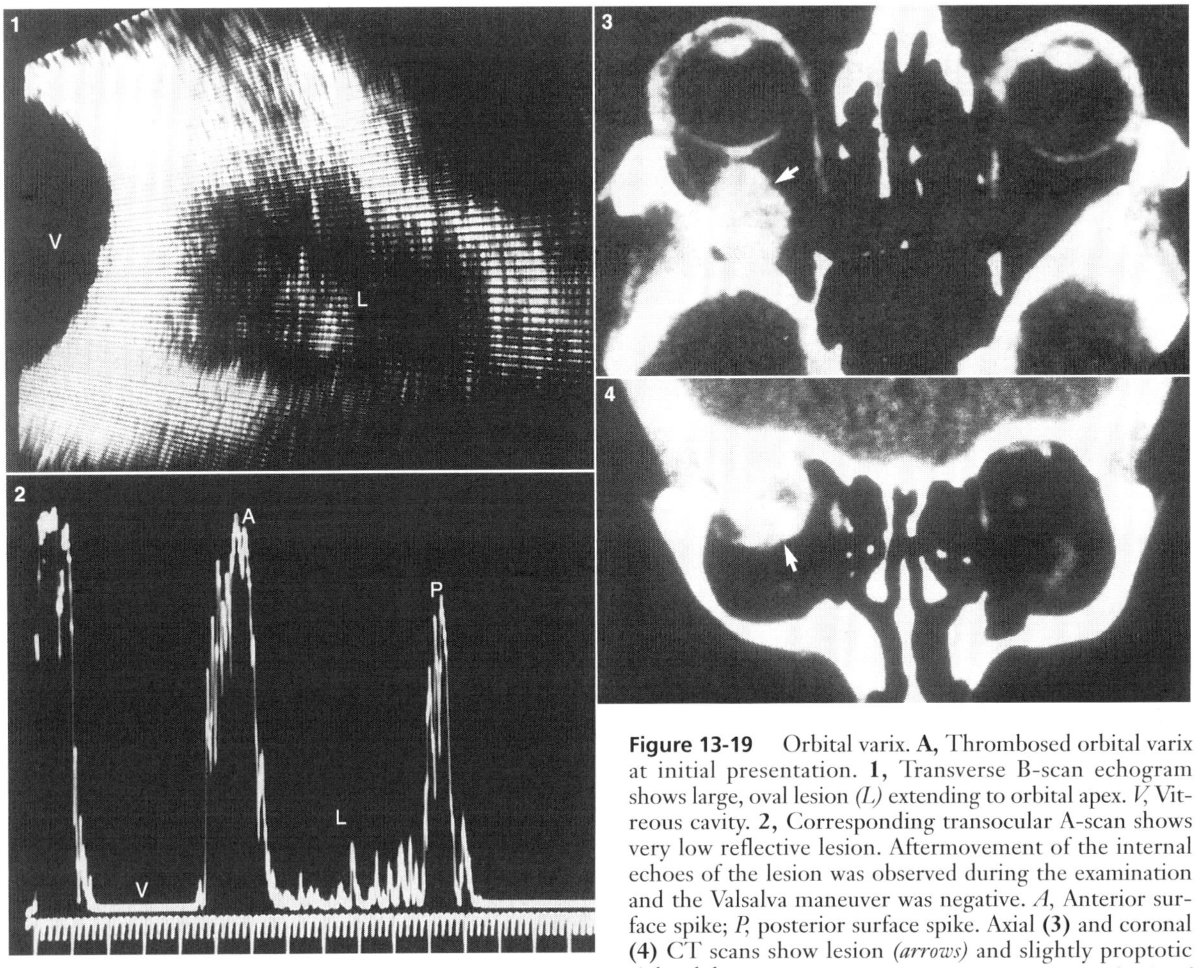

Figure 13-19 Orbital varix. **A,** Thrombosed orbital varix at initial presentation. **1,** Transverse B-scan echogram shows large, oval lesion *(L)* extending to orbital apex. *V,* Vitreous cavity. **2,** Corresponding transocular A-scan shows very low reflective lesion. Aftermovement of the internal echoes of the lesion was observed during the examination and the Valsalva maneuver was negative. *A,* Anterior surface spike; *P,* posterior surface spike. Axial **(3)** and coronal **(4)** CT scans show lesion *(arrows)* and slightly proptotic right globe. *Continued*

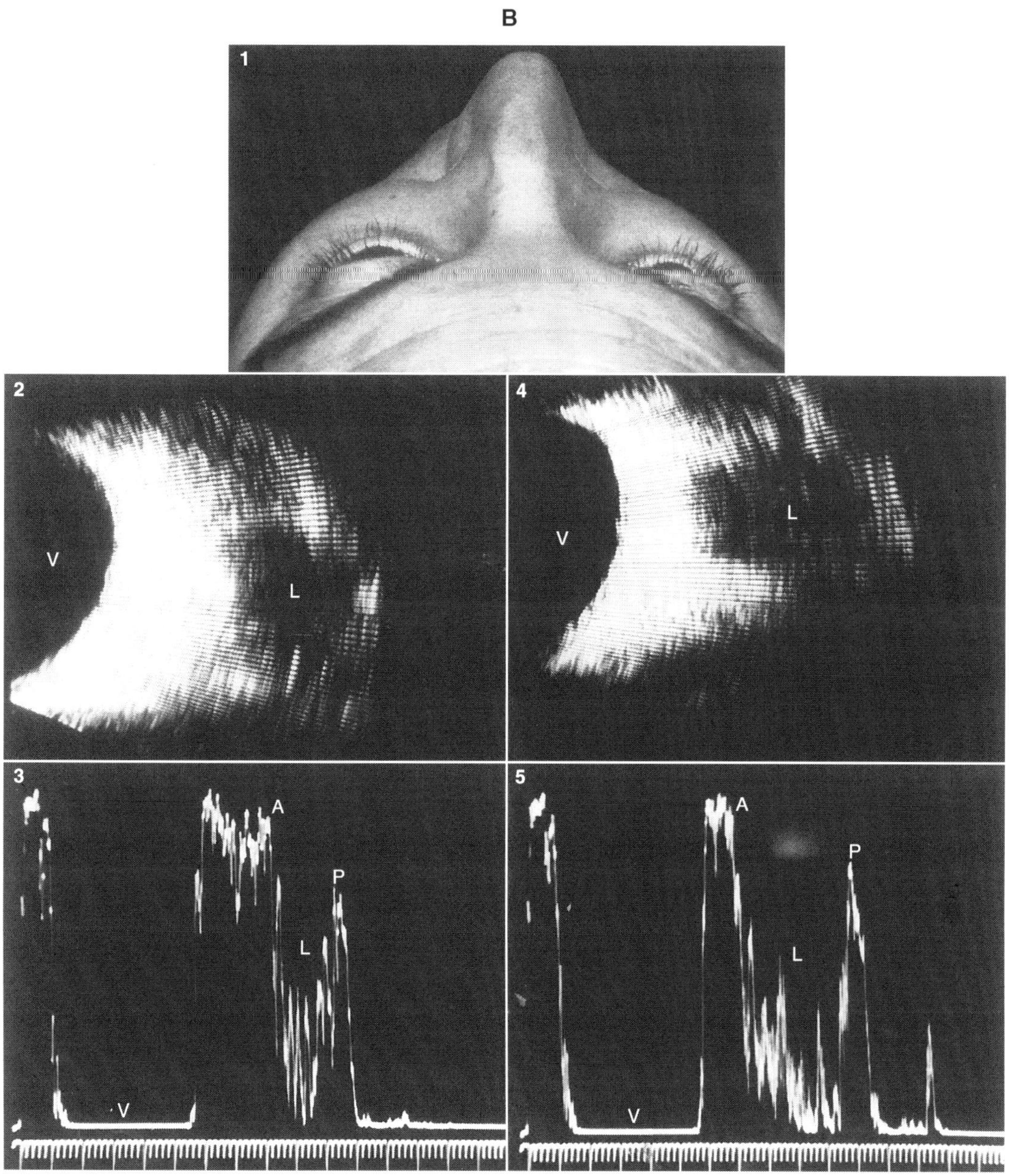

Figure 13-19, cont'd **B,** Follow-up examination of orbital varix 6 weeks after initial examination. **1,** External photograph now shows enophthalmos on right side. Transocular echograms (**2** to **5**) show lesion *(L)*. **2,** Transverse B-scan echogram displays marked decrease in size of mass compared with **1** in figure **A.** *V,* Vitreous cavity. **3,** Corresponding A-scan shows smaller size and higher reflectivity compared with **2** in part **A.** *A,* Anterior and *P,* posterior surface spikes. **4** and **5** show expansion of lesion during Valsalva maneuver (compared with **2** and **3**). This indicates varix is no longer completely thrombosed.

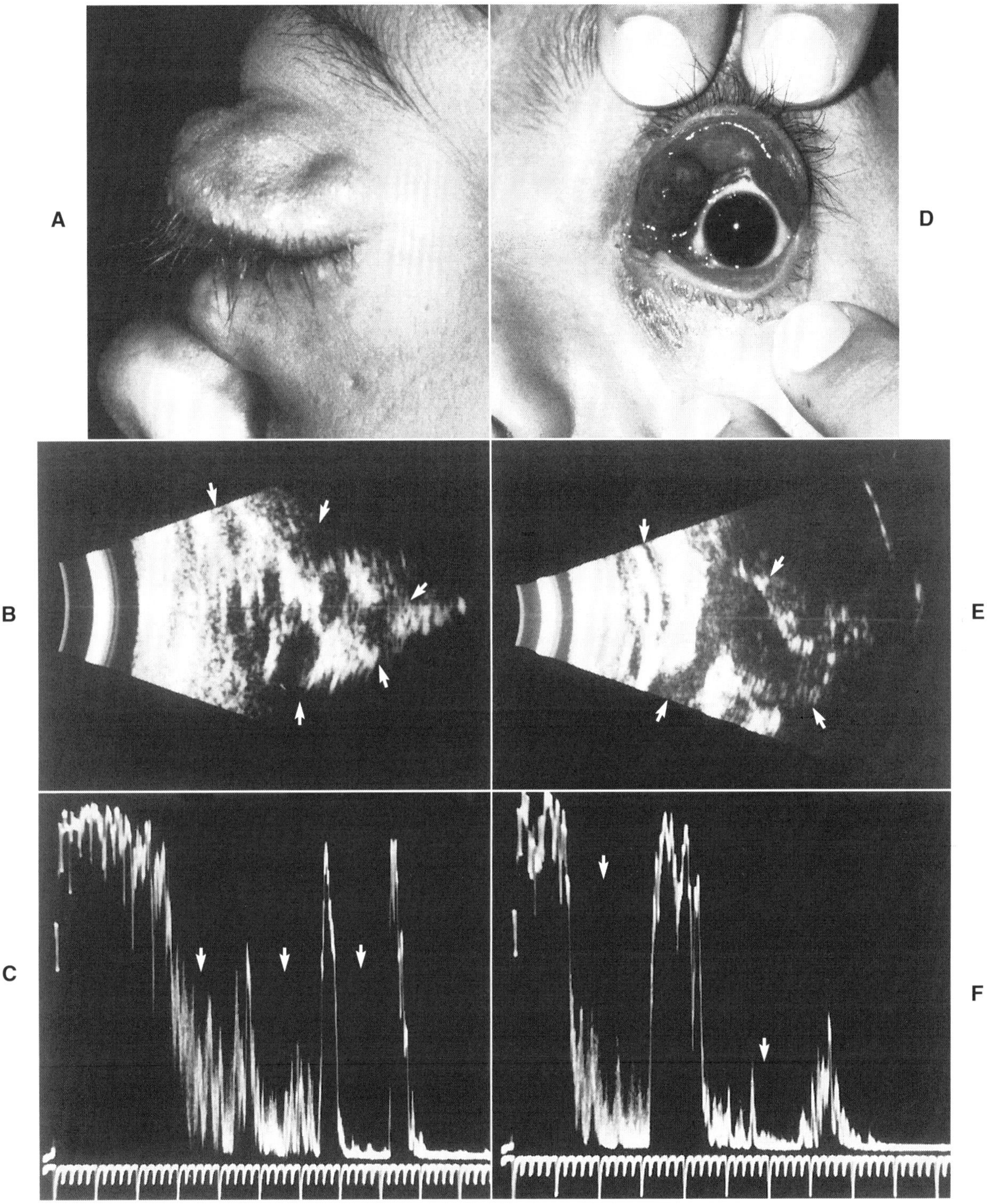

Figure 13-20 Congenital arteriovenous malformation involving left lids and orbit. External photographs (**A** and **D**) show marked thickening and irregularity of lids as well as hyperemia, injection, and swelling of conjunctiva. Paraocular echograms (**B, C, E,** and **F**) show extensive mass with irregular internal structure *(arrows)*. Blurring of A-scan spikes (**C** and **F**) indicates marked internal blood flow. (Clinical photographs courtesy Dr. Latif Hamed, Gainesville, Florida.)

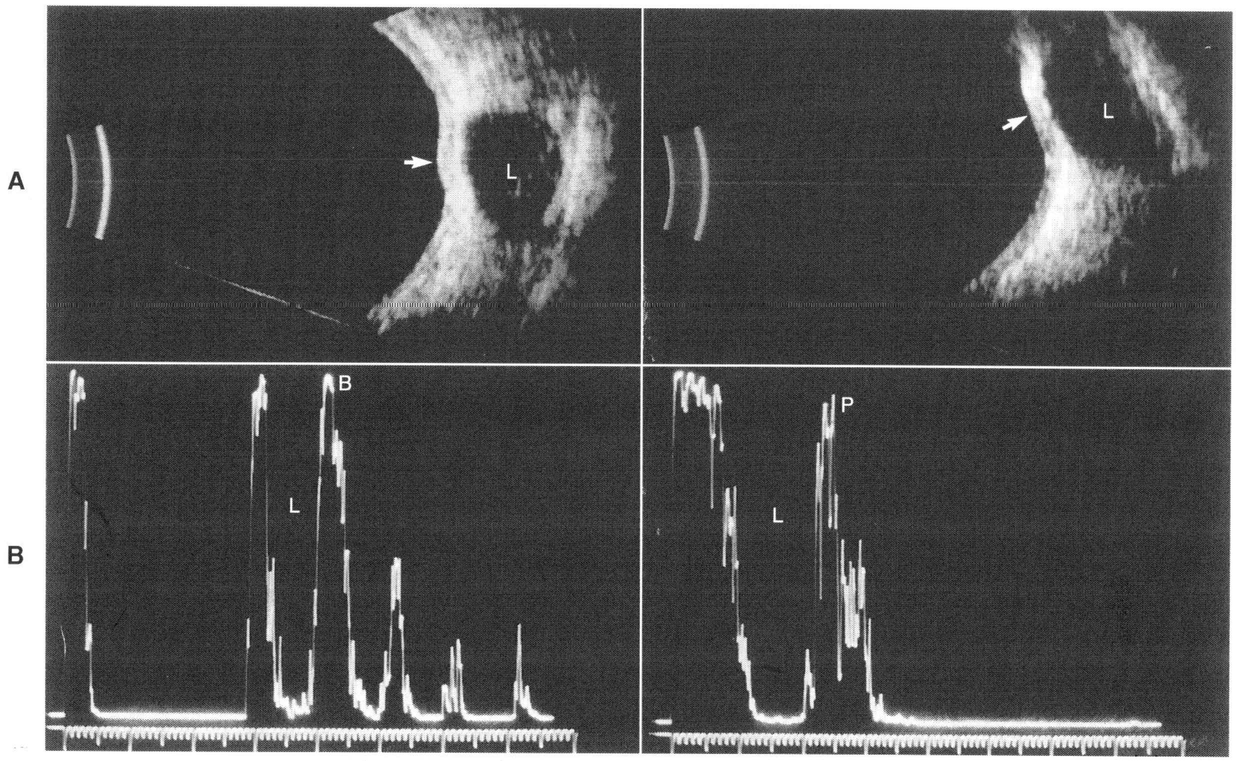

Figure 13-21 Large orbital aneurysm. Transocular (**A** to **C**) and paraocular (**D**) echograms show orbital lesion *(L)*. **A,** Transverse B-scan echogram shows well-outlined mass that is slightly indenting globe *(arrow)*. **B,** Transocular A-scan shows very low reflective, well-outlined lesion. *B,* Bone. **C,** Longitudinal B-scan view shows lesion indenting globe *(arrow)*. **D,** Paraocular A-scan shows very low reflective, well-outlined lesion. *P,* Posterior surface spike.

Arteriovenous Malformation

Arteriovenous malformations can be congenital, or they may develop spontaneously following trauma.[8] These lesions are often diffuse and irregularly shaped because they can be composed of "tangled malformed arteries and veins."[9] The internal structure of these lesions is typically irregular because of the very low reflective, fast flowing blood and the higher reflectivity of the vessel walls. The marked blood flow can normally be observed on A-scan (Figure 13-20) and can be demonstrated on both audio Doppler and color Doppler imaging (see Color Plate 15). These highly vascularized lesions are soft and compressible. Other associated findings can include generalized swelling of the orbital soft tissue and secondary glaucoma. Serous choroidal detachments sometimes occur in association with these lesions.

Orbital Aneurysm

Orbital arterial aneurysms are well outlined and low reflective, with regular internal structure (Figure 13-21). These lesions are usually highly vascularized on both A-scan and Doppler and are slightly compressible. Although they can have a tubular shape and contain fast blood flow similar to that of a carotid-cavernous sinus fistula, aneurysms normally can be differentiated by their course in the orbit. In a fistula, the dilated superior ophthalmic vein extends from the anterior aspect of the supranasal orbit to the orbital apex. In contrast, an orbital aneurysm is more localized and is usually situated in the anterior aspect of the orbit.[16]

REFERENCES

1. Atta HR, Dick AD, Hamed LM, et al: Venous stasis orbitopathy: a clinical and echographic study. *Br J Ophthalmol* 1996;80:129.
2. Bettelheim H, Till P: Diagnosis of orbital vascular disorders by ophthalmodynamography, in Thijssen JM, Verbeek AM (eds): *Ultrasonography in Ophthalmology.* Dordrecht, Dr W Junk, 1981, p 299.
3. Byrne SF: Standardized echography in the diagnosis of hemangioendothelioma, in Hillman JS, Lemay MM (eds): *Ophthalmic Ultrasonography.* Dordrecht, Dr W Junk, 1984, p 347.
4. Byrne SF, Glaser JS: Orbital tissue differentiation with standardized echography. *Ophthalmology* 1983;90:1081.
5. Bullock JD, Goldberg SH, Connelly PJ: Orbital varix thrombosis. *Ophthalmology* 1990;97:251.
6. Coleman DJ, Jack RL, Franzen LA: High resolution B-scan ultrasonography of the orbit. II: Hemangiomas of the orbit. *Arch Ophthalmol* 1972;88:368.
7. Dutton JJ, Byrne SF, Proia AD: *Diagnostic Atlas of Orbital Diseases.* Philadelphia, WB Saunders Co, 2000.

8. Henderson JW: *Orbital Tumors*, ed 2, New York, Thieme-Stratton, 1980.
9. Jakobiec FA, Font RL: Orbit, in Spencer WH: *Ophthalmic Pathology: An Atlas and Textbook*, ed 3. Philadelphia, WB Saunders Co, 1986, p 2546.
10. Lieb WE: Color Doppler imaging of the eye and orbit. *Radiol Clin North Am* 1998;36:1059.
11. MacNeill JR: Standardized echography in C.C. fistulas, in Ossoinig KC (ed): *Ophthalmic Echography*. Dordrecht, Dr W Junk, 1987, p 521.
12. Moster MR, Kennerdell JS: B-scan ultrasonic evaluation of a dilated superior ophthalmic vein in orbital and retro-orbital arteriovenous anomalies. *J Clin Neuroophthalmol* 1983;3:105.
13. Ossoinig KC: Die ultraschalldiagnostik orbitaler gefassprozesse. *Klin Monatsbl Augenheillkd* 1971;158:526.
14. Ossoinig KC: Standardized echography: Basic principles, clinical applications and results. *Int Ophthalmol Clin* 1979;19(4):127.
15. Ossoinig KC: Echographic differentiation of vascular tumors in the orbit, in Thijssen JM, Verbeek AM (eds): *Ultrasonography in Ophthalmology*. Dordrecht, Dr W Junk, 1981, p 283.
16. Ossoinig KC: *Standardized Ophthalmic Echography of the Eye, Orbit and Periorbital Region. A Comprehensive Slide Set and Study Guide*, ed 3. Iowa City, Goodfellow, 1985.
17. Ossoinig KC, Frieling E, Tamburrelli C, et al: Superior ophthalmic vein thrombosis—an echographic diagnosis, in Ossoinig KC (ed): *Ophthalmic Echography*. Dordrecht, Dr W Junk, 1987, p 529.
18. Ossoinig KC, Keenan TP, Bigar F: Cavernous hemangioma of the orbit: A differential diagnosis in clinical echography. *Bibl Ophthalmol* 1975;83:236.
19. Phelps CD, Thompson HS, Ossoinig KC: The diagnosis and prognosis of atypical carotid-cavernous fistula (red-eyed shunt syndrome). *Am J Ophthalmol* 1982;93:423.
20. Rootman J: Frequency and differential diagnosis of orbital disease, in Rootman J: *Diseases of the Orbit*. Philadelphia, JB Lippincott Co, 1988, p 131.
21. Rootman J, Graeb D: Vascular lesions, in Rootman J: *Diseases of the Orbit*. Philadelphia, JB Lippincott Co, 1988, p 525.
22. Rootman J, Hay E, Graeb DA, et al: Orbital-adnexal lymphangiomas: A spectrum of hemodynamically isolated vascular hamartomas. *Ophthalmology* 1986;93:1558.
23. Shields JA: *Diagnosis and Management of Orbital Tumors*. Philadelphia, WB Saunders Co, 1989.
24. Skalka HW, Callahan MA: Ultrasonically aided percutaneous orbital aspiration. *Ophthalmic Surg* 1979;10(11):41.
25. Sklar EL, Quencer RM, Byrne SF, et al: Correlative study of the computed tomographic, ultrasonographic, and pathological characteristics of cavernous versus capillary hemangiomas of the orbit. *J Clin Neuroophthalmol* 1986;6:14.
26. Spoor TC, Kennerdell JS, Dekker A, et al: Orbital fine needle aspiration biopsy with B-scan guidance. *Am J Ophthalmol* 1980;89:274.

Wolfgang E. Lieb

14

Color Doppler Imaging of the Eye and Orbit

Color Doppler imaging (CDI) is one of the most important developments of the last decade in ultrasonography. It allows for simultaneous, two-dimensional structural imaging (B-scan), as well as Doppler evaluation of blood flow. Doppler ultrasound detects changes in the frequency of sound reflected from flowing blood, allowing estimation of flow velocity. In medicine, CDI has come to play a role in the assessment of blood vessels, organ perfusion, and tumor neovascularity. Use of CDI in ophthalmology was first introduced in the late 1980s.

With CDI, it is possible to display indirectly the fine orbital vessels, including the ophthalmic artery (OA) and its branches, the central retinal artery (CRA), the posterior ciliary artery (PCA), and the lacrimal artery. In addition, venous structures, such as the superior ophthalmic vein (SOV), the vortex veins, and the central retinal vein (CRV) can be demonstrated. Aside from this qualitative assessment, CDI can also assess the hemodynamics of these vessels by measuring flow velocities during various phases of the cardiac cycle (Doppler spectrum analysis).

CDI is now being used in ophthalmology to evaluate vascular lesions and tumors in the eye and orbit. It can also document hemodynamic changes in patients with retinal vascular disease (e.g., CRA occlusion [CRAO], CRV occlusion [CRVO], and diabetic retinopathy) and enable study of the effects of drugs on these hemodynamics. In addition, CDI can evaluate the carotid arteries and periorbital vessels in patients with ischemic ocular disease (Box 14-1).

Color-Duplex Scanning

CDI incorporates the use of color with conventional duplex scanning. The technology of duplex scanning allows for simultaneous B-mode imaging and Doppler spectral analysis. Doppler spectral analysis is a means of assessing blood vessel flow characteristics. In conventional duplex scanning of the eye and orbit, the Doppler information is displayed graphically as a waveform on the screen, separate from the B-scan image. The Doppler spectra are obtained without precise localization of the vessel being studied because the diameter of intraocular and orbital vessels is too small to be imaged with conventional B-scan. With CDI, the Doppler blood flow information is encoded in color and superimposed on the B-scan echogram in real time to localize vascular structures (Figure 14-1). Since the ability to display a color Doppler image is not limited by the resolution of the B-scan echogram, CDI can detect very small vessels and depict their course.* A complete Doppler spectrum analysis is performed by evaluating both the superimposed color display and the more quantitative graphic waveform.

A new, important step in CDI technology is "power Doppler." This technology improves sensitivity, allowing the study of very small or very slow flowing vessels.†

PHYSICAL BACKGROUND AND IMAGING DEVICES

The physical principles of the Doppler effect were first described by C. J. Doppler in the early 19th century.[91,113,124,158,169] The *Doppler effect* (i.e., *Doppler shift*) is defined as a change in the frequency of the sound wave caused by movement of a reflector (e.g., blood). If reflector motion is toward the transducer, the frequency of the returning echo is greater than that of the emitted frequency. Conversely, if reflector motion is away from the transducer, the frequency of the returning echo is lower than that of the emitted sound beam. The greater the velocity of the reflector (e.g., the faster the blood flow), the greater the difference between the reflected and emitted frequencies. The magnitude of the frequency change (Doppler shift) depends on not only the velocity of the reflector (V) but also the sound velocity in the

*References 56, 57, 114, 117-119, 135, 136, 139.

†References 3, 6, 7, 9, 11, 58, 59, 65, 111, 121, 137, 144, 175, 182.

BOX 14-1

Indications for Color Doppler Imaging in the Eye and Orbit

- Evaluation of normal orbital and ocular vasculature
- Evaluation of other orbital vessels displaced by a mass lesion
- Primary evaluation and follow-up of orbital vascular lesions (e.g., varices, arteriovenous malformations, and carotid-cavernous sinus fistulas)
- Assessment of the vascular pattern of orbital and intraocular mass lesions
- Differentiation of intraocular tumors vs. hemorrhage and vitreous bands vs. retinal detachment
- Semi-quantitative assessment of perfusion in retinal and choroidal vascular disease

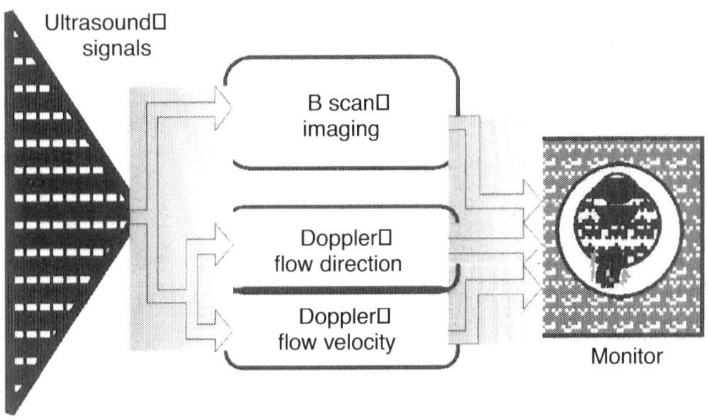

Figure 14-1 Schematic display of CDI system. (Modified from McDicken WN: *Diagnostic Ultrasonics. Principles and Use of Instruments.* ed 3, Edinburgh, Churchill Livingstone, 1990, p 228.)

medium (C) and the frequency of the sound source (e.g., transducer) (F_0). The detected frequency change (ΔF) is as follows:

$$\Delta F = 2VF_0/C$$

This equation shows that the greater the transducer frequency, the greater the frequency change for a given reflector velocity. This equation can also be converted to determine the flow velocity of the reflector. This equation is only valid, however, when the transducer and the reflector are parallel. If they are not parallel, a correction factor must be introduced, taking into account the angle (α) between the vessel and the axis of the sound beam (Doppler angle). Note, however, that as the angle increases, there is greater uncertainty in the accuracy of the velocity measurement. More recent CDI equipment displays the velocity directly and includes the angle of correction in the calculation:

$$V = \varnothing FC/(2F_0 \cos\alpha)$$

The maximum velocities of flowing blood usually encountered clinically range from 1 to 100 cm/sec and result in a frequency shift from 40 Hz to 11 kHz, depending on the transducer frequency. The nominal sound velocity of tissue is approximately 1,540 m/sec. In clinical practice, transducers range in frequency from 1 to 10 MHz. In ophthalmology, higher frequency transducers, with a range of 7.5 to 10 MHz, are preferred to achieve better resolution. Note that CDI instruments use linear array transducers. A linear array transducer consists of a group of closely spaced piezoelectric elements (see p 5) that are excited sequentially. This is in contrast to conventional ophthalmic B-scan, in which a single transducer element mechanically oscillates within the probe (see p 9).

With conventional duplex scanning, a pulsed Doppler signal is detected from only one area of an imaged blood vessel (sample volume). In this type of scanning, the examiner needs to evaluate multiple sample volumes along the two-dimensional image of the vessel to rule out pathologic Doppler signals. CDI, on the other hand, provides Doppler information from multiple sample volumes throughout the image simultaneously. Different color codes are used for flow direction with various color shades grossly indicating mean flow velocities. In this manner, blood flow is depicted in real time throughout the image. Direction of the flow is usually encoded in red (toward the transducer) or blue (away from the transducer), with the higher flow velocities represented by lighter hues. Since sensitivity for detecting very small blood vessels exceeds the gray scale image resolution of most B-scan instruments, vessels of very small size can be identified only indirectly by the color depiction of the Doppler shifts along the vessel course. With a color Doppler unit equipped with a 7.5 MHz linear array transducer, even very low Doppler shifts of 37.5 Hz (i.e., 0.385 cm/sec with a Doppler angle of 0 degrees or 0.77 cm/sec in 60 degrees) can be depicted.

Several modifications of CDI have greatly enhanced its clinical applicability. The most important of these is power Doppler.[26,58,65] For a given sample volume, power Doppler estimates the total strength of the Doppler signal, ignoring the blood flow velocity information. The power Doppler signal is primarily related to the number of red blood cells moving within the sample volume. In addition, the power Doppler is not significantly affected by the Doppler angle and varies little with the direction of the flow. Because the power Doppler signal is unaffected by the blood flow velocity, vessels that are very small or contain slow flow can be detected. In the power Doppler display, the total strength of the Doppler signal is indicated in yellow as opposed to the red and blue used for the CDI image. However, in newer instruments, some of the power Doppler information is depicted in red and blue. Other modifications include tissue harmonic imaging,[46] three-dimensional CDI,[88,134] and the use of contrast agents.[32,38,126,145]

CLINICAL APPLICATIONS OF COLOR DOPPLER IMAGING

Blood Vessel Evaluation

CDI can detect and measure arterial stenosis and flow-restricting or flow-disturbing abnormalities. Blood vessels that can be evaluated include large abdominal vessels (e.g., aorta and iliac) as well as femoral, popliteal, and other peripheral arteries. The large vessels of the head and neck, the carotid bifurcation, and the vertebral arteries can also be studied.

Organ Perfusion

CDI is used to visualize the perfusion of abdominal organs,[97,129,174] such as liver, kidneys,[167,176] spleen, testes,[116] and placenta,[96] as well as the heart,[164] the skeletal system,[154] and the brain.[147] CDI is used as a guide to obtain selective Doppler information and to allow better assessment of the hemodynamics in those organs. The major use in this category is the assessment of perfusion in renal and hepatic transplants.[74,95,141]

Tumor Neovascularity

CDI adds a new dimension to the ultrasound evaluation of mass lesions.* This technique is already being employed successfully in some cases to differentiate benign from malignant tumors of the liver,[31,54,71,87,156] tumors of the female breast,[35] and tumors of the testicles,[73] as well as tumors of the eye and orbit.†

OPHTHALMIC EXAMINATION TECHNIQUE

The CDI probe is applied against the closed eyelids using sterile ophthalmic methylcellulose as a coupling gel. During the examination, the patient is kept in a supine position. Care is taken to avoid pressure on the eye that might produce artifacts. Horizontal and vertical scans through the eye and orbit are performed. Depending on the direction of flow with respect to the transducer, the blood flow data is displayed in either red or blue. The colors can be arbitrarily assigned, but in this chapter, flow toward the transducer is depicted as red and away from the transducer as blue. The color saturation in the image represents the average frequency shifts from a spectral analysis performed at each sample site. These frequencies are converted into velocities by the CDI instrument by solving the Doppler equation for velocity (see p 368).

When the eye and orbit are examined through the eyelids, the ultrasound beam is essentially parallel to the orbital and ocular vessels; thus, most arterial flow is depicted in red and most veins are depicted in blue. Arteries can also usually be distinguished from veins by noting their pulsatility. Pulsed Doppler spectral analysis also helps to distinguish between the pulsatile arterial flow and the usually more continuous or minimally pulsatile venous flow. This difference allows for the quantification of data. Note, however, that when the ultrasound beam is at a 90-degree angle to a vascular structure or if a vessel contains only stagnant blood, no Doppler flow information is obtained and the structure is shown in gray scale display only.

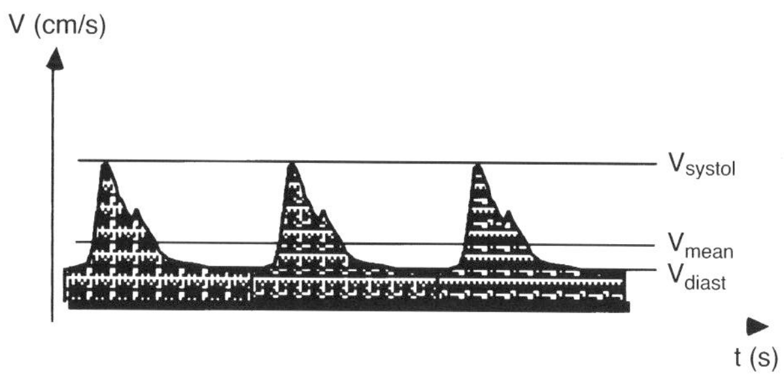

Figure 14-2 Schematic display of the Doppler spectrum (frequency-time display) from an arterial vessel. The peak systolic, the mean, and the end diastolic velocity can be measured from the Doppler spectrum.

CDI instruments offer different flow settings for studying different types of vessels. Examinations are first performed using a low or medium flow setting to allow for optimal detection of low to medium Doppler frequency shifts of the slow flowing blood in the small orbital vessels. Medium to high flow settings are applied for the OA since flow in this vessel is faster. Color threshold levels are adjusted to minimize artifacts caused by movement of the eyelid or involuntary eye movements. To then perform Doppler spectral analysis of a particular vessel, a sample volume of approximately 0.2×0.2 mm is chosen within the vessel. The proximal and distal portions of the vessel are imaged to determine the Doppler flow angle for estimation of velocity. The maximal systolic (V_{syst}) and end diastolic (V_{diast}) velocity (EDV) are two points on the waveform used to characterize this spectrum. The mean flow velocity is calculated from the spectral band as a frequency weighted mean (V_{mean}) (Figure 14-2).

It is also possible to use indices in the assessment of blood flow velocities. Doppler indices yield information about blood flow and vascular resistance that cannot be obtained from blood flow velocities alone. Various indices have been defined, including ratios of maximum systolic, end-diastolic, and mean velocity throughout a cardiac cycle. These indices are independent of the Doppler angle. In healthy individuals, the pulsatility (i.e., the ratio of systolic to diastolic velocity) can be used to assess vascular resistance distal to the area of measurement. The higher the vascular resistance, the lower the end-diastolic flow velocities. The three most commonly used indices are:

Ratio of $V_{syst}/V_{diast} = V_{syst}/V_{diast}$

Resistance index of Pourcelot (RI) $= (V_{syst} - V_{diast})/V_{syst}$

Pulsatility index (Gosling) $= (V_{syst} - V_{diast})/V_{mean}$

*References 127, 128, 130, 151, 155, 157, 159.

†References 18, 33, 45, 61, 62, 80, 99, 103-105, 143, 160, 178, 179, 183.

Color Doppler Imaging

Dept. of Ophthalmology, Julius-Maximilians-University, Würzburg

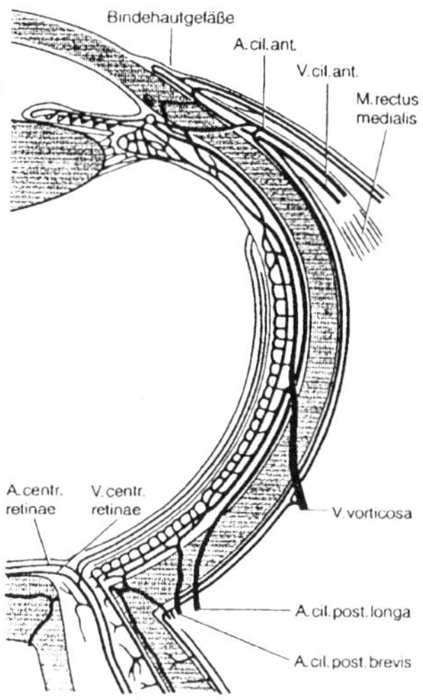

name, first name

date of birth

O M
O F

date

weight

RR

pulse rate

diagnosis

diabetes O yes O no

hypertension O yes O no

hyperlipidemia O yes O no

other

	OD (cm/sec)	P.R.	OS (cm/sec)	P.R.
CRA syst.				
CRA diast.				
CRA mean				
CRV max.				

	OD lat.	OD med.	P.R.	OS lat.	OS med.	P.R.
PCA short syst.						
PCA short diast.						
PCA short mean						
PCA long syst.						
PCA long diast.						
PCA long mean						

	OD	P.R.	OS	P.R.
ophthalmic art. syst.				
ophthalmic art. diast.				
ophthalmic art. mean				
sup. ophthalmic vein max.				

	OD lat.	OD med.	OS lat.	OS med.
vortex veins sup. max.				
vortex veins. inf. max.				

Comment

Figure 14-3 Sample sheet for documentation of ophthalmic CDI examinations.

The scan images can be recorded on videotape for later review, using cine-loop and frame-by-frame analysis of selected segments. During cine-loop replay, images can be photographed with a 35-mm camera directly from an isolated onboard color monitor. Quantitative measurements, as well as ratios for the various vessels, can be documented online or on a documentation sheet (Figure 14-3). The examination takes 20 to 30 minutes.*

VASCULAR TOPOGRAPHY OF THE NORMAL EYE AND ORBIT

Horizontal and vertical sections of the globe and normal orbit at the level of the optic nerve display Doppler signals along the course of the CRA and the CRV (see Color Plate 1, *A* and *B*).

The CRA and the CRV can be depicted within the anterior 2 mm of the optic nerve shadow (void). In some instances, these vessels can be traced to their entry point into the optic nerve. The CRV usually runs next to the CRA. It can be differentiated from the artery not only by its color coding but also by its Doppler characteristics and its continuous flow in systole and diastole. The spectrum of the CRA usually shows a venous overlap from the CRV (see Color Plate 1, *C*). The short and long PCAs can be identified on either side of the optic nerve, slightly posterior to the CRA. Several research groups have published their experiences and normal values with good overall reproducibility.*

*References 2, 13, 14, 18, 25, 40, 60, 63, 100-102, 143, 173.

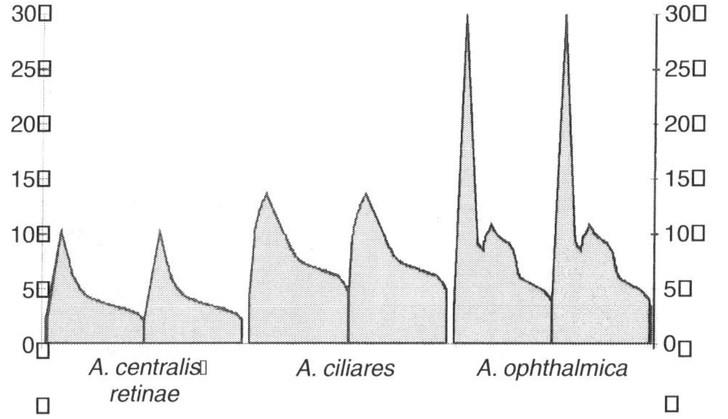

Figure 14-4 Schematic depiction of Doppler pulse curves (frequency-time spectra) for the CRA *(A. centralis retinae)*, ciliary artery *(A. ciliares)*, and the OA *(A. ophthalmica)*.

The Doppler spectrum of the PCAs shows velocity-time spectra similar to those of the CRA. However, the end-diastolic flow in the PCAs is higher, indicating the low resistance vascular channels of the choroid[98,103] (Figure 14-4). Segments of the main OA can be seen in the posterior orbit. The OA can be traced temporally to the optic nerve to the point where it usually crosses over the optic nerve toward the medial orbit.[67,68,93]

The flow velocity waveform of the OA is similar to that of the internal carotid artery, showing a high maximum peak systolic flow and low diastolic flow velocity (see Color Plate 2). Sometimes the superior orbital artery and the lacrimal artery can be identified. The SOV can be identified at the posterior aspect of the globe and in the supranasal orbit (see Color Plate 3, *A*). The SOV can be traced posteriorly until it crosses over the optic nerve.[22,40,98,173] Flow in the vortex veins can be demonstrated in all four quadrants. The spectrum with the continuous nonpulsatile flow pattern together with the blue color-coding is characteristic of venous flow (see Color Plate 3, *B*).

Several authors have performed reproducibility studies for quantitative velocity measurements of the various orbital vessels (Table 14-1). The most reliable and reproducible results were for the OA, the CRA, and the CRV. Greater variation was noted in the posterior ciliary vessels, whereas both the detection and velocity measurement of the SOV were unreliable.[14] When performing a more detailed analysis for quantitative measurements, the best intraindividual reproducibility, expressed as the relative error, was found for the peak systolic velocity (PSV) and the resistance index (RI) measured in the OA (PSV 5.9%, RI 3.1%) and the CRA (PSV 7.7%, RI 4.7%). The PSV and RI were less reproducible for the PCAs but were similar to

*References 1, 13, 14, 17, 18, 25, 40, 51, 52, 70, 82, 98, 100, 102, 125, 148, 161, 172, 173.

TABLE 14-1

Blood Flow Velocities (cm/sec) in Orbital Vessels (n = 222 Normal Eyes)

	Mean (STD) Peak Systolic	Mean (STD) End Diastolic
Central retinal artery (CRA)	9.6 ± (1.4)	2.4 ± (0.8)
Central retinal vein (CRV)	−4.2 ± (0.8)	—
Ophthalmic artery (OA)	37.7 ± (7.0)	8.8 ± (2.8)
Posterior ciliary artery (PCA)	11.3 ± (2.2)	3.6 ± (1.2)
Superior ophthalmic vein (SOV)	−7.6 ± (1.8)	—
Vortex vein (VV)	−8.5 ± (2.2)	—

the reproducibility of the EDV measured in the OA (11.8%) and CRA (19.9%). No systematic trend could be found between the first and second measurements of flow velocities in various orbital vessels, but consistent trends were observed when multiple measurements were taken.[148] For comparative measurements, it is quite important to measure at similar portions of the vessels. For the CRA, some authors noted significant changes according to the depth of measurement. The maximum velocity was found at 1.98 mm behind the optic disc surface.[39]

RETINAL, RETINAL VASCULAR, AND OTHER VASCULAR DISEASES OF THE EYE

Few reports have dealt with CDI in the evaluation of retinal disorders. Wells et al[170] and others have used CDI to depict a patent hyaloid artery in a case of persistent hyperplastic primary vitreous (see p 185). Wong et al[180] used the vascularity in the retinal vessels of detached retinas as an additional criterion to distinguish a detached retina from dense vitreous strands (Figure 14-5; see also Color Plate 4 and p 56). In a study of the flow velocities of the CRA and OA of patients with arterial hypertension and carotid artery disease, Cesarone and coworkers found significantly reduced systolic and end-diastolic flow velocities compared to a normal control group.[28] One group of patients with proliferative diabetic retinopathy was found to have significantly decreased PSV end-diastolic flow velocity of the CRA. The blood flow velocities in the PCAs and OA were unchanged compared with age-matched controls.[53] Other groups had similar results; however, this technique does not predict the course of an individual patient with diabetic retinopathy.[32,43,64,146]

Fluorescein angiography is the preferred technique for the study of retinal vascular disorders; however, CDI can add valuable information about CRA and PCA circulation by examining these vessels posterior to the retina and choroid.

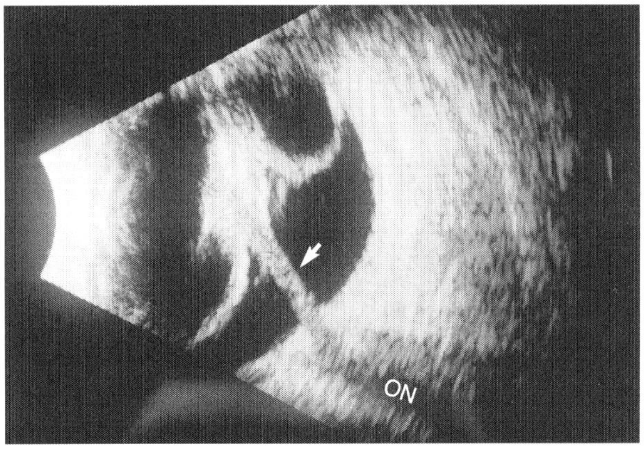

Figure 14-5 Total retinal detachment in a patient with stage V retinopathy of prematurity. Longitudinal B-scan shows a tight, closed funnel posteriorly *(arrow)* inserting into the optic nerve *(ON)*. See Color Plate 4 for CDI findings.

When CDI was used to examine patients with CRAOs, blood flow in the CRA was either absent or markedly decreased compared to normal controls.[69] Both maximum systolic amplitude and diastolic flow were decreased. Massive calcifications of the vessel walls of the intraocular retinal vessels can be detected in CRAO. The technique can also be used to study the extracranial vascular system, which might be a source of emboli to the retina.

CDI can answer several questions in patients with arterial occlusion of the retinal vessels:

- Are there emboli along the course of the CRA behind the optic disc?
- Are the flow velocities in the OA, CRA, and ciliary artery reduced?
- Are there collaterals from the external carotid circulation?
- Is there atherosclerotic disease of the carotid and vertebral artery system?

Ho et al[72] published the first study using CDI for the investigation and diagnosis of ocular ischemic syndrome (OIS). These investigators demonstrated reduced ocular blood flow in the OA, PCAs, or CRA in eyes with OIS. Furthermore, in some eyes with OIS, CDI showed undetectable or reversed blood flow velocities in the corresponding PCAs or OA (see Color Plate 5).[84,168,177,181] In general, lower flow values represent compromised blood flow proximal to the point of sampling by CDI or increased resistance distal to the sampling point.*

Although the posterior ciliary circulation can be difficult to assess, some reports indicate decreased flow velocities in patients with anterior ischemic optic neuropathy.[48] Several authors studying arteritic optic neuropathy found that no blood flow could be detected in up to three arteries in the affected (ipsilateral) orbit of six patients with giant cell arteritis (GCA) at presentation. Five of these patients also had undetectable blood flow in the PCAs of the contralateral orbit. Serial CDI examination revealed blood flow alterations in arteritic patients, despite treatment. Return of normal blood flow was slow and was related to the clinical features. By contrast, only one patient with nonarteritic anterior ischemic optic neuropathy showed undetectable blood flow in a PCA. These studies thus demonstrate that GCA leads to widespread and prolonged alterations in orbital blood flow. CDI allows the detection and monitoring of alterations in orbital blood flow that correlate with the clinical features of GCA. Serial CDI examinations in GCA may be used to aid management decisions.[50,81]

A characteristic Doppler spectrum pattern can be seen in patients with CRVO. Flow velocity in the CRA during systole is decreased, the peak systolic waveform is blunted, and diastolic flow is absent or markedly reduced. This decreased flow is an indication of the high resistance caused by the blockage of venous outflow in CRVO (see Color Plate 6).[15,86]

A highly turbulent flow with extremely high Doppler

*References 36, 49, 75, 76, 94, 112.

shifts and a high resistance flow pattern within the CRA have been found in several patients with drusen of the optic nerve and visual field defects. These findings support a direct compromise of the vasculature in the optic nerve head and a mechanical compression of the nerve fibers.

Belfort[19] and Baxter et al[16] used CDI to investigate the influence of pharmacological factors on flow parameters. Belfort detected a significant reduction in pulsatility and Pourcelot's index of the CRA and PCAs in a group of preeclamptic women treated with magnesium sulfate. Baxter and coworkers studied the effect of posture and topical β-blockers on the hemodynamics of orbital vessels. They found no postural effect, but there was a fall in Pourcelot's index. Since the orbital vessels are difficult to identify in these studies, caution should be used when interpreting this information as an indication that CDI can demonstrate subtle pharmacologic effects on orbital hemodynamics.

Decreased flow velocities in the long and short posterior ciliary vessels have been found in patients with primary open angle glaucoma (POAG). These findings support the theory that POAG causes vascular changes in the ciliary and choroidal vascular system.* CDI also provides a greater understanding of normal-tension glaucoma (see p 215).

INTRAOCULAR TUMORS

Effective vasculature is essential for all tumor growth. New vessels form and existing host vessels are incorporated into the tumor mass. Other than the qualitative information provided by intravenous fluorescein angiography and real-time conventional ultrasound, there has been no technique to assess tumor-associated blood flow in the eye and orbit.

Several groups have used conventional duplex scanning and CDI to assess intraocular tumors.† These researchers demonstrated flow within the intraocular tumors and noted a decrease in Doppler shift after radiotherapy. One group found vascular changes not only within the tumor but also in the normal ocular vessels after gamma knife therapy for choroidal melanoma.[165]

The abnormal Doppler signals reported from breast carcinomas,[35,140] hepatomas,[10,55,74,77,78] and renal tumors[29,97,133,138] are useful for differential diagnosis. Histopathologic examination of tumor vessels often reveals primitive vascular channels, lacking smooth muscle and consisting of an endothelial layer and connective tissue alone.[130] Low resistance to flow is expected since the vessels in most neoplasms lack normal arteriolar smooth muscle, the recognized site of peripheral vascular resistance.

High sensitivity to minimal flow is necessary to detect fine tumor vascularity (see Color Plate 7). Since lesions that can simulate uveal melanomas, such as large subretinal hemorrhages, usually do not have a distinctive blood supply, they can be differentiated from melanomas based on the absence of Doppler flow (Figure 14-6; see also Color Plate 8).

*References 30, 41, 42, 44, 66, 149, 161, 162.

†References 61, 62, 71, 105, 132, 178, 179.

The initial hope of differentiating various tumors based on their vascularity pattern and flow characteristics has not been fulfilled. The detection of low blood flow in neoplasms has been improved with the use of ultrasound contrast agents such as Levovist* and the power Doppler mode.[92,152]

ORBITAL DISORDERS

CDI has been used to study orbital vascular lesions, such as carotid-cavernous sinus fistulas and orbital varices, as well as orbital mass lesions. The use of conventional ophthalmic ultrasound for the evaluation of orbital tumors and vascular lesions is described in Chapters 12 and 13.

Carotid-Cavernous Sinus Fistulas

Various diagnostic modalities can be used to evaluate carotid-cavernous sinus fistulas (CCSF) or dural-cavernous arteriovenous malformations (DCAVM), also referred to as dural-cavernous sinus fistulas. These modalities include A- and B-scan ultrasonography,[120,131] (see pp 355 and 359), orbital and cranial computed tomography (CT) scanning,[85] carotid angiography, magnetic resonance imaging (MRI),[150] and orbital venography.[166] In these patients, CDI clearly shows the

*References 5, 12, 23, 24, 27, 87, 137, 142, 145, 163.

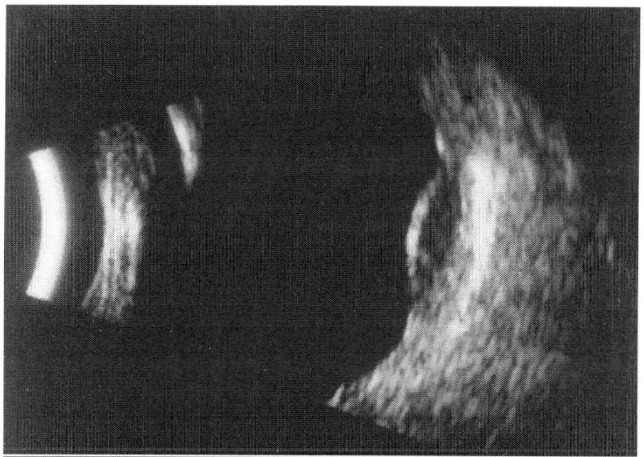

A

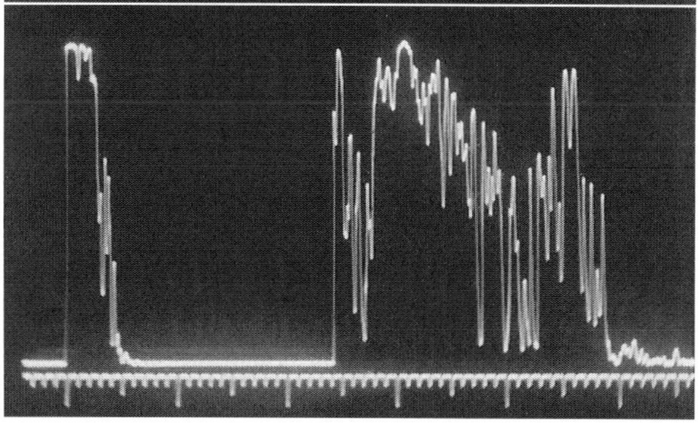

B

Figure 14-6 Dome-shaped choroidal melanoma. **A,** B-scan at reduced gain shows moderately elevated dome-shaped tumor. **B,** A-scan at Tissue Sensitivity shows medium-low internal reflectivity. See Color Plate 8 for CDI findings.

dilated, arterialized SOV with high velocity blood flow toward the transducer, indicative of a CCSF (see Color Plate 9, *A*).[47,90] Furthermore, CDI depicts the high preseptal vascularity and the thickened extraocular muscles characteristic of this entity.[8,37,110,122] The Doppler spectrum is similar to that typically seen with arteriovenous shunts, i.e., high systolic and diastolic flow velocities (see Color Plate 9, *B*). A recent report from Soulier-Sotto et al[153] confirmed these findings and stressed that CDI can also be used to monitor the clinical course of CCSF and/or to document the effect of embolization or balloon occlusion (see Color Plate 9, *C*).

The insidious onset of a red eye and elevated intraocular pressure in older women suggests a DCAVM. Often, however, the diagnosis cannot be made since CT fails to show a dilated SOV. Using CDI, the examiner can diagnose DCAVM by the presence of arterialized flow in the SOV together with the clinical signs.

Orbital Varix

In contrast to CCSF, orbital varices demonstrate relatively low blood flow velocities with CDI. In addition, dynamic evaluation of a varix during inspiration and Valsalva maneuver shows both inflow and outflow of blood (see Color Plate 10 and p 359).[83,99,171]

Orbital Mass Lesions

CDI adds a new dimension to the study of orbital mass lesions. Although CT, MRI, and conventional ultrasound provide an excellent topographic display of these lesions and some indication of vascularity (see p 306 and Chapter 13), CDI directly displays active blood flow when contrast enhancement or signal intensities are studied.

After studying several tumors, Jain and coworkers[80] reported that they were unable to attribute specific vascularity patterns to individual tumors. Others have reported that cavernous hemangiomas of the orbit usually show very little to almost no flow and that venous flow velocities are extremely low throughout the lesion (see Color Plate 11). In contrast, lymphomas, metastatic lesions, and highly vascular tumors such as hemangiopericytomas (see Color Plate 12) contain large arterial and venous vessels that supply the tumor.[98] Compression of the CRA has been shown in a case of gaze-induced amaurosis caused by a cavernous hemangioma.[89]

In patients with optic nerve sheath meningioma, CDI demonstrates progressive compression of the optic nerve and its vasculature. In advanced stages, a high resistance flow pattern is found in the CRA (Figure 14-7; see also Color Plate 13).

Several groups have found CDI quite helpful, in conjunction with CT and MRI, in planning the surgical approach to a tumor[79,183] and in the treatment of patients with thyroid ophthalmopathy.[20,21,123] Using CDI for the preoperative evaluation of orbital lesions, the surgeon can predict large arterial or venous vessels that might be encountered during the surgical procedure (Figure 14-8; see Color Plates 14 and 15).

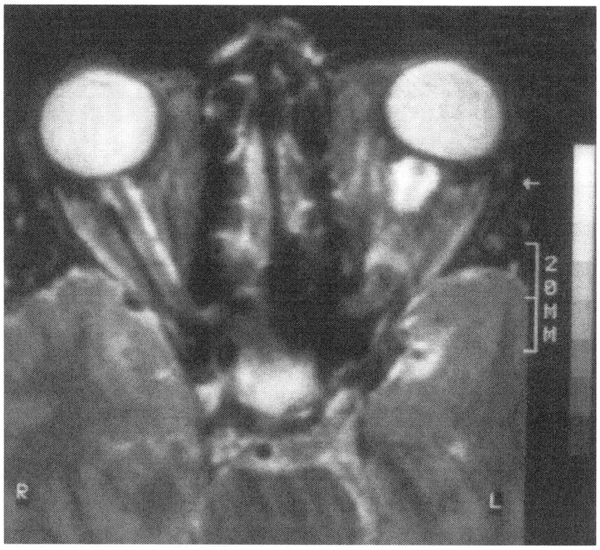

Figure 14-7 Optic nerve sheath meningioma. T2-weighted MRI of the orbit demonstrates the dilated left optic nerve. See Color Plate 13 for CDI findings.

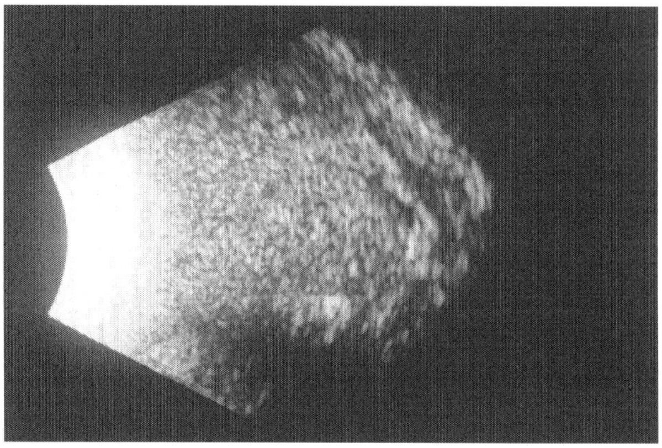

Figure 14-8 Capillary hemangioma located in the anterior orbit of a child. Paraocular B-scan shows diffuse orbital mass. See Color Plate 14 for CDI findings.

SAFETY CONSIDERATIONS

As with any diagnostic test, there may be some risk in diagnostic ultrasound. The potential risks are primarily related to the intensity of energy output by the ultrasound instrument. The measurement of energy output in ultrasound, referred to as the *spatial peak temporal average* (SPTA), is expressed in mW/cm^2. The SPTA is the highest intensity of energy occurring within the ultrasound field average over an entire scan frame period.

The American Institute of Ultrasound in Medicine (AIUM) has reviewed reports and issued a statement about the bioeffects of ultrasound on in vivo mammalian tissue.[4] According to the AIUM statement, with low frequency transducers (0.5-10 MHz) there is no independently confirmed significant biological effect on mammalian tissue exposed in vivo to unfocused ultrasound with intensities below 100 mW/cm^2 or focused ultrasound with intensities below 1000 mW/cm^2.[107,115] Currently, in the United States the Food and Drug Administration (FDA) has established limits for the ultrasound intensities (17 mW/cm^2) used for various clinical applications that are significantly lower than the limits indicated by the AIUM. These limits are linked to the measured output of instruments produced for ophthalmic and certain other particular applications prior to the enactment of the 1976 Medical Device Amendment. These parameters are not based on the assessment of risks published today.

For instruments currently used by the author of this chapter (QAD 1, QAD 2000, Siemens Elegra Siemens-Quantum Inc., Issaquah, Washington, USA), the estimated SPTA in the color imaging mode is 2 to 3 mW/cm^2 for the 7.5 MHz transducer. During spectral analysis, the SPTA is approximately 50 to 100 mW/cm^2. Although this measurement is within the AIUM safety limits, it exceeds the upper limits of the FDA guidelines.

Depending on the device settings for commercially available color Doppler units, even the AIUM limits of safety may be exceeded, especially during pulsed Doppler spectral analysis. However, the SPTA intensities of 100 mW/cm^2 should not be treated as a magic number. Lizzi et al[106,108,109] and Coleman et al[34] performed intensive experiments on bioeffects of ultrasound on ocular tissues. According to these studies, the intensities used for diagnostic imaging are significantly lower than those that would be expected to cause unwanted ocular side effects, especially chorioretinal lesions and cataract formation.

REFERENCES

1. Aburn NS, Sergott RC: Color Doppler imaging of the ocular and orbital blood vessels. *Curr Opin Ophthalmol* 1993;4:3.
2. Aburn NS, Sergott RC: Orbital colour Doppler imaging. *Eye* 1993; 7:639.
3. Adler RS, Rubin JM, Fowlkes JB, et al: Ultrasonic estimation of tissue perfusion: A stochastic approach. *Ultrasound Med Biol* 1995; 21:493.
4. AIUM: Bioeffects considerations for the safety of diagnostic ultrasound. *J Ultrasound Med* 1988:7(suppl):S4.
5. Albrecht T, Patel N, Cosgrove DO, et al: Enhancement of power Doppler signals from breast lesions with the ultrasound contrast agent EchoGen emulsion: Subjective and quantitative assessment. *Acad Radiol* 1998;5:195.
6. Allard L, Cloutier G: Power Doppler ultrasound scan imaging of the level of red blood cell aggregation: An in vitro study. *J Vasc Surg* 1999;30:157.
7. Allard L, Cloutier G, Guo Z, Durand LG: Review of the assessment of single level and multilevel arterial occlusive disease in lower limbs by duplex ultrasound. *Ultrasound Med Biol* 1999;25:495.
8. Aung T, Oen FT, Fu ER: Orbital colour Doppler imaging in carotid-cavernous sinus fistula. *Aust N Z J Ophthalmol* 1996;24:121.
9. Babcock DS, Patriquin H, LaFortune M, et al: Power Doppler sonography: Basic principles and clinical applications in children. *Pediatr Radiol* 1996;26:109.
10. Bartolozzi C, Lencioni R, Paolicchi A, et al: Differentiation of hepatocellular adenoma and focal nodular hyperplasia of the liver: Comparison of power Doppler imaging and conventional color Doppler sonography. *Eur Radiol* 1997;7:1410.
11. Bascom PA, Cobbold RS: Origin of the Doppler ultrasound spectrum from blood. *IEEE Trans Biomed Eng* 1996;43:562.
12. Bauer A, Hauff P, Lazenby J, et al: Wideband harmonic imaging: A novel contrast ultrasound imaging technique. *Eur Radiol* 1999; 9(suppl 3):S364.
13. Baxter GM, Williamson TH: Colour flow imaging of the orbit—concept or diagnostic tool? [editorial]. *Clin Radiol* 1994;49:845.
14. Baxter GM, Williamson TH: Color Doppler imaging of the eye: Normal ranges, reproducibility, and observer variation. *J Ultrasound Med* 1995;14:91.
15. Baxter GM, Williamson TH: The value of serial Doppler imaging in central retinal vein occlusion: Correlation with visual recovery. *Clin Radiol* 1996;51:411.
16. Baxter GM, Williamson TH, McKillop G, et al: Color Doppler ultrasound of orbital and optic nerve blood flow: Effects of posture and timolol 0.5%. *Invest Ophthalmol Vis Sci* 1992;33:604.
17. Bayramlar H, Totan Y, Cekic O, et al: Evaluation of hemodynamic changes in the ophthalmic artery with color Doppler ultrasonography after strabismus surgery. *J Pediatr Ophthalmol Strabismus* 2000;37:94.
18. Belden CJ, Abbitt PL, Beadles KA: Color Doppler US of the orbit. *Radiographics* 1995;15:589.
19. Belfort MA: The effect of magnesium sulphate on blood flow velocity in the maternal retina in mild pre-eclampsia: A preliminary colour flow Doppler study. *Br J Obstet Gynaecol* 1992;99:641.
20. Benning H, Lieb W, Kahaly G, et al: Farbduplexsonographische Befunde bei Patienten mit endokriner Orbitopathie. *Der Ophthalmologe* 1993 im Druck.
21. Benning H, Lieb W, Kahaly G, et al: Farbkodierte Duplexsonographie bei Patienten mit endokriner Orbitopathie. *Ophthalmologe* 1994;91:20.
22. Berges O: Colour flow imaging of the orbital veins. *Acta Ophthalmol Suppl* 1992;204:55.
23. Bogers HA, Sedelaar JP, Beerlage HP, et al: Contrast-enhanced three-dimensional power Doppler angiography of the human prostate: Correlation with biopsy outcome. *Urology* 1999;54:97.
24. Brown JM, Quedens CC, Alderman JL, et al: Contrast-enhanced sonography of tumor neovascularity in a rabbit model. *Ultrasound Med Biol* 1998;24:495.
25. Bucci M, Quaranta L, Ripandelli G, et al: Orbital blood flow assessment by color Doppler imaging in normal human subjects [abstract]. *Invest Ophthalmol Vis Sci* 1992;33:807.
26. Bude RO, Rubin JM: Power Doppler sonography [editorial comment]. *Radiology* 1996;200:21.
27. Cennamo G, Rosa N, Vallone GF, et al: First experience with a new echographic contrast agent. *Br J Ophthalmol* 1994;78:823.
28. Cesarone MR, Laurora G, Steigerwalt R, et al: Retinal duplex scanning in cerebrovascular disease and hypertension. *Vasa* 1992;21:163.
29. Chen P, Maklad N, Redwine M: Color and power Doppler imaging of the kidneys. *World J Urol* 1998;16:41.
30. Chiou HJ, Chou YH, Liu CJ, et al: Evaluation of ocular arterial changes in glaucoma with color Doppler ultrasonography. *J Ultrasound Med* 1999;18:295.
31. Choi BI, Kim TK, Han JK, et al: Power versus conventional color Doppler sonography: Comparison in the depiction of vasculature in liver tumors [comment]. *Radiology* 1996;200:55.
32. Cianci R, Mander A, Santarelli G, et al: Color-Doppler sonography in ophthalmology. *Minerva Cardioangiol* 2000;48:61.
33. Cioffi GA, Wang L: Optic nerve blood flow in glaucoma. *Semin Ophthalmol* 1999;14:164.
34. Coleman DJ, Lizzi F, Silverman R, et al: Therapeutic ultrasound. *Ultrasound Med Biol* 1986;12:633.
35. Cosgrove D, Bamber J, Davey J, et al: Color Doppler signals from breast tumors. *Radiology* 1999;176:175.
36. Costa VP, Kuzniec S, Molnar LJ, et al: The effects of carotid endarterectomy on the retrobulbar circulation of patients with severe occlusive carotid artery disease. An investigation by color Doppler imaging. *Ophthalmology* 1999;106:306.
37. Costa VP, Molnar LJ, Cerri GG: Diagnosing and monitoring carotid cavernous fistulas with color Doppler imaging. *J Clin Ultrasound* 1997;25:448.
38. Delcker A, Turowski B: Diagnostic value of three-dimensional transcranial contrast duplex sonography. *J Neuroimaging* 1997;7:139.
39. Dennis K, Dixon R, Winsberg F, et al: Variability in measurement of the central retinal artery velocity using color Doppler imaging. *J Ultrasound Med* 1995;14:463.
40. Erickson SJ, Hendrix LE, Massaro BM, et al: Color Doppler flow imaging of the normal and abnormal orbit. *Radiology* 1989;173:511.
41. Evans DW, Harris A, Cantor LB: Primary open-angle glaucoma patients characterized by ocular vasospasm demonstrate a different ocular vascular response to timolol versus Betaxolol. *J Ocul Pharmacol Ther* 1999;15:479.

42. Evans DW, Harris A, Chung HS, et al: Effects of long-term hypotensive therapy with nonselective beta-blockers on ocular hemodynamics in primary open-angle glaucoma. *J Glaucoma* 1999;8:12.
43. Evans DW, Harris A, Danis RP, et al: Altered retrobulbar vascular reactivity in early diabetic retinopathy. *Br J Ophthalmol* 1997;81:279.
44. Evans DW, Harris A, Garrett M, et al: Glaucoma patients demonstrate faulty autoregulation of ocular blood flow during posture change. *Br J Ophthalmol* 1999;83:809.
45. Falco L, Esente S, Fantani S, et al: Our experience in the diagnosis of intraocular tumors by a B-scan system and angiodynography (Doppler). Preliminary results. *Acta Ophthalmol Suppl* 1992;204:76.
46. Fish PJ, Hoskins PR, Moran C, et al: Developments in cardiovascular ultrasound. Part 1: Signal processing and instrumentation. *Med Biol Eng Comput* 1997;35:561.
47. Flaharty PM, Lieb WE, Sergott RC, et al: Color Doppler imaging. A new noninvasive technique to diagnose and monitor carotid cavernous sinus fistulas. *Arch Ophthalmol* 1991;109:522.
48. Flaharty PM, Sergott RC, Lieb WE, et al: Optic nerve sheath decompression may improve blood flow in anterior ischemic optic neuropathy. *Ophthalmology* 1993;100:297.
49. Geroulakos G, Botchway LT, Pai V, et al: Effect of carotid endarterectomy on the ocular circulation and on ocular symptoms unrelated to emboli. *Eur J Vasc Endovasc Surg* 1996;11:359.
50. Ghanchi FD, Dutton GN: Current concepts in giant cell (temporal) arteritis. *Surv Ophthalmol* 1997;42:99.
51. Gillies WE, Brooks AM, Scott M, et al: Comparison of colour Doppler imaging of orbital vessels in elderly compared with young adult patients. *Aust N Z J Ophthalmol* 1999;27:173.
52. Giovagnorio F, Quaranta L, Bucci MG: Color Doppler assessment of normal ocular blood flow. *J Ultrasound Med* 1993;12:473.
53. Goebel W, Lieb WE, Ho A, et al: Color Doppler imaging: A new technique to assess orbital blood flow in patients with diabetic retinopathy. *Invest Ophthalmol Vis Sci* 1995;36:864.
54. Goldberg BB, Hilpert PL, Burns PN, et al: Hepatic tumors: Signal enhancement at Doppler US after intravenous injection of a contrast agent. *Radiology* 1990;177:713.
55. Goldberg BB, Liu JB, Burns PN, et al: Galactose-based intravenous sonographic contrast agent: experimental studies. *J Ultrasound Med* 1993;12:463.
56. Grant E, Tessler F, Perrella R: Clinical Doppler imaging. *AJR Am J Roentgenol* 1989;152:707.
57. Grant EG, Schiller VL, Millener P, et al: Color Doppler imaging of the hepatic vasculature. *AJR Am J Roentgenol* 1992;159:943.
58. Griewing B, Doherty C, Kessler C: Power Doppler ultrasound examination of the intracerebral and extracerebral vasculature. *J Neuroimaging* 1996;6:32.
59. Griewing B, Doherty C, Zeller JA, et al: Power Doppler—a new tool for transcranial duplex assessment of intracranial vasculature. *Bildgebung* 1996;63:35.
60. Guthoff R: Ultraschall in der ophthalmologischen Diagnostik, in Guthoff R: *Ein Leitfaden für die Praxis*. Stuttgart, Germany, Enke, 1988.
61. Guthoff R, Berger RW, Helmke K, et al: Doppler sonographische Befunde bei intraokularen Tumoren. *Fortschr Ophthalmol* 1989; 86:239.
62. Guthoff RF, Berger RW, Winkler P, et al: Doppler ultrasonography of malignant melanomas of the uvea. *Arch Ophthalmol* 1991;109:537.
63. Guthoff RF, Berger RW, Winkler P, et al: Doppler ultrasonography of the ophthalmic and central retinal vessels. *Arch Ophthalmol* 1991;109:532.
64. Guven D, Ozdemir H, Hasanreisoglu B: Hemodynamic alterations in diabetic retinopathy. *Ophthalmology* 1996;103:1245.
65. Hamper UM, DeJong MR, Caskey CI, et al: Power Doppler imaging: Clinical experience and correlation with color Doppler US and other imaging modalities. *Radiographics* 1997;17:499.
66. Harris A, Spaeth GL, Sergott RC, et al: Retrobulbar arterial hemodynamic effects of betaxolol and timolol in normal-tension glaucoma. *Am J Ophthalmol* 1995;120:168.
67. Hayreh SS: Arteries of the orbit in the human being. *Br J Surg* 1963;50:938.
68. Hayreh SS, Dass R: The ophthalmic artery. II: Intra-orbital course. *Br J Ophthalmol* 1962;46:165.
69. Hedges T, Reichel E, Duker J, et al: Color Doppler imaging identifies different mechanisms of central retinal artery occlusion [abstract]. *Invest Ophthalmol Vis Sci* 1993;34:842.
70. Heggerick PA, Hedges T: Color Doppler imaging of the eye and orbit. *J Ophthalmic Nurs Technol* 1995;14:249.
71. Hirai T, Ohishi H, Yamada R, et al: Three-dimensional power Doppler sonography of tumor vascularity. *Radiat Med* 1998;16:353.
72. Ho AC, Lieb WE, Flaharty PM, et al: Color Doppler imaging of the ocular ischemic syndrome. *Ophthalmology* 1992;99:1453.
73. Horstman WG, Melson G, Middleton W, et al: Testicular tumors: Findings with color Doppler US. *Radiology* 1992;185:733.
74. Hosten N, Puls R, Bechstein WO, et al: Focal liver lesions: Doppler ultrasound. *Eur Radiol* 1999;9:428.
75. Hu H, Sheng WY, Yen MY, et al: Color Doppler imaging of orbital arteries for detection of carotid occlusive disease. *Stroke* 1993; 24:1196.
76. Hu HH, Luo CL, Sheng WY, et al: Transorbital color Doppler flow imaging of the carotid siphon and major arteries at the base of the brain. *Am J Neuroradiol* 1995;16:591.
77. Imamura M, Shiratori Y, Shiina S, et al: Power Doppler sonography for hepatocellular carcinoma: factors affecting the power Doppler signals of the tumors. *Liver* 1998;18:427.
78. Ishiguchi T, Shimamoto K, Fukatsu H, et al: Radiologic diagnosis of hepatocellular carcinoma. *Semin Surg Oncol* 1996;12:164.
79. Ivekovic R, Lovrencic HA, Novak LK, et al: Value of color-Doppler imaging in diagnosis of intrabulbar and intraorbital tumors. *Coll Antropol* 2000;24:205.
80. Jain R, Sawhney S, Berry M: Real-time sonography of orbital tumours. Colour Doppler characterization: Initial experience. *Acta Ophthalmol Suppl* 1992;204:46.
81. James CB, Smith SE: The effect of posture on the intraocular pressure and pulsatile ocular blood flow in patients with non-arteritic anterior ischaemic optic neuropathy. *Eye* 1991;5:309.
82. Kaiser HJ, Schotzau A, Flammer J, et al: Blood-flow velocities in the extraocular vessels in normal volunteers. *Am J Ophthalmol* 1996; 122:364.
83. Kawaguchi S, Nakase H, Noguchi H, et al: Orbital varix diagnosed by color Doppler flow—case report. *Neurol Med Chir (Tokyo)* 1997;37:616.
84. Kawaguchi S, Sakaki T, Morimoto T, et al: Effects of bypass on ocular ischaemic syndrome caused by reversed flow in the ophthalmic artery [letter]. *Lancet* 1999;354:2052.
85. Keltner JI, Satterfield D, Dublin AB, et al: Dural and carotid cavernous sinus fistulas. *Ophthalmology* 1987;94:1585.
86. Keyser BJ, Flaharty PM, Sergott RC, et al: Color Doppler imaging of arterial blood flow in central retinal vein occlusion. *Ophthalmology* 1994;101:1357.
87. Kim AY, Choi BI, Kim TK, et al: Hepatocellular carcinoma: Power Doppler US with a contrast agent—preliminary results. *Radiology* 1998;209:135.
88. Kimura K, Yasaka M, Koga M, et al: Successful application of three-dimensional transcranial power Doppler imaging in two stroke patients. *Intern Med* 1998;37:770.
89. Knapp ME, Flaharty PM, Sergott RC, et al: Gaze-induced amaurosis from central retinal artery compression. *Ophthalmology* 1992; 99:238.
90. Kotval PS, Weitzner IJ, Tenner MS: Diagnosis of carotid-cavernous fistula by periorbital color Doppler imaging and pulsed Doppler volume flow analysis. *J Ultrasound Med* 1990;9:101.
91. Kremkau FW: *Diagnostic Ultrasound. Principles, Instruments, and Exercises*. ed 3. Philadelphia, WB Saunders, 1989.
92. Kurjak A, Kupesic S, Breyer B, et al: The assessment of ovarian tumor angiogenesis: What does three-dimensional power Doppler add? *Ultrasound Obstet Gynecol* 1998;12:136.
93. Lang J, Reiter U, Reiter W: Topographie des Orbitainhaltes. Teil I: Musculi bulbi, Orbitawände und-inhalt. *Neurochirurgie* 1990;33:91.
94. Lee HM, Fu ER: Orbital colour Doppler imaging in chronic ocular ischaemic syndrome. *Aust N Z J Ophthalmol* 1997;25:157.
95. Lerner RM, Mevorach RA, Hulbert WC, et al: Testicular imaging. *Curr Opin Radiol* 1991;3:694.
96. Levine D, Hulka CA, Ludmir J, et al: Placenta accreta: Evaluation with color Doppler US, power Doppler US, and MR imaging. *Radiology* 1997;205:773.
97. Lewis BD, James EM: Current applications of duplex and color Doppler ultrasound imaging: Abdomen. *Mayo Clin Proc* 1989; 64:1158.
98. Lieb W, Flaharty P, Göbel W, et al: Color Doppler imaging—a technique to study the hemodynamics of ocular and orbital veins [abstract]. *Invest Ophthalmol Vis Sci* 1992;33:1047.

99. Lieb W, Merton D, Shields J, et al: Color Doppler imaging in the demonstration of an orbital varix. *Br J Ophthalmol* 1990;74:305.
100. Lieb WE: Color Doppler imaging of the eye and orbit. *Radiol Clin North Am* 1998;36:1059.
101. Lieb WE, Cohen SM, Merton DA, et al: Darstellung von intraokularen und orbitalen Gefäßen mittels Angiodynographie. *Fortschr Ophthalmol* 1990;87:537.
102. Lieb WE, Cohen SM, Merton DA, et al: Color Doppler imaging of the eye and orbit. Technique and normal vascular anatomy. *Arch Ophthalmol* 1991;109:527.
103. Lieb WE, Flaharty PM, Ho A, et al: Color Doppler imaging of the eye and orbit. A synopsis of a 400 case experience. *Acta Ophthalmol Suppl* 1992;204:50
104. Lieb WE, Flaharty PM, Sergott RC, et al: Color Doppler imaging provides accurate assessment of orbital blood flow in occlusive carotid artery disease. *Ophthalmology* 1991;98:548.
105. Lieb WE, Shields JA, Cohen SM, et al: Color Doppler imaging in the management of intraocular tumors. *Ophthalmology* 1990;97:1660.
106. Lizzi F, Coleman D, Driller J, et al: Effects of pulsed ultrasound on ocular tissue. *Ultrasound Med Biol* 1981;7:245.
107. Lizzi F, Mortimer A: Bioeffects considerations for the safety of diagnostic ultrasound. *J Ultrasound Med* 1988;7:1.
108. Lizzi F, Packer A, Coleman D: Experimental cataract production by high frequency ultrasound. *Ann Ophthalmol* 1978;10:934.
109. Lizzi FL, Coleman DJ, Driller J, et al: Experimental ultrasonically induced lesions in the retina, choroid, and sclera. *Invest Ophthalmol* 1978;17:350.
110. Martin TJ, Troost BT, Ginsberg LE, et al: Left dural to right cavernous sinus fistula. A case report. *J Neuroophthalmol* 1995;15:31.
111. Martinoli C, Derchi LE, Rizzatto G, et al: Power Doppler sonography: General principles, clinical applications, and future prospects. *Eur Radiol* 1998;8:1224.
112. Mawn LA, Hedges TR, Rand W, et al: Orbital color Doppler imaging in carotid occlusive disease. *Arch Ophthalmol* 1997;115:492.
113. McDicken WN: *Diagnostic ultrasonics. Principles and Use of Instruments.* ed 3, Edinburgh, Churchill Livingstone, 1991.
114. Merritt C: Doppler color-flow imaging. *J Clin Ultrasound* 1987;15:591.
115. Merritt CRB: Ultrasound safety. What are the Issues? *Radiology* 1989;173:304.
116. Middleton W, Thorne D, Melson G: Color Doppler ultrasound of the normal testis. *Am J Roentgenol* 1989;152:293.
117. Mitchell DG: Color Doppler imaging—principles, limitations, and artifacts. *Radiology* 1990;177:1.
118. Mitchell DG, Merton D, Needleman L, et al: Neonatal brain: Color Doppler imaging. Part I: Technique and vascular anatomy. *Radiology* 1988;167:303.
119. Mitchell DG, Merton DA, Mirsky PJ, et al: Circle of Willis in newborns: Color Doppler imaging of 53 healthy full-term infants. *Radiology* 1989;172:201.
120. Moster MR, Kennerdell JS: B-scan ultrasonic evaluation of a dilated superior ophthalmic vein in orbital and retroorbital arteriovenous anomalies. *J Clin Neuroophthalmol* 1983;3:105.
121. Murphy KJ, Rubin JM: Power Doppler: It's a good thing. *Semin Ultrasound CT MR* 1997;18:13.
122. Nagy ZZ, Nemeth J, Suveges I, et al: A case of paradoxical worsening of dural-sinus arteriovenous malformation syndrome after neurosurgery. *Eur J Ophthalmol* 1995;5:265.
123. Nakase Y, Osanai T, Yoshikawa K, Inoue Y: Color Doppler imaging of orbital venous flow in dysthyroid optic neuropathy. *Jpn J Ophthalmol* 1994;38:80.
124. Nelson R, Pretorius D: The Doppler signal: Where does it come from and what does it mean? *AJR Am J Roentgenol* 1988;151:439.
125. Niwa Y, Yamamoto T, Kawakami H, et al: Reproducibility of color Doppler imaging for orbital arteries in Japanese patients with normal-tension glaucoma. *Jpn J Ophthalmol* 1998;42:389.
126. Orden MR, Gudmundsson S, Kirkinen P: Intravascular ultrasound contrast agent: An aid in imaging intervillous blood flow? *Placenta* 1999;20:235.
127. Orr NM, Taylor KJW: Doppler detection of tumor vascularity. *Clin Diagn Ultrasound* 1990;26:149.
128. Park KS, Choi BI, Won HJ, et al: Intratumoral vascularity of experimentally induced VX2 carcinoma: Comparison of color Doppler sonography, power Doppler sonography, and microangiography. *Invest Radiol* 1998;33:39.
129. Parro A, Philpot EF, Czuwala PJ, et al: Amplitude information from Doppler color flow mapping systems: A preliminary study of the power mode. *J Am Coll Cardiol* 1991;18:997.
130. Paweletz N, Knierim M: Tumor related angiogenesis. *Crit Rev Oncol Hematol* 1989;9:197.
131. Phelps CD, Thompson HS, Ossoinig KC: The diagnosis and prognosis of atypical carotid-cavernous fistula (red-eye shunt syndrome). *Am J Ophthalmol* 1982;93:423.
132. Pineda RN, Theodossiadis PG, Gonzalez VH, et al: Establishment of a rabbit model of extrascleral extension of ocular melanoma. *Retina* 1998;18:368.
133. Polascik TJ, Hamper U, Lee BR, et al: Ablation of renal tumors in a rabbit model with interstitial saline-augmented radiofrequency energy: Preliminary report of a new technology. *Urology* 1999;53:465.
134. Postert T, Braun B, Pfundtner N, et al: Echo contrast-enhanced three-dimensional power Doppler of intracranial arteries. *Ultrasound Med Biol* 1998;24:953.
135. Powis R: Color flow imaging. Understanding its science and technology. *J Diagnostic Med Sonog* 1988;4:234.
136. Pozniak MA, Zagzebski JA, Scanlan KA: Spectral and color Doppler artifacts. *Radiographics* 1992;12:35.
137. Pugh CR, Arger PH, Sehgal CM: Power, spectral, and color flow Doppler enhancement by a new ultrasonographic contrast agent. *J Ultrasound Med* 1996;15:843.
138. Ramos I, Taylor K, Kier R, et al: Tumor vascular signals in renal masses: Detection with Doppler ultrasound. *Radiology* 1988;168:633.
139. Ranke C, Hendrickx P, Roth U: Color and conventional image-directed Doppler ultrasonography: Accuracy and sources of error in quantitative blood flow measurements. *J Clin Ultrasound* 1992;20:187.
140. Raza S, Baum JK: Solid breast lesions: Evaluation with power Doppler US. *Radiology* 1997;203:164.
141. Rifkin M, Sudakoff G, Alexander A: Prostate—techniques, results, and potential applications of Color Doppler US scanning. *Radiology* 1993;186:509.
142. Rizzatto G, Chersevani R, Abbona M, et al: High-resolution sonography of breast carcinoma. *Eur J Radiol* 1997;24:11.
143. Rosa N, Cennamo G, Breve MA, et al: Power Doppler ultrasonography in ocular and orbital diseases. *Ophthalmologica* 1998;1:99.
144. Rubin JM, Bude RO, Fowlkes JB, et al: Normalizing fractional moving blood volume estimates with power Doppler US—defining a stable intravascular point with the cumulative power distribution function. *Radiology* 1997;205:757.
145. Schlief R: Ultrasound contrast agents. *Curr Opin Radiol* 1991;3:198.
146. Schmetterer L, Muller M, Fasching P, et al: Renal and ocular hemodynamic effects of insulin. *Diabetes* 1997;46:1868.
147. Seibert JJ, Avva R, Hronas TN, et al: Use of power Doppler in pediatric neurosonography: A pictorial essay. *Radiographics* 1998;18:879.
148. Senn BC, Kaiser HJ, Schotzau A, et al: Reproducibility of color Doppler imaging in orbital vessels. *Geron J Ophthalmol* 1996;5:386.
149. Sergott RC, Aburn NS, Trible JR, et al: Color Doppler imaging: Methodology and preliminary results in glaucoma [published erratum]. *Surv Ophthalmol* 1994;39:165.
150. Sergott RC, Grossman RI, Savino PJ, et al: The syndrome of paradoxical worsening of dural cavernous sinus arteriovenous malformations. *Ophthalmology* 1987;94:205.
151. Shimamoto K, Sakuma S, Ishigaki T, et al: Intratumoral blood flow: Evaluation with color Doppler echography. *Radiology* 1987;165:683.
152. Silverman RH, Kruse DE, Coleman DJ, et al: High-resolution ultrasonic imaging of blood flow in the anterior segment of the eye. *Invest Ophthalmol Vis Sci* 1999;40:1373.
153. Soulier-Sotto V, Beaufrere L, Laroche JP, et al: Diagnostic par écho-Doppler-couleur d'une fistule durale de la loge caverneuse à révélation ophtalmologique. *J Fr Ophthalmol* 1992;15:38.
154. Strouse PJ, DiPietro MA, Adler RS: Pediatric hip effusions: Evaluation with power Doppler sonography. *Radiology* 1998;206:731.
155. Sumi S, Yamashita Y, Mitsuzaki K, et al: Power Doppler sonography assessment of tumor recurrence after chemoembolization therapy for hepatocellular carcinoma. *AJR Am J Roentgenol* 1999;172:67.
156. Tanaka S, Kitamura T, Fujita M, et al: Color Doppler flow imaging of liver tumors. *AJR Am J Roentgenol* 1990;154:509.
157. Taylor GA, Perlman EJ, Scherer LR, et al: Vascularity of tumors in children: Evaluation with color Doppler imaging. *AJR Am J Roentgenol* 1991;157:1267.

158. Taylor K, Holland S: Doppler ultrasound. Part I: Basic principles, instrumentation, and pitfalls. *Radiology* 1990;174:297.
159. Taylor K, Ramos I, Carter D, et al: Correlation of Doppler ultrasound tumor signals with morphologic features. *Radiology* 1988; 166:57.
160. Thorn KM, Arrue P, Delisle MB, et al: Cavernous hemangiomas of the orbit: MR imaging. *J Neuroradiol* 1999;26:79.
161. Trible JR, Anderson DR: Factors associated with retrobulbar hemodynamic measurements at variable intraocular pressure. *J Glaucoma* 1998;7:33.
162. Trible JR, Sergott RC, Spaeth GL, et al: Trabeculectomy is associated with retrobulbar hemodynamic changes. A color Doppler analysis. *Ophthalmology* 1994;101:340.
163. Uggowitzer MM, Kugler C, Mischinger HJ, et al: Echo-enhanced Doppler sonography of focal nodular hyperplasia of the liver. *J Ultrasound Med* 1999;18:445.
164. Ungerleider RM, Greeley WJ, Sheikh KH, et al: Routine use of intraoperative epicardial echocardiography and Doppler color flow imaging to guide and evaluate repair of congenital heart lesions. A prospective study. *J Thorac Cardiovasc Surg* 1990;100:297.
165. Vecsei PV, Kircher K, Nagel G, et al: Ocular arterial blood flow of choroidal melanoma eyes before and after stereotactic radiotherapy using Leksell gamma knife: 2 year follow up. *Br J Ophthalmol* 1999; 83:1324.
166. Vignaud J, Clay C, Bilaniuk LT: Venography of the orbit: an analytical report of 413 cases. *Radiology* 1974;110:373.
167. Visser MOJM, Leighton JO, van de Bor M, et al: Renal blood flow in neonates: Quantification with color flow and pulsed Doppler ultrasound. *Radiology* 1992;183:441.
168. Ward JB, Hedges T, Heggerick PA: Reversible abnormalities in the ophthalmic arteries detected by color Doppler imaging. *Ophthalmology* 1995;102:1606.
169. Wells PNT: Basic principles of Doppler physics, in Taylor KJW, Wells PNT (eds): *Clinical Applications of Doppler Ultrasound.* New York, Raven Press, 1988, p 1.
170. Wells RG, Miro P, Brummond R: Color-flow Doppler sonography of persistent hyperplastic primary vitreous. *J Ultrasound Med* 1991; 10:405.
171. Wildenhain P, Lehar S, Dastur K, et al: Orbital varix: Color flow imaging correlated with CT and MR studies. *J Comput Assist Tomogr* 1991;15:171.
172. Williamson T, Lowe GDO, Baxter GM: Influence of age, systemic blood pressure, smoking, and blood viscosity on orbital blood velocities. *Br J Ophthalmol* 1995;79:17.
173. Williamson TH, Harris A: Color Doppler ultrasound imaging of the eye and orbit. *Surv Ophthalmol* 1996;40:255.
174. Wilson SR, Thurston WA: Gastrointestinal sonography. *Curr Opin Radiol* 1992;4:69-77.
175. Winsberg F: Power Doppler US [letter]. *Radiology* 1992;195:473.
176. Winters WD: Power Doppler sonographic evaluation of acute pyelonephritis in children. *J Ultrasound Med* 1996;15:91.
177. Wolf S, Körper N, Reim M, et al: Ocular blood supply in internal carotid obstructions, in *Ocular Circulation and Neovascularization.* Dordrecht, Dr W Junk, 1987, p 37.
178. Wolff-Kormann PG, Kormann B, Hasenfratz GC, et al: Duplex and color Doppler ultrasound in the differential diagnosis of choroidal tumors. *Acta Ophthalmologica Suppl* 1992;204:66.
179. Wolff-Kormann PG, Kormann B, Riedel KG, et al: Quantitative color Doppler imaging in untreated and irradiated choroidal melanoma. *Invest Ophthalmol Vis Sci* 1992;33:1928.
180. Wong AD, Cooperberg PL, Ross WH, et al: Differentiation of detached retina and vitreous membrane with color flow Doppler. *Radiology* 1991;178:429.
181. Wong YM, Clark JB, Faris IB, et al: The effects of carotid endarterectomy on ocular haemodynamics. *Eye* 1998;12:367.
182. Wu SJ, Shung KK: Cyclic variation of Doppler power from whole blood under pulsatile flow. *Ultrasound Med Biol* 1996;22:883.
183. Zuravleff JJ, Johnson MH: An ophthalmic surgeon's view of orbital imaging techniques. *Semin Ultrasound CT MR* 1997;18:395.

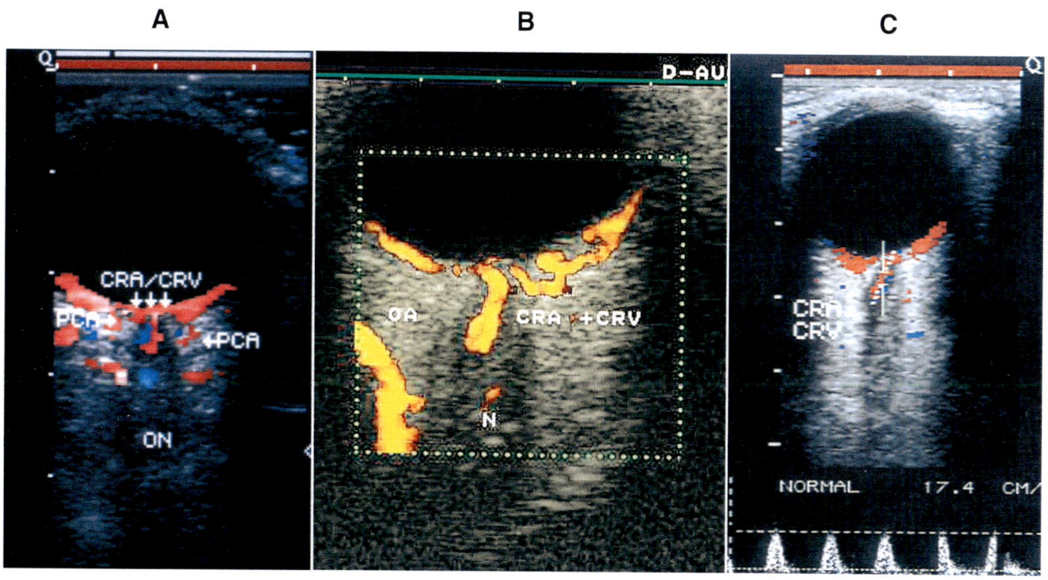

Color Plate 1, *A*, *B*, and *C*

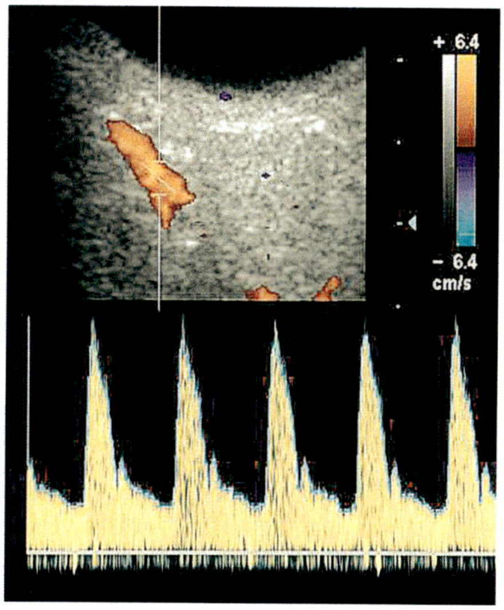

Color Plate 2

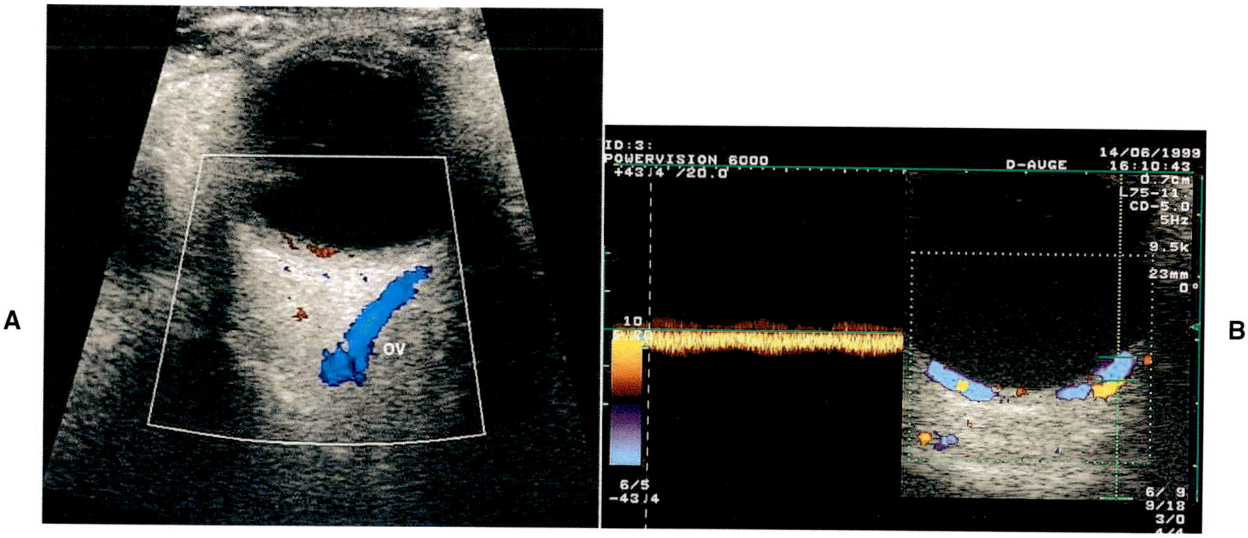

Color Plate 3, *A* and *B*

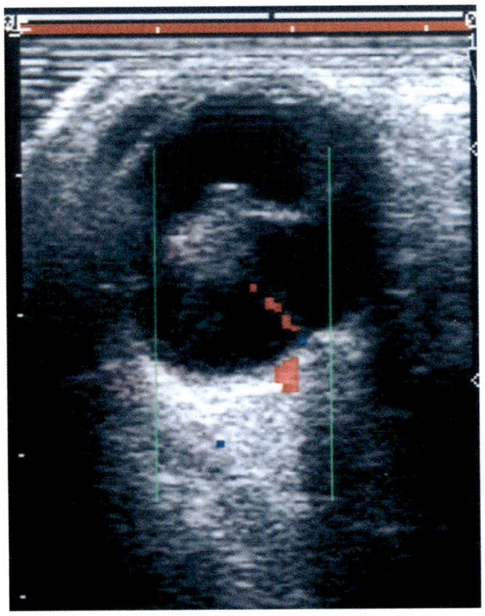

Color Plate 4

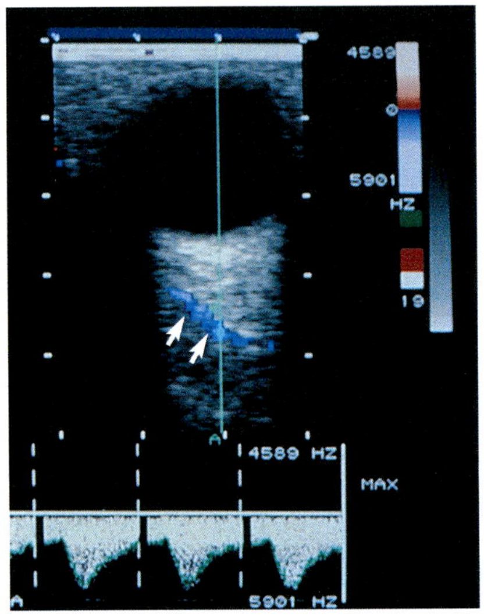

Color Plate 5

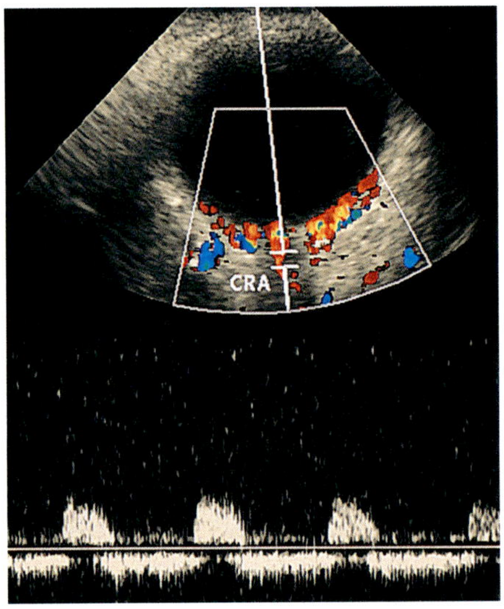

Color Plate 6

A

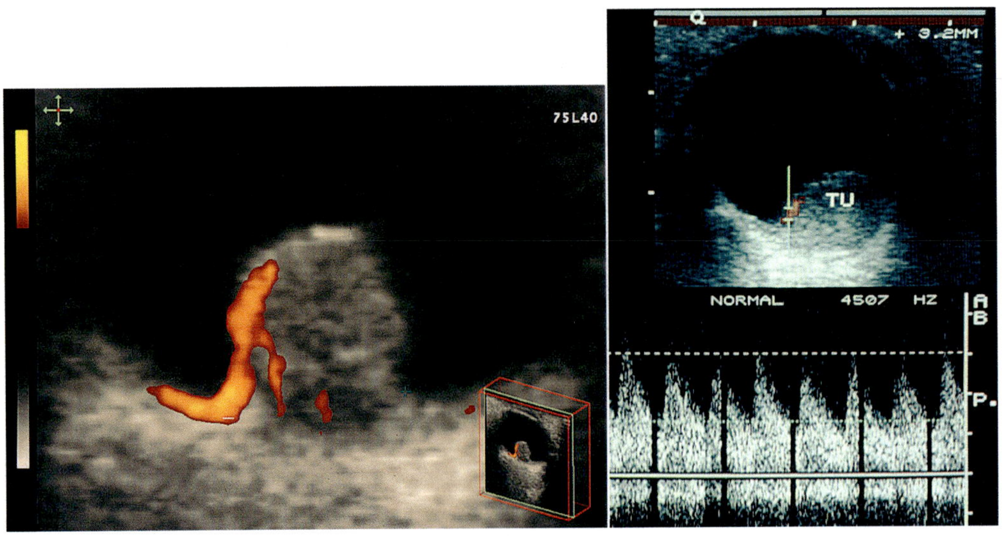

B

Color Plate 7, *A* and *B*

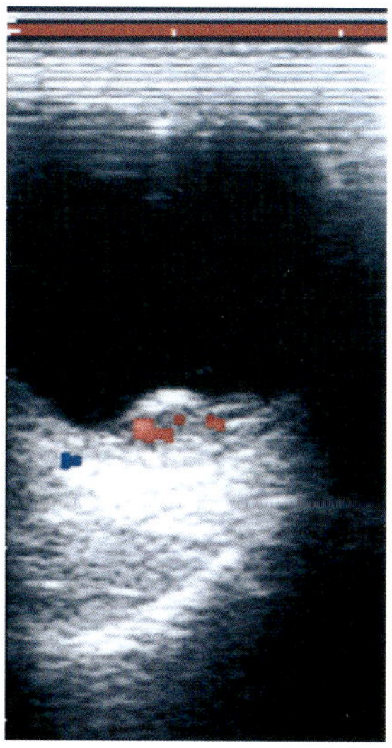

Color Plate 8

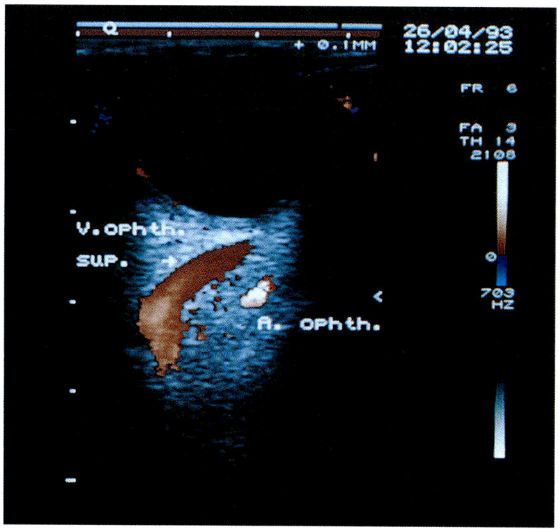

A

Color Plate 9, *A*

B

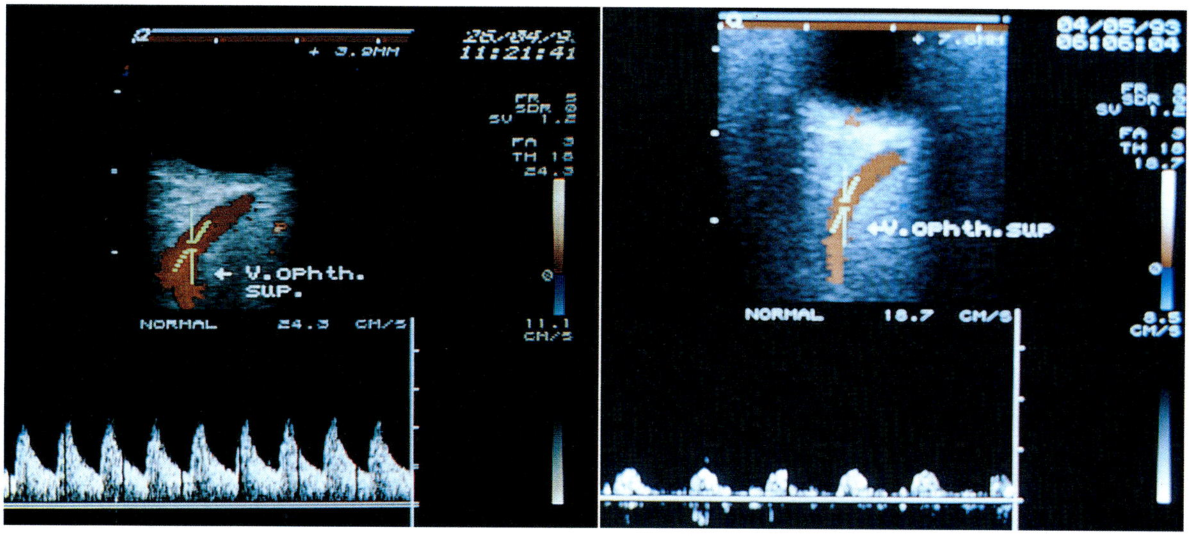

C

Color Plate 9, *B* and *C*

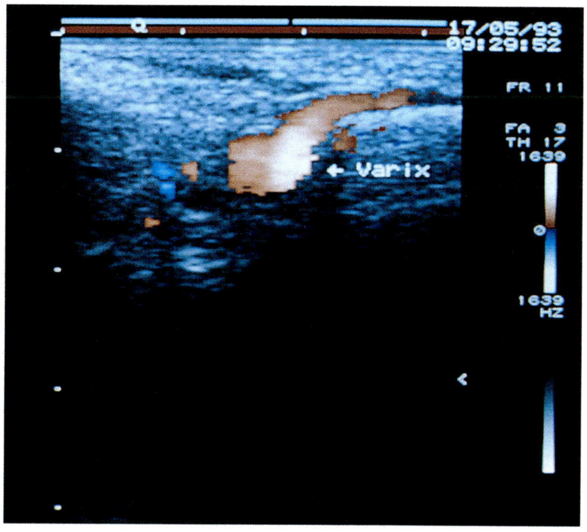

Color Plate 10

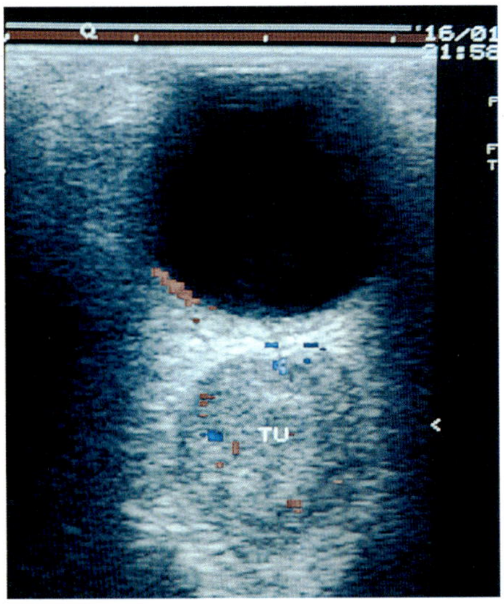

Color Plate 11

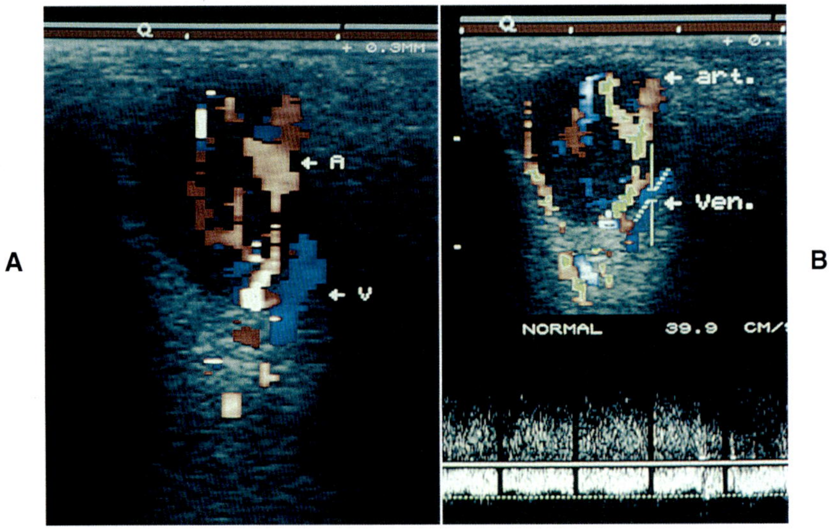

Color Plate 12, *A* and *B*

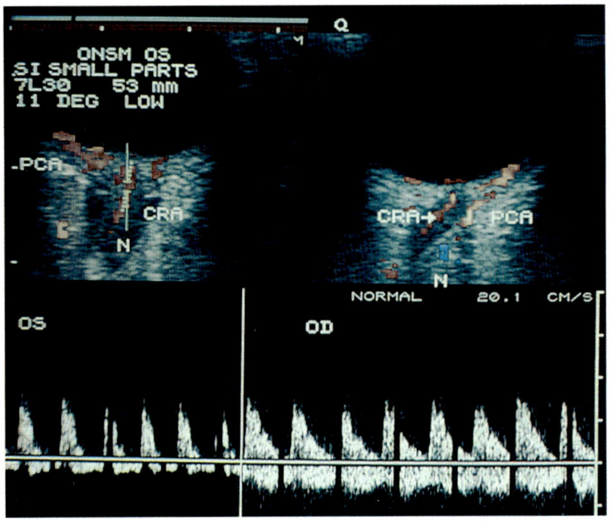

Color Plate 13

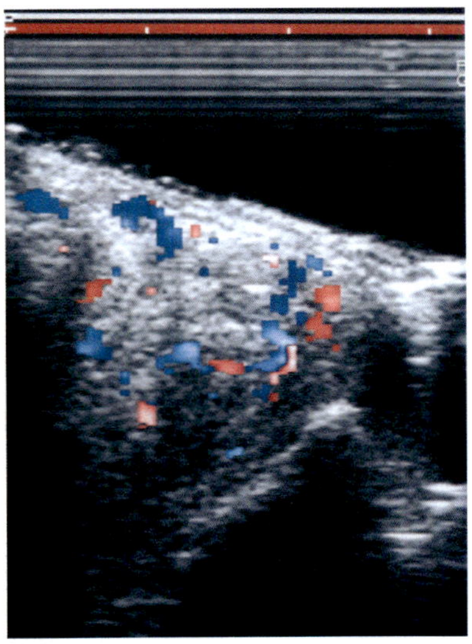

Color Plate 14

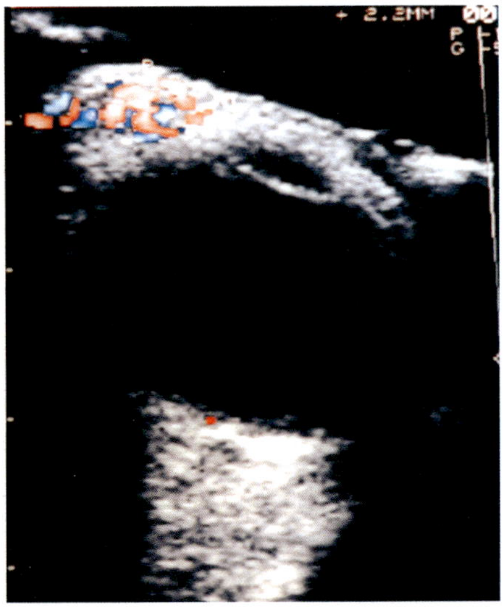

Color Plate 15

William D. Bates

Color Plates

Color Plate 1 CDI of normal eye and orbit. **A,** Horizontal section through the globe at the level of the optic nerve *(ON)*. The central retinal artery *(CRA)*, central retinal vein *(CRV)* and temporal short posterior ciliary arteries *(PCA)* are shown. **B,** Power spectrum display of the optic nerve region. The CRA, PCA, CRV and the ophthalmic artery *(OA)* are detectable without coding for flow direction. The sensitivity for detecting small vessels or low flow is higher than in the CDI mode. *N,* Optic nerve. **C,** Analysis of the Doppler spectrum. A cursor is placed on the vessel, and the angle is corrected according to the vessel course. The spectrum of the CRA usually shows venous overlap caused by the nearby CRV. (**A** and **C** courtesy Paula Heggerick, RVT, RDMS, Boston, Massachusetts.)

Color Plate 2 CDI showing course and Doppler spectrum of the ophthalmic artery.

Color Plate 3 CDI of normal superior ophthalmic vein and vortex veins. Blood flow in venous structures is directed away from the transducer and is thus coded in blue. **A,** The superior ophthalmic vein *(OV)* is demonstrated. **B,** Vortex veins with spectrum analysis showing characteristic continuous flow pattern below the baseline.

Color Plate 4 CDI of total retinal detachment in stage V retinopathy of prematurity. Blood flow within the detached retina is demonstrated. See B-scan of same case in Figure 14-5.

Color Plate 5 76-year-old patient with clinical signs of ocular ischemic syndrome *(OIS)*. CDI shows significantly reduced flow velocity in the CRA and a flow reversal *(blue)* in the OA *(arrows)*. The Doppler spectrum shows typical collateral high-end diastolic flow velocities as a sign of low vascular resistance.

Color Plate 6 Doppler signal from the CRA in a patient with a complete CRVO. There is a plump spectrum in systole and an absence of flow in diastole. The calculated Pourcelot's ratio is 1.

Color Plate 7 CDI of a large choroidal melanoma at the posterior pole. **A,** The tumor shows large feeding vessels. **B,** Spectrum analysis of tumor vessels demonstrating neoplastic vasculature with low resistance flow characteristics. *TU,* Tumor.

Color Plate 8 CDI of dome-shaped choroidal melanoma. Blood flow is shown within the tumor. See B- and A-scans of same case in Figure 14-6.

Color Plate 9 CDI of carotid-cavernous sinus fistula (high flow). **A,** A dilated, arterialized superior ophthalmic vein *(V. ophth.sup.)* is demonstrated. Flow reversal within the vein is depicted in red. **B,** Spectrum analysis of the arterialized vein shows characteristic high flow shunt pattern with high-end diastolic flow velocities. **C,** Spontaneous partial thrombosis of the vein. The blunted spectrum within the vessel is a sign of diminished flow.

Color Plate 10 CDI of superficial orbital varix. The paraocular image was captured during a Valsalva maneuver. Note that venous inflow appears red due to a change in flow direction during Valsalva maneuver. The venous nature of this flow can be confirmed by demonstrating the continuous venous pattern on spectrum analysis.

Color Plate 11 CDI of cavernous hemangioma within the muscle cone. There is only minimal vascularity within the tumor (*Tu*).

Color Plate 12 CDI of hemangiopericytoma (paraocular scans). **A,** The tumor shows significant vascularity in arterial *(A)* and venous *(V)* vessels. **B,** The Doppler spectrum clearly identifies a draining venous vessel *(Ven.)* with a continuous flow spectrum. An artery *(art.)* is shown in the anterior aspect of the lesion.

Color Plate 13 CDI of optic nerve sheath meningioma. The Doppler spectrum of the CRA in the eye with the meningioma *(OS)* is lower and has a higher Pourcelot's ratio than the uninvolved side *(OD)*. *N,* Optic nerve; *PCA,* posterior ciliary artery. See MRI scan of same case in Figure 14-7.

Color Plate 14 CDI of capillary hemangioma located in the anterior orbit (paraocular scan). Note the highly vascular nature of the tumor. See B-scan of same case in Figure 14-8.

Color Plate 15 CDI of superficial arteriovenous malformation. Note significant blood flow within mass involving the lid and anterior orbit.

William D. Bates

15 Extraocular Muscles

Extraocular muscle thickening is the most common abnormality encountered in orbital echography. Although other imaging techniques are very useful in showing moderate to marked muscle enlargement, echography is more effective for detecting subtle or early changes in muscle size.[15,34]

Occasionally, a slightly oblique section on computed tomography (CT) or magnetic resonance imaging (MRI) can result in misinterpretation regarding muscle enlargement. This is less likely to occur with ultrasound because the examiner constantly adjusts the probe position to prevent oblique sectioning. Echography is also useful for differentiating the various causes of muscle enlargement, for detecting associated orbital abnormalities, and for follow-up during therapy.

The most common cause of extraocular muscle thickening, both clinically and echographically, is Graves' disease.[17,27] Some of the other more common causes include idiopathic orbital myositis, venous congestion, tumors (e.g., metastatic carcinoma), and hematoma.[7]

The extraocular muscles are surrounded by a smooth sheath that produces distinct, highly reflective interfaces. The muscle fibers are relatively compact and homogeneous. As a result, the normal muscle is medium-high reflective on A-scan and less echo-dense than surrounding orbital soft tissue on B-scan (Figure 15-1). B-scan is very useful for documenting the gross size and contour of a muscle, whereas A-scan evaluation allows precise measurement of thickness. A-scan also can be useful for differentiating the various causes of muscle enlargement.[3,15,24]

Comparison of contralateral muscles always should be performed. This should be carried out using the same gain setting with both eyes fixating similarly. If strabismus is present, fixation should be adjusted so that the eye being examined is as close as possible to primary gaze. However, if one globe is either esotropic or exotropic and cannot be brought to primary gaze, the contralateral muscle should be measured using a similar gaze.

The rectus muscles, with their similar course and insertions into the globe, are all examined with the same basic techniques. The oblique muscles, on the other hand, necessitate different examination techniques due to their varied course and broad insertions (Figure 15-2).

EXAMINATION TECHNIQUES FOR RECTUS MUSCLES

B-Scan Technique

The B-scan examination is usually performed at a medium gain setting. The examiner may wish, however, to display the muscle at a high gain level initially and then decrease the setting until the muscle is clearly shown (Figure 15-3). The patient usually fixates in primary gaze or approximately 10 degrees toward the muscle being examined. The muscle is evaluated with both transverse and longitudinal approaches.

Transverse Scans

Transverse scans display a muscle in cross-section. For this approach, the probe is placed on the globe near the equator, on the side of the globe opposite from the muscle being evaluated. With a transverse probe position, the sound beam cuts across a muscle, imaging it as an oval-shaped defect within the echo-dense orbital soft tissue. The inserting tendon is first displayed as a thin defect adjacent to the sclera. Then, as the probe is angled posteriorly toward thicker portions of the muscle, the defect enlarges and approaches the bone line on the right side of the echogram (Figure 15-4).

The marker is directed superiorly for vertical scans (to evaluate the medial or lateral rectus muscles) and nasally for horizontal scans (to evaluate the superior rectus/levator complex or the inferior rectus muscle).

Longitudinal Scans

Longitudinal scans usually are performed with the patient fixating slightly away from the probe, toward the muscle being examined. The probe is placed on the side of the globe opposite to the muscle. For this approach, the probe is rotated 90 degrees from the position of the transverse scan. The marker is always directed toward the center of the cornea and the muscle being scanned. In longitudinal scans, the transducer oscillates perpendicular to the limbus, and the sound beam moves back and forth along the examined muscle, thus showing it in long section. This produces an echogram with the insertion of the muscle displayed at the upper portion of the screen and the wider muscle belly displayed at the lower portion (Figure 15-5).

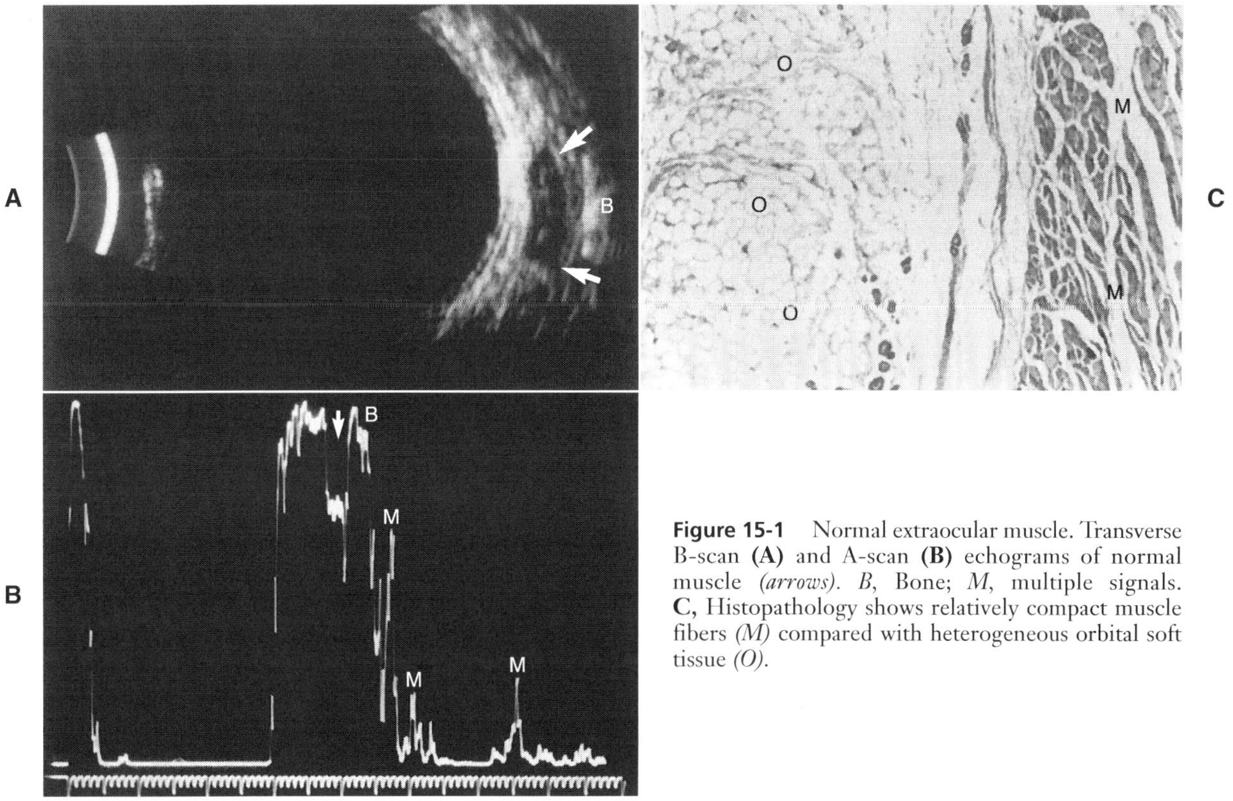

Figure 15-1 Normal extraocular muscle. Transverse B-scan **(A)** and A-scan **(B)** echograms of normal muscle *(arrows)*. *B*, Bone; *M*, multiple signals. **C,** Histopathology shows relatively compact muscle fibers *(M)* compared with heterogeneous orbital soft tissue *(O)*.

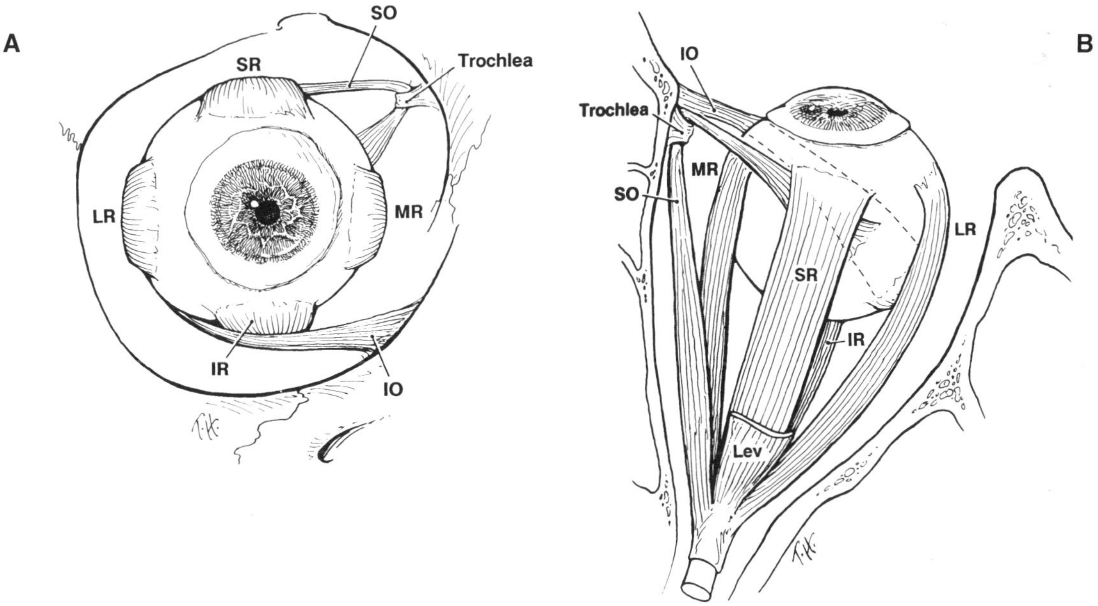

Figure 15-2 Schematic drawings indicate course of rectus and oblique muscles. Frontal **(A)** and axial **(B)** views. *SR*, Superior rectus; *MR*, medial rectus; *LR*, lateral rectus; *IR*, inferior rectus; *SO*, superior oblique; *IO*, inferior oblique; *Lev*, levator muscle.

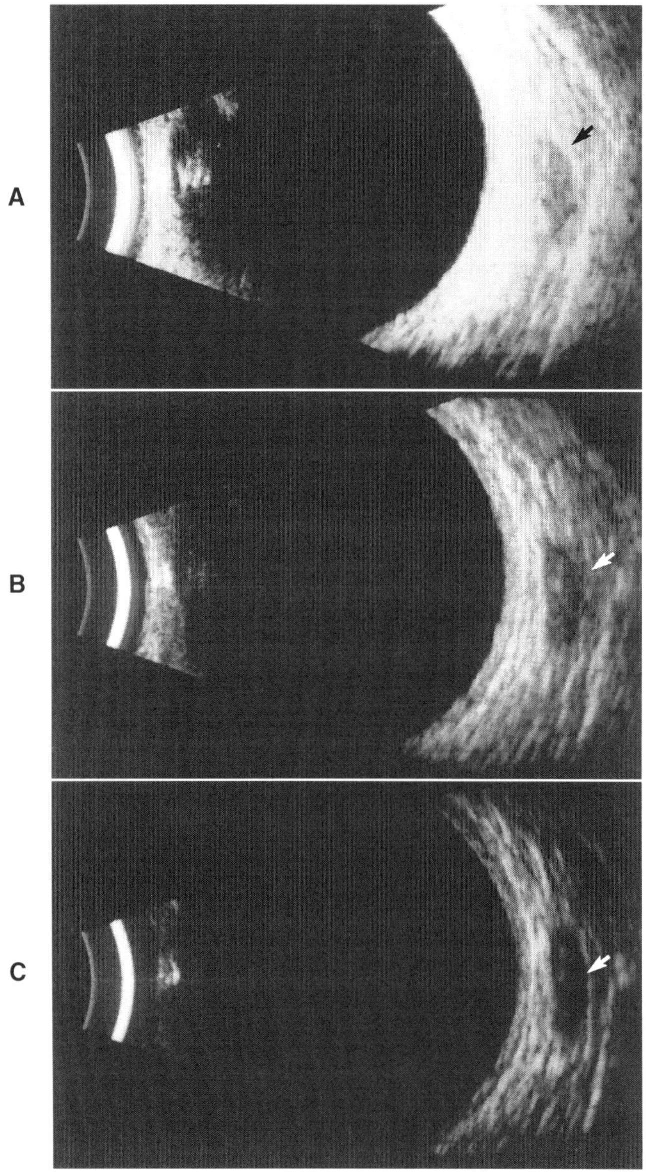

Figure 15-3 Transverse B-scan echograms of rectus muscle at various gain settings. **A,** Muscle *(arrow)* first located with high gain setting. **B,** Muscle at medium gain setting. **C,** Gain is reduced further until muscle is clearly delineated.

A-Scan Technique

For A-scan examination, the Tissue Sensitivity setting is used, and the patient fixates at or near primary gaze. With the globe in this position, it is easiest to direct the sound beam perpendicular to the muscle sheath. The A-scan probe is placed on the globe near the equator, opposite the muscle to be examined. The sound beam is aimed anteriorly toward the inserting tendon, which produces a small defect just to the right of the scleral spike. Once the insertion is demonstrated, the probe is angled more posteriorly, thereby shifting the sound beam along the muscle belly. As the sound beam progresses more posteriorly, the defect widens with the display of thicker portions of the muscle belly. At the same time, the muscle defect moves from left to right in the echogram, i.e., away from the scleral spike and toward the bone spike (Figure 15-6). As the sound beam is shifted along the muscle, it may be necessary to angle the probe somewhat to maintain perpendicular sound beam incidence to the muscle sheath. Perpendicularity is achieved when maximally high, steeply rising, double-peaked sheath spikes are displayed (Figure 15-7).

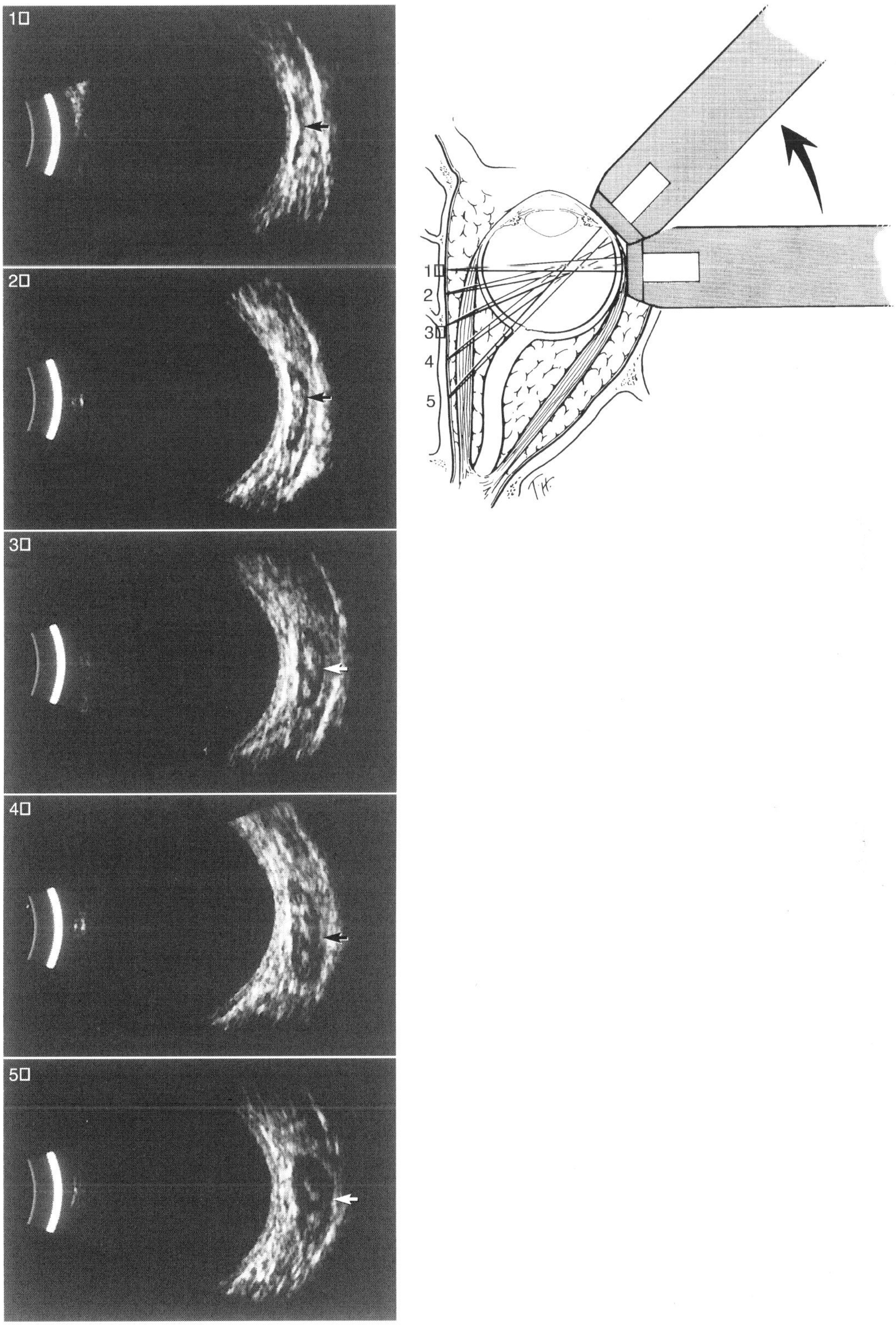

Figure 15-4 Dynamic B-scan evaluation of rectus muscle using transverse approach. With medium gain setting, probe is angled so that the muscle *(arrows)* is scanned from its insertion anteriorly *(1)* toward orbital apex posteriorly *(5)*. Note that muscle defect moves from left to right, gradually widens, and approaches the bone as the sound beam sweeps posteriorly.

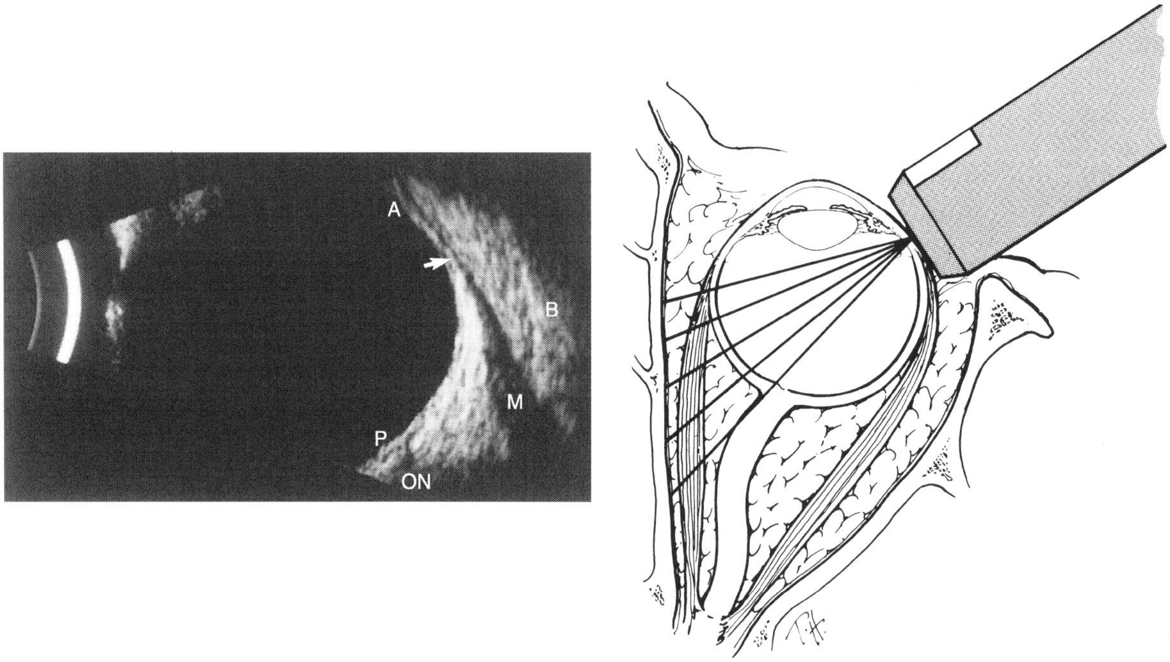

Figure 15-5 Longitudinal B-scan technique for evaluation of rectus muscle. The probe marker is directed toward the cornea. The muscle *(M)* is imaged in long section from its insertion anteriorly *(arrow)* toward the posterior orbit. *A*, Anterior aspect of globe; *B*, bone; *ON*, optic nerve; *P*, posterior aspect of globe.

One should always try to display the widest portion of the muscle. Because some muscles are thickest near the orbital apex (where it can be difficult to be perpendicular), the apparent maximum width may not truly represent the widest portion of the muscle. Despite this shortcoming, A-scan can reveal whether mid-portions of the muscle are abnormally thickened, which is usually sufficient for detecting muscle enlargement.

Measurements can be obtained from the screen using electronic cursors or taken directly from photoechograms by using calipers and conversion tables (with sound velocity of 1,550 m/sec) (Figure 15-8; see Appendix A). It is recommended that at least two measurements be taken of each muscle, using the widest measurement of the best quality echograms.

Normal values for the rectus muscles have been determined by two different studies: one by McNutt et al[20,21] (University of Iowa) and a second study by Byrne et al[3] (University of Miami) (Table 15-1). It should be pointed out, however, that these normal values may not truly reflect all age and population groups. More importantly, it may be best for individual echographers to establish their own control values to account for variability in technique.

To determine whether an individual muscle is enlarged, its thickness can be compared with the normal values shown in Table 15-1. In thyroid disease, it is useful to add the values for all four rectus muscles together and to compare this total to a normal overall value (see Table 15-1).

Often, the determination of whether a muscle is enlarged is easily made by comparing its thickness with that of the contralateral muscle (see Table 15-1). If, however a difference is found, it is important to be certain that the apparent difference is not the result of examiner error. Sources of possible error include lack of perpendicularity (see Figure 15-7) and failure to obtain measurements from the widest portions of the muscle.

Internal structure and reflectivity also should be assessed. Because of sound attenuation, reflectivity should be evaluated within the anterior one-third to one-half of the muscle (see Figure 15-6). As with thickness, reflectivity should be compared with that of the contralateral muscle.

EVALUATION OF INDIVIDUAL MUSCLES

Rectus Muscles

Medial Rectus

The medial rectus is best examined as the patient fixates in primary gaze with the A- or B-scan probe placed at the equator temporally. The medial is the easiest of the four recti to examine because temporally the recessed orbital rim allows easy probe positioning. Also, the medial rectus is the thickest of the four rectus muscles (Figure 15-9).

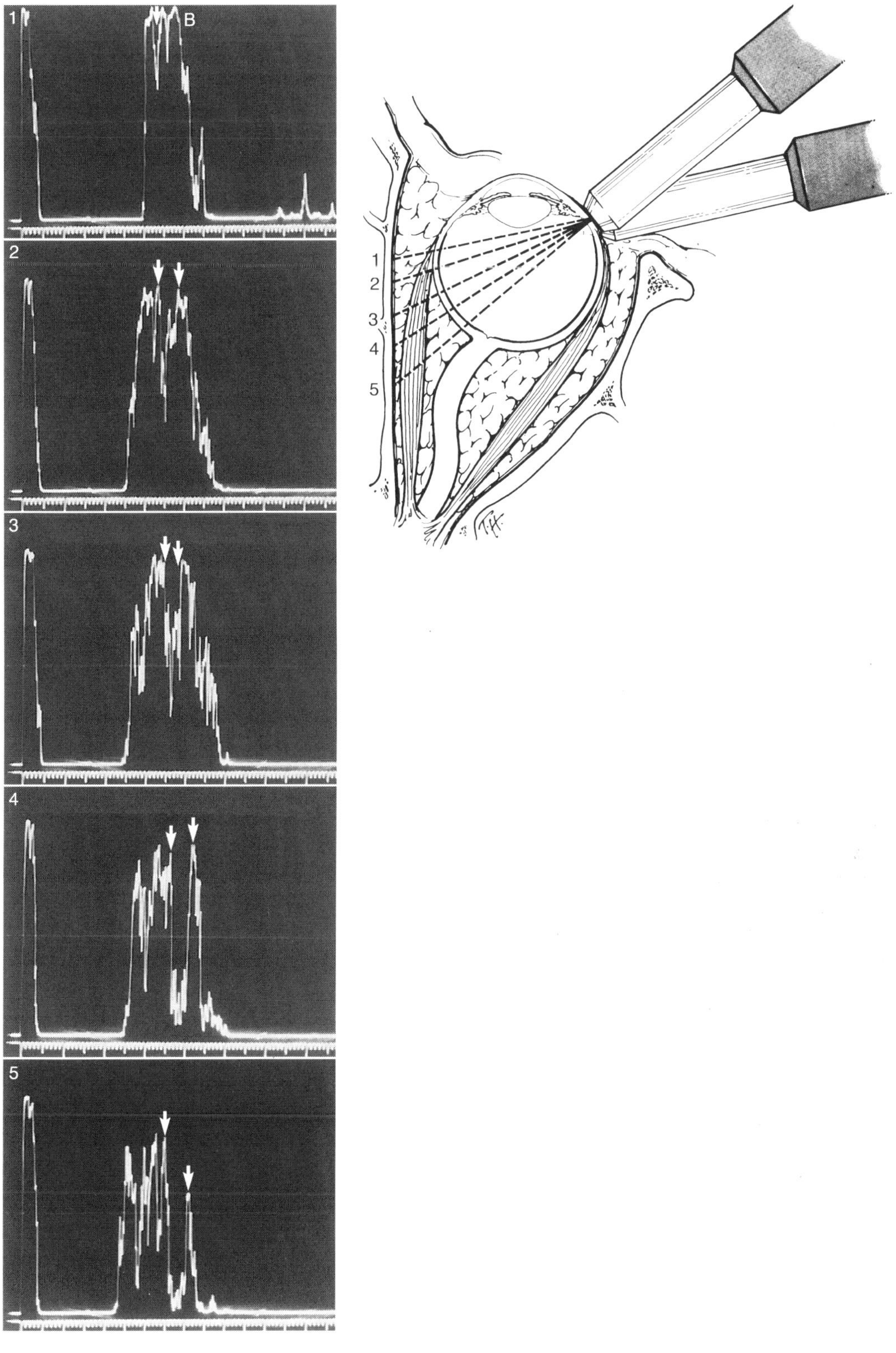

Figure 15-6 Dynamic A-scan evaluation of medial rectus muscle. As probe is angled posteriorly, the muscle *(arrows)* is examined from its insertion *(1)* toward the orbital apex *(5)*. The muscle defect moves from left to right as it extends back into the orbit. Note decrease in reflectivity of muscle more posteriorly as a result of sound attenuation. Maximal thickness of muscle is measured between the steeply rising sheath spikes *(arrows)*. *B*, Bone.

A 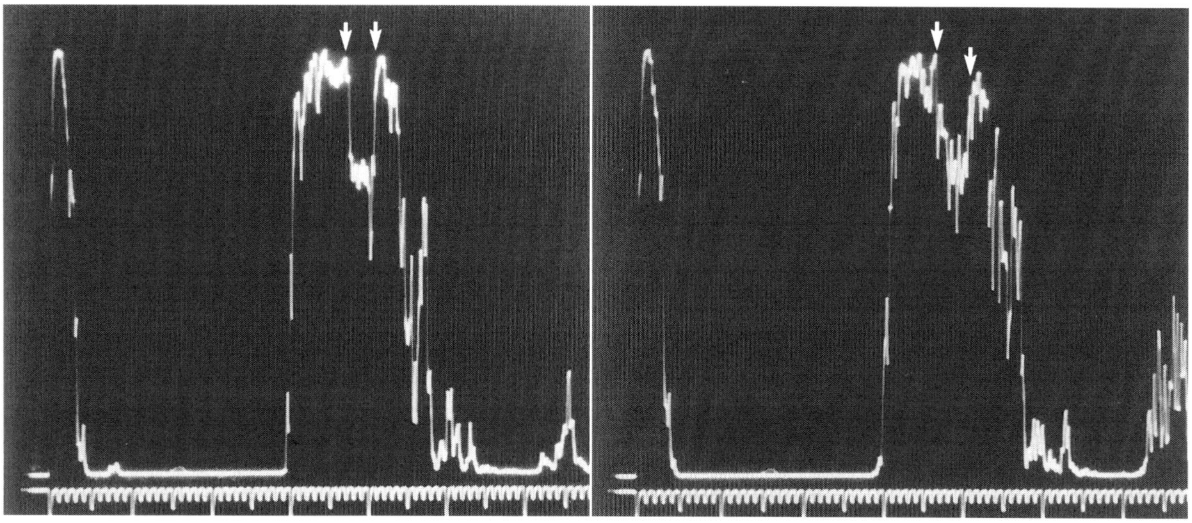 B

Figure 15-7 A-scan echograms of extraocular muscle displayed with perpendicular (correct) and oblique (incorrect) sound beam incidence. **A,** Steeply rising, distinct sheath spikes indicate perpendicular sound beam incidence *(arrows)*. **B,** Sheath spikes are indistinct because of oblique sound beam incidence.

A 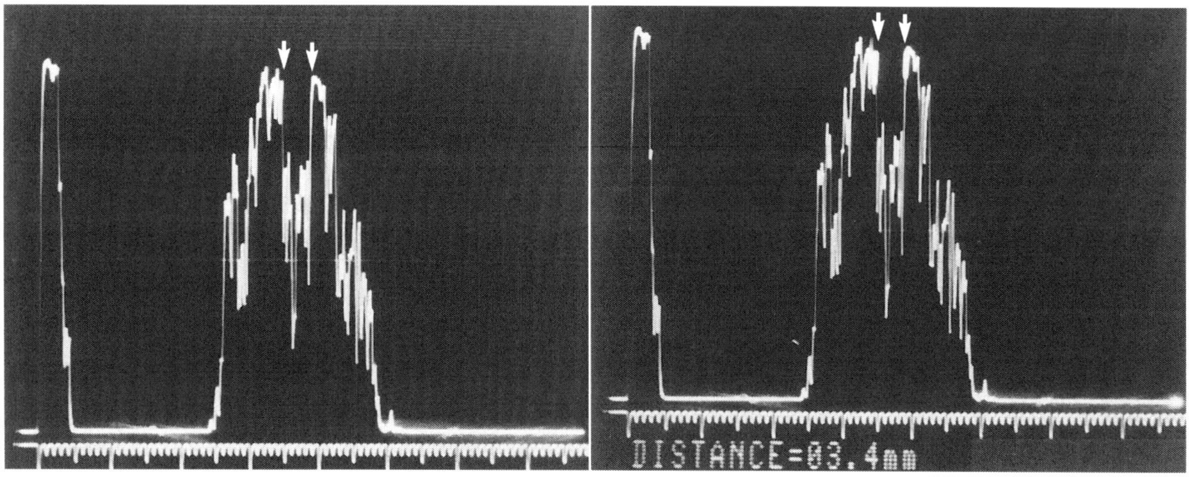 B

Figure 15-8 Measurement of muscle thickness with A-scan. **A,** Echogram with no gates. *Arrows,* Muscle sheath. **B,** Electronic gates (cursors) on sheath spikes indicate muscle thickness (3.4 mm).

TABLE 15-1
Normal Extraocular Muscle Values*

Muscle	Normal Range (mm)	Difference Between Contralateral Muscles
Superior rectus/levator complex	3.9-6.8	0.8
Lateral rectus	2.2-3.8	0.4
Inferior rectus	1.6-3.6	0.4
Medial rectus	2.3-4.7	0.5
Sum of all muscles	11.9-16.9	1.2

From Byrne SF, Gendron EK, Glaser JS, et al: Diameter of normal extraocular recti muscles with echography. *Am J Ophthalmol* 1991;112:706.
*This table indicates 95% confidence limits for the diameter of normal rectus muscles as well as the difference in the diameter of contralateral fellow muscles.

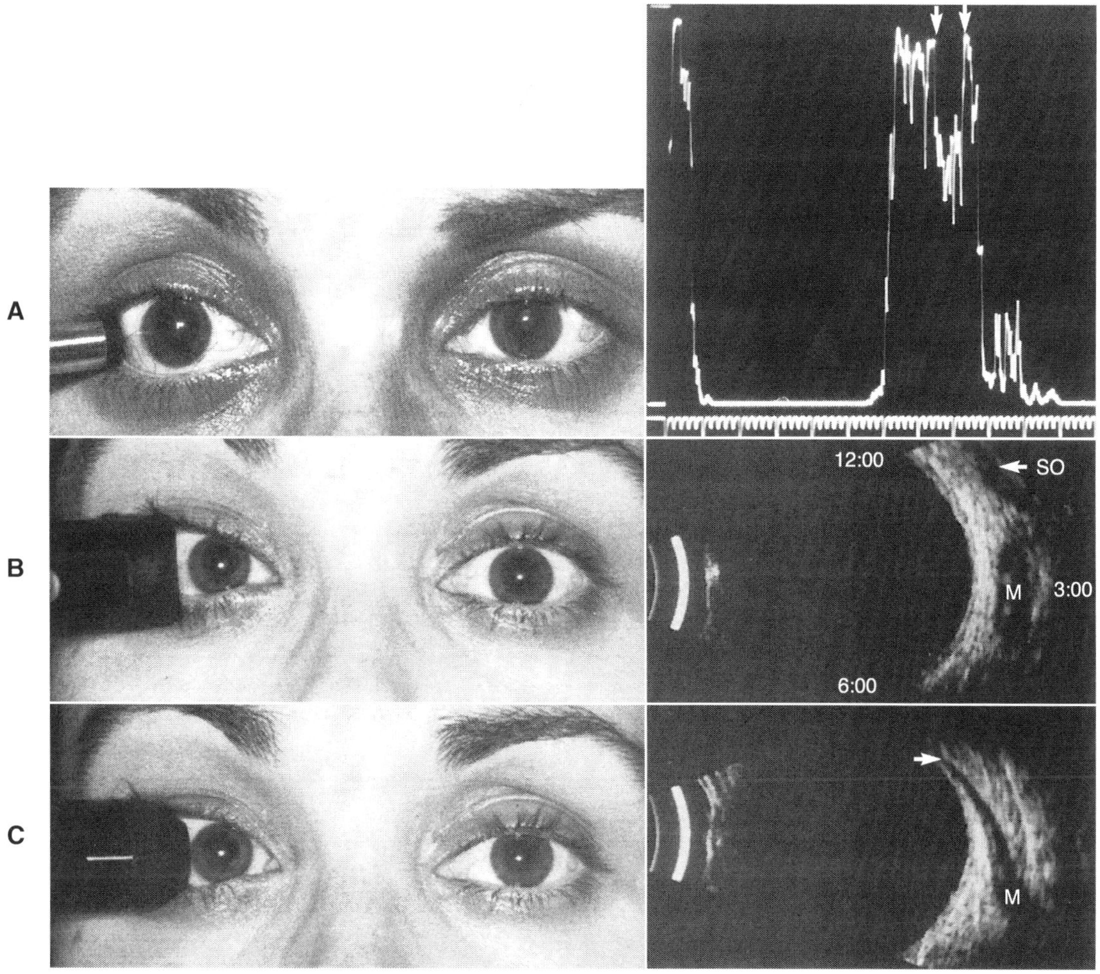

Figure 15-9 Technique for evaluation of medial rectus muscle with A-scan **(A)** and B-scan **(B** and **C)**. **A,** A-scan probe is placed at 9-o'clock near the equator, and sound beam is directed perpendicular to sheath of medial rectus *(arrows)*. **B,** Vertical transverse B-scan displays cross-section of medial rectus muscle *(M)*. Probe marker is oriented toward 12-o'clock. *SO*, Superior oblique muscle. **C,** Longitudinal scan displays long section of muscle *(M)*. Probe marker is directed toward cornea and 3-o'clock meridian. Muscle insertion *(arrow)* is displayed at top of echogram.

Lateral Rectus

The lateral rectus is examined with the A- or B-scan probe placed medially. When examining this muscle, the patient's nose may sometimes interfere with probe movement. This problem usually can be alleviated, however, by having the patient fixate approximately 10 degrees temporally (Figure 15-10).

Inferior Rectus

The inferior rectus may be particularly difficult to examine because of the prominent superior orbital rim. Consequently, this muscle is most easily evaluated when the globe is somewhat proptotic. Fixation normally should be approximately 10 degrees inferior to primary gaze in order to provide enough room for the probe (A- or B-scan) to be

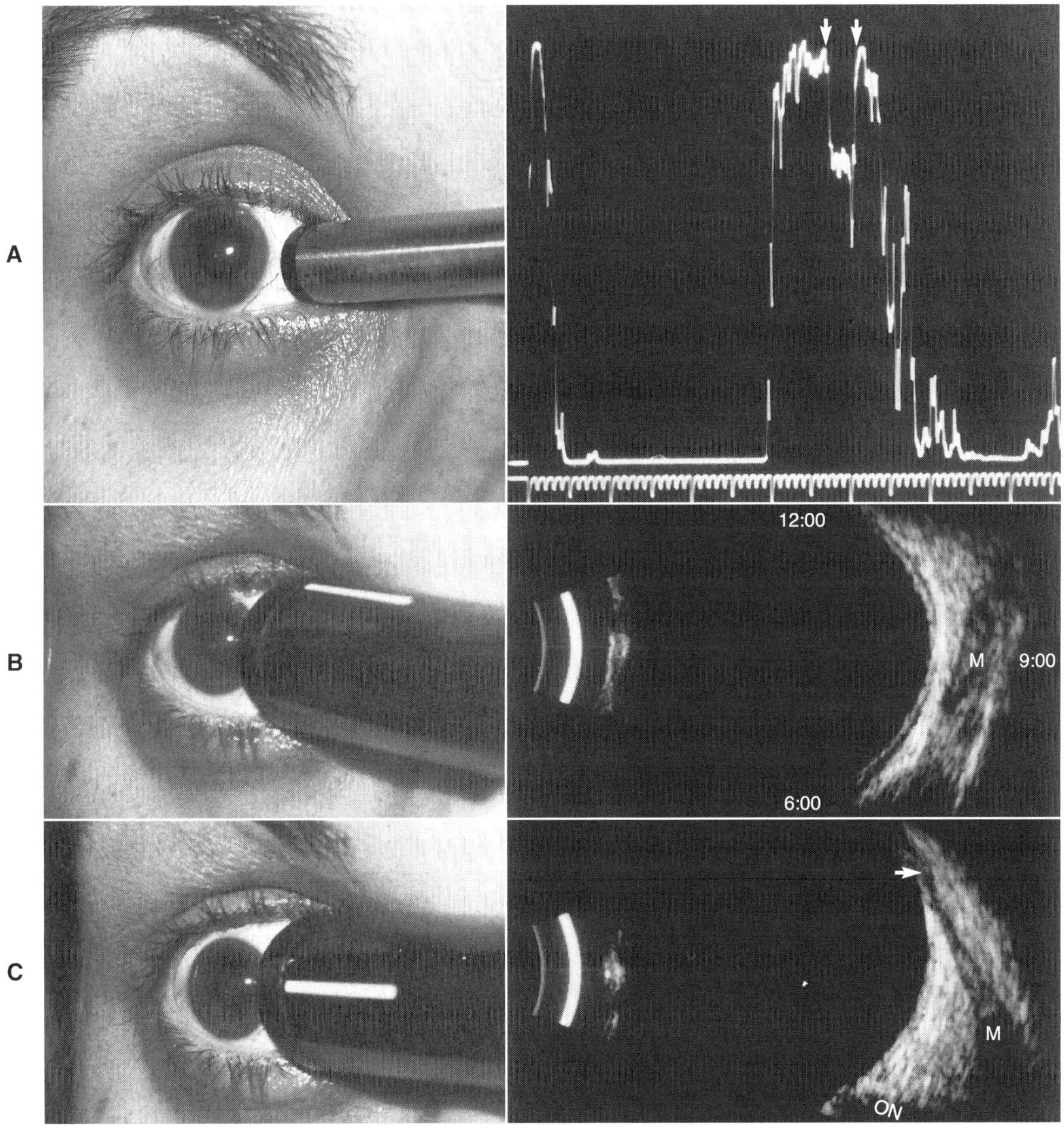

Figure 15-10 Technique for evaluating lateral rectus muscle with A-scan **(A)** and B-scan (**B** and **C**). **A,** A-scan probe is placed near equator at 3-o'clock nasally, and sound beam is directed perpendicular to sheath of lateral rectus muscle *(arrows)*. **B,** Vertical transverse scan displays cross-section of lateral rectus muscle *(M)*. Probe marker is oriented toward 12-o'clock. **C,** Longitudinal scan displays long section of muscle. Probe marker is directed toward cornea and 9-o'clock meridian. Muscle insertion *(arrow)* is displayed at top of echogram.

maneuvered on the superior aspect of the globe (Figure 15-11). If the orbital rim is particularly prominent, it may be easier to place the B-scan probe on the lid.

Superior Rectus and Levator Palpebrae Superioris

Although the superior rectus and levator muscles often can be imaged as separate structures on B-scan, these two muscles are usually displayed and measured as one complex on A-scan, thereby yielding a considerably larger normal value than the other muscles. The muscle complex is examined with the patient fixating in primary gaze or slightly superiorly for both A- and B-scan (Figure 15-12).

In transverse view, B-scan may show the two muscles to be separate anteriorly but as one large complex posteriorly. The tendon of the superior rectus muscle is thin and oval-shaped as it inserts into the globe anteriorly, whereas the levator aponeurosis produces a broad, umbrella-like lucency above the superior rectus muscle. The longitudinal view shows both the insertion of the superior rectus into the globe and the levator extending forward into the lid (see Figure 15-12, *C*). If the patient blinks, the levator muscle can be seen to move back and forth above the superior rectus muscle. In some cases, an extremely thick levator muscle may produce a defect during the paraocular examination when the A-scan probe is placed supratemporally.

Oblique Muscles

A different approach is needed to evaluate the oblique muscles because of their varied course and broad insertions[39,40] (Figure 15-13). Routinely, gross thickening of the oblique muscles is best detected with B-scan. Then, if an abnormality is suspected, A-scan can be used to more carefully assess thickness and reflectivity.

A

B

C

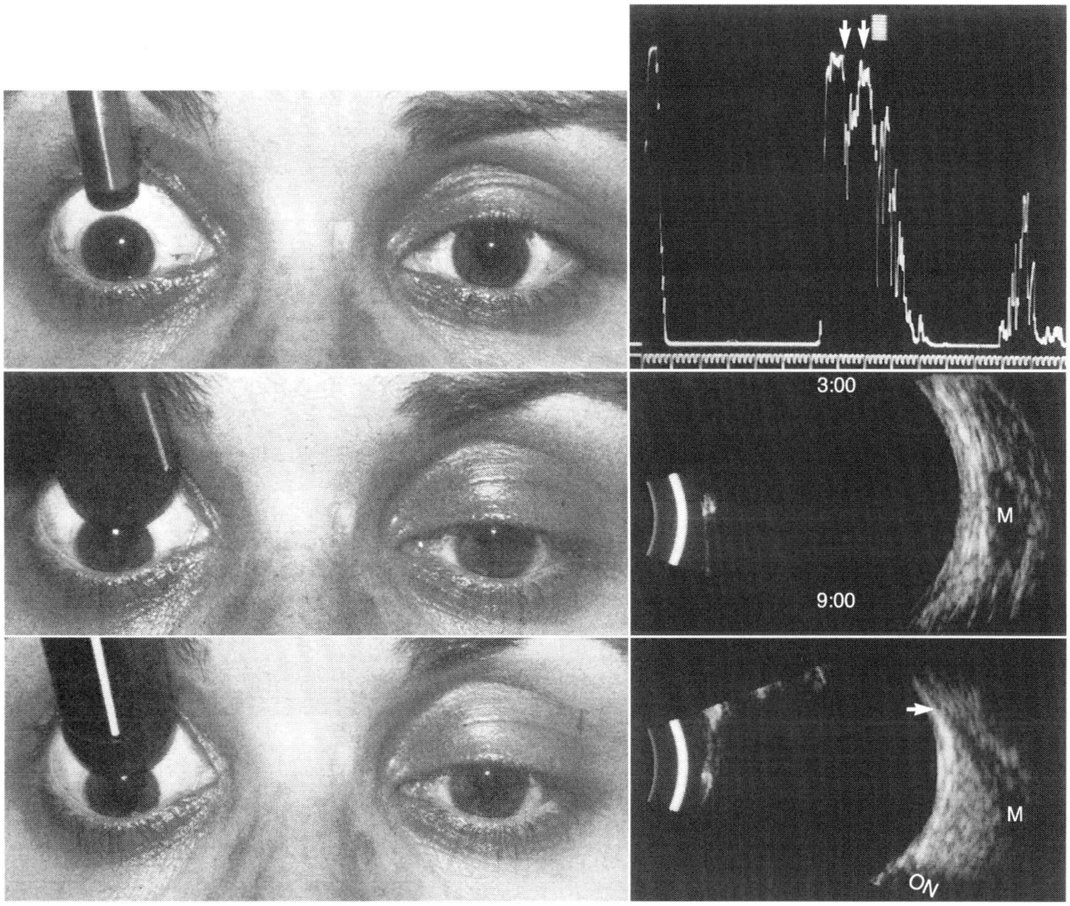

Figure 15-11 Technique for evaluating inferior rectus muscle with A-scan **(A)** and B-scan **(B** and **C)**. **A,** A-scan probe is placed near equator at 12-o'clock, and sound beam is directed perpendicular to sheath of inferior rectus muscle *(arrows)*. **B,** Horizontal transverse scan displays cross-section of inferior rectus muscle *(M)*. Probe marker is directed toward 3-o'clock meridian. **C,** Longitudinal scan displays long section of muscle. Probe marker is directed toward cornea and 6-o'clock meridian. Muscle insertion *(arrow)* is displayed at the top of the echogram. *ON*, Optic nerve.

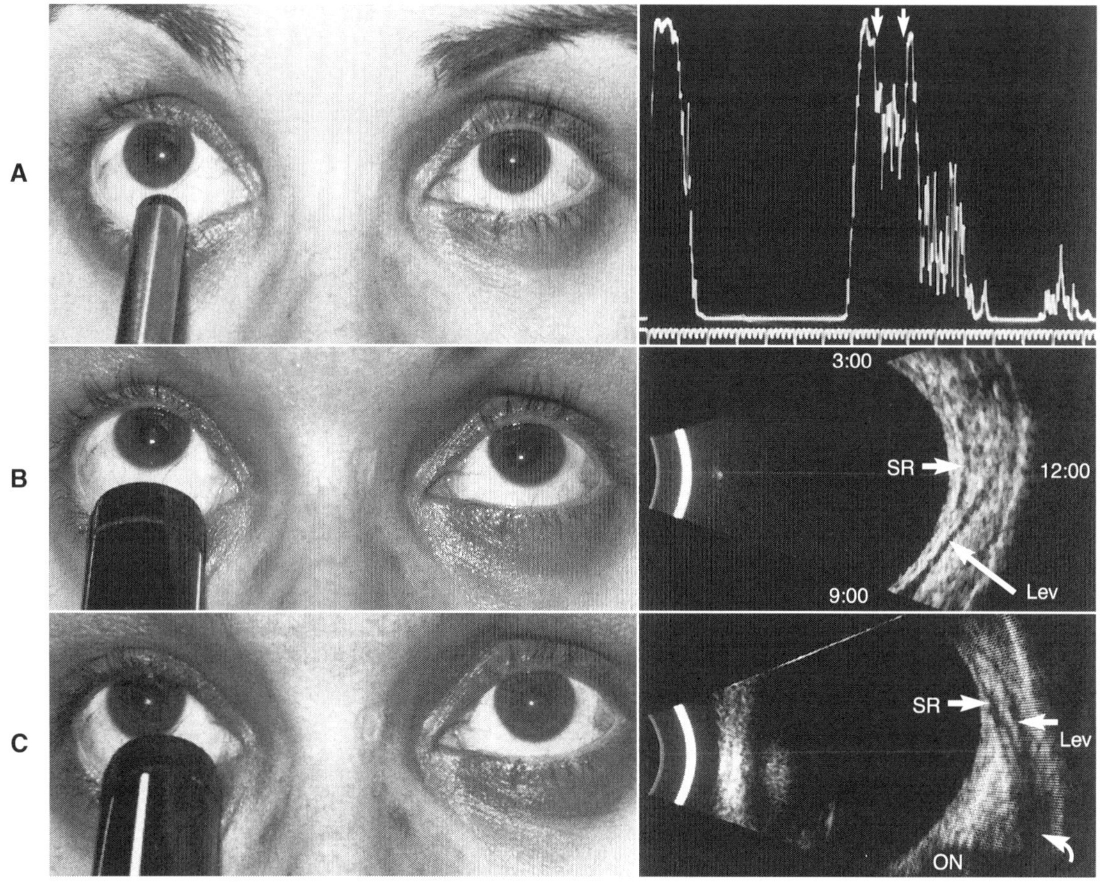

Figure 15-12 Technique for evaluation of superior rectus and levator muscles with A-scan **(A)** and B-scan (**B** and **C**). **A,** A-scan probe is placed near equator at 6-o'clock, and sound beam is directed perpendicular to sheaths of superior rectus/levator complex *(arrows)*. **B,** Horizontal transverse scan shows cross-section of superior rectus *(SR)* and levator *(Lev)* muscles. Note the broad, umbrella-like appearance of levator aponeurosis compared to the superior rectus muscle in this very anterior section. Probe marker is directed toward 3-o'clock meridian. **C,** Longitudinal scan shows long section of the superior rectus *(SR)* and levator *(Lev)* muscles. Probe marker is directed toward cornea and 12-o'clock meridian. Note levator muscle extending anteriorly, beyond insertion of superior rectus muscle. *ON,* Optic nerve; *curved arrow,* muscles appear to merge more posteriorly.

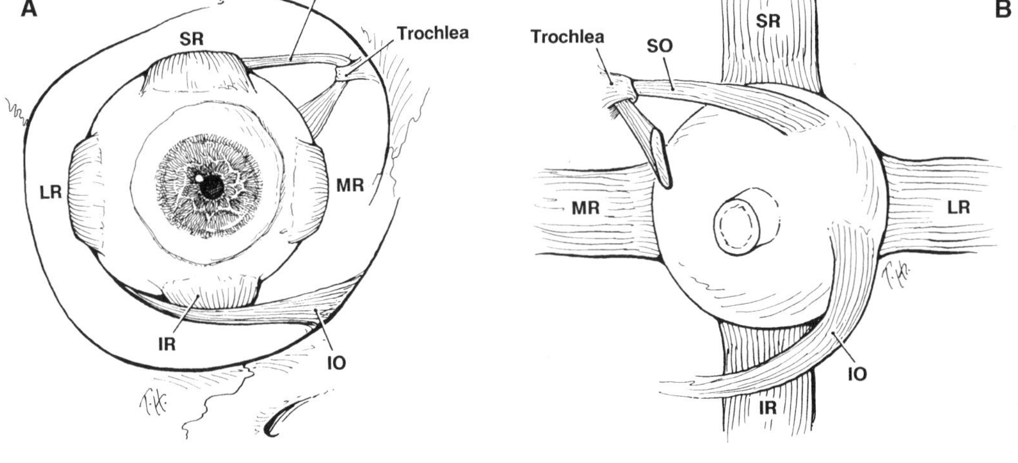

Figure 15-13 Schematic drawings illustrate the insertions and course of the superior oblique *(SO)* and inferior oblique *(IO)* muscles in frontal view **(A)** and posterior view **(B).** Note the more posterior insertions of the oblique muscles and their varied courses as they pass inferior to the superior and inferior rectus muscles. *SR,* Superior rectus; *MR,* medial rectus; *IR,* inferior rectus; *LR,* lateral rectus; *SO,* superior oblique; *IO,* inferior oblique.

Superior Oblique

Because the tendon and belly of the superior oblique muscle course through the orbit at different angles, separate techniques are necessary for displaying each of them. On B-scan, the tendon is best shown with a horizontal transverse scan through the superior orbit, using a similar but more anterior approach than that used for displaying the superior rectus muscle complex (Figure 15-14). The tendon also can be imaged with a longitudinal view, but it usually cannot be displayed entirely in one echogram. A-scan evaluation of the normal tendon is difficult; therefore, it is only performed when enlargement has been noted on B-scan.

A-scan evaluation of the superior oblique muscle is easiest to perform by first displaying the belly of the medial rectus. The sound beam is then shifted slightly upward until the superior oblique defect appears (Figure 15-15, *A*). The muscle belly then can be evaluated by scanning anteroposteriorly along this area, from trochlea toward the posterior orbit. Unlike that of the other muscles, the belly of this muscle remains close to the orbital bone at all times.

The muscle belly can be shown with both transverse and longitudinal B-scan approaches. A vertical transverse view of the medial orbit demonstrates a cross-section of the superior oblique muscle, which is located above the medial rectus muscle near the orbital bone (Figure 15-15, *B;* see also Figure 15-9, *B*). However, a better view of the muscle can be obtained by centering it in the echogram with an oblique transverse scan of the supranasal orbit. A longitudinal scan is also performed to provide a long section of the muscle (Figure 15-15, *C*).

Although the trochlea cannot be demonstrated under normal conditions, it often can be displayed if inflammation (e.g., trochleitis) is present. In such cases, a longitudinal B-scan view may show the muscle looping around the trochlea[40] (Figure 15-16).

Inferior Oblique

The inferior oblique muscle inserts into the globe inferior to the macula. It courses along the ocular wall, then extends horizontally beneath the inferior rectus to its origin at the orbital bone (see Figure 15-13).

The insertion of this muscle is easily demonstrated with B-scan instruments. A vertical transverse scan of the lateral rectus muscle is performed. With this approach, the tendon of

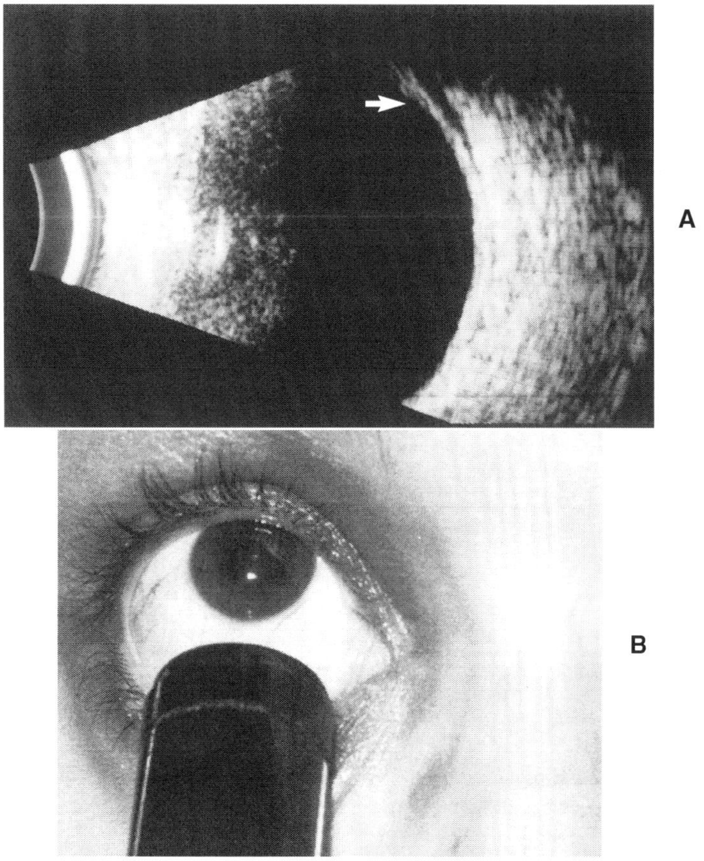

Figure 15-14 Horizontal transverse B-scan technique to display superior oblique tendon. **A,** Note slitlike defect *(arrow)* at upper aspect of echogram (supranasally). **B,** Probe marker is directed toward 3-o'clock.

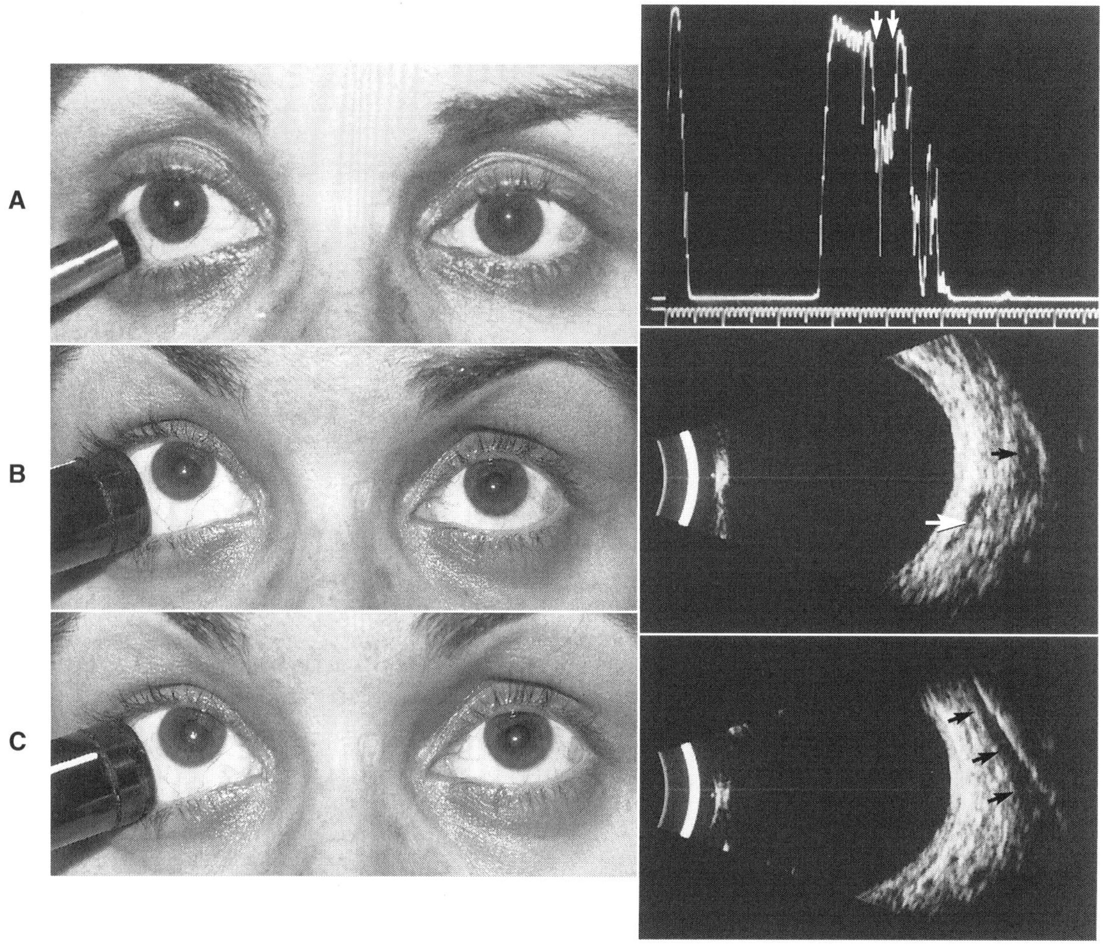

Figure 15-15 Technique for evaluation of the superior oblique muscle with A-scan **(A)** and B-scan (**B** and **C**). **A,** A-scan probe is placed near equator at 7:30 o'clock position, and sound beam is directed perpendicular to sheath of superior oblique muscle *(arrows)*. **B,** Oblique transverse scan displays cross-section of superior oblique muscle *(black arrow)*. *White arrow*, Medial rectus muscle. Note that probe marker is oriented toward the 10:30-o'clock meridian. **C,** Longitudinal scan displays long section of superior oblique muscle *(black arrows)*. Probe marker is directed toward cornea and 1:30 clock meridian. Note how muscle belly lies adjacent to orbital bone throughout its course.

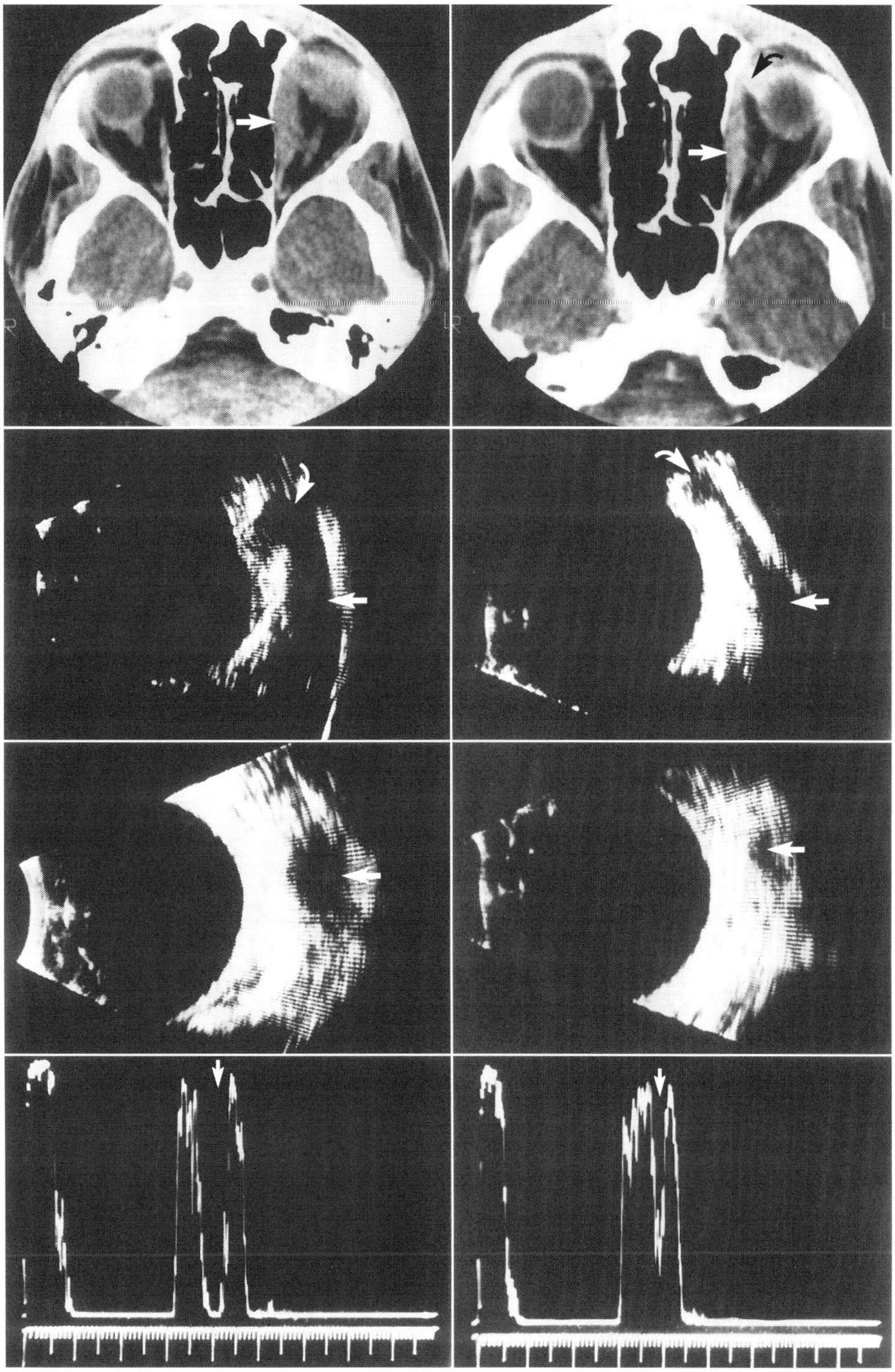

Figure 15-16 Echograms and CT scans showing left superior oblique myositis at initial presentation (**A** to **D**) and following corticosteroid therapy (**E** to **H**). **A,** Axial CT scan demonstrates irregular mass *(arrow)* in supranasal orbit. **B,** Longitudinal B-scan shows thickened superior oblique muscle *(straight arrow)* passing anteriorly around trochlea *(curved arrow)* and enlarged tendon that courses to the globe. **C,** Oblique transverse B-scan shows cross-section of thickened muscle *(arrow)*. **D,** A-scan shows low reflective thickening of muscle *(arrow)*. **E,** Axial CT scan shows decreased size of muscle *(straight arrow)* and now clearly delineated tendon *(curved arrow)*. **F, G,** and **H,** Corresponding B- and A-scans show decreased size of muscle following therapy. (From Wan WL, Cano MR, Green RL: Orbital myositis involving the oblique muscles: An echographic study. *Ophthalmology* 1988;95:1522.)

the inferior oblique is displayed as a thin defect located just below the insertion of the lateral rectus muscle (Figure 15-17, *A*). The tendon can be centered in the echogram by performing an oblique transverse scan through the inferotemporal orbit (Figure 15-17, *B*). A longitudinal scan along the inferotemporal meridian also can show the tendon (Figure 15-18).

The belly of the inferior oblique muscle is generally difficult to display because of its anterior, inferior location. If, however, this muscle is thickened, it can be more easily imaged. This muscle is usually best displayed with horizontal transverse scans. The sound beam is directed through the most anterior aspect of the inferior orbit. As with the inferior rectus muscle, it may be necessary to place the B-scan probe on the closed lid with the patient fixating slightly away from the probe (Figure 15-19).

The easiest way to detect a thickened inferior oblique muscle with A-scan is to use a paraocular approach with the probe positioned inferotemporally. If the muscle is enlarged, a defect will be apparent as the sound beam is directed just next to the globe wall. If extremely large, the thickened muscle also may be seen with a paraocular B-scan approach (Figure 15-20).

A
B
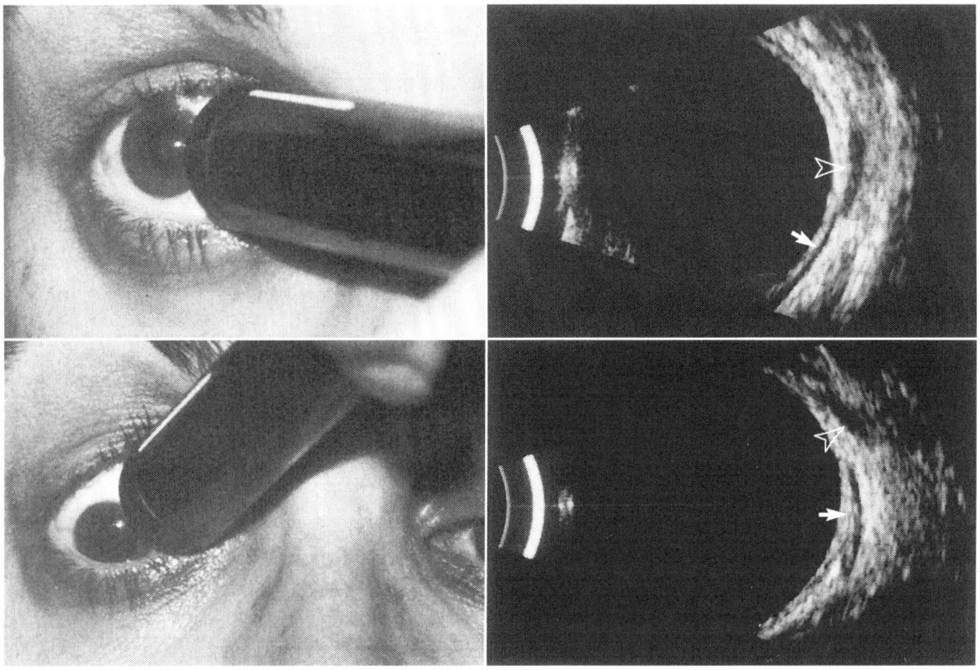

Figure 15-17 Transverse B-scan technique for displaying cross-section of inferior oblique tendon. **A,** Vertical transverse scan with patient fixating slightly temporally. Probe marker is directed toward the 12-o'clock meridian. Insertion of the lateral rectus muscle *(open arrow)* and tendon of the inferior oblique *(closed arrow)* are both displayed. **B,** Oblique transverse scan with patient fixating slightly inferotemporally. Probe marker is directed toward 10:30 o'clock meridian. Lateral rectus muscle *(open arrow)* is displayed near top of echogram and inferior oblique tendon *(closed arrow)* is centered in echogram.

A
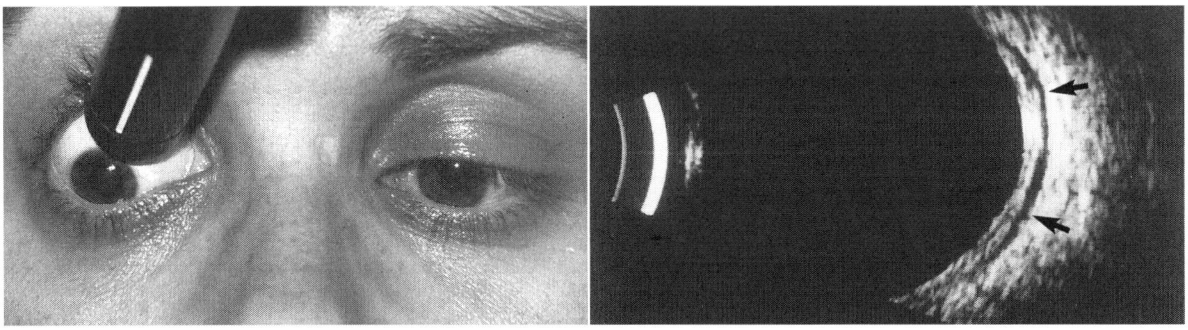
B

Figure 15-18 Longitudinal B-scan technique for displaying long section of inferior oblique tendon. **A,** Patient fixates slightly toward inferotemporal quadrant, and probe is placed at 1-o'clock. Probe marker is directed toward cornea and 7-o'clock meridian. **B,** The tendon produces a long, thin echolucent pattern adjacent to the sclera *(arrows)*.

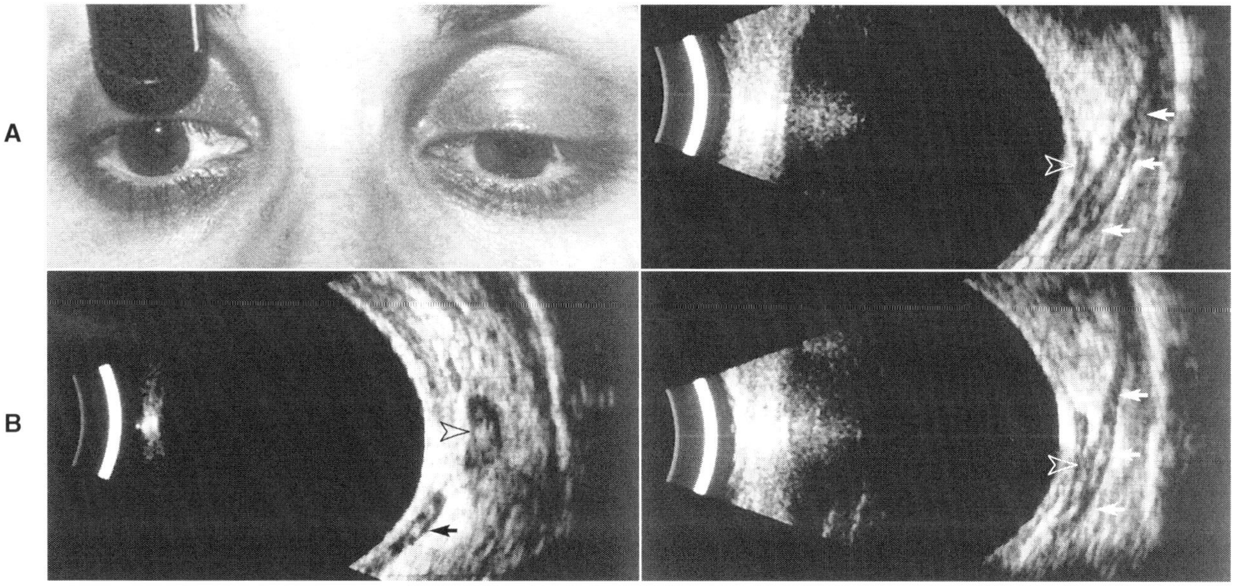

Figure 15-19 Dynamic B-scanning of thickened inferior oblique muscle belly. **A,** Horizontal transverse approach is used with probe placed on lid. Patient fixates slightly downward, and marker is oriented toward 3-o'clock meridian. **B,** Cross-section of inferior rectus muscle *(open arrow)* and inferior oblique muscle *(closed arrow)*. **C,** Slightly more anterior section. Inferior rectus *(open arrow)* inserts into globe, and inferior oblique *(closed arrows)* courses toward nasal orbit. **D,** Very anterior section shows inferior oblique muscle *(closed arrows)* extending toward nasal orbit. *Open arrow,* Insertion of inferior rectus muscle.

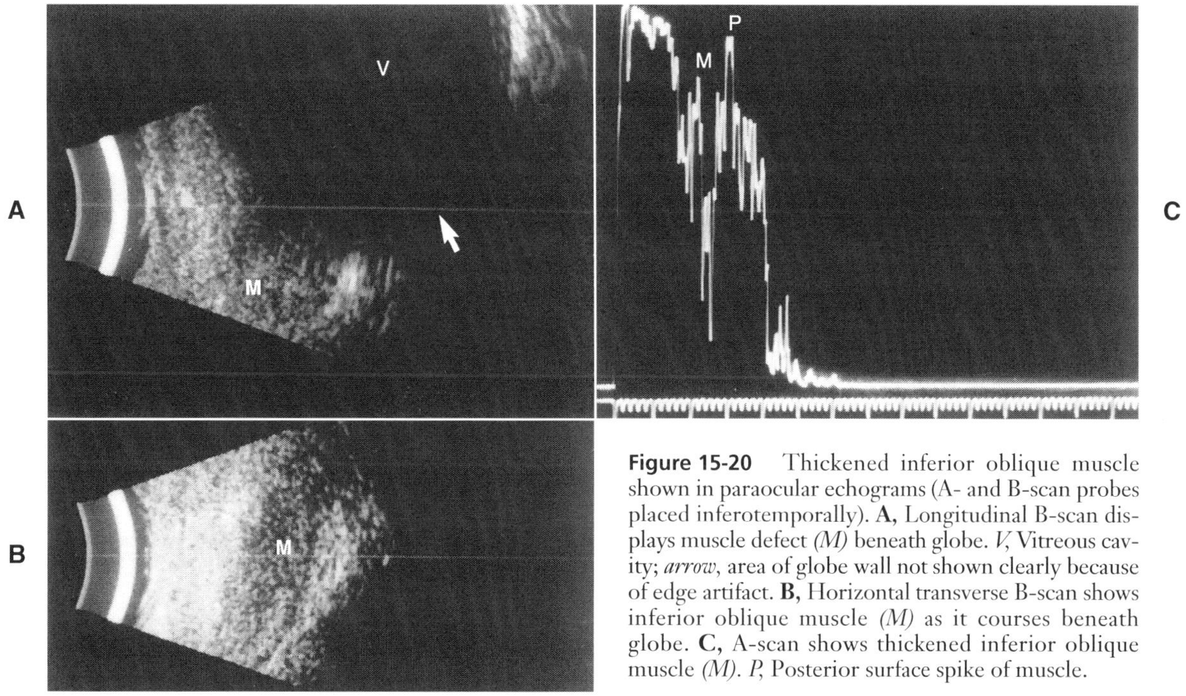

Figure 15-20 Thickened inferior oblique muscle shown in paraocular echograms (A- and B-scan probes placed inferotemporally). **A,** Longitudinal B-scan displays muscle defect *(M)* beneath globe. *V,* Vitreous cavity; *arrow,* area of globe wall not shown clearly because of edge artifact. **B,** Horizontal transverse B-scan shows inferior oblique muscle *(M)* as it courses beneath globe. **C,** A-scan shows thickened inferior oblique muscle *(M)*. *P,* Posterior surface spike of muscle.

EXTRAOCULAR MUSCLE DISORDERS

Thyroid Ophthalmopathy (Graves' Disease)

Thyroid ophthalmopathy is the most common cause of extraocular muscle enlargement (Box 15-1).[27,37] Many of these patients are referred for echography with unilateral proptosis of unknown etiology. In other cases, thyroid dysfunction may be suspected based on clinical findings, but blood studies or radiologic findings are normal. Echography can be very helpful in establishing or confirming the diagnosis of thyroid ophthalmopathy in these patients.*

Thyroid ophthalmopathy is typically a bilateral condition that affects multiple extraocular muscles.[7,27] It may, however, be very asymmetric, with marked changes in one orbit and only very subtle changes in the other. Even when the condition appears to be unilateral, echography often reveals mild changes in the clinically uninvolved orbit. In rare cases, however, only unilateral findings can be detected.

Muscle thickening in thyroid ophthalmopathy usually has a very characteristic appearance. In most cases the inserting tendon is spared while the mid- and posterior portions of the muscle belly are involved. The internal reflectivity of the thickened muscles in thyroid disease is typically medium to high, and the structure is quite irregular[23] (Figure 15-21 and Table 15-2). This appearance results from large interfaces within the muscles that are created by the separation of muscle fibers due to edema and inflammatory cells.[27] Other associated findings can include swelling of the orbital fat and lid tissues, thickening of the periorbita (Figure 15-22), and enlargement of the lacrimal gland.

In cases of marked apical muscle swelling, the superior ophthalmic vein (or other orbital veins) can be enlarged and the optic nerve sheaths thickened or distended (i.e., increased subarachnoid fluid) secondary to compression (Figure 15-23; see also Figure 16-22).[11,22,26,27,36] In rare cases of acute thyroid ophthalmopathy, thickening of the tendon may occur and fluid may be noted in the episcleral space.

As stated previously, bilateral, asymmetric muscle thickening is the rule in thyroid ophthalmopathy and is the key finding in the diagnosis of this condition with echography. On follow-up examination, these muscles often fluctuate in size, with some being larger and others being smaller than on previous examinations. The muscles found to be most commonly enlarged with echography are the superior rectus/levator complex and the medial rectus, followed by the inferior and lateral rectus muscles. This differs from the clinical presentation of Graves' disease, in which the inferior rectus muscle is most frequently affected.[30] Thickening of the levator muscle very often corresponds to the clinical presence of lid retraction,[38] and in mild cases may be the primary or even the only abnormal echographic finding (Figure 15-24). In some instances, there can be difficulty in distinguishing the highly reflective thickened muscle from surrounding orbital tissues, thus making accurate measurements hard to obtain. To avoid this problem, it can be helpful to decrease the gain by a few decibels to better delineate the muscle sheath.

*References 3, 6, 11-13, 20, 25, 34, 41.

BOX 15-1

Extraocular Muscle Disorders

Thyroid eye disease (Graves' ophthalmopathy)
Myositis
Tumors
Venous congestion
Trauma
Muscle thinning

Myositis

Myositis is an inflammatory condition of the extraocular muscles[31] that produces specific echographic findings that are quite different from those seen in thyroid ophthalmopathy. This condition can be acute and associated with severe pain and restrictive extraocular movements, or it can be more chronic, with less severe clinical symptoms.[18] Myositis can be primary, without associated changes in other orbital structures, or it can occur along with other orbital processes such as scleritis or an inflammatory mass (i.e., pseudotumor). Although some clinicians use the terms *myositis* and *pseudotumor of the orbit* interchangeably, the authors designate an inflamed, thickened muscle as *myositis* and reserve the term *pseudotumor* for an orbital mass of inflammatory etiology (see p 310).

Myositis can be unilateral or bilateral, and it can affect one or all of the extraocular muscles.[18,31,32] Typically, the muscle is diffusely thickened, with involvement of both the muscle tendon and belly fibers. In thyroid disease, however, the tendon is classically spared, and more posterior aspects

Text continued on p 402.

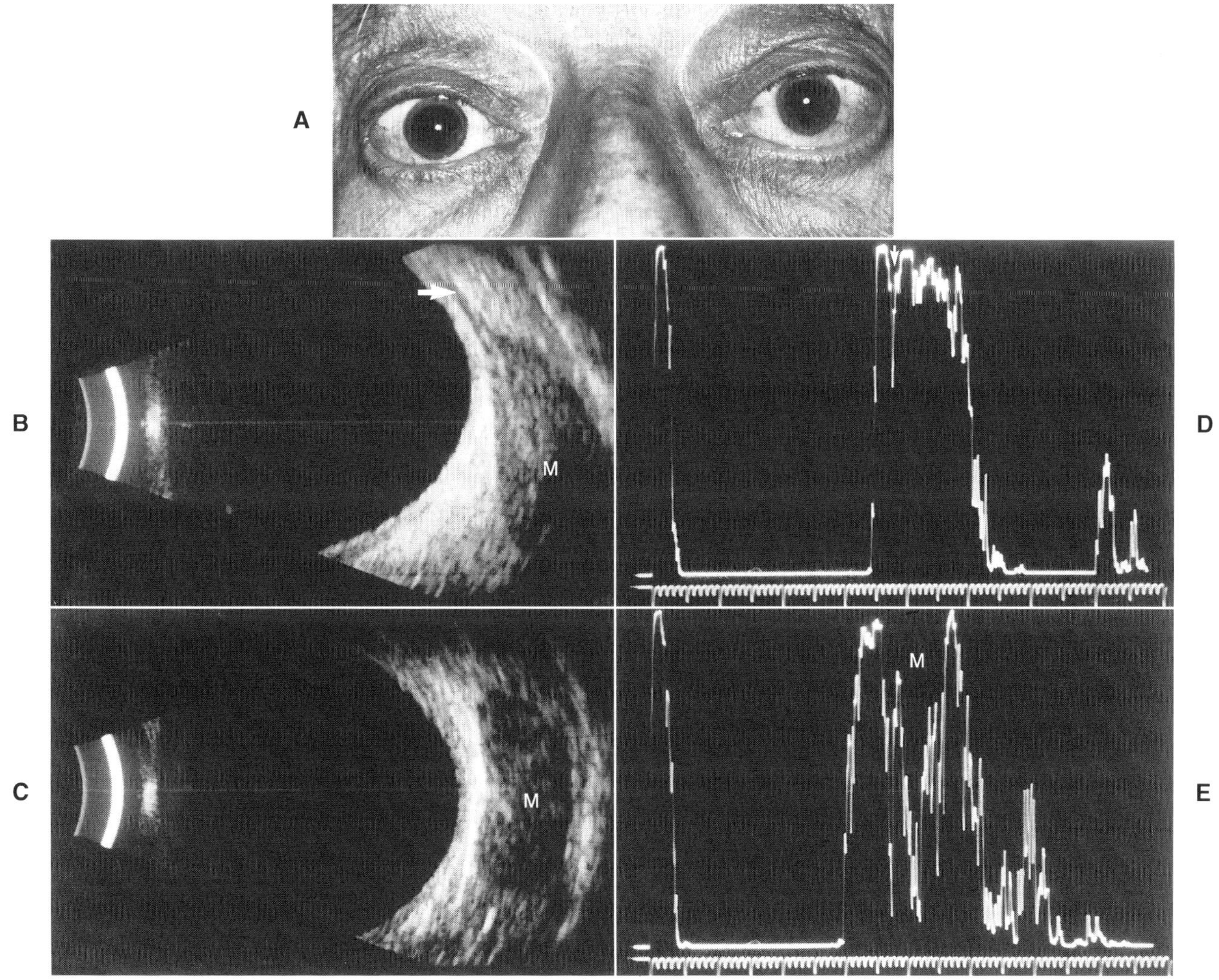

Figure 15-21 Thickening of medial rectus muscle in thyroid ophthalmopathy. **A,** External photograph shows bilateral exophthalmos and lid retraction. **B,** Longitudinal B-scan echogram of muscle *(M)* displays thin insertion *(arrow)*. **C,** Vertical transverse B-scan of thickened muscle. **D,** A-scan shows normal insertion of muscle *(arrow)*. **E,** A-scan through thickened muscle belly shows typical medium to high internal reflectivity and irregular structure.

TABLE 15-2

Differential Diagnosis of Extraocular Muscle Disorders*

Disorder	Reflectivity	Internal Structure	Insertions
Thyroid ophthalmopathy	Medium-high	Irregular	Normal
Myositis	Low	Regular	Thickened
Tumors	Low-medium	Regular	Normal
Venous congestion	Medium-high	Variable	Normal
Hematoma	Low-medium	Regular	Variable

*This table is a summary of the most typical echographic features of disorders causing thickening of the extraocular muscles.

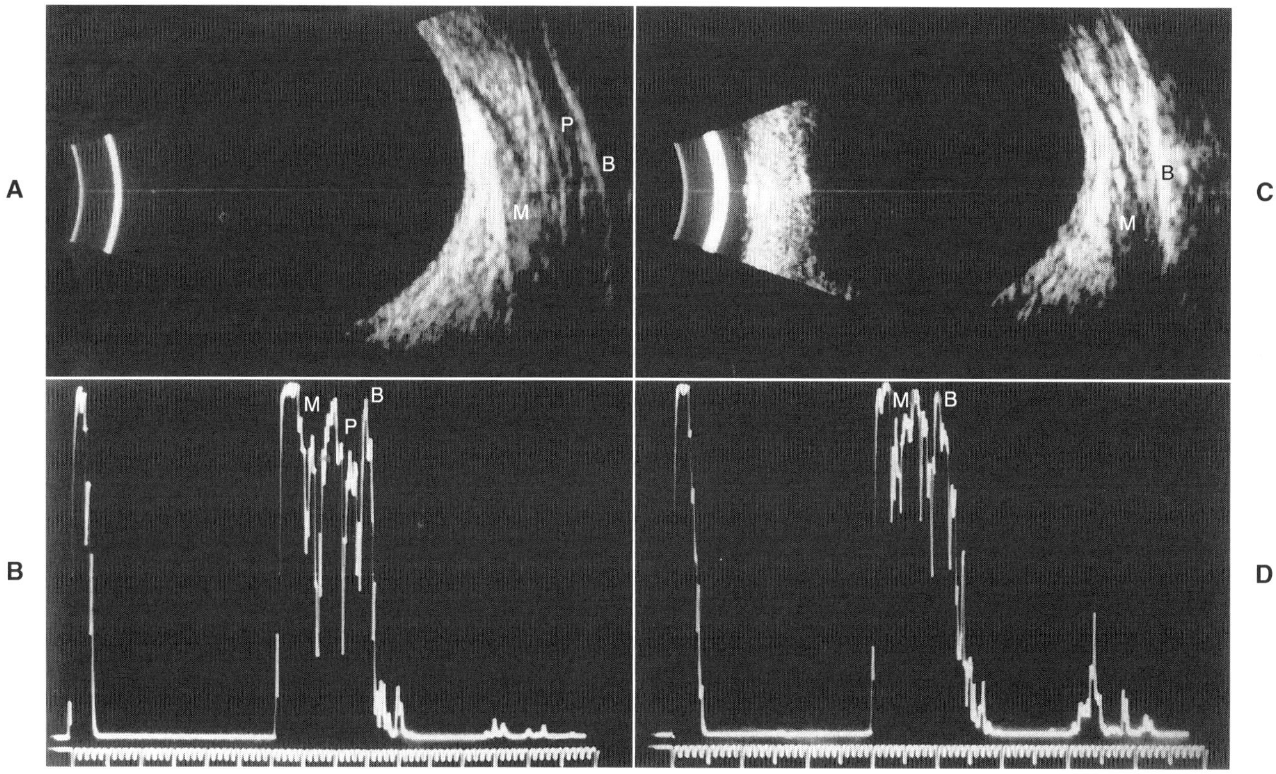

Figure 15-22 Thickening of periosteum in patient with thyroid ophthalmopathy (**A** and **B**) compared to normal orbit (**C** and **D**). **A,** Longitudinal B-scan through medial orbit shows periosteal thickening *(P)*. *B,* Bone; *M,* medial rectus muscle. **B,** Corresponding A-scan. **C,** Longitudinal B-scan through medial aspect of a normal orbit. **D,** Corresponding A-scan.

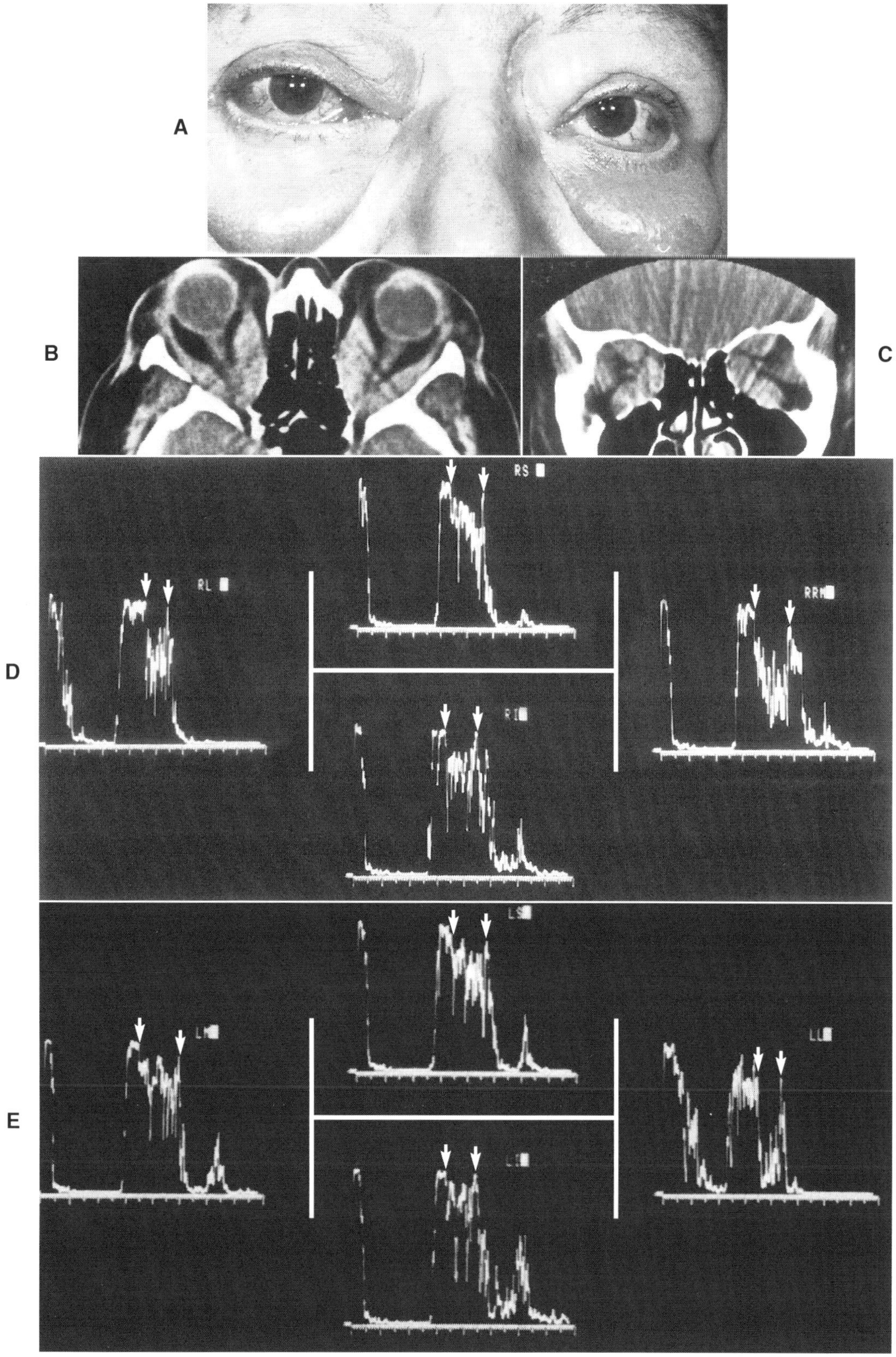

Figure 15-23 Advanced thyroid ophthalmopathy. **A,** External photograph shows bilateral lower lid retraction, injection, and lid swelling. Axial **(B)** and coronal **(C)** CT scans show marked bilateral extraocular muscle enlargement. A-scan montage of very thick rectus muscles in right orbit **(D)** and left orbit **(E).** *I,* Inferior rectus; *L,* lateral rectus; *M,* medial rectus; *S,* superior rectus/levator complex; *arrows,* muscle sheaths. See left optic nerve in Figure 16-22.

A

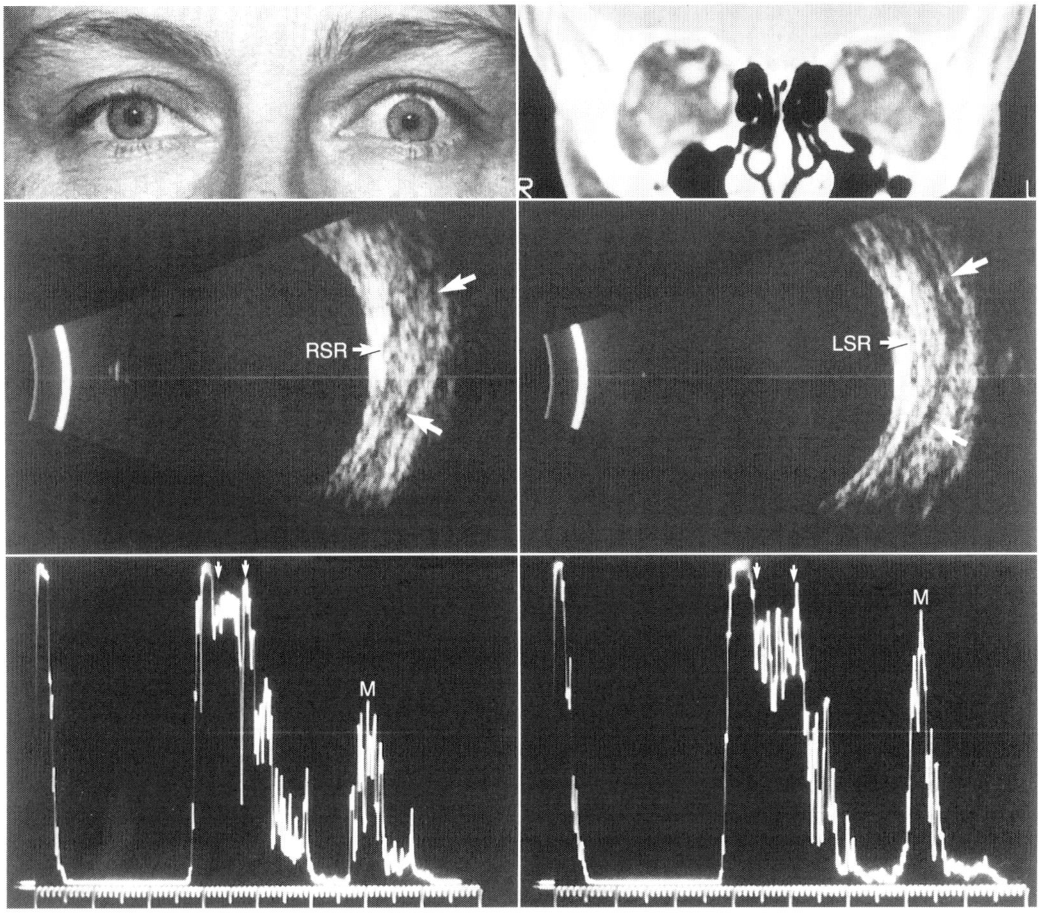

Figure 15-24 Thyroid ophthalmopathy. **A** *(1)*, External photograph shows mild left upper lid retraction. Echograms display normal right superior rectus/levator complex *(2* and *3)* and thickened left superior rectus/levator complex *(5* and *6)*. *2*, Horizontal transverse B-scan of right superior rectus *(RSR)* and levator muscle *(arrows)*. *3*, A-scan shows muscle complex as one defect. *M*, Multiple signals; *arrows*, muscle sheath. *4*, Coronal CT scan shows normal, symmetric appearance of muscles in the two orbits. *5*, Horizontal transverse B-scan of left superior rectus *(LSR)* and levator muscle *(arrows)*. Note that the left levator muscle is thicker than the right levator muscle. *6*, A-scan shows widened muscle complex. *Continued*

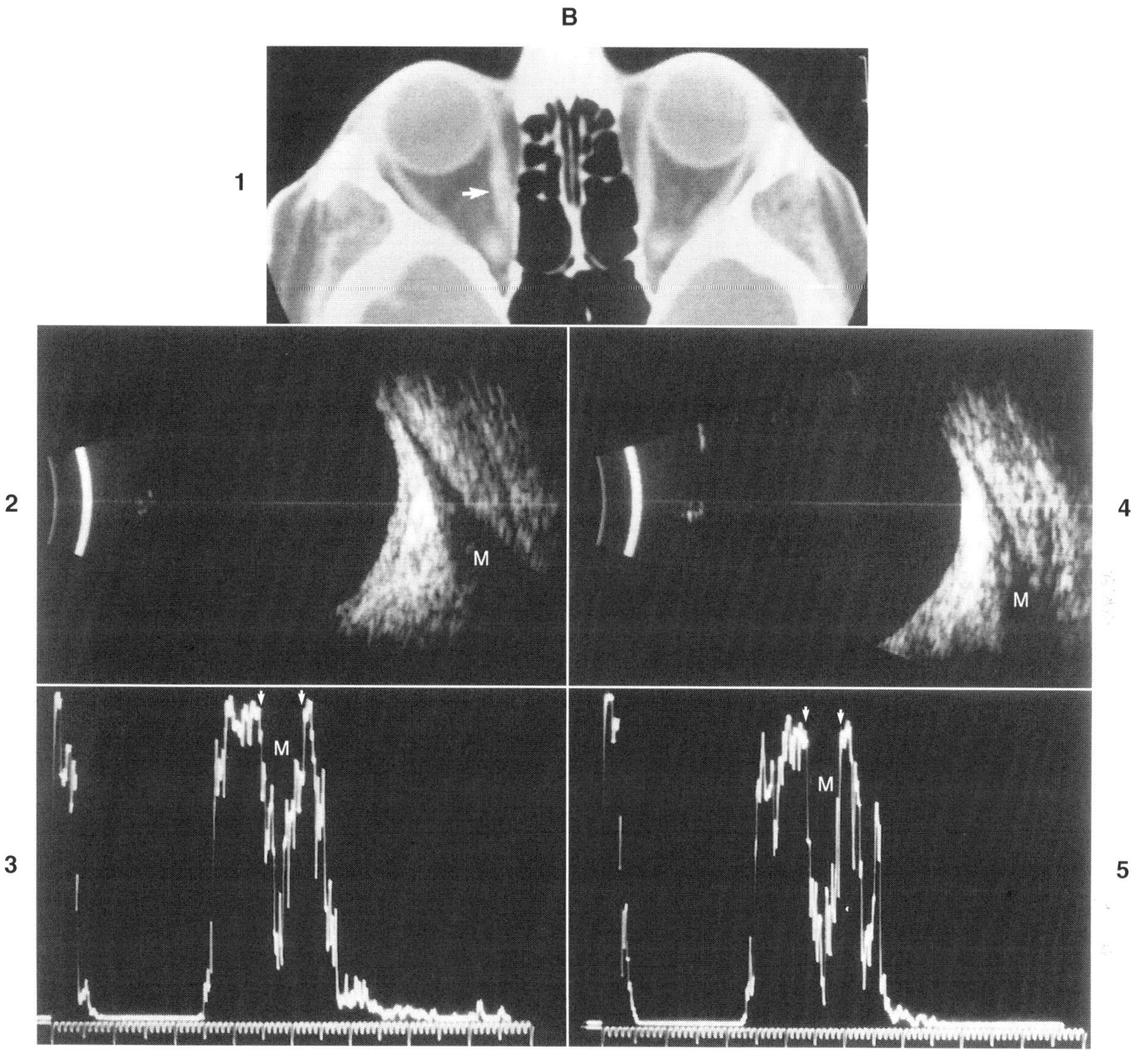

Figure 15-24, cont'd B *(1)*, Axial CT scan suggests possible slight enlargement of right medial rectus muscle *(arrow)*. Longitudinal B-scan *(2)* and A-scan *(3)* show enlargement of right medial rectus *(M)*. *Arrows*, Muscle sheath. Normal left medial rectus is shown in longitudinal B-scan *(4)* and A-scan *(5)*.

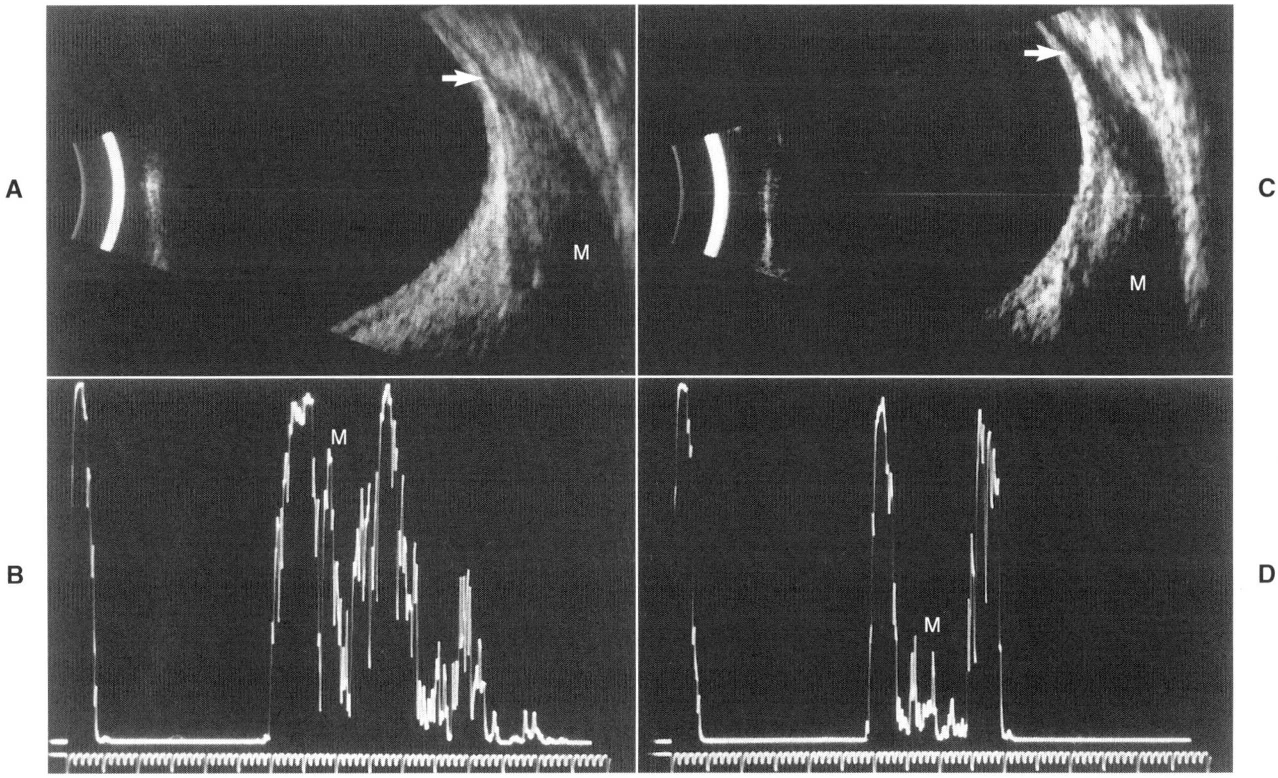

Figure 15-25 Thickened muscles due to thyroid ophthalmopathy (**A** and **B**) and orbital myositis (**C** and **D**). Longitudinal B-scan echograms (**A** and **C**) show enlarged muscles *(M)* with normal insertion in thyroid disease **(A)** and thickened insertion in myositis **(C)** *(arrows)*. A-scans **(B** and **D)** show thickened muscle to be irregular and medium-high reflective in thyroid **(B)** but regular and low reflective in myositis **(D)**.

of the muscle are affected[27] (Figure 15-25; see also Table 15-2). The internal reflectivity in myositis is usually low, owing to diffuse invasion of muscle fibers by inflammatory cells, which renders the tissue more homogeneous than normal[28] (Figure 15-26). There may be a number of associated findings, such as episcleritis or scleritis adjacent to the inserting tendon of the muscle, swelling of surrounding orbital fat and lid tissues, or inflammation and thickening of the lacrimal gland or optic nerve. In situations in which myositis is secondary to scleritis or episcleritis, muscle thickening can be limited primarily to the region of the tendon[35] (Figure 15-27).

Echography is an effective way of following and monitoring the response to therapy. A positive therapeutic response results in decreasing thickness of the inflamed muscle and a gradual increase in reflectivity to normal (Figure 15-28).

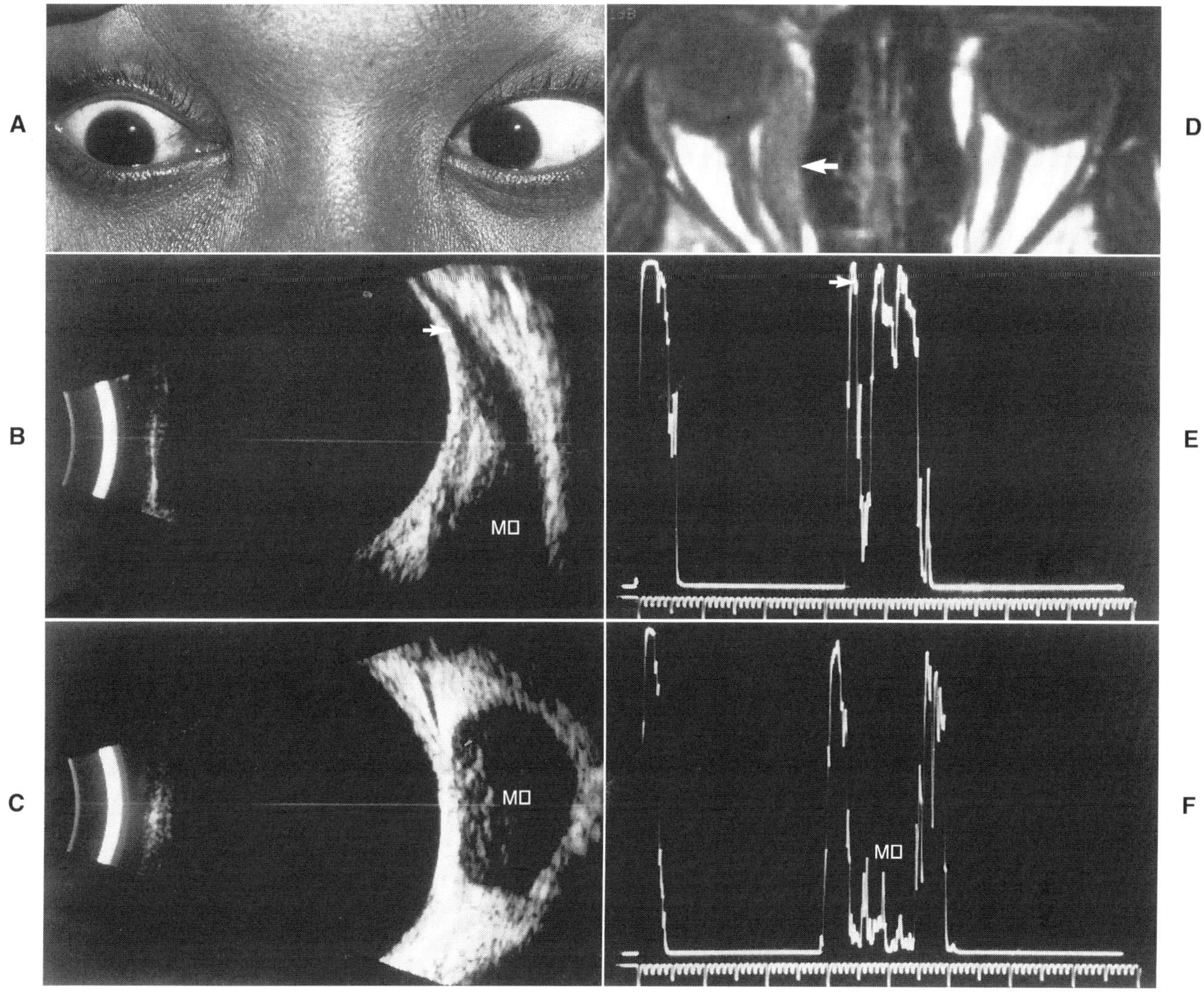

Figure 15-26 Myositis of right medial rectus muscle. **A,** External photograph demonstrates restricted abduction of right eye. **B,** Longitudinal B-scan echogram shows enlarged muscle *(M)* with thickened insertion *(arrow)*. **C,** Vertical transverse B-scan shows cross-section of markedly enlarged muscle. **D,** Axial MRI scan demonstrates pronounced enlargement of medial rectus muscle *(arrow)*. **E,** A-scan echogram displays low reflective, thickened insertion *(arrow)*. **F,** A-scan shows marked, low reflective enlargement of muscle belly.

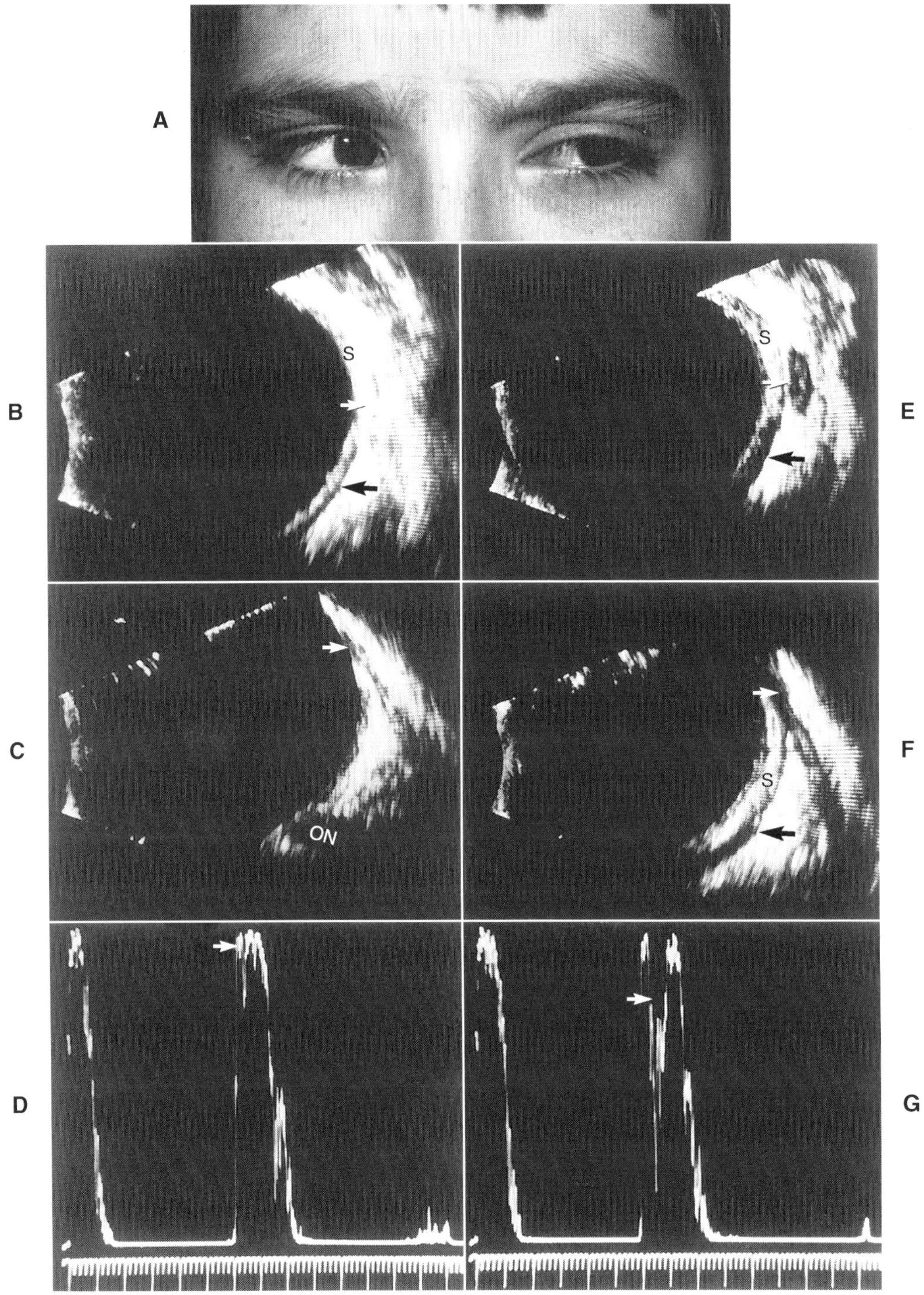

Figure 15-27 Myositis secondary to scleritis. **A,** External photograph shows child with ptosis and injection of left eye (patient complained of severe pain). Echograms are from normal right eye and orbit (**B** to **D**) and corresponding echograms from left eye and orbit with scleritis and myositis (**E** to **G**). **B,** Vertical transverse B-scan echogram shows thin insertion of normal right lateral rectus muscle *(white arrow)*, inferior oblique muscle *(black arrow)*, and sclera *(S)*. **C,** Longitudinal B-scan shows thin insertion of normal lateral rectus muscle *(white arrow)*. *ON*, Optic nerve. **D,** Corresponding A-scan shows thin insertion of normal lateral rectus muscle *(arrow)*. **E,** Vertical transverse B-scan view shows thickening of left lateral rectus muscle insertion *(white arrow)*, inferior oblique muscle *(black arrow)*, and sclera *(S)*. **F,** Longitudinal B-scan shows thickening of left lateral rectus muscle insertion *(white arrow)*. Note thickening of sclera *(S)* and edema in sub-Tenon's space *(black arrow)*. **G,** Corresponding A-scan shows thickened insertion of lateral rectus muscle *(arrow)*.

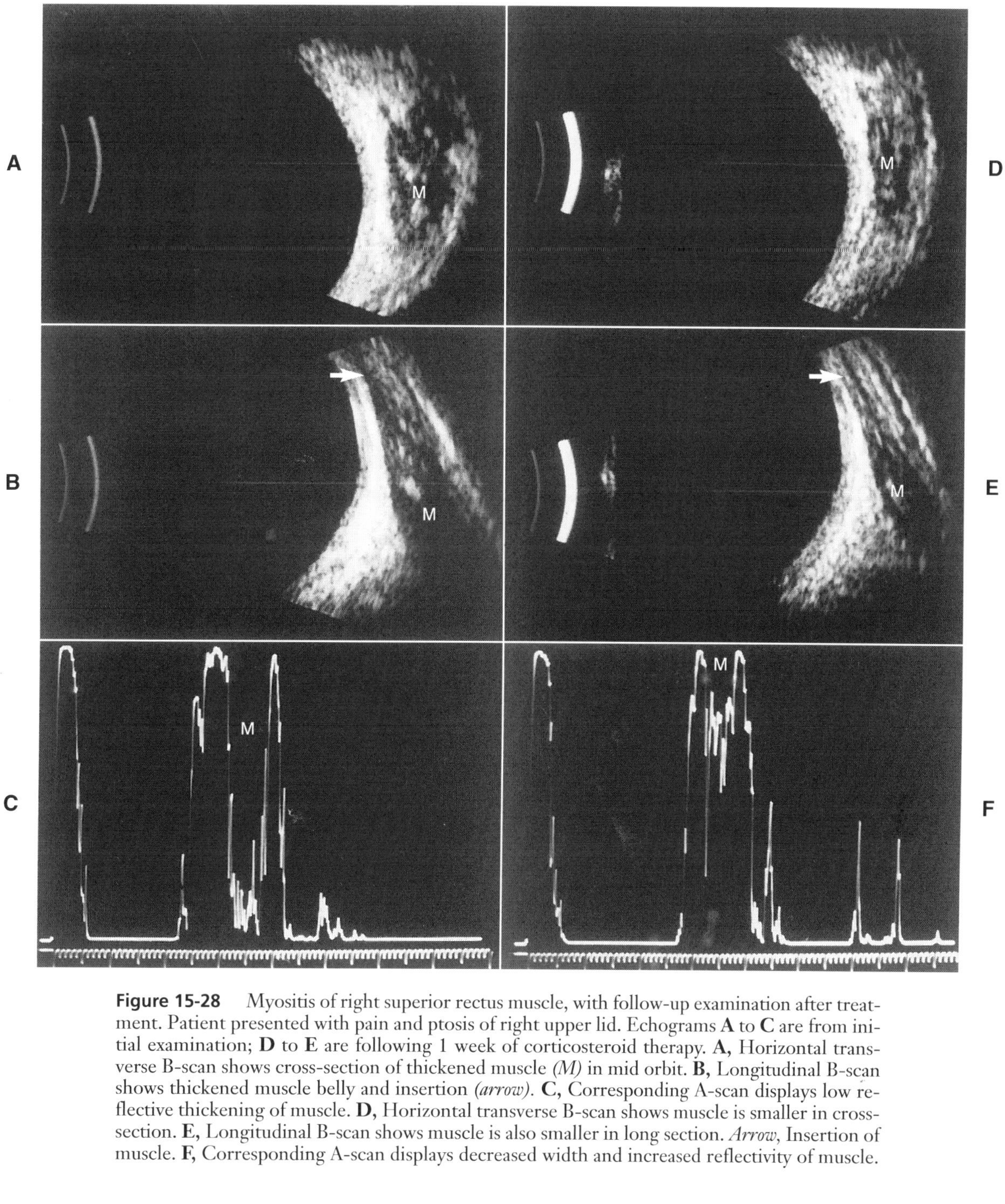

Figure 15-28 Myositis of right superior rectus muscle, with follow-up examination after treatment. Patient presented with pain and ptosis of right upper lid. Echograms **A** to **C** are from initial examination; **D** to **E** are following 1 week of corticosteroid therapy. **A,** Horizontal transverse B-scan shows cross-section of thickened muscle *(M)* in mid orbit. **B,** Longitudinal B-scan shows thickened muscle belly and insertion *(arrow)*. **C,** Corresponding A-scan displays low reflective thickening of muscle. **D,** Horizontal transverse B-scan shows muscle is smaller in cross-section. **E,** Longitudinal B-scan shows muscle is also smaller in long section. *Arrow,* Insertion of muscle. **F,** Corresponding A-scan displays decreased width and increased reflectivity of muscle.

Tumors

Various types of tumors can infiltrate the extraocular muscles.* Although infiltration by tumor is an uncommon finding, enlarged muscles due to metastatic carcinoma, lymphoma, sarcoma, metastatic melanoma, and amyloidosis may occur.[7,11]

*References 4, 6, 7, 10, 14, 16, 31, 32, 37.

Metastatic carcinoma to the extraocular muscles may be unilateral or bilateral and may affect one or more muscles. The tumor may involve the entire muscle, including the tendon, but is more commonly localized to the mid- and posterior portions of the muscle belly. Internal reflectivity is generally low to medium, with regular structure (Figure 15-29; see also Table 15-2). Differentiation between myositis and metastatic carcinoma sometimes can be difficult, both clinically and echographically, because both conditions

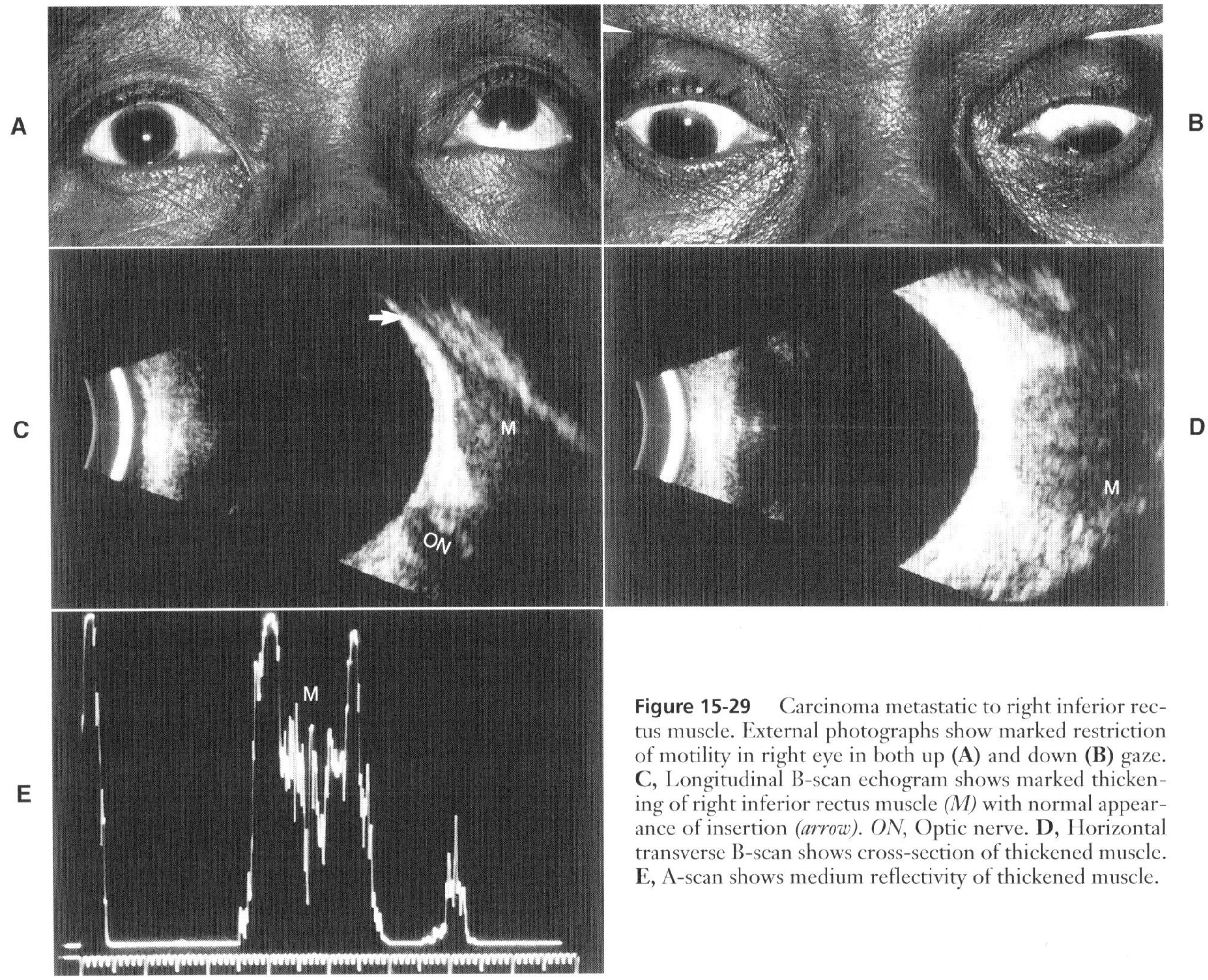

Figure 15-29 Carcinoma metastatic to right inferior rectus muscle. External photographs show marked restriction of motility in right eye in both up **(A)** and down **(B)** gaze. **C,** Longitudinal B-scan echogram shows marked thickening of right inferior rectus muscle *(M)* with normal appearance of insertion *(arrow)*. *ON,* Optic nerve. **D,** Horizontal transverse B-scan shows cross-section of thickened muscle. **E,** A-scan shows medium reflectivity of thickened muscle.

can be associated with pain and a thickened, low reflective muscle. Extraocular muscle enlargement may also be produced by metastatic melanoma from skin[6,32] (Figure 15-30), as well as by lymphoma that may involve the rectus and/or levator muscles (Figure 15-31).

Venous Congestion

Extraocular muscles can become thickened as a result of venous congestion.[1,29] This condition can be observed in orbits affected by carotid-cavernous or dural-cavernous sinus fistulas, diffuse inflammatory disease, and compression by a lesion located in the orbital apex or the cavernous sinus. Congestion is most often a unilateral condition that involves all muscles on the affected side to a mild or moderate degree. Internal reflectivity of the thickened muscles can be normal or moderately high (see Table 15-2). In addition, there is usually orbital soft tissue swelling as well as enlargement of the optic nerve (see p 428). Also, dilated orbital veins are often present, either secondary to compression or to arteriovenous fistula (see Figure 13-15). In patients with dural-cavernous sinus fistula, diffuse, mild thickening of the extraocular muscles and orbital soft tissues is sometimes the only finding.

In venous congestion, the enlarged muscles can appear similar to those of thyroid ophthalmopathy. Therefore, echographic differentiation between the two disorders sometimes can be difficult.

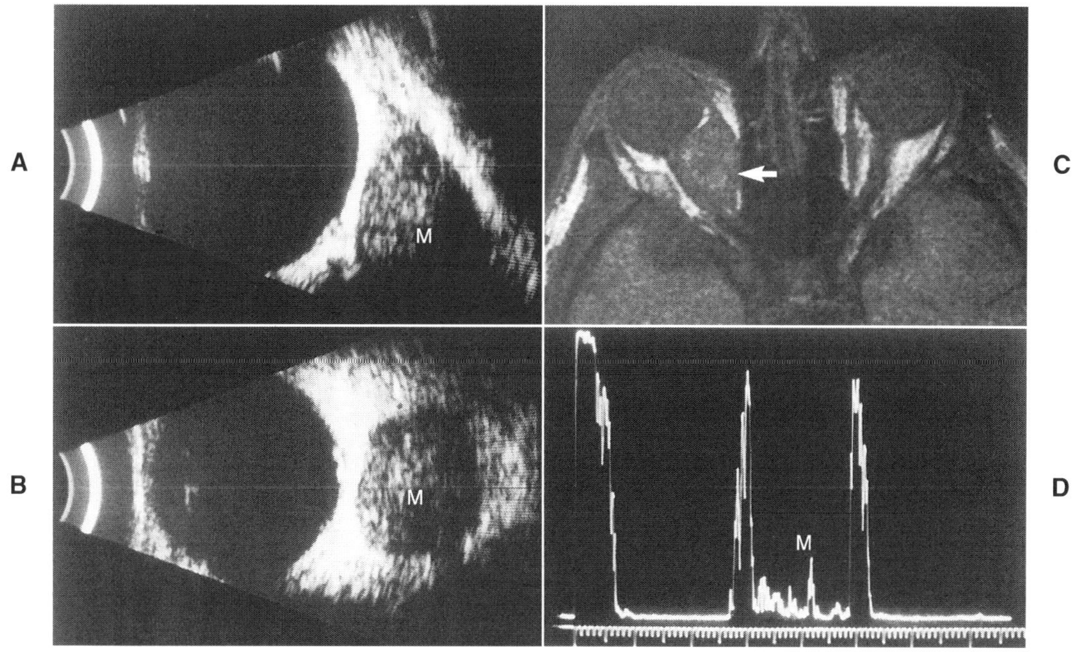

Figure 15-30 Melanoma metastatic to right medial rectus muscle. **A,** Longitudinal B-scan echogram shows markedly thickened muscle *(M)* with rounded appearance of anterior border. **B,** Vertical transverse B-scan shows cross-section of thickened muscle. **C,** Axial MRI scan shows very large right medial rectus muscle *(arrow)*. **D,** A-scan shows very low reflectivity of thickened muscle.

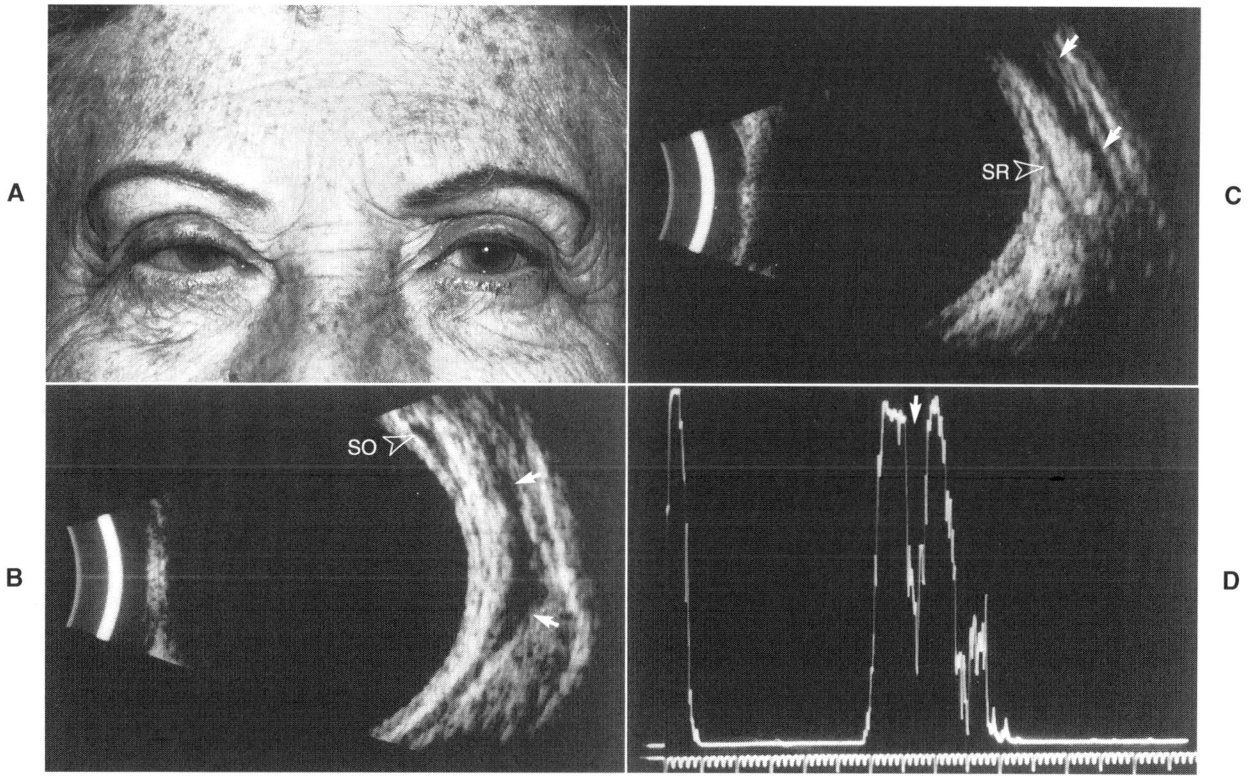

Figure 15-31 Lymphoma involving right levator muscle. **A,** External photograph shows bilateral upper lid ptosis (OD > OS) in patient with biopsy-proved orbital lymphoma. Transocular echograms from the right orbit show lesion involving the levator muscle *(closed arrows)*. **B,** Horizontal transverse B-scan through the anterior aspect of the superior orbit shows lesion involving the levator muscle *(arrows)*. *SO,* Superior oblique tendon. **C,** Longitudinal B-scan showing thickening of the levator muscle, especially anteriorly as it extends into the upper lid. *SR,* Superior rectus muscle. **D,** A-scan through very anterior aspect of levator muscle shows low to medium reflectivity.

Trauma

Hematoma occurring within the muscle sheath can occur secondary to trauma.[4] Internal reflectivity is low when swelling is pronounced, and the inserting tendon may or may not be thickened. Hemorrhage also can be present elsewhere in the orbit. Confirmation of the diagnosis is usually made by noting a decrease in the size of the muscle over time; some change often is apparent within a few days.

Muscle slippage following strabismus surgery or transection by trauma can result in retraction of the muscle into the posterior orbit.[19] In such cases, ultrasound can

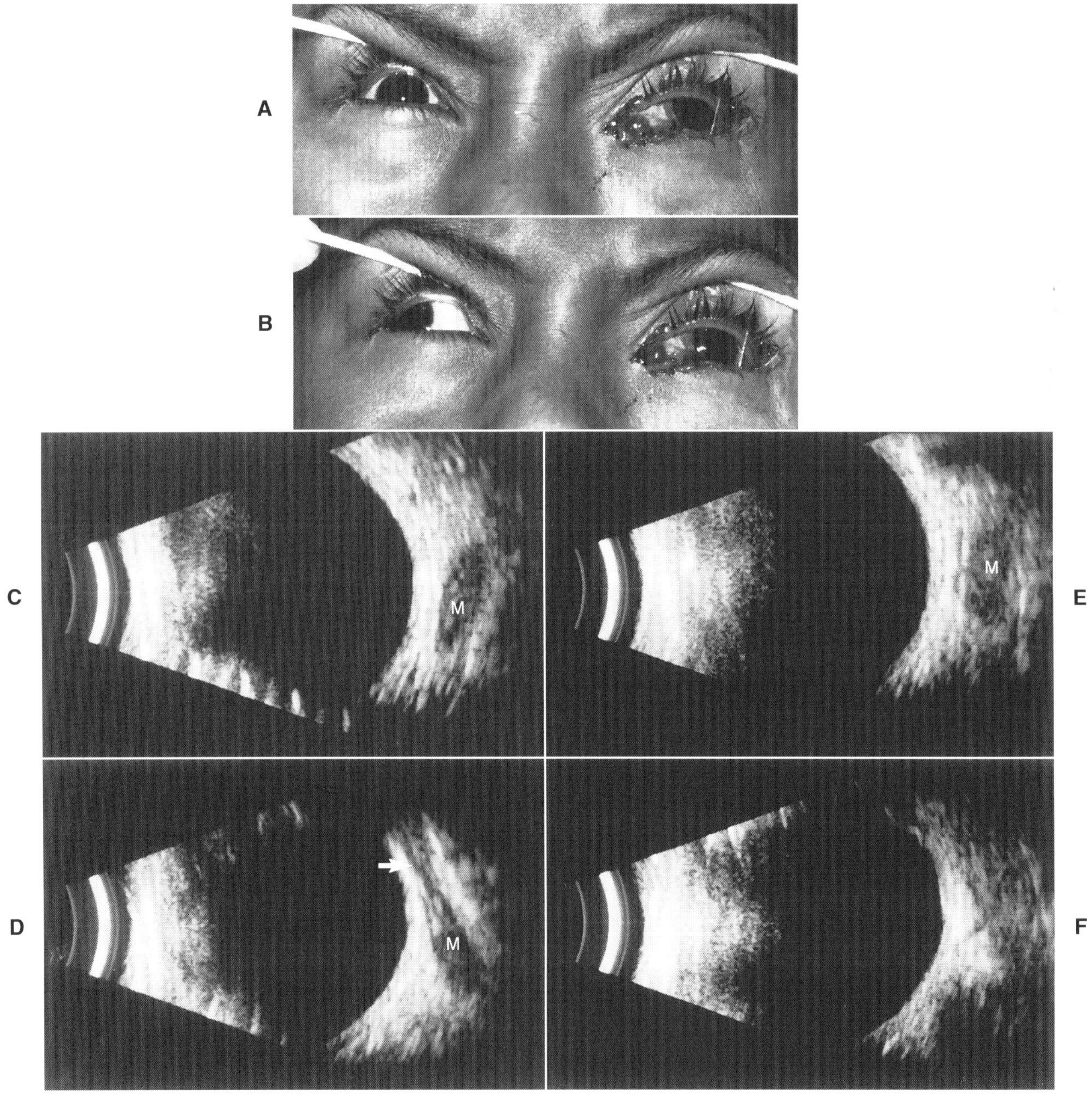

Figure 15-32 Severed left medial rectus muscle following penetrating trauma. External photographs (**A** and **B**) show chemosis, subconjunctival hemorrhage, and no horizontal movement of the left eye. Normal right medial rectus muscle *(M)* is shown in vertical transverse **(C)** and longitudinal **D)** views. *Arrow*, Insertion of muscle. Severed left medial rectus muscle is shown well in transverse view **(E)**, but the muscle is not identifiable in longitudinal section **(F)**.

sometimes show gross disinsertion from the globe (Figure 15-32). Very mild retraction or muscle slippage, however, may be undetectable with ultrasound. Incarceration of an extraocular muscle following trauma or sinus surgery also can occur[2,9] and can be shown with echography (Figure 15-33; see also Figure 17-13).

Muscle Thinning

Extraocular muscles can be abnormally thin in some situations. This is most commonly seen in very long globes with large posterior staphylomas[5,33] (Figure 15-34). Thinning of the extraocular muscles can occur due to congenital fibrosis, as well as from longstanding thyroid ophthalmopathy (Figure 15-35).

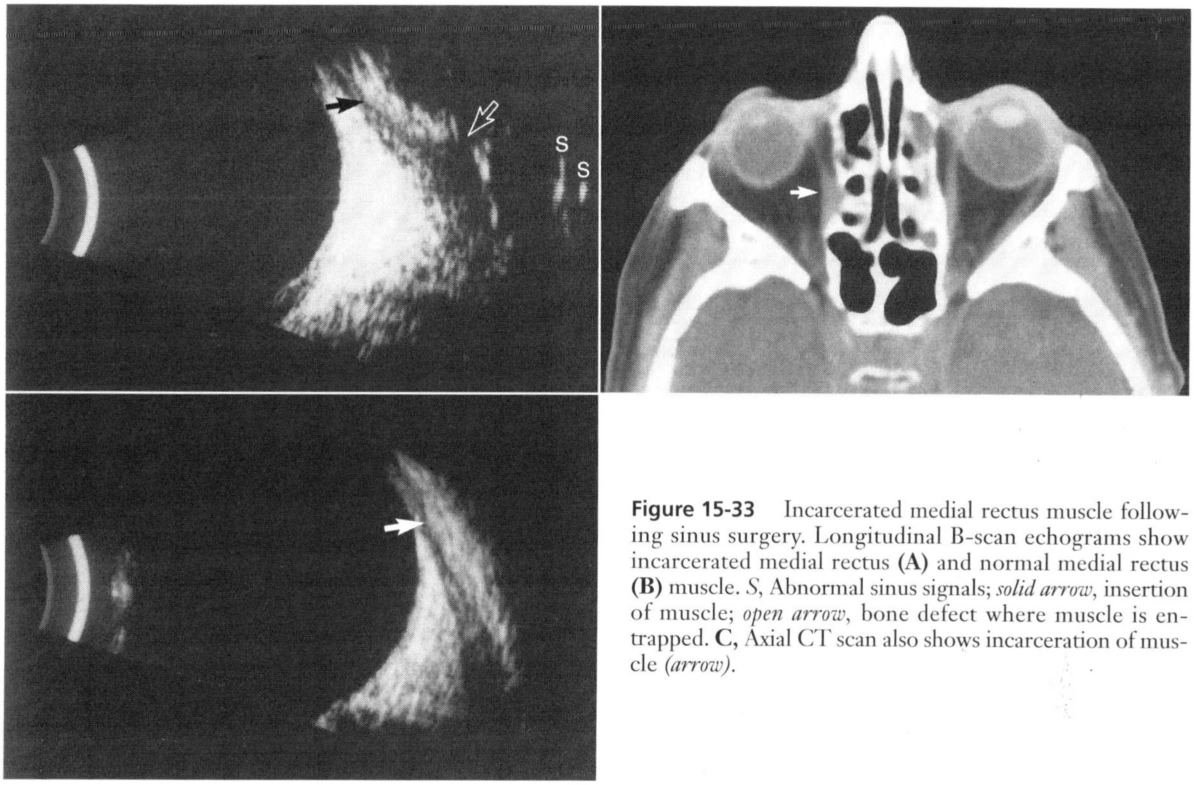

Figure 15-33 Incarcerated medial rectus muscle following sinus surgery. Longitudinal B-scan echograms show incarcerated medial rectus **(A)** and normal medial rectus **(B)** muscle. *S*, Abnormal sinus signals; *solid arrow*, insertion of muscle; *open arrow*, bone defect where muscle is entrapped. **C,** Axial CT scan also shows incarceration of muscle *(arrow)*.

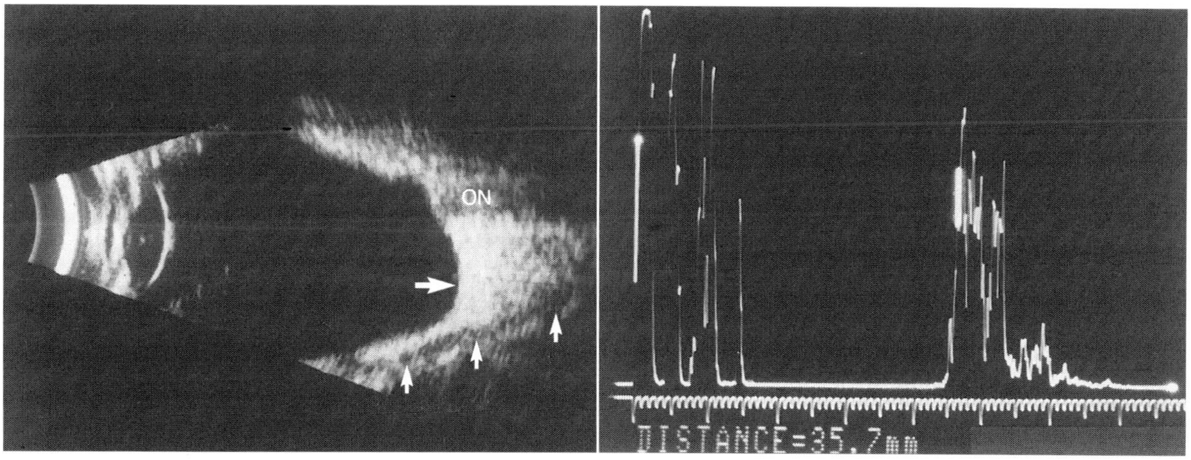

Figure 15-34 Posterior staphyloma in eye with restricted motility. Patient had refractive error of -18 diopters OU and restricted eye movement. **A,** Horizontal axial B-scan echogram of left eye shows large posterior staphyloma *(large arrow)* and thin lateral rectus muscle *(small arrows)*. *ON*, Optic nerve. **B,** A-scan contact axial length measurement = 35.7 mm.

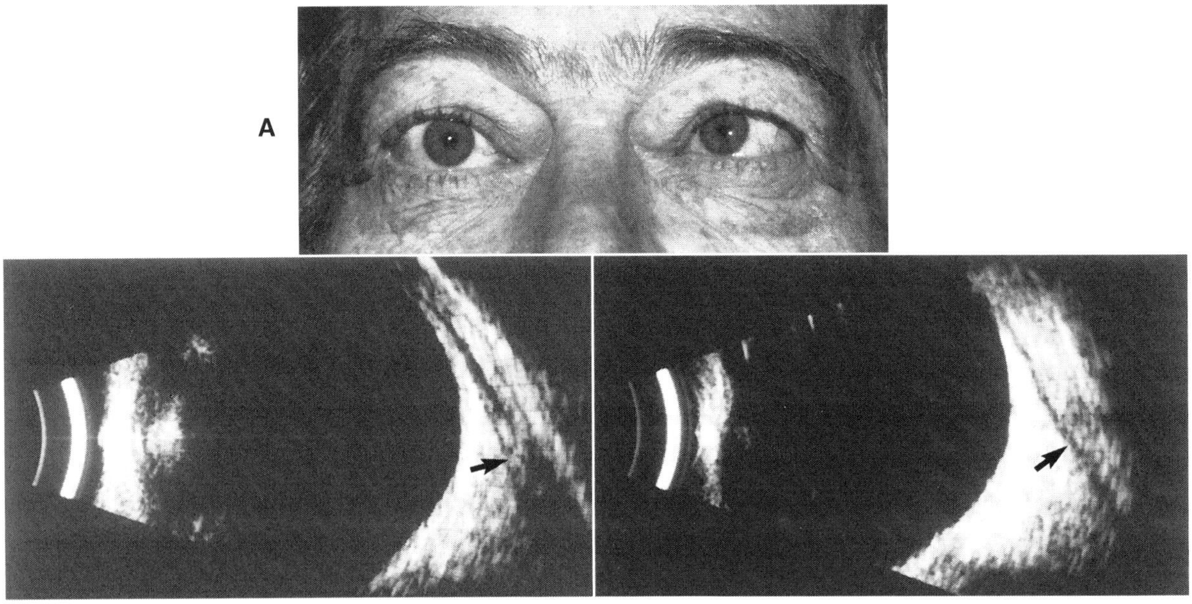

Figure 15-35 Thinning of left lateral rectus muscle in patient with longstanding thyroid ophthalmopathy. **A,** External photograph shows hypertropia of left eye. Longitudinal B-scans display normal right lateral rectus muscle **(B)** and very thin left lateral rectus muscle **(C).** *Arrows,* Muscle.

REFERENCES

1. Atta HR, Dick AD, Hamed LM, et al: Venous stasis orbitopathy—a clinical and echographic study. *Br J Ophthalmol* 1996;80:129.
2. Buus DR, Tse DT, Farris BK: Ophthalmic complications of sinus surgery. *Ophthalmology* 1990;97:614.
3. Byrne SF, Gendron EK, Glaser JS, et al: Diameter of normal extraocular recti muscles with echography. *Am J Ophthalmol* 1991;112:706.
4. Capone A Jr, Slamovits TL: Discrete metastasis of solid tumors to extraocular muscles. *Arch Ophthalmol* 1990;108:237.
5. Demer JL, von Noorden GK: High myopia as an unusual cause of restrictive motility disturbance. *Surv Ophthalmol* 1989;33:281.
6. DiBernardo CL, Pacheco EM, Hughes JR, et al: Echographic evaluation and findings in metastatic melanoma to extraocular muscles. *Ophthalmology* 1996;103:1794.
7. Dutton JJ, Byrne SF, Proia AD: *Diagnostic Atlas of Orbital Diseases.* Philadelphia, WB Saunders, 2000.
8. Fledelius HC, Gyldensted C: Ultrasonography and computer tomography in orbital diagnosis with special reference to dysthyroid ophthalmopathy. *Acta Ophthalmol* 1978;56:751.
9. Flynn JT, Mitchell KB, Fuller DG, et al: Ocular motility complications following intranasal surgery. *Arch Ophthalmol* 1979;97:453.
10. Friedman J, Karesh J, Rodrigues M, et al: Thyroid carcinoma metastatic to the medial rectus muscle. *Ophthalmic Plast Reconstr Surg* 1990;6:122.
11. Glaser JS: Orbital diseases and neuro-ophthalmology: An overview, in Glaser JS (ed): *Neuro-ophthalmology.* ed 2. Philadelphia, JB Lippincott, 1990, p 453.
12. Hasenfratz G: Standardized echography in Graves' disease, in Ossoinig KC (ed): *Ophthalmic Echography.* Dordrecht, Dr W Junk, 1987, p 557.
13. Hodes BL, Stern G: Contact B-scan echographic diagnosis of ophthalmopathic Graves' disease. *J Clin Ultrasound* 1975;3:255.
14. Holstrumom GE, Nyman KG: Primary orbital amyloidosis localised to an extraocular muscle. *Br J Ophthalmol* 1987;71:32.
15. Holt JE, O'Connor PS, Douglas JP, et al: Extraocular muscle size comparison using standardized A-scan echography and computerized tomography scan measurements. *Ophthalmology* 1985;92:1351.
16. Hornblass A, Jakobiec FA, Reifler DM, et al: Orbital lymphoid tumors located predominantly within extraocular muscles. *Ophthalmology* 1987;94:688.
17. Jakobiec FA, Font RL: Orbit, in Spencer WH: *Ophthalmic Pathology—An Atlas and Textbook.* ed 3. Philadelphia, WB Saunders, 1986, p 2766.
18. Kennerdell JS, Dresner SC: The nonspecific orbital inflammatory syndromes. *Surv Ophthalmol* 1984;29:97.
19. Mark LE, Kennerdell JS: Medial rectus injury from intranasal surgery. *Arch Ophthalmol* 1979;97:459.
20. McNutt L: Ultrasound of Graves' orbitopathy [seminar]. Iowa City, Iowa, Department of Ophthalmology, University of Iowa Hospitals, 1975.
21. McNutt LC, Kaefring SL, Ossoinig KC: Echographic measurement of extraocular muscles, in White D, Brown RE (eds): *Ultrasound in Medicine.* New York, Plenum Press, 1977, p 927.
22. Neigel JM, Rootman J, Belkin RI, et al: Dysthyroid optic neuropathy: The crowded orbital apex syndrome. *Ophthalmology* 1988; 95:1515.
23. Ossoinig KC: Standardized echography: Basic principles, clinical applications and results. *Int Ophthalmol Clin* 1979;19(4):127.
24. Ossoinig KC: The technique of measuring the extraocular muscles, in Gernet H (ed): *Diagnostica Ultrasonica in Ophthalmologica.* Meunster, RA Remy, 1979, p 166.
25. Ossoinig KC: The role of standardized ophthalmic echography in the management of Graves' ophthalmopathy. *Dev Ophthalmol* 1989;20:28.
26. Ossoinig KC: Early detection of compressive optic neuropathy in Graves' disease with standardized A-scan, in Ossoinig KC (ed): *Ophthalmic Echography.* Dordrecht, Dr W Junk, 1987, p 569.
27. Ossoinig KC: Ultrasonic diagnosis of Graves' ophthalmopathy, in Gorman CA, Waller RD, Dyer JA (eds): *The Eye and Orbit in Thyroid Disease.* New York, Raven Press, 1984.
28. Ossoinig KC, Hermsen VM: Myositis of extraocular muscles diagnosed with standardized echography, in Hillman JS, Lemay MM (eds): *Ophthalmic Ultrasonography.* Dordrecht, Dr W Junk, 1984, p 383.
29. Phelps CD, Thompson HS, Ossoinig KC: The diagnosis and prognosis of atypical carotid-cavernous fistula (red-eyed shunt syndrome). *Am J Ophthalmol* 1982;93:423.
30. Rootman J: Graves' orbitopathy, in Rootman J: *Diseases of the Orbit.* Philadelphia, JB Lippincott, 1988, p 248.
31. Rootman J, Robertson W, Lapointe: Inflammatory diseases, in Rootman J: *Diseases of the Orbit.* Philadelphia, JB Lippincott, 1988, p 165.

32. Rootman J, Ragaz J, Cline R, et al: Tumors (orbital metastasis, in Rootman J: *Diseases of the Orbit.* Philadelphia, JB Lippincott, 1988, p 426.
33. Ruttum MS, Lloyd MA, Lewandowski MF: Echography in the diagnosis of restrictive motility caused by severe myopia. *Am J Ophthalmol* 1990;109:350.
34. Shammas HJF, Minckler DS, Ogden C: Ultrasound in early thyroid orbitopathy. *Arch Ophthalmol* 1980;98:277.
35. Siatkowski RM, Capo H, Byrne SF, et al: Clinical and echographic findings in idiopathic orbital myositis. *Am J Ophthalmol* 1994; 118:343.
36. Skalka HW: Perineural optic nerve changes in endocrine orbitopathy. *Arch Ophthalmol* 1978;96:468.
37. Slamovits TL, Burde RM: Bumpy muscles. *Surv Ophthalmol* 1988; 33:189.
38. Small RG: Enlargement of levator palpebrae superioris muscle fibers in Graves' ophthalmopathy. *Ophthalmology* 1989;96:430.
39. Tychsen L, Tse DT, Ossoinig K, et al: Trochleitis with superior oblique myositis. *Ophthalmology* 1984;91:1075.
40. Wan WL, Cano MR, Green RL: Orbital myositis involving the oblique muscles: An echographic study. *Ophthalmology* 1988;95:1522.
41. Werner SC, Coleman DJ, Franzen LA: Ultrasonographic evidence of a consistent orbital involvement in Graves' disease. *N Engl J Med* 1974;290:1446.

William D. Bates

16 Optic Nerve

One of the most important uses of echography in the orbit is evaluation of the optic nerve. Techniques have been developed to evaluate subtle abnormalities of the optic nerve. Echography can sometimes provide information that is not apparent with other imaging modalities. This chapter addresses techniques and findings in the assessment of the retrobulbar optic nerve and the optic disc.

RETROBULBAR OPTIC NERVE

The intraorbital portion of the optic nerve is a distinct, homogeneous, tubular structure that courses through the orbit in a sinuous fashion. Using appropriate examination techniques, echography can enable one to detect, and often differentiate, optic nerve abnormalities associated with or caused by inflammation, tumor or trauma (Box 16-1).

B-Scan Technique

B-scan is used to evaluate general topography of the retrobulbar optic nerve. Additionally, B-scan can show the relationship of the optic nerve to normal structures such as the globe, extraocular muscles, and orbital bones, as well as to retrobulbar lesions. Other associated changes, such as abnormalities of the optic disc (e.g., disc edema) and alterations in contour of the globe wall (e.g., thickening and flattening) also can be well shown.

The B-scan examination is usually performed with a medium gain setting. The examiner may wish, however, to display the nerve at a high gain level initially and then decrease the gain setting until the optic nerve is clearly shown (Figure 16-1). Comparison with the contralateral optic nerve should always be performed at a similar gain setting. Axial, longitudinal, and transverse views can be used to display the optic nerve.

For the axial approach, the patient fixates in primary gaze, and the probe is centered on the cornea, with the sound beam directed through the lens toward the optic nerve. This approach displays the optic nerve as a wedge-shaped, echolucent defect (acoustic void) inserting into the back of the globe (Figure 16-2). This wedge-shaped appearance is due partially to the homogeneous nature of the optic nerve, as well as to artifact from oblique sound beam incidence to the nerve borders. Consequently, the axial approach provides only limited information and is primarily of value for documenting marked enlargement of the optic nerve. The transverse and longitudinal views provide more perpendicular sound beam incidence and therefore a more accurate display of the nerve.

With the longitudinal approach, the sound beam bypasses the lens and is directed more perpendicular to the optic nerve than the axial approach. Longitudinal scans are typically performed as the patient fixates slightly nasally with the probe placed on the temporal, horizontal meridian (i.e., longitudinal scan of the 3-o'clock meridian of the right orbit, and the 9-o'clock meridian of the left orbit). With the marker oriented toward the cornea, the probe is positioned close to the limbus and the nerve is thus displayed at the lower aspect of the echogram (Figure 16-3).

BOX 16-1

Optic Nerve Abnormalities

Retrobulbar Optic Nerve

- Increased subarachnoid fluid (e.g., pseudotumor cerebri)
- Optic neuritis
- Glioma
- Optic nerve sheath meningioma
- Tumors
- Arachnoid cyst
- Compressive optic neuropathy
- Trauma
- Vascular occlusive disease
- Optic atrophy

Optic Disc

- Cupping
- Coloboma
- Elevation
- Drusen
- Pit

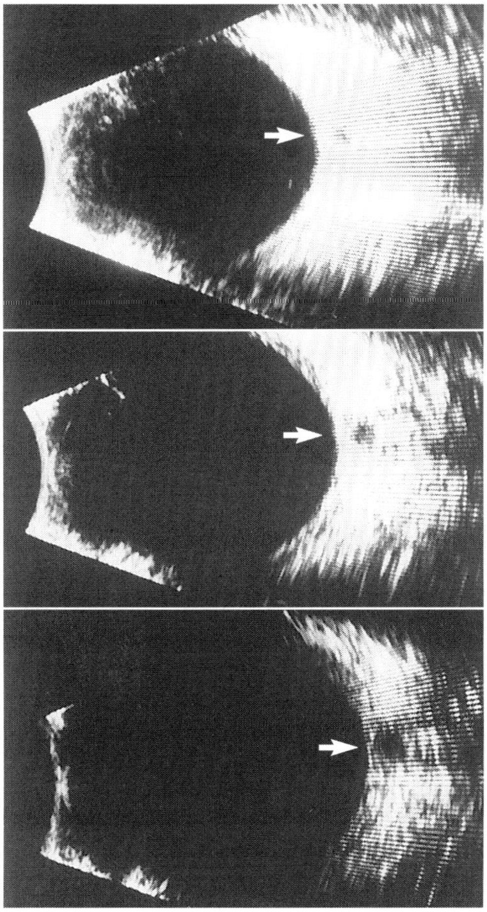

Figure 16-1 Transverse B-scan montage of normal optic nerve at high, medium, and low gain settings. **A,** Optic nerve *(arrow)* is detected but is not shown well at high gain. **B,** Nerve is more apparent as gain is decreased. **C,** Nerve is well delineated at medium-low gain setting. Note that the optic nerve defect enlarges as gain is reduced. (From Byrne SF: Evaluation of the optic nerve with standardized echography, in Smith JL [ed]: *Neuroophthalmology Now!* New York, Field, Raicha and Associates, 1986, p 54.)

The vertical transverse approach, also bypassing the lens, provides a cross-section of the optic nerve anteriorly, near the globe. This scan allows relative perpendicularity to the optic nerve, presumably because of refraction that occurs at or near the perineural sheaths. Gross enlargement, as well as abnormalities within the optic nerve, can be shown with this approach.[4,5] This scan is performed with the patient fixating in primary gaze with the probe placed temporally (marker directed superiorly). This results in the display of a circular echolucent defect just behind the globe. In some instances, edge artifacts (see p 466) are produced at the edge of the optic nerve when it is viewed in cross-section (Figure 16-4).

A-Scan Technique

A-scan provides cross-sectional measurements of the optic nerve and is used to analyze internal reflectivity and structure of the nerve and its sheaths.[1,4,5,17,35] The instrument is set at Tissue Sensitivity, and the examination is carried out initially with the patient fixating in primary gaze. The probe is placed on the globe temporally near the equator (9-o'clock position right eye, 3-o'clock position left eye), and the sound beam is directed across the globe anteriorly toward the insertion of the medial rectus muscle. The probe is then slowly angled posteriorly and slightly superiorly until the optic nerve pattern appears just behind the globe. When the sound beam is directed perpendicular to the optic nerve, a distinct defect is displayed. This defect, the optic nerve parenchyma, is low to medium reflective, and the bordering perineural sheaths are highly reflective (Figure 16-5). As previously explained for B-scan, perpendicular sound beam incidence presumably occurs due to refraction at or near the surface of the perineural sheaths.[24,34]

The optic nerve is first evaluated anteriorly. The probe is then slowly angled toward the orbital apex to enable evaluation of the nerve as far posteriorly as possible. During this procedure, it may be necessary to tilt the probe slightly up or down to maintain perpendicular sound beam incidence to the perineural sheaths. Also, as the nerve is traced back into the orbit, the sheath spikes tend to decrease in height because of oblique sound beam incidence and sound attenuation. Consequently, the sheath spikes should first be identified anteriorly (where perpendicularity is easiest to achieve) before tracing the nerve back into the orbit (Figure 16-6).

Measurements are made between the inner aspect of the two steeply rising, high sheath spikes, which are typically thick and double peaked. The inner peaks correspond to the pia mater and/or arachnoid sheath and the outer peaks to the dural sheath. The diameter of the optic nerve should be measured both anteriorly (a few millimeters behind the globe) and posteriorly (as close as possible to the orbital apex). Measurements can be made from the screen with electronic cursors (gates), or by hand from photographs using calipers (Figure 16-7). Regardless of the method used, calculations of nerve size should be made based on a velocity of 1,550 m/sec (see Appendix A).

The normal optic nerve measures approximately the same thickness anteriorly as posteriorly and is usually symmetric with the fellow optic nerve. The difference between the two nerves is generally within 0.5 mm; larger differences indicate probable abnormal thickness of one nerve. It is important, however, to be certain that these differences are not the result of examination error such as measurement of incorrect spikes or nonperpendicularity (Figure 16-8). Whenever a significant difference is detected between the two nerves, repeat measurements should be performed to confirm the findings.

The most important factor in detecting optic nerve disease is comparison of size with that of the fellow nerve. If, however, there is bilateral disease or if the fellow optic nerve cannot be measured, it can be helpful to refer to normal, standard values. One study has shown normal optic

Text continued on p 418

A

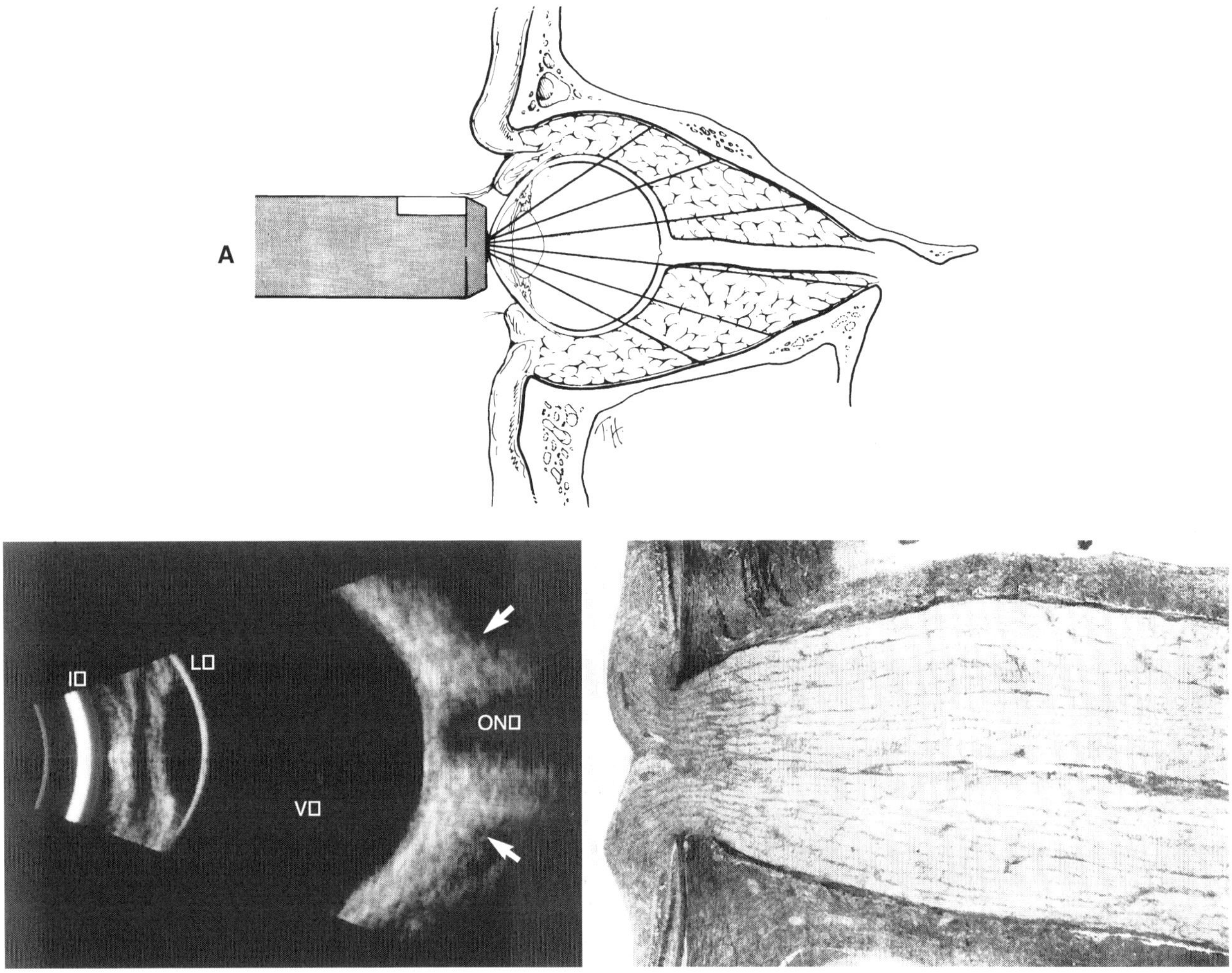

B C

Figure 16-2 Axial B-scan of normal optic nerve. **A,** Probe is centered on cornea, and sound beam sweeps through posterior pole and optic nerve. **B,** Axial B-scan echogram shows normal wedge-shaped acoustic void behind the globe. *I,* Initial line corresponding to probe face on cornea; *L,* lens; *V,* vitreous cavity; *ON,* optic nerve; *arrows,* orbital soft tissue. **C,** Gross pathologic specimen of normal optic nerve.

A B

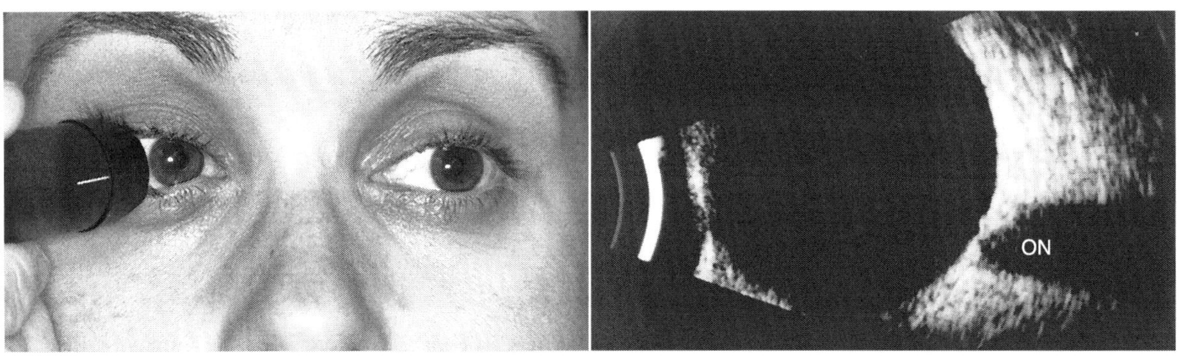

Figure 16-3 Longitudinal B-scan examination of normal optic nerve. **A,** Patient fixates slightly nasally and probe is placed temporally, with the marker directed toward the cornea. **B,** Echogram shows long section of normal optic nerve *(ON).*

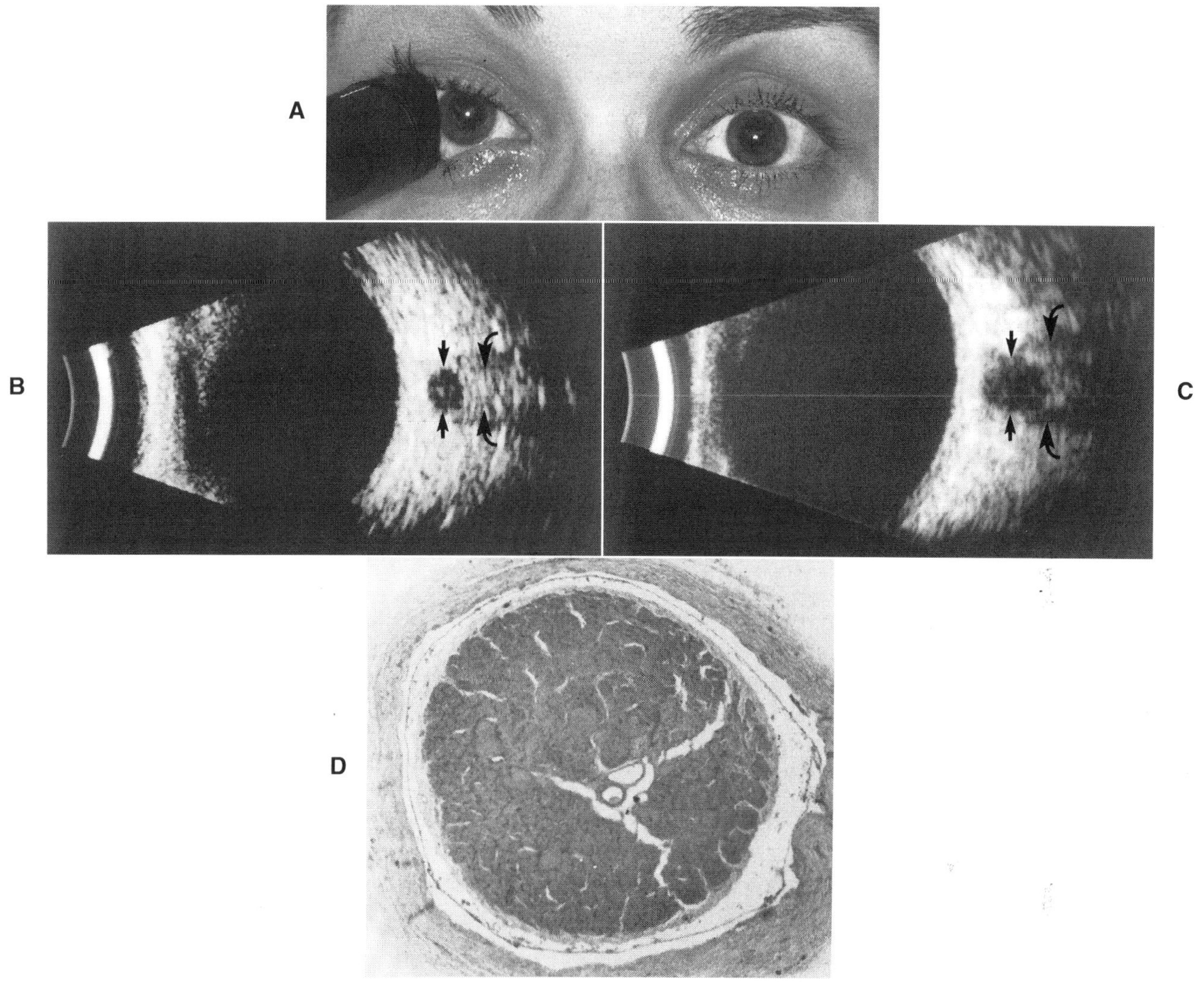

Figure 16-4 Vertical transverse B-scan examination of the optic nerve. **A,** Patient fixates in primary gaze, and probe is placed temporally with marker directed superiorly. **B,** Echogram shows cross-section of normal optic nerve *(arrows).* **C,** Cross-section of enlarged optic nerve. **D,** Pathologic specimen showing cross-section of normal optic nerve. Note edge artifact in **B** and **C** *(curved arrows).*

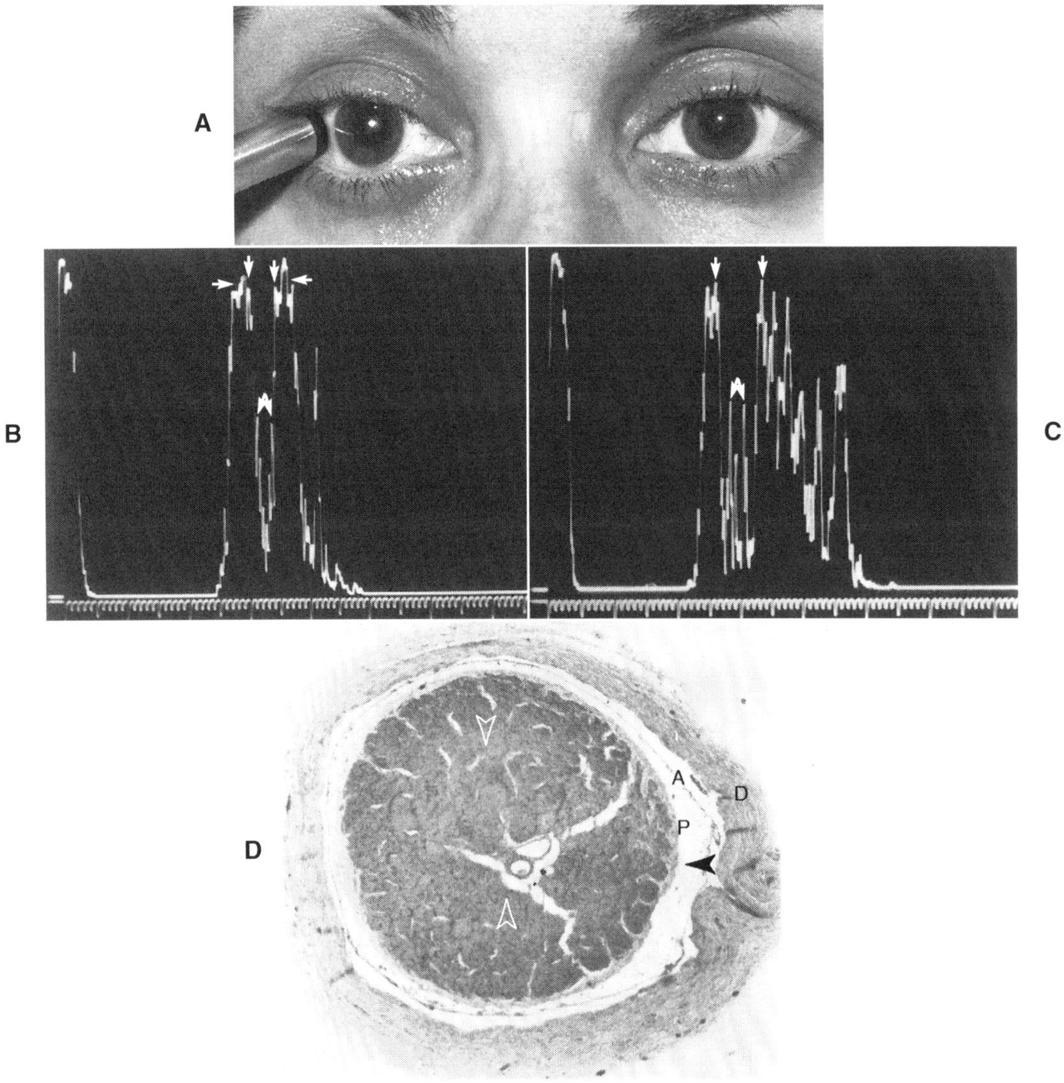

Figure 16-5 A-scan examination of the optic nerve. **A,** Patient fixates in primary gaze, and probe is placed temporally near the equator. **B,** Cross-section of normal optic nerve. *Horizontal arrows,* Dural sheath; *vertical arrows,* arachnoid sheath; *connected arrows,* surface of optic nerve parenchyma (pia mater). **C,** Cross-section of thickened nerve. **D,** Pathologic specimen showing cross-section of normal optic nerve and surrounding sheaths. *Open arrows,* Optic nerve parenchyma; *P,* pia mater; *black arrowhead,* subarachnoid space; *A,* arachnoid sheath; *D,* dural sheath.

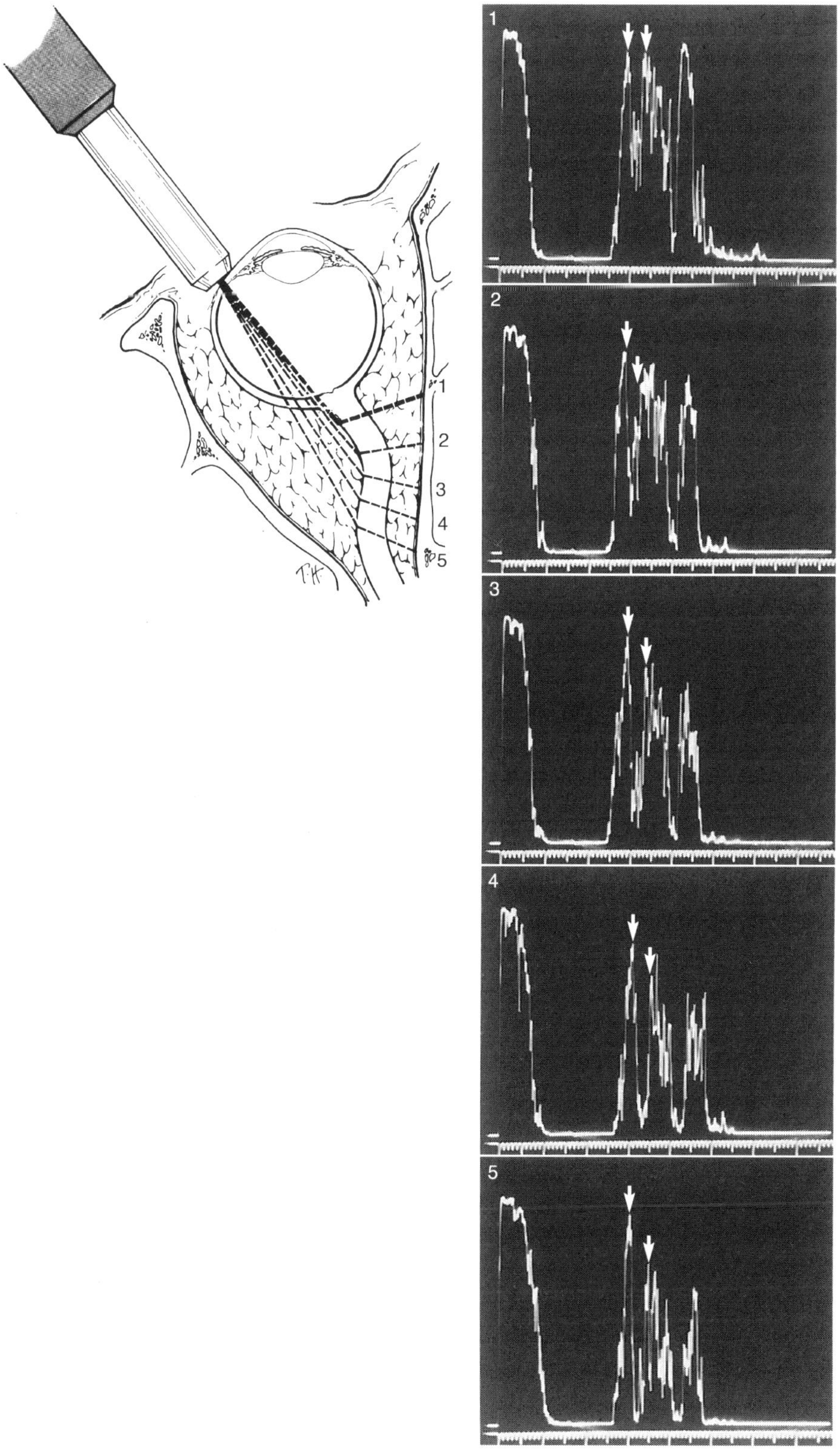

Figure 16-6 Dynamic A-scan screening of the optic nerve. Drawing demonstrates how movement of probe allows more posterior examination of optic nerve. Note that refraction at or near the nerve surface produces perpendicular sound beam incidence to the perineural sheaths. Once the optic nerve defect is detected anteriorly *(1)*, the probe is angled to display the nerve defect as far posteriorly as possible *(5)*. The steeply rising, high sheath spikes *(arrows)* indicate perpendicularity. Because amplitude of nerve and sheath spikes decreases as the sound beam progresses posteriorly, assessment of reflectivity should be made anteriorly (*1* and *2*).

A

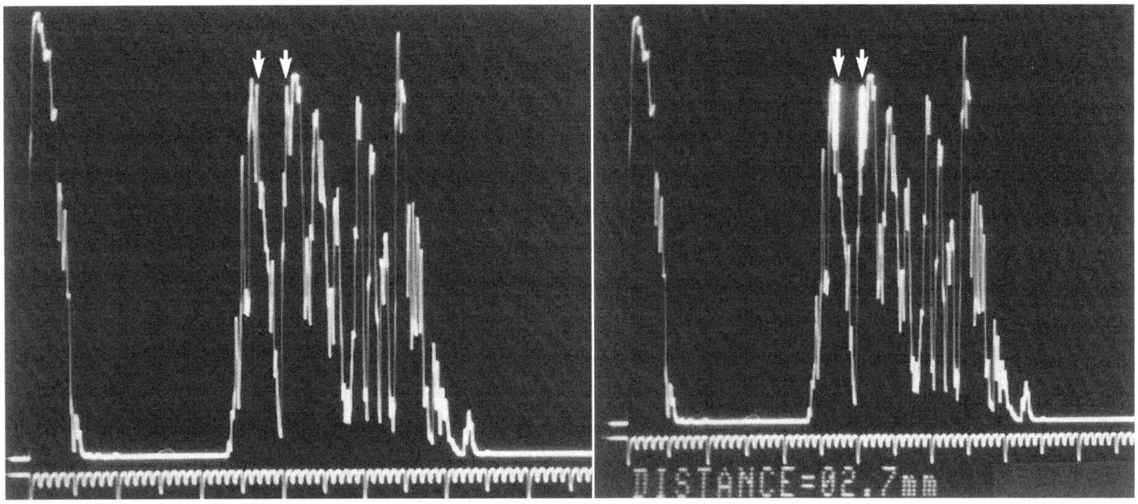

B

Figure 16-7 Measurement of optic nerve thickness with A-scan. **A,** Echogram with no gates. *Arrows,* Perineural sheaths. **B,** Electronic gates on sheath spikes *(arrows)* indicate optic nerve thickness.

A

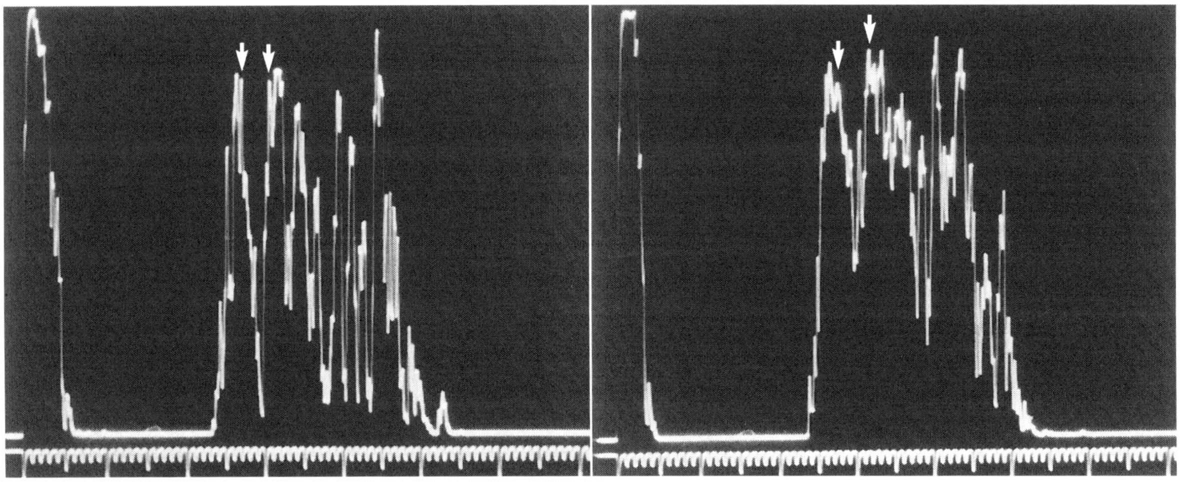

B

Figure 16-8 Optic nerve displayed with perpendicular (correct) and oblique (incorrect) sound beam incidence on A-scan. **A,** Steeply rising, distinct perineural sheath spikes indicate perpendicular sound beam incidence *(arrows).* **B,** Indistinct sheath spikes *(arrows)* due to oblique sound beam incidence.

nerve diameters to range between 2.2 and 3.3 mm, with a mean value of 2.5 mm.[17] However, it may be useful for individuals to establish their own control values, because techniques may differ somewhat among various examiners.

Internal reflectivity and structure of the optic nerve can be assessed at the same time that the nerve is measured. The normal optic nerve produces low to medium internal reflectivity with regular structure, as shown in Figure 16-5. It is important, however, that reflectivity be evaluated primarily in the anterior one-half of the optic nerve because sound attenuation typically causes lower reflectivity in the posterior orbit (see Figure 16-6).

The optic nerve is normally displayed best with the probe placed on the globe temporally, although placement of the probe in other areas is sometimes necessary. In some cases, the optic nerve may be better displayed with the probe placed nasally or, less frequently, inferiorly near the fornix. The optimal approach may, in part, depend on how the optic nerve courses in the orbit, which can vary among patients. Moreover, a different probe position may be required if the optic nerve is displaced by an orbital mass (see Figure 13-3). Regardless of the approach used, a similar probe orientation should be employed when comparing with the contralateral optic nerve.

RETROBULBAR OPTIC NERVE DISORDERS

Echography is very useful for the detection and differentiation of disorders that cause enlargement of the optic nerve or its sheaths[12,17] (Table 16-1). The optic nerve pattern may be widened as a result of thickening of the optic nerve parenchyma (e.g., tumor or inflammation), increased subarachnoid fluid (e.g., pseudotumor cerebri, inflammatory or vascular disorders), and thickening of the perineural sheaths (e.g., tumor or inflammation).[4,6,17] In some instances, echography is also useful for differentiating optic nerve enlargement from a separate orbital mass located adjacent to the optic nerve (Figure 16-9).

The differentiation of optic nerve lesions is based primarily on the degree of thickening, internal reflectivity, and structure of the nerve, as well as outcome of the thirty-degree test.[4,17,34] When thickening of the optic nerve is detected, the internal reflectivity and structure are first evaluated. If the A-scan pattern is regular and low reflective and B-scan shows a homogeneous defect, thickening of the optic nerve parenchyma is most likely present (Figure 16-10). Conversely, irregularity of echograms is more indicative of sheath thickening and/or increased subarachnoid fluid. On A-scan examination, irregularity is indicated by the presence of two or more high spikes between the sheath spikes (i.e., sheathing phenomenon).[34] On B-scan, a vertical transverse view can demonstrate a crescent-like configuration of the optic nerve pattern (see Figure 16-10). Furthermore, a longitudinal or, less frequently, an axial approach, may show optic nerve doubling[10] or sheath accentuation.[4-6] These signs, however, are nonspecific since they can be seen in both normal and abnormal optic nerves (Figure 16-11).

Increased Subarachnoid Fluid

Increased subarachnoid fluid, most commonly seen in patients with pseudotumor cerebri, is a frequent cause of a widened optic nerve pattern.[27,42] Other causes include optic neuritis, compressive optic neuropathy, trauma, and uveal effusion syndrome (see p 82).[16] When mild to moderate increased subarachnoid fluid (ISAF) is present, the optic nerve pattern may appear slightly widened and A-scan examination typically displays an irregular structure (see Figure 16-10, *D*). When sheath distention is marked, the subarachnoid space surrounding the optic nerve appears very low reflective on A-scan and as an echolucent crescent or circle around the parenchyma of the nerve on B-scan (i.e., "doughnut sign") (Figure 16-12). To confirm the presence of ISAF, however, the thirty-degree test can be performed with A-scan.

The Thirty-Degree Test

The thirty-degree test, developed by Ossoinig et al,[34] is a dynamic A-scan technique for differentiating ISAF from thickening of the optic nerve parenchyma or the perineural sheaths. The thirty-degree test is based on the assumption that when the eye is turned, the optic nerve and its sheaths are stretched, thus distributing the increased subarachnoid fluid over a greater area.

Once a widened optic nerve pattern has been detected, the maximum thickness of the nerve is documented both anteriorly and posteriorly as the patient fixates in primary gaze. The patient then re-fixates 30 degrees or more toward the probe, and the nerve is measured again (both anteriorly and posteriorly). If increased subarachnoid fluid is present, measurements of the optic nerve pattern will decrease in size as compared with those obtained with the patient in primary gaze (Figure 16-13). If a large volume of fluid is present, the nerve pattern may decrease by as much as 25% to 30%, whereas a reduction of as little as 10% may occur in mild sheath distention. The thirty-degree test is considered positive when the nerve pattern decreases by at least 10% at 30-degree gaze compared with the measurement at primary gaze. When ISAF is present, movement of the eye back and forth may cause the widened optic nerve pattern to decrease temporarily when the patient re-fixates in primary gaze. The examiner should be aware that this can occur and may therefore need to wait a few minutes before repeating measurements in primary gaze. Optic nerves of normal size and nerves that are enlarged as a result of solid infiltration of the nerve parenchyma or its sheaths have a negative thirty-degree test. B-scan can also be used to demonstrate a positive thirty-degree test in

TABLE 16-1

Differential Diagnosis of Optic Nerve Disorders*

Disorder	Reflectivity	Internal Structure	Thirty-degree Test
Increased subarachnoid fluid†	Variable	Irregular	Positive
Glioma	Low-medium	Regular	Negative
Meningioma	Medium-high	Irregular	Negative

*This table summarizes the most typical echographic features of the disorders that most often cause enlargement of the retrobulbar optic nerve.
†Some of the more common conditions associated with increased subarachnoid fluid include benign intracranial hypertension, optic neuritis, compressive optic neuropathy, and trauma.

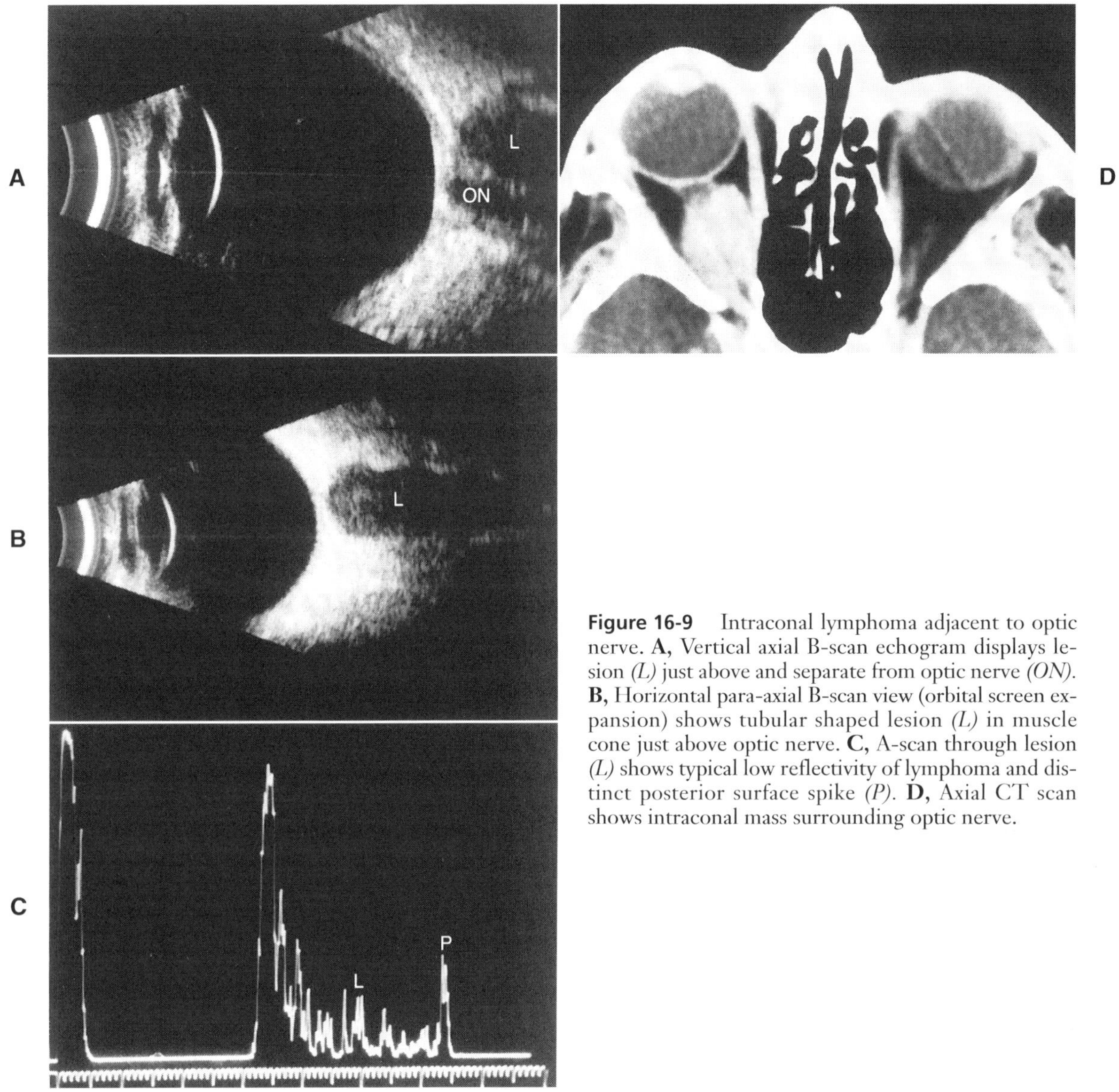

Figure 16-9 Intraconal lymphoma adjacent to optic nerve. **A,** Vertical axial B-scan echogram displays lesion *(L)* just above and separate from optic nerve *(ON).* **B,** Horizontal para-axial B-scan view (orbital screen expansion) shows tubular shaped lesion *(L)* in muscle cone just above optic nerve. **C,** A-scan through lesion *(L)* shows typical low reflectivity of lymphoma and distinct posterior surface spike *(P).* **D,** Axial CT scan shows intraconal mass surrounding optic nerve.

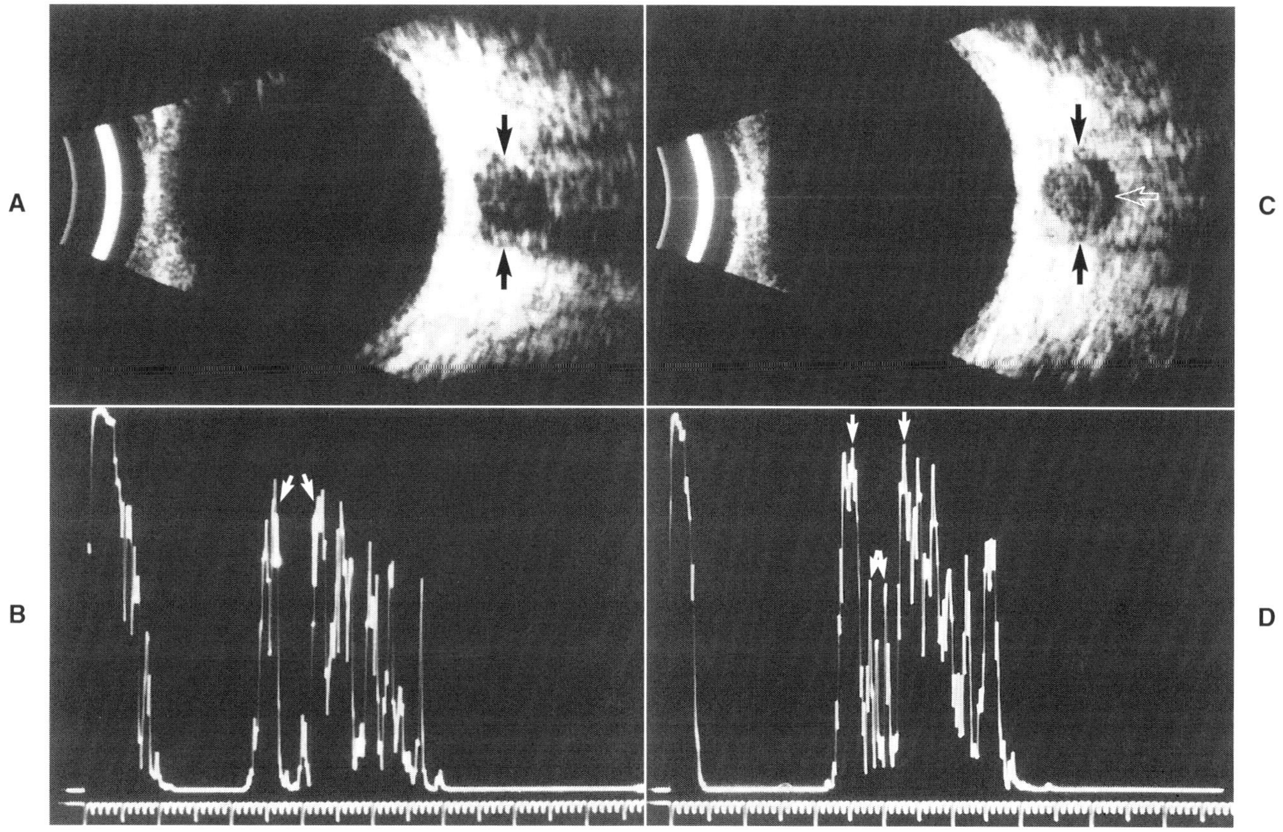

Figure 16-10 Echograms of enlarged optic nerve show regular internal structure in optic neuritis (**A** and **B**) and irregular structure in pseudotumor cerebri (**C** and **D**). **A,** Vertical transverse B-scan shows echolucent optic nerve void *(arrows)*. **B,** A-scan pattern is regular and low reflective. *Arrows,* Perineural sheaths. **C,** Vertical transverse B-scan shows crescent sign due to subarachnoid fluid *(open arrow)* between optic nerve parenchyma *(black arrows)* and perineural sheaths. **D,** A-scan pattern is irregular because of fluid around optic nerve parenchyma *(connected arrows)*. *Vertical arrows,* Perineural sheaths.

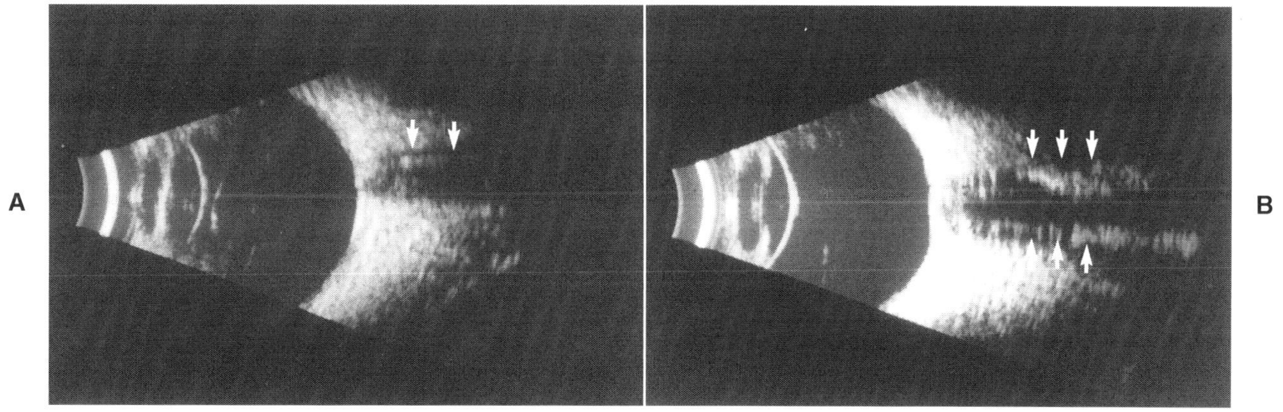

Figure 16-11 Axial B-scan echograms show optic nerve doubling (sheath accentuation). **A,** Normal optic nerve showing mild sheath accentuation *(arrows)*. **B,** Sheath accentuation *(arrows)* is more obvious when nerve is surrounded by increased subarachnoid fluid.

A

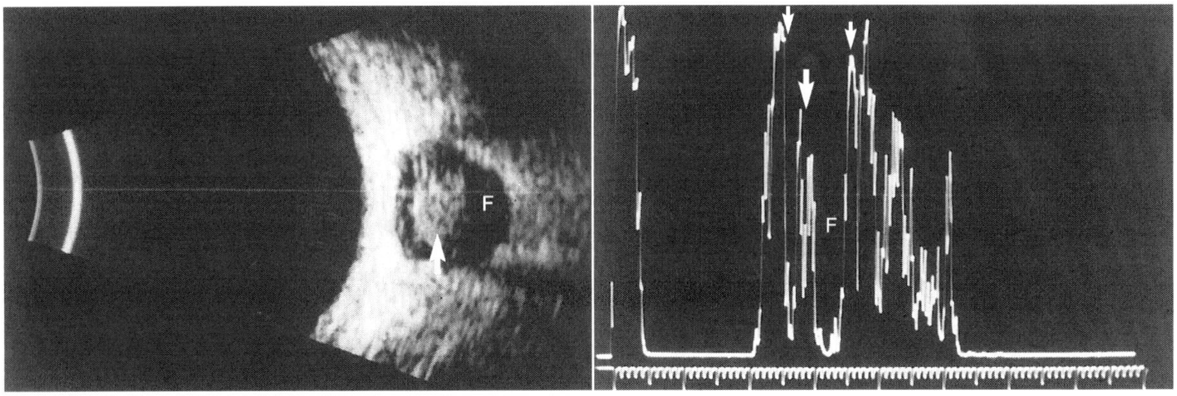

B

Figure 16-12 Marked increased subarachnoid fluid surrounding optic nerve of patient with pseudotumor cerebri. This results in doughnut sign on B-scan and irregular structure on A-scan. **A,** Vertical transverse B-scan shows doughnut sign. Optic nerve parenchyma *(arrow)* is completely surrounded by subarachnoid fluid *(F)*. **B,** A-scan shows marked distention of arachnoid sheaths *(small arrows)* and medium-high reflectivity from surfaces of optic nerve parenchyma *(large arrow)*. *F,* Fluid around optic nerve parenchyma.

A

B

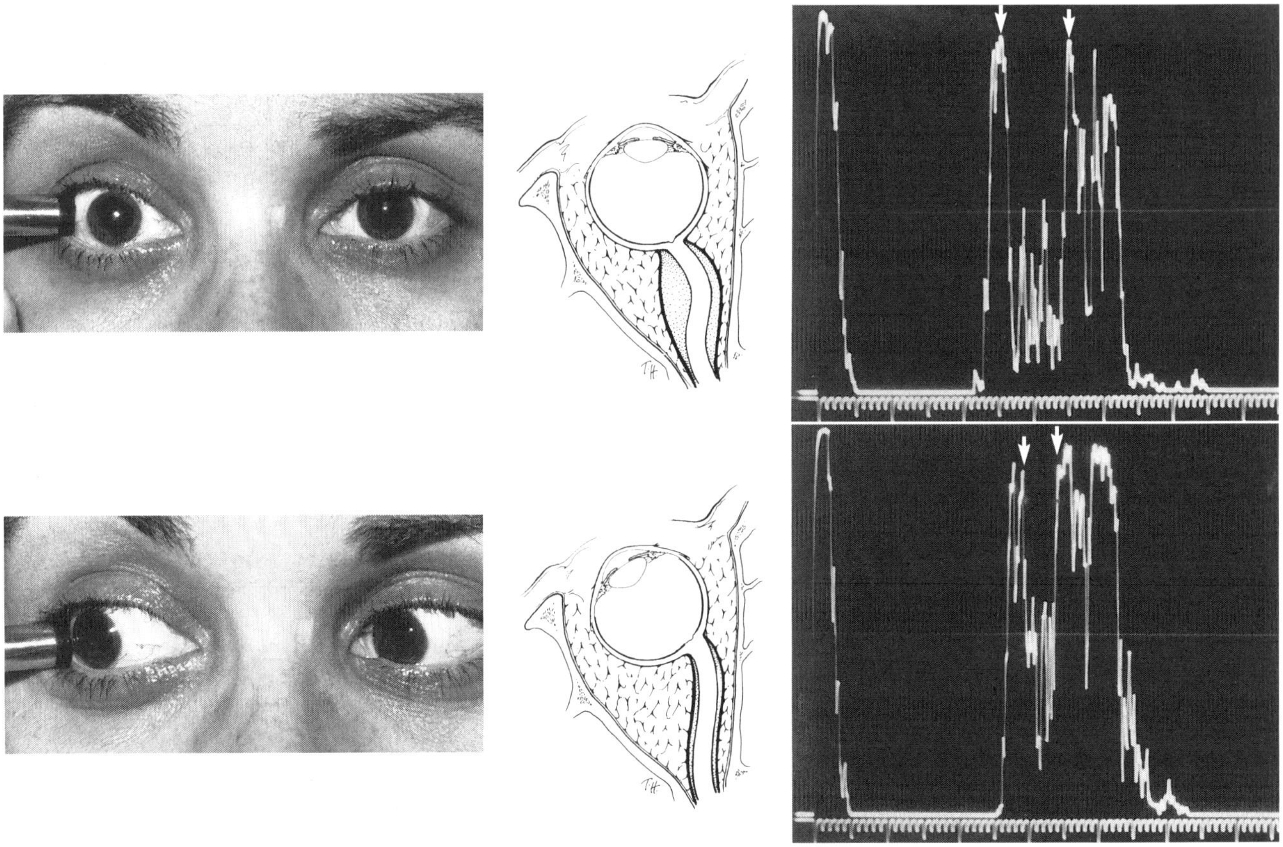

Figure 16-13 Positive thirty-degree test with A-scan. **A,** Patient fixates in primary gaze, which allows maximal fluid accumulation beneath the arachnoid sheath. Top echogram shows corresponding widening of optic nerve pattern between arachnoid sheath spikes *(arrows)*. **B,** Patient's gaze is redirected to at least 30 degrees toward the probe causing subarachnoid fluid to be redistributed over a longer area, thus decreasing effective diameter of the nerve and its echogram.

some cases, but it is not as reliable as is the A-scan (Figure 16-14).

In some cases, an optic nerve tumor that is located posteriorly can be associated with increased fluid around the anterior portion of the nerve. This can result in a positive thirty-degree test anteriorly and a negative test posteriorly. Consequently, it is important that the thirty-degree test routinely be performed both anteriorly and posteriorly.

Optic Nerve Lesions

Lesions involving the optic nerve parenchyma or the perineural sheaths often can be differentiated with echography. When there is solid thickening of the optic nerve pattern of at least twice normal size, a tumor should be suspected.[17,34] In contrast, inflammatory processes of the optic nerve typically produce only mild to moderate enlargement of the nerve pattern. This type of thickening, however, can be difficult to differentiate from smaller tumors involving the nerve or sheaths.

Optic Neuritis

In optic neuritis (either infectious or noninfectious), the optic nerve pattern is enlarged because of swelling of the optic nerve parenchyma, thickening of the perineural sheaths, or most often, ISAF.[21,41] Consequently, internal structure can be regular or irregular, and results of the thirty-degree test can vary from patient to patient. The authors have found that inflammation of the optic nerve and/or its sheaths can be secondary to other conditions such as scleritis, myositis, orbital cellulitis, or an inflammatory mass. In addition, syphilitic optic neuritis has been shown to cause marked enlargement of the optic nerve[28,41] (see Figure 6-26).

Optic Nerve Glioma

An optic nerve glioma often appears as a smooth, fusiform, or ovoid mass that replaces the normal optic nerve void. A-scan shows regular internal structure and low to medium reflectivity (Figure 16-15). In some cases, the nerve can appear very convoluted behind the globe before

A

B

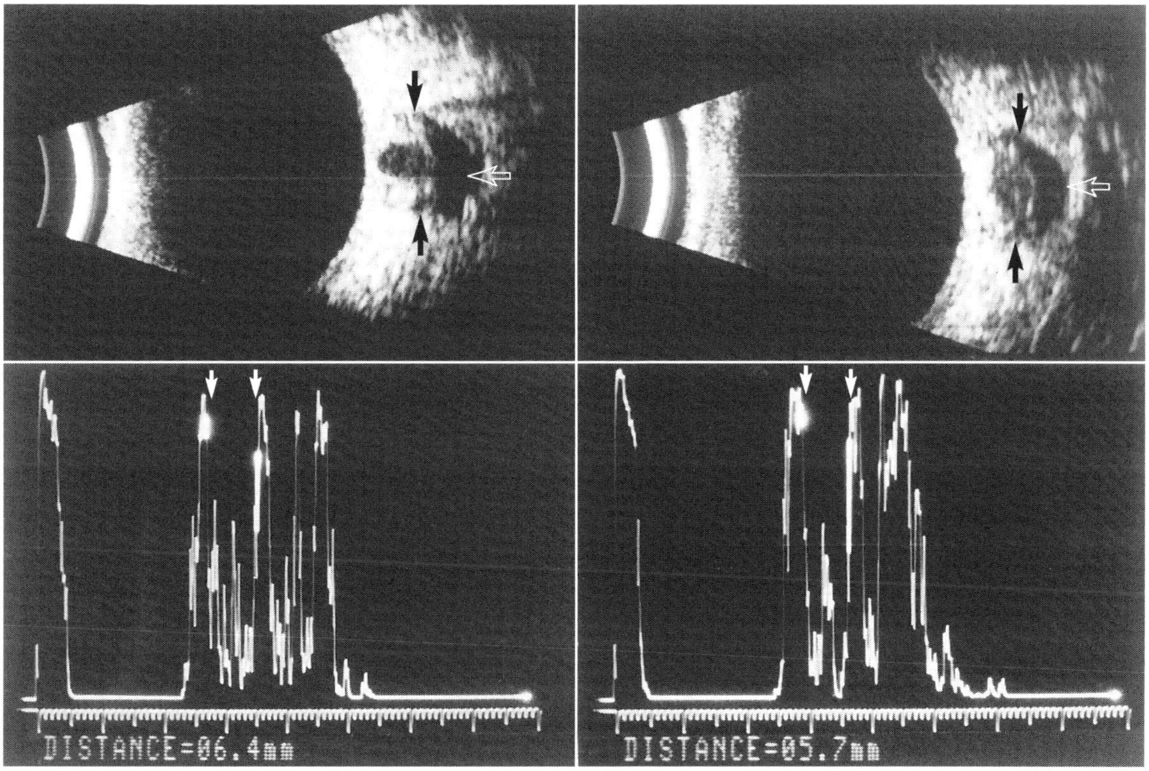

C

D

Figure 16-14 Positive thirty-degree test with B- and A-scan. Echograms with patient fixating in primary gaze (**A** and **B**) and 30 degrees temporally (**C** and **D**). **A,** Vertical transverse B-scan echogram shows widened optic nerve pattern *(closed arrows)* with crescent sign. *Open arrow,* Subarachnoid fluid. **B,** Corresponding A-scan shows widened optic nerve pattern *(arrows)*, measuring 6.4 mm. **C,** Vertical transverse B-scan shows decrease in size of optic nerve pattern and smaller crescent sign, suggesting positive thirty-degree test. **D,** Corresponding A-scan shows decrease in optic nerve pattern (now 5.7 mm), indicating positive thirty-degree test (11% decrease).

expanding into a more smooth, fusiform-shaped mass (Figure 16-16).

The thirty-degree test is usually negative unless ISAF has accumulated around or anterior to the tumor. In long-standing cases, cystic degeneration may result in small echolucent spaces on B-scan and areas of very low reflectivity on A-scan.

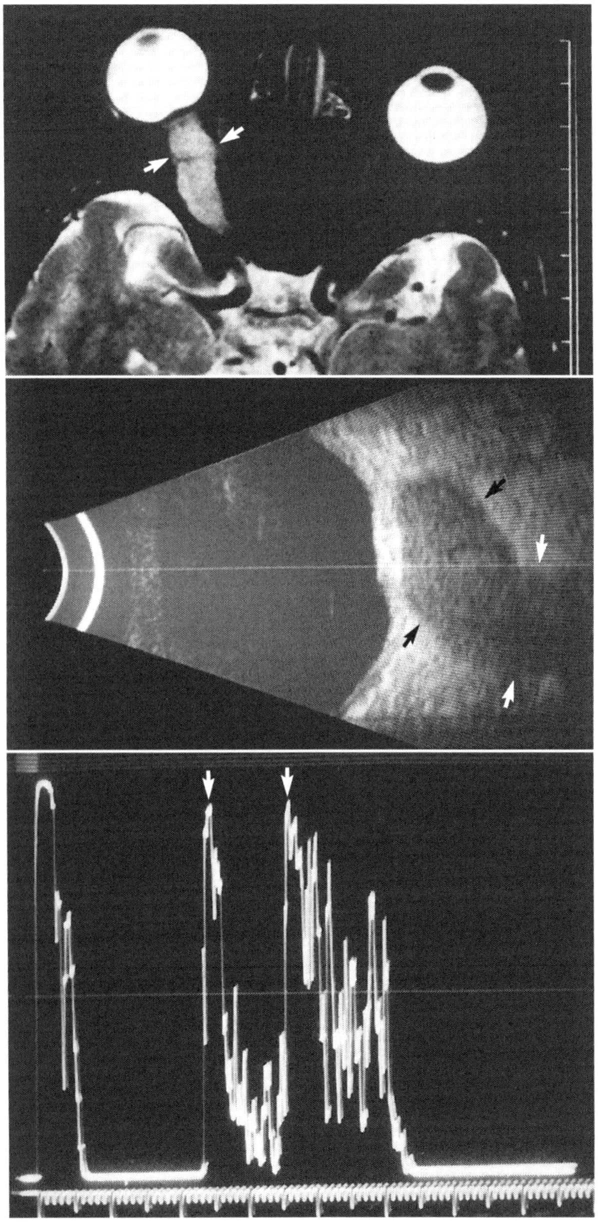

Figure 16-15 Large optic nerve glioma. **A,** Axial MRI scan shows large glioma *(arrows)*. **B,** Para-axial B-scan at medium-high gain setting demonstrates large tumor *(arrows)* replacing normal optic nerve void. **C,** A-scan shows cross-section of thickened optic nerve *(arrows)* with regular internal structure and low to medium reflectivity. (**A** courtesy Dr. Steve Feldon, Rochester, New York.)

Optic Nerve Sheath Meningioma

Optic nerve sheath meningiomas are irregularly structured, with predominantly medium to high reflectivity on A-scan (Figure 16-17). The thirty-degree test is negative in the area of tumor, but it can be positive in cases in which fluid is present anterior to the tumor (Figure 16-18). In contrast to gliomas, large meningiomas tend to appear irregular and nodular on B-scan. Abnormalities within the optic nerve pattern, such as sheath accentuation and/or calcification, also may be apparent[4-6, 8-10] (Figure 16-19). Color Doppler imaging can also be used to evaluate optic nerve sheath meningiomas (see Figure 14-7 and Color Plate 13).

Secondary and Metastatic Tumors

Tumors arising from the globe, such as retinoblastomas and melanomas, can extend into the retrobulbar optic nerve. Such extension, however, has been reported to occur more commonly with retinoblastomas than with melanomas.[37] However, the extension of retinoblastoma can be very difficult to detect echographically because of the calcification that is usually present within these tumors. This is an area where other imaging methods, such as CT scan, can be very useful.

Invasion of the optic nerve also can occur from neoplasms located within the orbit, periorbital sinuses, nasopharynx, and intracranial cavity.[43] Moreover, metastatic processes (e.g., leukemia and carcinoma) can infiltrate the optic nerve or its sheaths.[37,38] All of these conditions can cause thickening of the optic nerve, the perineural sheaths, or ISAF (Figure 16-20). As a result, these various processes can be difficult to differentiate echographically from primary lesions of the optic nerve.

Arachnoid Cyst of the Optic Nerve

Arachnoid cyst is a rare lesion that can affect the retrobulbar optic nerve.[37] B-scan shows a well-outlined, roundish,

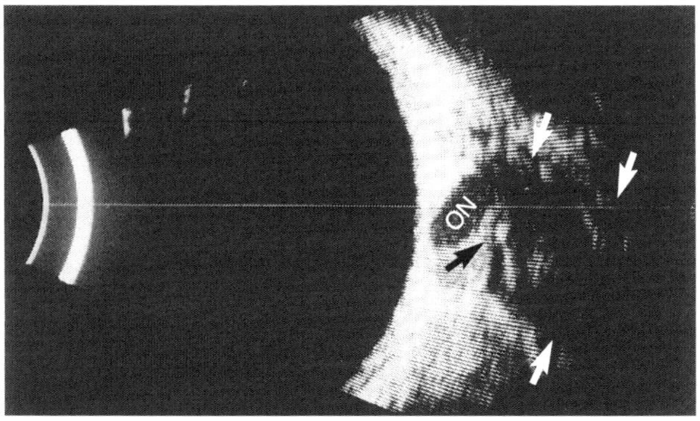

Figure 16-16 Vertical transverse B-scan echogram shows kinked appearance of optic nerve secondary to optic nerve glioma. The anterior portion of the optic nerve *(ON)* angles superiorly and then bends inferiorly as it expands from the glioma *(arrows)*.

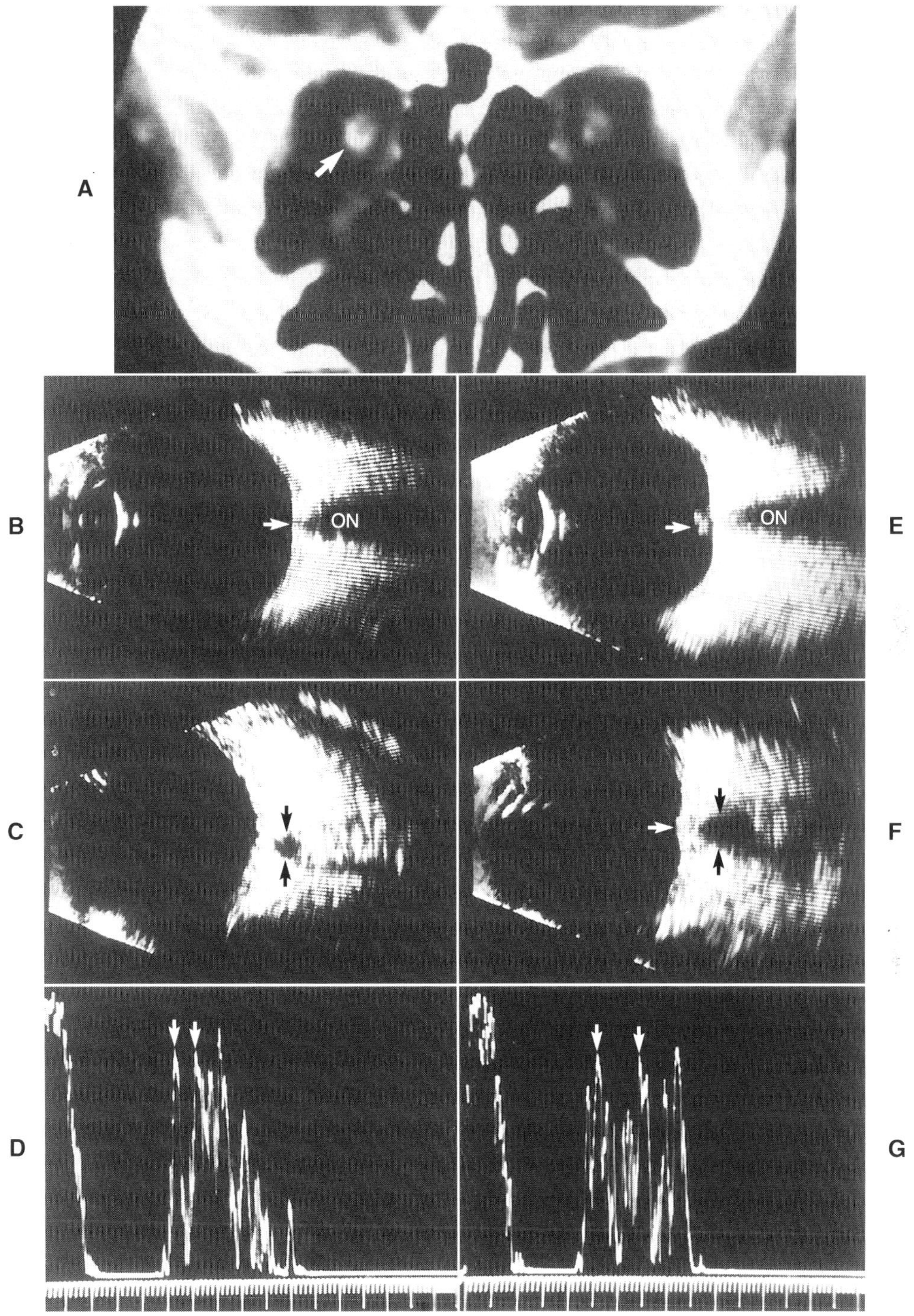

Figure 16-17 Right optic nerve sheath meningioma. **A,** Coronal CT scan shows enlarged right optic nerve *(arrow)*. Echograms are from normal left orbit (**B** to **D**) and meningioma in right orbit (**E** to **G**). **B,** Axial B-scan of normal left optic nerve *(ON)*. *Arrow* shows normal, flat optic disc. **C,** Vertical transverse B-scan shows cross-section of normal optic nerve *(arrows)*. **D,** A-scan cross-section of normal optic nerve. *Arrows,* Perineural sheaths. **E,** Axial B-scan of abnormal right optic nerve shows optic disc elevation *(arrow)* but no obvious abnormality of retrobulbar optic nerve *(ON)*. **F,** Vertical transverse B-scan through anterior aspect of right optic nerve shows enlarged nerve pattern *(black arrows)* and disc elevation *(white arrow)*. **G,** A-scan cross-section of widened right optic nerve echogram shows irregular internal structure that is typical of meningioma. *Arrows,* Perineural sheaths.

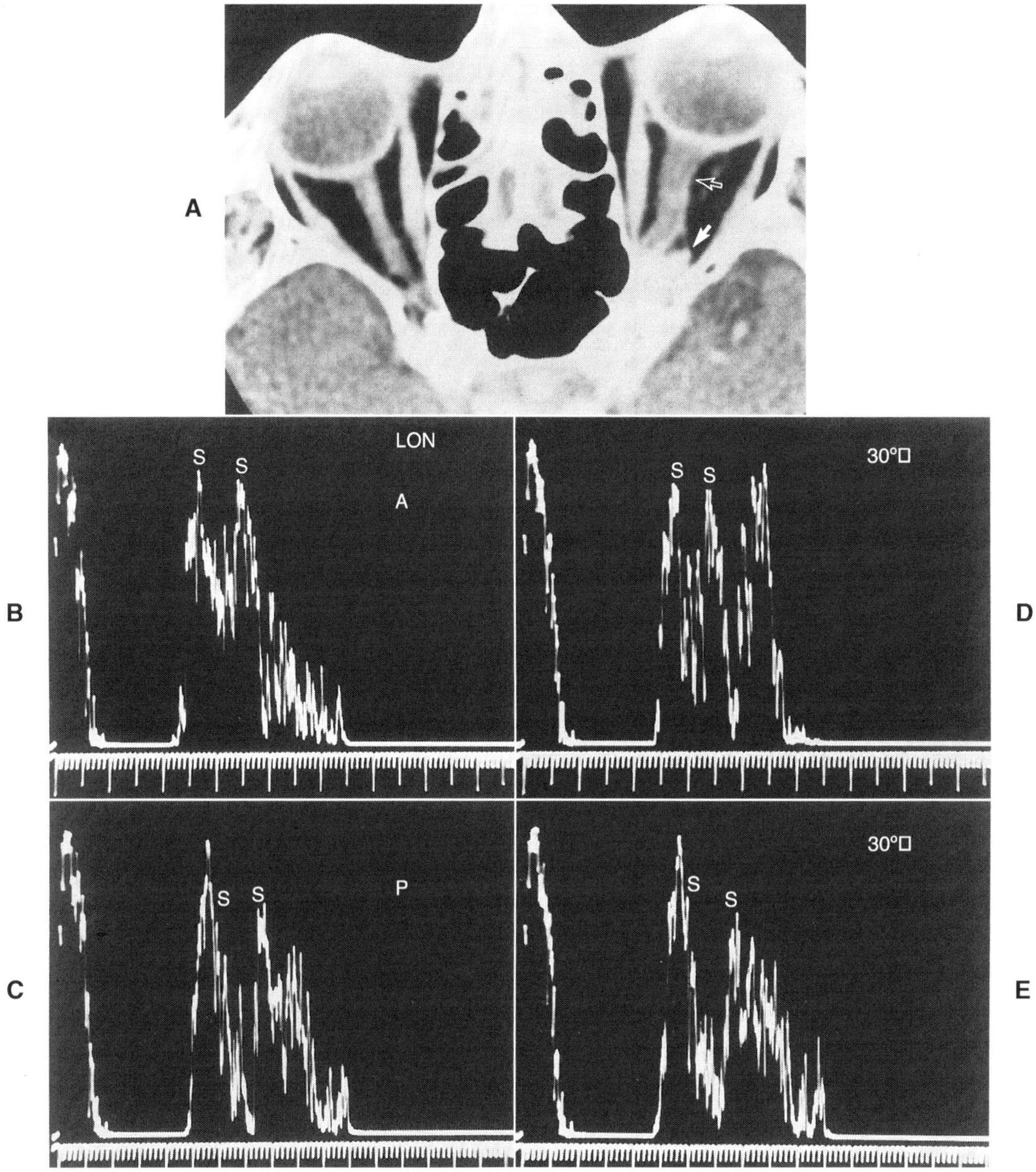

Figure 16-18 Optic nerve sheath meningioma located in orbital apex, with increased subarachnoid fluid anteriorly. **A,** Axial CT scan shows enlarged left optic nerve *(open arrow)* with maximum enlargement posteriorly *(closed arrow)*. A-scans of enlarged optic nerve were taken in primary gaze (**B,** anteriorly and **C,** posteriorly) and at 30 degrees (**D,** anteriorly and **E,** posteriorly). *S,* Peri-neural sheaths. Note that remeasurement of optic nerve at 30 degrees shows narrowing of pattern and thus positive thirty-degree test anteriorly **(D)** but no change and thus negative test posteriorly **(E).** This indicates increased subarachnoid fluid anteriorly but solid nerve posteriorly near orbital apex. (From Byrne SF: Evaluation of the optic nerve with standardized echography, in Smith JL [ed]: *Neuro-ophthalmology Now*! New York, Field, Raicha and Associates, 1986, p 57.)

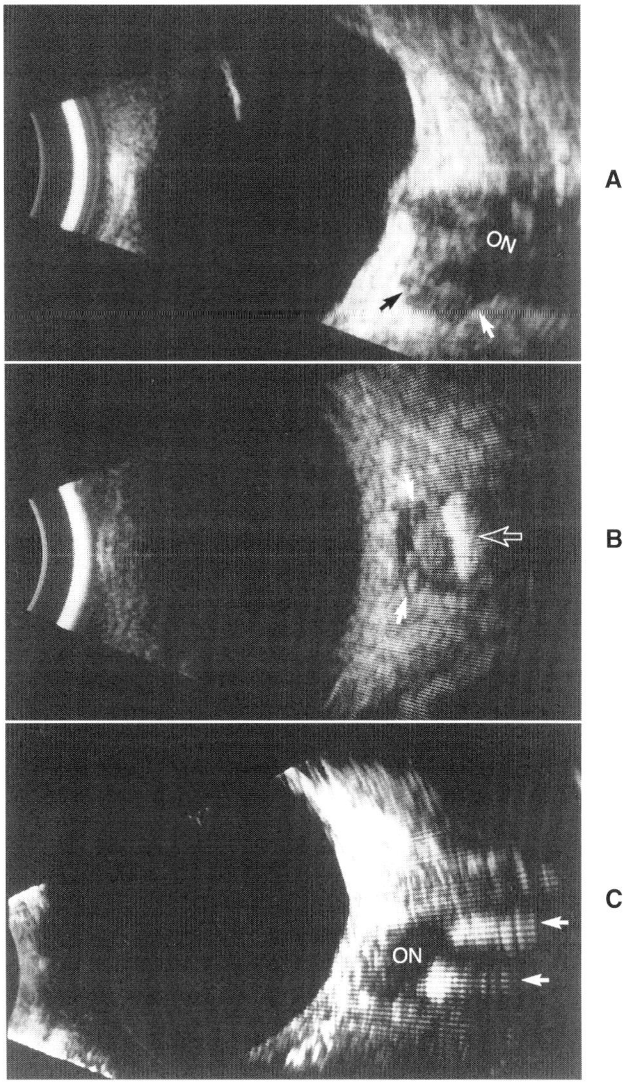

Figure 16-19 Various abnormalities in B-scan echograms of different optic nerve sheath meningiomas. **A,** Longitudinal scan demonstrates nodular enlargement *(arrows)* of optic nerve pattern *(ON)*. **B,** Vertical transverse view of optic nerve *(closed arrows)* shows large focus of calcium *(open arrow)*. **C,** Longitudinal view shows sheath accentuation *(arrows)*. *ON,* Optic nerve.

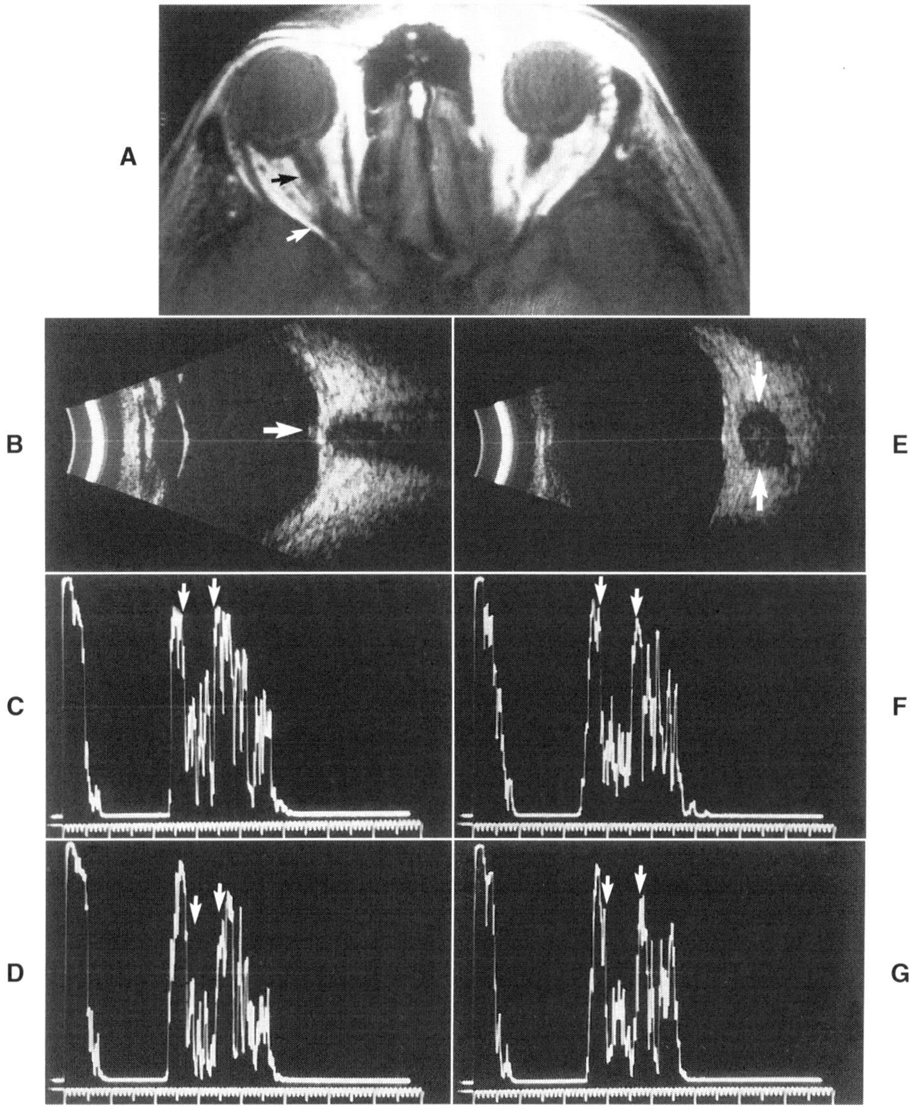

Figure 16-20 Metastatic carcinoma from lung to optic nerve. **A,** Axial MRI scan shows thickened right optic nerve *(arrows)*. **B,** Axial B-scan echogram shows elevation of optic disc *(arrow)*. A-scan echograms in primary gaze (**C** and **D**) and at 30-degree gaze (**F** and **G**) show widened optic nerve *(arrows)*, with negative thirty-degree test. **C,** Optic nerve anteriorly. **D,** Optic nerve posteriorly. **E,** Vertical transverse B-scan at low gain setting shows marked enlargement of the optic nerve *(arrows)*. Thirty-degree test is negative because there is no significant change in size of optic nerve pattern either anteriorly **(F)** or posteriorly **(G).**

echolucent lesion adherent to the optic nerve. In some cases, actual communication with the nerve can be appreciated (Figure 16-21). The lesion is very low reflective on A-scan, and the optic nerve may be enlarged with ISAF.

Compressive Optic Neuropathy

The optic nerve can become secondarily enlarged as the result of compression by a lesion that is located at or near the orbital apex; this can be due to injury, tumor, or inflammation.[36] The most common cause of this condition is thyroid ophthalmopathy, in which very large extraocular muscles can cause apical compression (see p 396).[29,32,33,39] Compression typically results in widening of the optic nerve pattern with increased subarachnoid fluid (Figure 16-22). Other conditions that cause extraocular muscle thickening (e.g., myositis, tumors, and venous congestion) also can produce compression of the optic nerve. Additionally, large orbital tumors within the muscle cone can markedly displace and stretch the optic nerve (see Figure 13-3).

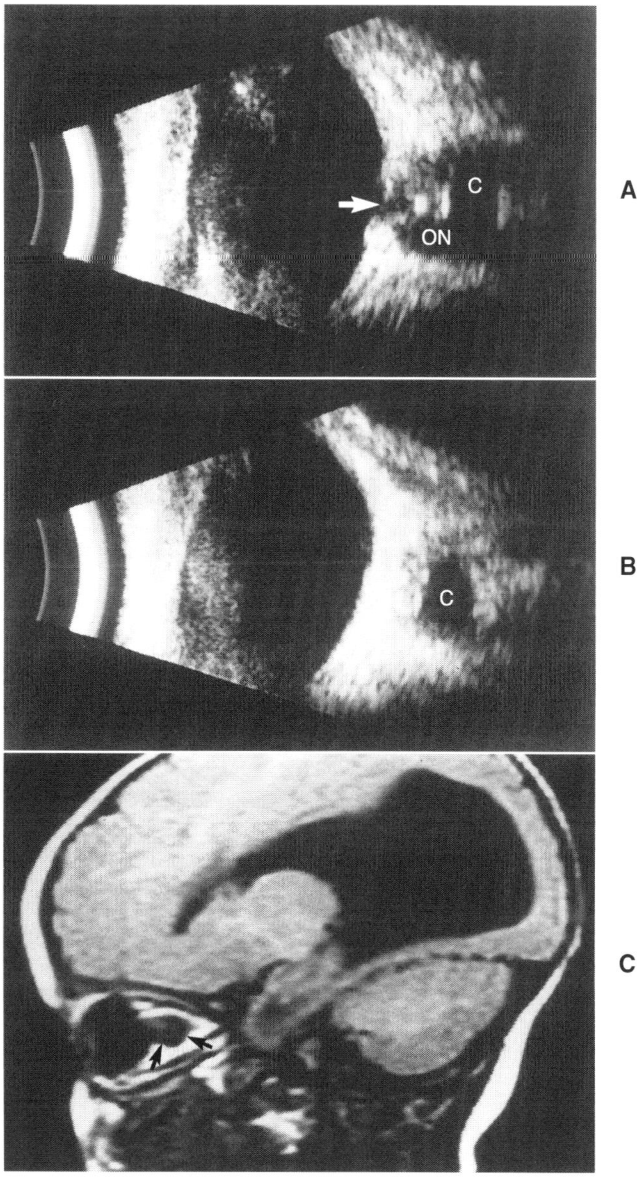

Figure 16-21 Optic disc coloboma and arachnoid cyst associated with Aicardi's syndrome. **A,** Optic disc coloboma *(arrow)*. Cyst *(C)* is shown communicating with optic nerve *(ON)*. **B,** Horizontal transverse scan with sound beam directed just above optic nerve through the cyst *(C)*. The optic nerve was enlarged with a positive thirty-degree test on the A-scan. **C,** Sagittal MRI scan shows enlarged optic nerve *(arrows)*.

Optic Nerve Trauma

Traumatic or spontaneous hemorrhage can occur in the subarachnoid space,[6,43] resulting in an enlarged optic nerve pattern with a positive thirty-degree test. Hemorrhage can be present elsewhere in the orbit, as well as in the globe.

Avulsion of the optic nerve produces various findings. In an acute injury, vitreous hemorrhage can be present and B-scan may show an actual break in the sclera near the optic disc (see Figure 4-10). Additionally, there can be enlargement of the retrobulbar optic nerve with a positive thirty-degree test. In more longstanding cases, there may be proliferative tissue at the optic disc, as well as an unusual appearance of the nerve insertion into the globe[20] (see Figure 4-11).

Vascular Occlusive Disease

The retrobulbar optic nerve is usually not enlarged in central retinal vein or artery occlusion, or in anterior ischemic

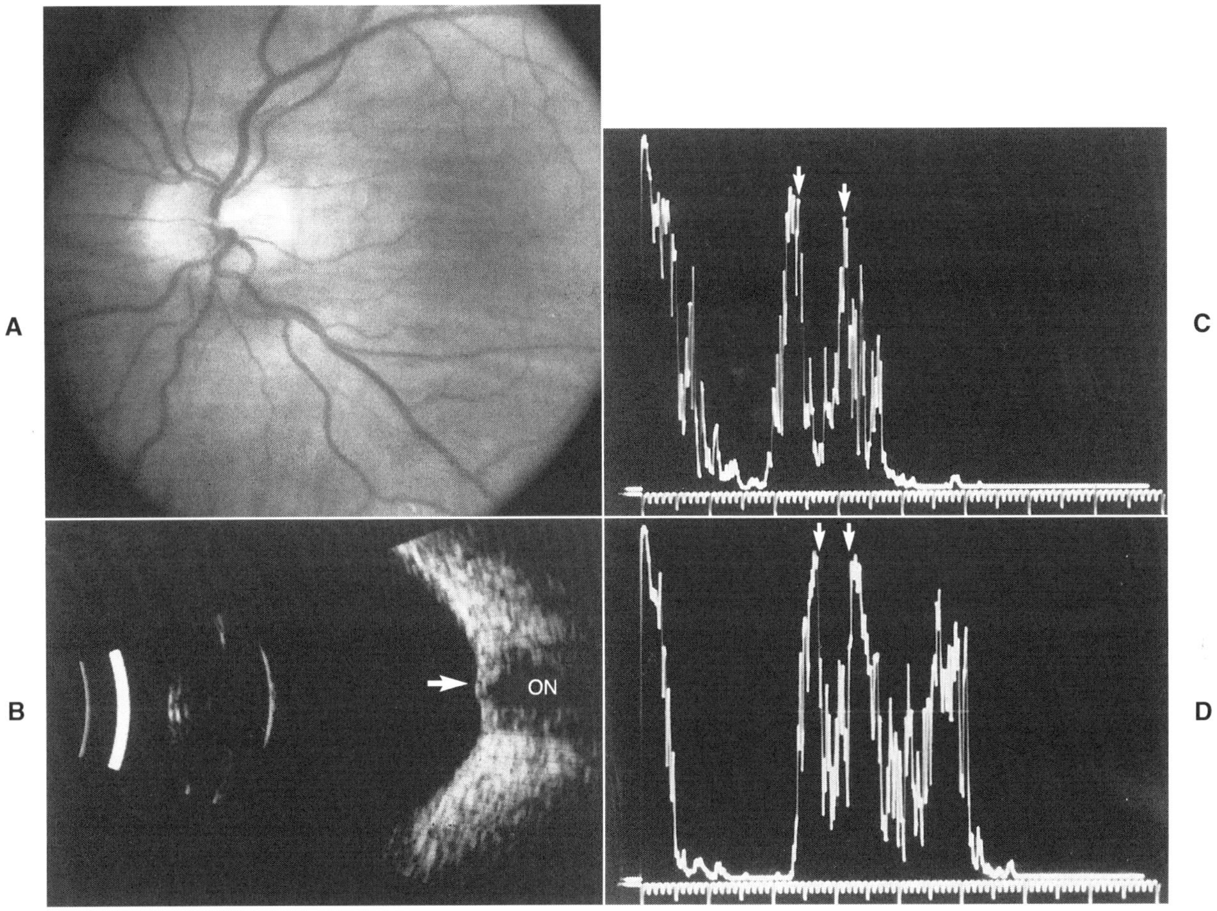

Figure 16-22 Compressive optic neuropathy in patient with advanced thyroid ophthalmopathy (same patient as shown in Figure 15-23). **A,** Fundus photograph of left eye shows blurred disc margins and horizontal choroidal folds. Echograms show optic disc swelling and thickened optic nerve. **B,** Axial B-scan echogram shows optic disc elevation *(arrow)*. *ON,* Optic nerve. **C,** Optic nerve pattern is widened in primary gaze on A-scan *(arrows)*. **D,** Remeasurement at 30 degrees shows marked decrease in diameter of optic nerve pattern, indicating positive thirty-degree test.

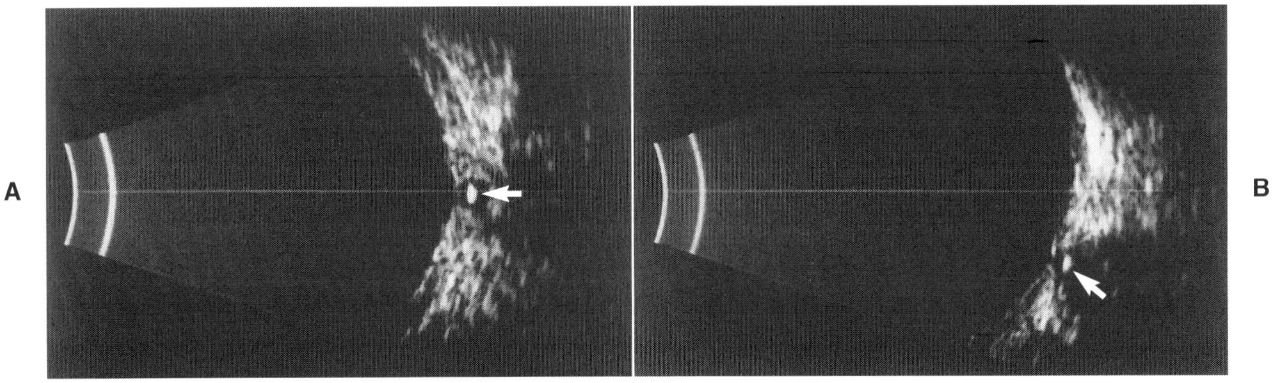

Figure 16-23 Calcification at level of lamina scleralis in eye with previous vascular occlusion. Small, bright nodule *(arrow)* shown in vertical transverse **(A)** and longitudinal **(B)** B-scan echograms.

optic neuropathy. However, both sheath thickening and ISAF have been observed occasionally in anterior ischemic optic neuropathy as well as central retinal artery occlusion.[26] Additionally, a small, calcified nodule may sometimes be observed within the optic nerve of patients with vascular occlusive disease.[3,30] These nodules have been demonstrated in the region of the lamina cribrosa, as well as a few millimeters posteriorly (Figure 16-23).

Optic Atrophy

Echography is indicated in eyes with optic atrophy to detect tumors or inflammatory lesions of the optic nerve or other compressive orbital mass lesions. When optic atrophy is present but no causative lesion is detected, the optic nerve is typically of normal size or smaller than normal; similar findings have been observed in orbits with hypoplasia of the optic nerve. In some cases, when optic atrophy is present, the internal reflectivity can be higher than is typically seen in the normal nerve.[4,5,34]

Postoperative Findings

It may be helpful to re-examine the optic nerve following decompression to determine whether there has been a decrease in ISAF surrounding the nerve. In one case of pseudotumor cerebri, a marked reduction in ISAF was documented echographically immediately following spinal tap[15] (Figure 16-24). In addition, re-examination following optic nerve sheath decompression frequently shows a decrease in ISAF that sometimes is also seen in the unoperated fellow nerve.[27] Another occasional finding on B-scan is a track of fluid located near the site of surgical incision. The fluid may develop into a lesion with a cystic appearance[23] (Figure 16-25).

OPTIC DISC

B-scan can be used to demonstrate excavation, elevation, and drusen of the optic disc (Box 16-1).[7,25] The axial, longitudinal, and vertical transverse approaches can be useful

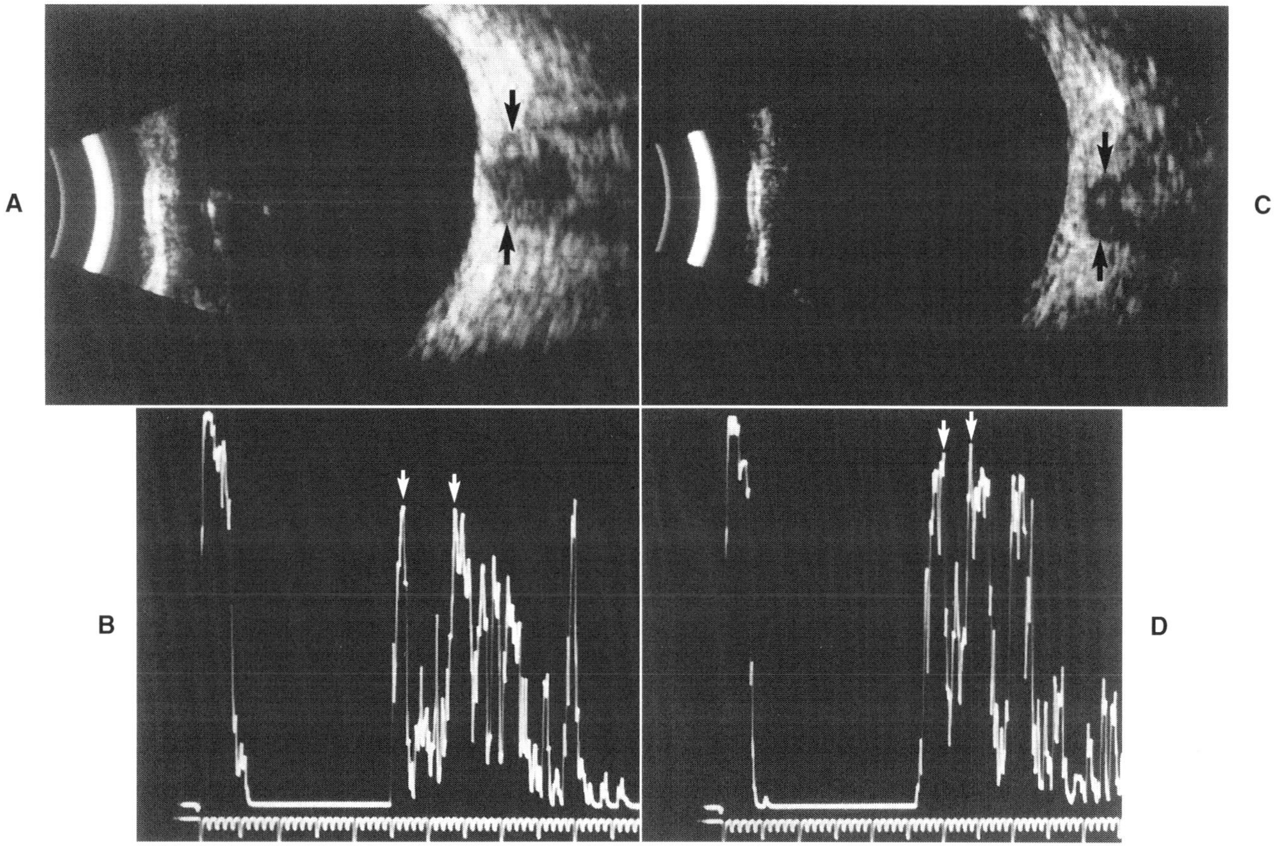

Figure 16-24 Echograms from patient with pseudotumor cerebri taken just before (**A** and **B**) and immediately following (**C** and **D**) lumbar puncture. **A,** Vertical transverse B-scan shows enlarged optic nerve pattern *(arrows)*. **B,** A-scan cross-section of optic nerve prior to procedure measures 4.9 mm. **C,** Vertical transverse B-scan after procedure shows decreased optic nerve pattern. **D,** A-scan cross-section of optic nerve following lumbar puncture measures 2.6 mm. (From Galetta S, Byrne SF, Smith JL: Echographic correlation of optic nerve sheath size and cerebrospinal fluid pressure. *J Clin Neuro-Ophthalmol* 1989;9:79.)

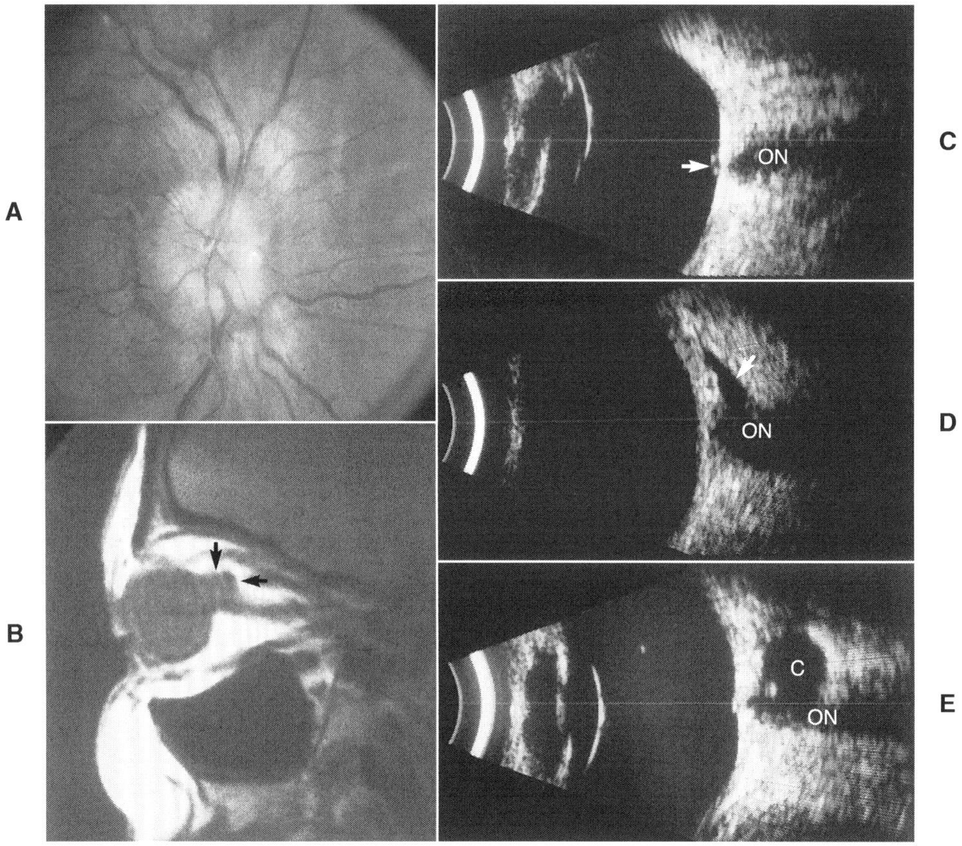

Figure 16-25 Pseudotumor cerebri with echograms taken before and after optic nerve sheath fenestration. **A,** Fundus photograph showing papilledema and choroidal folds. **B,** Sagittal MRI scan shows lesion in area of optic nerve near globe *(arrows)*. **C,** Preoperative axial B-scan shows optic disc elevation due to papilledema *(arrow)*. *ON*, Optic nerve. **D,** Vertical para-axial B-scan 10 days following fenestration shows echolucent fluid track *(arrow)* emanating from area of incision. **E,** Vertical axial B-scan 2 months after fenestration shows lesion with cystic appearance *(C)* in area where fluid track was previously seen.

for evaluating the optic disc (Figure 16-26). A-scan sometimes can be of additional use in assessing the reflectivity and height of certain lesions at the optic disc (e.g., drusen and tumors, see Figure 5-53).

Optic Disc Excavation

The optic cup is best displayed with a vertical transverse B-scan view, although a longitudinal scan performed along the 12-o'clock meridian sometimes helps to confirm cup size. Large, deep cups (glaucomatous or physiologic) are easily imaged with these views. A large cup may or may not be imaged in an axial view (see Figure 7-1).

Small to medium-sized cups can also be demonstrated, but detection is less reliable than with larger cups.[11] Large, shallow cups also can be difficult to detect. Whenever possible, comparison should be made with the fellow optic nerve. Such comparison is especially helpful when size of the cup in the other eye is known so it can be used as a reference.

Colobomas involving or adjacent to the optic disc are easily imaged with B-scan. These can be small and shallow (see Figure 16-21), or they can be large and deep, such as those associated with the morning glory syndrome[22,40,43] (Figure 16-27). Occasionally, a coloboma is associated with a cystic appearance of the retrobulbar optic nerve (Figure 16-28).

Optic pits are excavations of the optic nerve head and are probably a form of coloboma.[44] They appear as small circular or triangular depressions, usually located in the inferotemporal quadrant of the disc. They tend to be unilateral and are often associated with serous retinal detachments, often involving the macula. B-scan shows a distinct excavation at the optic nerve head (Figure 16-29).

Pseudocupping of the optic disc can be seen in eyes with marked, diffuse thickening of the retina and/or choroid surrounding the optic disc. In such cases, B-scan shows a cavity or depression overlying the optic nerve head that can simulate a large optic cup (see Figure 6-18). However, by comparing the thickness of the peripapillary retinochoroid

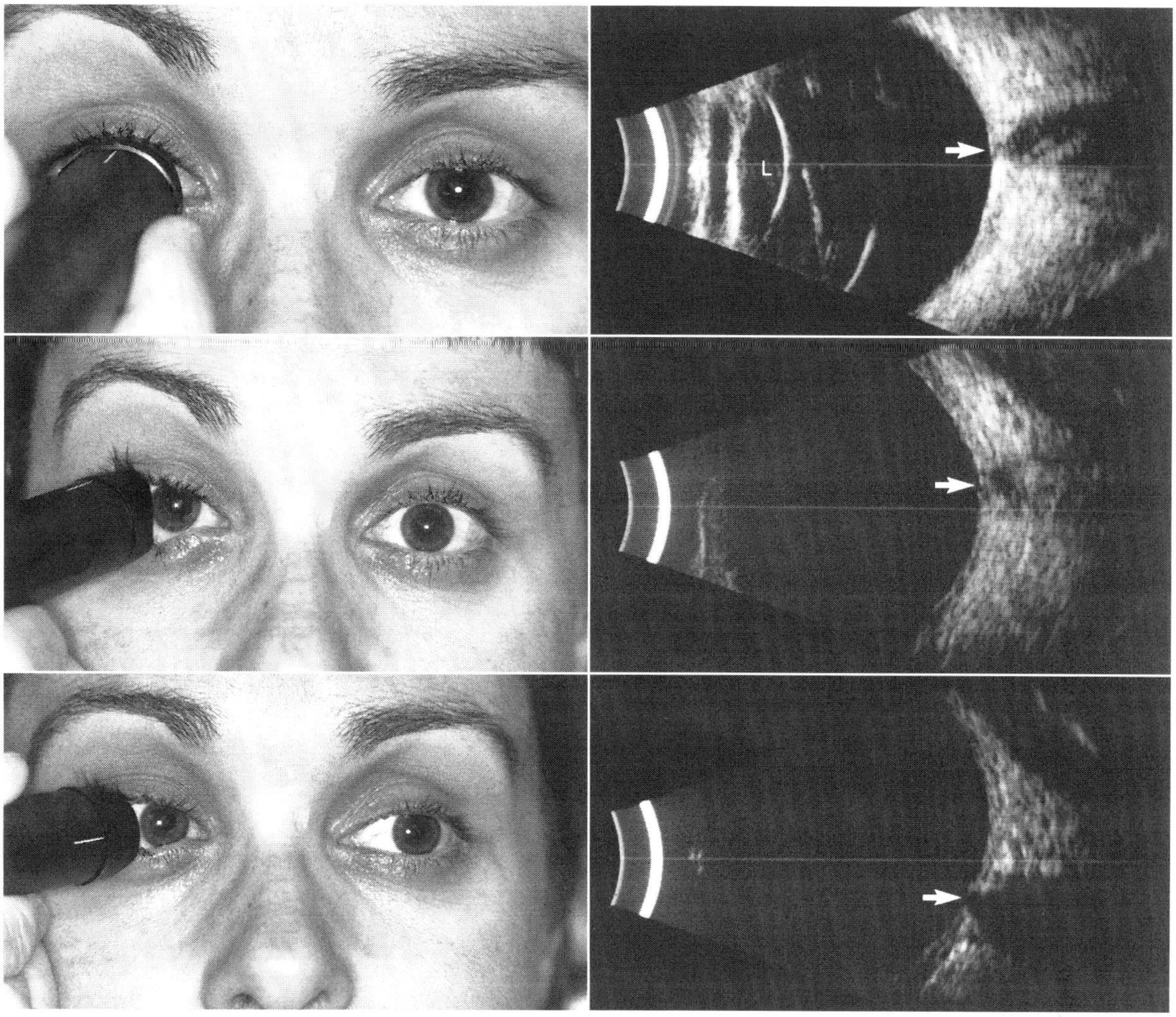

Figure 16-26 B-scan probe positions and corresponding echograms of normal optic disc. **A,** Vertical axial approach. The probe is centered on the cornea (marker up). A medium-high gain setting is used, and the sound beam is directed through the lens *(L)* toward the center of the optic nerve. Note flat appearance of normal optic disc *(arrow)*. **B,** Vertical transverse approach. The probe is positioned temporally (marker up). A medium gain setting is used, and the optic nerve is displayed in the center of the echogram *(arrow)*. **C,** Longitudinal approach (marker to cornea). A low-medium gain setting is used, and the optic disc is displayed at lower edge of echogram.

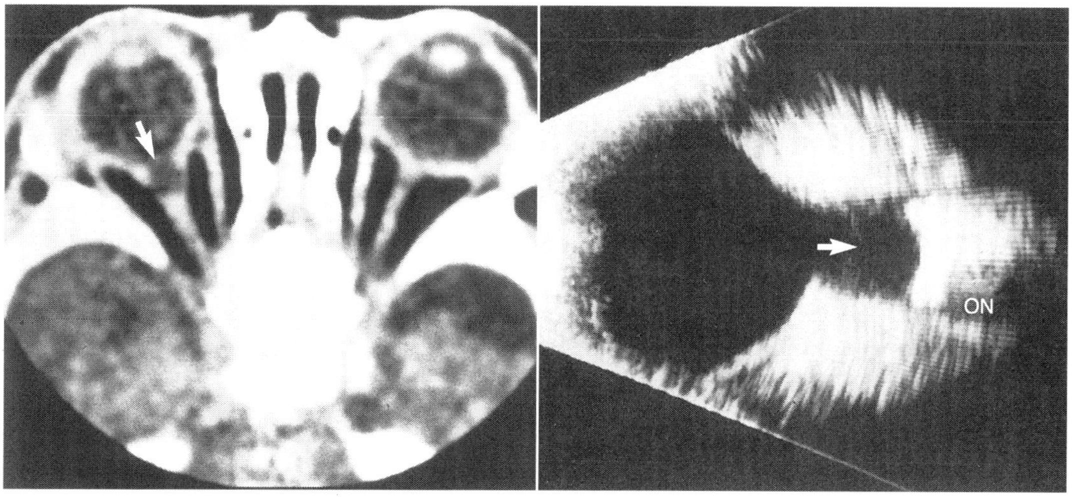

Figure 16-27 Large optic disc coloboma. Coloboma *(arrow)* is shown on axial CT scan **(A)** and B-scan **(B).** *ON,* Optic nerve. (From Byrne SF: Evaluation of the optic nerve with standardized echography, in Smith JL [ed]: *Neuro-ophthalmology Now*! New York, Field, Raicha and Associates, 1986, p 63.)

A

B

C

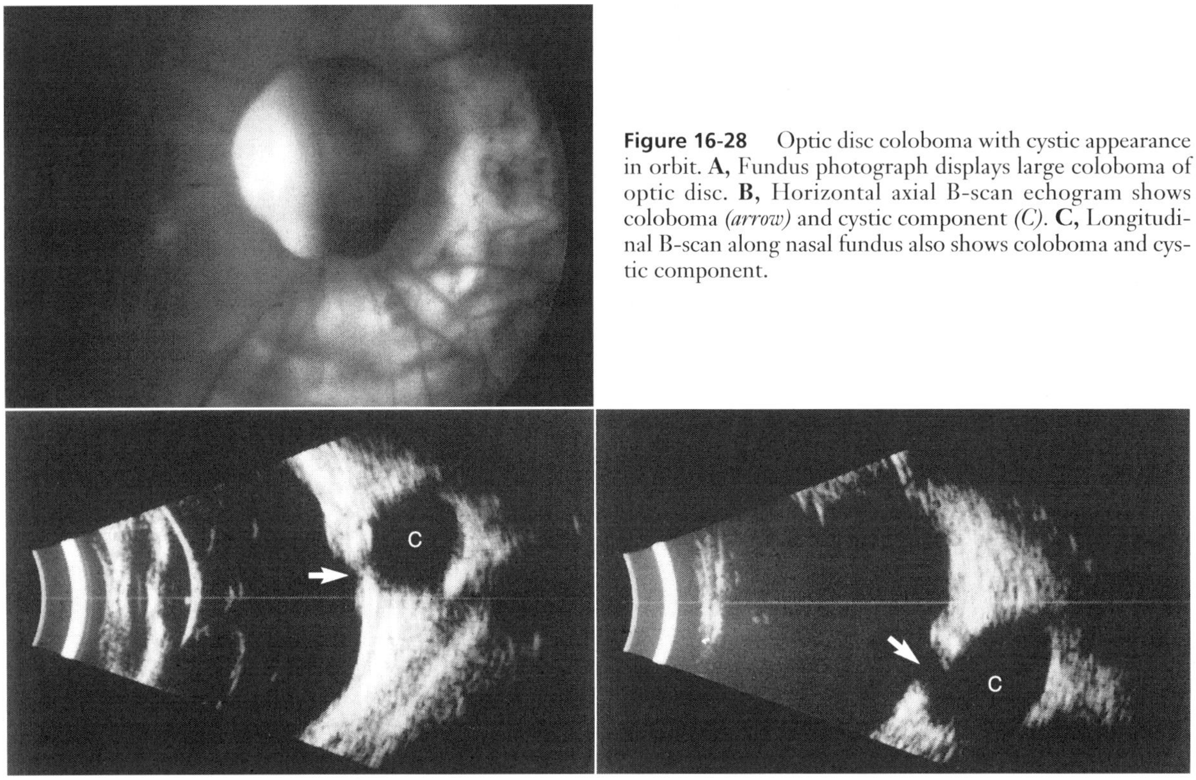

Figure 16-28 Optic disc coloboma with cystic appearance in orbit. **A,** Fundus photograph displays large coloboma of optic disc. **B,** Horizontal axial B-scan echogram shows coloboma *(arrow)* and cystic component *(C)*. **C,** Longitudinal B-scan along nasal fundus also shows coloboma and cystic component.

layer with other areas of the fundus and/or the fellow eye, differentiation from true optic cupping can usually be made.

Optic Disc Elevation

Elevation of the optic disc (e.g., edema, papilledema and tumor) can be easily shown with B-scan. Elevation usually can be detected with any of the three B-scan positions, but the axial approach is often best for documentation (Figure 16-30).

Optic Disc Drusen

Optic disc drusen can simulate papilledema clinically, or they can be buried and unappreciable with ophthalmoscopy.[3,19] These calcified nodules can be easily identified echographically, because they produce an echo of extremely high reflectivity at or within the optic nerve head[3,31] (Figure 16-31). Drusen can be large or small and are most often bilateral, although they may be asymmetric in size. Transverse and longitudinal B-scan approaches, which bypass the lens, often demonstrate the highly reflective calcified nodule more clearly than the axial approach (Figure 16-32).

Crowded Optic Disc (Pseudopapilledema)

Congenital anomalies of the optic disc can create an elevation of the optic nerve head and the appearance of pseudopapilledema (crowded optic disc) (see Figure 3-70, *A*). This appears to be due to narrow scleral canals through which the optic nerve enters the globe. It has been shown that the crowded disc appearance is associated with smaller hyperopic eyes, as well as some eyes of average length.[14,16] It is postulated that these anomalous optic discs are implicated in the pathogenesis of ischemic optic neuropathy.[2,13] B-scan examination of these eyes demonstrates that the posterior sclera is thickened and that the scleral optic nerve canals are elongated (see Figure 3-70, *B* and *C*). It should be noted, however, that it is usually very difficult to image the scleral optic nerve canals in eyes with normal posterior scleral thickness.

A

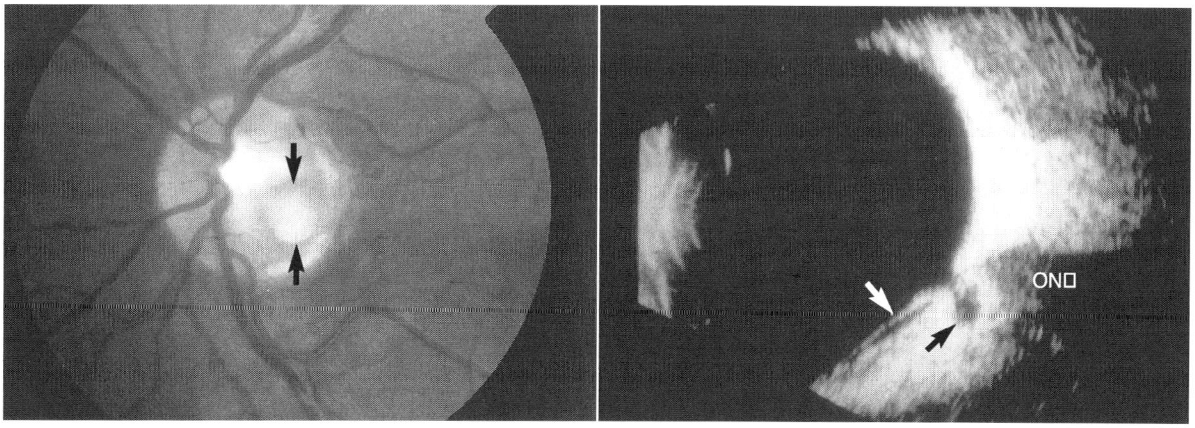

B

Figure 16-29 Optic nerve pit. **A,** Fundus photograph shows well-circumscribed pit in inferotemporal aspect of optic disc *(black arrows)*. **B,** Reverse longitudinal B-scan (see p 32) shows well-outlined, deep excavation corresponding to optic pit *(black arrow)*. Note shallow macular retinal detachment *(white arrow)* extending from edge of optic pit. *ON,* Optic nerve. (Courtesy Dr. Brian Leonard and Diane Chialant, COT, RDMS, Ottawa, Canada.)

A

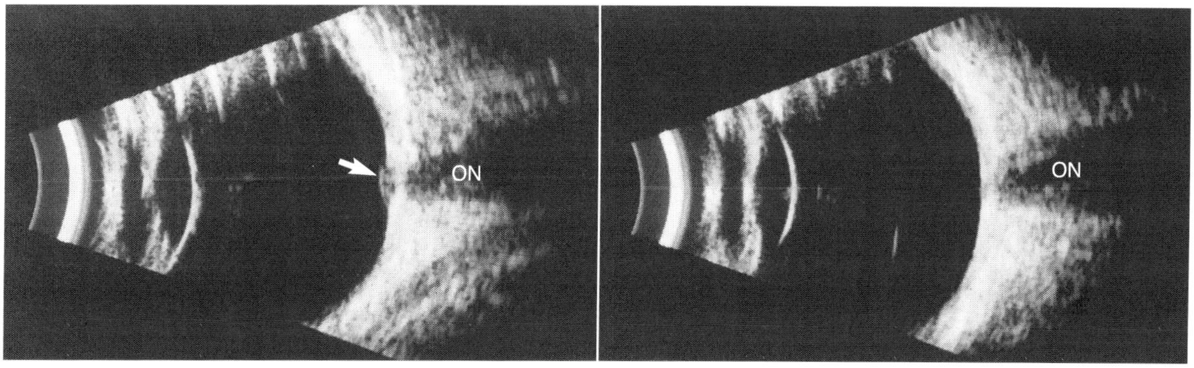

B

Figure 16-30 Axial B-scan echograms show elevated and normal optic discs. **A,** Elevated optic disc *(arrow)*. *ON,* Optic nerve. **B,** Normal flat optic disc.

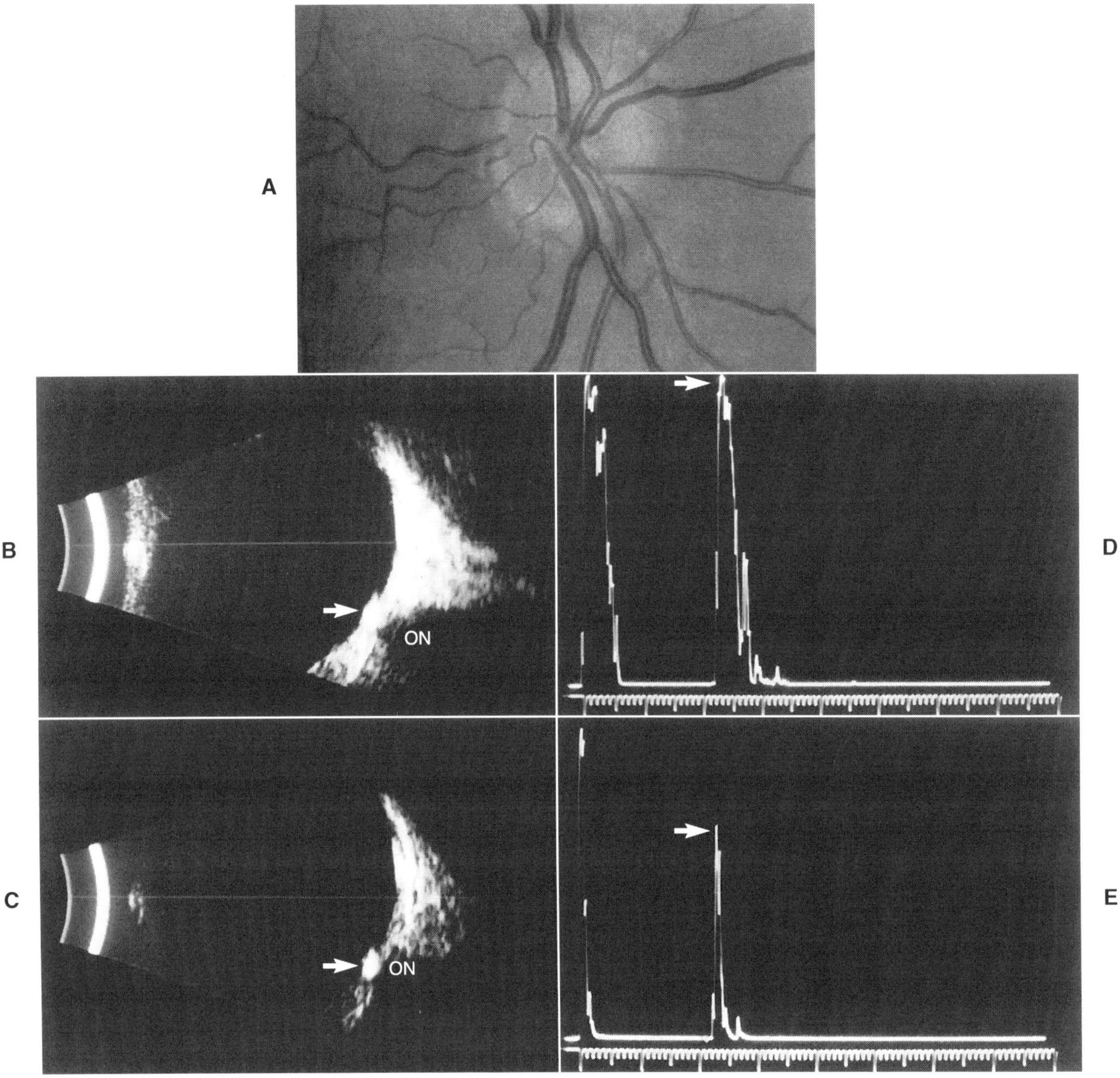

Figure 16-31 Large optic disc drusen. **A,** Fundus photograph shows elevated optic disc with small cup and no evidence of dilated vessels. Longitudinal B-scans (**B** and **C**) and A-scans (**D** and **E**) show calcified drusen *(arrows)*. **B,** B-scan at high gain setting shows elevation of optic disc. *ON,* Optic nerve. **C,** B-scan at lower gain setting shows drusen better than does **B. D,** A-scan at Tissue Sensitivity shows extremely high reflective spike from drusen. **E,** A-scan at reduced gain setting shows persistence of spike.

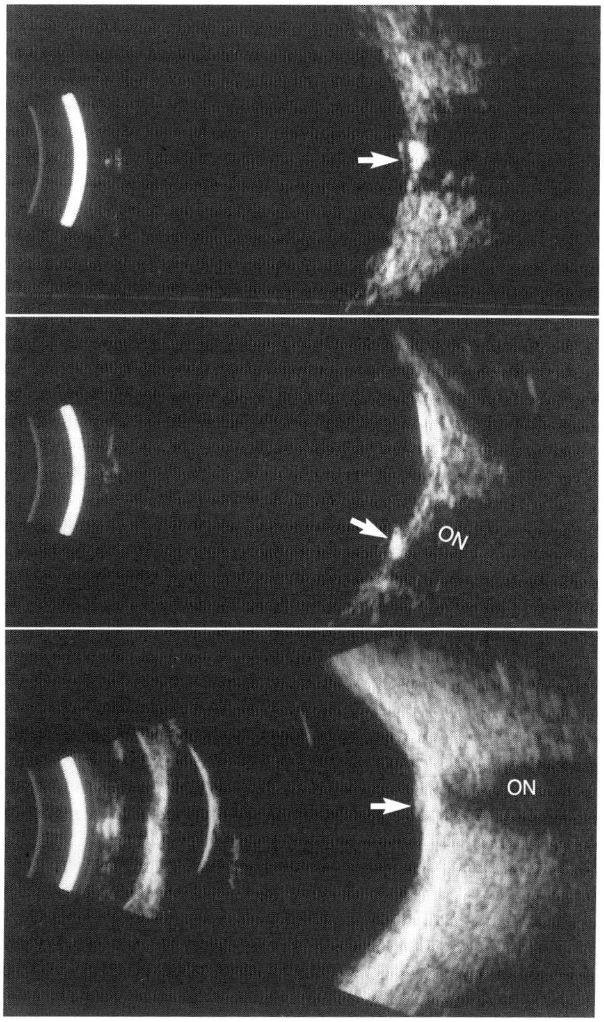

Figure 16-32 Optic disc drusen. Calcified drusen *(arrows)* is shown in vertical transverse **(A)** and longitudinal **(B)** B-scan views at low gain setting. *ON*, Optic nerve. **C,** Drusen is less apparent in axial B-scan echogram.

REFERENCES

1. Atta HR: Imaging of the optic nerve with standardised echography. *Eye* 1988;2:358.
2. Beck RW, Savino PJ, Repka MX, et al: Optic disc structure in anterior ischemic optic neuropathy. *Ophthalmology* 1944;91(2):1337.
3. Boldt HC, Byrne SF, DiBernardo CL: Echographic evaluation of optic disc drusen. *J Clin Neuro-Ophthalmol* 1991;11:85.
4. Byrne SF: Evaluation of the optic nerve with standardized echography, in Smith JL (ed): *Neuro-ophthalmology Now!* New York, Field, Raicha and Associates, 1986, p 45.
5. Byrne SF: The echographic measurement and differential diagnosis of optic nerve lesions (review), in Ossoinig KC (ed): *Ophthalmic Echography.* Dordrecht, Dr W Junk, 1987, p 571.
6. Byrne SF, Glaser JS: Orbital tissue differentiation with standardized echography. *Ophthalmology* 1983;90:1071.
7. Cohen JS, Stone RD, Hetherington J Jr: Glaucomatous cupping of the optic disk by ultrasonography. *Am J Ophthalmol* 1976;82:24.
8. Coleman DJ, Carroll FD: Evaluation of optic neuropathy with B-scan ultrasonography. *Am J Ophthalmol* 1972;74:915.
9. Coleman DJ, Jack RL, Franzen LA: High resolution B-scan ultrasonography of the orbit: Neurogenic tumors of the orbit. *Arch Ophthalmol* 1972;88:380.
10. Coleman DJ, Lizzi FL, Jack RL: *Ultrasonography of the Eye and Orbit.* Philadelphia, Lea & Febiger, 1977, p 331.
11. Darnley-Fisch DA, Byrne SF, Hughes JR, et al: Contact B-scan echography in the assessment of optic nerve cupping. *Am J Ophthalmol* 1990;109:59.
12. Dutton JJ, Byrne SF, Proia AD: *Diagnostic Atlas of Orbital Diseases.* Philadelphia, WB Saunders, 2000.
13. Feit RH, Tomsak RL, Ellenberger C Jr: Structural factors in the pathogenesis of ischemic optic neuropathy. *Am J Ophthalmol* 1984;98:105.
14. Feldon SE, Sadun AA, DuBois LG, et al: Echographic features pre- and post-optic nerve sheath fenestration for progressive aion. *Invest Ophthalmol Vis Sci* 1991;32(4):951.
15. Galetta S, Byrne SF, Smith JL: Echographic correlation of optic nerve sheath size and cerebrospinal fluid pressure. *J Clin Neuro Ophthalmol* 1989;9:79.
16. Gass JDM: *Stereoscopic Atlas of Macular Diseases*, ed 4, vol 2. St. Louis, Mosby, 1997, p 916.
17. Gans MS, Byrne SF, Glaser JS: Standardized A-scan echography in optic nerve disease. *Arch Ophthalmol* 1987;105:1232.
18. Glaser JS: Orbital diseases and neuro-ophthalmology: An overview, in Glaser JS (ed): *Neuro-ophthalmology*, ed 2, Philadelphia, JB Lippincott, 1990, p 454.

19. Glaser JS: Topical diagnosis: Prechiasmal visual pathways, in Glaser JS (ed): *Neuro-ophthalmology*, ed 2, Philadelphia, JB Lippincott, 1990, p 83.
20. Green RL, Byrne SF: Diagnostic ophthalmic ultrasound, in Ryan SJ (ed): *Retina*. St Louis, Mosby, 1989, p 191.
21. Haag JR, Smith JL, Susac JO, et al: Optic atrophy following jejunoileal bypass. *J Clin Neuro-Ophthalmol* 1985;5:14.
22. Haik BG, Greenstein SH, Smith ME, et al: Retinal detachment in the morning glory anomaly. *Ophthalmology* 1984;91:1638.
23. Hamed LM, Byrne SF, Tse D: Neuro-imaging of the optic nerve following fenestration for pseudotumor cerebri. *Ophthalmology* 1989; 96(Sept suppl):97.
24. Hasenfratz G: Experimental studies on the display of the optic nerve, in Ossoinig KC (ed): *Ophthalmic Echography*. Dordrecht, Dr W Junk, 1987, p 590.
25. Hodes BL: Ultrasonographic demonstration of glaucomatous optic nerve excavation. *J Clin Ultrasound* 1975;3:255.
26. Hupp SL, Buckley EG, Byrne SF, et al: Post traumatic venous obstructive retinopathy associated with enlarged optic nerve sheath. *Arch Ophthalmol* 1984;102:254.
27. Hupp SL, Glaser JS, Byrne SF: Optic nerve sheath decompression: Review of 17 cases. *Arch Ophthalmol* 1987;105:3867.
28. Kronish JW, Johnson TE, Gilberg SN, et al: Orbital infections in patients with human immunodeficiency virus infection. *Ophthalmology* 1996;103:1483.
29. Neigel JM, Rootman J, Belkin RI, et al: Dysthyroid optic neuropathy. The crowded orbital apex syndrome. *Ophthalmology* 1988; 95:1515.
30. Nobe JR, Cano MR, Borchert M, et al: Congested papillopathy: Echographic and radiologic evidence of calcified phleboliths. *Ophthalmology* 1987;94(Oct suppl):138.
31. Noel LP, Clarke WN, MacInnis BJ: Detection of drusen of the optic disc in children by B-scan ultrasonography. *Can J Ophthalmol* 1983;18:266.
32. Ossoinig KC: Early detection of compressive optic neuropathy in Graves' disease with standardized A-scan, in Ossoinig KC (ed): *Ophthalmic Echography*. Dordrecht, Dr W Junk, 1987, p 568.
33. Ossoinig KC: The role of standardized ophthalmic echography in the management of Graves' ophthalmopathy, in Pickardt CR, Boergen KP (eds): *Graves' Ophthalmopathy: Developments in Diagnostic Methods and Therapeutic Procedures*. Basel, Karger, 1989, p 28.
34. Ossoinig KC, Cennamo G, Byrne SF: Echographic differential diagnosis of optic nerve lesions, in Thijssen JM, Verbeek AM (eds): *Ultrasonography in Ophthalmology*. Dordrecht, Dr W Junk, 1981, p 327.
35. Ossoinig KC, Kaefring SL, McNutt LC, et al: Echographic measurement of the optic nerve (summary), in White D, Brown RE (eds): *Ultrasound in Medicine*. New York, Plenum Press, 1977;3A:1065.
36. Rootman J, Neigel J: Structural lesions—trauma, in Rootman J: *Diseases of the Orbit*. Philadelphia, JB Lippincott, 1988, p 510.
37. Rootman J, Robertson WD: Tumors—neurogenic tumors, in Rootman J: *Diseases of the Orbit*. Philadelphia, JB Lippincott, 1986, p 281.
38. Siatkowski RM, Byron LL, Schatz, et al: Optic neuropathy in Hodgkin's disease. *Am J Ophthalmol* 1992;114:625.
39. Skalka HW: Perineural optic nerve changes in endocrine orbitopathy. *Arch Ophthalmol* 1978;96:468.
40. Slamovits TL, Kimball GP, Friberg TR, et al: Bilateral optic disc colobomas with orbital cysts and hypoplastic optic nerves and chiasm. *J Clin Neuro Ophthalmol* 1989;9:172.
41. Smith JL, Byrne SF, Cambron CR: Syphiloma/gumma of the optic nerve and human immunodeficiency virus seropositivity. *J Clin Neuro-Ophthalmol* 1990;10:175.
42. Smith JL, Tse DT, Byrne SF, et al: Optic nerve sheath distention in Leber's optic neuropathy and the significance of the "Wallace mutation." *J Clin Neuro Ophthalmol* 1990;10:231.
43. Spencer WH: Optic nerve, in Spencer WH: *Ophthalmic Pathology: An Atlas and Textbook*, ed 3, Philadelphia, WB Saunders, 1986, p 2337.
44. Yanoff M, Fine BS: *Ocular Pathology*, ed 4, London, Mosby-Wolfe, 1996, p 464.

17

William D. Bates

Orbital Trauma and Periorbital Disease

Orbital echography can be useful for evaluating the orbit following trauma and for detection of abnormalities secondary to periorbital disorders.

TRAUMA

Blunt or penetrating injury to the eye or lids can result in a variety of orbital abnormalities and lesions[27] (Box 17-1). The orbital fat can become edematous or infiltrated by hemorrhage or pus; the optic nerve and extraocular muscles can become thickened from inflammation or hemorrhage, or they can be avulsed or transected; foreign bodies can lodge in any aspect of the orbit or within an adjacent sinus cavity. Severe trauma can result in a fracture of the orbital bone. In addition, air (e.g., emphysema) can enter the orbital tissue from an adjacent sinus cavity as the result of a fracture. Although examination of the traumatized patient may be quite difficult as a result of lid swelling and pain, in most cases, useful information can be obtained with ultrasound.

Orbital Cellulitis

Cellulitis may result in diffuse swelling of all orbital structures. In this condition, echograms of the orbital fat are widened but reflectivity remains predominantly high (Figure 17-1). If, on follow-up examination there is a progressive decrease of reflectivity in certain areas, abscess formation should be suspected.[8]

Orbital Hematomas/Abscesses

Echography can be used to detect and localize hemorrhage or abscess that is present within the orbital cavity. These low to medium reflective lesions can appear multiloculated (Figure 17-2) or as a solitary mass[13] (Figure 17-3). Compressibility may be difficult to evaluate in these patients due to pain and lid swelling.

Blood and pus may be difficult to distinguish from one another by ultrasound. Blood, however, has a tendency to layer more than pus (see p 309 and Figure 11-32). In some cases, this subtle difference may be helpful in attempting to differentiate between the two. In other situations, follow-up examination may be the only way of distinguishing between these two conditions. Over time, hematomas usually decrease in size, whereas abscesses tend to enlarge. In certain instances, needle aspiration may be necessary for diagnosis. Ultrasound can be helpful to guide the insertion of the needle into the abscess cavity[31,32] (Figure 17-4).

Hemorrhage or abscess can occur in the subperiosteal space following trauma to the orbit or periorbital sinuses.[27] Additionally, subperiosteal abscess may develop secondary to sinus infection[29,33] (Figure 17-5). These lesions are well outlined, located adjacent to the orbital wall, and are sharply demarcated from the orbital soft tissue by the smooth, highly reflective periosteum.[15,33] On B-scan, these lesions have a tapered (fusiform) appearance when examined in longitudinal orientation. This fusiform shape results in the display of a weakly reflective posterior border spike on A-scan. Reflectivity of the subperiosteal fluid is typically very low and the internal structure is regular (Figure 17-6). When compression testing is possible, these lesions are quite firm. Subperiosteal hematomas may persist for weeks or months (Figure 17-7).

Orbital Foreign Bodies

Echography can be used to evaluate foreign bodies within the orbit.[9,21,22,30] The echographic appearance of foreign

Text continued on p 446

BOX 17-1

Orbital Trauma

Orbital cellulitis
Orbital hematomas/abscesses
Orbital foreign bodies
Emphysema
Orbital fractures
Extraocular muscle trauma
Optic nerve trauma

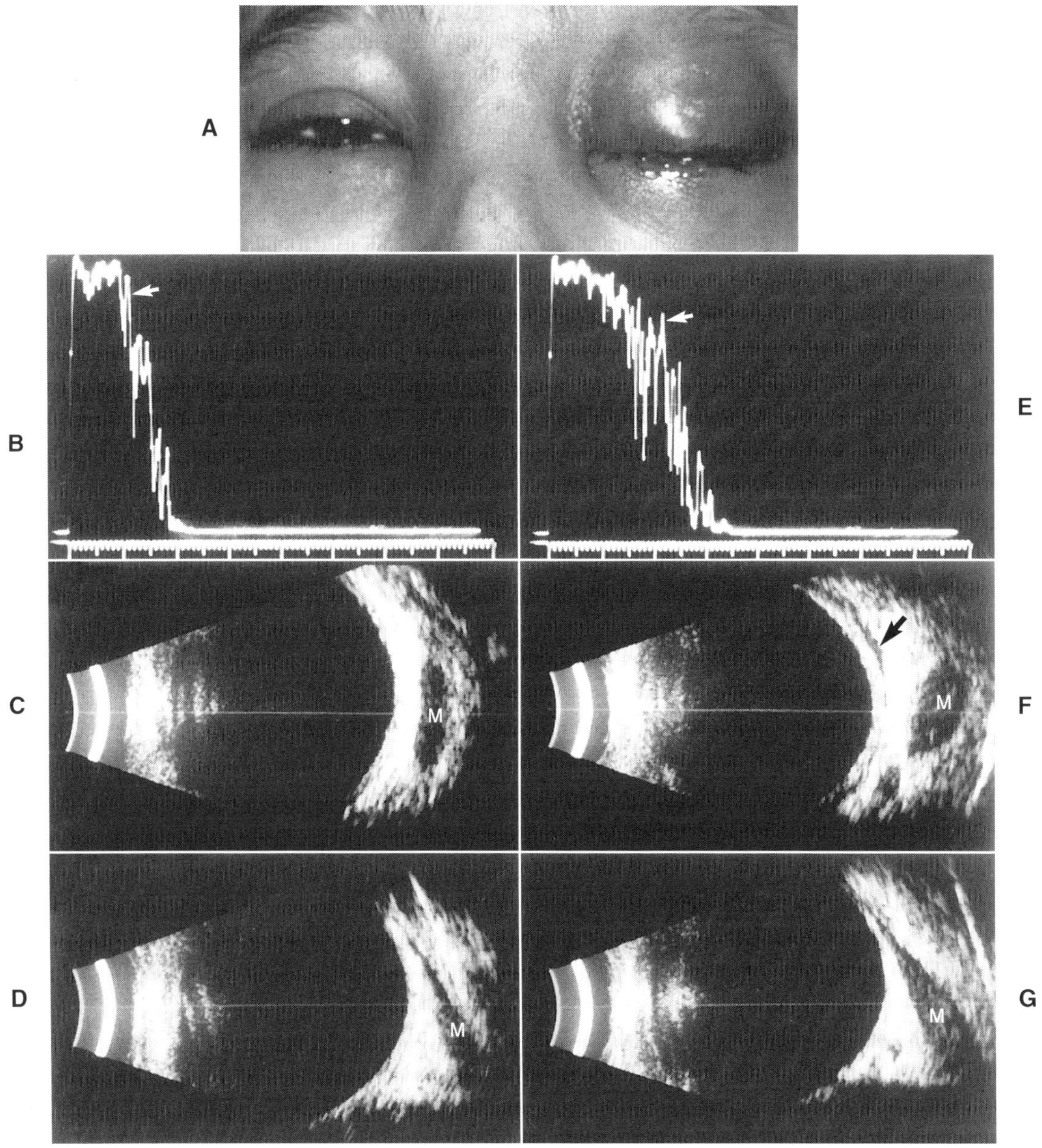

Figure 17-1 Orbital cellulitis. **A,** External photograph shows marked lid swelling and proptosis of left eye. Echograms are of normal right orbit (**B** to **D**) and abnormal left orbit (**E** to **G**). Diffuse swelling of orbital structures was detected in the left orbit. **B,** Normal paraocular A-scan pattern *(arrow)*. **C,** Vertical transverse B-scan echogram of nasal orbit shows normal orbit and medial rectus muscle *(M)* in cross-section. **D,** longitudinal B-scan view of nasal orbit shows normal orbit and medial rectus muscle *(M)* in long section. **E,** Widened paraocular A-scan pattern from cellulitis *(arrow)*. **F,** Vertical transverse B-scan view of nasal orbit shows widened orbital soft tissue, thickened medial rectus muscle *(M)*, and fluid in sub-Tenon's space *(arrow)*. **G,** Longitudinal B-scan echogram of nasal orbit shows widened orbital soft tissue and medial rectus muscle *(M)* in long section.

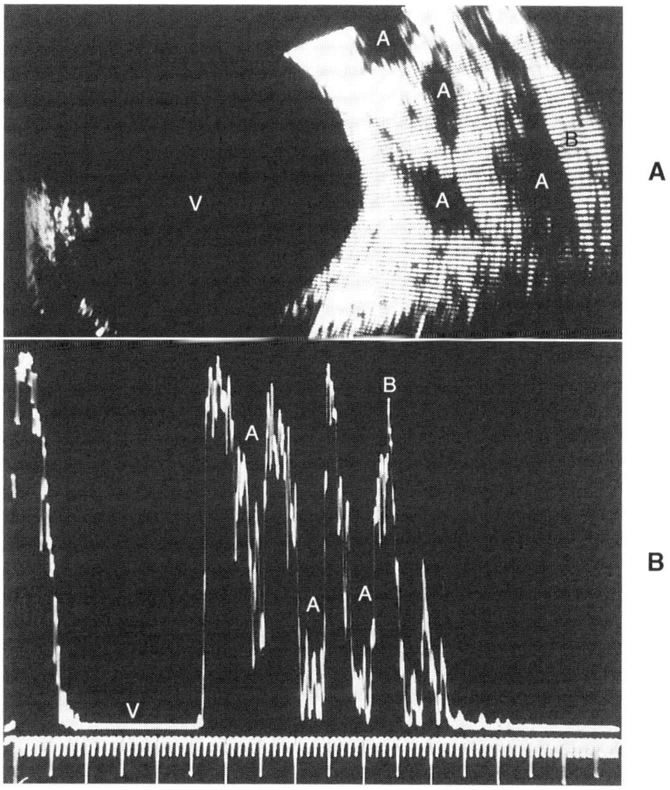

Figure 17-2 Loculated orbital abscess. **A,** Transocular B-scan echogram shows multifocal pockets of abscess *(A)* in orbital cavity. *V,* Vitreous cavity. **B,** Transocular A-scan shows multiple low to medium reflective abscess cavities *(A)*. *B,* Bone.

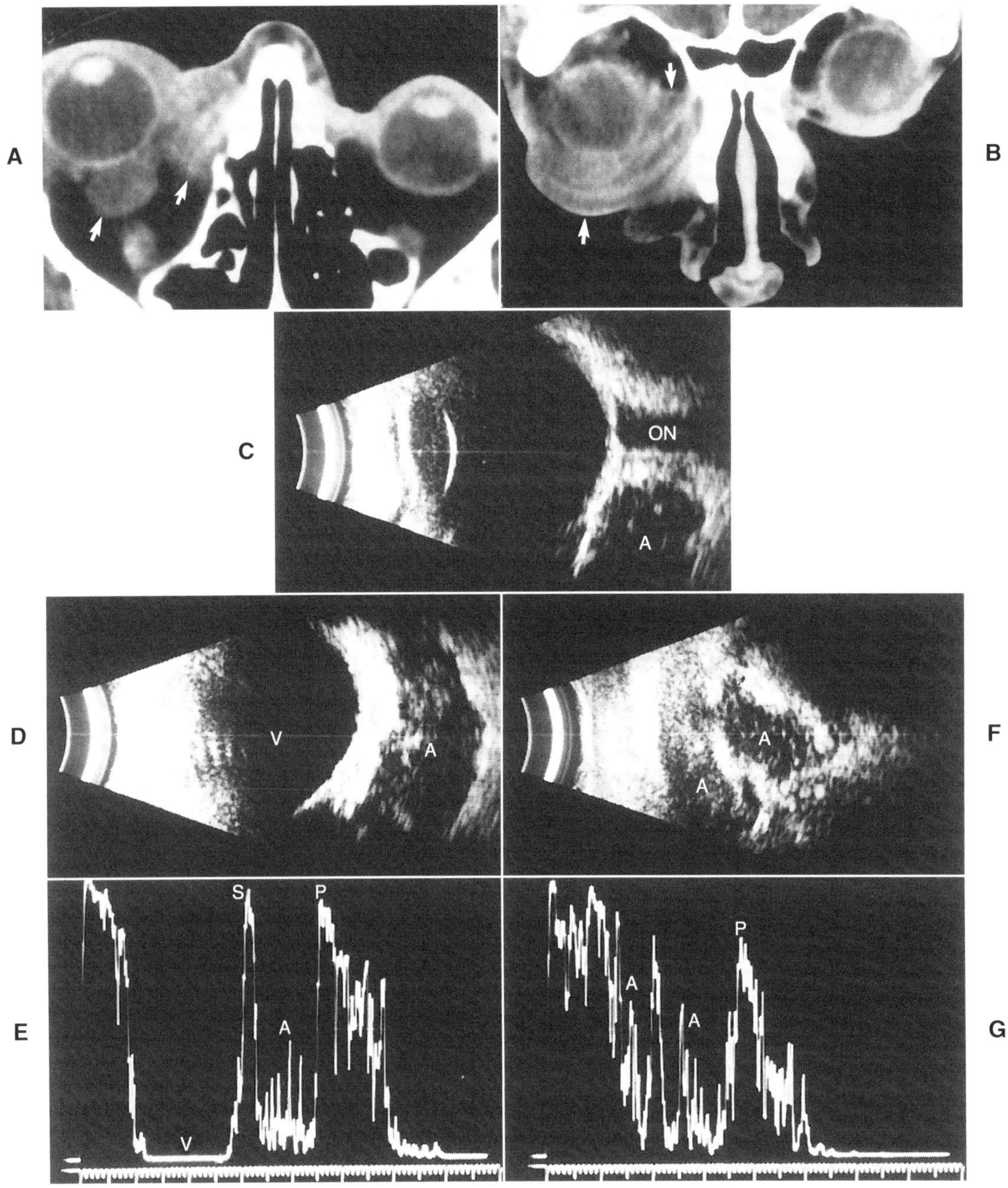

Figure 17-3 Large orbital abscess. Axial **(A)** and coronal **(B)** CT scans show large orbital abscess located inferonasally *(arrows)*. Transocular (**C** to **E**) and paraocular (**F** and **G**) echograms show large inferior orbital abscess *(A)*. **C,** Vertical axial B-scan reveals abscess behind globe and beneath optic nerve *(ON)*. **D,** Transverse B-scan shows extensive mass with irregular contour. *V,* Vitreous cavity. **E,** Corresponding A-scan shows low reflectivity of abscess. *V,* Vitreous cavity; *S,* sclera; *P,* posterior surface spike. **F,** Transverse paraocular B-scan displays irregular shape and loculated appearance of abscess in this view. **G,** Corresponding paraocular A-scan shows more irregular structure in this view as a result of loculation. *P,* Posterior surface spike.

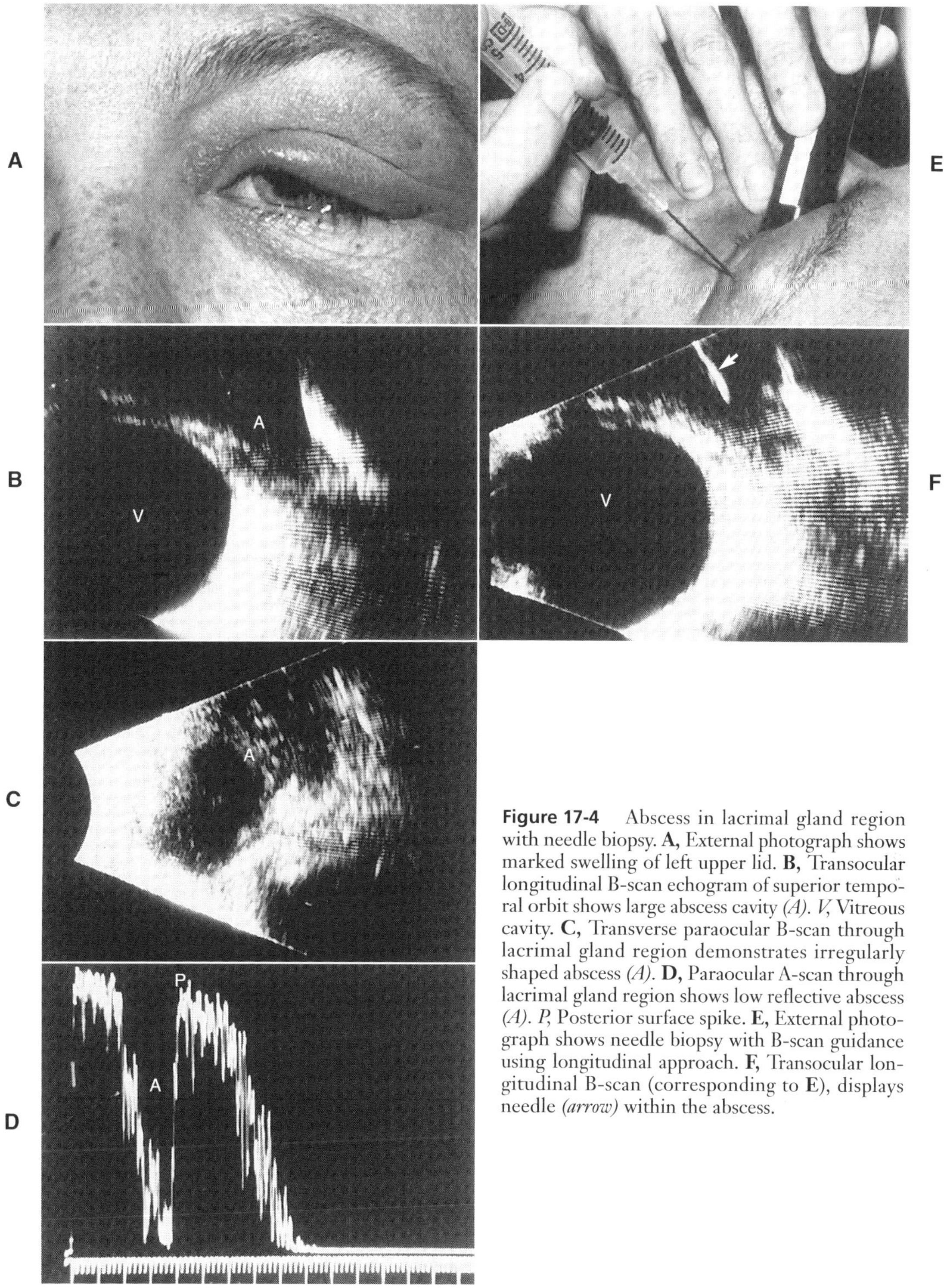

Figure 17-4 Abscess in lacrimal gland region with needle biopsy. **A,** External photograph shows marked swelling of left upper lid. **B,** Transocular longitudinal B-scan echogram of superior temporal orbit shows large abscess cavity *(A)*. *V,* Vitreous cavity. **C,** Transverse paraocular B-scan through lacrimal gland region demonstrates irregularly shaped abscess *(A)*. **D,** Paraocular A-scan through lacrimal gland region shows low reflective abscess *(A)*. *P,* Posterior surface spike. **E,** External photograph shows needle biopsy with B-scan guidance using longitudinal approach. **F,** Transocular longitudinal B-scan (corresponding to **E**), displays needle *(arrow)* within the abscess.

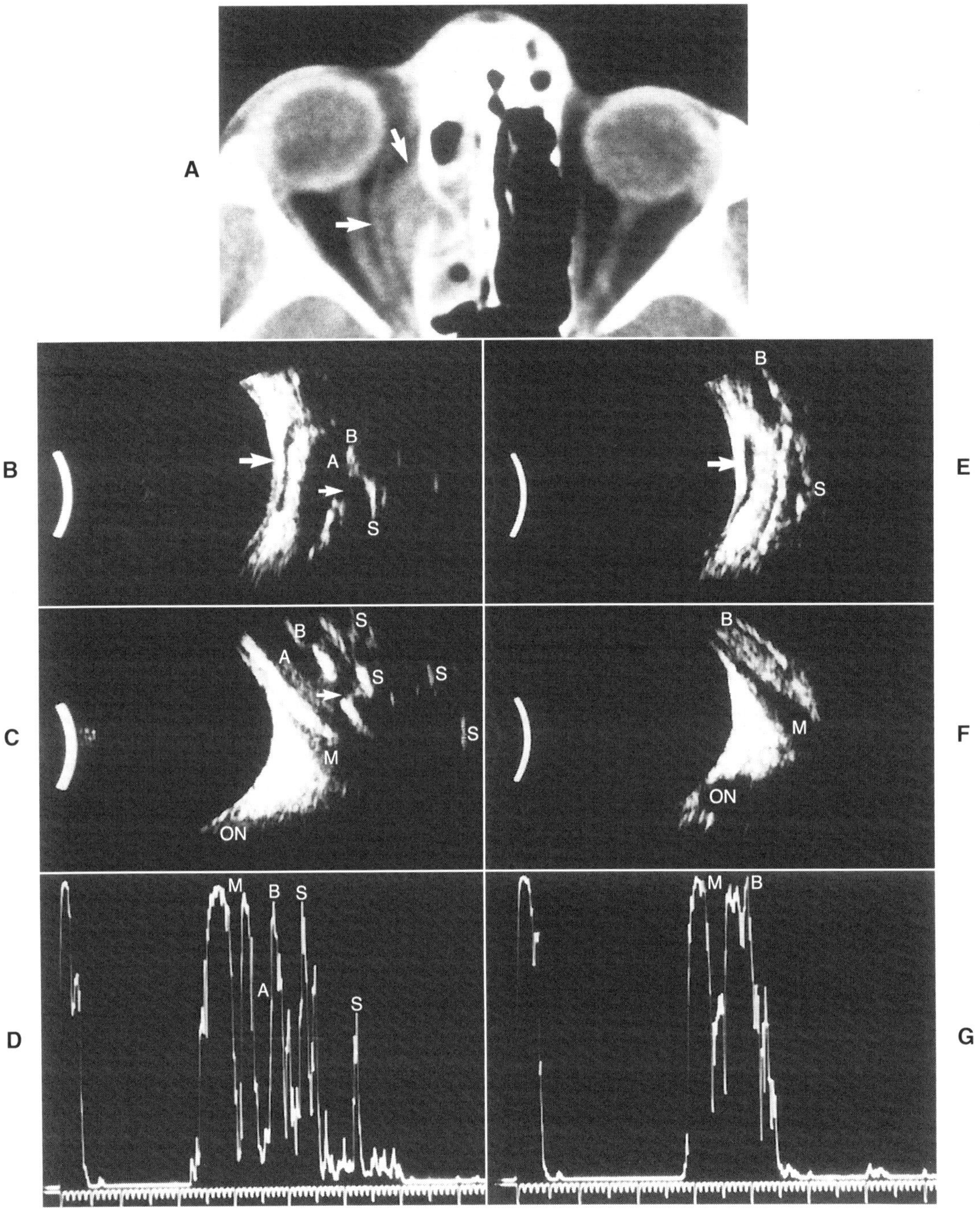

Figure 17-5 Subperiosteal abscess with follow-up examination. **A,** Axial CT scan shows abscess in right ethmoid sinus *(arrows)* extending through bone defect into subperiosteal space. Transocular echograms display abscess *(A)* at initial examination (**B** to **D**) and at follow-up after antibiotic therapy (**E** to **G**). **B,** Transverse B-scan shows subperiosteal abscess between medial rectus muscle *(large arrow)* and orbital bone *(B)*. Abscess extends into orbit from sinus through large bone defect *(small arrow)*. *S,* Echo in sinus. **C,** Longitudinal B-scan shows subperiosteal abscess between medial rectus *(M)* and bone *(B)*. Abscess extends from sinus through bone defect. *ON,* Optic nerve. **D,** Corresponding A-scan displays subperiosteal abscess between medial rectus muscle *(M)* and bone *(B)*. Note echoes within sinus *(S)*. **E,** Transverse B-scan shows marked reduction of subperiosteal abscess as compared with initial examination. Defect in bone *(B)* is much less apparent. *Arrow,* Medial rectus muscle; *S,* echo in sinus. **F,** Longitudinal B-scan shows marked reduction of abscess as well as sinus echoes. **G,** Corresponding A-scan displays resolution of abscess; only medial rectus muscle *(M)* is shown. Also, note that sinus echoes are no longer present. *B,* Bone.

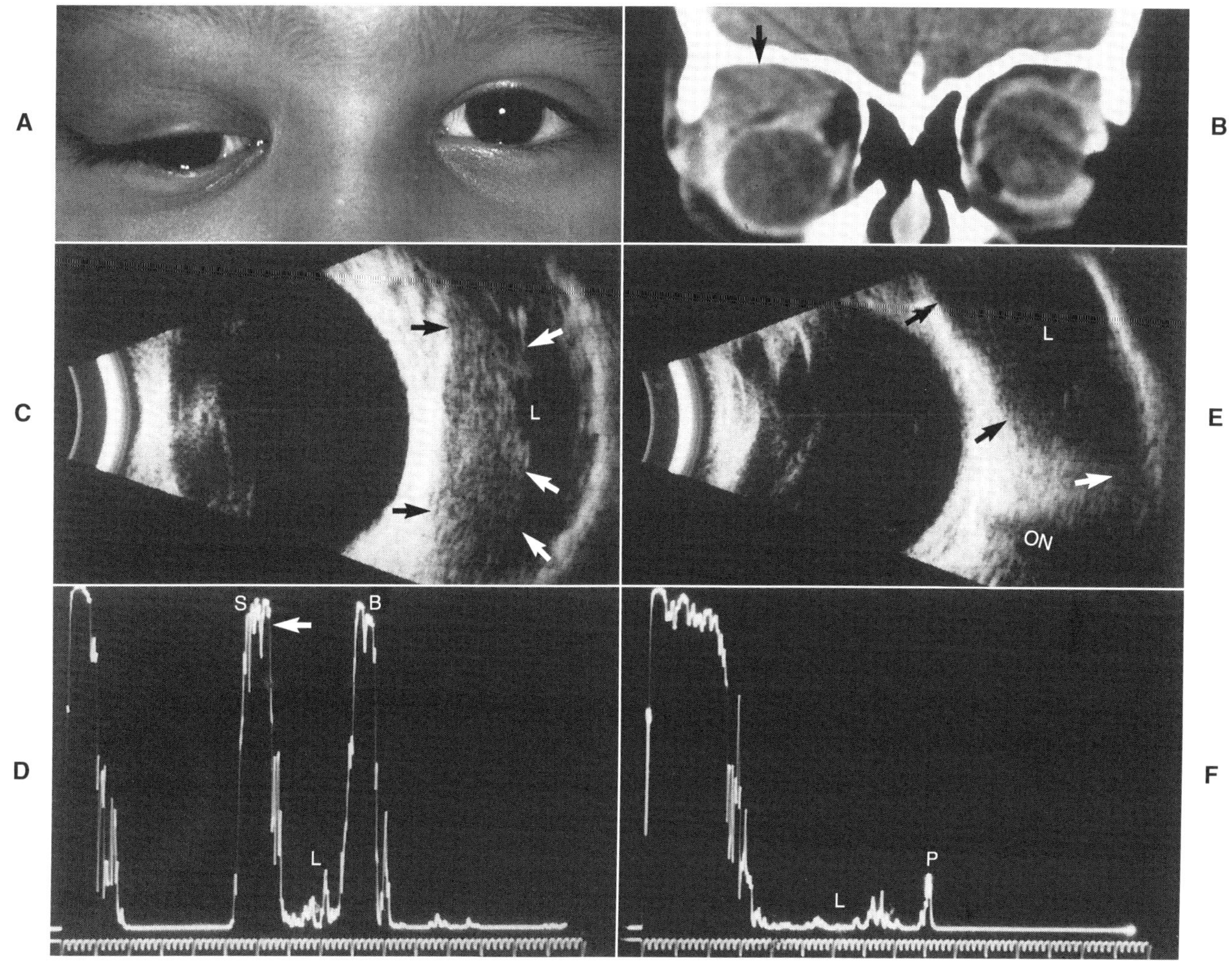

Figure 17-6 Subperiosteal hematoma following trauma. **A,** External photograph shows right upper lid swelling and ptosis, as well as downward displacement of globe. **B,** Coronal CT scan shows lesion in superior aspect of right orbit *(arrow)*. Transocular (**C** to **E**) and paraocular (**F**) echograms show lesion *(L)*. **C,** Transverse B-scan shows extensive lesion beneath smooth periosteum *(black arrows)* with layering of contents *(white arrows)*. Patient was examined in upright position so that blood layered toward periosteum rather than bone. **D,** Corresponding A-scan shows well-demarcated, extremely low reflective lesion beneath periosteum *(arrow)*. *S,* Sclera; *B,* bone. **E,** Longitudinal B-scan shows typical fusiform shape of subperiosteal lesion with pointed appearance posteriorly *(white arrow)*. *Black arrows,* Periosteum; *ON,* optic nerve. **F,** Paraocular A-scan shows very low reflectivity of lesion and weakly reflective posterior surface spike *(P)*.

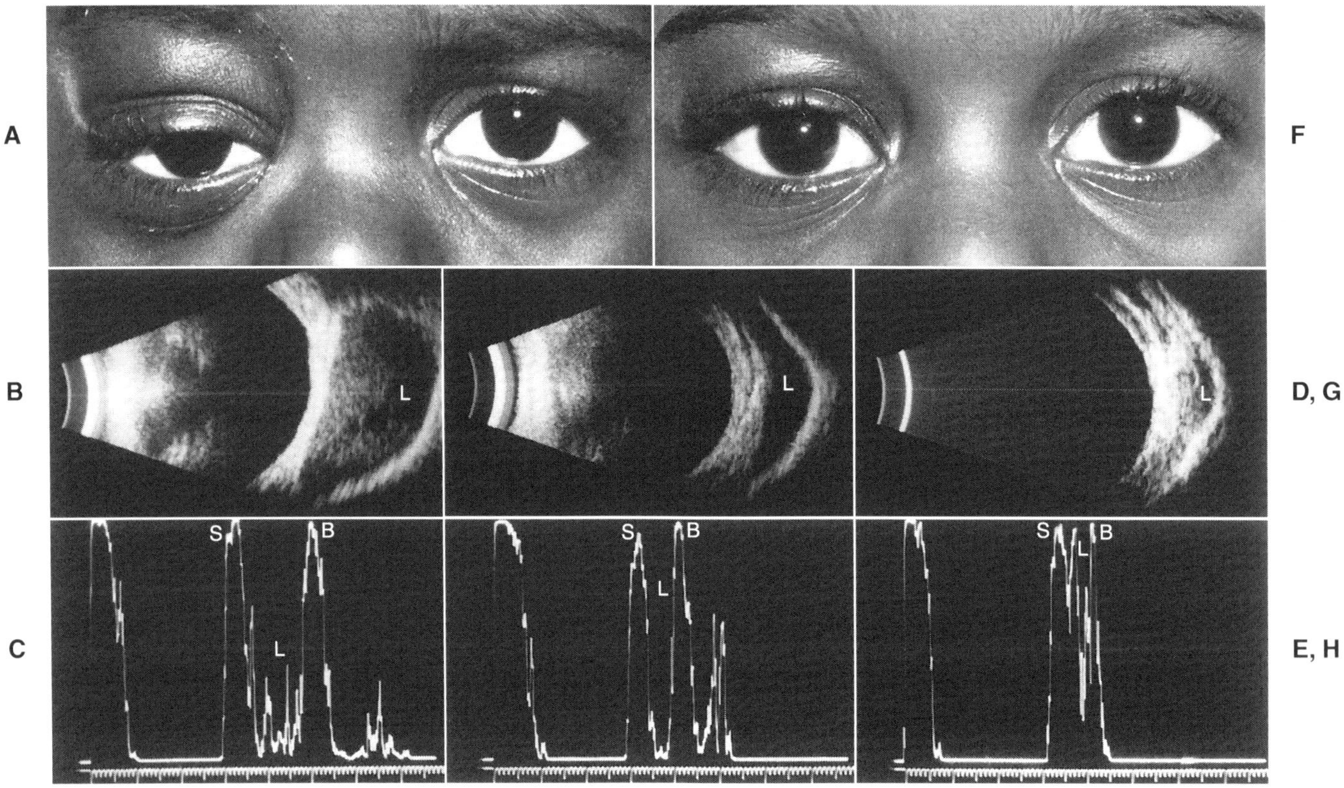

Figure 17-7 Subperiosteal hematoma occurring spontaneously in child with sickle cell disease. **A,** External photograph shows lid swelling, proptosis, and downward displacement of the right eye at initial presentation. Transocular echograms show subperiosteal lesion *(L)* at presentation (**B** and **C**), at 5 days (**D** and **E**), and 15 days (**G** and **H**). **B** and **C** show large subperiosteal hematoma with low internal reflectivity. *S,* Sclera; *B,* bone. **D** and **E** show marked reduction in size of lesion at 15 days. Also note much lower reflectivity on A-scan because of decreased density of hemorrhage. **F,** External photograph taken at 15 days shows marked improvement. **G** and **H** (corresponding to **F**) show almost complete resolution of hematoma at 15 days.

bodies has been described in Chapter 4. Most foreign bodies (e.g., glass, metal, and stone) have a very echo-dense appearance on B-scan (Figure 17-8) and are very high reflective on A-scan. Foreign bodies occurring within the orbit are, however, generally much more difficult to detect than intraocular foreign bodies because the foreign body signal may be masked by surrounding highly reflective orbital structures (fat, bone, and so forth). As a general rule, foreign bodies that are located anteriorly are more readily detected than those closer to the orbital apex. In some cases, however, those foreign bodies located more posteriorly may produce a hemorrhagic track through the orbital soft tissues that can be easily identified with ultrasound[11] (Figure 17-9; see also Figures 4-18 and 4-19). The detection of an orbital foreign body can be enhanced if it is surrounded by a homogeneous material such as blood or abscess[9] (Figure 17-10). Wooden foreign bodies often can be detected soon after the injury, but over time they may become more soft and thereby less distinguishable from surrounding orbital soft tissue.[22] In addition, spherical foreign bodies, that produce a characteristic chain of multiple signals, are relatively easy to detect[21] (Figure 17-11).

Emphysema

Air may enter the orbit from a paranasal sinus following a fracture.[16,18] A large volume of air may result in proptosis and crepitus.[27] Marked narrowing of the orbital pattern can be seen echographically (Figure 17-12). When air bubbles are small, they appear echographically similar to spherical foreign bodies, thus producing extremely high reflective, pointlike echoes followed by multiple signals (Figure 17-13).

Orbital Fractures

Orbital fractures can be due to direct trauma to the orbital bones or can occur indirectly as a result of a blowout

Text continued on p 450.

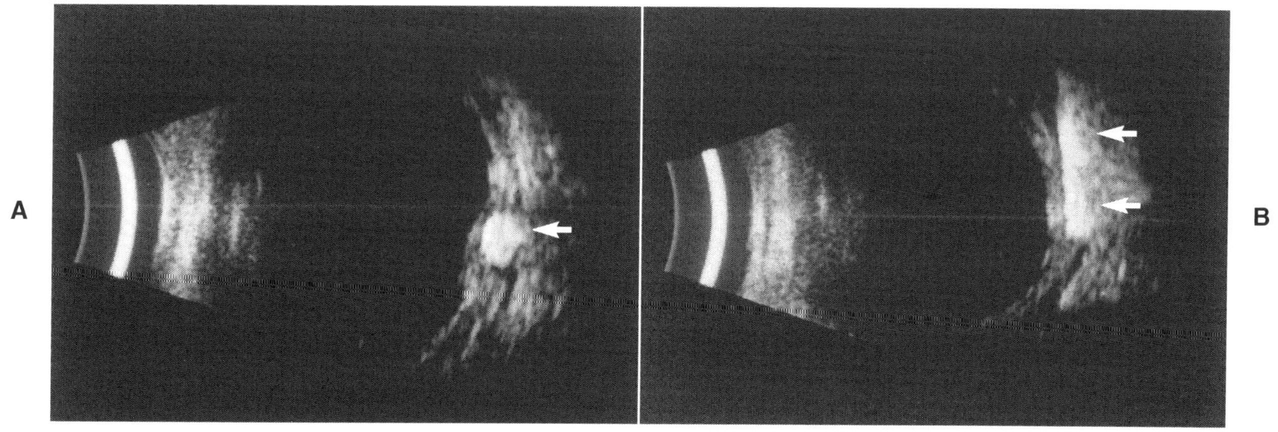

Figure 17-8 Shell casing located in orbit next to globe. **A,** Transverse B-scan echogram shows cross-section of foreign body *(arrow)* and slight indentation of globe. **B,** Longitudinal B-scan view shows long section of shell casing adjacent to sclera *(arrows)*.

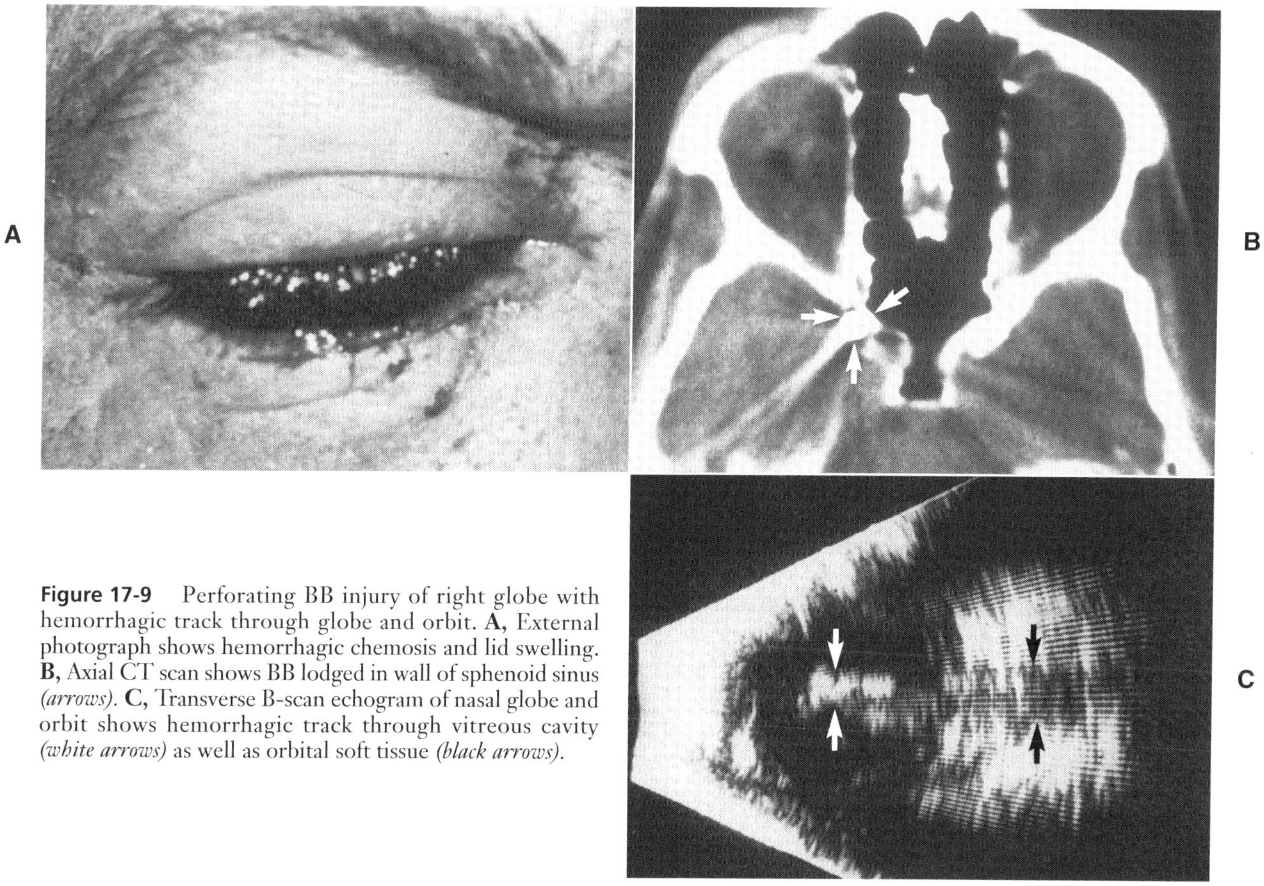

Figure 17-9 Perforating BB injury of right globe with hemorrhagic track through globe and orbit. **A,** External photograph shows hemorrhagic chemosis and lid swelling. **B,** Axial CT scan shows BB lodged in wall of sphenoid sinus *(arrows)*. **C,** Transverse B-scan echogram of nasal globe and orbit shows hemorrhagic track through vitreous cavity *(white arrows)* as well as orbital soft tissue *(black arrows)*.

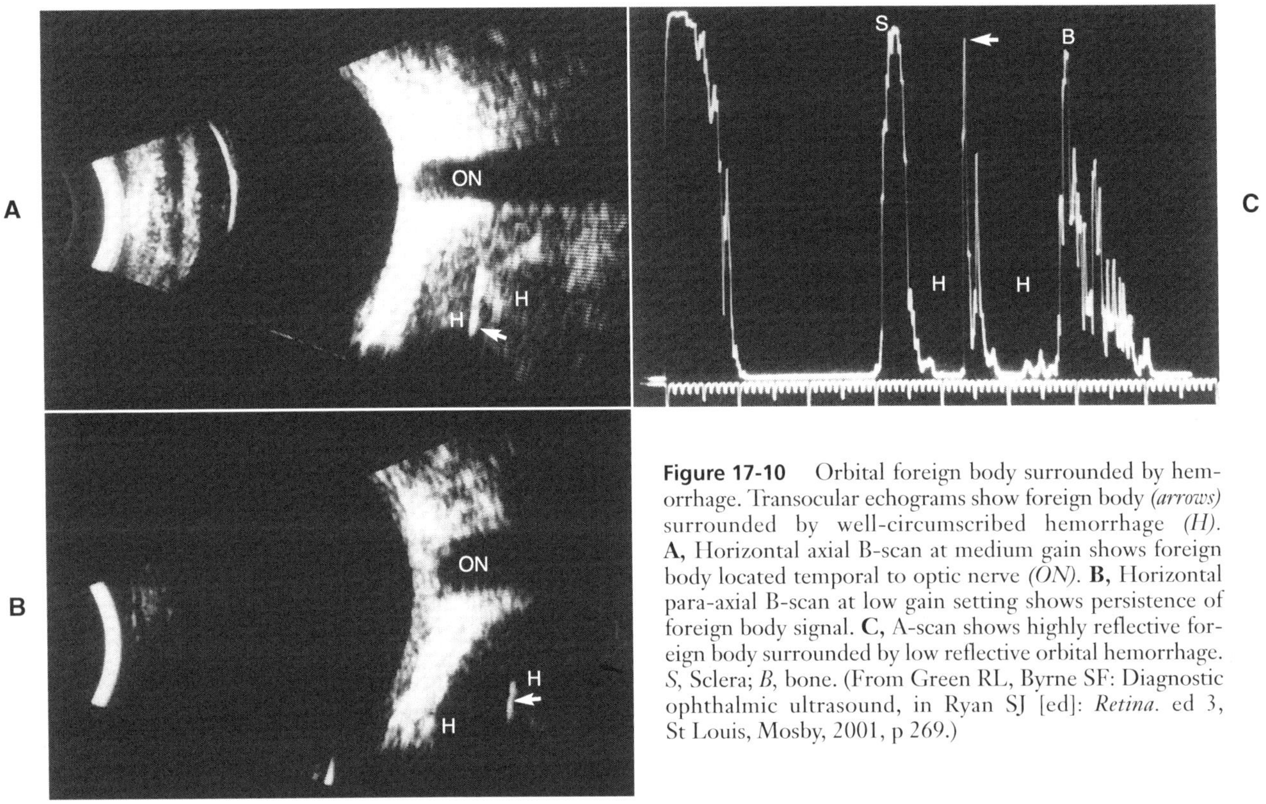

Figure 17-10 Orbital foreign body surrounded by hemorrhage. Transocular echograms show foreign body *(arrows)* surrounded by well-circumscribed hemorrhage *(H)*. **A,** Horizontal axial B-scan at medium gain shows foreign body located temporal to optic nerve *(ON)*. **B,** Horizontal para-axial B-scan at low gain setting shows persistence of foreign body signal. **C,** A-scan shows highly reflective foreign body surrounded by low reflective orbital hemorrhage. *S,* Sclera; *B,* bone. (From Green RL, Byrne SF: Diagnostic ophthalmic ultrasound, in Ryan SJ [ed]: *Retina*. ed 3, St Louis, Mosby, 2001, p 269.)

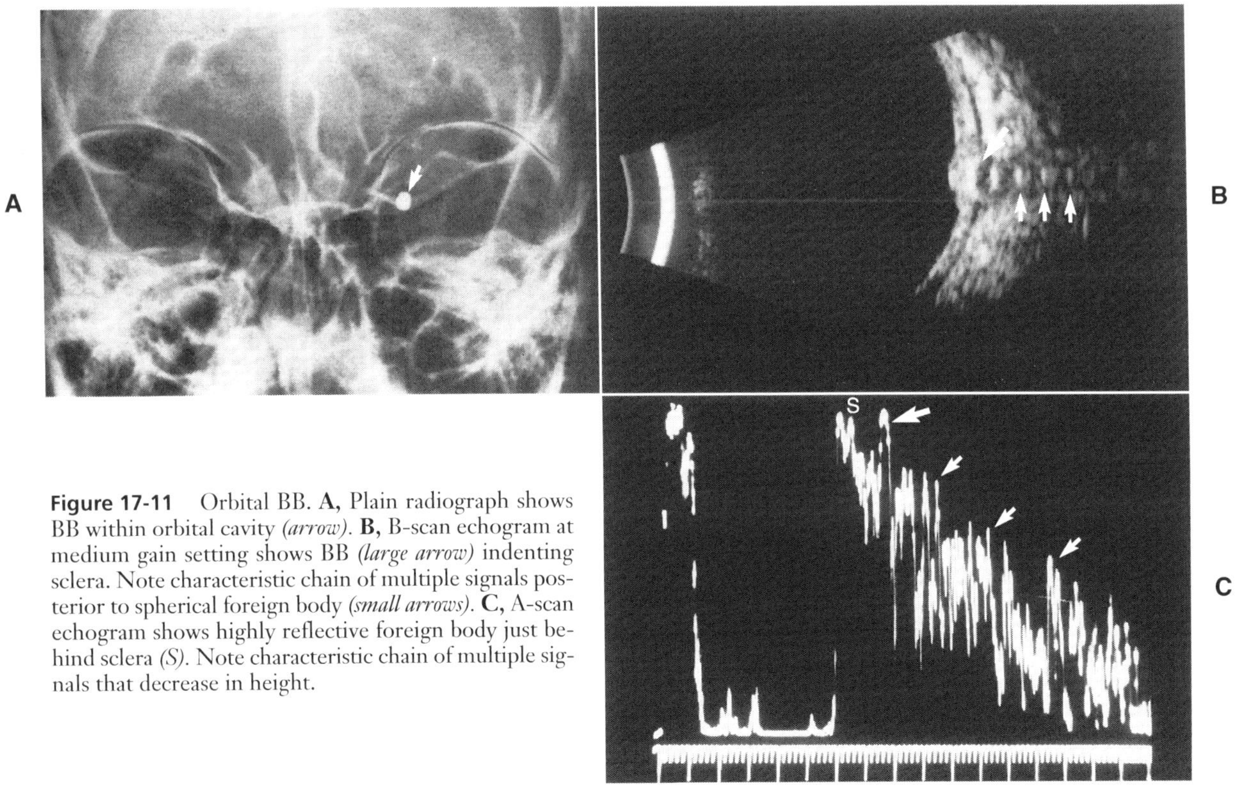

Figure 17-11 Orbital BB. **A,** Plain radiograph shows BB within orbital cavity *(arrow)*. **B,** B-scan echogram at medium gain setting shows BB *(large arrow)* indenting sclera. Note characteristic chain of multiple signals posterior to spherical foreign body *(small arrows)*. **C,** A-scan echogram shows highly reflective foreign body just behind sclera *(S)*. Note characteristic chain of multiple signals that decrease in height.

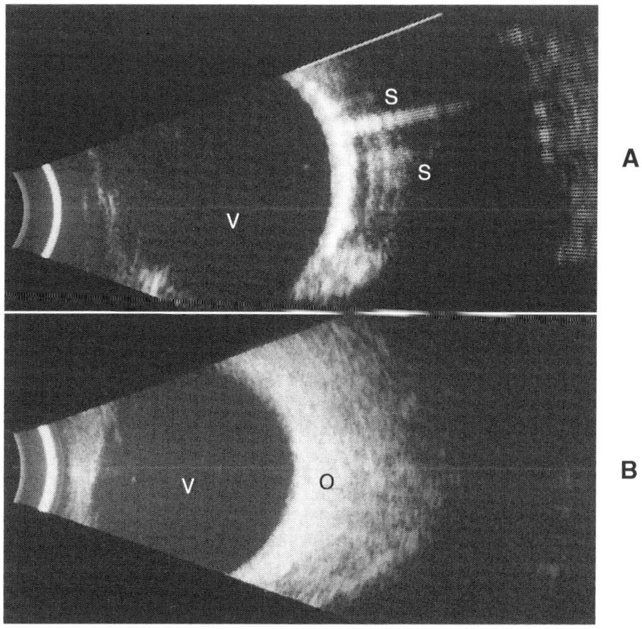

Figure 17-12 Air in sub-Tenon's space following retrobulbar injection. **A,** B-scan shows marked shadowing *(S)* of orbital soft tissue due to sub-Tenon's air. *V,* Vitreous cavity. **B,** Corresponding B-scan echogram from normal orbit. *O,* Orbital soft tissue.

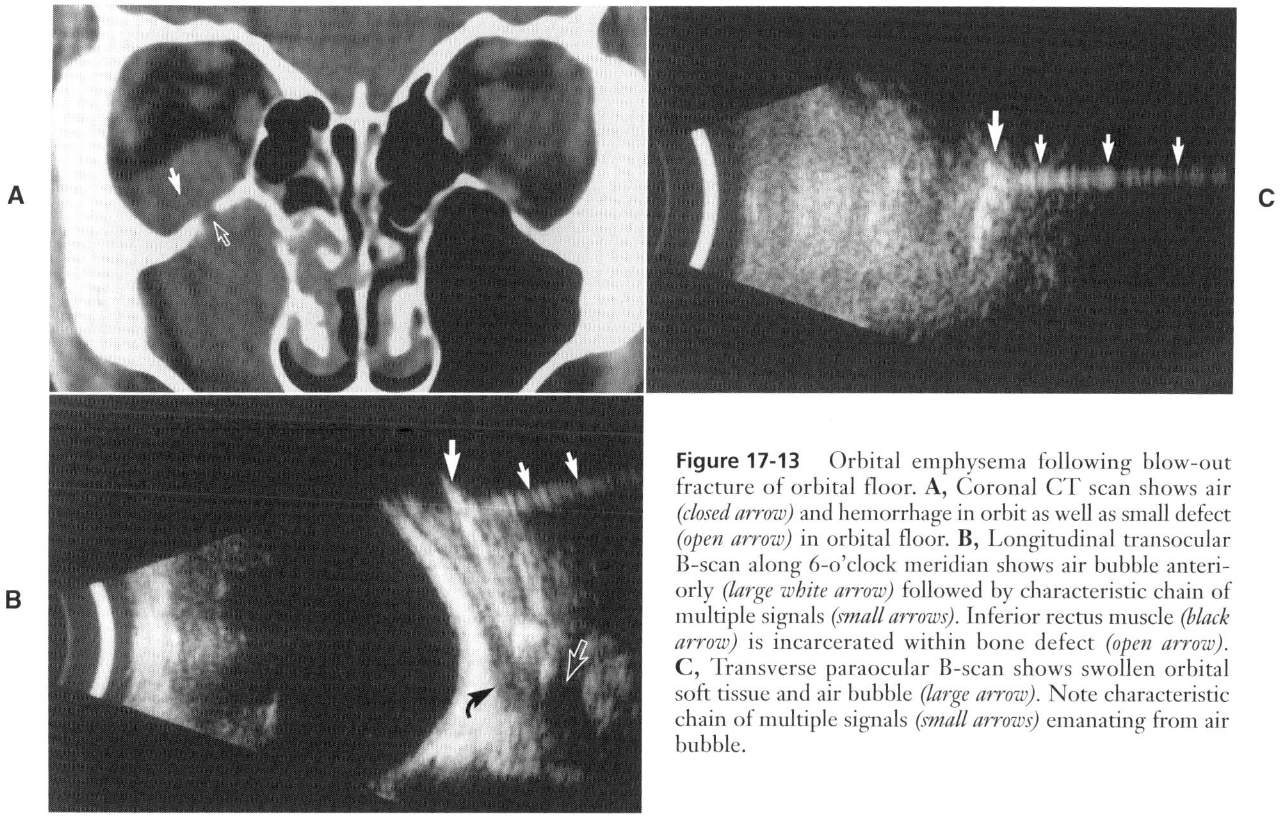

Figure 17-13 Orbital emphysema following blow-out fracture of orbital floor. **A,** Coronal CT scan shows air *(closed arrow)* and hemorrhage in orbit as well as small defect *(open arrow)* in orbital floor. **B,** Longitudinal transocular B-scan along 6-o'clock meridian shows air bubble anteriorly *(large white arrow)* followed by characteristic chain of multiple signals *(small arrows)*. Inferior rectus muscle *(black arrow)* is incarcerated within bone defect *(open arrow)*. **C,** Transverse paraocular B-scan shows swollen orbital soft tissue and air bubble *(large arrow)*. Note characteristic chain of multiple signals *(small arrows)* emanating from air bubble.

fracture.[27] In these cases, echography may be unable to image the actual fracture but the fracture often can be indirectly diagnosed by detecting incarceration of orbital tissue (see Figure 17-13). Other findings that can be associated with fractures include orbital and subperiosteal hematomas, emphysema, and bony fragments.

A bony fragment may lodge within the orbit following severe injury to the orbital wall.[1] In one case, the fragment was surrounded by a large orbital hematoma and there was marked indentation of the ocular wall (Figure 17-14).

Extraocular Muscle Trauma

Hemorrhage within the muscle sheath can occur following trauma.[4] This results in thickening of the muscle and a decrease in the normal internal reflectivity. Follow-up examination typically shows a gradual decrease in size.

Incarceration of an extraocular muscle (especially the inferior or medial rectus muscles) has been observed following sinus surgery (see Figures 17-13 and 15-33).[2,7] If a muscle tendon is disinserted from the globe as a result of strabismus surgery or other trauma, the muscle may retract

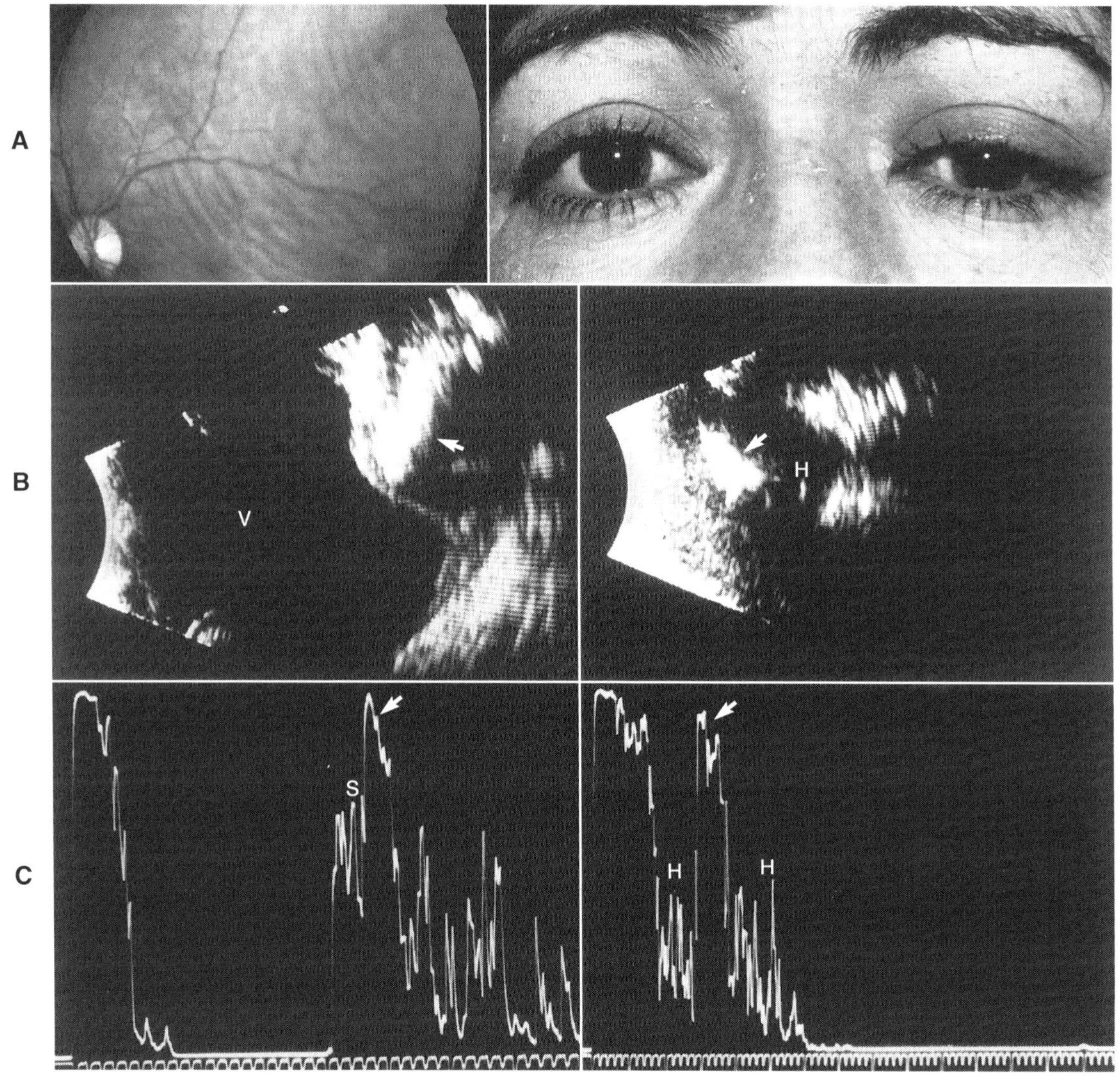

Figure 17-14 Bone fragment and orbital hematoma following trauma. **A,** Fundus photograph shows deep choroidal folds extending from the superotemporal quadrant. Transocular (**B** and **C**) and paraocular (**E** and **F**) echograms show bony fragment *(arrow)*. **B,** Longitudinal B-scan along 1:30-o'clock meridian shows marked indentation of ocular wall by fragment. *V,* Vitreous cavity. **C,** A-scan of 1:30 meridian at reduced gain setting shows very high reflective spike from bony fragment and thickened retinochoroid/scleral layer *(S)*. **D,** External photograph shows proptosis, ptosis, and downward displacement of left globe. **E,** Transverse paraocular B-scan shows bright signal from fragment surrounded by echolucent hemorrhage *(H)*. **F,** Paraocular A-scan shows low reflective hemorrhage adjacent to highly reflective bony fragment. (**A** to **D** from Atta HR, Byrne SF: The findings of standardized echography for choroidal folds. *Arch Ophthalmol* 1988;106:1236.)

into the orbit.[17] In these cases, echography may show that the inserting tendon is not located in its proper position at the globe (see Figure 15-32).

Optic Nerve Trauma

Hematomas of the optic nerve have also been detected following severe ocular or orbital injury.[3,12] The optic nerve pattern is widened and the thirty-degree test is positive (see p 419). Avulsion of the optic nerve produces various findings that are dependent on whether the injury is acute or longstanding (see p 92 and Figures 4-10 and 4-11).

PERIORBITAL DISEASE

Echography can be useful for evaluating periorbital disorders and diseases of the orbital bones.[19,20] Computed tomography and magnetic resonance imaging are the procedures of choice for assessments of the bony orbital wall, periorbital sinuses, and the retro-orbital region. There are many situations, however, in which echography can provide additional information (Box 17-2). In these cases, it is particularly important to be familiar with the appearance of the normal bony orbital walls and sinuses.

Normal Bone and Sinuses

The normal orbital wall has a smooth contour and appears either straight or slightly concave, except inferiorly, where the concavity is more pronounced. The bone produces an echo-dense line on B-scan and a highly reflective spike on A-scan (see Figure 11-2). In some areas of the orbit, normal small irregularities of the bone are present (Figure 17-15). Abnormalities of bone include defects, excavation and hyperostosis (see Figure 11-22). It is important to always compare the appearance of the bone being elevated with that of the same area in the fellow orbit.

BOX 17-2

Periorbital Disease

- Mucocele
- Sphenoid wing meningioma
- Periorbital malignancy
- Eosinophilic granuloma
- Fibrous dysplasia
- Hematic cyst (see p 340)

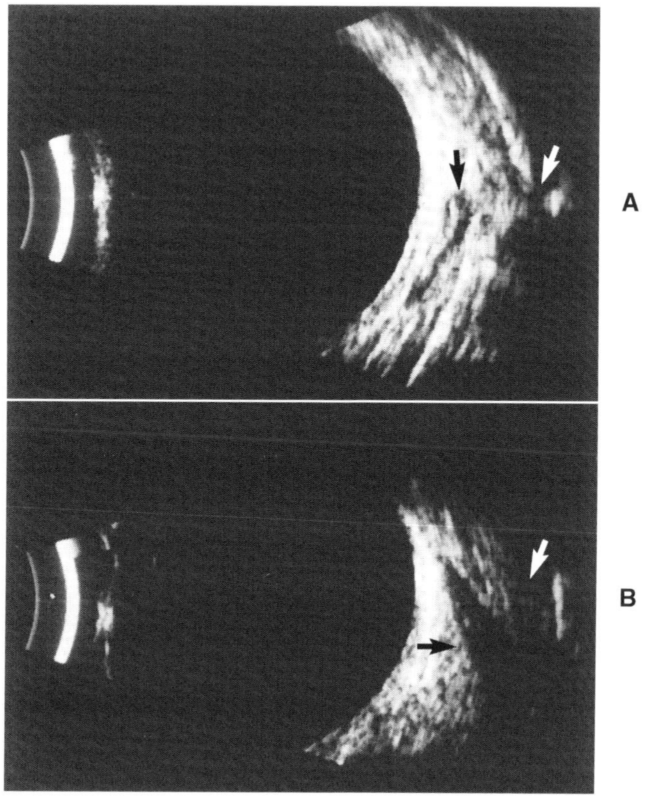

Figure 17-15 Normal irregularity of medial orbital wall. Small discontinuity in bone *(white arrows)* is shown in vertical transverse **(A)** and longitudinal **(B)** B-scan echograms through midportion of nasal orbit. This irregularity is presumably due to a vessel communicating between ethmoid sinus and orbit. Medial rectus muscle is indicated by *black arrows.*

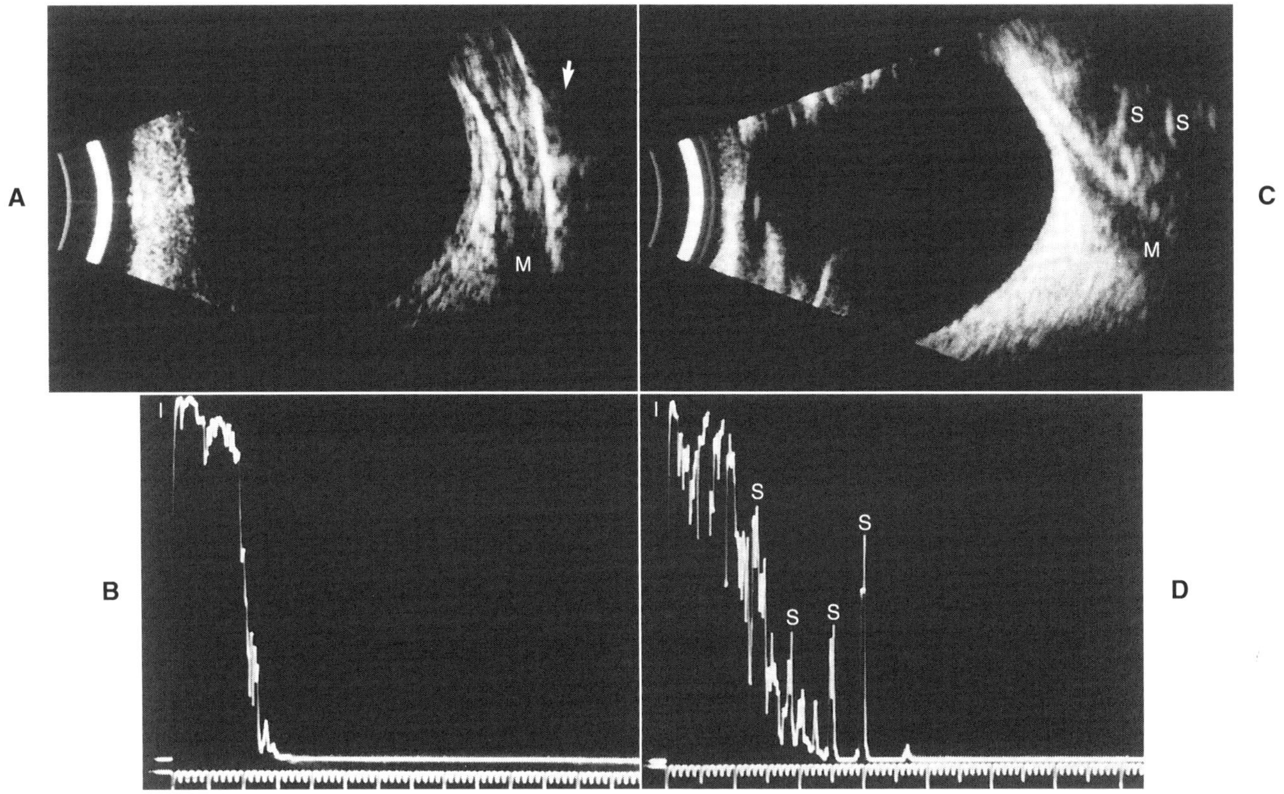

Figure 17-16 Severe ethmoid sinusitis compared with a normal sinus. Normal echograms are shown in **A** and **B** and sinusitis is shown in **C** and **D. A,** Longitudinal transocular B-scan shows medial rectus muscle *(M)*, orbital bone, and characteristic absence of signals from normal air-filled sinus *(arrow)*. **B,** Paraocular A-scan with sound beam directed toward sinus shows normal highly reflective echogram and lack of echoes from air-filled sinus. **C,** Longitudinal transocular B-scan through abnormal sinus shows abnormal echoes *(S)*. *M,* Medial rectus muscle. **D,** Paraocular A-scan shows abnormal spikes within sinus *(S)*.

The normal sinus is air filled and totally reflects the sound waves so that no echoes are usually detected. However, mucosal swelling, fluid accumulation, or tissue within a sinus create abnormal echoes (Figures 17-16 and 17-17).

Bone Defects

Bone defects can be solitary or multiple. In addition, they can be secondary to benign processes or related to malignant tumors. On B-scan, a large bone defect appears as a discontinuity of the bone line (see Figure 11-22). This may be seen in transocular and/or paraocular views, depending on the size and location of the defect (Figure 17-18). On A-scan, a zig-zag movement of the bone spike[10] may be apparent during the dynamic examination; this up-and-down motion of the spike is observed when the sound beam is shifted back and forth across the defect (Figure 17-19). When numerous bone defects are present, the bone may appear very irregular on B-scan and less reflective on A-scan.

Excavation

Excavation, or remolding, of a bony wall is due to pressure exerted by a mass of longstanding duration[26] (e.g., benign mixed tumor or dermoid cyst). B-scan echograms show a concave indentation of the bone line (see Figure 11-22).

Hyperostosis

Thickening of the orbital bone (e.g., fibrous dysplasia and sphenoid wing meningioma) usually produces an expansion of the bone into the orbit (see Figure 11-22). This expansion may, in turn, cause narrowing of the orbital soft tissue pattern in the space between the thickened bone and the globe.

Periorbital Lesions

Mucocele

Mucoceles are sinus lesions of a cystic nature that are caused by obstruction of the normal sinus drainage openings.[24] This leads to a build up of pressure within the sinus,

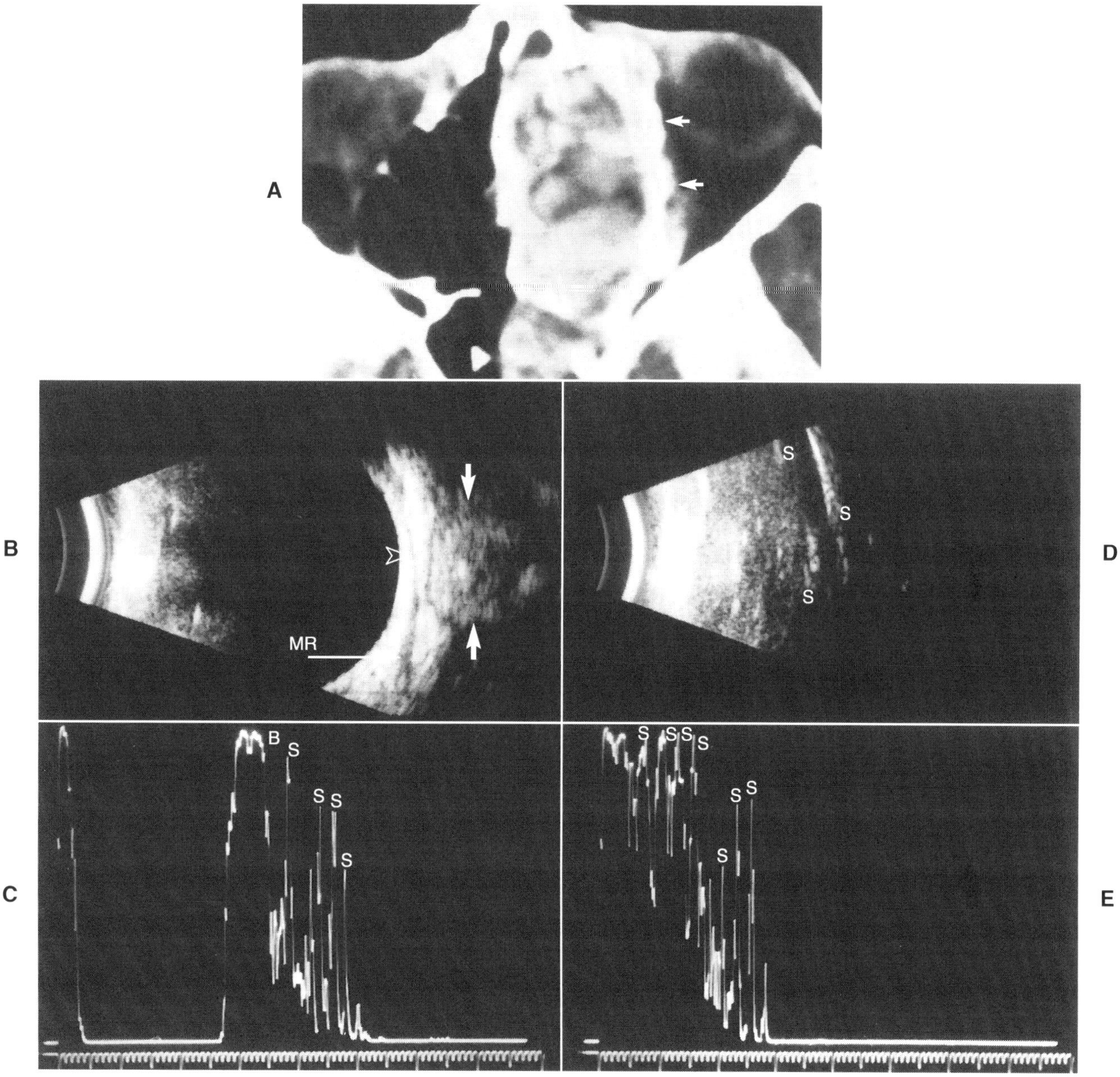

Figure 17-17 Polyposis of left ethmoid sinus. **A,** Axial CT scan shows mass filling left ethmoid sinus *(arrows)* with expansion of medial orbital wall toward orbit. Transocular (**B** and **C**) and paraocular (**D** and **E**) echograms show abnormal echoes from polyps within sinus. **B,** Vertical transverse B-scan of medial orbit and ethmoid sinus. Roundish polyp within sinus *(vertical arrows)* is causing lateral displacement of medial orbital wall *(open arrow)* and compression of orbital soft tissue. *MR,* Cross-section of medial rectus muscle. **C,** Corresponding A-scan through medial orbit and ethmoid sinus shows orbital bone *(B)* followed by abnormal sinus spikes *(S)* from polyps. **D,** Transverse paraocular B-scan shows abnormal echoes from polyposis in sinus *(S)*. **E,** Corresponding paraocular A-scan shows numerous abnormal spikes from polyposis in sinus *(S)*.

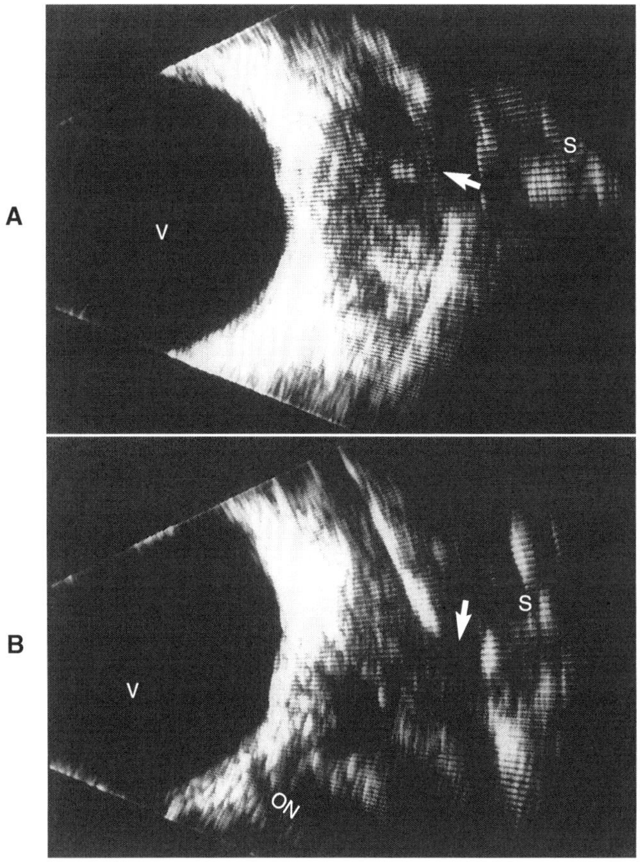

Figure 17-18 Bone defect secondary to periorbital malignancy. **A,** Transverse B-scan echogram of medial orbit displays mass extending through large defect in orbital wall *(arrow)* into ethmoid sinus *(S)*. This view demonstrates the superior and inferior edges of the defect. *V,* Vitreous cavity. **B,** Longitudinal B-scan of medial orbit also shows mass extending through bone defect into sinus. This view demonstrates the anterior and posterior edges of bone defect. *ON,* Optic nerve.

which results in enlargement and eventually extension of the mucocele into the orbit. Although frontoethmoidal mucoceles occur most commonly, these lesions also can originate in the sphenoid and, less frequently, in the maxillary sinus.[14,24]

Echographically, a mucocele appears usually as a large, very low reflective, nonvascular mass[5] that is most often located in the supranasal quadrant (frontoethmoidal).[10] Mucoceles in this region most often produce outward and downward displacement of the globe.[25] Typically, these lesions are very well outlined, producing highly reflective borders. In most instances, they have a very firm consistency and often compress the globe. The key diagnostic finding is a large, solitary bone defect through which the lesion extends from the sinus into the orbit. However, difficulty in diagnosis may arise when the bone defect is so large that it cannot be readily identified. In such situations, the echographer may not appreciate that the lesion is actually extending from the sinus into the orbit, and may mistakenly determine that the lesion lies totally within the orbit (Figure 17-20). Such errors can be avoided, however, by remembering to compare the area of investigation with the fellow orbit. Additionally, if the mucocele originates in the frontal sinus and is located far anteriorly, the bone defect may be best detected with a paraocular approach (Figure 17-21).

When it appears that the lesion extends laterally in the subperiosteal space, a mucopyocele may be present. These patients also may have inflammation of the orbital soft tissue[24] (Figure 17-22).

Sphenoid Wing Meningioma

Intracranial meningiomas can secondarily involve the orbit.[23] Of these lesions, the sphenoid wing meningioma is the most common and is the most amenable to detection by echography. Typically, these tumors cause hyperostosis

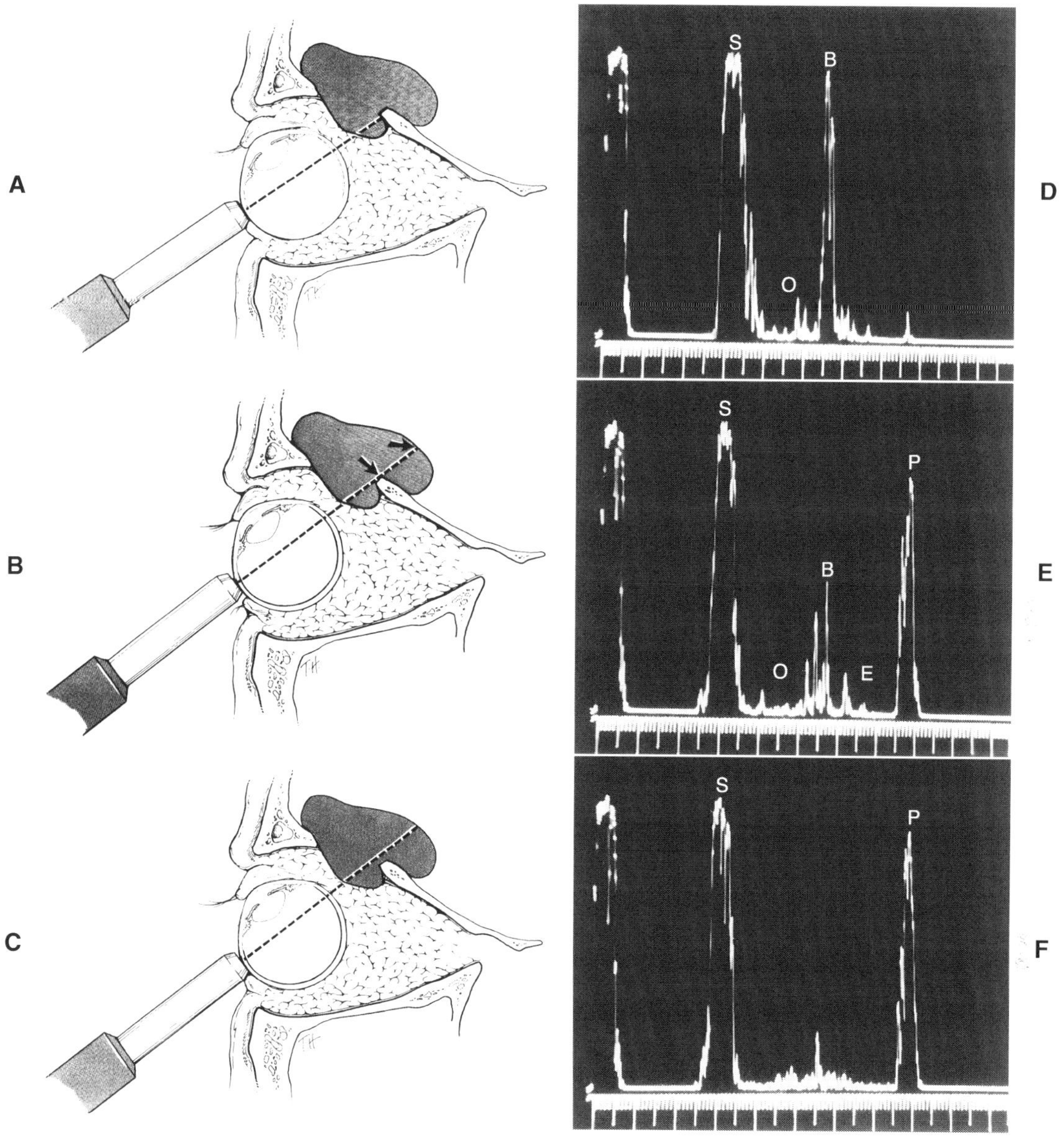

Figure 17-19 Drawings and corresponding A-scan echograms of large periorbital lesion demonstrating zigzag phenomenon. **A** and **D,** Sound beam directed through orbital portion of low reflective lesion *(O)* and perpendicular to orbital bone *(B)* at edge of bone defect. *S,* Sclera. **B** and **E,** Probe is shifted slightly so that sound beam now strikes edge of bone defect *(B)* and posterior bony wall of sinus *(P)*. Both orbital *(O)*, and extraorbital *(E)* portions of lesion are now shown. **C** and **F,** Further movement of probe now directs sound beam entirely through bone defect, bypassing edge of orbital bone.

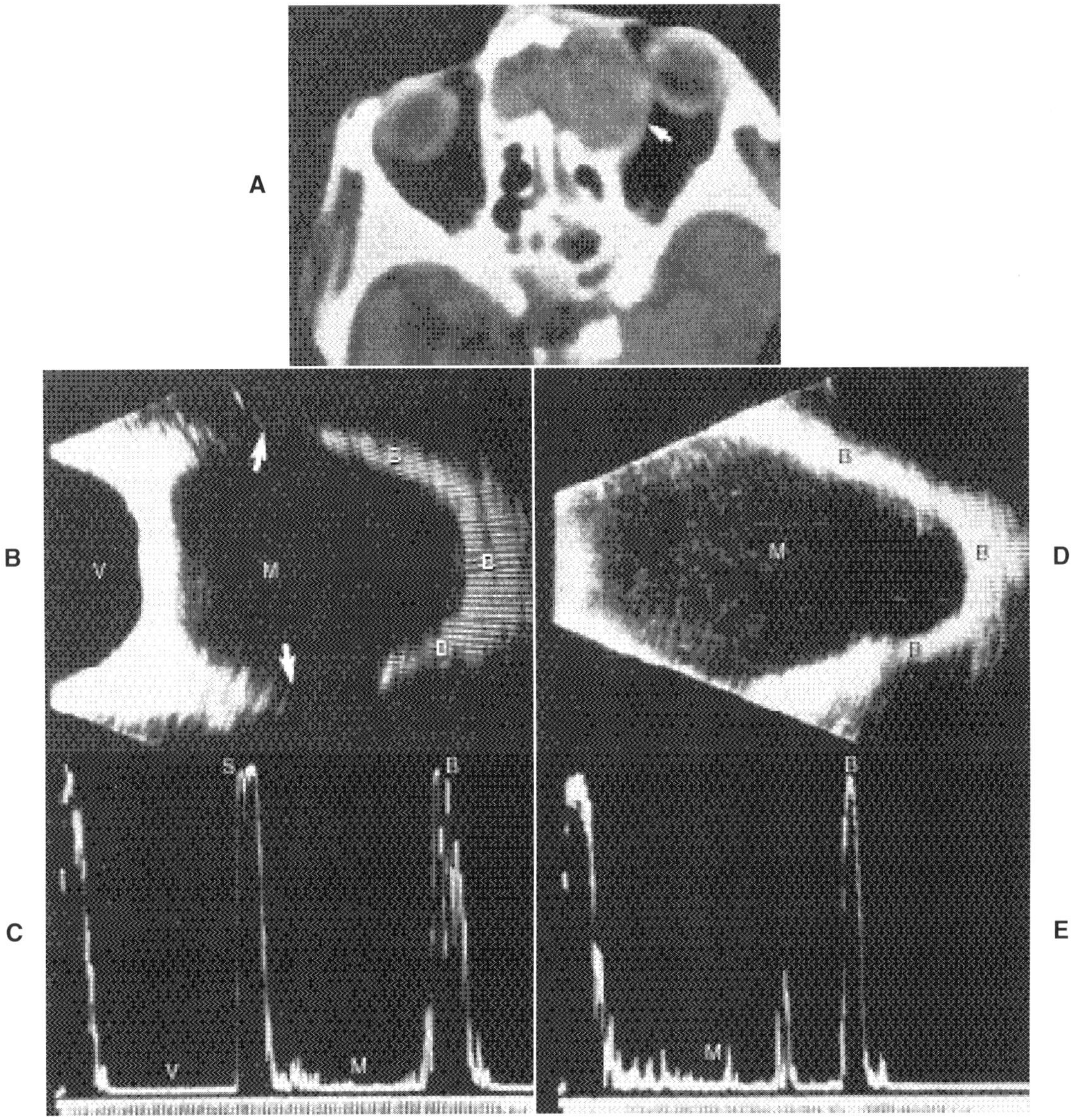

Figure 17-20 Frontoethmoidal mucocele extending into orbit. **A,** Axial CT scan shows large mucocele extending from sinus into orbit *(arrow)*. Transocular (**B** and **C**) and paraocular (**D** and **E**) echograms show large mucocele *(M)*. **B,** Transverse B-scan shows mucocele extending from sinus into orbit through very large bone defect *(arrows)*. *V,* Vitreous cavity; B, bone within sinus. **C,** Corresponding A-scan shows very low reflective lesion with regular internal structure between sclera *(S)* and posterior bony wall of sinus *(B)*. **D,** Transverse paraocular B-scan with sound beam directed through bone defect into sinus shows mass extending from sinus into orbit. **E,** Corresponding paraocular A-scan with sound beam directed through bone defect into sinus shows very low reflectivity of lesion.

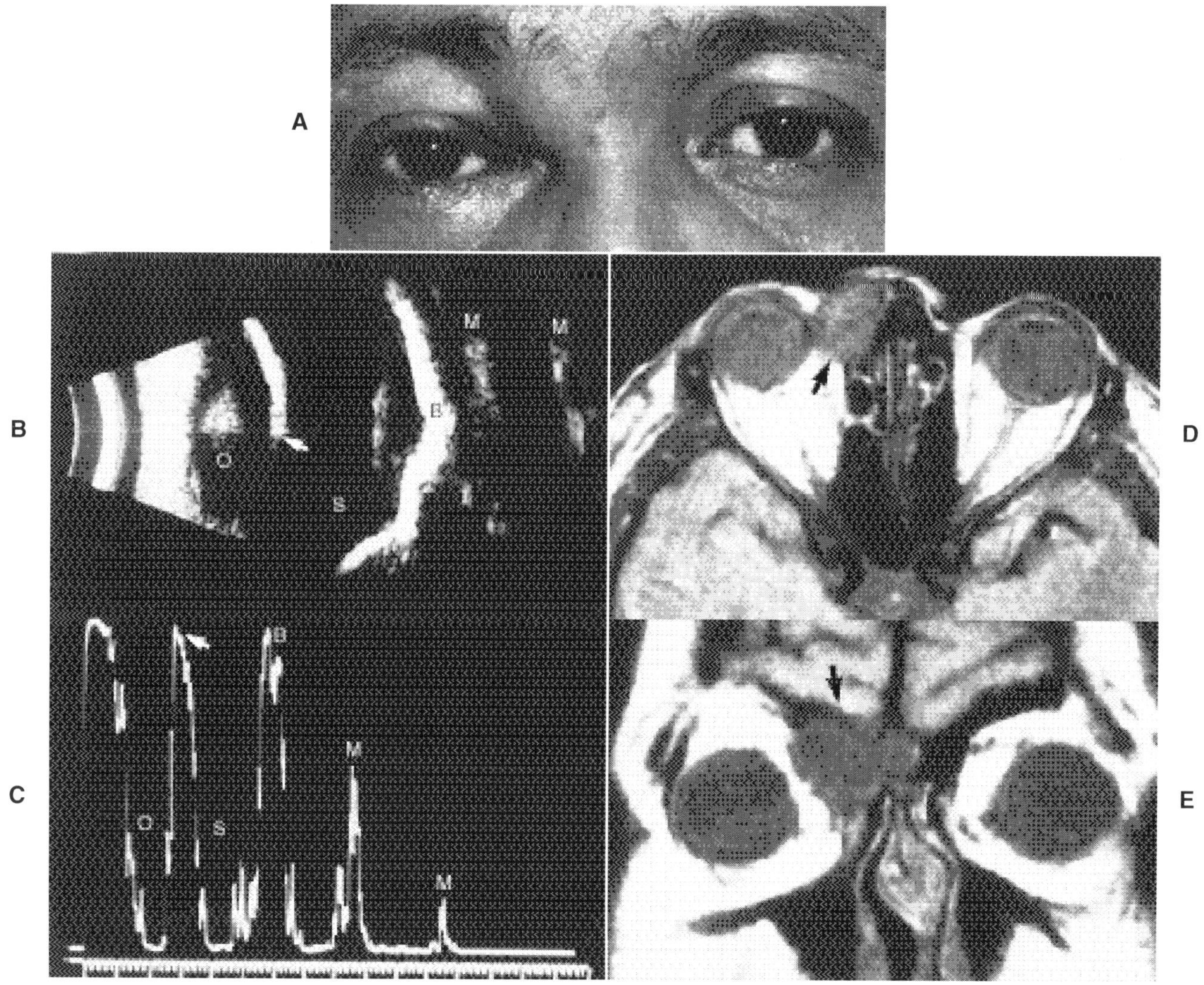

Figure 17-21 Frontal mucocele extending into orbit through large anterior bone defect. **A,** External photograph shows swelling of nasal aspect of right upper lid and ptosis. **B,** Transverse paraocular B-scan echogram shows large mass extending through bone defect into orbit *(O)* from sinus *(S)*. *Arrow,* Edge of large defect in orbital bone; *B,* posterior bony wall of sinus; *M,* multiple signals. **C,** Paraocular A-scan with sound beam directed through both orbital *(O)* and sinus *(S)* portions of lesion as well as edge of bone defect *(arrow)*. *B,* Posterior bony wall of sinus; *M,* multiple signals. Axial **(D)** and coronal **(E)** MRI scans demonstrate large frontal mucocele *(arrows)* extending into orbit. (MRI scans courtesy Dr. Myron Tannenbaum, Miami, Florida.)

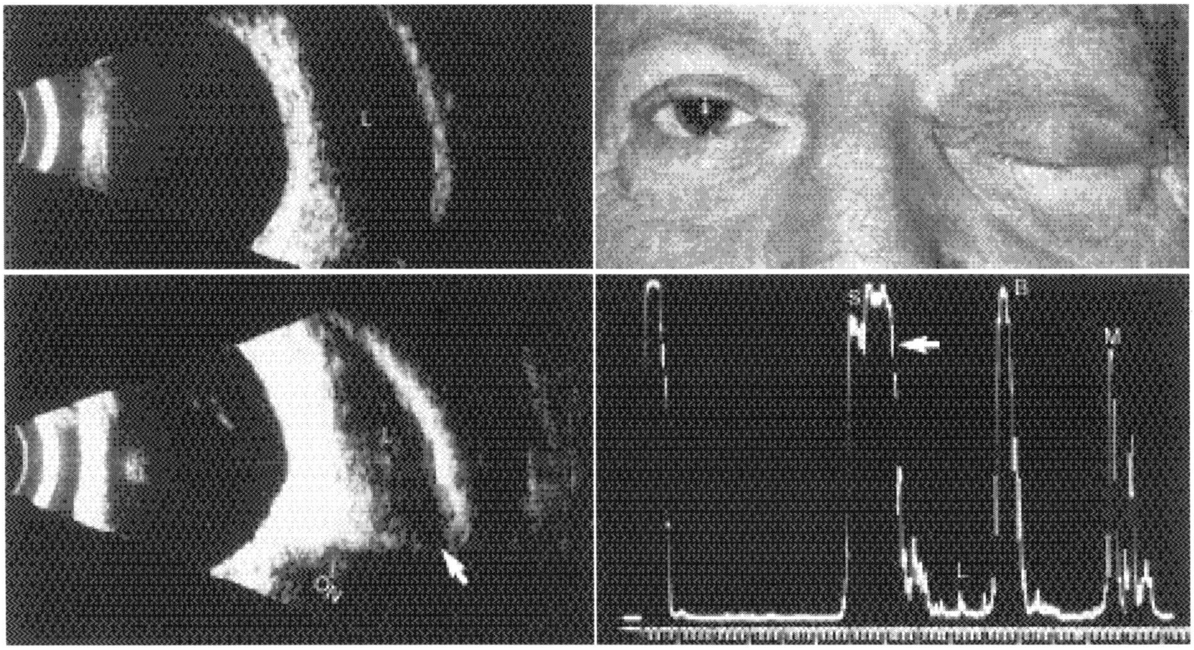

Figure 17-22 Left frontoethmoidal mucopyocele with subperiosteal extension. Transocular echograms (**A**, **B**, and **D**) show orbital portion of lesion *(L)* extending beneath smooth periosteum (bone defect not shown). **A**, Transverse B-scan shows large, smooth subperiosteal lesion. **B**, Longitudinal B-scan shows posterior extent of mucocele. Note typical tapered appearance *(arrow)* of subperiosteal lesion. *ON*, Optic nerve. **C**, External photograph shows complete ptosis of left upper lid. Globe was proptotic and displaced downward. **D**, A-scan shows very low reflective subperiosteal lesion. *Arrow*, Surface of periosteum; *S*, sclera; *B*, bone; *M*, multiple signal.

or irregularity of the orbital bone in the supratemporal quadrant (Figure 17-23). In some cases, a low to medium reflective soft tissue mass (i.e., en plaque meningioma) can be demonstrated adjacent to the orbital wall supratemporally (Figures 17-24 and 17-25).

Periorbital Malignancy and Bony Metastasis

Malignant tumors that invade the orbit from periorbital cavities are usually associated with multiple bony defects. Once these lesions reach the orbit, they tend to grow expansively, often in the subperiosteal space. These tumor extensions typically have low internal reflectivity and are sharply demarcated from the normal orbital soft tissue, as are all subperiosteal lesions. The overall structure may appear irregular because of the numerous bone defects and the echoes received from the tumor within the extraorbital space (Figure 17-26). These lesions usually have a very hard consistency and are typically not highly vascularized.

Tumors that metastasize to orbital bone often result in the bone appearing irregularly shaped, thickened and less reflective than normal. If such a lesion is detected in the supratemporal, posterior orbit, a sphenoid wing meningioma should be considered in the differential diagnosis.

Eosinophilic Granuloma

This rare disorder, usually seen in the supratemporal orbit of children and teenagers, can be associated with inflammation.[6] The lesion is normally low reflective, hard, slightly vascularized, and relatively well circumscribed, with a roundish or somewhat irregular shape. Eosinophilic granuloma is almost always associated with a bone defect superiorly (Figure 17-27).

Fibrous Dysplasia

Fibrous dysplasia occurs typically in children and causes abnormal expansion of the orbital bone.[28] This bony expansion decreases the size of the orbital cavity and thus compresses the orbital soft tissue. Echographically, such compression is most evident when comparing the involved orbit with the normal fellow orbit (Figure 17-28).

Text continued on p 465

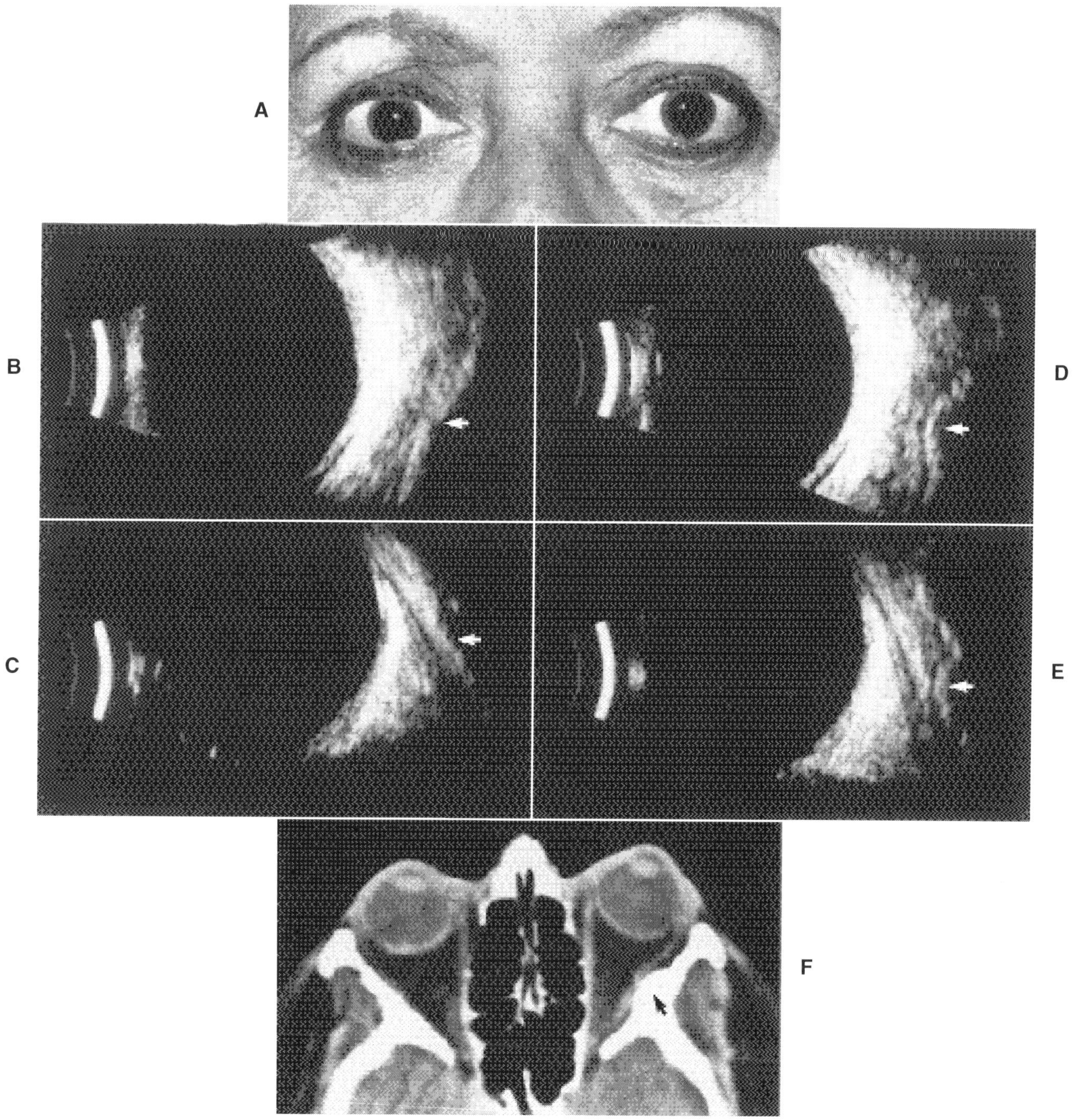

Figure 17-23 Left sphenoid wing meningioma. **A,** External photograph shows proptosis of left eye and slight lid retraction (patient had history of thyroid disease). Transocular B-scans are of normal right orbit (**B** and **C**) and abnormal left orbit (**D** and **E**). Vertical transverse **(B)** and longitudinal **(C)** B-scans of right temporal orbit show normal contour of lateral orbital wall *(arrows)*. Vertical transverse **(D)** and longitudinal **(E)** B-scans of left temporal orbit show localized convexity of orbital wall due to hyperostosis of sphenoid bone *(arrows)*. **F,** Axial CT scan shows hyperostosis of sphenoid wing *(arrow)*.

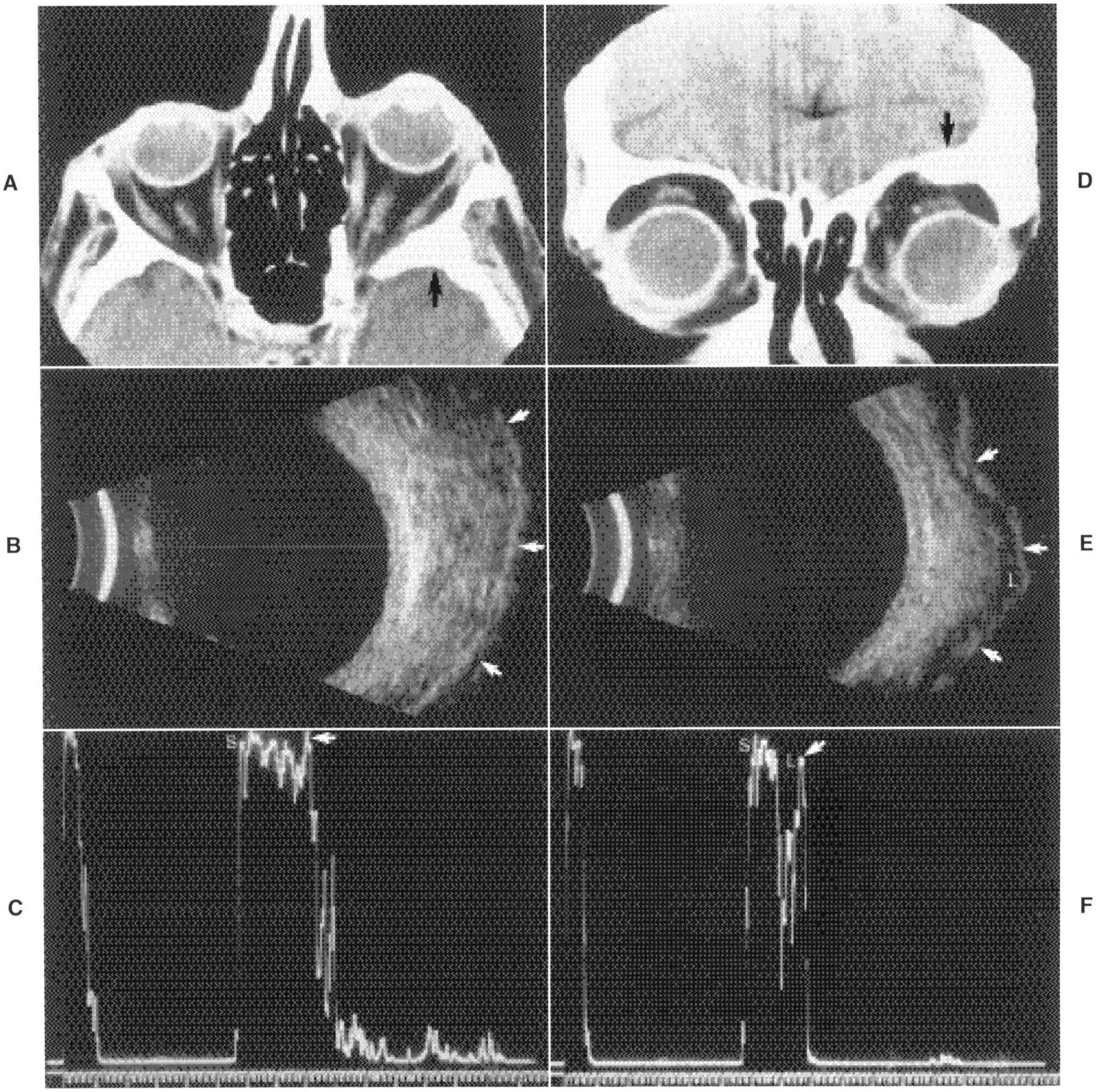

Figure 17-24 Sphenoid wing meningioma (en plaque). Axial **(A)** and coronal **(D)** CT scans display hyperostosis of left orbital roof and sphenoid bone *(arrows).* Transocular echograms are from superior aspect of normal right orbit (**B** and **C**) and abnormal left orbit (**E** and **F**). **B,** Horizontal transverse B-scan shows normal orbital soft tissue and orbital bone *(arrows).* **C,** Corresponding A-scan shows normal highly reflective orbital soft tissue. *S,* Sclera; *arrow,* bone. **E,** Horizontal transverse B-scan shows convex-shaped indentation of the orbital roof *(arrows)* and thin soft tissue mass lesion *(L)* adjacent to roof. **F,** Corresponding A-scan shows narrowing of orbital soft tissue pattern, as compared with **E.** Also note medium reflective lesion *(L)* adjacent to orbital bone *(arrow). S,* Sclera.

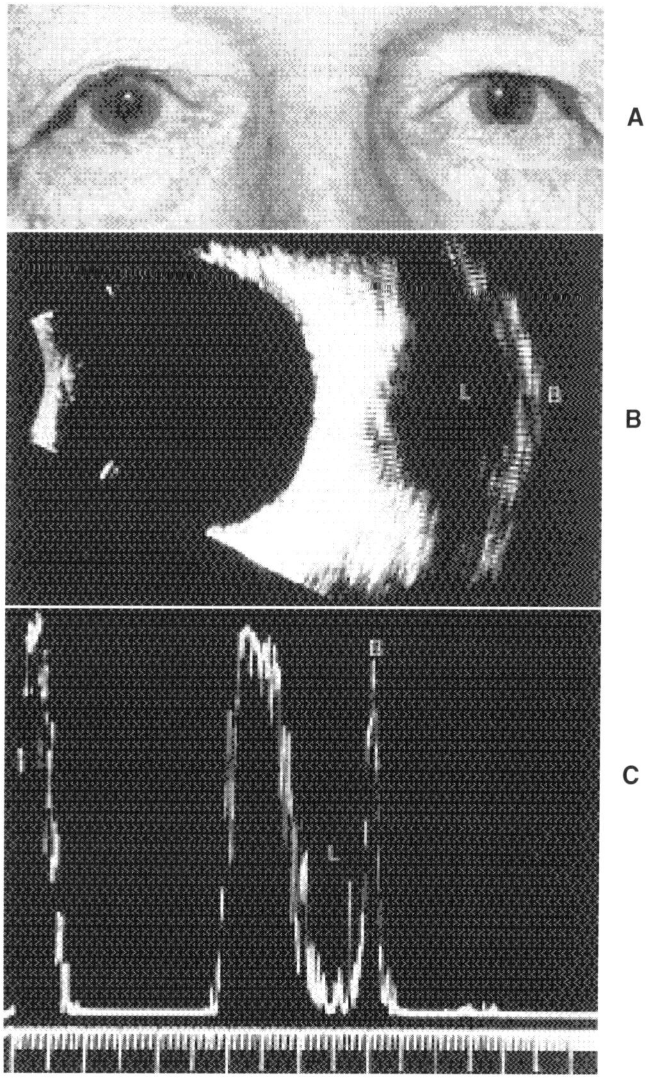

Figure 17-25 Sphenoid wing meningioma (en plaque). **A,** External photograph shows left upper lid swelling and ptosis as well as downward displacement of eye. **B,** Transocular B-scan echogram of temporal posterior orbit shows large lesion *(L)* and irregularity of orbital bone *(B)*. **C,** Transocular A-scan shows low internal reflectivity of lesion.

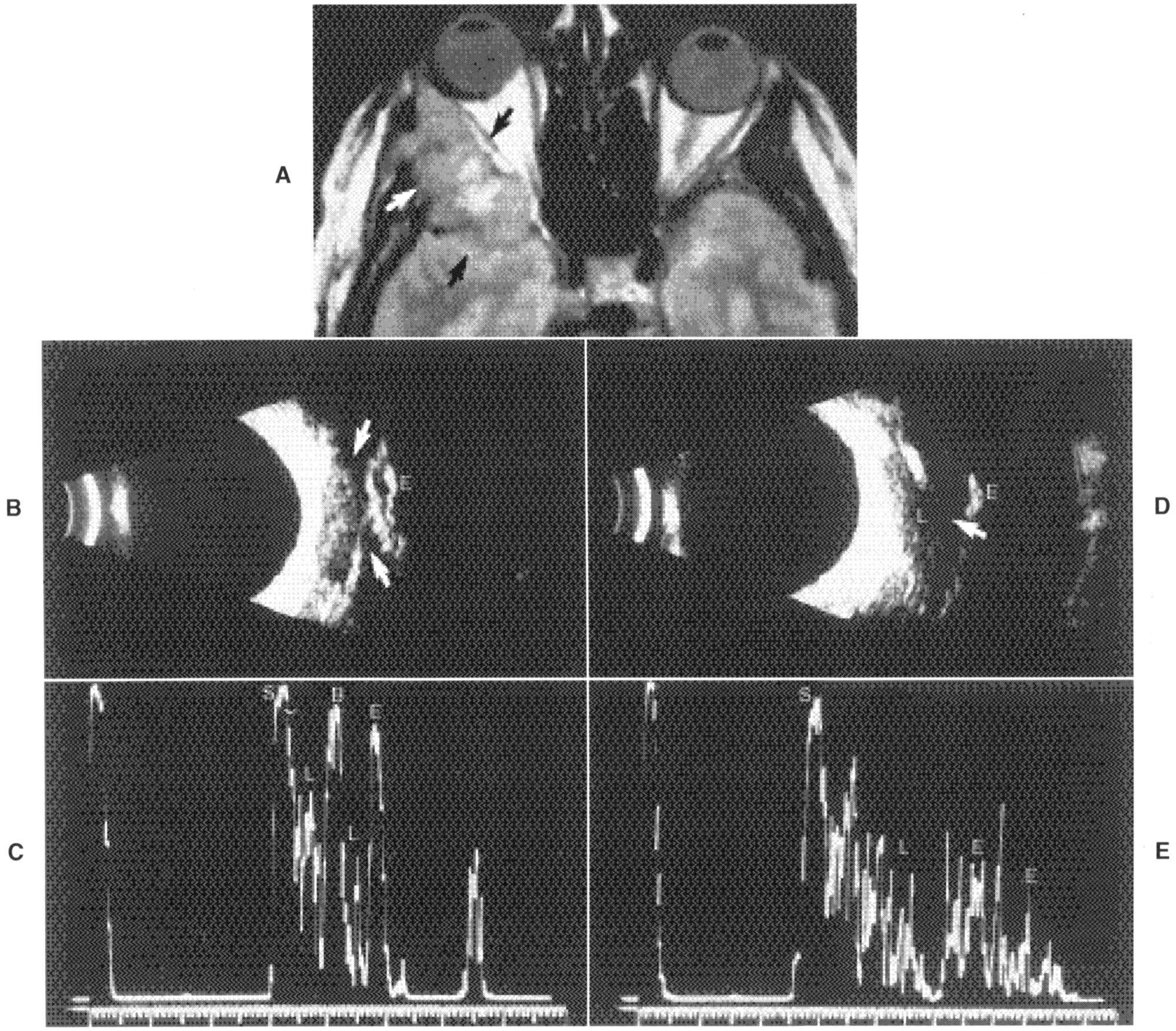

Figure 17-26 Metastatic breast carcinoma to right orbit. **A,** Axial MRI scan shows mass involving temporal aspect of orbit with erosion of lateral orbital wall and extension into frontal lobe *(arrows)*. Transocular echograms show subperiosteal lesion *(L)* extending through bone defect in lateral orbital wall. **B,** Transverse B-scan shows subperiosteal lesion, irregular bone defects *(arrows)* and extraorbital echoes *(E)*. **C,** Corresponding A-scan shows tumor involving both subperiosteal and extraorbital regions. *S,* Sclera; *B,* orbital bone. **D,** Longitudinal B-scan also shows tumor, bone defect, and extraorbital echo. **E,** A-scan with sound beam directed through bone defect in lateral orbital wall. Note markedly different appearance and much larger size of lesion in this echogram compared with **C,** thus emphasizing extraorbital involvement and irregular internal structure of lesion.

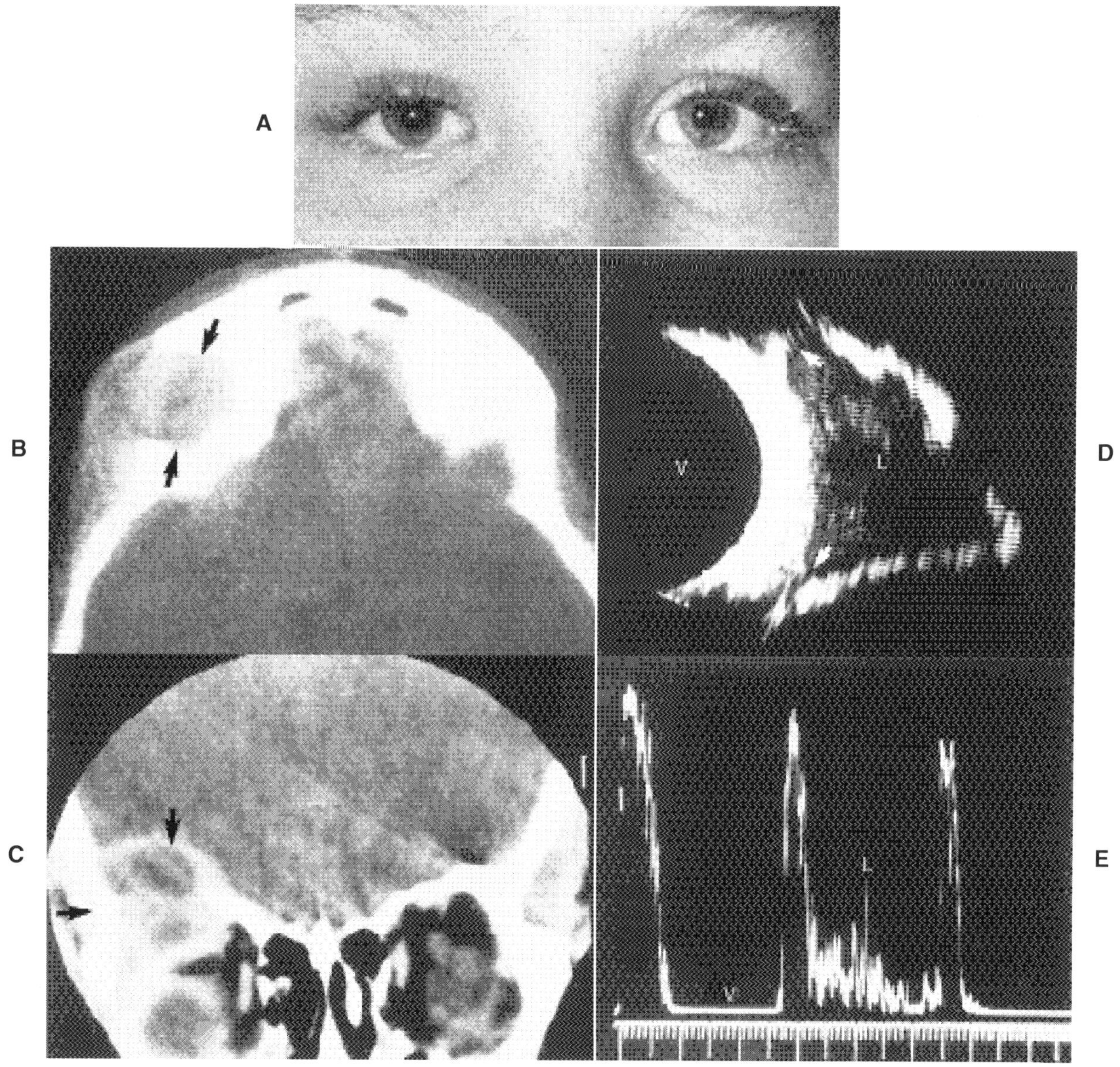

Figure 17-27 Eosinophilic granuloma in a child. **A,** External photograph shows proptosis and downward displacement of right eye. Axial **(B)** and coronal **(C)** CT scans show supratemporal orbital mass extending through large bone defect into anterior cranial fossa *(arrows)*. **D,** Transocular B-scan shows orbital lesion *(L)* located superiorly associated with large defect in orbital roof *(arrows)*. Note that majority of the mass is located above the orbital roof. *V,* Vitreous cavity. **E,** Transocular A-scan shows low reflectivity of large lesion.

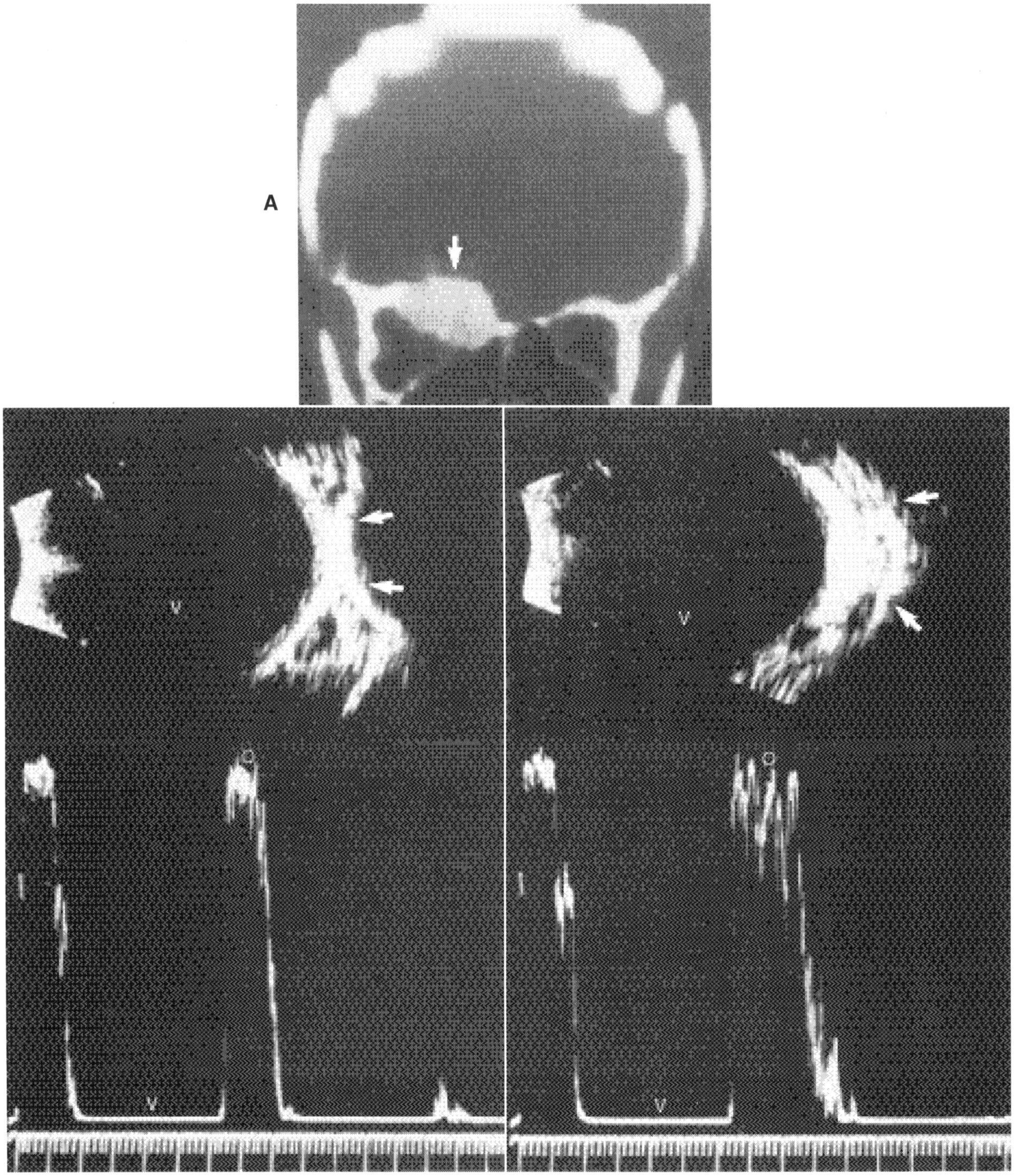

Figure 17-28 Fibrous dysplasia involving roof of right orbit. **A,** Coronal CT scan shows hyperostosis of orbital roof *(arrow)*. Transocular echograms are from superior aspect of abnormal right orbit (**B** and **C**) and normal left orbit (**D** and **E**). Transverse B-scans shows convex indentation of orbital roof *(arrows)* in area of mass in **B** compared with normal concave appearance of bone in **D.** *V,* Vitreous cavity. **C,** A-scan shows narrowed orbital soft tissue pattern *(O)* due to compression by protruding bone compared with normal orbital pattern in **E.**

Other periorbital disorders that may be encountered include hematic cyst (see p 340), osteoma, meningocele and encephalocele, osteomyelitis, and osteosarcoma.

REFERENCES

1. Atta HR, Byrne SF: The findings of standardized echography for choroidal folds. *Arch Ophthalmol* 1988;106:1236.
2. Buus DR, Tse DT, Farris BK: Ophthalmic complications of sinus surgery. *Ophthalmology* 1990;97:614.
3. Byrne SF, Glaser JS: Orbital tissue differentiation with standardized echography. *Ophthalmology* 1983;90:1071.
4. Capone A, Slamovits TL: Discrete metastasis of solid tumors to extraocular muscles. *Arch Ophthalmol* 1990;108:241.
5. Coleman DJ, Jack RL, Franzen LA: B-scan ultrasonography of orbital mucoceles. *Eye Ear Nose Throat Mon* 1972;51:207.
6. Feldman RB, Moore DM, Hood CI, et al: Solitary eosinophilic granuloma of the lateral orbital wall. *Am J Ophthalmol* 1985;100:321.
7. Flynn JT, Mitchell KB, Fuller DG, et al: Ocular motility complications following intranasal surgery. *Arch Ophthalmol* 1979;97:453.
8. Goodwin WJ Jr, Weinshall M, Chandler JR: The role of high resolution computerized tomography and standardized ultrasound in the evaluation of orbital cellulitis. *Laryngoscope* 1982;92:729.
9. Green RL, Byrne SF: Diagnostic ophthalmic ultrasound, in Ryan SJ (ed): *Retina.* St Louis, Mosby, 1989, p 191.
10. Hasenfratz G, Ossoinig KC: The diagnosis of orbital mucoceles and pyoceles with standardized echography, in Hillman JS, LeMay MM (eds): *Ophthalmic Ultrasonography.* Dordrecht, Dr W Junk, 1984, p 407.
11. Hughes RL, Byrne SF: Detection of posterior ruptures in opaque media, in Ossoinig KC (ed): *Ophthalmic Echography.* Dordrecht, Dr W Junk, 1987 p 331.
12. Hupp SL, Buckley EG, Byrne SF, et al: Post traumatic venous obstructive retinopathy associated with enlarged optic nerve sheath. *Arch Ophthalmol* 1984;102:254.
13. Jacobson DM, Itani K, Digre KB, et al: Maternal orbital hematoma associated with labor. *Am J Ophthalmol* 1988;105:547.
14. Jakobiec FA, Font RL: Orbit, in Spencer WH: *Ophthalmic Pathology; An Atlas and Textbook.* ed 3, Philadelphia, WB Saunders, 1986, p 2746.
15. Katz RS, Abrams G: Orbital subperiosteal hematoma (epidural hematoma of the orbit). *J Clin Neuro Ophthalmol* 1981;1:45.
16. Linhart WO: Emphysema of the orbit: A study of seven cases. *JAMA* 1943;123:89.
17. Mark LE, Kennerdell JS: Medial rectus injury from intranasal surgery. *Arch Ophthalmol* 1979;97:459.
18. Murray RS: Orbital emphysema following fracture of nasal sinuses. *J Fac Radiol* 1949;1:121.
19. Ossoinig KC: A-scan echography and orbital disease. *Mod Probl Ophthalmol* 1975;14:203.
20. Ossoinig KC: Echography of the eye, orbit, and periorbital region, in Arger PH (ed): *Orbit Roentgenology.* New York, J Wiley & Sons, 1977, p 221.
21. Ossoinig KC, Bigar F, Kaefring SL, et al: Echographic detection and localization of BB shots in the eye and orbit. *Bibl Ophthalmol* 1975;83:109.
22. Reshef DS, Ossoinig KC, Nerad JA: Diagnosis and intraoperative localization of a deep orbital organic foreign body. *Orbit* 1987;6:3.
23. Rootman J: Secondary tumors of the orbit, in Rootman J: *Diseases of the Orbit.* Philadelphia, JB Lippincott, 1988, p 433.
24. Rootman J, Allen L: Acquired lesions, in Rootman J: *Diseases of the Orbit.* Philadelphia, JB Lippincott, 1988, p 496.
25. Rootman J, Allen L: Acquired lesions, in Rootman J: *Diseases of the Orbit.* Philadelphia, JB Lippincott, 1988, p 499.
26. Rootman J, Lapointe JS: Tumors of the lacrimal gland, in Rootman J: *Diseases of the Orbit.* Philadelphia, JB Lippincott, 1988, p 394.
27. Rootman J, Neigel J: Trauma, in Rootman J: *Diseases of the Orbit.* Philadelphia, JB Lippincott, 1988, p 504.
28. Rootman J, Robertson WD: Orbital tumors originating in bone, in Rootman J: *Diseases of the Orbit.* Philadelphia, JB Lippincott, 1988, p 356.
29. Rootman J, Robertson W, Lapointe JS: Inflammatory diseases, in Rootman J: *Diseases of the Orbit.* Philadelphia, JB Lippincott, 1988, p 144.
30. Skalka HW: Ultrasonography in foreign body detection and localization. *Ophthalmic Surg* 1976;7(2):27.
31. Skalka HW, Callahan MA: Ultrasonically aided percutaneous orbital aspiration. *Ophthalmic Surg* 1979;10(11):41.
32. Spoor TC, Kennerdell JS, Dekker A, et al: Orbital fine needle aspiration biopsy with B-scan guidance. *Am J Ophthalmol* 1980;89:274.
33. Tannenbaum M, Tenzel J, Byrne SF, et al: Medical management of orbital abscess. *Surv Ophthalmol* 1985;30:211.

William D. Bates

18

Artifacts

Acoustic artifacts may be encountered during the course of an ultrasound examination (Box 18-1). Awareness of these artifacts allows accurate interpretation of the ultrasound findings.[1,2] Certain artifacts can be avoided simply by changing the position of the probe or by applying more methylcellulose to the probe tip. Other artifacts will always be present, but they can usually be identified when their cause is understood and their typical appearance is recognized. Some artifacts, such as those produced by a BB, can actually aid in the interpretation of echograms.

MULTIPLE SIGNALS (REVERBERATIONS)

Multiple signals are artifactual echo signals produced by reverberations of the sound wave between interfaces. It is important that multiple signals be distinguished from true echoes. Two types of multiple signals can occur: external and internal. External multiple signals are due to reverberations of the sound wave between the probe tip and a highly reflective acoustic interface. Internal multiple signals result from reverberations within a solid object (e.g., metallic or glass foreign body), as well as within small gas bubbles.

External Multiple Signals

External multiple signals result from reverberations between the transducer (probe tip) and an acoustic interface, such as the surface of the crystalline lens, an intraocular lens, a foreign body, an air bubble, the sclera, or the orbital bone. These types of interfaces reflect a portion of the sound wave back to the transducer (true echo), resulting in the display of a strong signal in the echogram. If the true echo is of significant magnitude, it is partially reflected at the transducer surface (probe tip) and redirected back toward the originating acoustic interface. The originating acoustic interface then produces a second echo (reverberation echo) that appears in the echogram distal to the true echo. Thus, a reverberation echo is produced when the sound wave travels back and forth twice (two round trips) between the transducer and the acoustic interface.[1,2] In the echogram, the first reverberation echo is displayed in a position corresponding to twice the distance between the probe tip and the originating acoustic interface. Subsequent reverberation signals may be caused by additional round trips of the sound wave between the transducer and the originating acoustic interface. It is of note that the true echo and the subsequent reverberation echoes are equidistant and generally decrease in strength (Figure 18-1; see also Figures 2-30, 4-42, 10-12, and 10-16). In addition, movement of this type of multiple reverberation signal, when the probe is gently pressed against the eye or lid tissues, is different from that of true echoes. Multiple signals move to a much greater degree than do true echoes.

Internal Multiple Signals

Internal multiple signals are artifactual echoes caused by reverberations (ringing) within certain types of foreign bodies. They most commonly occur when the sound beam strikes a spherical foreign body, such as a BB, gunshot pellet, or small bubble of air or gas. They can also be produced by certain nonspherical, flat foreign bodies with closely spaced, parallel surfaces, such as a glass sliver. The echo pattern for this type of foreign body is unique in that it appears as a chain of closely spaced signals emanating from the foreign body echo. This echo complex is sometimes referred to as the comet tail artifact.[1,2] It occurs because some of the energy is trapped when the sound wave enters the object. The trapped energy then bounces back and forth like echoes within a silo.[2] As the sound wave bounces back and forth within the object, a portion of the wave escapes and returns to the probe. This results in a chain of echoes of decreasing amplitude that extends from the foreign body echo (see Figure 4-26). In many instances, the comet tail artifact can be useful for identifying the location and type of foreign body (see Figures 2-34, 4-26, 4-27, 4-28, and 4-47).

SHADOWING

Shadowing is caused by strong sound attenuation. Partial shadowing can result in the diminution of echoes posterior to a lesion, such as a large choroidal melanoma. Complete shadowing causes an absence of echoes posterior to an extremely dense interface such as bone, calcium, a large foreign body, or a large bubble of air/gas. In some cases, this artifact can prevent the evaluation of structures and lesions located posterior to the source of shadowing (see

BOX 18-1

Common Artifacts

Reverberations (multiple signals)
- External
- Internal (comet tail)

Shadowing
- Sound attenuation
- Refraction (edge)

Enhancement

Perpendicularity

Baum's bumps

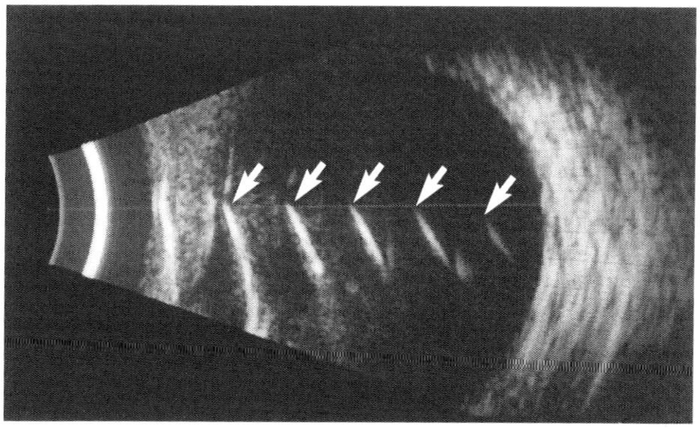

Figure 18-1 External multiple signals. Artifacts are due to insufficient contact between the B-scan probe and the eye. B-scan echogram shows multiple signals *(arrows)* from air located between the probe face and the eye. (From Green RL, Byrne SF: Diagnostic ophthalmic ultrasound, in Ryan SJ [ed]: *Retina.* ed 3, St Louis, Mosby, 2001, p 300.)

Figure 4-46 and p 109). Conversely, the presence of shadowing can help diagnose the lesion being examined, such as in an osteoma (see Figure 5-48), a retinoblastoma (see Figure 5-95), or an intraocular foreign body (see Figure 4-24).

Another type of shadowing is caused by refraction at the edges of smooth, curved interfaces rather than by sound attenuation. This artifact, sometimes referred to as refraction or edge artifact, commonly occurs from the surface of the globe (see Figures 11-9 and 12-34) or from a cystic lesion in the orbit, or it can be caused by a scleral fold (see Figure 4-23). This type of shadowing also partially explains the wedge-shaped appearance of the optic nerve when displayed with an axial B-scan approach.

ENHANCEMENT

Enhancement is the increased amplitude of echoes located posterior to a very weakly attenuating structure or lesion. This explains why the soft tissue and bone of the orbit are so well demonstrated when examined through the very low reflective vitreous cavity (see Figure 11-1) or through a serous orbital cyst (see Figure 12-37).

PERPENDICULAR SOUND BEAM INCIDENCE

A specific echographic finding caused by perpendicular sound beam incidence can occur in B-scan echograms. It may be observed when the sound beam is directed perpendicular to a very smooth, highly reflective interface. This finding appears as a bright, focal signal in the center of the echogram when a medium or low gain setting is used. It is commonly produced by the surface of the retina in the normal eye, although it can occur at any very smooth surface (see Figure 2-13, *B*). To avoid confusion of this echo signal with a foreign body or a localized area of calcification, the probe can be reoriented to display the area in question at the periphery rather than in the center of the echogram. The sound beam then engages the area in question obliquely rather than perpendicularly.

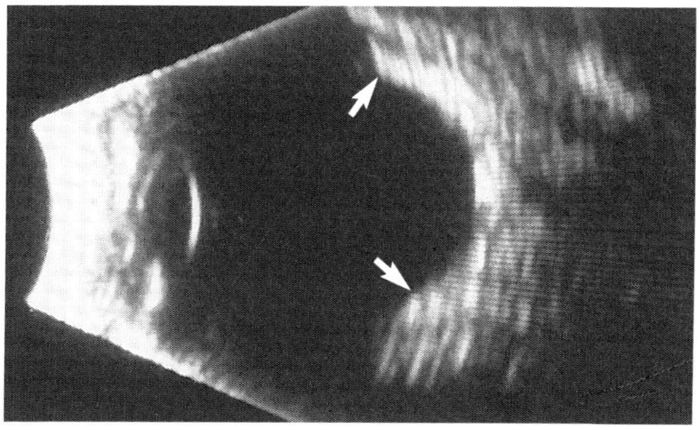

Figure 18-2 Baum's bumps. Axial B-scan shows mild elevations at the posterior fundus *(arrows)*, caused by refraction of the sound beam by the peripheral lens. (From Green RL, Byrne SF: Diagnostic ophthalmic ultrasound, in Ryan SJ [ed]: *Retina.* ed 3, St Louis, Mosby, 2001, p 300.)

BAUM'S BUMPS

Baum's bumps are B-scan artifacts that appear as elevations of the fundus. These artifacts are typically caused by refraction of the sound beam as it sweeps through the peripheral aspect of the lens when an axial approach is used. Baum's bumps can be misinterpreted as tumors, or they may give the impression of a posterior staphyloma (Figure 18-2; see also p 263). To eliminate these artifacts, the probe can be repositioned peripheral to the limbus to avoid the lens.

REFERENCES

1. Kremkau FW: *Diagnostic Ultrasound—Principles, Instruments and Exercises,* ed 3, Philadelphia, WB Saunders, 1989, p 147.
2. Zagzebski AA: *Essentials of Ultrasound Physics.* St. Louis, Mosby, 1996.

Glossary

Absorption The loss of sound energy as it passes through a medium due to heat conversion.

Acoustic Impedance The sound velocity of a medium multiplied by its density.

Acoustic Interface A surface separating two media of differing acoustic impedance.

A-scan Time amplitude display. A one-dimensional display where echoes are depicted as vertical deflections from a baseline. The strength of an echo is indicated by the amplitude (height) of the spike.

Attenuation A decrease in the strength (amplitude) of ultrasound energy as it passes through a medium.

Axial Resolution The minimum distance between two interfaces (located along the axis of the sound beam) that can be displayed separately.

Biometry The measurement of distances within the eye and orbit.

B-scan Brightness intensity-modulated display. A two-dimensional display where echoes are depicted as dots. The strength of an echo is indicated by the brightness of the dot.

Color Doppler Imaging (CDI) An imaging modality that incorporates the use of color with conventional duplex scanning (see Duplex scanning)

Decibel A relative unit that measures ultrasound intensity.

Doppler Effect A change in the frequency of the sound wave that is caused by movement of a reflector (e.g., blood) either away from or toward the transducer.

Duplex Scanning Ultrasound modality that combines Doppler spectral analysis with simultaneous B-scan imaging.

Dynamic Range The range of echo intensities (minimum to maximum) that an instrument can display.

Echo-dense Highly echogenic.

Echogenic A medium (e.g., tissue) that is capable of producing echoes.

Echography The utilization of ultrasound as a diagnostic modality (also known as ultrasonography).

Echolucent An absence of echoes (anechoic).

Edge Artifact A type of shadowing caused by refraction at the edges of smooth, curved interfaces.

Enhancement An artifact whereby the reflectivity of a tissue that is located behind a weakly attenuating medium is increased.

Frequency Oscillations (cycles) of ultrasound waves per unit of time. 1 Hertz (Hz) = 1 cycle/sec.

Gain The echo amplification, expressed in decibels, of an ultrasound system (also known as sensitivity setting).

Gray Scale The gradation of brightness levels (shades of gray) between minimum and maximum intensities on B-scan.

Impedance See Acoustic impedance.

Internal Reflectivity The amplitude of echoes within a tissue (e.g., tumor).

Internal Structure The degree of uniformity of internal echoes, correlating with histologic architecture of a tissue (e.g., tumor).

Kinetic Echography A technique that is used to assess the motion of or within a lesion.

Lateral Resolution The minimum distance between interfaces that can be resolved when the interfaces are located perpendicular to the sound beam.

Longitudinal Scan B-scan probe orientation where the moving sound beam is directed along a given meridian, in an anterior-posterior direction (also known as radial scan).

Multiple Signals Artifacts caused by reverberations of the sound waves. These usually occur between the probe and a highly reflective interface or between two highly reflective interfaces (also known as reverberations).

Piezoelectric Element An element that converts electrical to mechanical energy and vice versa.

Probe A device containing a piezoelectric element that is used to scan the eye or orbit (also known as a transducer).

Pulse-echo Technique A system that emits pulses of ultrasound and detects returning echoes between the pulses.

Quantitative Echography A technique that is used to assess the reflectivity, internal structure, and sound attenuation of a lesion.

Real-time The ability of an ultrasound instrument to display movement of structures within the body as it is occurring.

Reflectivity The strength or amplitude of an echo produced by an interface.

Refraction The bending of a sound wave as it passes from one medium to another.

Resolution The smallest distance between two interfaces that can be displayed.

Reverberations See Multiple signals.

Scattering The spreading of sound waves in multiple directions, occurring primarily from small or coarse interfaces.

Sensitivity The ability of the ultrasound system to detect echoes.

Sensitivity Setting See Gain.

Shadowing The reduction in echo amplitude posterior to a strongly reflecting or attenuating interface.

Sound Attenuation A decrease in the amplitude of ultrasound energy as it passes through a medium; caused by scattering, reflection or absorption.

Sound Beam The directed sound waves produced by an ultrasound transducer.

Sound Velocity The speed at which ultrasound energy travels through a given medium.

Sound Wave A mechanical vibration of particles in a medium.

Spectral Analysis A process by which a complex signal is broken down or analyzed into simple frequency components (e.g., distribution of frequencies in a Doppler signal).

Three-dimensional Ultrasonography (3DUS) A technique that combines sequential two-dimensional (2D) digital image acquisition (tomograms) with computerized reconstruction software. This image processing allows ocular pathology to be viewed in "3D."

Topographic Echography The shape, location, and extension of a lesion.

Transducer See Probe.

Transverse Scan B-scan probe orientation where the moving sound beam is directed across a given meridian. This probe orientation displays the lateral extent of a structure or a lesion.

Ultrasonography See Echography.

Ultrasound An acoustic wave that consists of an oscillation of particles within a medium with a frequency greater than 20,000 Hertz (cycles/sec).

Ultrasound Biomicroscopy (UBM) High resolution B-scan ultrasound technology using frequencies in the 40-100 MHz range. This technique provides imaging of ocular tissue at microscopic resolution.

Vector A-scan An A-scan that is derived simultaneously from one portion of a B-scan echogram.

Velocity See Sound velocity.

Wavelength The distance between any two similar points on two consecutive cycles of a sound wave.

Appendices

APPENDIX A

Table for Converting Microseconds (μsec) to Millimeters (mm)

μsec	Aqueous/Vitreous* (1,532 m/sec)	Tissues† (1,550 m/sec)	Lens‡ (1,631 m/sec)
0.1	0.08	0.08	0.08
0.2	0.15	0.16	0.16
0.3	0.23	0.23	0.25
0.4	0.31	0.31	0.33
0.5	0.38	0.39	0.41
0.6	0.46	0.47	0.49
0.7	0.54	0.54	0.57
0.8	0.61	0.62	0.66
0.9	0.69	0.70	0.74
1.0	0.77	0.78	0.82
2.0	1.53	1.55	1.64
3.0	2.30	2.33	2.46
4.0	3.06	3.10	3.28
5.0	3.83	3.88	4.11
6.0	4.60	4.65	4.93
7.0	5.36	5.43	5.75
8.0	6.13	6.20	6.57
9.0	6.89	6.98	7.39
10.0	7.66	7.75	8.21

*Aqueous/vitreous: μsec × 0.766.
†Tissues: μsec × 0.775.
‡Lens: μsec × 0.821.

APPENDIX B

Basic B-Scan Screening: Probe Orientation*

	Areas Examined	Gaze	Probe Position	Marker
A	Superior	Up	Horizontal	Nasal
B	Nasal	Nasal	Vertical	Superior
C	Inferior	Down	Horizontal	Nasal
D	Temporal	Temporal	Vertical	Superior

*These transverse probe positions are used to evaluate the eye during the basic screening examination.

OD

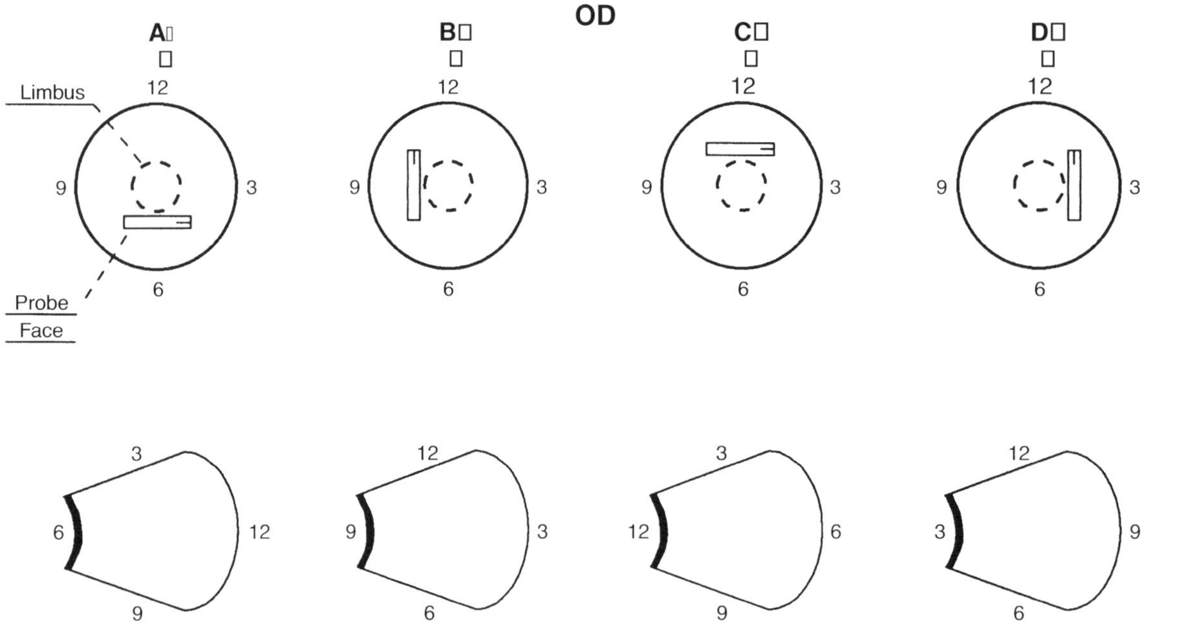

OS

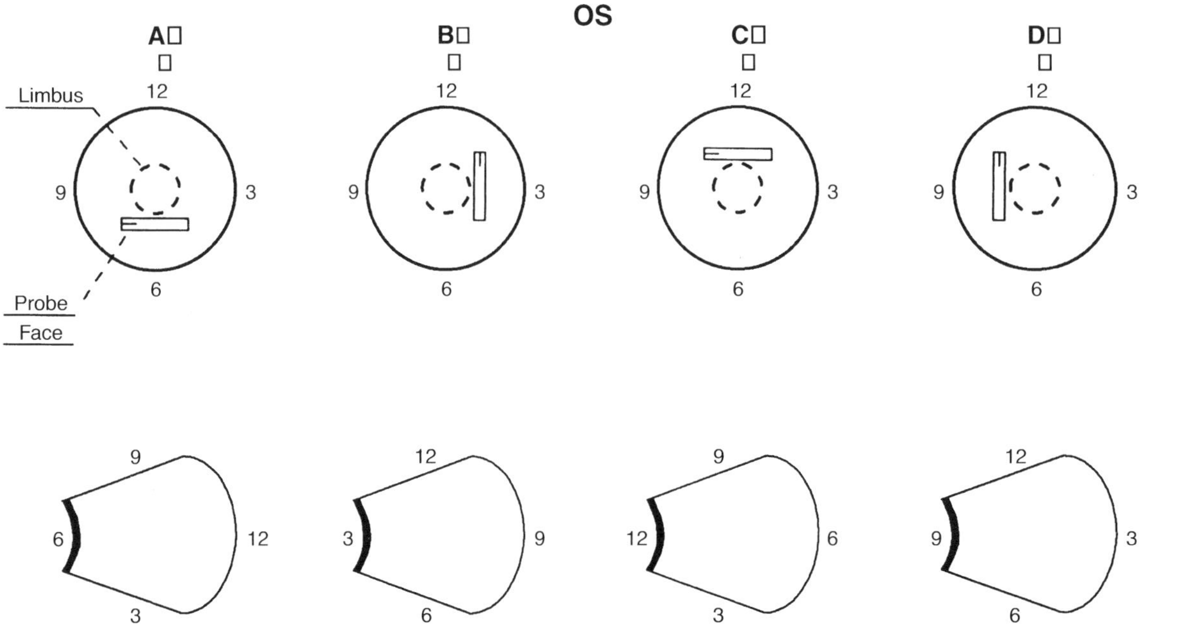

APPENDIX C

Topographic Evaluation of Intraocular Lesions with A- and B-Scan

Four different types of intraocular lesions (pointlike, membranelike, bandlike, and masslike) can be distinguished with topographic echography. This can be achieved with both A- and B-scan by using varied probe positions.

In the B-scan echograms, the lesion is displayed with transverse *(column 1)* and longitudinal *(column 2)* probe positions. Note that all lesions have the same general configuration in both transverse and longitudinal views except for the bandlike lesion that produces a pointlike echo in one view and a line in the other.

The A-scan echograms are obtained with the sound beam directed perpendicular to the lesion *(column 3)* and with the probe repositioned approximately 90° from the first position *(column 4)*. Note that echograms for the pointlike and masslike lesions have a similar appearance in both sound beam directions. For both membranelike and bandlike lesions, however, a single spike is obtained when the sound beam is directed perpendicular to the lesion and a chain of spikes is displayed when the sound beam is directed along the lesion's surface.

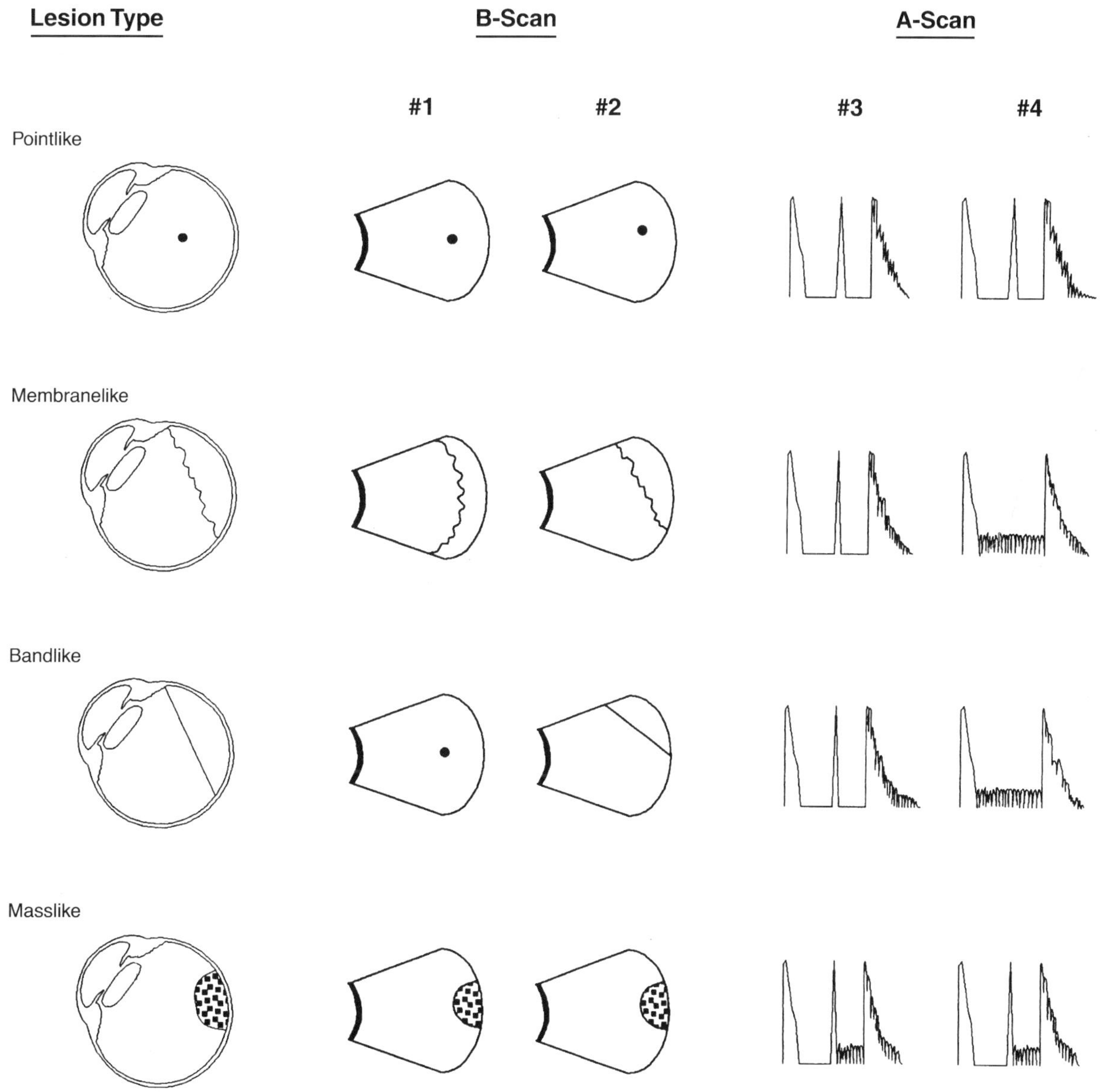

APPENDIX D

Scleral Shells for Use with the Immersion Technique

Darling Shell (Conventional A- or B-scan probes)
Laurie Darling, C.O.T.
Eye Associates Medical Group, Inc.
P.O. Box 1777
6880 Palm Avenue
Sebastopol, California 95472

Eye Cups (Ultrasound biomicroscope)
Paradigm
2355 South 1070 west
Salt Lake City, Utah 84119

Flanged Shells (I^3 High resolution B-scan [20 MHz] probe)
Innovative Imaging, Inc
9940 Business Park
Sacramento, California 95827

Hansen Shells (A- or B-scan probes)
Hansen Ophthalmic Development Laboratories
2412 Towncrest Drive
Iowa City, Iowa 52240

Prager Shell (A-scan biometry probe)
Tom Prager, PhD
1819 North Rainbow Ranch Road
Wimberely, Texas 78676

APPENDIX E
Echogram Labeling

Schematic fundus drawings *(top)* and sagittal sections *(bottom)* of normal eye *(left)* and fundus lesion *(right)*. These diagrams indicate the labeling system for localizing a lesion in the posterior segment of the eye. *P,* Posterior; *PE,* posterior-equator; *EP,* posterior to equator; *E,* equator; *EA,* anterior to equator; *O,* ora serrata; *CB,* ciliary body; and *AX,* axial. *Right,* Lesion centered on 10 o'clock meridian at the equator (i.e., 10 E).

Echograms are labeled according to the area of the eye where the sound beam is directed (rather than where on the globe the probe is positioned). Labeling of A- and B-scan photoechograms for the lesion shown above would be as follows: A-scan, 10E; transverse B-scan, 10E; longitudinal B-scan, L10; axial B-scan, 10AX.

In orbital examinations, a similar procedure is used for labeling transocular scans. Paraocular scans are labeled according to where the probe is positioned on the closed eyelid.

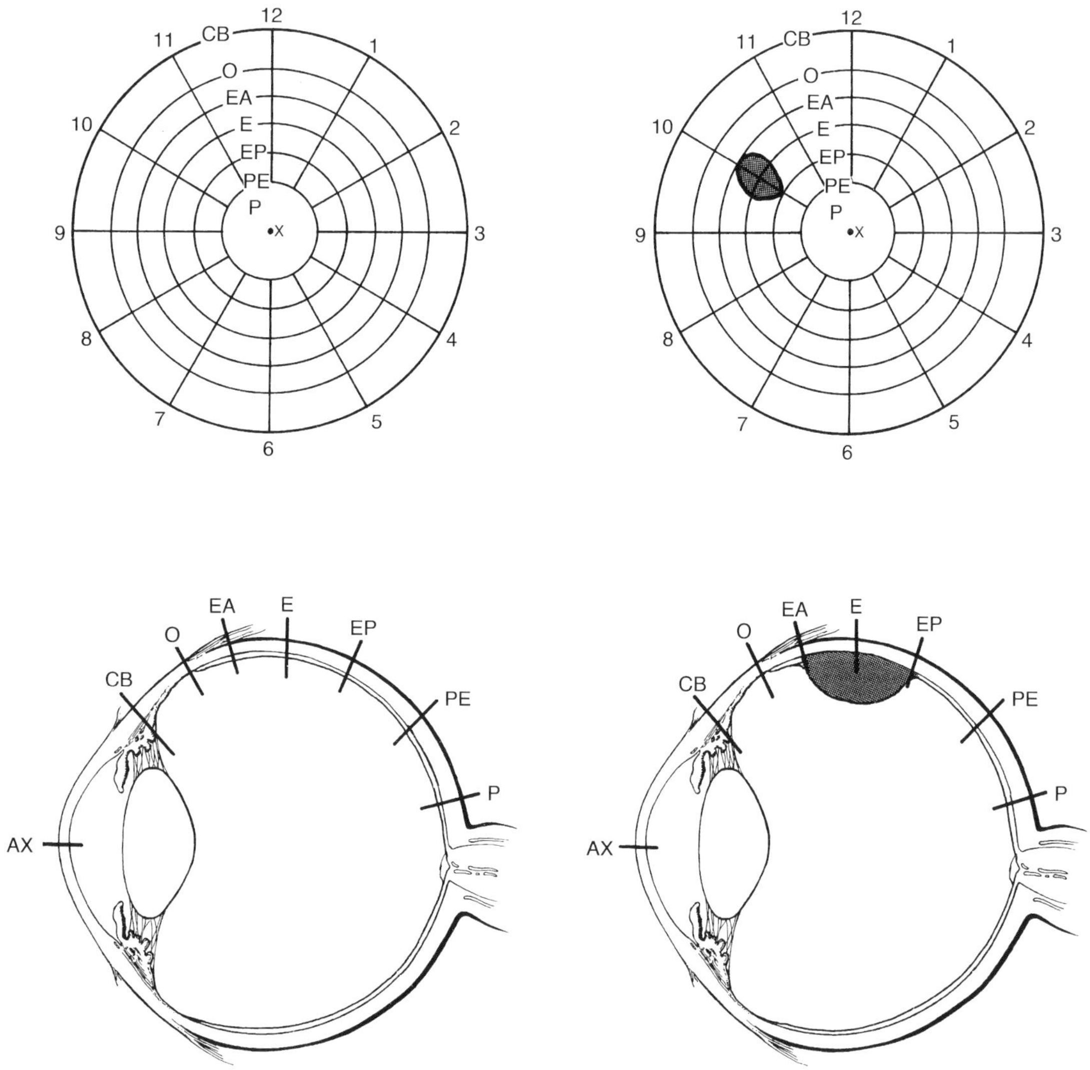

APPENDIX F

Method for Obtaining Measurements from B-Scan Echograms*

1. With the B-scan running, set the gain level to zero and then switch to the vector A-scan (without the B-scan)
2. Place the vector through the center and freeze the screen.
3. Perform measurement A: display the two electronic cursors and position them centrally, so that they measure approximately 10 mm apart *(arrows)*. Note that the measurement is 9.9 mm in this example.
4. Perform measurement B: take a photograph of the screen and, using a millimeter ruler, measure the distance between the two cursors on the photograph.
5. Determine conversion factor (CF): divide measurement A by measurement B (A/B = CF). This factor will then allow millimeter measurements to be obtained directly from B-scan photographs (e.g., if A = 9.9 mm and B = 19.8 mm, then the conversion factor = 9.9/19.8 = 0.50).
6. To obtain a final measurement, multiply the measurement obtained from the photograph (in millimeters) by the conversion factor. This value will provide an approximate measurement that correlates with A-scan measurements. This method may be used for any given instrument/probe/camera combination. If any of these three components is changed, the conversion factor should be recalculated.

*This method is only necessary for B-scan instruments that do not have a measuring scale but have a vector factor A-scan with electronic cursors for measurements (e.g., Ophthascan S, Alcon Surgical, Inc).

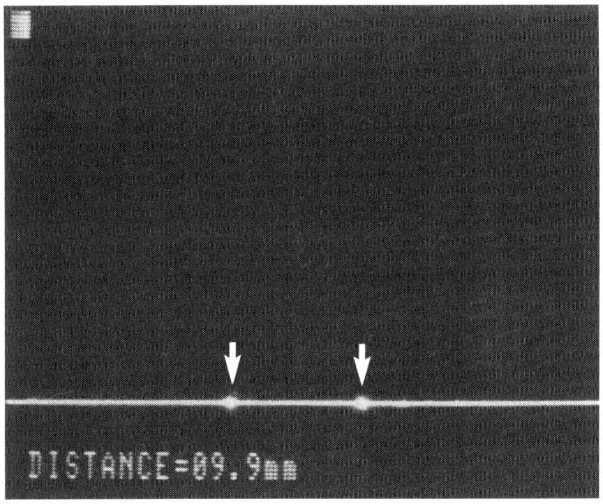

Index

Page references followed by *f*, *t*, and *b* indicate figures, tables, and boxes, respectively.

B

C